Stephen J. Ro...
'95

W9-ADB-723

HANDBOOK OF
PAIN MANAGEMENT

SECOND EDITION

HANDBOOK OF PAIN MANAGEMENT

SECOND EDITION

Editor

C. DAVID TOLLISON, PH.D.

Director
Pain Therapy Center of Greenville
Greenville Hospital System
Greenville, South Carolina
Associate Clinical Professor
Department of Anesthesiology
Medical College of Georgia
Augusta, Georgia

Associate Editors

John R. Satterthwaite, M.D.

Medical Director
Pain Therapy Center of Greenville
Greenville Hospital System
Greenville, South Carolina

Joseph W. Tollison, M.D.

Professor and Chairman, Department of Family Medicine, Medical College of Georgia,
Augusta, Georgia

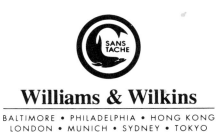

Williams & Wilkins

BALTIMORE • PHILADELPHIA • HONG KONG
LONDON • MUNICH • SYDNEY • TOKYO

A WAVERLY COMPANY

Editor: John P. Butler
Managing Editor: Linda S. Napora
Copy Editor: John M. Daniel
Designer: Ann Rebecca Feild
Illustration Planner: Wayne Hubbel
Production Coordinator: Charles E. Zeller

Copyright (c) 1994
Williams & Wilkins
428 East Preston Street
Baltimore, Maryland 21202, USA

All rights reserved. This book is protected by copyright. No part of this book may be reproduced in any form or by any means including photocopying, or utilized by any information storage and retrieval system without written permission from the copyright owner.

Accurate indications, adverse reactions, and dosage schedules for drugs are provided in this book, but it is possible that they may change. The reader is urged to review the package information data of the manufacturers of the medications mentioned.

Printed in the United States of America

First Edition 1989

Library of Congress Cataloging in Publication Data

Handbook of pain management / editor, C. David Tollison : associate editors, John R. Satterthwaite, Joseph W. Tollison. — 2nd ed.
    p.   cm.
    Rev. ed. of: Handbook of chronic pain management. c1989.
    Includes bibliographical references and index.
    ISBN 0-683-08332-5
    1. Intractable pain—Handbooks, manuals, etc. 2. Pain—Handbooks, manuals, etc. 3. Analgesia—Handbooks, manuals, etc.   I. Tollison, C. David, 1949–   . II. Satterthwaite, John R.   III. Tollison, Joseph W.
    [DNLM: 1. Pain—therapy.   WL 704 H2437 1994]
RB127.H353 1994
616'.0472—dc20
DNLM/DLC
for Library of Congress
    92-48553
    CIP

93 94 95 96 97
1 2 3 4 5 6 7 8 9 10

To my wife,
Linda Surett Tollison,
and children,
Courtney Louise Tollison
and
Charles David Tollison, Jr.

FOREWORD

THE HANDBOOK of Chronic Pain Management is a tribute to progress in medicine. The chapters highlight the tremendous growth of pain research and provide a basis for its clinical application by the many kinds of health professionals who are necessarily involved in treating the chronic pain patient. This text features the complexities of comprehensive multidisciplinary care in such a way that the practitioner can understand and effectively apply this knowledge in the practice of chronic pain management.

Diagnostic and therapeutic difficulties are further complicated by the fact that each patient's problem is unique. This individuality is substantiated by asking, "How many people in the world have the same thumbprint?" The answer, of course, is "None." Not even look-alike twin monkeys have identical thumbprints. This is an anatomic variation. Thus, no two people are alike anatomically, biochemically, or in life-style. Treatment of any diagnosed medical disease or disorder must therefore be tailored to fit each unique individual.

No cookbook recipe for therapy should be employed, nor is the tunnel vision of any single medical specialty adequate, as a rule, for successful chronic pain management. Every practitioner should have the broad background of knowledge that this book supplies.

The superlative chapters of this text review first the classification of pain, its theoretical pathways and mechanisms, and its social, cultural, and psychological aspects. Chapters then focus attention on the diagnosis and management of chronic pain due to many causes, including neurologic lesions of spinal and peripheral nerves, malignancy, visceral and vascular diseases, various forms of joint degeneration and joint locking, and pain as a variant of depression.

One frequent and often overlooked source of chronic pain, the myofascial pain syndrome, receives ample and practical discussion. This condition can be demonstrated objectively by palpation of the muscles for trigger points and by recognition of their related referred pain patterns. The myofascial pain syndrome responds well to specific local therapy if its multiple perpetuating factors are recognized and corrected. Stresses that are both physical and emotional usually must be dealt with if trigger point therapy is to succeed. In addition, systemic perpetuating factors such as chronic infection and parasitic infestation, endocrine disorders (especially marginal (subclinical) hypothyroidism), borderline anemia, vitamin inadequacies, and deficiencies of other nutrients may play a role in maintaining chronicity. Evaluation of these multicausal factors requires unhurried time, detective work, and both skill and humility in communicating with the patient in chronic misery.

The largest organ in the body is the skeletal musculature, comprising nearly half the body weight. The myofascial pain syndrome may be the most common affliction of the human race. Muscles are different from other tissues. When the skin is cut or a bone is broken, it heals. When a muscle is injured or strained, it learns to guard that part. The better the person's athletic ability and coordination, the more likely the muscle is to continue its protective splinting with restricted motion, pain, and weakness for years, until the muscle is taught otherwise. Neuromuscular reeducation may be accomplished by passive stretching to full length during inhibition of reflex contraction, and by other techniques such as the Karel Lewit isometric contraction procedure.

The book's chapters present a large choice of therapeutic modalities, invasive and noninvasive, together with detailed consideration of the pharmacology of antiinflammatory, analgesic and antidepressant drugs. Prescription of such medications may be necessary, with caution, when other management approaches fail.

The broad range and practical view of the *Handbook for Chronic Pain Management* make it an important working manual for effective clinical care that can improve the quality of life of the suffering patient.

Janet G. Travell, M.D.
Emeritus Clinical Professor of Medicine
The George Washington University
Washington, D.C.

PREFACE

Much has evolved in the diagnosis and treatment of pain since the first edition of this text was published in 1989. A respected senior colleague, still actively practicing at age 76, has even offered the opinion that "More has been learned about pain in the past 10 years than in the 50 years preceding!"

Given the relative infancy and recent focus of pain management as a formal clinical discipline, perhaps these welcomed advances should come as little surprise. Today there are more health professionals of various disciplines with an interest in pain than in any time before, more continuing research into causes and cures, and more clinics and centers offering diagnosis and treatment. Perhaps no human condition other than pain has before brought together such a wide range of scientific and clinical disciplines into cooperative efforts and practice. George Bernard Shaw wrote in *Back to Methuselah*: " 'You see things, and you say, 'Why?' But I dream things that never were; and I say, 'Why not?' " Professionals with an interest in pain have repeatedly asked, "Why?" More importantly, many of these individuals and groups have stepped forward to develop those dreams of "Why not?" into realities. As a result, both our diagnostic skills and treatment techniques are increasing, practice methodology and market trends are appropriately changing, and our science is maturing. Though many miles of mystery lie ahead, we have begun a journey with a destination of conquering one of humankind's oldest and most dreaded maladies—*Pain!*

In the planning and development of the second edition of this text, every effort has been made to incorporate the recently established and the emerging clinical advances in pain diagnosis and treatment. Readers will note major text changes throughout, beginning with the retitling of the book. *Handbook of Chronic Pain Management* has been changed to *Handbook of Pain Management*. This new title accurately reflects the emphasis of the second edition on the treatment of the wide spectrum of pain, rather than chronic pain alone. In addition, five chapters from the original text have been eliminated, and ten new chapters have been added. Of particular interest is a new major section on "Pharmacologic Interventions." This section contains five chapters that discuss the use of various medications in clinical pain practice as well as an excellent chapter on "Drug Detoxification Protocols." Furthermore, the section on "Pain Clinics" has been expanded to detail the various types of clinical pain practice—Office and Hospital Pain Consultations, Office-Based Outpatient Treatment Programs, Hospital-Based Inpatient Treatment Programs, and Occupational Rehabilitation Programs. Finally, a new major section on "Medical-Legal Issues" has been added, which includes chapters designed to assist the practitioner in the evaluation and rating of both physical and psychological impairment. Chapters retained from the first edition have been updated to reflect current clinical research and practice.

The primary objective in developing this text was to collect the considerable expertise of many recognized authorities, representing various disciplines, and to orchestrate that expertise into a comprehensive clinical resource for the diagnosis and treatment of pain. Our appreciation is extended to the many colleagues who offered constructive criticism of the first edition and helpful suggestions for this, the second edition. The significant changes that are obvious in this second edition reflect, in large part, their collective recommendations.

The complaint of pain remains the single greatest catalyst for seeking medical attention. Despite increased knowledge and scientific advances, the diagnosis and effective treatment of human suffering remains one of health care's most formidable challenges. It is hoped that this text will equip practitioners with the knowledge, skills, and enthusiasm required to continue the battle against pain.

C. David Tollison, Ph.D.

CONTRIBUTORS

HENRY E. ADAMS, PH.D.
(Chapter 21)
University of Georgia
Athens, Georgia

EBEN ALEXANDER, M.D.
(Chapter 7)
Department of Surgery
Division of Neurosurgery
Duke University Medical Center
Durham, North Carolina

JOHN ARYANPUR, M.D.
(Chapter 26)
Department of Neurosurgery
The Johns Hopkins Hospital
Baltimore, Maryland

J. HAMPTON ATKINSON, M.D.
(Chapter 16)
Department of Psychiatry
University of California at San Diego
School of Medicine
La Jolla, California

MAHMOUD A. AYOUB, PH.D.
(Chapter 48)
Department of Industrial Engineering
North Carolina State University
Raleigh, North Carolina

DAVID BOYD, M.D., F.R.C.P.(C)
(Chapter 2)
Victoria Hospital
London, Ontario, Canada

RONALD BRISMAN, M.D.
(Chapter 23)
College of Physicians and Surgeons of Columbia
  University
Department of Neurological Surgery
New York, New York

KIM J. BURCHIEL, M.D.
(Chapter 22)
School of Medicine
Division of Neurosurgery
Oregon Health Sciences University
Portland, Oregon

JEFFREY BURGESS, D.D.S., M.S.D.
(Chapter 22)
Department of Oral Medicine
Department of Anesthesiology
Division of Neurosurgery
Oregon Health Sciences University
Portland, Oregon

JEROME D. BUXBAUM, D.D.S., F.A.G.D.
(Chapter 24)
Department of Physiology
The University of Maryland
Baltimore College of Dental Surgery
Baltimore, Maryland

STANLEY CHAPMAN, PH.D.
(Chapter 50)
Center for Pain Medicine
Emory Clinic, South
Atlanta, Georgia

ANDREW J. COLE, M.D.
(Chapters 9 and 30)
Baylor University Medical Center
Department of Physical Medicine & Rehabilitation
Dallas, Texas

STEPHEN R. CONWAY, M.D.
(Chapter 38)
Department of Neurology
Hartford Hospital
Hartford, Connecticut

DAVID R. CORNBLATH, M.D.
(Chapter 37)
Department of Neurology
The Johns Hopkins Hospital
Baltimore, Maryland

PENNY LOZON CROOK, J.D.
(Chapter 54)

BENJAMIN L. CRUE, JR., M.D., F.A.C.S.
(Chapter 29)
Neurology-Neurosurgery Associates and
  Nondiagnostic Laboratory
Durango, Colorado

MERLE L. DIAMOND
(Chapter 19)
Diamond Headache Clinic, Ltd.
Chicago, Illinois

SEYMOUR DIAMOND, M.D.
(Chapter 19)
Diamond Headache Clinic, Ltd.
Chicago, Illinois

THOMAS B. DUCKER, M.D.
(Chapter 26)
Department of Neurosurgery
The Johns Hopkins Hospital
Baltimore, Maryland

RICHARD E. EAGLESTON
(Chapter 30)
Health South Physical Therapy
Portola Valley, California

TERESA FERRER-BRECHNER, M.D.
(Chapter 33)
Southern California Pain Consortium
Bakersfield, California

MICHAEL FEUERSTEIN, PH.D.
(Chapter 1)
Psychiatry and Anesthesiology
University of Rochester Medical Center
Westfall Medical Office Park
Rochester, New York

DAVID A. FISHBAIN, M.D.
(Chapter 18)
Department of Psychiatry and Neurological Surgery
Comprehensive Pain and Rehabilitation Center
South Shore Hospital and Medical Center
Miami Beach, Florida

RICHARD H. FITZGERALD, JR.
(Chapter 36)
Radiation Oncology Department
Roper Hospital
Charleston, South Carolina

DON E. FLINN
(Chapter 11)
Professor and Vice Chairman
Department of Psychiatry
Assistant Dean
UCLA School of Medicine
Los Angeles, California

STEPHEN R. FREIDBERG, M.D.
(Chapter 35)
Chairman, Department of Neurosurgery
Lahey Clinic Medical Center
Burlington, Massachusetts

R. MICHAEL GALLAGHER, D.O.
(Chapter 15)
University Headache Center
Moorestown, New Jersey

LARRY A. GAUPP, PH.D.
(Chapter 11)
Psychology Service
V.A. Medical Center
Newington, Connecticut

JERALD B. GILBERT
(Chapter 32)
Section of Urology
University of Pennsylvania
Philadelphia, Pennsylvania

JONATHAN D. GLASS
(Chapter 37)
Department of Neurology
The Johns Hopkins Hospital
Baltimore, Maryland

J. LEONARD GOLDNER, M.D.
(Chapter 28)
Division of Orthopaedic Surgery
Duke University Medical Center
Durham, North Carolina

JAMES L. HALL, PH.D.
(Chapter 3)
College of Medicine
Department of Anatomy and Cell Biology
University of Cincinnati Medical Center
Cincinnati, Ohio

NELSON HENDLER, M.D., M.S.
(Chapter 39)
Mensana Clinic
Stevenson, Maryland

THOMAS K. HENTHORN, M.D.
(Chapter 46)
Department of Anesthesia
Northwestern University Medical School
Chicago, Illinois

STANLEY A. HERRING
(Chapter 9)
Puget Sound Sports Physicians
Seattle, Washington

MARC HERTZMAN, M.D.
(Chapter 47)
Department of Psychiatry and Behavioral Sciences
The George Washington University Medical Center
Washington, D.C.

DONALD W. HINNANT, PH.D.
(Chapters 4 and 56)
Saint Francis Medical Center
Cape Girardeau, Missouri

STEVEN M. HONIG, M.D.
(Chapter 14)
The Hospital for Joint Diseases
New York University School of Medicine
New York, New York

MICHAEL HOUSTON
(Chapter 47)
The George Washington University Medical Center
Washington, D.C.

PATRICIA HOWSON, M.D.
(Chapter 28)
Fellow in Hand Surgery
Division of Orthopaedic Surgery
Duke University Medical Center
Durham, North Carolina

ANTHONY IEZZI, PH.D.
(Chapter 21)
Department of Psychology
Victoria Hospital
London, Ontario, Canada

J. GREG JOHNSON, M.D.
(Chapter 31)
Greenville OB-GYN Associates
Greenville, South Carolina

H. ROYDEN JONES, JR., M.D.
(Chapter 38)
Department of Neurosurgery
Lahey Clinic Medical Center
Burlington, Massachusetts

TOM C. KREJCIE, M.D.
(Chapter 46)
Department of Anesthesia
Northwestern University Medical School
Chicago, Illinois

JERRY C. LANGLEY, D.C.
(Chapter 10)
Private Practice
Greenville, South Carolina

VICTOR C. LEE, M.D.
(Chapter 49)
Pain Management Center
Department of Anesthesiology
University of Virginia
Health Sciences Center
Charlottesville, Virginia

TERRENCE MALLOY, M.D.
(Chapter 32)
Section of Urology
University of Pennsylvania
Philadelphia, Pennsylvania

EDGAR MARIN
(Chapter 55)

LEONARD N. MATHESON, PH.D.
(Chapter 52)
Employment and Rehabilitation Institute of California
Santa Ana, California

G. WAYNE MCCALL, M.ED., C.R.C.
(Chapter 53)
Vocational Diagnostics Laboratory
Stone Mountain, Georgia

JOHN A. MCCULLOCH, M.D.
(Chapter 27)
Summit Orthopaedic Group, Inc.
Akron, Ohio

MARILOU MOSCHETTI
(Chapter 30)
AquaTechnics Consulting Group
Aptos, California

NORBERT R. MYSLINSKI, PH.D.
(Chapter 24)
Associate Professor
Orafacial Neuroscience Group
Department of Physiology
School of Dentistry, University of Maryland

JAMES R. B. NASHOLD
(*Chapter 7*)
Division of Neurosurgery
Duke University Medical Center
Durham, North Carolina

BLAINE S. NASHOLD, JR., M.D.
(*Chapter 7*)
Division of Neurosurgery
Duke University Medical Center
Durham, North Carolina

JAMES NITKA, M.D.
(*Chapter 28*)
Resident, Orthopaedic Surgery
Division of Orthopaedic Surgery
Duke University Medical Center
Durham, North Carolina

RICHARD NORTH, M.D.
(*Chapter 8*)
Department of Neurosurgery
The Johns Hopkins Hospital
Baltimore, Maryland

ROBERT N. PILON, M.D.
(*Chapter 21*)
Athens Regional Medical Center
Athens, Georgia

SRINIVASA N. RAJA
(*Chapter 39*)
Department of Anesthesiology
The Johns Hopkins School of Medicine
Baltimore, Maryland

ROSLYN RAKOFF
(*Chapter 47*)

CARLA RODGERS, M.D.
(*Chapter 45*)
Department of Psychiatry and Human Behavior
Jefferson Medical College
Philadelphia, Pennsylvania

HUBERT L. ROSOMOFF, M.D., D.Sc.
(*Chapter 51*)
Department of Neurological Surgery
University of Miami School of Medicine
Miami, Florida

RENEE STEELE ROSOMOFF, B.S.N.
(*Chapter 51*)
Comprehensive Pain and Rehabilitation Center
Miami, Florida

KAREN RUCKER, M.D.
(*Chapter 55*)
Chairman and Associate Professor
Department of Physical Medicine and Rehabilitation
Medical College of Richmond
Richmond, Virginia

THOMAS E. RUDY, M.D.
(*Chapter 12*)
Pain Evaluation and Treatment Institute
Pittsburgh, Pennsylvania

JOHN D. RYBOCK, M.D.
(*Chapter 6*)
Assistant Professor of Neurosurgery
Johns Hopkins School of Medicine
Baltimore, Maryland

JOEL R. SAPER, M.D., F.A.C.P.
(*Chapter 20*)
Michigan Headache and Neurological Institute
Ann Arbor, Michigan

JOHN R. SATTERTHWAITE, M.D.
(*Chapter 41*)
Pain Therapy Center of Greenville
Greenville, South Carolina

JULIE SAWYER, M.S., C.B.E., C.R.C., O.T.R./L.
(*Chapter 55*)
Pro Active Therapy, Inc.
Greenville, North Carolina

DAVID G. SIMONS, M.D.
(*Chapters 43 and 44*)
Department of Physical Medicine and Rehabilitation
University of California
Irvine, California

LOIS STATHAM SIMONS, M.S., R.P.T.
(*Chapter 44*)
Physical Therapist
Huntington Beach, California

BRUCE SMOLLER, M.D.
(*Chapter 47*)
Medical Director
Washington Pain Assessment Group
Washington, D.C.

GLEN D. SOLOMON, M.D.
(*Chapter 13*)
Section of Headache
Department of Internal Medicine
Cleveland Clinic Foundation
Cleveland, Ohio

HENRY A. SPINDLER, M.D.
(Chapter 5)
Rehabilitation Medicine
Franklin Square Hospital
Baltimore, Maryland

BLAKE H. TEARNAN, PH.D.
(Chapter 34)
Nevada Occupational Health Clinic
Sparks, Nevada

TROY L. THOMPSON II, M.D.
(Chapter 45)
Department of Psychiatry and Human Behavior
Jefferson Medical College
Philadelphia, Pennsylvania

BRUCE TOBEY, M.D.
(Chapter 28)
Fellow in Hand Surgery
Division of Orthopaedic Surgery
Duke University Medical Center
Durham, North Carolina

C. DAVID TOLLISON, PH.D.
(Chapter 56)
Pain Therapy Center of Greenville
Greenville, South Carolina
Department of Anesthesiology
Medical College of Georgia
Augusta, Georgia

JOSEPH W. TOLLISON, M.D.
(Chapter 17)
Department of Family Medicine
Medical College of Georgia
Augusta, Georgia

ROGER B. TRAYCOFF, M.D.
(Chapter 42)
Division of Rheumatology
Southern Illinois University School of Medicine
Springfield, Illinois

DENNIS C. TURK, PH.D.
(Chapter 12)
Center for Pain Evaluation and Treatment
University of Pittsburgh Medical Center
Pittsburgh, Pennsylvania

SANFORD H. VERNICK, M.D., PH.D.
(Chapter 55)
East Carolina University School of Medicine
Department of Physical Medicine and Rehabilitation
Regional Rehabilitation Center
Greenville, North Carolina

CLAY H. WARD, M.S.
(Chapter 34)
Psychiatry Service
Veterans Administration Medical Center
Reno, Nevada

CLARK WATTS, M.D.
(Chapter 25)
Division of Neurological Surgery
University of Missouri-Columbia
Columbia, Missouri

RICHARD L. WEDDIGE, M.D.
(Chapter 11)
Chairman
Department of Psychiatry
Texas Tech University Health Sciences Center
Lubbock, Texas

PETER G. WILSON, M.D.
(Chapter 40)
Department of Psychiatry
Cornell University Medical College
New York, New York

CHARLES WITTEN, M.D.
(Chapter 32)
Section of Urology
University of Pennsylvania
Philadelphia, Pennsylvania

CONTENTS

Foreword by Janet G. Travell, M.D. .... *vii*
Preface .... *ix*
Contributors .... *xi*

SECTION I
FOUNDATIONS

CHAPTER **1**   Definitions of Pain 3
Michael Feuerstein

CHAPTER **2**   Taxonomy and Classification of Pain 7
David B. Boyd

CHAPTER **3**   Anatomy of Pain 11
James L. Hall

CHAPTER **4**   Psychological Evaluation and Testing 18
Donald W. Hinnant

CHAPTER **5**   Medical Electrodiagnostics 36
Henry A. Spindler

SECTION II
THERAPEUTIC MODALITIES

CHAPTER **6**   Diagnostic andTherapeutic Nerve Blocks 51
John D. Rybock

CHAPTER **7**   Neurosurgical Treatment of Deafferentation Pain 62
Blaine S. Nashold, Jr., James R. B. Nashold, and Eben Alexander

CHAPTER **8**   Neural Stimulation Techniques for Chronic Pain 74
Richard B. North

CHAPTER **9**   Role of the Physiatrist in Management of Musculoskeletal Pain 85
Andrew Cole and Stanley A. Herring

CHAPTER **10** Spinal Manipulation and Physical Rehabilitation 96
Jerry C. Langley

CHAPTER **11** Adjunctive Treatment Techniques 108
Larry A. Gaupp, Don E. Flinn, and Richard L. Weddige

CHAPTER **12** A Cognitive-Behavioral Perspective on Chronic Pain: Beyond the Scalpel
and Syringe 136
Dennis C. Turk and Thomas E. Rudy

SECTION III
PHARMACOLOGIC INTERVENTIONS

CHAPTER **13** Analgesic Medications 155
Glen D. Solomon

CHAPTER **14** Nonsteroidal Anti-Inflammatory Drugs 165
Stephen M. Honig

CHAPTER **15** Muscle Relaxant Medications 173
R. Michael Gallagher

CHAPTER **16** Psychopharmacologic Agents in the Treatment of Pain Syndromes 181
Joseph H. Atkinson, Jr., Mark A. Slater, Jason N. Doctor, and Joshua C. Klapow

CHAPTER **17** Special Considerations in Pharmacologic Pain Management 215
Joseph W. Tollison

CHAPTER **18** Drug Detoxification Protocols 224
David A. Fishbain

SECTION IV
PAIN MANAGEMENT IN SELECTIVE DISORDERS

CHAPTER **19** Differential Diagnosis of Headache Pain 239
Seymour Diamond and Merle L. Diamond

CHAPTER **20** Medical Management of Headache Pain 253
Joel R. Saper

CHAPTER **21** Psychological Management of Headache Pain 268
Anthony Iezzi, Henry E. Adams, and Robert N. Pilon

CHAPTER **22** Differential Diagnosis and Management of Orofacial Pain 280
Kim J. Burchiel and Jeffrey A. Burgess

CHAPTER **23** Medical/Neurosurgical Management of Orofacial Pain 294
Ronald Brisman

CHAPTER **24** Dental Management of Orofacial Pain 306
Jerome D. Buxbaum and Norbert R. Myslinski

CHAPTER **25** Spinal Surgery for Pain Management 328
Clark Watts

CHAPTER **26** Differential Diagnosis and Management of Cervical Spine Pain ... 331
John Aryanpur and Thomas B. Ducker

CHAPTER **27** Differential Diagnosis of Low Back Pain 347
John A. McCulloch

CHAPTER **28** Painful Arthropathies 369
J. Leonard Goldner, James Nitka, Patricia Howson, and Bruce Tobey

CHAPTER **29** Neuritis, Neuropathy, and Neuralgia 377
Benjamin L. Crue, Jr.

CHAPTER **30** Lumbar Spine Aquatic Rehabilitation: A Sports Medicine Approach 386
Andrew J. Cole, Marilou Moschetti, and Richard E. Eagleston

CHAPTER **31** Gynecologic Pain 401
J. Greg Johnson

CHAPTER 32 Pain in the Male Genitalia 409
Terrence R. Malloy, Charles Witten, and Jerald B. Gilbert

CHAPTER 33 Physical Management of Malignant Pain 419
Theresa Ferrer-Brechner

CHAPTER 34 Psychological Management of Malignant Pain 431
Blake H. Tearnan and Clay H. Ward

CHAPTER 35 Neurosurgical Treatment of Pain Related to Cancer 447
Stephen R. Freidberg

CHAPTER 36 Palliation of Pain Secondary to Malignancy by Radiation Therapy 454
Richard H. Fitzgerald, Jr.

CHAPTER 37 Peripheral Neuropathy 463
David R. Cornblath and Jonathan D. Glass

CHAPTER 38 Entrapment and Compression Neuropathies 470
Stephen R. Conway and H. Royden Jones, Jr.

CHAPTER 39 Reflex Sympathetic Dystrophy and Causalgia 484
Nelson Hendler and Srinivasa N. Raja

CHAPTER 40 Phantom Pain 497
Peter G. Wilson

CHAPTER 41 Post-Herpetic Neuralgia 503
John R. Satterthwaite

CHAPTER 42 Chronic Joint and Connective Tissue Pain 523
Roger B. Traycoff

CHAPTER 43 Single-Muscle Myofascial Pain Syndromes 539
David G. Simons

CHAPTER 44 Chronic Myofascial Pain Syndrome 556
David G. Simons and Lois Statham Simons

SECTION V
SELECTED TOPICS

CHAPTER 45 Pain Problems in Primary Care Medical Practice 581
Carla Rodgers and Troy L. Thompson, II

CHAPTER 46 Postoperative Pain Management 600
Thomas K. Henthorn and Tom C. Krejcie

CHAPTER 47 Early Recognition of the Chronic Pain Syndrome 623
Michael Houston, Marc Hertzman, Roslyn Rakoff, and Bruce Smoller

CHAPTER 48 Ergonomic Conditions in the Workplace 640
Mahmoud A. Ayoub

CHAPTER 49 Office and Hospital Pain Consultations 667
Victor C. Lee

CHAPTER 50 Outpatient Chronic Pain Management Programs 676
Stanley Chapman

CHAPTER 51 Hospital-Based Inpatient Treatment Programs 686
Renee Steele Rosomoff and Hubert L. Rosomoff

CHAPTER 52 Occupational Rehabilitation Treatment Programs 694
Leonard N. Matheson

CHAPTER **53** Legal Aspects of Pain and Social Security Disability 712
G. Wayne McCall

APPENDIX 53.1: Physical Demands 716

APPENDIX 53.2: Working Conditions 719

APPENDIX 53.3: Training Time 720

CHAPTER **54** Workers' Compensation 722
Penny Lozon Crook

CHAPTER **55** Evaluation and Rating of Physical Disability 732
Sanford H. Vernick, Julie Sawyer, Edgar Marin, and Karen Rucker

CHAPTER **56** Assessment of Psychological Impairment and Disability 742
C. David Tollison and Donald W. Hinnant

INDEX 757

FOUNDATIONS

CHAPTER 1
DEFINITIONS OF PAIN
MICHAEL FEUERSTEIN

Pain, although a common experience to most of us, remains an enigma. Pain is a construct or concept. As a construct, its definition is a function of the theoretical orientation one takes with regard to pain. For example, to some neurosurgeons pain is the description of a sensation by a patient that can best be conceptualized within a strictly neuroanatomic and neurophysiologic framework. Anything that does not fall within this model is not pain but a "psychiatric disorder." Clearly, while secular trends in medicine are moving away from such a position, I am certain many readers have consulted with various surgeons and indeed patients who continue to hold such a "definition" of pain.

In fairness to our neurosurgeon colleagues, there are the proponents of the exclusive psychological definition(s) or conceptualizations of pain who are perhaps equally biased in their viewpoint. These clinicians, frequently psychologists or psychiatrists, often disregard the neurophysiologic, anatomic, or disease process potentially involved in persistent pain because as they conceive it such an approach has not proved useful in the management of many chronic pain disorders. Their definition of pain reflects some integration of psychological and social factors and conceptualizes pain as modulated by a complex set of emotional, environmental, and psychophysiologic variables.

As is the case with most matters, the "truth" probably lies somewhere at the midpoint of this neurophysiologic-behavioral continuum. The purpose of this brief chapter is not to provide a scholarly review of this debate, nor to provide a historic perspective of various views of pain; rather, my intention is to provide the reader with the most recent generally accepted definition of pain proposed by the International Association for the Study of Pain, along with some key definitions related to functional changes associated with pain. Finally, the chapter provides a brief summary of an operational definition of chronic pain that the author has found useful in his practice in providing a framework for conceptualizing the patient with chronic pain.

THE INTERNATIONAL ASSOCIATION FOR THE STUDY OF PAIN DEFINITION

Perhaps the most widely accepted definition of pain by pain specialists is that proposed by the International Association for the Study of Pain (IASP). This definition is as follows:

> **An unpleasant sensory and emotional experience associated with actual or potential tissue damage, or described in terms of such damage.**
>
> *Note:* Pain is always subjective. Each individual learns the application of the word through experiences related to injury in early life. Biologists recognize that those stimuli which cause pain are liable to damage tissue. Accordingly, pain is that experience which we associate with actual or potential tissue damage. It is unquestionably a sensation in a part or parts of the body, but it is also always unpleasant and therefore also an emotional experience. Experiences which resemble pain, e.g., pricking, but are not unpleasant should not be called pain. Unpleasant abnormal experiences (dysaesthesiae) may also be pain but are not necessarily so because, subjectively, they may not have the usual sensory qualities of pain.
>
> Many people report pain in the absence of tissue damage or any likely pathophysiological cause; usually this happens for psychological reasons. There is usually no way to distinguish their experience from that due to tissue damage if we take the subjective report. If they regard their experience as pain and if they report it in the same ways as pain caused by tissue damage, it should be accepted as pain. This definition avoids tying pain to the stimulus. Activity induced in the nociceptor and nociceptive pathways by a noxious stimulus is not pain, which is always a psychological state, even though we may well appreciate that pain most often has a proximate physical cause.
>
> Taxonomy Committee of the International Association for the Study of Pain (1)

The emphasis of this definition is on pain as a sensory and emotional experience in which pain is not exclusively defined in terms of nociceptive input but is rather a *psychological state*. This is particularly the case with chronic pain, the focus of this handbook. Indeed, the exclusive emphasis on a nociceptive generator, disease process, and its "associated pain" can impede the pain management process with certain patients. Clearly, the need to assess both nociceptive and psychological processes represents the state of the art approach to pain and its management.

DEFINITIONS OF FUNCTIONAL CAPACITY

Given the recent emphasis in pain management on restoration of functioning with or without reduction of pain itself (2), discussion of definitions of pain should also consider definitions of function. The Committee on Pain, Disability and Chronic Illness Behavior of the Institute of Medicine recently delineated three broad categories that are frequently used to define alterations in functional capacity (3). These terms are *impairment, functional limitation*, and *disability*. Using the World Health Organization's definitions as a framework, the committee defined these terms in the following way:

> **Impairment:** "*Any* loss or abnormality of psychological, physiological or anatomical structure or function" (3). Functions that may be affected by chronic pain include walking, standing, sitting, reaching, lifting, bending, attentional abilities, mood, and social interaction, to name but a few.
> **Functional Limitation:** "*Any* restriction or lack of ability to perform an activity in the manner or within the range considered normal for a human being that results from an impairment (World Health Organization's definition of "disability")" (3). This definition indicates that any loss of capabilities because of an inability to integrate physical and psychosocial functions because of pain, disease, or impairment represents a functional limitation. The limitation can include any combination of physical and psychosocial functions (e.g., housecleaning, operating a drill press, helping one's children get off to school).
> **Disability:** "A disadvantage for a given individual (resulting from an impairment or a functional limitation) that *limits* or *prevents* the fulfillment of a role that is normal (function of age, sex, social and cultural factors) for that individual (World Health Organization's definition of "handicap")" (3). This definition indicates that if pain limits or prevents one from fulfilling an appropriate role in life, the pain is associated with a disability.

The use of such terms as impairment, functional limitation, and disability is found on the numerous forms one is asked to complete daily for patients with chronic pain, yet there remains little consensus as to what these terms mean. Also, each definition includes the term *normal* or *abnormal*, and until there is a sufficient data base to statistically define such terms, the "objective determination" of such states resulting from pain will

Table 1.1.
Components of an Operational Definition of Chronic Pain

Pain sensation
Pain behavior
Functional status at work
Functional status at home
Emotional state
Somatic preoccupation

continue to be influenced by a complex set of social, economic, interpersonal, and medical variables. This current situation places many patients with chronic pain and resultant impairment, functional limitation, or disability in a precarious position. Fortunately, efforts are underway to more carefully define and quantify the functional capabilities necessary to perform various job tasks and activities in daily living that should assist in more definitive determination of these indices of ability.

OPERATIONAL DEFINITION OF PAIN

As will be discussed in Chapter 2 ("Taxonomy and Classification of Pain"), a classification system has been developed by the IASP that defines pain in a given patient along five axes: (*a*) regions, or general anatomic location for pain; (*b*) systems, or the primary organ system in the body associated with the pain (e.g., cardiovascular, nervous); (*c*) temporal characteristics of the pain or its pattern of occurrence (e.g., single episode, recurrent regular, continuous/nonfluctuating); (*d*) time since onset; and (*e*) suspected etiology (e.g., neoplasm, trauma, unknown) (1). Although such a framework should assist with research efforts and provide the clinician with a prognosis and treatment approach, the schema does not consider certain aspects of the presenting complaints.

The components of an operational definition of chronic pain the author uses in practice are presented in Table 1.1. This definition considers pain sensation, pain behavior, functional status at work and home, emotional state, and somatic preoccupation. Various contributors to this handbook will elaborate in detail on certain aspects of these components of chronic pain as they relate to each specific pain problem discussed. However, a brief overview of these components should help the clinician place most chronic pain problems within this general framework.

PAIN SENSATION

The pain sensation component of chronic pain is best described as the actual experience of pain as reported by the patient. This category can include actual sensory qualities of the pain as well as its location. A series of measurement devices are available to assist the clinician in evaluating this dimension of pain. However, it is not uncommon to rely on the patient's report of the qualities of pain at certain locations and, when appropriate, to recreate or reproduce the pain sensation during the physical exam. Pain maps are also used for identifying location.

PAIN BEHAVIOR

Pain behavior is a complex set of expressions and overt (observable) behaviors that suggest a patient is experiencing pain. The behaviors can include grimacing, use of supportive devices, vocalizations, continued medication use despite its apparent lack of effectiveness, and avoidance of movement for fear of increased pain, to name but a few. As with pain sensation, there are several direct observation techniques and self-report diaries of pain behavior and activity. Pain behavior represents an important component in defining chronic pain. As one might expect, the variation in such behavior is extensive and its specific manifestations can also vary considerably across patients.

FUNCTIONAL STATUS AT WORK

The area of functional capacity, important to rehabilitation for years, has only recently been a focus of interest in chronic pain. Consideration of this component of chronic pain is essential to its adequate definition. Although in the past much reliance was placed on what the employee and/or supervisor reported, recently direct observation using video techniques at the job site has been used more frequently. In addition, the use of simulated job tasks has represented an area of increased activity, potentially reducing the need for direct observation at the work site. This type of evaluation, coupled with isokinetic strength testing, has been used to provide a more quantitative index of functional abilities related to movements associated with specific job tasks. The influence of pain sensation and emotions in influencing job performance can now be more adequately determined in a given case, and baseline indices of abilities can be used as a point of departure for rehabilitation efforts.

FUNCTIONAL STATUS AT HOME

Consideration of the ability to perform functions related to the home also should be included in a comprehensive definition of chronic pain. Self-report questionnaires, direct observation of home-related functional capabilities, and reports from family members represent sources of data for this component. Although this area is generally limited to physical functioning within the home, such an evaluation should also consider the psychosocial functioning within the family. That is, the different roles that family members play, the communication and problem-solving skills the family possesses, and the role pain and illness plays in the family system should be considered when evaluating functional status at home.

EMOTIONAL STATE

An often-neglected area when considering chronic pain, particularly from the non-pain specialist's perspective, is the emotional component of pain. Many practitioners continue to search for the specific pain generator in patients and if such an "origin" is not found, the patient's pain is considered "not serious" or the patient is said to have psychogenic pain, or some variant of a psychiatric disorder. The all-or-none hypothesis related to chronic pain remains a significant force in health care despite definitions of pain such as that proposed by the IASP.

Emotional factors can play a significant role in the initiation, exacerbation, and maintenance of a variety of chronic pain disorders with or without observable pathophysiologic pain generators. Therefore, it is useful to evaluate the role of emotional factors and include such factors when defining pain.

Anxiety, depression, fatigue, and irritability can all play a complex role in the exacerbation of pain and pain behavior. The clear challenge for the clinician is to differentiate whether the emotional state of the patient is primary or secondary to chronic pain. It is important to obtain as clear a picture as possible as to the long-standing nature of a mood disturbance and/or personality disorder. This information can play an important role in determining various treatment options. As with each of the areas discussed, there are several methods one can use to assess the emotional factors associated with chronic pain.

SOMATIC PREOCCUPATION

Somatic preoccupation represents a cognitive component of chronic pain that can be defined as a heightened sensitivity and/or selective attention to bodily discomfort. This final component of chronic pain is one of the more resistent to modification. Pain reports can be significantly reduced (~50% reduction), pain behaviors can be eliminated, and functional status at work and home can be enhanced, while emotional distress can also be significantly reduced. Despite these changes, many patients, particularly those with strong disease convictions, continue to display a persistent sensitivity and selective attention to bodily sensations and discomfort.

Consideration of this component of chronic pain should help the clinician conceptualize the role of different treatment options for the patient. For example, if an overall goal in a treatment program was a reduction in pain, not its elimination, such a goal needs to be made explicitly clear to a patient with a high somatic preoccupation. Otherwise, patient expectations may not be consistent with those of the treating clinician. Another example would be in the area of neural blockade (e.g., epidural steroid injections for back pain with radicular component). A patient with high levels of somatic preoccupation should be clearly informed of what to expect in terms of short-term/long-term pain relief and whether the series of blocks represents a way to help the patient move into a rehabilitation program directed at behavioral pain management or the blocks are in themselves the treatment.

The view the patient has regarding his health and the role this view has taken in influencing his approach to health represents an important area with significant clinical implications. Somatic preoccupation can influence a chronic pain patient's view of the treatment plan, the treatment team, and treatment goals. Assessment of this component of chronic pain, therefore, can be quite important.

SUMMARY

Pain is clearly more than a sensation. Chronic pain should be considered in the context of the patient's abilities and disabilities. An operational definition of chronic pain potentially helpful to the practitioner should include consideration of pain sensation, pain behavior, functional status at work and home, emotional state, and somatic preoccupation. Assessment of these components of chronic pain can provide a working framework for evaluation and management of these complex patients.

REFERENCES

1. Merskey H: Classification of chronic pain: descriptions of chronic pain syndromes and definitions of pain terms. *Pain* Suppl 3, S217, 1986.
2. Mayer TG, Gatchel RJ, Kishino N, Keeley J, Mayer H, Capra P, Mooney V: A prospective short-term study of chronic low back pain patients utilizing novel objective functional measurement. *Pain* 25:53–68, 1986.
3. Osterweis M, Kleinman A, Mechanic D (eds): *Pain and Disability: Clinical, Behavioral, and Public Policy Perspectives.* Washington, DC, National Academy Press, 1987.

CHAPTER 2

TAXONOMY AND CLASSIFICATION OF PAIN

DAVID B. BOYD

PAIN CAN be classified in a variety of ways. With a rapidly expanding body of literature on chronic pain, it is inevitable that different classifications will be put forth by individuals and disciplines. Each approach has its virtues—and its criticisms. The symptom of "pain" is of interest to a wide spectrum of students and potential therapists. Each clinical discipline approaches the problem of pain from its own viewpoint, with its own body of knowledge, and with its own language biases. At times, these differing attitudes and languages make a cohesive approach seem almost impossible; and yet, most people involved with the study and treatment of chronic pain would agree that a multidisciplinary approach is best. In this second edition of the *Handbook of Pain Management* the need for a more or less universally accepted classification of pain is again stressed.

The "Classification of Chronic Pain" was published in 1986 as a supplement of *Pain*, the journal of the International Association for the Study of Pain, or IASP (1). The IASP subcommittee on taxonomy and classification is multidisciplinary and put together this classification after considering many different approaches. The result is not presented as the perfect endpoint. Any attempt at classification should be continually improved and remodeled as further information and understanding develop.

In discussing the need for and style of sorting and classifying, it becomes apparent that some people are "lumpers" (wanting a few large, rather mixed groups) and others are "splitters" (sometimes to the point of individualizing groups to just one). The IASP classification is reasonably complete in terms of complexity and length but it is still manageable. It has practical application to patients as they are seen. It should be adopted and used.

Examine some of the advantages of a unified approach. For research purposes, a homogeneous group of patients lends itself to good study design and more refined results that can reasonably be extrapolated to other patients with the same problem. To say that a patient has "chronic pain" is a start, but it is ludicrous to lump together, as if they are the same, a patient with metastatic bone pain, a patient with chronic migraine, a patient with postamputation phantom pain, and a patient with psychotic delusional pain. Little wonder that plans to manage pain sometimes, indeed all too frequently, fail. Pain, and especially chronic pain, is a vague and intrinsically difficult subject to measure and categorize. Pain is something everyone knows about regardless of whether we accept the definition as "pain is what hurts" or the more sophisticated definition of pain as "an unpleasant sensory and emotional experience associated with actual or potential tissue damage, or described in terms of such damage," as stated by Dr. Harold Merskey (1). Even within disciplines there is much disagreement about any particular pain with respect to etiology, pathophysiology, and treatment. Once different disciplines try to compare information, it becomes even more vital that an accepted pain syndrome be focused upon. For example, "chronic leg pain" might be more precise than simply "chronic pain" but less specific than "chronic leg pain from diabetic neuropathy." In the ideal situation the presenting pain would be sorted out specifically so that only those therapists who are really likely to be helpful need to become involved. At this point the situation is often unclear: Should the patient with low back pain see some or all of the following: physiotherapist, chiropractor, rheumatologist, anesthesiologist, neurosurgeon, orthopedic surgeon, or psychologist (to name but a few of the potential caregivers)?

If information is collected from all disciplines and put together in a framework that allows accurate comparison then it will be possible to gradually develop a system that expands current knowledge and correlates treatments to specific situations. Apart from knowledge that is immediately useful clinically, various groups ranging from government statisticians to insurance

Congenital

Acquired
   Infectious (viral, bacterial, fungal, or protozoal)
   Toxic—endocrine-metabolic
   Allergic/autoimmune
   Traumatic
   Collagen vascular
   Vascular
   Neoplastic
   Hematologic
   Neurologic
   Psychiatric
   Degenerative
   Iatrogenic
   Other
      sarcoid
      amyloid

Figure 2.1. Sample list classification often used in internal medicine—an example of a one-dimensional system.

	Biologic	Psychologic	Sociocultural
Predisposing			
Precipitating			
Perpetuating			

Figure 2.2. Sample grid classification often used in psychiatry—an example of a two-dimensional system.

Axis I: Region
Axis II: System
Axis III: Temporal characteristics of pain: pattern of
           occurrence
Axis IV: Patient's statement of intensity: time since onset of
           pain
Axis V: Etiology

Figure 2.3. Overview of the IASP Five Axis Pain Taxonomy.

Head, face, and mouth	000
Cervical region	100
Upper shoulder and upper limbs	200
Thoracic region	300
Abdominal region	400
Lower back, lumbar spine, sacrum, and coccyx	500
Lower limbs	600
Pelvic region	700
Anal, perineal, and genital region	800
More than three major sites	900

Figure 2.4. Axis I: Regions. Record main site first; record two important regions separately. If there is more than one site of pain, separate coding will be necessary. (From Mersky H: Classification of chronic pain, descriptions of chronic pain syndromes and definitions of pain terms. *Pain* Suppl 3, S10–S11, 1986.)

Nervous system (central, peripheral, and autonomic) and special senses; physical disturbance or dysfunction	00
Nervous system (psychological and social)	10
Respiratory and cardiovascular systems	20
Musculoskeletal system and connective tissue	30
Cutaneous and subcutaneous and associated glands (breast, apocrine, etc.)	40
Gastrointestinal system	50
Genito-urinary system	60
Other organs or viscera (e.g., thyroid, lymphatic, hemopoietic	70
More than one system	80

Figure 2.5. Axis II: Systems. The system coded is that in which abnormal functioning produces the pain (e.g., claudication = vascular). Similarly, the nervous system is to be coded only when a pathologic disturbance in it produces pain. Thus pain from a pancreatic carcinoma = gastrointestinal; pain from a metastatic deposit affecting bones = musculoskeletal. (From Mersky H: Classification of chronic pain, descriptions of chronic pain syndromes and definitions of pain terms. *Pain* Suppl 3, S10–S11, 1986.)

Not recorded, not applicable, or not known	0
Single episode, limited duration (e.g., ruptured aneurysm, sprained ankle)	1
Continuous or nearly continuous, nonfluctuating (e.g., low back pain, some cases)	2
Continuous or nearly continuous, fluctuating severity (e.g., ruptured intervertebral disc)	3
Recurring, irregularly (e.g., headache, mixed type)	4
Recurring, regularly (e.g., premenstrual pain)	5
Paroxysmal (e.g., tic douloureux)	6
Sustained with superimposed paroxysms	7
Other combinations	8
None of the above	9

Figure 2.6. Axis III: Temporal Characteristics of Pain, Pattern of Occurrence. (From Mersky H: Classification of chronic pain, descriptions of chronic pain syndromes and definitions of pain terms. *Pain* Suppl 3, S10–S11, 1986.)

companies to hospital medical records departments want data about diagnosis, epidemiology, and prognosis. Currently, the position to give much more than speculation about so many aspects of pain is weak. With improving communications systems worldwide and gradual computerization of data, an accepted backbone of structure is needed that is similar to post office zip codes or telephone books.

Throughout clinical medicine, one is confronted by attempts to classify. There is often a somewhat artificial effort to dichotomize: acute versus chronic, benign versus malignant, mild versus severe, treatable versus intractable. To avoid such oversimplification various one- or two-dimensional systems have been developed as

Not recorded, not applicable, or not known		.0
Mild—	1 month or less	.1
	1 month to 6 months	.2
	more than 6 months	.3
Medium—	1 month or less	.4
	1 month to 6 months	.5
	more than 6 months	.6
Severe—	1 month or less	.7
	1 month to 6 months	.8
	more than 6 months	.9

Figure 2.7. **Axis IV: Patient's Statement of Intensity, Time Since Onset of Pain.** (From Mersky H: Classification of chronic pain, descriptions of chronic pain syndromes and definitions of pain terms. *Pain* Suppl 3, S10–S11, 1986.)

Genetic or congenital disorders (e.g., congenital dislocation)	.00
Trauma, operation, burns	.01
Infective, parasitic	.02
Inflammatory (no known infective agent), immune reactions	.03
Neoplasm	.04
Toxic, metabolic (e.g., alcoholic neuropathy, anoxia, vascular, nutritional, endocrine), radiation	.05
Degenerative, mechanical	.06
Dysfunctional (including psychophysiologic)	.07
Unknown or other	.08
Psychological origin (e.g., conversion hysteria, depressive hallucination). (Note: No physical cause should be held to be present nor any pathophysiological mechanism.)	.09

Figure 2.8. **Axis V: Etiology.** (From Mersky H: Classification of chronic pain, descriptions of chronic pain syndromes and definitions of pain terms. *Pain* Suppl 3, S10–S11, 1986.)

lists or grids, as seen in Figures 2.1 and 2.2. Even these approaches leave out a lot—hence the development of systems with axes like that of the IASP taxonomy, which is similar to DSM-III as used by the American Psychiatric Association.

The IASP Taxonomy proposes a five-axis system (Fig. 2.3). Any patient's pain can be described by all five of these axes in sequence—for example, a low back pain (Axis I), of neurologic origin (Axis II), occurring continuously and severely (Axis III) for 6 months (Axis IV) from degenerative disk disease (Axis V). To allow numerical coding, if desired, each axis has been assigned a digit in an order of magnitude (Figs. 2.4 through 2.8). For complete discussions of taxonomy and pain syndromes the reader is referred to *Pain,* Supplement 3, 1986.

This classification takes into account a number of the well-recognized but perhaps poorly standardized approaches to pain, namely site, system, time course and duration, severity, and etiology. It also allows for fur-

Table 2.1.
Syndromes by Group According to IASP Taxonomy[a]

I.	Relatively Generalized Syndromes
II.	Neuralgias of the Head and Face
III.	Craniofacial Pain of Musculoskeletal Origin
IV.	Lesions of the Ear, Nose, and Oral Cavity
V.	Primary Headache Syndromes
VI.	Pain of Psychological Origin in the Head and Face
VII.	Suboccipital and Cervical Musculoskeletal Disorders
VIII.	Visceral Pain in the Neck
IX.	Pain of Neurologic Origin in Neck, Shoulder, and Upper Extremity
X.	Lesions of the Brachial Plexus
XI.	Pain in the Shoulder, Arm, and Hand
XII.	Vascular Disease of the Limbs
XIII.	Collagen Disease of the Limbs
XIV.	Vasodilating Functional Disease of the Limbs
XV.	Arterial Insufficiencies in the Limbs
XVI.	Pain in the Limbs of Psychological Origin
XVII.	Chest Pain
XVIII.	Chest Pain of Psychological Origin
XIX.	Chest Pain: Referred from Abdomen or Gastrointestinal Tract
XX.	Abdominal Pain of Neurologic Origin
XXI.	Abdominal Pain of Visceral Origin
XXII.	Abdominal Pain Syndromes of Generalized Diseases
XXIII.	Abdominal Pain of Psychological Origin
XXIV.	Disease of Uterus, Ovaries and Adnexa
XXV.	Pain in the Rectum, Perineum and External Genitalia
XXVI.	Backache and Pain of Neurologic Origin in Trunk and Back
XXVII.	Back Pain of Musculoskeletal Origin
XXVIII.	Back Pain of Visceral Origin
XXIX.	Low Back Pain of Psychological Origin
XXX.	Local Syndromes in the Leg or Foot—Pain of Neurologic Origin
XXXI.	Pain syndromes of Hip and Thigh of Musculoskeletal Origin
XXXII.	Musculoskeletal Syndromes of the Leg

[a]From Mersky H: Classification of chronic pain, descriptions of chronic pain syndromes and definitions of pain terms. *Pain* Suppl 3, S13–S24, 1986.

ther delineation along traditional questions: associated symptoms, aggravating factors, usual course, complications, social and physical disability, pathology, and differential diagnosis.

Table 2.1 overviews pain syndromes commonly seen clinically and discussed in greater detail in the IASP Taxonomy and Descriptions of Pain Syndromes.

The ideal classification system would have a specific location for each pain syndrome with no chance of omission or overlap. Clinical medicine rarely lends itself to such precise dissection. Nonetheless, by continual reexamination by various groups, even pain gradually becomes more understandable. The IASP pain classification proposed above has several noteworthy advantages. First of all, it was developed by a multidisciplinary association. Second, this association is widely based in terms of both geography and expertise. Third, it publishes a respected and well-circulated journal and has already published a proposed pain taxonomy. The five axes follow criteria that are currently used in pain problems, and so should be easy to adopt by most clinicians. This classification will be modified as knowledge expands but offers a firm starting point.

A lot of work is currently going into classification of low back pain. The attempt to make homogeneous pain patient groups identifiable (for purposes of research, investigation, and treatment) continues.

Reference

1. Merskey H: Classification of chronic pain, descriptions of chronic pain syndromes and definitions of pain terms. *Pain Suppl 3*, S10–S11, S13–S24, S217, 1986.

CHAPTER 3
ANATOMY OF PAIN
JAMES L. HALL

THE DESIRED objective of this chapter is to acquaint the reader with the principal central and peripheral anatomic structures involved in perception of painful stimuli. The mechanisms of pain are perhaps one of the more complex topics in medicine. In many areas complete anatomic and physiologic explanations are not yet known or are inadequate.

This, then, is an attempt by an anatomist to set forth the anatomic substrates that may be more exhaustively dealt with in subsequent sections. It is instructive to note that the word "pain" is derived from a Greek word meaning penalty. We can easily imagine a penalty in the form of pain being visited upon some poor mortal for his affrontries to the Gods of Mt. Olympus.

PERIPHERAL STRUCTURES

RECEPTORS

We are now aware that most receptors on the peripheral endings of afferent nerves respond to a variety of stimuli. However, their shape and location and field of reception indicate that they are able to perceive one type of stimulus more efficiently than many other types. The specific receptor type that is incriminated in the reception of the pain stimulus is said to be an unencapsulated nerve ending. Although this receptor, in many examples, has a thin myelin covering, it is usually referred to as an unmyelinated or naked nerve ending.

The pain receptor is a primitive, unorganized nerve ending and often has a weed-like appearance. It has many branches and often overlaps the territory of other nerve endings from cord segments above and below it. Here, it is important to realize that the strength of the stimulus is a critical factor in the production of pain in this and other types of receptors. When a certain threshold of intensity of the stimulus is surpassed, any stimulus can be interpreted as painful to most receptors. This specific threshold is referred to as a noxious stimulus, one that will elicit tissue damage. At that point the receptor is referred to as nociceptive. Pressure, for example, if increased can become painful, and an encapsu-

lated pacinian corpuscle, which is admirably modified by its onion-like capsule to have a large receptive field for pressure, can at a specific threshold level become a nociceptive receptor and generate an impulse of pain along its afferent nerve.

AFFERENT PAIN FIBERS

All nerve fibers are classified as to their age and conduction rate. They are called A, B, and C fibers, with A fibers being the largest in diameter and most rapid conducting fibers. B fibers are intermediate-sized fibers and have a somewhat slower conducting rate. C fibers are the smallest in caliber and the slowest conducting. There are apparently two types of pain-conducting fiber: an A-delta fiber, which is the most rapid of the pain-conducting fibers but the slowest of the alpha-conducting fibers, and C fibers, which are comparatively the slowest conducting fibers.

The pain conducted by the A-delta fibers is the quick, "bright" pain. It is often described as sharp, shooting, or even intense. C-fiber pain, on the other hand, is described as steady, slow, and constant.

SOMATIC PAIN CLASSIFICATION

Since the days of Henry Head in 1920, two other types of classifications of somatic pain have been used. Head proposed the terms of "epicritic" and "protopathic" to describe somatic pain. Head suggested that epicritic pain could be discriminated and localized; thus, such pain must usually come from the skin or more superficial areas. Protopathic pain, conversely, can only be discriminated in a generalized way and not definitely localized.

SPINAL OR DORSAL ROOT GANGLIA

Dorsal root ganglia are found on the dorsal or posterior root of all spinal nerves. These are the sensory roots conducting the central process of the spinal ganglion cell into the central nervous system. The spinal or segmental nerve conducts epicritic pain from a specific area of the skin called the *dermatome*.

There may be some individual variation in size and contours of the dermatome, but dermatomic areas are always segmental and have distinct boundaries. A given spinal ganglion supplies a specific dermatome in a one-to-one relationship, but there may be overlap between the sensory roots. A ganglion may carry some information from the dermatome above and below it; this is usually true in the conduction of pain. Thus, when a specific ganglion is destroyed, there may be only a slight loss of pain from the dermatome it supplies.

Protopathic or deep somatic and visceral pain are less rigidly related to the nerve roots. This is at least in part due to the migration of structures during embryonic development (e.g., the diaphragm, supplied by C3–C5 via the phrenic nerve). The segmental division of deep pain is called a *sclerotome*. Because the pain fibers from a sclerotome enter the cord through several posterior roots, a more generalized or nonlocalizing pattern results.

Visceral pain is conducted by the peripheral process of the dorsal root ganglia traveling with the autonomic fibers that supply the target tissue. If they are bound in the same sheath as the sympathetic fibers they may travel some distance from their origin in the spinal ganglia via the white ramus of the sympathetic chain and the very long preganglionic fibers before they reach the specific viscera they supply.

An example of this arrangement is the afferent fibers from spinal ganglia T5–T10 that travel with the greater splanchnic nerve to reach the celiac ganglia in the abdomen. The afferent fibers pass through the celiac ganglia without synapsing and supply the derivatives of embryonic foregut. It is useful to conceptualize the sympathetic innervation of viscera to be somewhat like a cascade or waterfall, with the viscera in the cavities being supplied by sympathetic fibers that originate at higher levels. The afferent fibers to these same viscera accompany the sympathetic fibers. Thoracic fibers cascade down into abdominal viscera, and fibers from lumbar sympathetic ganglia, called lumbar splanchnics, cascade down into pelvic viscera via the hypogastric fibers.

Although this concept also holds for afferents conducted in the parasympathetic vagus nerve, which is also supplying afferent innervation to some structures in the thorax and abdomen from its cranial origin via its two sensory ganglia, it is not entirely true for parasympathetic supply to the embryonic hindgut and pelvic splanchnic nerves. These arise from sacral segments S2–S4 and travel superiorly to supply the embryonic hindgut through the inferior mesenteric plexus. Nevertheless, the axiom that the efferent sympathetic response is regional or widespread and the parasympathetic response is usually local or confined has some validity when applied to afferent impulses as well. Cranial sympathetics, of course, arise at lower levels in the cord and ascend via the anterior and posterior cerebral circulation to higher levels. Thoracic sympathetics, usually above T5 or T6, supply thoracic viscera at those levels even though they may ascend in the chain some distance, as in the case of the cardioaccelerator nerves, to do so.

The relationship between pain-conducting afferent fibers and sympathetic efferent fibers is thought to be involved in the condition known as *causalgia*. The patient complains of a persistent and burning pain usually following the course of the nerve fibers in the region. It is thought that the integrity of the afferent pain fibers has been compromised so that the neurotransmitter of the afferent fibers (in this case, acetylcholine) is noxious to the sympathetic fiber, thus producing the burning sensation. The condition is usually relieved by a sympathectomy.

Receptors of pain are sparse in the viscera, and this generally contributes to a poorly localized sensation from most of the viscera. There are two notable exceptions to this rule. Distention of the gut and pain from the heart can readily be localized by the physician. However, the sensory innervation of the heart is now known to be much more elegant than was previously thought.

REFERRED PAIN

Referred pain is a troublesome topic in the interpretation and diagnosis of pain. In essence, it means that the originating pain from one region of the body is referred to another region of the body that is not receiving the noxious stimulus directly. A classic example is that of pain from the gallbladder being referred to the tip of the right shoulder, because the C3–C5 nerve roots are distributed to both the diaphragm and the shoulder area. Anatomically the usual reason given for referred pain is that the pain-conducting fibers are distributed to different localities by portions of the same spinal nerves. These pain fibers then converge on the same neurons in the dorsal gray horn of the spinal cord. There, based on the patient's past experience and the breakdown of the integrity of the neuronal pool, a message is sent to the cortex that the pain is coming from point ''A,'' which the cortex is preferentially structured to handle with ease, when the pain is really coming from point ''B,'' which it is not so well equipped to handle. The referred pain is finally localized correctly when somatic pain receptors are involved. Pain from the appendix, for example, may initially be perceived as originating from the umbilicus because the T10 nerve supplies both structures. Eventually when the pain involves the peritoneum or the anterior abdominal wall, which are more densely supplied with afferent receptors, the pain will be correctly perceived as coming from the appendix.

SPINAL CORD

Pain fibers enter the spinal cord in the medial portion of the dorsal roots of spinal nerves. They enter in the dorsolateral funiculus, just dorsal to the dorsal gray horn. Here they usually give off collaterals that descend in the dorsolateral funiculus or the tract of Lissauer for one or two cord segments. The main group of fibers, however, ascend in the tract of Lissauer for about two cord segments before entering the dorsal gray horn to synapse. They do so on cells lying in Rexed's laminae II, III, IV, and V on a group of small neurons called the nucleus proprius. The ascent in the cord prior to synapsing is the anatomic reason given as to why patients perceive somatic pain at a higher level than the origin of the spinal nerve that is involved.

The axons of the cells in the nucleus proprius, following the law of neurobiotaxis, leave diagonally opposite the point of the incoming stimulus and travel across the midline of the cord in the ventral gray and white commissures just below the central canal of the spinal cord.

As these fibers cross just below the central canal they are vulnerable to a condition in which the central canal enlarges or cavitates, known as *syringomyelia.* This would cause a loss of pain and temperature in the patient two cord segments below the cord segment in which the cavitation occurs. Typically this occurs in the cervical cord, and the deficit is a bilateral loss of pain and temperature in the upper extremities; usually other sensory modalities are spared.

The fibers then pass to the ventral lateral portion of the contralateral lateral funiculus, where they form two separate tracks or pathways to the thalamus. These are the classic ventral and lateral spinothalamic pathways. In the current literature these are also referred to as the paleo- and neospinothalamic tracts. The two tracts are joined, and some think that the fibers are mixed in each tract. The neospinothalamic or lateral tract is the more rapidly conducting tract that produces so-called bright, quick pain and the paleospinothalamic or ventral tract elicits dull aching pain. The ventral tract is sometimes thought to be clinically unimportant, but is now receiving more attention.

The spinothalamic tracts are the principal pain-conducting pathways in the cord, but not the only ones. A phylogenetically older tract that conducts visceral pain may be found closely applied to the gray matter of the cord in all funiculi. This is the fasciculus proprius, and its axons travel up or down one cord segment, then synapse in the dorsal gray horn to again travel up one more segment. The reticulospinal tract may also conduct pain impulses, again usually from the viscera, and its axons travel up or down the cord a few segments to eventually reach the thalamus and even the cerebral cortex itself. The fasciculus proprius system ends at the medulla and the impulses conducted by it are conducted rostrally by the reticular formation.

Pain of visceral origin, therefore, can be conducted rostrally in one of three alternative pathways. This is given as the anatomic explanation as to why visceral pain may persist after a surgical procedure to cut the lateral spinothalamic tract, as in a cordotomy.

It should be noted that within the spinal cord the lateral spinothalamic tract is topographically laminated. As the axons from the nucleus proprius in the sacral segments cross the midline and ascend, they take a dorsolateral position in the newly formed tract. Fibers from higher cord segments, as they assume their positions, become more medially placed. The final configuration of the tract would then have sacral segments represented most laterally and cervical segments more ventromedially. A space-occupying extramedulary neoplasm that compresses the ventrolateral spinal cord at any level therefore might compromise the conduction of pain and temperature from the sacral and lumbar regions of the body.

BRAINSTEM PAIN SYSTEMS

An exhaustive treatment of brainstem form systems is not within the intended scope of this chapter. Principal mechanisms and systems are presented with a view to elucidating a very voluminous and complex topic.

Spinothalamic Pathways in the Brainstem

We have seen that there are two spinothalamic tracts, a ventral or paleospinothalamic and a more significant lateral or neospinothalamic tract. Both conduct pain, although of different types, in the spinal cord. These two tracts diverge in the medulla, then come in close proximity in the lateral pons and are eventually associated with the medial lemniscus in either the rostral pons or the caudal mesencephalon. En route to this association both tracts are greatly diminished in size, with the ventral spinothalamic tract probably very modest in the mesencephalon.

The impulse from both tracts ends in the ventrobasal nuclear complex of the thalamus, with most fibers terminating in the ventral posterior lateral nucleus. Many studies have shown that the paleospinothalamic tract is polysynaptic and gives off many collaterals to reticular nuclei in the medulla, chiefly to the nucleus gigantoreticularis and the lateral reticular nucleus. These in turn project to the centromedian nucleus of the thalamus.

There are also many pain-conducting fibers of the reticular formation of both spinal and brainstem origin projecting to the intralaminar nuclei of the thalamus. The reticular formation of the brainstem is a monitoring or modulating mechanism. All modalities pass through its network and are in some way affected by it. It is thought that by its projections to the thalamus and the cortex directly the reticular formation contributes to a better total image of the body and its parts. Certainly, it accentuates or inhibits certain stimuli to produce a focus of attention or awareness of some impulses that are filtered through its all-encompassing network. Some specific reticular mechanisms, such as the nucleus of the median raphe in the pons, play down on other structures, such as the neurons in the IInd, IIIrd, IVth, and Vth lamina of the dorsal gray horn of the cord, to inhibit the transmission of pain. Other reticular nuclei around the periaqueductal gray of the midbrain do the same to the neo- and paleospinothalamic tracts as they pass through the midbrain.

A noteworthy relationship between the spinothalamic tracts and the spinal or descending nucleus of the trigeminal complex is found in the caudal medulla. The spinal nucleus of the trigeminal complex is a pain-conducting nucleus from the ipsilateral face. Its presence usually produces a small, but grossly visible, lateral bulge in the medulla called the tuberculum cinereum. Just ventral to the tuberculum cinereum is another smaller bulge or protuberance, called Monakow's area, that indicates the location of the spinothalamic tracts. At this level, in the medulla the spinothalamic tracts are conducting pain from the contralateral body, because all of the fibers originating from the dorsal gray horn have crossed the midline of the cord and are ascending contralaterally. Both of these areas are supplied by small branches of the posterior inferior cerebellar artery. Both structures are vulnerable to a deficit in the blood supply from the same artery. When this occurs (as the well-known lateral medullary syndrome), the patient complains of a loss of pain and temperature sensation from the ipsilateral face and the contralateral body. Other complaints, such as difficulty in swallowing or loss of taste on the ipsilateral side of the tongue, may also be present if the lesioned area is more extensive and involves the nucleus ambiguous and the nucleus of the solitary tract. This is a classic neuroanatomic deficit and is also known as Weber's syndrome.

Trigeminal System

Perhaps the most significant neuroanatomic structure involved in pain in the brainstem is the trigeminal system. The trigeminal nuclear complex has components in the midbrain, pons, and medulla, and even extends down into the upper cervical segments of the spinal cord. There are three sensory nuclei and one motor nucleus. The sensory nuclei are a mesencephalic nucleus lying along the cerebral aqueduct that is functionally associated with proprioception; the chief or principal sensory nucleus in the pons, which receives impulses of touch and pressure, but also some impulses of pain; and a long, attenuated spinal or descending nucleus that descends to the upper cervical segments as far as C4 to blend with the substantia gelatinosa of the cervical cord. The spinal nucleus is the nucleus usually associated with pain conduction. The motor nucleus also lies in the pons, and through reflex connections with the spinal nu-

cleus can produce activity of the muscles of mastication (e.g., clenching of the jaw or chattering of the teeth) in response to noxious stimuli to the face.

The sensory nuclei receive their input from the pseudounipolar neurons of the trigeminal gasserian ganglion lying in Meckel's cavity in the middle cranial fossa. The peripheral processes of the ganglion are distributed via the ophthalmic maxillary and mandibular divisions of the trigeminal nerve to those regions of the face anterior to the ears. All three divisions conduct pain from their area of distribution. An irritative lesion of one of these divisions may produce a severe episodic pain in the patient, a condition called *trigeminal neuralgia*. The mandibular division is very commonly affected; the patient would complain of severe pain from the region of the lower lip and jaw. The pain is so severe and debilitating that some patients have contemplated suicide to escape its ravages.

The descending fibers of the pseudounipolar cells in the ganglion descend along the lateral aspect of the spinal nucleus through the pons and the medulla. They enter the spinal nucleus as they descend to synapses on the secondary cells of the nucleus. They, too, descend as far caudally as the C4 segment of the spinal cord.

The spinal nucleus has been described as having a rostral portion called the nucleus oralis, a caudal portion called the caudalis or subcaudalis, and an intermediate portion called the interpolaris. The nucleus appears to be laminated or organized in both a rostral-to-caudal and a dorsal-to-ventral fashion. The nucleus oralis portion would be comprised mainly of secondary neurons receiving pain impulses from the mandibular division of the nerve, whereas the subcaudalis would be receiving much of its input from the ophthalmic division. Hence, the lamination represents an innervated face. Lesions involving the upper cervical cord may sometimes cause production of pain or loss of pain in the ophthalmic region of the face along with other manifestations of spinal cord involvement.

The secondary fibers then sweep caudally from their origin from the neurons in the elongated spinal nucleus and cross the midline. As they cross the midline in the pons and medulla, they are called the ventral central trigeminal tract and are anatomically and physiologically separate from the fibers originating from the principal sensory nucleus conducting primarily impulses of touch and pressure, some of which also cross the midline to ascend to the thalamus as the dorsal central trigeminal tract. The remainder of the fibers originating from the principal sensory nucleus do cross the midline and ascend ipsilaterally. Hence, touch and pressure impulses are found bilaterally represented above the location of the principal sensory nucleus, whereas pain-conducting fibers are found contralaterally only. Touch and pressure perception may often be perceived in a patient with a brainstem lesion because of its bilateral representation, while the pain-conducting pathway may be compromised.

As both pathways ascend to the thalamus they are called the trigeminal thalamic pathways. They will come to be so close to the medial lemniscus in the caudal midbrain that they cannot be anatomically distinguished from it. However, physiologically they maintain their integrity and can be identified. The medial lemniscus is located on the lateral aspect of the midbrain above the level of the inferior colliculus, which is the auditory relay nucleus; above this level the trigeminal thalamic or lemniscal fibers are vulnerable to compromise. They may be severed or compressed by the sharp and firm edge of the dura mater as it forms the incisura to allow the brainstem to pass through. The extensions of the tentorium cerebelli rostrally to the clinoid processes forming the incisura pass alongside the lateral surface of the midbrain to form a formidable presence if there should be any sudden movement of the midbrain such as might occur in some types of trauma. A meningioma at this point could slowly compress the laterally placed medial lemniscus, with the trigeminal fibers at first producing pain through irritation, and eventually causing a contralateral loss of pain in the face as the compression slowly destroyed integrity of the axons to conduct the impulses. The deficit produced by the destruction of the medial lemniscus would be loss of conscious proprioception: position sense, two-point discrimination, and vibratory sense.

The secondary pain and touch axons of the trigeminal thalamic pathway terminate in the posterior ventral medial nucleus of the thalamus. This conforms to a phylogenetic pattern: the older structures in the central nervous system have a more favored position, that is, they are more medially placed. Most neurologic structures concerned with the head and neck are phylogenetically older and more medially placed than others that have to do mainly with body parts.

THALAMUS

The two groups of thalamic nuclei that are of interest to us are in the posterior basal complex: the posterior ventral lateral and the posterior ventral medial nuclei. They are mainly concerned with the perception and integration of the pain impulse from the body and from the face, respectively. Other thalamic nuclei may be involved after the impulses reach these primary targets, but which nuclei and to what degree is not clear at the present time. Pain is perceived on a conscious level at the thalamus. However, it is not recognized there as completely as it is in the cortex. Thalamic pain perception is a low-level type of appreciation. The thalamus tends to synchronize all incoming stimuli and place them in some form of order for transmission to the ce-

rebral cortex. Otherwise, much of what we perceive would produce neurologic chaos.

The frailties of the thalamus are known to many. The *thalamic syndrome* can produce amplification of various stimuli so that many innocuous stimuli, such as putting a spoon to the lips, can be interpreted as a very painful experience. Patients may go to great lengths to prevent exposure to these stimuli and protect themselves from the very real pain produced by ordinary events. The thalamic syndrome is thought to be elicited by an altered blood supply to the nuclei involved. The blood supply is in the main from the thalamostriate branch of the posterior cerebral artery. It is presumed to be diminished but not completely absent, thus causing an improper functioning of the nuclei.

Reticular nuclei are found in the external and internal medullary lamina of the thalamus. These nuclei project to the various thalamic nuclei and modulate their activity. The reticular nuclei apparently can excite or inhibit the thalamic nuclei and the various impulses that are received by them. The reticular formation has also been modulating the impulses conducted through it by the specific pain-conducting tracts in the brainstem, that is, the spinothalamic and trigeminothalamic tracts. The attention of the thalamus can thereby be focused in on a specific stimulus or the stimulus could be significantly downgraded both at the brainstem and the thalamic level.

The reticular nuclei also receive input from the corticothalamic fibers arising from the cortex. These fibers are found in the anterior limb of the internal capsule. The thalamic nuclei also receive input from this feedback loop. The cortex then monitors, through this feedback loop, much of the information that comes to it both at the reticular and the thalamic level. The thalamocortical loop could play a major role in the patient's ability to tolerate pain at various thresholds.

INTERNAL CAPSULE

The pain impulse, along with other general sensory impulses, is projected to the cerebral cortex through the posterior limb of the internal capsule. At this point the exquisite orderliness of neurologic organization observed at the brainstem level breaks down. There is little or no organization to the arrangement of the general sensory-conducting fibers in the posterior limb of the internal capsule. The fibers are found alongside the lateral border of the thalamus in the posterior limb. The pain-conducting fibers are spread diffusely in this area. Lesions of the posterior limb of the internal capsule can produce either a diffuse loss of pain or general sensations in the case of irritative lesions such as edema or blood from hemorrhage eliciting the production of pain.

In either instance, the deficit may be puzzling to the diagnostician. The irritated fibers may represent conduction from a knee, a shoulder, a hand, or other widely separated parts of the body. The fact that the patient does have these very unusual deficits may be useful in localizing the lesion to the internal capsule.

It should also be recalled that portions of the optic radiations and the auditory radiations pass through the posterior limb as well as the corticobulbar and cortiocospinal portions of the voluntary motor system. The motor deficits, especially supranuclear facial paralysis, need no elaboration here. However, the possible involvement of the optic radiations, producing visual field deficits, or the auditory radiations, producing hearing deficits or hallucinations, might be useful to keep in mind when presented with patients with seemingly nonlocalizable signs.

CEREBRAL CORTEX

The general sensory impulses, including pain, project through the internal capsule and the corona radiata to the postcentral gyrus and posterior paracentral lobule of the cerebral cortex. Other areas of the cerebral cortex have also been incriminated in the pain pathway. The centromedian nucleus is thought to project some pain conducted by the reticular formation to the frontal lobe. Pain is also projected to the parietal operculum just posterior to the postcentral gyrus. It would appear that many cortical areas, not just the primary sensory strip, can be involved in pain. In this respect pain is unique as a general sensory sensation.

Visceral pain is projected to the insular cortex, which is hidden deep to the lateral fissure. The insular cortex, or island of Reil, is known to be associated with the autonomic nervous system and may produce autonomic responses such as nausea and vomiting when stimulated.

The model of the homunculus, or "little man," is laid out on the postcentral gyrus in an inverted fashion. The head, at the base of the gyrus, and the body parts are represented disproportionately as one moves superiorly along the gyrus to the superior longitudinal fissure. For example, the lower extremity below the knee is represented on the medial surface in the posterior part of the paracentral gyrus. The main portion of the lateral convexity of the hemisphere is supplied by the middle cerebral artery and its branches; this would include most of the postcentral gyrus. The superior aspect of the gyrus, however, is supplied by the anterior cerebral artery, as is the postcentral gyrus.

The pariental operculum and the insular cortex as well as the lateral aspect of the frontal lobe are also supplied by branches of the middle cerebral artery. The anterior and middle cerebral arteries are portions of the anterior cerebral circulation and are direct terminal branches of the internal carotid artery. It is worthy of note that cortical areas incriminated in the analytic recognition of pain are supplied by two different branches of the internal carotid, whereas some of the thalamic nuclei involved with relatively crude but conscious recognition of pain are supplied by branches of the posterior cerebral artery.

The thalamic relay nuclei, involved in the projection of pain, project to very specific areas of the cortex on a point-to-point basis. If the nuclei are destroyed there is degeneration of cortical neurons in the specific area to which that nucleus projects its axons.

The pain fibers from the thalamus project to the fourth layer of cortical cells of the postcentral gyrus, the posterior paracentral lobule, and the parietal operculum. Here the impulse is conducted first to the more superficial layers of the cortex for further integration. In a sensory cortex, the layers above the fourth layer or granule layer are perhaps more significant in processing the information that comes to that area of the cortex. Because they are superficial they are more vulnerable to some types of injuries and difficulties within the cranial cavity than the deeper layers (e.g., layers five and six in a mammalian neocortex).

The impulse for pain and other general sensations is then conducted to the superior parietal lobule on the ipsilateral side for integration. This is interpreted to mean the critical recognition of the stimulus, and the specific body part from which that stimulus has been perceived in the other areas of the cortex may be relevant to its significance to a given individual based on his/her past experiences. Interpretation of the stimulus or impulse above and beyond recognition is a function of the parietal lobe. Various forms of aphasia are examples of this type of activity. The primary cortical receptor area is intact, as are the secondary and perhaps tertiary areas. The stimulus is perceived correctly, but when conducted to the parietal lobe, as in the case of pain, its true meaning or significance may not be interpreted correctly.

Impulses are then conducted from the parietal lobe via association bundles in the white matter to other areas of the cortex and specifically to the frontal lobe for further cortical activity and perhaps decision making. The long association bundles of the cerebral hemisphere are very important in the production of a unified activity of the nervous system. The long association bundles involved in transmission, in this case, would be the superior fronto-occipital bundle and the superior longitudinal fasciculus. Lesions of these structures would not alter the perception of the pain or its meaning but would have an effect on the patients' response to it or their attitude toward the pain.

These same association bundles could also send collaterals to the medial portions of the limbic system and evoke an emotional or autonomic response to somatic pain.

DESCENDING PATHWAYS

The periaqueductal gray of the midbrain appears to have an ameliorative effect on pain. When stimulated, these neurons have an analgesic effect on ascending pain pathways.

SUMMARY

The elementary basis of neurologic structures involved in the conduction, recognition, and integration of pain have been identified. A difficulty with understanding the role of each of the anatomic entities involved in the process is that there is a duality or overlap of activities that makes clarification elusive.

There are two pathways for conduction of somatic and visceral pain in the spinal cord, the paleo- and neospinothalamic tracts. A third, the fasciculus proprius, conducts visceral pain. A fourth system, the reticular formation, can conduct either type of pain impulse rostrally or caudally. There are several brainstem structures involved: tracts, both ascending and descending, and cranial nerve nuclei and their secondary nuclear axons. All of these have differing arterial supplies that can, when compromised, involve one structure and spare another, and can cause production of pain or a loss of pain. These entities pass through the reticular formation, which monitors all impulses passing through to all-encompassing networks. This, in turn, can excite or inhibit the production of pain.

Two principal nuclei are involved at the thalamic level, but other nuclei participate. Their role is uncertain; however, they project to areas other than the postcentral gyrus and the paracentral lobule, the classic cortical centers for recognition of pain. In the cortex itself, there are many areas involved in pain perception and their roles differ from recognition to integration to attitudes and response. Even in the white matter two or more association bundles may be involved in even the most straightforward pathway.

An anatomic description of the structures involved in the pain pathway presents a picture that is very different from most other sensory pathways. The structures involved have evolved and been modified and enhanced over a very long period of time and probably are still being modified to deal with a specific type of stimulus that is disturbing to the usual functions of the brain. Yet as we learn more about the structures and their connections their role may become clearer, and more enlightened diagnoses and treatments should be forthcoming.

There cannot be many more causes in medicine more worthy of the attention and efforts of all physicians and scientists than the reflex of pain. The author hopes he has made a contribution to that cause.

SUGGESTED READINGS

Adams RD, Victor M: *Principles of Neurology.* New York, McGraw-Hill, 1977, p 1041.

Bond MR: *Pain: Its Nature and Treatment.* New York, Churchill Livingstone, 1979, p 185.

Gilman S, Newman SW: *Manter and Gatz's Essentials of Clinical Neuroanatomy and Neurophysiology,* ed 7. Philadelphia, FA Davis, 1987, p 256.

Hall JL: Peripheral pain pathways. In Lee JF (ed): *Pain Management.* Baltimore, Williams & Wilkins, 1977, pp 1–11.

Holden AV, Winlow N (eds): *The Neurobiology of Pain.* Manchester, England, Manchester University Press, 1983, p 414.

Kandel ER, Schwartz JH: *Principles of Neural Sciences.* New York, Elsevier, 1985, p 979.

Keller JT: The anatomy of central pain pathways. In Lee JF (ed): *Pain Management.* Baltimore, Williams & Wilkins, 1977, pp 12–24.

Pawl RP: *Chronic Pain Primer.* Chicago, Year Book, 1979, p 106.

CHAPTER 4
PSYCHOLOGICAL EVALUATION AND TESTING
DONALD W. HINNANT

Although sophisticated diagnostic technologic advances such as magnetic resonance imaging, myelography, computerized tomography, and technetium bone scanning have been developed, chronic pain remains a medical enigma. Results from diagnostic tests and efforts towards defining anatomic sites of pain often leave the clinician and the patient frustrated. Most treatment approaches have been based on the dichotomy between physiologic and psychological causes of pain. Pain assessment constitutes a primary basis for development of sound clinical judgment and formulation of treatment protocols. Although it may be argued that there is no direct way to measure pain, we do have the capacity to assess the behavioral-objective, subjective, and physiologic correlates of pain. Assessment of pain is strengthened by a combination of measures that involve these three basic components. The purpose of this chapter is to outline current assessment techniques and provide an overview of various methods for assessing pain and its psychological correlates. Although many of these assessment devices are used in the acute pain situation, they are also helpful in evaluating chronic pain status as well as in aiding the development of treatment strategies and outcome measures.

In acute pain physiologic and behavioral changes often occur that are correlated with nociceptive stimulation. In chronic pain, however, the clinician is confronted with extremely complex variables related to the pain syndrome. Assessment of the chronic pain patient involves evaluation of numerous interacting variables as highlighted by the work by Melzack and Wall (1). Their work in the development of the gate control theory suggests that pain assessment should include evaluation of various dimensions including the motivational-affective, sensory-discriminative, and cognitive-evaluative processes. Special attention is now being paid to pain evaluation with the development of guidelines issued by the United States Agency for Health Care Policy and Research (2) and The American Pain Society

(3). The importance of accurate assessment of the pain experience has been demonstrated by research that suggests that the failure of medical staff to accurately and routinely assess pain is the most common reason for inadequate pain management (4). Psychological evaluation is also a required component of the evaluation in pain treatment programs accredited by the Commission On Accreditation Of Rehabilitation Facilities (CARF) (5).

The gate control theory as defined by Melzack and Wall (1) has demonstrated the highly complex nature of pain perception and response, and has led to our appreciation of the interactive variables involved in the pain experience. We now know that nociceptive impulses at the level of spinal integration are affected by multiple pathways and interacting systems. The transmission of pain impulses may be inhibited by peripheral large fiber impulses. Descending spinal tracks involve neuropeptides and serotonergic mechanisms that have the capability of inhibiting the perception of painful sensation. At higher cortical levels, pharmacologic and lesion studies have demonstrated that the frontal and limbic systems can modify the meaning of an emotional reaction to nociceptive stimulation. This research shows that there is a varying correspondence between the subjective experience of pain and the physiologic functions involved in the somatosensory cortex, the limbic system, and the frontal lobes. These findings explain that there is no simple correlation between the degree of tissue damage and the degree of suffering expressed by the patient (1).

COMMON MISCONCEPTIONS IN PAIN EVALUATION

For the clinician who works in the medical setting, it is not unusual to hear medical personnel comment about whether they believe patients do indeed suffer the degree of pain that has been reported. It is defeating to discount a patient's report of pain or imply that he or she is exaggerating symptoms. McCaffery and Beebe

Table 4.1.
Misconceptions about Assessment of Patients Who Indicate They Have Pain[a]

Misconception	Correction
1. The health team is the authority about the existence and nature of the patient's pain sensation.	The person with pain is the only authority about the existence and nature of that pain, since the sensation of pain can be felt only by the person who has it.
2. Our personal values and intuition about the trustworthiness of others is a valuable tool in identifying whether a person is lying about pain.	Personal values and intuition do not constitute a professional approach to the patient with pain. The patient's credibility is not on trial.
3. Pain is largely an emotional or psychological problem, especially in the patient who is highly anxious or depressed.	Having an emotional reaction to pain does not mean that pain is caused by an emotional problem. If anxiety or depression is alleviated, the intensity of pain will not necessarily be any less.
4. Lying about the existence of pain, malingering, is common.	Very few people who say they have pain are lying about it. Outright fabrication of pain is considered rare.
5. The patient who obtains benefits or preferential treatment because of pain is receiving secondary gain and does not hurt as much as he says or may not hurt at all.	The patient who uses his pain to his advantage is not the same as a malingerer and may still hurt as much as he says he does. Also, secondary gain may be an inaccurate diagnosis.
6. All real pain has an identifiable physical cause.	All pain is real, regardless of its causes. Almost all pain has both physical and mental components. Pure psychogenic pain is rare.
7. Visible signs, either physiological or behavioral, accompany pain and can be used to verify its existence and severity.	Even with severe pain, periods of physiological and behavioral adaptation occur, leading to periods of minimal or no signs of pain. Lack of pain expression does not necessarily mean lack of pain. How must the patient act for us to believe he has pain?
8. Comparable physical stimuli produce comparable pain in different people. The severity and duration of pain can be predicted accurately for everyone on the basis of the stimuli for pain.	Comparable stimuli in different people do *not* produce the same intensities of pain. Comparable stimuli in different people will produce different intensities of pain that last different periods. There is no direct and invariant relationship between any stimulus and the perception of pain.
9. People with pain should be taught to have a high tolerance for pain. The more prolonged the pain or the more experience a person has with pain, the better is his tolerance for pain.	Pain tolerance is the individual's unique response, varying between patients and varying in the same patient from one situation to another. People with prolonged pain tend to have an increasingly low pain tolerance. Respect for the patient's pain tolerance is crucial for adequate pain control.
10. When the patient reports pain relief following a placebo, this means that the patient is a malingerer or that the pain is psychogenic.	There is not a shred of evidence anywhere in the literature to justify using a placebo to diagnose malingering or psychogenic pain.

[a]From McCaffery M, Beebe A: *Clinical Manual for Nursing Practice.* St. Louis, CV Mosby, 1989.

have highlighted common misconceptions that prevail with regard to pain and pain assessment (6). Please refer to Table 4.1. McCaffery and Beebe base their manual on their belief that pain control is a legitimate therapeutic goal and that effective management must rank high in the list of priorities in patient care. Although much of their work is focused on acute pain management, their general principles of pain assessment and pain management may be helpful in evaluation of the chronic pain patient.

PURPOSE OF PSYCHOLOGICAL ASSESSMENT WITH CHRONIC PAIN PATIENTS

The primary goal in performing a psychological evaluation is to assist in the delineation of emotional and behavioral factors that may be operating in the chronic pain syndrome. Often an evaluation is requested when the patient's symptoms are greater than would be expected based on the patient's physical findings. The psychological evaluation may also be helpful when patients demonstrate excessive use of the health care system and insist on continuing the search for a new doctor, diagnosis, or simple solution to their problem. An evaluation may be particularly important when there is evidence of psychological disorder, drug abuse or dependence, or insufficient coping mechanisms. For example, chronic back pain patients have been a major topic of study, and recent investigations have provided important information when these patients were compared with the general population. For example, an investigation by Polatin and colleagues found that psychological illness pre-existed development of chronic low back pain in a sample of 200 patients entering a functional restoration program (7). The most common pre-existing conditions were major depression (54%), substance abuse, and anxiety disorders. Fifty-one percent of their sample met the criteria for at least one personality disorder. Fifty-nine percent of the sample demonstrated current symptoms for at least one psychiatric diagnosis. The authors found patients with a prior history of substance abuse (94%) and anxiety disorders (95%) who manifested these symptoms prior to the onset of their back pain. Depression was found to develop either before or after the onset of chronic back pain. In support of these findings, Schofferman and colleagues reported on 101 consecutively evaluated chronic back pain patients (8). A childhood history of trauma including physical abuse, sexual abuse, psychological abuse, abandonment, and chemically dependent parents was present in both the failed back surgery group (n = 56) and the group who had not had surgery (n = 45). In the failed back surgery group, 48% had three or more of the abovementioned childhood traumas, and 77% had two or more of the childhood traumas. In the group of patients who had not had surgery, 58% had three or more of the abovementioned types of abuse, and 84% had two or more types of trauma in childhood. These startling results suggest that there is an extremely high percentage of chronic back pain patients who have a childhood history of psychological trauma and abuse.

Results of these recently presented investigations suggest that a thorough psychological evaluation is necessary in the treatment of the patient with chronic pain. Most importantly, the psychological evaluation is helpful in the development of specific treatment strategies and in facilitating implementation of an interdisciplinary comprehensive treatment plan.

Unfortunately, a psychological evaluation is often requested to determine whether a patient's pain and related symptoms are "organic" or "functional." Although many psychologists are willing to venture into this realm, one should remember that physical and psychological difficulties are not mutually exclusive. It is also helpful to avoid use of diagnostic labels such as "hypochondriacal," "hysterical," and "functional." Identifying a chronic pain syndrome as "psychogenic" may potentiate confusion and inappropriate treatment for the patient. Rather than resorting to these traditional labels, one will be much more helpful if environmental, emotional, cognitive, and behavioral factors are identified in the evaluation.

REFERRAL PROCESS

It is very important for physicians and psychologists to develop appropriate strategies for the referral of patients for a psychological and behavioral evaluation. Ideally, the psychological evaluation should be a preliminary component of the interdisciplinary pain eval-

uation. The way that the referral is conducted may dramatically affect the behavior and cooperation of the patient and provide an optimal environment for valid assessment. Unfortunately, many patients are defensive and frustrated by the time they actually undergo the evaluation because of the implicit message that "the doctor thinks the pain is all in my head." This of course leads to an angry and defensive stance on the part of the patient and distrust of the physician and psychologist. The following guidelines have been proposed by Cameron and Shapell (9):

1. Acknowledge the legitimacy of the problem, attempt to reassure the patient that his or her pain is considered real and that there is no suspicion of malingering. Again, the credibility of the evaluation may be enhanced if the psychological evaluation and the physical examination are performed concurrently. It is also helpful to attempt to educate the patient about symptoms, diagnosis, and findings during the evaluation.
2. Provide a positive rationale for the referral. The primary emphasis should be placed on communicating to the patient that the purpose of the evaluation is to provide thorough solutions to problems with the goal of obtaining the best possible care.
3. Inform other staff members of the general rationale. Both clinical and administrative-clerical staff members should have a clear understanding of the referral process and its rationale. In a clinic or medical setting patients are often exposed initially to the support staff. Many of patients' perceptions are made by the manner in which they are treated and how they are received.
4. Let the patient know that the referral is routine.
5. Personalize discussion of the referral. It may be helpful to present the psychologist as the professional who can determine effective ways of helping patients better cope with their pain and the stress caused by their problems. Most patients agree that their pain problems are creating numerous stressors in their lives, and that stress, insomnia, and pain are a vicious cycle.
6. Make it clear that the referral does not imply a transfer. Because many patients suffering from chronic pain are frustrated and feel as if their problems may never be resolved, they often think that a referral or request for consultation is actually a discharge or "dump." Although these patients are often problematic and a referral may actually be an attempt to transfer, it is helpful to reassure patients of the intention of the referral.

MULTIDIMENSIONAL NATURE OF PAIN

As mentioned previously, the gate control theory has led to the understanding of the multidimensional nature of pain. It is important to appreciate the variety of characteristics of the pain experience, and researchers in cancer pain have elucidated six dimensions, which are pre-

Table 4.2.
Multiple Dimensions of the Pain Experience[a]

Physiologic dimension
  Location
  Onset
  Duration
  Etiology
  Syndrome
Sensory dimension
  Intensity
  Quality
  Pattern
Affective dimension
  Mood state
  Anxiety
  Depression
  Well-being
Cognitive dimension
  Meaning of pain
  View of self
  Coping skills and strategies
  Previous treatment
  Attitudes and beliefs
  Factors influencing pain
Behavioral dimension
  Communication
  Interpersonal interaction
  Physical activity
  Pain behaviors
  Medications
  Interventions
  Sleep
Sociocultural dimension
  Ethnocultural background
  Family and social life
  Work and home responsibilities
  Recreation and leisure
  Environmental factors
  Attitudes and beliefs
  Social influences

[a]Adapted from McGuire DB: The multidimensional phenomenon of cancer pain. In McGuire DB, Yarbro CH (eds): *Cancer Pain Management*. Philadelphia, WB Saunders, 1987, pp 1–20.

Table 4.3.
Additional Assessment Instruments for Chronic Pain Patients

Millon Behavioral Health Inventory (Millon, Green, and Meahger, 1982[43])
Coping Strategies Questionnaire (Rosenstiel and Keefe, 1983[45])
Symptom Checklist 90 (Derogatis et al., 1973[46])
Illness Behavior Questionnaire (Pilowsky and Spence, 1975[28])
Sickness Impact Profile (Bergner et al., 1981[71])
Clinical Analysis Questionnaire, 16PF (Cattell et al., 1970, 1980[72])
Simultaneous Interview Technique (Jacobson et al., 1991[53])

of interdisciplinary care. Various dimensions of the pain experience will be presented in the following paragraphs, and their utilization in pain assessment will be discussed.

PAIN BEHAVIOR

Fordyce, in his seminal work on behavioral approaches with chronic pain patients, defined pain behavior as any overt behavior that is susceptible to conditioning and learning influences (11). Fordyce postulated that chronic pain patients demonstrate pain behavior that is maintained through the process of operant conditioning. Some pain researchers raise the possibility that pain behavior is actually a coping mechanism, and that these behaviors are not always maladaptive (12). Turk and Flor caution that an oversimplistic behavioral orientation in pain assessment may lead to a disservice to patients and the possibility of "blaming" the patient for his or her symptoms (13). Further, they raise the possibility of misapplication of pain behavior as a construct, and warn against reverting to the dangerous dichotomy of emotional as compared to physical or psychogenic causes versus real pain.

Pain behavior may be described as any verbal descriptions of pain and suffering as well as nonverbal behavior such as limping, grimacing, guarded movement patterns, taking medications, or avoidant behavior such as reclining or withdrawal from activity. As mentioned previously, Fordyce called interest to the susceptibility of a person having pain to conditioning and learning influences. Much attention has been paid to the fact that pain behavior may be maintained through operant conditioning effects in the patient's environment. Numerous treatment protocols have been developed with the operant conditioning model, in which reinforcers and other operant techniques such as extinction have been used to shape or eliminate pain behavior. More recently, cognitive-behavioral psychologists have promoted a more detailed assessment of overt and covert pain be-

sented in Table 4.2 (10). Although the six dimensions listed may appear difficult to separate, some dimensions are more relevant in particular types of pain. In chronic rheumatic arthritis, for example, the affective dimension has been found to distinguish this type of pain from postoperative pain. Particular dimensions may be more significant in the pain assessment, depending on the nature of the disease and the setting. Chronic pain is often found to influence the affective dimension as compared to the sensory characteristics found in postoperative pain. In most acute pain situations, the behavioral, sensory, and physiologic dimensions are most notable and helpful for the clinician with regard to pain control. A systematic approach to pain assessment is valuable in the development of treatment planning and the delivery havior. These techniques will be reviewed later in this chapter.

BEHAVIORAL AND OBSERVATIONAL ASSESSMENT OF CHRONIC PAIN

Measurement of pain behavior implies that data acquisition reveals the quantification, extent, and degree of pain in a standard objective manner without bias. In contrast, assessment implies a critical analysis of pain in which the nature and significance of pain behavior is judged. Although much has been written about pain evaluation in the last 45 years, controversy continues about the best techniques to use. Behavioral psychologists have continued their efforts toward objective, scientific evaluation of the chronic pain patient. Although the behavioral approach as originated by Fordyce has met with much criticism as being too simplistic, many researchers have continued their scientific elaboration of the problems inherent with behavioral observation of pain, and current investigations continue to help clinicians evaluate this most complex behavior.

Behavioral Data Collection

Self-Monitoring

Activity level is one of the major categories of behavior typically measured through self-monitoring. Daily activity diaries are commonly provided to patients, with the patient being asked to make hourly or daily entries of time spent reclining, sitting, standing, or moving about. The emphasis is on measurement of "downtime" and "uptime," which are often used as indicators of the effects of treatment. Improvement is usually considered to be correlated with an increase in uptime. Antecedent events and premonitory symptoms are usually recorded.

Follick and his colleagues have demonstrated the value of having pain patients keep a diary, both as an assessment technique and as a method for evaluating treatment outcome (14). Limitations of the self-reporting approach are obvious, however. As Craig has pointed out, patients often report in a biased manner in order to maximize personal benefits (15). Patient's memory and verbal skills may be poor and may distort accurate recordings. It has been recommended that steps should be taken towards enhancement of the accuracy of data from the self-report diary, including utilization of a standardized data sheet, clear instructions, and delivery of reinforcement for data collection efforts. The patient also should receive feedback on the accuracy of his or her reporting. Simplicity in data collection is critical for compliance.

Direct Observation

Overt pain behaviors can be assessed directly using specific observation methods. As pointed out by Keefe

and Crisson, clinical personnel such as physicians, nurses, and physical therapists often evaluate patients' behavior to gauge their clinical status (16). An attempt is made to judge whether or not the patient's pain reaction is consistent with the underlying physical condition. These researchers have examined the reliability and validity of structured observation methods through videotaped sessions in which patients were asked to sit, stand, walk, and recline. Five overt motor behaviors were recorded: guarded movement, bracing, rubbing or touching the painful area, grimacing, and sighing. The researchers have also extended their behavior observations to coincide with the medical evaluation. They have had nurses and other clinical staff record patient behavior. The use of trained observers working with the pain patient has been found to be a reliable, valid, and economical method for monitoring symptoms. The University of Alabama Pain Behavior Scale is an example of a systematic rating scale that has been reliably administered by a variety of pain team personnel in the clinical setting (17). See Figure 4.1.

Behavioral Assessment Guidelines

Several excellent papers have been published in the first volume of the Journal of the American Pain Society. Scholarly works by Keefe, Dunsmore, Merskey, Turk, and Matyas argue in detail the various aspects of the multifaceted nature of pain and pain behavior. Keefe and Dunsmore review pain behavior observation methods and common methods for sampling pain behavior in naturalistic settings, as well as in the clinical realm (18). They also provide a review of controversial issues and criticisms in pain behavior observation. They emphasize that the concept of pain behavior and its analysis recognizes the complexity of pain behavior. They caution against an oversimplification of pain behavior and emphasize the need for careful observation of pain behavior without careless interpretation. They offer the following suggestions for future research (18):

1. Developing functional analysis methods for identifying variables that control behavior
2. Conducting sequential analysis of interactions between chronic pain patients and individuals in their social environment
3. Sampling behavior during more complex, demanding, and personally relevant tasks
4. Investigating how pain behavior relates to indices of pain perception, such as pain threshold and tolerance

Merskey has pointed out limitations of the pain behavior concept (19). He argues that although pain behavior might be learned, the evidence of this notion is limited. He agrees with Keefe and Dunsmore when he says that "pain behavior is not simply controlled by environmental factors, but may be influenced by underlying nociceptive input, constitutional factors, and per-

Patient _____

Room # _____

Rater _____

1. <u>Vocal Complaints:</u> Verbal

2. <u>Vocal Complaints:</u> Nonverbal
   (moans, groans, gasps, etc.)

3. <u>Down-Time:</u>
   (Time spent lying down per day
   because of pain: 8 a.m.- 8 p.m.)

4. <u>Facial Grimaces:</u>

5. <u>Standing Posture:</u>

6. <u>Mobility:</u>

7. <u>Body Language:</u>
   (clutching, rubbing site of pain)

8. <u>Use of visible supportive equipment:</u>
   (braces, crutches, cane, leaning on
   furniture, TENS, etc.)
   Do not score if equipment prescribed.

9. <u>Stationary movement:</u>

10. <u>Medication:</u>

The UAB Pain Behavior Scale (0–10)

DATE		M	T	W	T	F	S	S	M	T	W	T	F	S	S	M	T	W	T	F	S	S
1. Vocal Complaints: Verbal	None	0	0	0	0	0	0	0	0	0	0	0	0	0	0	0	0	0	0	0	0	0
	Occasional	1/2	1/2	1/2	1/2	1/2	1/2	1/2	1/2	1/2	1/2	1/2	1/2	1/2	1/2	1/2	1/2	1/2	1/2	1/2	1/2	1/2
	Frequent	1	1	1	1	1	1	1	1	1	1	1	1	1	1	1	1	1	1	1	1	1
2. Vocal Complaints: Nonverbal	None	0	0	0	0	0	0	0	0	0	0	0	0	0	0	0	0	0	0	0	0	0
	Occasional	1/2	1/2	1/2	1/2	1/2	1/2	1/2	1/2	1/2	1/2	1/2	1/2	1/2	1/2	1/2	1/2	1/2	1/2	1/2	1/2	1/2
	Frequent	1	1	1	1	1	1	1	1	1	1	1	1	1	1	1	1	1	1	1	1	1
3. Down-Time	None	0	0	0	0	0	0	0	0	0	0	0	0	0	0	0	0	0	0	0	0	0
	0–60 min	1/2	1/2	1/2	1/2	1/2	1/2	1/2	1/2	1/2	1/2	1/2	1/2	1/2	1/2	1/2	1/2	1/2	1/2	1/2	1/2	1/2
	>60 min	1	1	1	1	1	1	1	1	1	1	1	1	1	1	1	1	1	1	1	1	1
4. Facial Grimaces	None	0	0	0	0	0	0	0	0	0	0	0	0	0	0	0	0	0	0	0	0	0
	Mild and/or infrequent	1/2	1/2	1/2	1/2	1/2	1/2	1/2	1/2	1/2	1/2	1/2	1/2	1/2	1/2	1/2	1/2	1/2	1/2	1/2	1/2	1/2
	Severe and/or frequent	1	1	1	1	1	1	1	1	1	1	1	1	1	1	1	1	1	1	1	1	1
5. Standing Posture	Normal	0	0	0	0	0	0	0	0	0	0	0	0	0	0	0	0	0	0	0	0	0
	Mildly impaired	1/2	1/2	1/2	1/2	1/2	1/2	1/2	1/2	1/2	1/2	1/2	1/2	1/2	1/2	1/2	1/2	1/2	1/2	1/2	1/2	1/2
	Distorted	1	1	1	1	1	1	1	1	1	1	1	1	1	1	1	1	1	1	1	1	1
6. Mobility	No visible impairment	0	0	0	0	0	0	0	0	0	0	0	0	0	0	0	0	0	0	0	0	0
	Mild limp and/or mildly impaired walking	1/2	1/2	1/2	1/2	1/2	1/2	1/2	1/2	1/2	1/2	1/2	1/2	1/2	1/2	1/2	1/2	1/2	1/2	1/2	1/2	1/2
	Marked limp and/or labored walking	1	1	1	1	1	1	1	1	1	1	1	1	1	1	1	1	1	1	1	1	1
7. Body Language	None	0	0	0	0	0	0	0	0	0	0	0	0	0	0	0	0	0	0	0	0	0
	Occasional	1/2	1/2	1/2	1/2	1/2	1/2	1/2	1/2	1/2	1/2	1/2	1/2	1/2	1/2	1/2	1/2	1/2	1/2	1/2	1/2	1/2
	Frequent	1	1	1	1	1	1	1	1	1	1	1	1	1	1	1	1	1	1	1	1	1
8. Use of visible supportive equipment	None	0	0	0	0	0	0	0	0	0	0	0	0	0	0	0	0	0	0	0	0	0
	Occasional	1/2	1/2	1/2	1/2	1/2	1/2	1/2	1/2	1/2	1/2	1/2	1/2	1/2	1/2	1/2	1/2	1/2	1/2	1/2	1/2	1/2
	Dependent: constant use	1	1	1	1	1	1	1	1	1	1	1	1	1	1	1	1	1	1	1	1	1
9. Stationary movement	Sits or stands still	0	0	0	0	0	0	0	0	0	0	0	0	0	0	0	0	0	0	0	0	0
	Occasional shifts of position	1/2	1/2	1/2	1/2	1/2	1/2	1/2	1/2	1/2	1/2	1/2	1/2	1/2	1/2	1/2	1/2	1/2	1/2	1/2	1/2	1/2
	Constant movement, position shifts	1	1	1	1	1	1	1	1	1	1	1	1	1	1	1	1	1	1	1	1	1
10. Medication	None	0	0	0	0	0	0	0	0	0	0	0	0	0	0	0	0	0	0	0	0	0
	Non-narcotic analgesic and/or psychogenic medications as prescribed	1/2	1/2	1/2	1/2	1/2	1/2	1/2	1/2	1/2	1/2	1/2	1/2	1/2	1/2	1/2	1/2	1/2	1/2	1/2	1/2	1/2
	Demands for increased dosage or frequency, and/or narcotics, and/or medication abuse.	1	1	1	1	1	1	1	1	1	1	1	1	1	1	1	1	1	1	1	1	1
	TOTAL																					

Figure 4.1. **The UAB Pain Behavior Scale. (From Richards JS, Nepomuceno C, Riles M, Suer Z: Assessing pain behavior: The UAB Pain Behavior Scale.** *Pain* **14:393–398, 1982.**

sonality factors (e.g., motivational trends or the effect of personality traits)" (19). He further points out his concern that sometimes treatment is offered for reducing pain behavior in lieu of attempts toward alleviating the pain. Also, a focus strictly on identifying pain behavior may lead to the possible erroneous inference that pain behavior suggests motivated illness, hypochondriacal behavior, or malingering. Most importantly, Merskey advises the pain clinician to be very cautious in interpreting pain behavior as a "functional" rather than a true physical illness. He cites the work of Slater and Glitheroe, which found that 60% of patients diagnosed with hysteria by qualified neurologists subsequently revealed physical disease that could account for their symptoms (20). It is therefore suggested that evaluation of pain behavior not be considered solely as a sign of psychological illness. A careful analysis of pain behavior is needed.

COMBINED BEHAVIORAL AND PHYSICAL ASSESSMENT

In an effort to improve evaluation of the chronic pain patient, which traditionally relies on the patient's self-report in addition to radiographic imaging and other diagnostic procedures, behavioral assessment procedures have been conducted in conjunction with the physical examination. Spratt et al. used a set of 21 tests, with 17 assessing organic and 4 assessing nonorganic signs with back patients (21). Their observations of pain behavior, in addition to patient self-reporting during examination maneuvers, were recorded. A rating of pain intensity was included and a score was produced that was found to be reliable and valid as a measure of low back dysfunction. Other researchers have used a functional capacity evaluation combined with psychological self-report measures to provide the clinician with a quantifiable measure of a patient's physical status as well as of psychological disturbance. This information can be useful in treatment planning and as a measure of treatment success and outcome. Pope and colleagues evaluated chronic back pain patients with traditional physical tests, a psychological test (the Minnesota Multiphasic Personality Inventory), and a test of pain tolerance (22). Significant correlations were found between low pain threshold and tolerance, restrictions in spinal mobility, and imbalances between muscle groups related to reconditioning.

Although psychologists have traditionally left the responsibility for all of the physical parameters to their medical colleagues, pain psychologists should possess a working knowledge of the nervous system and anatomy in addition to various pain syndromes and their physiologic correlates. I have found it helpful to evaluate patients with the physician as both clinicians look for traditional physical symptoms in relation to the patient's pain behavior and self-report of pain intensity. This degree of collaboration allows for more consistent and thorough treatment planning.

SPECIFIC ASSESSMENT DEVICES

SENSORY AND PHYSIOLOGIC ASSESSMENT DEVICES

Unidimensional instruments are designed to assess a single dimension of pain such as intensity, location, or degree of relief. The most commonly used instruments include pain drawings, visual analog scales, pain intensity scales, pain maps, and other simple devices. Please refer to Figure 4.2.

Three main categories of self-report devices include the Visual Analog Scale (VAS), which measures several dimensions of pain, the Graphic Rating Scale (GRS), which consists of words along a continuum of increasing value, and the Numerical Rating Scale (NRS), which utilizes a number span (e.g., 0 to 5, or 1 to 100) to reflect increasing degrees of pain. The greatest strengths of these scales are their clarity and simplicity. They are usually useable with children and the elderly population. The scales are also versatile in that they may be adapted to various cognitive levels and may be used in a variety of clinical settings. Administration and scoring are simple and straightforward.

Several limitations are associated with these devices, however. Most notably, it may be assumed that the scale is measuring a single dimension such as pain intensity, when in fact the rating is easily influenced by the emotional state of the patient and by numerous other factors that can influence the pain rating. In other words, these scales may be oversimplified, and changes in the scale over time may be influenced by a wide range of undetected variables. Another major criticism of the scales is the fact that self-reporting requires a patient to translate some aspect of what is being measured into a mark, ratio, or word in a linear manner. It is recommended that several scales that relate to various aspects of the pain experience be used to compensate for this limitation.

For research purposes, two conditions must be met for statistical interpretation. The scale ratings must be drawn from a normally distributed population, and the data points at which values are given to ratings of the scale must be equally spaced along the line. These two major requirements are often not included in various reports that use these scales as a dependent variable following treatment (23).

STRUCTURED TESTS AND QUESTIONNAIRES

The Minnesota Multiphasic Personality Inventory (MMPI) is the most frequently used psychological instrument in the assessment of chronic pain. The MMPI consists of 556 true/false questions that produce a profile with three validity scales and eight clinical scales. The original MMPI was normalized on a psychiatric population. For this reason MMPI profiles must be interpreted with caution. There are practical as well as empirical grounds for judicious use of the MMPI with chronic pain patients. Specific scales on the test have been reported to correlate with treatment outcome, with a particular emphasis on scales 1 and 3 (hypochondriasis and hysteria, respectively). Chronic pain patients often have elevations on other clinical scales as well. Fordyce presented a review of the MMPI with chronic pain patients that has become widely accepted (24). Fordyce attempted to utilize various scale configurations that may indicate the degree to which the patient finds pain rewarding or the degree to which he or she has some element of gain or reward by having the pain

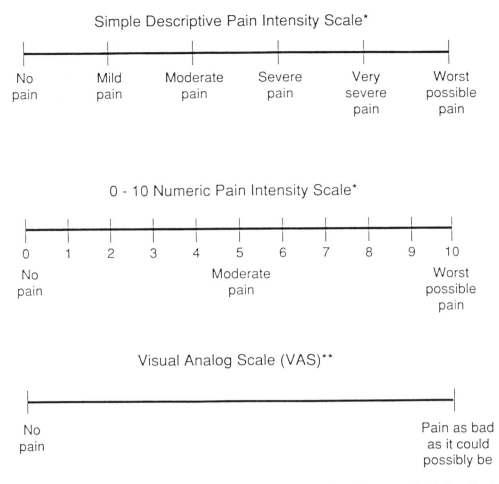

Figure 4.2. Sample unidimensional pain assessment devices. (From Acute Pain Management Guideline Panel: *Acute Pain Management: Operative or Medical Procedures and Trauma. Clinical Practice Guideline.* **Rockville, MD, Agency for Health Care Policy and Research, Public Health Service, U.S. Department of Health and Human Services, 1992.)**

problem. Fordyce predicted that the patient with a high score on scale 2 (depression) was less likely to find pain reinforcing than would the patient whose profile showed a very low scale 2. With elevations on scales 1 (hypochondriasis) and 3 (hysteria) in conjunction with a proportionately low scale 2 (depression), the patient typically reports pain and somatic distress, although there is a corresponding low level of emotional concern about the pain. Although this configuration is often referred to as the "Conversion V" the clinician is reminded that this test does not address the presence of physical abnormalities that may or may not be causing the pain. In addition, chronic pain patients may have elevations on scales that indicate paranoia (scale 6) or even schizophrenia (scale 8). Chronic pain patients may identify with these scales because of sensory disturbances, confusion due to medications, or bizarre interpretations of their symptoms.

Patients taking this test often identify with statements that describe apparently pathological experiences. Even

so, the test is useful as a gross screening instrument that may have some predictive utility toward treatment, and that may indicate emotional disturbance and significant psychopathology.

Fortunately, new norms for the MMPI have been developed, and the test has been revised and restandardized. The new version is known as the MMPI-2 and was designed to retain the most valuable traditional features of the test while addressing contemporary concerns. In addition to the basic validity and clinical scales, supplementary scales have been provided that address many specific content areas; several computerized interpretive packages are available to the clinician. Specifically tailored reports are available for numerous settings, including the chronic pain treatment program. Particular sections on diagnostic and treatment considerations are provided.

A study performed by Ahles and colleagues has shown that the typical psychopathologic profile often produced by the chronic pain patient on the original

MMPI tends to be reduced when the contemporary norms are used (25). This is fortunate because the misuse of the MMPI has been widespread, and because patients have often had treatment recommendations based entirely on their profiles on this test. I am aware of numerous cases in which surgical intervention was declined in spite of positive clinical findings because of MMPI results alone. Of course there are studies that purport to predict a poor response to physical treatment based on the MMPI. It is recommended that this test be used most cautiously in the decision-making process regarding treatment programming.

McGill Pain Questionnaire

Melzack developed the McGill Pain Questionnaire to measure multiple dimensions of the pain experience and help the patient to identify more accurately the subjective dimensions of pain (26). The questionnaire consists of 20 category scales of descriptors that are ranked according to intensity. The first 11 scales identify the patient's perceptions of the sensory dimension of pain. Scales 12 through 15 evaluate the affective dimension of the pain experience. Scale 16 identifies the intensity of the pain. The final four scales assess miscellaneous dimensions of the pain experience. Dubuisson and Melzack used the questionnaire to evaluate particular pain syndromes that were quantifiably different from one another so that patients with similar pain syndromes used similar words to communicate their pain experiences (27). They reported that the instrument may differentiate among groups of patients with various pain syndromes including neuralgia, arthritis, reflex dystrophy, and radiculopathy. Numerous studies have been performed that suggest that although the McGill Pain Questionnaire shows reliability and validity, there is significant disagreement over the accuracy of the test and its ability to discriminate diagnostic groups of patients. The McGill Pain Questionnaire combined with unidimensional rating scales has been found to be useful and valid for research and clinical applications (27). The questionnaire is depicted in Figure 4.3.

Assessment of Affective Disturbance

Because affective disturbances, typically depression and anxiety, are associated with chronic pain, several simplified scales are often useful in the psychological evaluation. The Beck Depression Inventory consists of 21 items with a cumulative scoring system based on questions common in depression, such as sleep disturbance, weight change, fatigue factors, sexual dysfunction, and cognitive components of depressive illness. The test requires only 5 minutes, and scoring requires less than 1 minute. The test may be used throughout a treatment program for the chronic pain patient as a measure of improvement. The incidence of depression varies greatly from study to study with chronic pain patients,

and may range from 10% to 100%. This significant discrepancy in the evaluation of depression as a component in chronic pain syndrome is thought to reflect differences in the definition and diagnostic criteria for depression as well as patient selection bias. Nevertheless, depression is considered a common component in the chronic pain syndrome. Other self-report instruments include the Hamilton Rating Scale for Depression, the Zung Depression Index, and the Illness Behavior Questionnaire (28).

Recently, a "distress and risk assessment" method, which was derived from a set of scales validated for use with patients suffering from low back pain, was developed by Main and colleagues (29). The scale combination classifies patients into those showing no significant psychological distress, those at high risk of developing major psychological overlay, and those clearly under significant distress. Four patient types were identified in the study, including descriptions of "normal," "at risk," "distressed-depressive," and "distressed-somatic" patients.

Cognitive Assessment in the Chronic Pain Patient

Cognitive distortions are common in chronic pain patients. These distortions typically include catastrophization, over-generalization, and selective abstraction. In other words, patients often anticipate the worst outcome following their experience, and there is a tendency to generalize symptoms to future experiences, which will be presumed to be negative. Selective abstraction refers to the tendency for patients to focus primarily on the negative aspects of their pain and symptoms. There is sufficient research with cognitive factors in chronic pain patients to suggest that evaluation of cognitive variables is important in treatment (30). Lefebvre developed the Cognitive Error Questionnaire, which helps to identify cognitive distortions in chronic pain patients who may benefit from treatment techniques such as cognitive restructuring and self-instructional training (31). The majority of current pain treatment programs utilize cognitive pain coping skill programs that teach distraction, relaxation, imagery, and rational interpretation of symptoms. In my experience, it is common to find the unsophisticated patient's perception of his or her symptoms to be discrepant with information provided by the patient's physicians. For example, chronic back pain patients often misinterpret their symptoms. Misinterpretation and catastrophization of continued pain is translated to mean "tissue damage." For these reasons, it is critical to implement an educational program for patients who suffer from chronic pain syndromes and to help them evaluate their symptoms realistically.

In addition to behavioral analysis and traditional psychological tests used in evaluation of chronic pain patients, it is occcasionally important to evaluate the pa-

Figure 4.3. The McGill Pain Questionnaire. The descriptors fall into four major groups. The rank value for each descriptor is based on its position in the word set. The sum of the rank values is the pain rating index (PRI). The present pain intensity (PPI) is based on a scale of 0 to 5. (From Melzack R: The McGill Pain Questionnaire. In Melzack R (ed): *Pain Measurement and Assessment.* New York, Raven Press, 1983.)

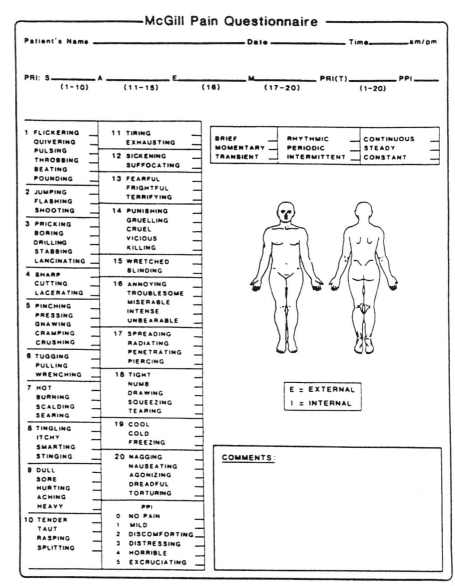

tient's cognitive status from a neuropsychological perspective. An evaluation of cognitive status in the patient who suffers from post-traumatic cervical pain or post-traumatic headaches is often indicated for delineation of specific symptoms that may appear to be psychological yet are a function of actual mild brain impairment. The evaluation may be helpful for the development of treatment strategies and rehabilitation planning efforts. Radanov and colleagues have identified two different syndromes often found among patients suffering from soft tissue cervical spine injuries (32). First these authors identified the "cervicoencephalic syndrome." This syndrome is characterized by headaches, fatigue, dizziness, poor concentration, disturbed accommodation, and an impaired adaptation to light intensity. The second syndrome was identified as a "lower cervical spine syndrome" characterized by cervical and cervicobrachial pain. The cervicoencephalic

syndrome patients demonstrated poor results on tests of divided attention and deficits in information processing. These symptoms are often overlooked characteristics of the "post-traumatic syndrome." This study indicated the need for thorough cognitive-intellectual assessment in patients who report persistent pain and other symptoms following whiplash and acceleration-deceleration injuries (32, 33).

OTHER MULTIDIMENSIONAL TESTS

Due to the current interest and popularity of the cognitive-behavioral perspective on the evaluation and treatment of chronic pain, several tests have been developed to encompass the wide array of variables that affect the pain patient. The Westhaven Yale Multidimensional Pain Inventory (WHYMPI) was developed by Kerns, Turk, and Rudy into a standardized questionnaire (34). This test consists of 12 scales designed to measure the impact of pain on the patient's life, communication of the pain experience, and the extent to which patients participate in activities of daily living. Turk and Rudy have also developed the Multiaxial Assessment of Pain (MAP), which integrates the medical, psychosocial, and behavioral characteristics of pain patients (35). Both of these tests are popular in chronic pain treatment centers, and have been found to be valid and reliable.

A relatively new instrument has been developed by Tearnan and Lewandowski that provides a multifactorial assessment of chronic pain. The behavioral assessment of pain questionnaire (BAP) is a comprehensive self-report test for the pain clinician.* This test offers excellent reliability and validity as well as internal consistency. These authors have used a biopsychosocial framework for the development of this test instrument, which includes important data often ignored by other assessment instruments. Various scales evaluate potential influences on the patient's pain problems, including physician influence, spousal influence, cognitive beliefs, and traditional scales of mood and activity level. The BAP should be implemented with other measures of psychological disturbance, as well as measures of physical capacity.

Psychophysiologic Assessment

The evaluation of the chronic pain patient is often enhanced by the addition of psychophysiologic responses. Caution is advised in the interpretation of specific psychophysiologic responses, such as electromyographic recordings of musculature, and other indicators of physical symptoms that may or may not be correlated with a specific pain syndrome. Chronic headache patients and low back pain patients have often been evaluated with surface electrode electromyographic (EMG) biofeedback, and assumptions have been made about the correlation between these findings and the patient's underlying pain syndrome. Although several studies have produced contradictory results (36–38), it is often helpful to utilize the physiologic data in treatment planning. It is well known that higher levels of autonomic reactivity may be associated with positive stress reactions as a result of pain. Biofeedback-assisted relaxation has been found to be extremely helpful in the treatment of chronic pain syndromes, especially back pain, as well as headaches and other disorders.

Another promising area for psychophysiologic assessment in chronic pain syndromes may be forthcoming with the use of specific corticosensory evoked potentials. Evoked potentials are currently being used extensively during spinal surgery, and dermatome-specific corticosensory potentials are useful as a diagnostic mo-

dality both pre- and intra-operatively in spinal surgical patients. Event-related potentials recorded from scalp areas, particularly the post-central cortex and the somatosensory cortex, have been found to correlate with the intensity of pain stimulation. Interestingly, it has been shown that both aspirin and morphine can lead to a reduction in the somatosensory evoked potentials produced by painful electrical shock. This type of advanced psychophysiologic evaluation may eventually enhance our current methods of pain assessment (39–41).

The P300 amplitude has been used as an index of levels of pain during real and feigned pain in normal subjects and is currently being studied as a direct physiologic measure of true pain. These physiologic measures will require correlation with subjective pain descriptors and analog scales (42). In addition, psychophysical scaling principles are currently being tested in clinical pain assessment. This research is important because it combines multiple judgments to provide more stable pain estimates and it provides an index of the individual's consistency in scaling the painful sensations. It is well known that inconsistencies in scaling pain have dramatic research and clinical implications. Treatment effects are often misconstrued or inconsistent in pain research performed with traditional pain scaling methods (39).

Other attempts at physiologic measurement of pain variables have included the ischemic-tourniquet technique, infrared heat, and the cold-pressor test. Although these methods of inducing pain are useful in the experimental setting, considerable variability is found on pain threshold and pain tolerance measures. It is suggested that chronic pain patients may seldom react to only a simple sensory signal. The experimental pain induction procedures used as assessment tools for evaluating the chronic pain patient's pain threshold and tolerance have not been shown to be reliable predictors of treatment outcome. The notion of "low pain threshold" on these tests as a predictor of treatment outcome is also questionable because experimental pain induction techniques are perceived by patients as temporary and time-limited experiences that cause them no permanent physical harm. Therefore, pain induction techniques as an assessment device for evaluating chronic pain require further study and validation (30).

Brief Overview of Additional Assessment Devices

The Millon Behavioral Health Inventory (MBHI) is a computerized questionnaire based on 20 clinical scales that assess physical concerns and behavioral reactions to disease or illness (43). The MBHI is a true/false test that takes a patient 20 to 30 minutes to complete. Several researchers have identified various scales associated with responses compared to chronic pain patients. Mayer and Gatchel have found that patients who score low on the cooperative style scale and high on the sen-

---

*For more information, see Tearnan DH, Lewandowski MJ: The Behavioral Assessment of Pain Questionnaire: The development and validation of a comprehensive self-report instrument. *Am J Pain Mgmt* 2:181–191, 1992.

sitive scale demonstrate poor outcome in their functional restoration program (44). Their preliminary research suggested that individuals who score high on the pre-morbid pessimism and forceful style scales may be prone to seek out surgical treatment as compared to subjects who do not show elevations on these scales.

Rosenstiel and Keefe developed the Cognitive Strategies Questionnaire while studying a population of chronic pain patients (45). This test consists of three major underlying dimensions including cognitive coping and suppression, helplessness, and diverting attention and praying. High levels of functional impairment were found on scales associated with cognitive coping and suppression and with diverting attention and praying.

The Symptom Checklist 90–revised (SCL-90R) has been found to be a good measure of psychopathology in psychiatric and medical patients (46). Kinney and colleagues have used the SCL-90R as an alternative to the MMPI for psychological screening of chronic low back pain patients (47). Although they found this test to be useful because of its brevity, they suggest that this instrument should be used as a screening device and correlated with more familiar instruments such as the MMPI.

Pilowsky developed the Illness Behavior Questionnaire, which provides a measure of seven aspects of illness behavior: general hypochondriasis, disease conviction, somatic versus psychological concern, affective inhibition, affective disturbance or dysphoria, denial, and irritability (48). The questionnaire could prove to be helpful for early detection of abnormal illness behavior associated with chronic pain. The questionnaire does not provide accurate information for a diagnosis or for distinguishing characteristics that may exist among chronic pain patients.

The Sickness Impact Profile (SIP) as developed by Bergner and colleagues measures mobility, social functions, and elements of self-management (49). This instrument may be helpful in developing treatment planning because of its emphasis on the functional status of the patient. The SIP discriminates psychosocial and physical dysfunction (50).

The Clinical Analysis Questionnaire (CAQ) was derived from the Sixteen Personality Factor Questionnaire (16PF) developed by Catell (51). This test provides traditional evaluation of the 16 personality factors, yet includes clinical scales similar to those described on the MMPI. Recently, Iacono and Baranchok presented a paper suggesting that the CAQ may be more appropriate than the MMPI for assessment in the rehabilitation setting with pain patients (52).

The Simultaneous Interview Technique (SIT) was recently presented by Jacobson and colleagues as a comprehensive interview strategy in which chronic pain patients are interviewed simultaneously by a psychologist and a physician (53). This structured interview instru-

ment proved successful because it appears to facilitate patient management by (1) emphasizing the multidimensional components of chronic pain, (2) encouraging acceptance of the psychological aspects of pain management, (3) developing consistency within the treatment facility, (4) avoiding misinformation and manipulation of healthcare providers by the difficult patient, (5) decreasing hostile situations, and (6) decreasing time required for duplication of interviews and questions by the medical staff and psychologist. Overall, the SIT was reported to help provide effective pain management.

PREDICTORS OF CONSERVATIVE TREATMENT OF CHRONIC PAIN: A BRIEF OVERVIEW

Maruta and colleagues developed an index of variables that were predictive of treatment outcome in a multidisciplinary pain program (54). The index compared admission and pre-admission information to treatment outcome. Variables included initial pain level, number of operations, duration of pain, amount of lost time from work, medication dependence, and the hypochondriasis and hysteria scales from the MMPI. In their original study, the researchers found significant differences in 34 successfully treated and 35 unsuccessfully treated patients who were evaluated at 1 year follow-up. The unsuccessful group typically had a longer pain history, lost more time from work, underwent more surgical procedures for pain, had a higher dependence on medication, and had higher pain ratings than the successfully treated group. In this study, significant differences were not found with regard to sex, age, marital status, number of medications, compensation, pain location, and diagnosis. Aronoff and Evans used the Maruta index with 104 subjects and found that the index was not predictive of treatment outcome in a multidisciplinary center. A recent investigation performed by Chandren and colleagues evaluated whether the MMPI was useful in predicting treatment outcome in a functional restoration program (56). Patients were contacted and evaluated 1 year after treatment, and successful and failed treatment groups were selected. The following array of MMPI scales significantly discriminated between the success and failure groups: lie, mania, psychopathy, introversion, anxiety, and the MacAndrews scales. This investigation, presented in 1992, may help to provide a basis for replication studies and clarify the contradictory results in predicting conservative treatment in previous research endeavors.

Research in this area is extremely difficult and interpretation of various studies is confusing because of methodologic flaws in clinical outcome measures. There is a notable lack of standardized treatment components, outcome measures, controls, and comparison groups, and many studies have a very small population sample. Roberts and Reinhardt evaluated the effectiveness of a chronic pain inpatient program with treatment and no-treatment groups (57). Guck et al. (58) used treatment and no-treatment groups while utilizing the Roberts and Rheinhardt criteria for success, which include the following:

1. Patients were employed or able to complete appropriate activities of daily living.
2. Patients were not receiving any compensation for pain.
3. Patients had no further hospitalizations or surgery for pain since their initial evaluation.
4. Patients were not taking any prescription pain medications.

Guck's research group used a discriminate analysis procedure that involved 14 commonly used demographic variables to predict membership in the successful and unsuccessful groups. They found that age, compensation, educational level, psychotropic medication use, and pain surgeries were predictive variables that categorized over 70% of their subjects. A follow-up study of treated versus nontreated groups was performed by Deardorff, Rubin, and Scott and was designed to overcome many of the weaknesses of previous studies by using a no-treatment comparison group, assessing relevant outcome variables, and meeting a high proportion of contacted follow-up patients at approximately 11 months after treatment (59). Their study demonstrated a positive response to multidisciplinary treatment, with measures demonstrating increased physical functioning, positive return-to-work rates, decreased medication use, and reduced pain ratings, although these reductions were statistically insignificant.

In addition to the predictive variables cited above, which include demographic data and patient statistics, other researchers have used pretreatment evaluation of chronic pain patients' beliefs about their pain and their perceptions of treatment in a pain clinic. A study by Shutty and colleagues included a pain clinic orientation videotape that detailed conservative approaches to pain management (60). In addition a questionnaire measuring recall of the video tape information and patient acceptance or rejection of the information was recorded. At 1 month after treatment, the extent of agreement with the videotape content was significantly correlated with lower pain ratings, improved physical ability measures, and higher degrees of treatment satisfaction. This novel assessment procedure prior to treatment permits categorization of patients who will probably not be satisfied with conservative treatment efforts, and supports the necessity for evaluation of patients' cognitions and attitudes about their pain and their expectations regarding conservative treatment. In this study, measures of psychological distress, as well as of age and other variables, were not predictive of treatment outcome. This study was consistent, however, with the expectations of a study performed by Schwartz and his colleagues, which suggested that the extent of patient agreement with videotaped content would be associated with short-term treatment outcome (61).

In summary, predictors of outcome in multidisciplinary programs for chronic pain have been weak because of methodologic problems. Research in this area must be carefully detailed, and characteristics of patient and outcome variables must be fully explained and must measure what they purport to measure. Increased population samples in these studies are critical for their statistical validation. Improved predictor and criterion variables must be identified, and replication studies with identical criteria are needed.

SPECIAL POPULATIONS: CHRONIC PAIN IN THE ELDERLY AND IN CHILDREN

PAIN ASSESSMENT WITH THE ELDERLY

It is unfortunate that elderly people often suffer from chronic and painful diseases and take multiple medications, yet little attention has been paid to pain management problems in this population. This is particularly true of the geriatric population in long-term medical settings. In fact, research in this area has shown that the prevalence of persistent pain is doubled in those patients over age 60 as compared with those individuals under the age of 60 (62). It appears that the priority in geriatric medicine has been the control of disease symptoms, enhanced comfort and, one hopes, the preservation of dignity. Because this population is the fastest-growing segment of our population, continued research is needed into this group of patients, who have specialized needs. I am reminded of the depiction of a participant who happened to be 101 years of age in a study on aging by Butler and Gastel (63). When the patient complained that his left leg was continuously painful, the physician suggested that perhaps it should be expected at his age. The wise older gentleman then asked the physician to explain why his right leg, which was also over 100 years old, did not hurt at all! Part of the problem with our lack of understanding and minimum of research with this population is more than likely due to the erroneous assumption that the aging process is synonymous with increased pain and disease. The consequence of this type of thinking may lead to undertreatment of the elderly patient regarding pain, as well as to the possibility of missed diagnostic indicators that are not pursued medically when the patient complains. The institutionalized older patient often has a stoic presentation with regard to pain; to make the situation more complex, such patients often demonstrate an altered presentation of diseases including "silent" myocardial infarctions and other medical emergencies (63). They often report pain very differently from the way younger patients do because of physiologic as well as psychological and cultural variables associated with the aging process. Experiments that purport to test pain threshold and tolerance in the elderly population have produced equivocal results. As we now know, experimentally induced pain may not be analogous to clinical pain (30, 40).

Conversely, we often are reminded of the elderly patient who has numerous medical complaints and seems to thrive on them. It appears as if they have nothing better to do than to speak of their medications, physicians, and diseases. Although this may be a common stereotypical generalization, recent research indicates a need for a more thorough and accurate assessment of pain and symptoms in this population. In a recent study by Ferrell et al., 97 subjects from a nursing home were interviewed, and charts were reviewed for pain problems and management strategies (64). Affective status, cognitive status, and functional status were evaluated. In this group of patients, 71% of the residents reported a minimum of one pain complaint, and 34% described continuous persistent pain. Sixty-six percent described intermittent pain, whereas 51% described pain on a daily basis. Interestingly, only 15% of those patients having persistent pain had received medications within the last 24 hours. This important study suggests that pain is an overlooked problem in the long-term care facility (64).

Common problems in the assessment of chronic pain in the elderly patient include cognitive impairment and dementia, delirium, and other specific problems such as visual and hearing impairment and motor impairment. These conditions may make pain assessment difficult because elderly patients may not be capable of communicating properly or understanding a pain assessment protocol. Often these patients have difficulty in understanding exactly what is being requested from them and, as in children, they may not understand the purpose of the assessment and its potential for bringing relief. Many of these patients have suffered for many years without lasting relief. There is a good probability that there is an element of "learned helplessness"; the institutionalized or frequently hospitalized elderly patient may simply have exhausted any efforts toward obtaining relief. They may have been told that they have an untreatable condition. Thus the elderly patient presents the unfortunate opportunity for both under- and over-treatment.

Although traditional evaluation approaches, including verbal descriptors, numerical ratings scales, and visual analog scales, may be helpful in those patients who do not have seriously impaired cognitive functioning, these instruments have not been thoroughly evaluated with the elderly population. Following are general recommendations for pain assessment in the elderly:

1. The pain patient may need to be prompted frequently regarding symptoms. If discussions are unproduc-

tive, the family may need to be interviewed. Observation of family and staff interactions is often beneficial to the assessment.

2. If the patient appears to have a significant degree of cognitive impairment and it is difficult to obtain a review of symptoms, it is often helpful to have a psychological or neuropsychological consultation to rule out cognitive symptoms due to depression or so-called "pseudo dementia" versus true dementia. Obviously, if the patient's inability to communicate and elaborate on pain problems is due to severe depression, appropriate treatment can then be rendered. Following improvement and/or clarification of symptoms, perhaps an evaluation of the patient's persistent pain problems will be more easily obtained.

3. As part of the assessment, a trial dose of pain medication may be implemented and the patient's behavior and response to the medications monitored. This practice may help to determine how much of the patient's problem is due to pain, depression, or cognitive disturbance.

4. In normally functioning patients, it is helpful to instruct them to keep a pain diary and daily pain rating scale. As with any pain assessment, the patient may be instructed to record antecedent behaviors or events that precipitate increased pain. If a patient is incapable of keeping such a record, perhaps family members or other caregivers could be of help.

For an excellent review of nursing considerations and pain management in the elderly patient, the reader is referred to the clinical manual developed by McCaffery and Beebe (6).

PAIN ASSESSMENT IN CHILDREN

Although it appears vital that assessment of pain be accurate to render proper diagnostic tests and subsequent treatment, characteristics specific to children further compound the evaluation process. Fortunately, most clinicians have moved away from the antiquated view that infants and very young children have an immature nervous system and therefore do not experience pain as the mature adult does. Nevertheless, there still remains the widespread problem of under-treatment of the pediatric patient. There is evidence that many children do not receive any opioid analgesics following painful surgical procedures (65). It is also well known that when analgesic medications are provided to children, doses are often inadequate, and the analgesics are commonly prescribed on an "as needed" basis. There is a tendency towards treatment of children with chronic pain only during an exacerbation. Chronic pain syndromes in children typically involve hematologic and oncologic diseases such as hemophilia, sickle cell anemia, the leukemias and solid tumors, and associated symptoms for these diseases. Other chronic pain syndromes include headaches, juvenile rheumatoid arthritis, and painful complications due to diseases such as cystic fibrosis. In addition, children may have persistent pain problems as a result of post-traumatic injuries and orthopedic or developmentally related abnormalities.

Assessment of pain in children involves not only the verbal report of pain intensity and location, but behavioral expressions such as grimacing, moaning, weeping, or withdrawal from regular activities. It is especially important to use assessment strategies that are consistent with the child's developmental-cognitive level. It is equally important to obtain a pain history from the child and the parents and to learn which types of pain behaviors and verbal descriptions the child uses with them. There may be specific cultural and familial beliefs about pain and medical care. The following general guidelines are suggested for the clinician:

1. Repeated estimates of the pain experience are needed. Knowing the child will optimize the assessment of the pain and will be of tremendous value in tailoring the pain management program.
2. Behavioral observations with preverbal and nonverbal children are critical and should compliment the report from parents and other caregivers. Particular pain behaviors and expressions, as well as posture, motor responses, and levels of agitation or withdrawal, should be included in the behavioral assessment. Interpretation of the behavior should be performed with caution because children may engage in activities such as sleeping or television watching that may actually be helping the child to cope with his or her discomfort.
3. Self-report measures are useful for most children 4 years of age and older. Children who are 8 years old or beyond typically are capable of understanding numerical scales and simple word descriptors for pain.
4. Specific developmental evaluation may be indicated in the child who does not appear to be capable of communicating his pain and other symptoms, and a developmental-psychological evaluation may be indicated. Traditional standardized tests such as the Wechsler Intelligence Scale for Children or the Leiter International Performance Scale for the nonverbal child may provide an accurate estimate of cognitive-developmental level.

Several assessment instruments have been developed specifically for the evaluation of pediatric pain. An adaptation of the visual analog scale has been developed with happy and sad faces to provide more meaningful representations for the younger child. Although most of these instruments have been developed for acute pain assessment, they also may play a valuable role in the assessment of ongoing persistent pain in children. Most of the chronic pain syndromes prevalent in childhood are those disorders which fluctuate in their severity. It is helpful to educate the child about the nature of his or her disease, reporting symptoms, and playing an active

role in pain management. Varni and Thompson developed a pediatric pain questionnaire, which is shown in Figure 4.4 (66). The three forms in the questionnaire are for the parent, child, and adolescent, respectively. Questions elicit descriptions of the pain and provide a visual analog scale for rating pain. A map is included on the child form that provides color choices for different intensities of pain. The adolescent form produces information with more emphasis on the psychosocial aspects of the pain and the child's life situation. This instrument appears to have satisfactory validity and reliability according to studies performed on children with juvenile rheumatoid arthritis (66). McGrath developed the Children's Comprehensive Pain Questionnaire (CCPQ), which is suitable for the clinical setting but also provides a comprehensive picture of the child's view of his pain (67). This questionnaire evaluates the child's coping strategies, possibilities for pain-related secondary gain, and the child's perception of family reactions to his or her pain and the potential for conditioning effects (68).

In addition to questionnaires and traditional visual and numerical rating scales, tools such as The Poker Chip Tool (69) and pain thermometers (70) have been developed.

The development of effective assessment tools is critical to the understanding and management of childhood pain. Although specific assessment instruments are limited in number, and many remain untested psychometrically, significant progress has been made in understanding chronic pain syndromes in children. Unfortunately, many children still undergo painful medical procedures without adequate treatment. Perhaps better assessment devices for childhood pain will help to validate their suffering and will result in more effective pain management.

CONCLUSIONS

This chapter has provided a basic overview of psychological assessment devices and current tests that may be helpful in evaluating chronic pain patients. A more exhaustive critical review of the literature was presented in the first edition of the *Handbook of Chronic Pain Management*. Thorough evaluation of the chronic pain patient should include multiple measures of subjective pain, cognitive variables, interpretations of the pain, overt behavior, affective and stress symptoms, and psychophysiologic responses associated with pain and distress. In addition, the evaluation may help identify possible compliance issues, hostility, and motivation. Because of the devastating social effects of chronic pain, many patients develop marital and family problems in addition to problems with employment. A thorough assessment with chronic pain patients requires acceptance of the bio-psychosocial model with an emphasis on

When did your present pain problem begin? Please also explain the symptoms.

What was your reaction to the pain at that time? Please explain.

Were any major changes in your life occurring then? Please explain.

If your pain were suddenly to disappear, how would it change your life?

How would it change your family relationships?

Assuming that the pain continues, what kinds of things do you think you should do <u>now</u>, which will help later on?

What words do you use to describe your pain?

What day of the week do you have the most pain?

Have you ever noticed something that tells you that you are about to experience a pain episode? (e.g., stiffness, particular thoughts or statements, physical sensations or irritability)

What do you call your pains? (e.g., "headache," "joint pain," "stomachache," "back-ache," etc.) Please list them in order of severity, #1 being the most severe pain.

On a scale of 0–10, (0 = no pain, 10 = severe pain), how severe is your pain at the following times of the day?
6 A.M. 9 A.M. 12 noon 3 P.M. 6 P.M. 9 P.M. 12 A.M. 3 A.M.

What do you currently do, besides taking medication, to relieve your pain?

Does your pain seem worse when you are (Yes/No to each):
tired, anxious, bored, happy, unhappy, angry, busy, lonely, arguing, upset.

Are there any other situations in which your pain is worse? If yes, what are they?

Please rate how much pain you are <u>having at the present time</u> by placing a mark some-where on the line.

Not Hurting
No Discomfort _____ Hurting a Whole Lot
No Pain   Very Uncomfortable
                                               Severe Pain

Figure 4.4. The pediatric pain questionnaire of Varni and Thompson. (From Varni JW, Thompson KL, Hanson V: The Varni/Thompson Pediatric Pain Questionnaire. *Pain* 28:27–38, 1987.)

functional restoration, pain reduction, and a return to a productive lifestyle.

REFERENCES

1. Melzak R: *The Puzzle of Pain.* New York, Basic Books, 1973.
2. *Acute Pain Management: Operative or Medical Procedures and Trauma. Clinical Practice Guideline.* Washington, D.C., Agency for Health Care Policy and Research, Public Health Service, U.S. Department of Health and Human Services, 1992.
3. American Pain Society: *Principles of Analgesic Use in the Treatment of Acute Pain and Cancer Pain,* ed 3. Skokie, IL, APS, 1992.
4. Donovan M, Dillon P, McGuire L: Incidents and characteristics of pain in a sample of medical-surgical inpatients. *Pain* 30:69–87, 1987.
5. Commission on Accreditation of Rehabilitation Facilities: *Standards Manual for Organizations Serving People with Disabilities.* Tuscon, Commission on Accreditation of Rehabilitation Facilities, 1986.
6. McCaffery M, Beebe A: *Pain: Clinical Manual for Nursing Practice.* St. Louis, CV Mosby, 1989.
7. Polatin PB, Kinney R, Gatchel RG, Mayer TG: Psychiatric Illness and Chronic Low Back Pain: The Mind and the Spine—Which Goes First? Paper presented at the Seventh Annual Meeting, North American Spine Society, Boston, July, 1992.
8. Schofferman J, Anderson D, Smith G, Hines R, Keane G: Childhood Psychological Trauma and Chronic Back Pain. Paper Presented at the Seventh Annual Meeting, North American Spine Society, Boston, July, 1992.
9. Cameron AJ, Shepell: Psychological assessment. In Kirkaldy-Willis WH (ed): *Managing Low Back Pain,* ed 2. New York, Churchill Livingstone, 1988.
10. McGuire DB: Comprehensive and multidimensional assessment and measurement of pain. *J Pain Symptom Mgmt.* 7:312–319, 1992.
11. Fordyce WE: *Behavioral Methods for Chronic Pain and Illness.* St. Louis, CV Mosby, 1976.
12. Turk DC, Meichenbaum D, Genest M: *Pain and Behavioral Medicine: A Cognitive-Behavioral Perspective.* New York, Guilford, 1983.
13. Turk DC, Flor H: Pain > Pain behaviors: The utility and limitations of the pain behavior construct. *Pain* 31:277–296, 1987.
14. Follick MJ, Ahern DK, Journal Laser-Wallston, N: Evaluation of a daily activity diary for chronic pain patients. *Pain* 19:373–382, 1984.

15. Craig KD: Echoes of pain. *APS J* 1:105–108, 1992.

16. Keefe FJ, Crisson JE: Assessment of behaviors. In Lynch TN, Vasudevan SV (eds): *Persistent Pain. Psychosocial Assessment Intervention.* Boston, Kluwer Academic Publishers, 1988.

17. Richards JS, Nepomuceno C, Riles M, Suer Z: Assessing pain behavior: The UAB Pain Behavior Scale. *Pain* 14:393–398, 1982.

18. Keefe FJ, Dunsmore J: Pain behavior concepts and controversies. *APS J* 1:92–100, 1992.

19. Merskey H: Limitations of pain behavior. *APS J* 1:101–104, 1992.

20. Slater E, Glitheroe: A follow-up of patients diagnosed as suffering from "hysteria." *J Psychosom Res* 9:9–13, 1965.

21. Spratt KF, Lehmann TR, Weinstein JN, Sayre HA: New approach to the low back physical examination: Behavioral assessment of mechanical signs. *Spine* 15:96–102, 1990.

22. Pope MH, Rosen JC, Wilder DG, Frymoyer JW: The relation between biomechanical and psychological factors in patients with low back pain. *Spine* 5:173–178, 1980.

23. Ross DM, Ross SA: *Childhood Pain: Current Issues, Research and Management.* Baltimore, Urban and Schwarzenberg, 1988, pp. 111–165.

24. Fordyce WE: Use of the MMPI in the assessment of chronic pain. In Clinical Notes on the MMPI. Butcher J, Dahlstrom G, Gynther W, Schofield W (eds): *Clinical Notes on the MMPI.* LaRoche NJ, Hoffman, 1979.

25. Ahles TA, Yunus MB, Gaulier B, Riley SD, Masi AT: The use of contemporary MMPI norms in the study of chronic pain patients. *Pain* 24:159–163, 1986.

26. Melzak R: The McGill Pain Questionnaire: Major properties and scoring methods. *Pain* 1:277–299, 1975.

27. Dubuisson D, Melzack R: Classification of clinical pain description by multiple group discriminate analysis. *Exp Neurol* 51:480–487, 1976.

28. Pilowsky I, Spence ND: Patterns of illness behavior in patients with intractable pain. *J Psychosom Res* 19:279–287, 1975.

29. Main CJ, Wood PLR, Hollis S, Spanswick CC, Waddell G: The distress and risk assessment method: A simple patient classification to identify distress and evaluate the risk of poor outcome. *Spine* 17:42–52, 1992.

30. Hinnant D: Cognitive Coping Strategies with Chronic Back Pain Patients. Doctoral Dissertation, North Texas State University, Denton, TX, 1985.

31. Lefebvre MF: Cognitive distortion and cognitive errors in depressed psychiatric and low back pain patients. *J Consult Clin Psychol* 49:517–525, 1984.

32. Radanov BP, Dvorak J, Valach L: Cognitive deficits in patients after soft tissue injury of the cervical spine. *Spine* 17:127–131, 1992.

33. Hinnant DW, Kade DH: Cognitive deficits following cervical trauma. In Tollison CD, Satterthwaite JR (eds): *Painful Cervical Trauma: Diagnosis and Rehabilitative Treatment of Neuro-Musculoskeletal Injuries.* Baltimore, Williams & Wilkins, 1992.

34. Kerns RD, Turk DC, Rudy TE: The Westhaven-Yale Multidimensional Pain Inventory (WHYMI). *Pain* 23:345–356, 1985.

35. Turk DC, Rudy TE: The robustness of an empirically derived taxonomy of chronic pain patients. *Pain* 43:27–25, 1990.

36. Cohen MJ, Swanson GA, Naliboff BD, Schandler SL, McArthur DL: Comparison of electromyographic response patterns during posture and stress tasks in chronic low back pain patterns and control. *J Psychosomat Med* 30:135–141, 1986.

37. Collins GA, Cohen MJ, Naliboff, Schandler EL: Comparative analysis of paraspinal and frontal EMG, heartrate, and skin conductants in chronic low back pain patients and normals to various postures and stress. *Scand J Rehabil Med* 14:36–46, 1982.

38. Cram JR, Steger JC: EMG Scanning in the diagnosis of chronic pain. *Biofeedback Self Regul* 8:229–241, 1983.

39. Buchsbaum MS, Davis GC, Coppolar, Naber D: Opiate pharmacology and individual differences: II: Somatosensory evoked potentials. *Pain* 6:121–130, 1981.

40. Chatrian GE, Canfield RC, Knauss TA, Lettich E: Cerebral responses to electrical tooth pulp stimulation in man: An objective correlate of acute experimental pain. *Neurology* 25:745–757, 1975.

41. Dowman R, Goashko L: Somatosensory Evoked Potential Scalp Topographies Elicited by Noxious Sural Nerve Stimulation in Men. Paper Presented at the Tenth Annual Meeting of the American Pain Society, New Orleans, November, 1991.

42. Rosenfeld JP, Koo J, Goldbloom E, Johnson MM: P300 Amplitude as an Index of Levels of Pain During Real (Ischemia) and Feigned Pain in Normals. Paper Presented at the Tenth Annual Meeting of the American Pain Society, New Orleans, November 1991.

43. Millon T, Green CJ, Meagher RB: *Millon Behavioral Health Inventory,* ed 3. Minneapolis, Interpretive Scoring System, 1982.

44. Mayer TG, Gatchel RJ: *Functional Restoration for Spinal Disorders: The Sports Medicine Approach.* Philadelphia, Lea & Febiger, 1988.

45. Rosenstiel AK, Keefe FJ: The use of coping strategies in chronic low back pain patients: Relationship to patient characteristics in current assessment. *Pain* 17:33–44, 1983.

46. Derogatis LR, Lipman RS, Covi L: The SCL-90: An outpatient psychiatric rating scale. *Psychopharmacol Bull* 9:13–28, 1973.

47. Kinney R, Catchell RJ, Mayer TG: The SCL-90R: An alternative to the MMPI for Psychological Screening of Chronic Low Back Pain Patients. Presented at the Annual Meeting of the International Society for the Study of the Lumbar Spine, Kyoto, Japan, May, 1989.

48. Pilowsky I: A general classification of the abnormal illness behavior. *Br J Med Psychology* 51:131–137, 1978.

49. Follick MJ, Smith TW, Ahern DK: The Sickness Impact Profile: A global measure of disability in chronic low back pain. *Pain* 21:67–76, 1985.

50. Bradley LA, Anderson KO, Young LD, Williams T: Psychological testing. In Tollison CD (ed): *Handbook of Chronic Pain Management.* Baltimore, Williams & Wilkins, 1989, pp 570–591.

51. Cattell RB: *Clinical Analysis Questionnaire.* Chicago, Institute for Personality and Ability Testing, Inc., 1982.

52. Iacono CU, Baranchok J: The Clinical Analysis Questionnaire: An Alternative to the MMPI for Personality Assessment for Chronic Pain Patients. Presented at the Tenth Annual Meeting of the American Pain Society, New Orleans, November, 1991.

53. Jacobson L, Mariano AJ, Chaney EF, Chabal C: Simultaneous Interview Techniques for patients with persistent pain. *Pain* 45:105–106, 1991.

54. Maruta, Swanson SW, Swerson WM: Chronic pain: Which patients may a pain-Management Program Help? *Pain* 7:321–329, 1979.

55. Aronoff GM, Evans WO: The prediction of treatment outcome at a multidisciplinary pain center. *Pain* 14:67–73, 1982.

56. Chandran S, Gatchel RJ, Mayer TG: *The MMPI as a predictor of treatment outcome in chronic low back pain patients.* Paper presented at the Seventh Annual Meeting of the North American Spine Society, Boston, July 1992.

57. Roberts AH, Reinhardt D: Behavioral management of chronic pain: Long-term follow-up with comparison groups. *Pain* 8:151–162, 1980.

58. Guck TP, Meilman PW, Skultety FM, Dowd ET: Prediction of long-term outcome of multidisciplinary pain treatment. *Arch Phys Med Rehabil* 67:295–306, 1986.

59. Deardorff WW, Rubin HF, Scott DW: Comprehensive multidisciplinary treatment of chronic pain: A follow-up study of treated and non-treated groups. *Pain* 45:35–43, 1991.

60. Shutty MS, DeGood DE, Tuttle DH: Chronic pain patients' beliefs about their pain and treatment outcomes. *Arch Phys Med Rehabil* 71:1990.

61. Schwartz DP, DeGood DE, Shutty MS: Direct assessment of beliefs and attitudes of chronic pain patients. *Arch Phys Med Rehabil* 66:806–809, 1985.

62. Crook J, Rideout E, Brown EG: The prevalence of pain complaints in a general population. *Pain* 18:299–314, 1984.

63. Butler RN, Gastel B: Care of the aged: Perspectives on pain and discomfort. In Ng, LK, Bonica J (eds): *Pain, Discomfort, and Humanitarian Care.* New York, Elsevier, North Holland, 1980, pp 297–311.

64. Ferrell BA, Ferrell BR, Osterweil D: Pain in the nursing home. *Jags* 38:409–414, 1990.

65. Thompson KL, Varni JW: A developmental cognitive-bio-behavioral approach to pediatric pain assessment. *Pain* 25:283–296, 1986.

66. Varni JW, Thompson KL, Hanson V: The Varni/Thompson Pediatric Pain Questionnaire: I. Chronic musculoskeletal pain in juvenile rheumatoid arthritis. *Pain* 28:27–38, 1987.

67. McGrath PA: *The Children's Comprehensive Pain Questionnaire* [unpublished manuscript]. London, University of Western Ontario, 1986.

68. McGrath PA, deVeber LL, Hearn MT: Multidimensional pain assessment in children. In Fields HL, Dubner R, Cervero F (eds): *Advances in Pain Research and Therapy,* vol. 9: *Proceedings of the Fourth World Congress on Pain.* New York, Raven Press, 1985, pp 387–393.

69. Hester NKO: The pre-operational child's reaction to immunization. *Nursing Res* 28:25–255, 1979.

70. Szyfelbein SK, Osgood PF, Carr DB: The assessment of pain in plasma beta B-endorphin in immunoactivity in burned children. *Pain* 22:173–182, 1985.

71. Bergner M, Bobbitt RA, Carter WB, Gibson BS: The Sickness Impact Profile: Development and final revision of a health status measure. *Med Care* 19:787–805, 1981.

72. Cattell RB, Krug SE: *Clinical Analysis Questionnaire.* Champaign, IL, IPAT.

CHAPTER 5

MEDICAL ELECTRODIAGNOSTICS

HENRY A. SPINDLER

P ATIENTS ARE referred for electrodiagnostic evaluation of a variety of complaints. These include pain, weakness, sensory complaints, gait disturbances, headache, and bowel and bladder disfunction (1). These electrical studies are frequently of great help in diagnosing acute and chronic pain involving the neck, back, and extremities. The most useful tests are electromyography (EMG) and nerve conduction studies (NCSs), including H reflex and F wave measurement. Somatosensory-evoked potentials may also sometimes be helpful in evaluating patients with pain syndromes. Older methods of electrodiagnosis (reaction of degeneration, chronaxie, rheobase, galvanic-tetanus ratio, strength-duration curves) are rarely, if ever, used for the evaluation of pain in a modern electrodiagnostic laboratory. However, they are certainly of historical interest, and nerve excitability studies continue to be used for evaluation of Bell's palsy (2, 3).

The primary function of an electrodiagnostic evaluation utilizing EMG and NCSs is to evaluate the functional integrity of the motor unit. The term *motor unit* was first used by Liddell and Sherrington in 1925 to describe the functional unit of the peripheral nervous system (4). The motor unit is defined as an anterior horn cell, its axon, and all the muscle fibers innervated by that axon. Electrodiagnostic studies attempt to localize sites of pathology within the motor unit (e.g., root, plexus, peripheral nerve) to diagnose the presence of a lesion causing the clinical pain syndrome.

ELECTROMYOGRAPHY

Electromyography is the technique of recording voltage changes within a muscle. Resting mammalian muscle fibers have a transmembrane potential of 70–90 mV in the resting state. The inside of the cell is negative with respect to the outside. This resting potential arises because the membrane is impermeable to the large organic anions within the cell and because of the active transport mechanism that maintains the internal sodium (Na^+) concentration at a low level. When a nerve impulse reaches the neuromuscular junction, acetylcholine is re-

leased across the end plate zone. This initiates an action potential, or reversal of polarity across the muscle membrane, which rapidly spreads over the length of the muscle fiber, initiating contraction. The amplitude of this voltage change may be 100 mV or more when measured with an intracellular electrode.

Intracellular muscle potential recording is technically difficult and unsuited to the clinical situation. Extracellular electromyographic recordings are performed clinically with a needle electrode. Adrian and Bronk in 1929 introduced the concentric needle electrode (5). This electrode consists of a hypodermic needle serving as the cannula with a wire located centrally in the needle but completely insulated from it. Voltage is recorded as the potential difference between the exposed tip of the central wire and the cannula. Because the recording is made extracellularly at a distance from the muscle fiber, the voltage changes recorded are much smaller, ranging from 500 μV to 5 mV. Also, with standard recording electrodes, the recording surface at the tip is quite large with respect to the muscle fiber, and potentials from several muscle fibers are recorded simultaneously. Specialized electrodes with very small recording areas have been developed for recording single muscle fiber potentials. Single fiber recordings, however, are quite specialized studies, and are not used routinely in the electrodiagnostic examination.

Today, the most commonly used needle electrode is of the monopolar type. This is a small-diameter wire electrode that is coated with insulating Teflon except at the tip, where recording is done. Potential measurements are made between the exposed tip of the needle within the muscle and a surface electrode taped to the skin. This electrode arrangement has largely replaced the concentric electrode in most clinical conditions because of the much greater patient comfort.

Electrical activity measured within the muscle is fed into a suitable amplifier and then displayed on an oscilloscope. The activity is also monitored through a loudspeaker, because the various potential changes encountered have characteristic sounds. Electromyographic activity is measured during needle insertion, during complete rest of the muscle without needle movement, and during various grades of active muscle contraction.

INSERTIONAL ACTIVITY

The electrical response seen when a needle electrode is inserted into resting muscle is termed the *insertional activity*. This appears as a burst of spike potentials which continues for 100 to 300 msec after needle motion has ceased. This electrical activity is produced by mechanical damage or deformation of the muscle membrane by the advancing needle. Although the evaluation of insertional activity may appear simple, it is actually a difficult procedure. With careful analysis a great deal of information may be gained by an experienced electromyographer.

The duration of insertional activity may be normal, increased, or decreased. The exact duration of normal insertional activity cannot be given because it depends on many factors, including the velocity of needle insertion and the degree of tissue deformation that occurs. Each electromyographer must therefore to some degree determine "normal" insertional activity with his equipment and technique. An increase in the duration of insertional activity may be the first or only sign of neuromuscular disease. A decrease in the duration of insertional activity is also significant. It most commonly indicates a loss of muscle tissue and is usually a late finding in neuromuscular disease.

The character of the electrical discharges seen with needle insertion must also be examined. Occasional positive sharp waves may be seen during insertional activity as the first sign of denervation.

Because abnormal insertional activity may not be uniform throughout the muscle, at least 10–20 needle insertions must be performed at various sites within the muscle. Electromyographers must be aware of the "end plate noise," which is the normal electrical activity seen in the end plate zone of the muscle, and not report this as abnormal insertional activity.

RESTING MUSCLE

With the needle electrode at rest in relaxed muscle, there is normally no electrical activity seen. Resting activity is observed during pauses between needle insertions. During this procedure, the electromyographer is searching for the presence of abnormal spontaneous activity at rest, but he may also encounter normal spontaneous activity that must be recognized as such.

Normal Spontaneous Activity

Normal spontaneous activity can be recorded if the needle electrode is near the motor end plate region (6). Two types of end plate noise are commonly seen. The first appears as a widening of the baseline, but at closer

inspection is a series of 8–10 μV negative potentials that exhibit a characteristic "seashell" sound over the loudspeaker. This electrical activity corresponds to the miniature end plate potentials caused by acetylcholine release. Occasionally, large spike potentials are seen superimposed on the end plate noise. These are most likely due to the needle electrode provoking enough acetylcholine release to depolarize the entire muscle membrane, resulting in the recording of a propogated single muscle fiber nerve action potential.

Abnormal Spontaneous Activity

Fibrillation Potentials

Fibrillation potentials are the electrical activity recorded from the spontaneous depolarization of single muscle fibers. They are usually bi- or tri-phasic potentials, 50–500 μV in amplitude, with a duration of less than 1.5 msec. The initial deflection is positive when recording away from the end plate zone. Each muscle fiber depolarizes at a regular rate varying from 1–30/sec, but in some cases the firing may be irregular (7). Because multiple fibrillations are usually seen simultaneously, however, an irregular pattern appears on the oscilloscope with a characteristic crackling, "rain on a tin roof" sound from the loudspeaker. Fibrillations have been most commonly associated with lower motor neuron disease such as anterior horn cell pathology, radiculopathies, and neuropathies. In these disorders muscle fiber has lost continuity with its motor nerve fiber, allowing spontaneous depolarization. It is now known that fibrillations can occur in the presence of myopathies, however, especially polymyositis, in which splitting of the muscle fiber occurs. Fibrillations may also be seen in electrolyte disorders such as hypokalemia or hyperkalemia. Fibrillations have also been reported in spinal cord injury and stroke, but this finding is still controversial (8, 9).

Positive Sharp Waves

Positive sharp waves are seen in the same conditions and have the same significance as fibrillation potentials. They are biphasic potentials with an initial sharp positive phase of 50 μV to 1 mV followed by a low-amplitude, long-duration negative phase commonly exceeding 10 msec before its return to baseline. Positive waves fire regularly, commonly at a rate of 2–10/sec. Positive waves are felt to arise from spontaneously depolarizing single muscle fibers that have been damaged by needle insertion.

Fasciculation Potentials

Fasciculation potentials are the electrical activity recorded from the spontaneous firing of a motor unit. When these occur near the surface of the muscle, a visible twitch can be seen. The neural discharge initiating the fasciculation is most commonly in the anterior horn cell, but it may be anywhere within the motor unit (10). Thus, although usually associated with motor neuron disease, fasciculations may be present in radiculopathies or peripheral neuropathies. They may be occasionally seen in otherwise normal muscle, especially with fatigue. Fasciculations are not seen in primary muscle disorders.

Complex Repetitive Discharges

Complex repetitive discharges (previously called bizarre high-frequency discharges) can be seen in many forms of lower motor neuron disorders or myopathies. These are trains of potentials that begin and end abruptly. Their amplitude may range from 50 μV to several millivolts. The individual potentials may assume many forms and range from 50–100 msec in duration. They may fire at rates ranging from 5–100 cycles/sec. These discharges most likely arise within a group of denervated muscle fibers in which one muscle fiber acts as a pacemaker with spread of dipolarization to the neighboring denervated muscle fibers (11). Myotonic discharges are felt to be distinct repetitive discharges due to muscle membrane instability, as seen in disorders such as myotonic dystrophy and myotonia congenita. These discharges wax and wane in frequency and amplitude, whereas complex repetitive discharges display constant rate and amplitude. Myotonic discharges also differ in that the trains of potentials slowly decrease in frequency until they stop, instead of suddenly ceasing.

VOLUNTARY MUSCLE CONTRACTION

After the muscle being examined has been studied at rest, the patient is asked to produce a minimal contraction with the needle electrode in place. The number of motor unit potentials seen is proportional to the strength of contraction; therefore, to examine individual motor unit potentials, the contraction must be kept minimal. The normal motor unit potential usually contains up to four phases. A potential with five or more phases is termed *polyphasic*. A small proportion of normal motor units may be polyphasic (5–15%). An increase in the percentage of polyphasic motor unit potentials is considered abnormal. This may occur with either neuropathic disease or with myopathy. In neuropathy, impaired conduction in the terminal nerve fibers of the motor unit will result in asynchrony of firing and an increase in the number of phases seen on electromyography (12). In primary muscle disorders, loss of muscle fibers contributing to the motor unit potential may result in an increased number of phases.

The amplitude of the normal motor unit action potential ranges from 500 μV to 5 mV. This amplitude will vary with the density of the muscle fibers in the region of the tip of the electrode as well as with the synchrony of firing of the individual muscle fibers in the unit. In lower motor neuron disorders, reinnervation frequently leads to an increase in fiber density, resulting in increased motor unit potential amplitudes. In myopathy, loss of muscle fibers from the unit will result in decreased amplitude. Normal motor unit potential duration ranges from 5–12 msec as defined from the first deviation from the baseline to the final return to baseline. In neuropathy, with slowing in terminal nerve fiber conduction, there will be an increase in the duration of the potential. In myopathy, the common finding is a decrease in potential duration.

As the strength of voluntary contraction increases, the number of motor units firing increases proportionally. The first recruited motor unit potentials fire at a rate of approximately 5/sec. As the strength of contraction increases, the initial unit begins firing at a higher rate, and simultaneously other motor units are recruited. In neuropathic disease, when fewer motor units are available for recruitment, the first unit will be seen firing at a higher-than-normal rate before the second unit appears. In myopathy, in which the strength produced by each motor unit is reduced, the second motor unit will be recruited much earlier. With maximal voluntary contraction in normal muscle, the oscilloscope will be obscured by electrical activity, and individual motor units cannot be seen (complete interference pattern). In neuropathic disorders, at maximal contraction there may not be a complete obliteration of the baseline with electrical activity (incomplete interference pattern); or, in severe cases, individual motor units may still be discernible (single-unit interference pattern). In myopathies, as previously discussed, there is decreased strength produced by contraction by each motor unit. Therefore, for a contraction of fixed strength, more motor units will need to be recruited than in normal muscle. This causes a complete interference pattern with less than maximal effort.

Although evaluation of the interference pattern is important, it must be interpreted with caution because lack of patient cooperation from anxiety or pain may influence the results.

NERVE CONDUCTION STUDIES

Nerve conduction studies are safe, reliable, and reproducible in assessing peripheral nerve function. They are used to determine the presence and type of neuropathy, to localize lesions, and to determine their severity. The nerve is stimulated electrically, and various parameters are measured to determine the nerve's ability to carry the impulse. Stimulation may be done with either needle or surface electrodes. In most laboratories, surface stimulation is the method of choice. However, with deeply placed nerves, such as the sciatic in the gluteal region, near-nerve needle stimulation is easier and more comfortable for the patient. At rest the nerve is charged with a 90-mV transmembrane potential, positive externally.

When the negatively applied stimulus exceeds threshold, an action potential is generated. This potential is then self-propagated proximally and distally.

Motor conduction studies are performed by stimulating the nerve and recording the evoked response from a distal muscle. The time from stimulation to the onset of the evoked response is termed the *latency*. Conduction velocity from the distal stimulation site to the muscle cannot be determined because of the presence of the neuromuscular junction. If the nerve is stimulated at two points, however, the velocity between these points is easily determined by subtracting the distal from the proximal latency and dividing this into the distance between the stimulus sites. Conduction velocities can thus be determined over multiple segments of the nerve to localize a lesion.

Sensory conduction studies are performed by placing recording electrodes directly over the sensory nerve being examined. The nerve may be stimulated either proximally (antidromic conduction) or distally (orthodromic conduction) to these electrodes. The time is measured from the onset of the stimulus to the onset of the action potential that is being recorded. Dividing this time into the distance between the recording and stimulating electrodes yields the sensory conduction velocity. The sensory nerve action potential is usually bi- or tri-phasic. Latency measurements are frequently made to both the onset and the peak of the first negative phase. As in motor studies, the amplitude of the evoked response is recorded.

Decrease in nerve conduction velocity is most commonly associated with disorders of the myelin. This may also occur with diseases affecting the large, rapidly conducting axons, however. Axonal disorders more commonly cause a decrease in the amplitude of the evoked motor and sensory responses because fewer fibers are available to contribute to the response.

Sensory nerves commonly studied include the median, ulnar, radial, medial and lateral antebrachial cutaneous, lateral femoral cutaneous, sural, superficial peroneal, and tibial. Motor studies may be done on the median, ulnar, radial, tibial, peroneal, and sciatic nerves. Motor latency studies may be done on the femoral, axillary, suprascapular, accessory, and facial nerves.

PROXIMAL CONDUCTION STUDIES

The conduction studies discussed thus far allow evaluation of peripheral nerve function in the extremities. Nerve root stimulation, H reflex, and F wave measurements allow examination of proximal segments at the root and plexus level.

Nerve Root Stimulation

Nerve root stimulation may be performed in either the cervical or lumbar region. In the cervical region, the C8 nerve root is the most frequently studied, but C6 and C7 may also be evaluated. In the lumbar region, L4, L5, or S1 may be examined. A stimulating needle cathode is placed into the paraspinal musculature at the proper level. The anode is placed on the skin. Recording of the evoked response from an appropriate muscle in the limb is made in the normal manner. Side-to-side latency comparisons are made to determine abnormality (13).

H Reflex

The H reflex, first discovered by Hoffman in 1918, was later named and further investigated by Magladery and associates in the 1950s (14). Since then hundreds of articles have been published on the further investigation and use of this reflex. Most investigators feel that this is the electrical counterpart of the muscle stretch reflex, but it differs in several ways. In infancy, an H reflex can be obtained from most nerves, but after age 2, it can reliably only be found in the tibial nerve. In spinal shock, when reflexes may be absent, the H reflex may still be present.

The tibial H reflex is normally obtained by stimulating the tibial nerve at the knee with recording from the gastrocnemius or soleus. It is felt that the impulse is carried proximally by the 1a fibers to the spinal cord. There they synapse with the alpha motor neurons and the impulse is conducted back to the muscle, resulting in a muscle twitch. The latency measurement between the stimulus and twitch is therefore a measure of the integrity of both the S1 motor and sensory roots. This study is most commonly used for evaluating S1 radiculopathies. It has also been described as useful in diagnosing C6–C7 lesions by stimulating the median nerve with recording from the flexor carpi radialisis, and with L3–L4 by stimulating the femoral nerve and recording from the vastus medialis.

F Wave

The F wave was first described by Magladery and McDougal (14). When any motor nerve is stimulated with recording from a distal muscle, a late response may be seen following the initial muscle response. The amplitude and latency of this late response is quite variable, and it may not be present with each stimulation. In contrast, the H reflex is identical with each stimulus. It is believed that the F wave results from antidromic conduction of the stimulus in the alpha motor neurons to the spinal cord. There they cause firing of the anterior horn cells. These impulses are then carried orthodromically by the alpha motor neurons, causing discharge of the muscle fibers that they innervate. The same alpha motor neurons may not fire with each stimulus, thus resulting in a variable response. Because only alpha motor neurons are involved, the F wave is a measurement of motor function only. F waves are commonly studied in the median, ulnar, peroneal, and tibial nerves.

They are most valuable in examining proximal nerve function in neuropathy and thoracic outlet syndrome, but they may also be abnormal in radiculopathy. If distal conduction studies are normal but the F wave latency is prolonged, it may be assumed that a proximal lesion exists. This is commonly helpful in evaluating proximal neuropathies such as Guillain-Barré syndrome.

Somatosensory-Evoked Potentials

Somatosensory potentials may be obtained by stimulating a peripheral nerve, usually the median or ulnar at the wrist or tibial or peroneal at the ankle, and recording wave forms from the contralateral scalp. It is felt that these potentials are carried by sensory fibers in the peripheral nerves and in the dorsal column–lemniscal system centrally. They can therefore be theoretically used to measure function distally or proximally in the peripheral nervous system or in the spinal cord or brain. They are most commonly used as an aid in diagnosing multiple sclerosis (15) along with auditory- and visual-evoked potentials. They have also proven useful in monitoring spinal cord function during spinal surgery.

Somatosensory-evoked potentials continue to undergo evaluation as to their clinical usefulness in diagnosing plexus and root lesions, especially when only sensory fibers are involved. Limited success has been achieved thus far, and the clinical usefulness of these studies in radiculopathy is controversial. Studies in several centers are presently underway to evaluate dermatomal cutaneous stimulation to better localize lesions to a single root, but these studies are still in an experimental stage. At this point, few electromyographers would be willing to base a diagnosis of radiculopathy on somatosensory abnormalities alone.

Magnetic Stimulation

Magnetic stimulation studies of the peripheral and central nervous system, although still investigational, deserve mention. Magnetic coils have been developed that induce current flow in tissue with essentially no patient discomfort. Deeply seated structures such as the brachial plexus can be stimulated with ease. The major problem with this technique is the inability to determine the exact point of nerve stimulation, because a broad area of current flow is induced. Therefore conduction velocities can not be accurately calculated, and the value of this procedure will be limited in peripheral nerve studies until more focused stimulators can be developed.

Transcranial stimulation of the motor cortex with magnetic coils has also been accomplished. Recording motor-evoked responses from appropriate contralateral muscles should provide another method of evaluating central and peripheral pathways complementary to somatosensory studies.

CLINICAL APPLICATIONS

Electrodiagnostic studies were originally developed for evaluation and localization of peripheral nerve injuries. Although this continues to be an important use of these studies, they are more frequently used to diagnose radiculopathies, peripheral neuropathies, entrapment syndromes, and myopathies in patients with acute and chronic pain, paresthesias, and weakness.

RADICULOPATHIES

Neck and low back pain are the most common forms of musculoskeletal disability. Cervical and lumbar radiculopathies may cause acute and chronic back pain, headaches, extremity pain, numbness, paresthesias, and weakness. Thoracic radiculopathies, although less common, may cause noncardiac chest pain and abdominal pain.

Electrodiagnostic studies have proven useful in the diagnosis of radiculopathy. Although myelography, computerized axial tomography, and magnetic resonance imaging (MRI) all examine the anatomy of the spine, spinal cord, and roots, electrical testing is the only widely accepted method of assessing the physiologic function of the nerve roots. Because 15–20% of asymptomatic patients will show evidence of disk herniation on MRI, electrodiagnostic studies are necessary to document which of these are causing significant neural compromise. Although radiculopathy is usually due to a compressive lesion, such as a herniated disk, it may also be due to a noncompressive lesion, as in diabetic radiculopathy. It has been found that electrodiagnostic studies and myelography are equal in their sensitivity and accuracy in diagnosing compressive root lesions (16). Comparisons with computerized tomography have shown electrical studies to be the more accurate study in localizing a radiculopathy (17). Most studies have shown that both anatomic and electrical studies have approximately a 75–80% accuracy, but when a combination of the two types of study are performed, a much higher degree of accuracy will be obtained. Therefore, when evaluating the patient with chronic pain, both imaging and physiologic studies should be employed.

In evaluating for a possible radiculopathy, the examiner performs EMG on multiple muscles innervated by each of the roots supplying the extremity involved. Although this will evaluate function in the anterior primary ramus, the corresponding paraspinal musculature must also be examined to evaluate the posterior primary ramus. If root compression is causing damage to motor fibers within the root, EMG abnormalities will be seen in the muscles supplied by that root, allowing the level of the lesion to be localized. In some cases, EMG abnormalities will be seen only in the paraspinal musculature. This localizes the lesion to the root level, but the exact root involved cannot be determined because there is a large overlap in innervation of the paraspinal musculature. In an acute nerve root lesion, EMG abnormalities in the paraspinal musculature will not occur until approximately 7–10 days after onset. In the extremity musculature, abnormalities such as fibrillations and positive waves may not occur for 3–4 weeks. If weakness is present, however, a decrease in motor unit recruitment may be seen in a myotomal pattern during this early phase. Medicolegally, it may be worthwhile performing EMG during the first week after injury to determine if abnormalities are present from a pre-existing lesion. This is especially true in the chronic pain patient who may have had multiple previous injuries or surgery. If no fibrillations are found on this initial examination, but are then present three weeks later, they can be ascribed to the present illness.

Because most peripheral nerves contain fibers from multiple nerve roots, standard peripheral NCSs are usually normal. They may be abnormal if multiple roots are involved with loss of a large number of nerve fibers, however. H reflex, F wave, and somatosensory studies in the affected nerve root distribution may show abnormalities and thus aid in the diagnosis.

Cervical Radiculopathy

The C7 nerve root is probably the most commonly involved in cervical radiculopathy, followed in order by C6, C8, and C5 (18). With C5 *radiculopathies*, pain is usually felt radiating into the shoulder. Weakness may be seen in the deltoid and possibly the biceps. The biceps reflex may be depressed. Sensory complaints are uncommon, but there may be some dysesthesias over the lateral aspect of the forearm. Electromyographic abnormalities may be seen in the rhomboids, Supraspinatus, infraspinatus, deltoid, and possibly the biceps. *C6 radiculopathies* give a similar pain pattern, but paresthesias are frequently complained of in the thumb. Electromyographic abnormalities are commonly seen in the biceps, pronator teres, and extensor carpi radialis, but may also be seen in the deltoid and supraspinatus. *C7 radiculopathy* frequently presents with pain radiating into the triceps, forearm, and hand. Paresthesias are commonly present in the index and long fingers. Weakness may be prominent in the triceps with an absent triceps reflex. Electromyographic abnormalities are likely to be found in the triceps, pronator teres, flexor carpi radialis, and extensor digitorum communis. A prolonged median H reflex latency to the flexor carpi radialis may be seen with C6–C7 lesions. With *C8 radiculopathy*, the patient frequenty presents with pain and paresthesias radiating down the ulnar aspect of the arm into the fourth and fifth digits. The triceps tendon reflex may be absent. Electromyographic abnormalities may be seen in the extensor digitorum communis, extensor and flexor carpi ulnaris, and all the intrinsic hand musculature. Median and ulnar F wave latencies may be prolonged to the thenar and hypothenar musculature respectively, but these findings must be interpreted with caution because thoracic outlet syndrome may also cause F wave abnormalities in the C8 distribution.

Although fibrillations and positive waves are the hallmark of an acute radiculopathy, increased insertional activity and an increased number of polyphasic motor unit potentials may be the only abnormality seen. With chronic radiculopathies, these are commonly the only abnormalities present (19).

Lumbosacral Radiculopathies

Electrodiagnostic studies are of great use in the evaluation of low back and leg pain. They can differentiate radiculopathy from the many other causes of back and leg pain such as vascular lesions, mechanical or muscular low back pain, arthritis of the spine, and hip or disk disease without nerve root compression.

In *L4 radiculopathy*, the patient commonly experiences pain in the hip radiating into the groin, anterior thigh, and knee. Sensory complaints are not common, but paresthesias may be experienced over the medial aspect of the knee. The patient may complain of buckling of the knee on weight bearing. Interestingly, the patient with primary hip pathology will have many of these same complaints. On physical examination, the knee jerk may be decreased and weakness may be appreciated in the quadriceps. Electromyography may show abnormalities in the quadriceps and femoral adductors. The femoral H reflex latency to the vastus medialis may be prolonged. Femoral motor conduction should be normal to differentiate this from a femoral neuropathy.

With *L5 radiculopathies*, the patient will commonly complain of pain radiating from the back to the lateral hip and thigh and anterior tibial region. Paresthesias may be felt over the dorsum of the foot, and weakness may be noted in the ankle. On physical examination, weakness in the ankle and toe dorsiflexors may be appreciated. There may also be weakness of hip abduction. The medial hamstring reflex may be reduced. Electrically, EMG abnormalities will be seen in the ankle and toe dorsiflexors, flexor digitorum longus, medial hamstrings, tensor fascia lata, and hip abductors. The peroneal F wave latency recorded from the extensor digitorum brevis may be prolonged on the affected side. Differentiation from peroneal neuropathy is made by normal peroneal conduction and by EMG abnormalities in the proximal L5 innervated musculature at the hip.

In *S1 radiculopathy*, the patient experiences pain radiating to the hip, posterior thigh, and calf. There may be complaints of paresthesias over the lateral aspect of the foot. Weakness is uncommon, but there may be some difficulty with toe standing on the affected side. Electrical abnormalities are most commonly found in the gastrocnemius and soleus. They may also be found in the lateral hamstrings and gluteus maximus, as well as the intrinsic foot musculature. Findings localized to the foot musculature must be interpreted with caution, however, because the extensor digitorum brevis is subject to much trauma, and tarsal tunnel syndrome may cause abnormality in the tibial innervated foot musculature. The tibial H reflex latency will commonly be prolonged or absent with stimulation of the tibial nerve at the knee recording from the gastrocnemius or soleus. Normal tibial motor conduction will indicate that this tibial H reflex abnormality is due to a proximal lesion. Normal sural sensory conduction will confirm that the sensory abnormalities on the lateral aspect of the foot are due to a proximal lesion.

In all patients who have undergone spinal surgery, EMG abnormalities found in the paraspinal musculature must be interpreted with caution. Electrical abnormalities may persist in these muscles for years after surgery. Some researchers feel that performing the EMG needle examination at 3 cm from the scar at a 3–5 cm depth will avoid abnormalities due to the trauma of surgery. In most circumstances it is safest to avoid examination of these muscles once surgery has been performed, however. In the distribution of the anterior primary ramus, EMG abnormalities tend to subside faster than clinical abnormalities (20). With severe root lesions, however, EMG abnormalities may persist as long as 3–4 years after surgery. Therefore, in examining a patient with recurrent back or leg pain, it is helpful to have a preoperative examination for comparison of the distribution of the abnormalities.

Thoracic Radiculopathies

Thoracic radiculopathies are much less common than cervical or lumbosacral radiculopathies. They may be the cause of chest or abdominal pain, which usually begins in the spine and radiates anteriorly, or spinal pain may be the only symptom. Compressive root lesions can occur with a herniated disk or tumor, but the lesion may also be the result of herpes zoster or diabetes. In patients with abdominal pain but an otherwise normal examination, a radiculopathy must be considered, especially in diabetics. The classic findings in diabetic thoracic radiculopathy include mild peripheral nerve conduction abnormalities with fibrillation in the thoracic paraspinal musculature on the symptomatic side (21).

Entrapment Syndromes

Peripheral nerve entrapment syndromes are a frequent cause of extremity paresthesias, pain, and weakness (22). Median nerve entrapment at the wrist, or carpal tunnel syndrome, is the most commonly encountered nerve entrapment syndrome, but many others have been described. Both the median and ulnar nerves may be entrapped at the wrist and elbow. The radial nerve may be entrapped at the elbow, and its superficial sensory branch may be entrapped in the forearm. The

sensory division of the musculocutaneous nerve may be entrapped at the elbow. The femoral, lateral femoral cutaneous, and tibial nerves may be entrapped in the lower extremities.

The classic electrodiagnostic finding in an entrapment syndrome is segmental slowing of conduction across the area of entrapment. Conduction in segments proximal and distal to the lesion are frequently normal, but with a severe nerve compression, conduction in the distal segment may also be affected. Sensory conduction is commonly affected before motor conduction is. Electromyographic abnormalities may be found in the muscle supplied by the entrapped nerve, but this is usually a late finding.

Median Nerve

Median nerve entrapment at the wrist, or *carpal tunnel syndrome,* is by far the most common median nerve entrapment, but it must be differentiated from entrapment at the elbow. Patients with carpal tunnel syndrome usually present with paresthesias in the hand. This should be confined to the thumb, index finger, long finger, and radial half of the ring finger. Many patients have difficulty localizing their symptoms and complain of generalized numbness in the entire hand, however. Although this should alert the examiner to consider other lesions, carpal tunnel syndrome is frequently the only problem found. There may be pain in the hand and wrist with radiation up the arm to the shoulder. Occasionally, shoulder pain is prominent, and it may be confused with cervical radiculopathy. In a small group of patients, shoulder pain will be the only symptom. There are frequent complaints of weakness in the hand and of dropping small objects. Patients commonly complain that their symptoms awaken them at night or are most severe on arising in the morning. The symptoms may be brought on by use of the hand as in knitting, driving, or any repetitive activity. Complaints are often bilateral, with the dominate hand more involved. Carpal tunnel syndrome may be associated with such conditions as trauma, arthritis and connective tissue disease, or hypothyroidism, but is frequently idiopathic.

Hundreds of articles have been written on the electrodiagnostic evaluation of carpal tunnel syndrome. Many methods exist for evaluating median conduction across the wrist, and each laboratory will have its preferred procedure. Because carpal tunnel syndrome is often bilateral and associated with other entrapment neuropathies, median, ulnar, and radial sensory studies as well as median and ulnar motor conduction studies should be performed in both hands. Slowing of median sensory and motor conduction across the wrist with normal conduction proximal and distal to the transverse carpal ligament is the classic finding in carpal tunnel syndrome. Sensory conduction will be abnormal before motor conduction is in the vast majority of patients. Frequently, in early cases, the absolute values of median conduction may be within the normal range, but comparison to the asymptomatic hand or to radial or ulnar conduction in the same hand will yield evidence of relative slowing of median conduction, which may be diagnostic (23). Again, it can not be emphasized too strongly that when assessing a patient for possible carpal tunnel syndrome, conduction studies should not be limited to the median nerve. In addition to finding other entrapments it is not at all unusual for the electromyographer to discover an unsuspected peripheral polyneuropathy.

Electromyography must always be performed along with NCS for a complete evaluation. Electromyography may sometimes show denervation of the thenar musculature in carpal tunnel syndrome, but usually only in severe cases. In addition to the hand musculature, the entire extremity should be examined to rule out the presence of a radiculopathy simulating carpal tunnel syndrome, or coexisting with it. Persistent symptoms after carpal tunnel release may be due to a root lesion that was not recognized.

In very early or mild carpal tunnel syndrome, all electrical studies may be normal in a small percentage of patients. This occurs because significant demyelinization or axonal damage may not have taken place. Detailed cutaneous sensory testing, when combined with the electrical studies, may improve the diagnostic yield (24), but there still may be the exceptional case with no abnormal findings. In this event, the exam should be repeated at a later date to differentiate psychogenic symptoms from neuropathology.

Median nerve entrapments in the proximal forearm are rare, but they may be confused with carpal tunnel syndrome. At the elbow, the median nerve may be entrapped within the pronator teres (pronator syndrome) or, very rarely, by the ligament of Struthers at the level of the medial epicondyle. Patients with these proximal entrapments may have symptoms very similar to those of carpal tunnel syndrome, but pain in the forearm is more prominent. These patients frequently perform work that requires repetitive pronation of the forearm, but other cases have been related to fractures, dislocations, and trauma to the elbow. Electrodiagnostically, median conduction slowing may be seen across the elbow or in the forearm. In the pronator syndrome, EMG abnormalities may be seen in the forearm musculature distal to the innervation of the pronator teres. More proximal entrapment at the ligament of Struthers would be necessary for EMG abnormalities to be seen in the pronator teres. In both of these elbow entrapments, EMG abnormalities have been reported to be of more diagnostic significance than NCSs (25).

The anterior interosseous nerve is a motor branch of the median nerve that arises below the pronator teres. The nerve may be entrapped at this point or, more commonly, may be involved in trauma. Clinically, weakness is found in the pronator quadratus, flexor pollicis longus, and flexor digitorum profundus to the index and long fingers. Electromyographic abnormalities will be seen in these muscles, whereas the remainder of the median musculature will be normal. Standard median motor and sensory conduction studies will be normal because they bypass the anterior interosseous nerve. Stimulation of the median nerve at the elbow and recording from the flexor pollicis longus will occasionally reveal a prolonged latency, but this is not frequent (26).

Ulnar Nerve Entrapments

Entrapment of the ulnar nerve at the elbow is the second most common entrapment neuropathy. The ulnar nerve may also be entrapped at the wrist and in the palm, however. Although not truly an entrapment neuropathy, *thoracic outlet syndrome* commonly causes symptoms primarily in the ulnar distribution.

Ulnar neuropathy at the elbow may be the result of a long-standing deformity of the elbow (*tardy ulnar palsy*) or entrapment of the nerve under the aponeurosis connecting the two heads of the flexor carpi ulnaris (*cubital tunnel syndrome*) (27). Patients commonly complain of pain in the elbow with numbness and paresthesias in the fourth and fifth digits as well as of weakness in the hands. These symptoms are often bilateral. Nerve conduction studies will classically show slowing of ulnar motor and/or sensory conduction velocity across the elbow as compared to the proximal and distal segments or as compared to the opposite ulnar nerve. This slowing should be at least 10 m/sec (28). There will usually be a decrease in the amplitude of the ulnar sensory nerve action potential recorded from the fifth digit when stimulating at the wrist. In severe ulnar neuropathies, there may be slowing in the distal segments as well as across the elbow because of wallerian degeneration. Electromyographic abnormalities in advanced cases will be seen in the ulnar portion of the flexor digitorum profundus and the ulnar innervated intrinsic hand musculature. The flexor carpi ulnaris will be spared because this muscle is innervated by a branch of the ulnar nerve arising above the elbow.

The ulnar nerve may also be compressed at the wrist in Guyon's canal. The sensory complaints and weakness in the hand are similar to lesions at the elbow, but discomfort proximal to the wrist is unusual. Electrical studies will show slowing of ulnar motor and sensory conduction across the wrist, and there may be EMG changes in the ulnar innervated intrinsic hand musculature. Proximal ulnar conduction studies should be normal.

The deep motor branch of the ulnar nerve may also be traumatized or compressed by a ganglion distal to Guyon's canal. In this case ulnar motor distal latency from the wrist to the abductor digiti quinti may be normal while conduction to the first dorsal interosseous may be prolonged. Sensory conduction to the fifth digit may be normal or abnormal depending on the site of the lesion.

Thoracic outlet syndrome is defined as compression of the neurovascular bundle in the thoracic outlet that results in pain, dysesthesias, and occasionally weakness in the arm. In most cases, this is a vascular syndrome, but in a small percentage of patients neurologic symptoms are prominent. When this occurs, paresthesias are most prominent in the ulnar distribution and weakness may be seen in the hand. Because this syndrome is usually primarily vascular, electrodiagnostic studies frequently yield normal results. When there is neurologic involvement, slowing of ulnar conduction through the thoracic outlet may occur. The best method to detect this is controversial, however. It has been proposed that stimulation of the ulnar nerve in the supraclavicular fossa and in the axilla will allow for measurement of ulnar motor conduction velocity through the thoracic outlet (29). Other authors have found this unreliable, however, because stimulation at the supraclavicular fossa may be distal to the actual area of compression (30). Nerve root stimulation may be a better method of demonstrating slowing of conduction through the thoracic outlet. Well-documented electrical abnormalities found in patients with clear-cut neurogenic thoracic outlet syndrome include reduced ulnar sensory- and motor-evoked amplitudes with denervation of the median and ulnar innervated intrinsic hand musculature in the presence of normal distal median and ulnar motor conduction (31). The ulnar F wave latency may also be prolonged on the affected side as compared to the normal side (32).

Thoracic outlet syndrome has classically been considered rare, but in recent years this syndrome has been invoked in patients involved in minor trauma, especially when litigation is involved. They usually have vague, poorly documented neck and extremity pain as well as paresthesias. Objective studies are usually normal. Many of these patients are subjected to first rib resection, when conservative treatment until the litigation is resolved would appear to be more appropriate.

Because the ulnar nerve may be injured or entrapped at many points along its course, patients with symptoms in an ulnar distribution should receive segmental conduction studies throughout the course of the nerve to best localize the lesion. Also, studies should be done in both arms because these symdromes are frequently bilateral. Electromyography should also be performed on the extremities and cervical paraspinals to rule out a C8 cervical radiculopathy, which may give a clinical picture identical to that of an ulnar neuropathy.

Radial Nerve

Although not a true entrapment neuropathy, the radial nerve is most commonly injured in the spiral groove. Prolonged pressure in this area results in the classic "Saturday night palsy." Triceps strength and the reflex will be normal, whereas the brachioradialis and all distal radial innervated muscles will be weak. There may be sensory loss over the radial aspect of the dorsum of the hand. Radial motor conduction studies may show slowing across the spiral groove, and radial sensory conduction may also be abnormal. Electromyographic abnormalities will be found from the brachioradialis distally in the radial distribution.

True entrapments of the radial nerve occur in the region of the elbow. Compression of the recurrent branch of the radial nerve at the elbow gives rise to local pain and is felt to be one of the causes of "tennis elbow." This is a rather small branch, and it cannot be tested electrically.

The *posterior interosseous syndrome* is entrapment of the terminal motor branch of the radial nerve as it passes through the arcade of Froshe between the two heads of the supinator. A lesion at this level will cause weakness of the extensor carpi ulnaris and finger extensors, but the extensor carpi radialis will be spared. Because the superficial radial sensory nerve has already exited the main trunk at this level, there should be no sensory complaints. Motor nerve conduction studies may show slowing in the distal portion with normal proximal conduction. Electromyography will show abnormalities distal to the innervation of the extensor carpi radialis longus and brevis.

Compression of the radial nerve at the wrist (*cheiralgia paresthetica*) by a wrist band is well documented, and radial sensory conduction studies are useful in demonstrating this lesion (33). Entrapment of the radial sensory nerve in the forearm has been described (34). These patients usually present with pain or burning over the dorsoradial aspect of the forearm and wrist. The cause is felt to be local trauma, twisting injuries, or repetitive pronation-supination movements at work. On physical examination, there is usually a positive Tinel's sign over the radial sensory nerve in the distal forearm. There is often a "positive Finklestein's test" that may lead to a misdiagnosis of de Quervain's syndrome. Sensation may be impaired in the radial distribution of the hand, but strength should be normal. Hyperpronation of the forearm may reproduce the symptoms. It is felt that the superficial radial sensory nerve is compressed between the tendons of the extensor carpi radialis longus and brachioradialis when the wrist is pronated. Radial sensory conduction studies may be abnormal with slowing of radial sensory conduction in the forearm, but with normal conduction from the wrist to the thumb. Comparison to musculocutaneous sensory conduction is often helpful because the two conditions have a similar course. Decrease in the amplitude of the radial sensory nerve action potential may be the only abnormality found. Radial motor conduction studies should be normal, and no EMG abnormalities should be seen.

Suprascapular Nerve

The suprascapular nerve is composed of nerve fibers from the C5 and C6 roots. This nerve leaves the upper trunk of the brachial plexus and passes under the trapezius muscle, eventually passing through the suprascapular foramen to innervate the supraspinatus and infraspinatus muscles. The nerve may be entrapped in this foramen under the transverse scapular ligament, or it may be subjected to a stretch injury at this site. Entrapment of this nerve will result in shoulder pain, which may be misdiagnosed as bursitis or cervical radiculopathy. Nerve conduction studies may show prolongation of the suprascapular nerve latency from Erb's point to the supraspinitus or infraspinatus. Electromyography will show abnormalities confined to the supraspinitus and infraspinatus with no other C5–C6 innervated muscles involved.

Musculocutaneous Nerve

The musculocutaneous nerve is occasionally injured with local trauma, but can also be damaged by heavy exercise. Rarely, the musculocutaneous nerve is entrapped by the coracobrachialis. Weakness will be seen in the biceps with sensory loss over the lateral aspect of the forearm. The biceps stretch reflex should be absent. This diagnosis may be confirmed by musculocutaneous motor conduction with stimulation in the axilla and at Erb's point. Sensory conduction may also be abnormal. Electromyographic abnormalities will be seen in the biceps, brachialis, and coracobrachialis muscles.

A recently described lesion of the musculocutaneous nerve at the elbow involves only the sensory division, the lateral antibrachial cutaneous nerve. These patients experience pain in the region of the biceps tendon insertion with paresthesias over the radial aspect of the forearm. The biceps tendon reflex and strength will be normal. There is frequently tenderness over the tendonous insertion of the biceps with clinical sensory loss in the distribution of the sensory branch. Musculocutaneous sensory conduction will be abnormal, whereas motor conduction is within normal limits (35, 36). No EMG abnormalities will be present.

Lateral Femoral Cutaneous Nerve

The lateral femoral cutaneous nerve arises from the L2 and L3 nerve roots. It emerges through the inguinal ligament near the anterior superior iliac spine to innervate the skin over the lateral thigh from the hip to the knee. Compression of this nerve in the inguinal ligament results in burning pain and paresthesias over the lateral thigh (*meralgia paresthetica*). Objective sensory loss can usually be demonstrated in this area. Because the nerve is purely sensory, there will be no weakness. Nerve conduction studies may show abnormalities in this nerve (37). Comparison should always be made between the symptomatic and asymptomatic legs, because conduc-

tion in this nerve is frequently difficult to obtain in obese patients. Electromyography must be performed to rule out a lumbar radiculopathy.

Femoral Nerve

The femoral nerve may be compressed within the pelvis by tumor, psoas abscess, retroperitoneal lymphadenopathy, or hemorrhage into the iliacus or psoas muscles. The nerve may also be entrapped at the level of the inguinal ligament. These patients complain of pain, paresthesias, and weakness in the groin and anterior thigh. Femoral motor conduction studies may show abnormal distal latencies, and it may be possible to demonstrate slowing across the inguinal ligament (38). Abnormalities on EMG will be confined to the femoral distribution. Commonly, L3–L4 radiculopathies or plexopathies, especially in diabetics, mimic femoral neuropathy; EMG of the entire extremity with emphasis on the quadriceps, femoral adductors, and lumbar paraspinals should make this differentiation.

Obturator Nerve

The obturator nerve is most commonly injured during labor, but may also be injured with pelvic fractures and pelvic surgery. Obturator hernias may entrap the nerve in the obturator canal. Patients complain of pain in the groin radiating along the medial aspect of the thigh. There may be dysesthesias in the medial aspect of the upper thigh. Reproducible obturator conduction studies have not been reported. Electromyographic examination will show abnormalities confined to the femoral adductors, however.

Peroneal Nerve

The peroneal nerve is commonly injured at the level of the fibular head, where it is very superficial. The nerve may also be compressed at the level of the biceps femoris tendon after prolonged squatting. Pain and numbness may be experienced in the anterior aspect of the leg and foot. Weakness of the ankle and toe dorsiflexors is prominent. Peroneal motor conduction studies may show segmental slowing across the fibular head. With more severe lesions, distal peroneal motor conduction will also be abnormal. Superficial peroneal sensory conduction may also be affected. Electromyographic abnormalities should be confined to the peroneal innervated musculature. Because this may easily be confused with an L5 radiculopathy, the entire extremity must be examined. Electromyography should always be performed on the short head of the biceps femoris, because this is innervated by a branch from the common peroneal nerve. Involvement of this muscle suggests a lesion proximal to the fibular head.

The deep peroneal nerve is commonly traumatized at the ankle. Many patients may have a prolonged distal peroneal motor latency with no symptoms whatsoever. Fibrillations may be found in the extensor digitorum brevis in approximately 25% of otherwise normal patients, and in older patients the muscle may be completely atrophied. The deep peroneal nerve has been reported to be involved in an entrapment neuropathy at the ankle (39); this was termed the *anterior tarsal tunnel syndrome.* Patients complain of pain on the dorsum of the foot with numbness between the first and second toes. Because, as previously mentioned, many "normal" individuals have electrical abnormalities in this segment, this diagnosis must only be made when the clinical picture is compatible.

Tibial Nerve

The tibial nerve may be entrapped in the tarsal tunnel, which lies posterior to the medial malleolus and is covered by the lancinate ligament. This entrapment is termed the *tarsal tunnel syndrome* (40). This may be idiopathic or follow fractures of the ankle. The patient will frequently complain of pain in the ankle, heel, and foot with paresthesias on the sole of the foot and toes. A positive Tinel's sign will be present over the tarsal tunnel. Motor or sensory tibial distal latencies may be abnormal in either the medial or lateral plantar division. This is not analogous to carpal tunnel syndrome, however. Frequently the conduction studies are normal, even when comparing to the asymptomatic side. Electromyography of the abductor hallucis and abductor digiti minimi may help establish this diagnosis (41). Fibrillations confined to these muscles on the involved side with normal extensor digitorum brevis examination (peroneal innervated) and a normal examination of the opposite foot suggest tarsal tunnel syndrome. Positive waves alone are not enough to establish this diagnosis because these are frequently seen in otherwise normal patients. In all patients being evaluated for possible tarsal tunnel syndrome, EMG should be performed on the entire extremity and lumbar paraspinals to rule out a radiculopathy, which may give a similar clinical picture.

PERIPHERAL POLYNEUROPATHY

Peripheral polyneuropathy may be a cause of severe acute or chronic pain, especially in diabetics. It may also be a prominent cause of pain with alcoholic neuropathy, vasculitis, or nutritional neuropathies, however. The clinical and electrical findings may be diffuse and symmetric or more localized. In mononeuritis multiplex, one nerve may be severely abnormal with other nearby nerves relatively spared. If the basic pathology is axonal loss, the EMG will show abnormalities, and NCSs will show decreased amplitude of the evoked responses. If the myelin sheath is primarily affected, nerve conduction slowing will be the most prominent finding. Commonly both types of pathology are seen together. Occasionally, small fiber–type neuropathies are seen in which no electrical abnormalities can be demonstrated.

This occurs because nerve conduction studies primarily measure conduction in the large myelinated fibers. In addition to the naturally occurring neuropathies, iatrogenic peripheral neuropathies or plexopathies may be due to chemotherapy or radiation.

MYOPATHIES

Myopathies are generally not considered when evaluating a patient with chronic pain. However, dermatomyositis and polymyositis may result in chronic pain and weakness. Electromyographic examination would demonstrate fibrillations, positive waves, and repetitive discharges at rest. Motor unit action potentials tend to be polyphasic, with decreased amplitude and duration. Proximal muscles are involved more than distal muscles, and the paraspinal musculature is also involved. Myopathy may also be associated with other connective tissue diseases such as scleroderma or rheumatoid arthritis. It may also be secondary to chronic steroid treatment.

ELECTRODIAGNOSTIC EXAMINATION

Most patients approach the electrodiagnostic examination with some degree of fear and anxiety, because many have some fear of needle puncture and/or electrical stimuli. Frequently patients have been subjected to "horror stories" involving electrodiagnostic studies by their acquaintances. This may have been either in jest or in an attempt to gain sympathy. Because patient cooperation is important to a successful examination, the electromyographer must be able to allay the patient's fears. Although some complaints of discomfort are to be expected, most patients will agree that their fears were unwarranted and that many other medical diagnostic and therapeutic procedures are much more uncomfortable.

Timing is very important when ordering and interpreting electrodiagnostic studies. After a nerve is severed, conduction velocity in the distal segment will remain normal for 7–10 days. However, during that time the amplitude of the evoked response will begin to decline. Electromyography will not show fibrillations for 3–4 weeks following injury. With radiculopathy the paraspinal EMG may begin to show abnormalities 7–10 days after onset, but the extremity musculature will probably be normal until 4–6 weeks later. Most electromyographers will usually prefer to postpone electrical studies until the full development of electrical abnormalities can be expected. If a patient presents with both an old and an acute injury, however, it may be advisable to perform an immediate exam and another in 4 weeks to differentiate the age of the findings.

An electrodiagnostic examination, unlike other studies such as electrocardiography or electroencephalography, cannot be performed in a preset, routine manner.

Each examination must be individualized according to the clinical picture. To properly plan the study, a complete history and physical examination must be done by the physician performing the study. The structure of the examination may be changed several times during the procedure as new information is gained. A patient may have initially been felt to have an entrapment neuropathy, but further examination may reveal the presence of a polyneuropathy, radiculopathy, or similar finding. Screening nerve conduction studies are performed on the symptomatic extremity as the first step in most examinations. If abnormalities are found, the opposite extremity is also studied. Should abnormal findings again be present, the other limbs may be examined. Electromyography is then conducted on the symptomatic extremity and corresponding paraspinal musculature. Again, other areas will need to be studied if the first limb is abnormal. The results of the examination must then be interpreted in light of the history and clinical findings.

Ideally, the clinical neurophysiologist performing the electrodiagnostic study will have met the minimal training criteria established by the American Association of Electromyography and Electrodiagnosis (42). These criteria recognize that the electrodiagnostic examination is essentially a neuromuscular disease consultation utilizing electrophysiologic methods. The examiner must, therefore, have special expertise in the diagnosis of neuromuscular disease. Completion of an approved residency in neurology or physical medicine and rehabilitation is recommended. This training should include adequate instruction in anatomy and physiology of muscle and nerve, electrophysiology, and clinical aspects of neuromuscular disease as they pertain to electrodiagnostic studies. A minimum of 6 months' supervised training with performance of at least 200 examinations is recommended. In spite of these recommendations, one can find electrodiagnostic studies being performed by physicians with little or no formal training. In some states, these studies may legally be performed by technicians. It therefore behooves the physician requesting the electrodiagnostic examination to know the qualifications of the examiner. If an experienced clinical neurophysiologist is to perform the examination, it is best to allow him to plan and carry out the examination as he feels is appropriate to the clinical picture. In this chapter I have specifically not mentioned normal values for most studies because each clinical neurophysiologist will have established these for his own laboratory and will be able to advise the referring physician as to the outcome of his examination. If the electrodiagnostic study is to be performed by a technician, a detailed outline of the examination requested should be given to the technician. All of the diagnostic possibilities should be outlined, and the specific nerves and muscles to be examined must be listed. If a detailed outline is not provided for the technician, an incomplete examination may well be done. This is illustrated by the following case reports.

CASE 1

A 54-year-old female received electrodiagnostic studies because of a 1-month history of numbness in the right thumb and index finger. She also complained of pain in the hand and shoulder, but no neck pain. Right median sensory conduction to the index finger could not be obtained, whereas ulnar sensory conduction and median motor conduction were normal. Electromyography of the thenar musculature was also normal. This was the full extent of the examination, and on the basis of these findings the diagnosis of carpal tunnel syndrome was made.

On admission to the hospital for surgery, a new exam was requested. In addition to the studies outlined above, radial and musculocutaneous conduction were measured, and EMG was performed on the entire extremity and cervical paraspinal musculature. Both median and musculocutaneous sensory conduction were absent while all other conduction studies were normal. Electromyography showed the presence of fibrillations and positive waves in the right biceps, brachialis, and pronator teres with sparing of the paraspinals. These findings indicated that the lesion was in the lateral cord of the brachial plexus, rather than at the wrist. Further workup revealed a metastatic breast carcinoma to the plexus.

This case points out that the study should not be cut short as soon as one abnormality is found, or the clinical impression is "confirmed." Multiple lesions may be missed, or an incorrect diagnosis made.

CASE 2

A 62-year-old female patient was referred to a technician for nerve conduction studies because of weakness. She had fallen on several occasions and fractured her right hip. Extensive motor and sensory conduction studies were done on the upper and lower extremities with no abnormalities found. This was reported as a "normal study." This patient was later seen in another laboratory where the normal conduction studies were confirmed. Electromyography was also done, however, and showed the presence of diffuse fibrillations and fasciculations that led to the diagnosis of amyotrophic lateral sclerosis.

This case illustrates the need to know your examiner. The initial referring physician assumed his patient would be seen by physician/clinical neurophysiologist and used the term "nerve conduction study" in a generic sense. Unfortunately the technician took him literally, and hence the inadequate study and delay in diagnosis.

In summary, routine performance of only brief, limited electrical studies is analogous to ordering a limb radiograph and examining only the bones while ignoring the soft tissue structures. Since so much information is to be gained, especially in the evaluation of the patient with chronic pain, the full potential of the electrodiagnostic examination should be utilized.

REFERENCES

1. Johnson EW: Use of the electrodiagnostic examination in a university hospital. *Arch Phys Med Rehabil* 46:573, 1965.
2. Rogoff J: Traditional electrodiagnosis. In Johnson EW (ed): *Practical Electromyography.* Baltimore, Williams & Wilkins, 1980, p 326.
3. Licht S: History. In Johnson EW (ed): *Practical Electromyography.* Baltimore, Williams & Wilkins, 1980, p 403.
4. Liddell E, Sherrington C: Recruitment and some other features of reflex inhibition. *Proc Roy Soc London (Biol)* 97:488–518, 1925.
5. Adrian E, Bronk D: The discharge of impulses in motor nerve fibers. Part II. The frequency of discharge in reflex and voluntary conduction. *J Physiol (Lond)* 67:119–151, 1929.
6. Brown W, Varkey G: The origin of spontaneous electrical activity at the endplate zone. *Ann Neurol* 10:557–570, 1981.
7. Buchthal F, Rosenfalk P: Spontaneous electrical activity of human muscle. *Electroencephalo Clin Neurophysiol* 20:321–326, 1966.
8. Johnson EW, Denny ST, Kelley JP: Sequence of electromyographic abnormalities in stroke syndrome. *Arch Phys Med Rehabil* 56:468, 1975.
9. Chokroverty S, Medina T: Electrophysiological study of hemiplegia. *Arch Neurol* 35:360, 1978.
10. Wettstein A: The origin of fasciculations in motor neuron disease. *Ann Neurol* 5:295, 1979.
11. Stalberg E, Trontel JV: *Single Fiber Electromyography:* Old Woking, Surrey U.K., Mirvalle Press Limited, 1979.
12. Borenstein S, Desmedt J: Range variations in motor unit potentials during reinnervation after traumatic nerve lesions in humans. *Ann Neurol* 8:460, 1980.
13. MacLean I: Nerve root stimulation to evaluate conduction across the brachial and lumbosacral plexuses. *Third Annual Continuing Education Course, American Association of Electromyograph and Electrodiagnosis,* Philadelphia, Sept. 25, 1980.
14. Magladery JW, McDougal DB: Electrophysiological studies of nerve and reflex activity in normal man: I. Identification of certain reflexes in electromyogram and conduction velocity of peripheral nerve fibers. *Bull Johns Hopkins Hosp* 86:265, 1950.
15. Namerow HS: Somatosensory evoked responses in multiple sclerosis patients with varying sensory loss. *Neurology* 18:1197, 1968.
16. Knutson B: Comparitive values of electromyographic, myelographic and clinical-neurological examinations of lumbar root compression syndromes. *Acta Orthop Scand Suppl* 49:1, 1961.
17. Khatri B, Baruah J, McQuillen P: Correlation of electromyography with computed tomography in evaluation of lower back pain. *Arch Neurol* 41:594, 1984.
18. Marinacci A: *Applied Electromyography.* Philadelphia, Lea & Febiger, 1968.
19. Waylonis G: Electromyographic findings in chronic cervical radicular syndrome. *Arch Phys Med Rehabil* 49:407, 1968.
20. Johnson E, Burkhart J, Earl W: Electromyography in post-laminectomy patients. *Arch Phys Med Rehabil* 53:4047, 1972.
21. Langstreth G, Newcomer A. Abdominal pain caused by diabetic radiculopathy. *Ann Intern Med* 86:166, 1977.
22. Kopell HP, Thompson WA: *Peripheral Entrapment Neuropathies.* Baltimore, Williams & Wilkins, 1963.
23. Felsenthal G: Median and ulnar distal motor and sensory latencies in the same normal subject. *Arch Phys Med Rehabil* 58:297, 1977.
24. Spindler H, Dellon AL: Nerve conduction studies and sensibility testing in carpal tunnel syndrome. *J Hand Surg* 7:260, 1982.
25. Hartz CR: The pronator teres syndrome: Compressive neurology of the median nerve. *J Bone Joint Surg [Am]* 3:885, 1981.
26. Nakano KK: Anterior interosseous nerve syndrome. *Arch Neorol* 34:477, 1977.
27. Feindel W, Stratford J: The role of the cubital tunnel in tardy ulnar palsy. *Can J Surg* 1:287, 1958.
28. Eisen A: Early diagnosis of ulnar nerve palsy. An electrophysiological study. *Neurology* 24:256, 1974.
29. Caldwell JW, Crane CR, Krasen EM: Nerve conduction studies: An aid in the diagnosis of thoracic outlet syndrome. *South Med J* 64:210, 1971.
30. Daube JR: Nerve conduction studies in the thoracic outlet syndrome. *Neurology* 25:347, 1975.
31. Gilliat RW: Peripheral nerve conduction in patients with a cervical rib or band. *J Neurol Neurosurg Psychiatry* 33:615, 1970.
32. Dorfman LJ: F-wave latency in the cervical rib-and-band syndrome [Lett]. Muscle Nerve 2:158, 1979.
33. Dorfman LJ, Jayaram AR: Handcuff neuropathy. *JAMA* 239:957, 1978.
34. Dellon AL, MacKinnon SE: Radial sensory nerve entrapment. *Arch Neurol* 43:833, 1986.
35. Spindler HA, Felsenthal G: Sensory conduction in the musculocutaneous nerve. *Arch Phys Med Rehabil* 59:70, 1978.
36. Felsenthal G, Mondell DL: Forearm pain secondary to compression syndrome of lateral cutaneous nerve of the forearm. *Arch Phys Med Rehabil* 65:139, 1984.
37. Butler ET, Johnson EW, Kaye ZA: Normal conduction velocity in the lateral femoral cutaneous nerve. *Arch Phys Med Rehabil* 55:31, 1974.
38. Johnson EW, Wood P, Pomeus J: Femoral nerve conduction studies. *Arch Phys Med Rehabil* 49:528, 1968.
39. Krause KH, Witt T, Ross A: The anterior tarsal tunnel syndrome. *J Neurol* 217:67, 1977.
40. Delisa JA, Saeed MA: AAEE case report #8: The tarsal tunnel syndrome. *Muscle Nerve* 6:664, 1983.
41. Gatens PF, Saeed MA: Electromyographic findings in the intrinsic muscles of normal feet. *Arch Phys Med Rehabil* 63:317, 1982.
42. *Guidelines in Electrodiagnostic Medicine.* Rochester, MN, American Association of Electromyography and Electrodiagnosis, 1984.

THERAPEUTIC MODALITIES

CHAPTER 6
DIAGNOSTIC AND THERAPEUTIC NERVE BLOCKS
JOHN D. RYBOCK

NEURAL BLOCKADE, the interruption of a nerve's function by the injection of a local anesthetic agent or other drug, is one of the most powerful tools in the diagnosis of chronic pain problems, and, in many cases, its application can also be a useful form of therapy. Used in a haphazard manner, it can lead to entirely erroneous diagnoses and totally inappropriate treatment.

ROLE OF NERVE BLOCKS IN CHRONIC PAIN MANAGEMENT

Nerve blocks are of no value in many cases of chronic pain. Although virtually any body region can be anesthetized, temporarily abolishing a patient's pain neither adds much insight into the underlying problem nor leads to a long-term solution. Nerve block therapy should be used to answer specific questions resulting from a careful evaluation of the patient's pain problem.

When certain diagnoses seem possible, such as intercostal neuralgia or lumbar facet syndrome, nerve blocks can provide a definitive answer. When there is a discrepancy between the demonstrated pathology and the complaints or findings, such as an L4 disk bulge with an S1 root syndrome, selective blockade will clarify the situation. When multiple sources of pain are present, such as arm pain with both signs of root dysfunction and causalgia-like symptoms, or knee pain with an old knee injury and midlumbar disk disease, selective blocks can help determine the relative contribution of each component. When it is unclear if the pain is central or peripheral, as in leg pain following spinal cord injury, nerve blocks can quickly define the source of the pain.

Careful patient evaluation is necessary not just to pose the questions to be resolved by nerve block, but also to understand the patient's means of describing his pain, as well as how the pain varies over time and with various activities. Such information is necessary to make a meaningful evaluation of the patient's block since it is only through his verbal description that the result can

be determined. It must be kept in mind that a patient describing chronic pain is not providing an objective assessment of a noxious sensation but is expressing his suffering in organic terms. The relative contributions of organic dysfunction, psychological abnormalities, and social factors in the patient's complaint of "pain" are only apparent after careful evaluation has been carried out. If the patient's pain complaint is assumed to be a simple description of the nociceptive input, confusion often results from nerve blockade. A successful block, significantly reducing the nociceptive input, may not be reported as giving significant pain relief if significant psychological and social factors are playing a role in the pain. In other cases a block totally ineffective at reducing the pain input may be perceived by a patient as highly effective. To take these results at face value would interfere with future therapy, either causing the true organic lesion to be "ruled out," and therefore ignored once the other factors are dealt with, or leading the patient to further interventional therapy that is inappropriate and ineffective.

Once a patient's complaint of pain is viewed as more than a source of nociceptive input awaiting definition, nerve blockade becomes a much more useful test. It is no longer simply a test to be ordered from an anesthesiologist that returns a yes/no answer; rather, it is a complex interaction between the clinician and the patient that not only explores the specific organic factors but also provides further insight into the patient's sensitivity to pain and means of responding to it. With a fairly brief amount of experience, a clinician can become sensitive to the usual amount of discomfort caused by any particular block and the usual pattern of pain and sensory changes. The response of each subsequent patient can then be measured against this standard, and tendencies toward exaggerated pain behavior, stoicism, or bizarre descriptions of sensations can be recognized. Therefore, rather than a nerve block being a simple test providing a simple answer, it becomes much more a meaningful period of interaction and observation extending from preparation of the patient for the block until the period of complete recovery from its effects.

In addition to careful patient selection, skill in evaluating the results of a block is required. There are two aspects to be evaluated: the adequacy of interruption of nerve function and the effect of that blockade on the patient's pain. The effectiveness of the actual nerve blockade must be evaluated by objective means at the neural level. Even with the best technique, inadequate blockade will occasionally be obtained. With sympathetic nerve blockade, for example, temperature changes in the extremity as well as signs of hyperemia should be documented following the block. With somatic nerve blockade, peripheral motor and sensory loss must be noted and its time course specified.

Once an effective block can be confirmed, then the patient's report of the effect on his pain must be carefully interpreted. If the patient is simply asked to evaluate whether the block helped his pain or not, the result may not be meaningful. For example, even with the best preblock instruction, patients will sometimes report the block to have failed to work if, at the time of questioning, the pain has returned. The best way to carry out evaluation is to either question the patient or have the patient record in writing at 15–30 min intervals following the block the level of his pain, the activities being performed, and any observations concerning weakness, numbness, or other signs of neural blockade. A careful review of these data then allows meaningful interpretation of the result of the block.

It must also be realized that many patients will slant reports of effectiveness in an attempt to please the physician and that the placebo effect does occur with nerve blocks as with other medications. If any doubt exists as to the true effectiveness of the block, the physician should be prepared to repeat the block several times, in some cases using blocking agents of different durations or blocking different nerves on subsequent blocks. In occasional complex cases, it may be helpful to consider the use of placebo injections.

BASIC EQUIPMENT FOR PERFORMING NERVE BLOCKS

ANESTHETIC AGENTS

Although virtually any anesthetic agent can be used for a diagnostic or therapeutic nerve block, a consideration of the goals of the nerve block can lead to the selection of an optimal agent. The large variety of agents and concentrations available are useful in allowing the surgical anesthesiologist to deal with a variety of situations requiring varying durations, varying degrees of muscle paralysis, and differing toxicity risks. The majority of nerve blocks used in chronic pain diagnosis and treatment require only a single injection of a small quantity of medication, and therefore toxicity and absorption rate are minor considerations. Because, in most diagnostic blocks, patient observation and feedback are the means through which the result is assessed, the longer a block is effective the more likely a meaningful evaluation will be made. A short-acting agent may wear off before the patient has adequately recovered from the stress of the injection itself to evaluate the result. In addition, for most blocks, it is desirable to use a concentration that will provide partial to complete motor blockade, since the appearance of a motor deficit is often used to determine the technical adequacy of the block.

Acceptably long durations of action can be obtained by using lidocaine with the addition of epinephrine. The epinephrine, by causing local vasoconstriction, delays the absorption of anesthetic in the area of injection and therefore prolongs the period of time in which nerve fibers are exposed to the active agent. However, some authors believe that such vasoconstriction causes local ischemic necrosis and therefore, at least in injection into muscle, recommend against its use.

Long-acting effects without the use of added epinephrine may be obtained by using bupivacaine (Marcaine, Sensorcaine). This naturally long-acting anesthetic has a rapid onset of action and a duration of action 2–3 times that of lidocaine. Good motor blockade can usually be obtained with a 0.5% concentration, and this is generally the preferred agent for most blocks. For lumbar sympathetic and celiac blocks, requiring large volumes of agent, 0.25% bupivacaine, which will provide good autonomic blockade, is generally used.

In spinal anesthesia, a shorter acting agent may be appropriate since close monitoring is required throughout the entire period of anesthesia. Tetracaine (Pontocaine) is often the preferred agent for spinal anesthesia. It must be kept in mind that, whatever agent is used for spinal (or even epidural) anesthesia, because of the risk of inadvertent intrathecal injection) a single-use vial of drug, with no preservatives, must be used.

NEEDLES

A needle long enough to reach the desired target with length to spare should be selected. For deep blocks, where adjustments in the trajectory have to be made as the needle is advanced, a 21-gauge or larger needle should be used. For more superficial blocks, a 23-gauge needle can be employed. Since many blocks involve advancing the needle to or near a bony prominence, it is best to use a relatively short beveled needle, which is less likely to bend and form a hook that would damage tissue on removal. For the majority of blocks, a disposable 21-gauge 3½-inch needle will be quite satisfactory. For lumbar sympathetic and celiac plexus blocks, a 5- or 6-inch needle is required.

Neurolytics

Because of widespread nonspecific and poorly controllable destruction, the caustic lytics used in the past are seldom indicated. Except in very specific circumstances, phenol and absolute alcohol have no role to play in chronic pain therapy.

For reasons not fully understood, depository steroids can be effective in cases in which extremely long-lasting blockade is desired. In some cases, this agent may be effective because of its anti-inflammatory properties, such as in greater occipital nerve entrapment secondary to chronic spasm in the neck muscles. In other situations, where no cause for local inflammation can be easily defined, such as monoradicular pain with negative studies, the observed prolonged effect is more difficult to understand. The possibilities include disruption of a self-perpetuating cycle of inflammation, swelling, and compression or possible minor toxic effects of steroid on small nerve fibers.

In most cases, 40 mg (1 ml) of methylprednisolone acetate (Depo-Medrol, Depo-Predate) suspended in 1 ml of local anesthetic agent is the effective dosage. Although 40 mg is a relatively small dosage and is absorbed over a prolonged period of time, frequent repeated dosage must be avoided to prevent systemic effects. As a basic rule, a dose should not be repeated in less than 30 days.

In cases in which neurolysis is indicated and in which loss of the nerve's function is acceptable, a radiofrequency electrode allows controllable nerve destruction. It is most useful for facet joint denervation but can also be used in difficult cases of greater occipital neuralgia or intercostal neuralgia, and its use has been described in differential denervation of spinal nerve roots.

A radiofrequency electrode is a sharply pointed metal rod approximately the size of an 18-gauge needle. It is insulated except for the very tip, and its hub is connected by cable to a radiofrequency control unit. When a radiofrequency current is passed down the electrode, heating occurs at the interface between the uninsulated tip and the surrounding tissue. The current returns to the machine through a standard patient grounding pad. A thermistor within the tip of the electrode monitors the temperature and provides a continuous readout on the control unit; the operator regulates the tip temperature by adjusting the intensity of current flow. Most control units also allow passage of a stimulating current to provide physiologic confirmation of adequate electrode placement prior to lesion generation.

Fluoroscope

Most nerve blocks can be performed without the use of radiographic control. The early textbooks describe elaborate methods of triangulation based on surface features to allow placement of a needle tip in most lo-cations. However, the use of fluoroscopy, particularly those units with on-line memory storage to provide freeze-frame display, allow for a much more accurate and speedy needle or electrode placement with minimal radiation exposure. Fluoroscopy is now considered essential for properly carrying out nerve root blocks, facet blocks, and lumbar sympathetic and celiac blocks.

SPECIFIC BLOCKS

Spinal

Subarachnoid

By injecting a substance whose density differs from that of spinal fluid into the subarachnoid space and subsequently positioning the patient appropriately, a region of several contiguous dermatomes can be anesthetized or otherwise affected. Because of the cervical origin of the phrenic nerve, such blockade is generally confined to the midthoracic levels or caudally.

Purpose

Diagnostically, this approach may be used to distinguish central from peripheral pain. Such a distinction can usually be made on clinical grounds, but occasionally the clinical signs are too indefinite to yield a firm conclusion. Poorly characterized pain in a leg that is hypesthetic as a result of a stroke might, for example, present such difficulty that a subarachnoid block could be used to clarify the situation.

Therapeutically, subarachnoid injection is generally useful only for malignant pain, because of both its nonspecific destruction of neural tissue and the eventual return of sensation or dysesthesia. The most common use is in pelvic pain due to cancer, especially since midline pain is difficult to control with percutaneous cordotomy.

Anatomy and Technique

The injection site and patient position is dependent upon the area to be affected and the agent to be injected. Both tetracaine in distilled water and absolute alcohol are hypobaric to spinal fluid, therefore rising to the top of the subarachnoid space; tetracaine in 5–10% dextrose and phenol and glycerol are hyperbaric, settling to the bottom of the subarachnoid space. The patient must therefore be positioned so that the target area is either uppermost or lowermost, depending upon the agent. Awareness of the slope of the path toward cervical levels is important to prevent dangerous migration of the agent cranialward. Although it seems easier to keep the head and neck higher than the point of injection, making hypobaric agent injection easier, upper lumbar blockade can lead to sympathetic outflow disruption, vasoparalysis in the lower extremities, and a fall in blood pressure. A hypobaric agent, however, prevents treatment by Trendelenburg positioning, so alternatives, including leg elevation without head lowering and fluid infusion, must be available. In fact, it light of the potential widespread effects, desired or otherwise, of subarachnoid agents, such injections are most safely done by or with the assistance of an anesthesiologist, in a fully equipped anesthesia room with the patient screened and prepared as if undergoing general anesthesia. These blocks are not casual undertakings and are inappropriate in the office or clinic block room.

Epidural

Purpose

Injection into the epidural space allows blockade of spinal nerve roots over a more limited area than does subarachnoid injection and allows placement of depository agents that can give prolonged effects. Although the risk of penetrating the spinal cord generally limits selection of the site of subarachnoid injection, and hence its area of major effect to the region of L2–L5, epidural drugs can be placed at virtually any point along the spinal axis.

Diagnostically, epidural injection is seldom of use. Although it is easier to confine the medication injected into a limited area, bilateral effects usually occur and controlled manipulation of its area of action is difficult. Unlike subarachnoid drugs, epidural fluids do not flow freely or predictably with changes in the patient position.

Therapeutically, long-lasting relief of nerve root irritation, as occurs in small disk herniations, can be obtained by epidural steroid injection. One theory postulates that the radicular pain of disk herniation is the result of dural irritation due to leakage of the abundant intradiskal degradative enzymes through an anular tear, whereas neurologic deficit results from migration of nuclear fragments through that tear with secondary nerve root compression. Epidural depository steroids, slowly releasing active agent, counter the inflammation, decreasing the pain and increasing mobility.

Although some practitioners recommend epidural steroids as the primary treatment for classic lumbar disk herniation, with definite neurologic deficit and strongly positive nerve root tension signs (straight leg raise test), one must be cautious of increasing the root dysfunction by injecting a volume of nonsoluble material into an already compromised lateral spinal canal. Surgical therapy remains the best solution for clinically classic disk herniation, especially with a stenotic lateral recess or large disk fragment. In less classic cases, where radicular pain is prominent but neurologic findings are minimal, epidural steroids are a reasonable treatment if standard conservative therapy fails. In the latter group of patients, surgical results can be disappointing, and neuroradiologic studies often show only minor structural abnormalities.

Anatomy and Technique

A needle can be placed into the epidural space either in the midline or 1 cm lateral to the midline on the side of the affected root. Paramedian insertion is in fact slightly easier as well as more effective at delivering agent to the root desired. The needle is advanced to strike the superior portion of the lamina below the interlaminar space to be injected. It is then advanced cranially to step off the bone. Gentle pressure on a saline-filled syringe will allow detection of the passage of the tip through the dense ligamentum flavum into the nonresistent epidural space. The entrance into the epidural space can also be detected by placing a drop of fluid in the needle hub and observing its disappearance as the negative pressure of the epidural space is encountered. One milliliter of agent is adequate to bathe the target nerve root and the surrounding area.

PERIPHERAL NERVE BLOCK

The need for a well-defined approach and goal is never more apparent than when carrying out blockade of peripheral nerves. Virtually any peripheral nerve or nerve root can be located and blocked, but, in the majority of cases, this serves no useful purpose. Even if blockade of a specific nerve gives temporary pain relief, this seldom leads to any form of useful long-term therapy. If the nerve that is blocked is a major mixed nerve, which is usually the case, the loss of motor function and sensation that would result from permanent interruption is seldom acceptable. Even if sacrifice of the nerve can be justified, surgical section or other maneuvers designed to permanently interrupt its function may fail to provide pain relief and may be followed by the formation of a painful neuroma. If the pain is due to soft tissue or joint injuries in the nerve's peripheral field, dermatomal overlap or subsequent collateral sprouting usually results in return of the painful sensation within 6–12 months. Except in the case of specific syndromes that involve focal nerve root irritation or peripheral nerve entrapment, peripheral nerve blockade has a very minor role in chronic pain therapy.

Selective Root

With the aid of fluoroscopic imaging, it is not difficult to place a needle tip adjacent to the lateral margin of a neuroforamen, allowing selective reproducible blockade of a specific nerve root with a small amount of agent. Any nerve root from C3 through S5 can be selectively blocked utilizing a posterior approach, and the cervical roots can also be blocked by an anterior approach.

Purpose

Diagnostically, nerve root blockade is particularly useful in three situations. First, when the patient's pain appears to be due to a classic monoradiculopathy but the neuroradiologic studies fail to provide a structural explanation, selective nerve root blockade will usually clarify the situation. If blocking the suspected nerve root totally abolishes the pain, this provides strong argument that the pain is indeed monoradicular and a closer look at the adjacent disk and neuroforamen would be warranted. On the other hand, if the patient gets a good pattern of numbness, but some pain persists, this effectively rules out a radicular source of the pain and a search more distally, in both neural and nonneural tissue, needs to be carried out. Second, in some cases of classic monoradicular pain, the radiologic studies may demonstrate an abnormality related to an adjacent nerve root only. Whether this is a false-positive finding or a case of anatomic variation, as occurs in a postfixed plexus, can be determined by selective nerve root blockade. If blockade of the structurally affected nerve root abolishes the pain, this confirms the clinically significant role of the imaged abnormality. If it does not, additional nerve roots should be explored with selective blockade, with the recognition that a neuroradiologic study can be simultaneously falsely positive at one level and falsely negative at another. The third situation in which selective nerve root blockade is useful diagnostically is in those cases in which the clinical picture is suggestive of, but not typical for, both nerve root and distal nerve or joint disease. Blockade of a single root is very unlikely to completely abolish pain with a distal origin because of dermatomal overlap. In this situation, careful questioning of the patient is necessary to make sure that complete pain relief has been obtained before concluding that there is a radicular origin to the pain. A good pattern of sensory and motor loss with some persistence of the pain warrants a further search for a peripheral source.

Therapeutically, selective nerve root blockade is most useful in treating postsurgical radicular pain that is presumed to be due to scarring as well as monoradicular pain, confirmed by diagnostic blockade, in which no surgical lesion can be identified. In both cases, injection of depository steroid will often provide lasting relief. Radiofrequency lesions can be made in the nerve roots, but since the nerve roots commonly affected by surgery or injured by disk herniations contain significant motor components, such destructive lesions are seldom of use.

Anatomy

Selective nerve root blockade is carried out by placing a needle tip just lateral to the bony neuroforamen at the desired level. Placement is confirmed fluoroscopically and the patient generally will report paresthesias in the anatomically appropriate region with needle placement or at the beginning of injection.

Technique

Cervical   Cervical nerve roots may be blocked by either an anterior or a posterior approach. Although the an-

terior approach can be performed without x-ray control, using palpation of the transverse processes as landmarks (particularly the bony projection known as Chassaignac's tubercle on the transverse process of C6), the vertebral artery is relatively vulnerable from this approach and we recommend a posterior approach for cervical nerve root blockade. From the back, the vertebral artery is largely protected by the articular masses and, using fluoroscopy control, needle placement lateral to the lateral margin of the neuroforamen can be obtained, so that the needlepoint is in fact well away from the vertebral artery. With the fluoroscope in an anteroposterior direction, local infiltrative anesthesia is obtained directly posterior to the lateral mass on the desired side at approximately the level of the disk space. It should be recalled that in the cervical area, nerve roots exit at approximately the level of the disk above the same numbered vertebral body. Therefore, the C6 nerve root would be exiting at approximately the level of the C5–C6 disk space. The needle is advanced under fluoroscopic control to impinge on the lateral mass at approximately the inferior margin of the appropriate space. The needle is then gradually walked off the lateral edge of the lateral mass. The patient will often report paresthesias in the appropriate area, indicating impingement upon the nerve root, but if he does not, shifting of the fluoroscopic beam toward an oblique position to allow visualization of the neuroforamen will allow precise positioning. Careful aspiration must be carried out, since the subarachnoid space may occasionally continue out the nerve root and be entered by a needle in the described position. Once it is clear that the subarachnoid space has not been entered, 0.5–1 ml of the appropriate agent is injected and the needle removed.

Thoracic   In general, selective thoracic nerve root blocks are not carried out, since the problems affecting that region of the body are more commonly distal, in the intercostal nerves, and because intercostal nerve block can be carried out much more easily and safely. If selective thoracic nerve root block is desired, an approach similar to cervical nerve root blockade is performed. In the thoracic area, each numbered root exits through a neuroforamen that is over the superior half of the same numbered body and that also corresponds to the inferior margin of the same numbered rib. Blockade is most easily achieved by inserting the needle toward the junction of the transverse process and lamina at the desired level and then carefully marching the needle caudally and slightly laterally until it drops into the superior portion of the intercostal space. A shift of the fluoroscope to a lateral projection will help control the depth of insertion at this point and minimize the risk of puncturing the pleura with the needle.

Lumbar   Selective nerve root block in the lumbar area is simplified by the easy visualization of the pedicle on anteroposterior fluoroscopy. The pedicles appear as oval densities on either side of the upper half of the vertebral body and form the superior margin of the neuroforamen. Each nerve root is closely approximated to the medial surface of the pedicle of the same numbered body and then turns lateralward to enter the neuroforamen. It passes just below the most inferior point on the pedicle and then continues in an approximately 45° angle caudally and laterally to join the lumbar plexus or lumbosacral trunk. Direct insertion of the needle into a position slightly caudal and lateral to the inferior edge of the pedicle will place it in the lateral opening of the neuroforamen. Lateral fluoroscopy should then be used to confirm placement and regulate depth of insertion, since there is a significant amount of variation in the distance from skin to neuroforamen in various patients. One milliliter of agent is adequate for complete root block.

Sacral Selective sacral nerve root blockade is carried out by passing a needle through the appropriate posterior neuroforamen. The foramina can be visualized on fluoroscopy, although at times some repositioning of the patient or reangling of the tube is necessary because of the slope of the sacrum and because of the multiple radiologic lines on the sacrum. The location of the S1 neuroforamen, the one most commonly subjected to selective nerve root block, is approximately the same distance from the inferior margin of the pedicle of L5 as that point is from the inferior margin of the pedicle of L4 and just slightly lateral to a line running through those points. When a needle enters the posterior neuroforamen, a sudden give in resistance can be felt. It should be remembered that this block is in fact carried out in the epidural space and therefore spread of anesthetic to adjacent roots and to contralateral nerve roots may occur. Therefore, injection should be confined to 1 ml of agent.

Greater Occipital Nerve

Occipital neuralgia, resulting from injury to the greater occipital nerve or entrapment of that nerve in its passage to the scalp, is a fairly well-defined cause of headaches. Head pain that radiates from the base of the skull over the posterior two-thirds of the scalp, often with a retro-orbital component, is typical of this condition. The pain may be unilateral or bilateral and may be constant or intermittent. In some cases, occipital neuralgia results from greater occipital nerve injury due to a blow to the back of the head or a direct trauma to the nerve from a scalp laceration. However, in most cases, occipital neuralgia results from entrapment of the greater occipital nerve in its course from this origin from the C2 nerve root to its entrance into the scalp through the midportion of the superior nuchal line. Its course carries it just external to the skull, through the fibrous insertions of the cervical musculature into the pericranium. The passageway through the fibrous tissues forms a tunnel and the nerve is accompanied by the occipital artery.

In some cases, it appears that occipital neuralgia may represent a neurovascular compression syndrome as the result of a continual pulsation of the occipital artery against the nerve. In the majority of cases, however, occipital neuralgia appears to be secondary to chronic spasm of the neck muscles, as a result of either myofascial syndrome or underlying cervical spine disease.

Purpose

Diagnostically, blockade of the greater occipital nerve can confirm the clinical impression of occipital neuralgia, particularly if the clinical picture is not entirely typical. Therapeutically, injection of depository steroids along the greater occipital nerve in its course just proximal to its exit from the cervical musculature can give lasting relief, particularly if chronic muscle spasm appears to be present. When pain results from closed or open trauma to the posterior scalp, radiofrequency denervation of the greater occipital nerve can be carried out, although surgical section under direct vision and local anesthesia may be no more difficult and more effective.

Technique

In order to carry out injection of the greater occipital nerve, the patient is placed in a seated position with the head flexed forward. The greater occipital nerve exits just below the superior nuchal line, in the interval between the insertion of the trapezius and the sternocleidomastoid muscles. In lean individuals, this location can often be visualized. More commonly, the location can be approximated by selecting the midpoint between the external occipital protuberance in the midline and the mastoid process. Exploration of that region with digital pressure, localizing the area of maximum tenderness, most accurately defines the site for needle placement. For diagnostic block, 2–3 ml of anesthetic agent are injected. If depository steroid is to be injected, 40 mg of methylprednisolone acetate in 1–2 ml of local anesthetic are used. Following injection, the patient should be reassured that a lump palpable in the area for several hours is not unusual. If radiofrequency denervation is to be performed, an anesthetic wheal is raised on the skin overlying the presumed target and the electrode is inserted through the skin. Stimulation is carried out through the electrode while it is moved in a medial and lateral plane until the point of lowest threshold for scalp paresthesias is located. With the electrode held in place, infiltrative anesthesia in the area of its tip is obtained and a radiofrequency lesion at 75°C for 2 min is made.

Suprascapular Nerve

Entrapment of the suprascapular nerve as it passes through the suprascapular notch can produce a syndrome of aching pain within the shoulder in the absence of other evidence of joint dysfunction as well as weakness of the supraspinatus and infraspinatus muscles, characterized by weakness of abduction of the shoulder as well as lateral rotation. The suprascapular nerve, after arising from the superior cord of the brachial plexus, passes posteriorly through the scapular notch, a V-shaped wedge in the superior border of the scapula at the medial border of the coracoid process. An overlying ligament converts the notch into a canal and entrapment can occasionally result. If the diagnosis is suspected, suprascapular nerve block leading to relief of pain can confirm the diagnosis, and injection of depository steroid can sometimes provide lasting relief.

Technique

Although there are techniques for injection in the scapular notch based upon trigonometric relationships of the notch to certain palpable landmarks, the block is very easily done under fluoroscopic control. With the patient prone on a fluoroscopy table and a folded sheet placed under the shoulder on the appropriate side, to place the scapula in approximately horizontal position, the scapula can be visualized in an anteroposterior direction. The scapular notch at the base of the coracoid process can then be localized and an anesthetic wheal raised above it. A needle can then be inserted directly into the notch. Since it is difficult to visualize the notch with lateral fluoroscopy, it is preferable to advance the needle to the scapula medial to the notch and then walk the needle into the notch. Once the notch is reached, the needle is advanced to 2–3 mm, aspiration is carried out, and 2 ml of agent are injected.

Intercostal Nerve

Intercostal pain generally results from direct injury to the intercostal nerve, as a result of either a rib fracture or injury from a thoracotomy incision. Although the pain pattern is quite diagnostic, it is sometimes difficult to be certain of which intercostal nerve or nerves are involved, and selective intercostal nerve blockade is useful for completing the definition of the patient's syndrome. Once the specific nerve or nerves have been identified, radiofrequency denervation or surgical section of the nerve can give lasting relief. Intercostal nerve destruction often causes no detectable neurologic deficit, because of the limited motor distribution of the nerve to the intercostal muscles and a small portion of the serratus muscles only, and the marked dermatomal overlap on the thorax.

Anatomy

Each intercostal nerve is the main continuation of the ventral primary ramus of the same numbered thoracic nerve root. From its origin at the nerve root to the angle of the rib, the intercostal nerve runs on top of the pleura. At the angle of the rib, the nerve assumes a course between the internal and external intercostal muscles in a

groove along the inferior surface of its rib and stays in that position until well past the anterior axilliary line. Therefore, intercostal nerve blockade can usually be carried out anywhere in the interval from the angle of the rib to the anterior axillary line, by placement of the needle into the groove on the inferior surface of the rib.

Technique

The appropriate rib is defined by palpation at the point selected for injection. An anesthetic wheal is raised over the lower half of the rib and a needle inserted normal to the skin in order to contact the lower half of the rib. The needle is then walked caudally on the rib until the inferior margin is detected. The needle is then advanced approximately 3 mm under the rib and the injection carried out after a negative aspiration. One to 2 ml of anesthetic agent are satisfactory for blockade. If radiofrequency denervation is to be carried out, the needle is removed and the electrode is inserted in the same manner, first contacting the rib and then being marched caudally until it slips over the inferior edge of the rib and can be advanced several millimeters. A radiofrequency lesion at 75°C for 90 sec is then made. At the time of denervation, a vascular blush may be noted in the field of distribution of the nerve anterior to the electrode. Following completion of the denervation, digital pressure is maintained over the electrode track for 30 sec to allow soft tissue to shift back into place and obliterate the track. This will prevent a pneumothorax in the rare event of a breach in the parietal pleura by the needle or electrode.

Lateral Femoral Cutaneous Nerve

Meralgia paresthetica, a dull aching pain of the anterolateral thigh often associated with dysesthetic cutaneous sensation, results from entrapment of the lateral femoral cutaneous nerve as it traverses a fibrous tunnel in the lateral inguinal region. The diagnosis can usually be easily made on clinical grounds, but blockade of the lateral femoral cutaneous nerve is confirmatory in unclear cases. Lasting relief can often be obtained with injection of depository steroid in the area of entrapment.

Anatomy

The lateral femoral cutaneous nerve arises from the ventral primary rami of the second and third lumbar nerve roots and runs internal to the ilium and iliacus muscle until it reaches the anterior superior spine of the iliac crest. The nerve then passes through a fibrous tunnel along the inferior edge of the inguinal ligament just medial to the anterior superior spine, entering the subcutaneum of the thigh in the interval between the inguinal ligament and sartorius muscle insertion. It then distributes to the skin overlying the anterolateral thigh, not quite reaching the knee. Chronic local trauma in the region of the anterior superior spine, as from a corset or belt; chronic traction on the inguinal ligament, as in obesity or pregnancy; or a change in stress on the inguinal ligament, as follows abdominal surgery, can lead to lateral femoral cutaneous nerve entrapment, presumably due to inflammation and edema of the encasing fibrous tissues. Burning or aching pain along with hypesthesia or dysesthesia in the nerve's distribution then results.

When abnormal sensation is present, it is usually very sharply demarcated and can be outlined on the skin. With temporary blockade of the lateral femoral cutaneous nerve, anesthesia is obtained that closely approximates that pattern and relief of the pain occurs. When the symptoms persist despite treatment of the precipitating condition, injection with depository steroids can often give lasting relief.

Technique

To carry out blockade of the lateral femoral cutaneous nerve, the anterior superior spine of the iliac crest is palpated. In lean individuals, with the hip extended and slightly rotated internally, the sartorius muscle can often be visualized or palpated, and the triangle formed by the insertion of the inguinal ligament and that muscle can be used as a landmark. Otherwise, a point approximately 2 cm medial and 2 cm inferior to the anterior superior spine is used. A wheal of anesthetic is raised and a needle inserted through the skin. The needle is angled superiorly and laterally, to strike the medial edge of the anterior superior spine of the iliac crest. The needle is then withdrawn a few millimeters and 5 ml of anesthetic, with or without added depository steroid, are injected.

AUTONOMIC NERVOUS SYSTEM

Visceral Efferent (Sympathetic) Blockade

Hyperactivity of sympathetic outflow is demonstrable in a variety of well-defined but poorly understood pain conditions. The most common form is known as causalgia and usually results from a partial penetrating injury of a major mixed nerve. It is thus most commonly a wartime injury. It is characterized by a severe burning pain throughout the affected extremity, usually appearing a short time after the injury. The limb tends to be so hyperpathic that the patient usually cannot bear the contact of clothing on the skin. Even a light breeze blowing across the extremity can elicit severe pain, as does a drop in environmental temperature. The extremity is pale and cool to the touch and the skin quickly loses secondary appendages, becoming shiny and glossy, and occasionally discolored and dusky. The pain relief following sympathetic blockade is usually dramatic, and often a series of three to six sympathetic blocks with local anesthetic alone will give lasting relief. If blocks give only transient relief, sympathectomy is usually curative.

A much more common pain problem is a less dramatic version of causalgia, referred to as causalgia minor or, preferably, post-traumatic sympathetic dystrophy. This condition most commonly comes on after an injury, sometimes trivial, to soft tissues or joints of the extremity. Sympathetic hyperactivity follows, although the findings are generally less dramatic than those in true causalgia. Whereas the diagnosis of true causalgia is easy because of the presence of a functionally useless extremity that the patient is continually protecting, the presence of post-traumatic sympathetic dystrophy may not be recognized until an abnormal thermogram is obtained, documenting the less obvious temperature difference. Although sympathetic blockade can give significant relief, the results are seldom as dramatic as with true causalgia, and much more caution must be taken in proceeding beyond blocks to surgical sympathectomy. In essence, one should make sure that repeated blocks predictably give excellent relief and placebo blocks give no relief before progressing further.

The sympathetic nerve fibers exit the spinal cord along the nerve roots from T1 to L2. After passing laterally a short distance, the fibers leave the nerve roots and enter the paravertebral sympathetic chains, made up of interconnected sympathetic ganglia that traverse the length of the spinal axis, giving up postganglionic fibers to each of the spinal nerves. Therefore, since all sympathetic output to the upper extremity must pass up the sympathetic chain from the thoracic to the cervical region, blockade of the stellate ganglion, a fusion of the inferior cervical ganglion and the first thoracic ganglion, will effectively block all sympathetic output to the limb. Similarly, since all output to the leg arises at L2 and above, blockade of the sympathetic chain at the L3 level will effectively interrupt all sympathetic outflow to the limb.

Anatomy and Technique

Stellate Ganglion Block Although a stellate ganglion block is a technically easy bedside procedure, it has the highest complication rate of any form of nerve block and should therefore be carried out in a facility that is adequately equipped to diagnose and treat the complications. The complication rate is due to the large number of important structures located in the area of the ganglion. Just lateral to the stellate ganglion are the carotid artery and jugular vein, which must be displaced laterally prior to needle insertion. Deep to the ganglion and sympathetic chain is the vertebral artery. The dome of the pleural cavity often rises close to the stellate ganglion, and the recurrent laryngeal nerve, controlling the vocal cords, and the phrenic nerve, innervating the diaphragm, run nearby.

The block is most easily carried out with the patient supine with a pillow placed under the shoulders so that the head falls back into a gently extended position. The target is approximately two finger-breadths above the sternal notch and two finger-breadths lateral to the midline. The nondominant index and middle finger are applied at that location and the carotid bundle gently displaced laterally. Palpation is used to detect Chassaignac's tubercle, a bony prominence on the transverse process of C6. A wheal is then raised overlying the tubercle and a needle inserted to strike just medial to the tubercle. Bone should be contacted and the needle slightly withdrawn, aspiration carried out, and 3–5 ml of anesthetic agent injected. If there is slight angulation of the needle, the transverse process will be missed and the vertebral artery might be struck. If arterial blood is obtained with aspiration, it is recommended that the procedure be terminated and not reattempted for several hours. If needle placement produces paresthesias down the extremity, this suggests that the needle has passed lateral to the transverse process and is striking the brachial plexus. The needle should then be repositioned before injection.

If sympathetic blockade is obtained, the patient will develop ipsilateral Horner's syndrome, characterized by pupillary miosis and a mild ptosis of the eyelid. If Horner's syndrome is not obtained, it should be concluded that blockade did not occur.

The most common complication is pneumothorax produced by striking the apex of the pleura. In most cases, only a small pneumothorax will occur, producing only mild breathing discomfort and requiring no specific treatment. However, the patient should be alerted to the possibility of an increase in the size of a pneumothorax and should immediately report increasing dyspnea.

Lumbar Sympathetic Block   Lumbar sympathetic blockade is obtained by injection of a relatively large quantity of anesthetic agent into the retroperitoneal space anterolateral to the lumbar vertebral column. Since the lowest sympathetic outflow is at the L2 level, injection at the L3 level will effectively block all sympathetic fibers destined for the lower extremity.

With the aid of fluoroscopy, lumbar sympathetic block is easy to perform. The patient is positioned prone on the x-ray table. A wheal of anesthesia is raised over the tip of the L3 transverse process on the side to be blocked. A 6-inch needle is then inserted normal to the skin to contact the transverse process. Depth of insertion is then noted; the final depth achieved will be 3–4 cm deeper. Under fluoroscopic control, the needle is backed out slightly, angled in a slightly caudal direction to pass below the inferior edge of the transverse process, and angled medially 10–15°. There is a tendency to angulate the needle too far medially, causing the tip to strike the posterior half of the vertebral body or enter the neuroforamen. Until one is comfortable with the procedure, it is therefore wise to advance the needle just to the edge of the vertebral body in anteroposterior projection and then to check a lateral view to make sure the tip overlies the anterior half of the vertebral body. The needle is then

advanced further until, on lateral view, the tip is even with the anterior surface of the L3 vertebral body.

Careful aspiration needs to be carried out, since the great vessels lie nearby. Ten to 20 ml of anesthetic agent are then injected; there should be minimal resistance to injection. The needle is then removed and the patient placed in a sitting position so that gravitational forces will encourage the anesthetic agent to bathe the lower lumbar sympathetic plexus, maximizing the sympathetic blockade. The extremity is observed for evidence of blockade, in the form of warming to touch and flushing as cutaneous vasodilatation occurs.

In advancing the needle into position, after stepping off the inferior edge of the transverse process, the patient may report paresthesias or pain radiating into the anterolateral thigh, a sign that the needle has impinged upon the L3 nerve root. Slight reangulation in one direction or another should be carried out after the needle is backed out slightly to avoid that sensation. Since the needle does pass close to the L3 nerve root, migration of anesthetic agent along the needle track will occasionally give a partial L3 root block in conjunction with the sympathetic nerve block.

Visceral Afferent Blockade

Visceral pain sensation from the stomach, small intestine, colon, and up to the splenic flexure, liver, gallbladder, pancreas, kidneys, and ureters is conducted through fibers that run along with the sympathetic fibers and traverse the celiac plexus. Temporary relief of abdominal visceral pain can therefore be obtained by blockade of the celiac plexus. This is sometimes most useful diagnostically in sorting out a pain whose characteristics do not allow classification otherwise. A specialized technique, with the injection of a lytic agent into the area of the celiac ganglion, has been used to temporarily treat visceral pain of malignant disease also.

Anatomy and Technique

Celiac Ganglion Block   The celiac ganglion is located at the level of the first lumbar vertebra and lies ventral and lateral to the aorta. The technique for celiac plexus block is similar to that of lumbar sympathetic block except that the needle placement is more medial. The skin wheal is therefore raised opposite the body of L1, 10 cm lateral to the midline. The needle is inserted at approximately a 30° angle and advanced under fluoroscopic control to just contact the anterolateral body of L1. The needle is then walked off the body and advanced an additional 2 cm. On anteroposterior filming, the needle point will be just short of the midline. Aortic pulsations may be transmitted through the needle and visible. Very careful aspiration needs to be carried out and a small test injection performed. There should be no resistance to injection; if there is, repositioning of the needle should be carried out until a resistance-free injection site is identified. Fifteen to 20 ml of anesthetic agent are then injected and the needle withdrawn. Since sympathetic blockade to both lower extremities as well as the abdominal cavity may occur, the patient is only brought gradually to the sitting position because of the possibility of orthostatic hypotension.

Because this technique involves injection of agent into the space surrounding the aorta, it is recommended that the injection of lytic agents such as alcohol be carried out only by those who have been specifically trained in the technique.

Facet Joint Block and Denervation

Most back and leg pain is not due to disk herniation. Failure to recognize this fact has led to an inordinately high rate of lumbar disk surgery with overall poor results. In the search for other etiologies for back pain, attention became focused upon the facet joints as a possible source. These diarthrodial joints, well supplied with pain fibers, are placed in a state of constant compression with the development of the usual lumbar lordosis early in infancy. Throughout life they are subjected to great forces, and the development of hypertrophic arthropathy of the facet joints is a frequent occurrence in the fifth and sixth decades. It has been postulated that a traumatic arthritis of the facet joints can occur and accounts for some cases of back pain. Furthermore, there appears to be referred pain arising from each of the lower three lumbar facet joints, which explains the occurrence of pain beyond the local area of the facet joint per se. Stimulation of the L3–L4 facet joint often yields sensations rising into the posterior thoracic area; stimulation of the L4–L5 facet produces sensations radiating into the hip and thigh, and L5–S1 facet stimulation produces sensations radiating into the buttock and sacral region.

Facet joint pain is difficult to diagnose, since the joints are not accessible to close examination, and lumbar facet blocks are usually necessary to make the diagnosis. However, the diagnosis can be suspected if the back pain does not have a strong radicular component, does not have associated neurologic deficit, and is aggravated by hyperextension of the spine, which stresses the facet joints. If the diagnosis of facet syndrome is confirmed, long-lasting relief can be obtained by means of lumbar facet denervation using a radiofrequency electrode.

Anatomy and Technique

The technique of lumbar facet denervation has undergone a progressive evolution. The initial procedures used a thin scalpel to make a deep stab incision in the approximate location of the facet joint. The knife was then swept cranially and caudally to interrupt the facet innervation. Finding this excessively traumatic, Shealy developed a technique of insertion of a radiofrequency electrode under fluoroscopic control to the inner trans-

verse ligament, where a heat lesion would be made (1). Anatomic dissections by Bogduk and Long have led to the definition of a more specific target, at the junction of the transverse process and the articular facet (2). Further attempts to refine the target are being made.

Needle placement and electrode placement for facet block and facet denervation, respectively, are identical. The general practice has been to carry out blockade and denervation of the lowest three facet joints bilaterally unless there is specific evidence of injury to a single facet joint. At L4 and L5, the target is the junction of the transverse process with the superior articular process. An anesthetic wheal is raised above the lateral portion of the transverse process and the needle inserted under fluoroscopic control to the above-defined target. A slight medialward angulation of the needle that this approach provides allows the needle to slip under a hypertrophic facet joint and approach the articular branch of the posterior primary ramus directly. At the S1 level, the target is defined by the superior edge of the sacrum at the point where it joins the superior articular process of S1, forming a notch on anteroposterior fluoroscopy. At each location, 1 ml of anesthetic agent is injected. One must avoid injecting large quantities of agent lest blockade of multiple other structures, including the nearby nerve roots, be obtained. If denervation is to be carried out, the needle is removed and replaced by an electrode along the same course. When the tip of the electrode is resting in the proper position, striking the posterior surface of the transverse process, the nerve root itself is shielded from the heat of the electrode. A radiofrequency lesion at 75°C for 90 sec is then made and the electrode removed.

After facet denervation, the patient is advised that he may note some aggravation of his usual pain after the anesthetic wears off. It is normally difficult to draw a definite conclusion as to how helpful a procedure will be until approximately 1 week has elapsed, during which time the associated soft tissue injury will heal and any muscle spasm triggered by needle insertion will have resolved.

References

1. Bogduk N, Long DM: Percutaneous lumbar medial branch neurotomy: A modification of facet denervation. *Spine* 5:193–200, 1980.
2. Shealy CN: Percutaneous radiofrequency denervation of spinal facets. *J Neurosurg* 43:448–451, 1975.

Suggested Readings

Camins M, O'Leary P: *The Lumbar Spine.* New York, Raven Press, 1987.
Carron H, Korbon GA, Rowlingson JC: *Regional Anesthesia.* Orlando, FL, Grune & Stratton, 1984.

Finneson B: *Low Back Pain*, ed. 2. Philadelphia, JB Lippincott, 1980.

Hendler NH, Long DM, Wise TN: *Diagnosis and Treatment of Chronic Pain.* Littleton, MA, John Wright & Sons, 1982.

Rothman R, Simeone F: *The Spine,* ed 2. Philadelphia, WB Saunders, 1982.

Stanton-Hicks M, Boas R: *Chronic Low Back Pain.* New York, Raven Press, 1982.

White JC, Sweet WH: *Pain and the Neurosurgeon.* Springfield, IL, Charles C Thomas, 1969.

Youmans JR: *Neurological Surgery,* ed 2. Philadelphia, WB Saunders, 1982.

CHAPTER 7

NEUROSURGICAL TREATMENT OF DEAFFERENTATION PAIN

BLAINE S. NASHOLD, JR.
JAMES R. B. NASHOLD
EBEN ALEXANDER

"DOCTOR, WHY do I have burning pain in my numb arm?" This question not only puzzles the patient but also the physician. The patient may be describing deafferentation pain if he suffers from brachial plexus avulsion or paraplegia. The diagnosis of deafferentation pain is not difficult, but its cause is unknown and treatment can be difficult. Numerous authors have characterized deafferentation pain as did Tasker et al. (1), whose clinical definition was "a state of dysesthetic pain resulting from neural injury," whereas Wall, a neurophysiologist, defined it as "Not only a loss of input but actually degeneration so that the spinal cord cells were free to act in a pathologic way" (2). There remains no adequate pathophysiologic explanation of deafferentation pain. We classify deafferentation pain into three clinical types: (1) a dysesthesia due to lesions that involve the peripheral nerve and/or the dorsal root ganglion, (2) dysesthesia with lesions rostral to the dorsal root ganglion but including the spinal cord, and (3) dysesthetic pain with lesions of the spinal axis, brainstem, and/or thalamus. This latter type of pain is often designated as a central pain and was described in the early neurological literature as associated with the thalamic syndrome. The best clinical examples of the deafferentation pain syndrome include brachial plexus avulsion, avulsion of spinal roots from the conus medullaris, and dysesthesia following spinal cord injury with paraplegia, as well as a variety of other pathologic insults of the brainstem and/or thalamus.

The patient with the deafferentation syndrome often describes severe pain in a partial or completely anesthetic area of the body. The pains are intractable to treatment. On neurologic examination, there is always alteration of the various sensory modalities, with the pain described as disagreeable and/or burning. The pain may or may not be intensified by cutaneous stimulation of the painful area, but there may exist cutaneous trigger points found in areas of the body at some distance from the original region of dysesthesia. Touching the trigger points will activate the pain. For example, a patient with a brachial plexus avulsion and an associated anesthetic arm may have trigger spots on the skin of the neck or abdomen, usually several dermatomal levels away from the site of the original injury. Touching the trigger spot will excite the pain in the deafferented, anesthetic limb.

Every pathologic lesion involving the central sensory pathways does not necessarily result in a central pain syndrome. In fact, only 10–15% of avulsion injuries to the brachial plexus or spinal cord exhibit this pain syndrome. In the thalamic syndrome, the number of patients who suffer from pain is probably smaller. When the onset of deafferentation pain occurs early in the course of the disease or following trauma, it then becomes intractable, and it is in this group of patients that medical and surgical treatment has been so difficult. In this chapter we will confine our discussion to four types of deafferentation pain—the thalamic syndrome and three others due to pathologic changes in the spinal cord: brachial/conus medullaris nerve root avulsions, post-herpetic pain involving either the trigeminal or spinal nerve roots, and traumatic paraplegia with pain.

DORSAL ROOT ENTRY ZONE PHYSIOLOGY AND NEUROANATOMY

The successful neurosurgical operation for relief of pain depends on the careful selection of the patient along with the choice of a therapeutic lesion that involves specific neuroanatomic structures, in this case the dorsal entry area. It is well known that a surgical section of the lateral spinothalamic tract will result in the loss of pain and thermal sensation on the contralateral side of the body; therefore, a lateral spinothalamic tractotomy deprives large regions of the body of these two sensory modalities even though the pain may be confined to a smaller region of the body. The ideal pain operation would be performed at a specific site in the central nervous system that would result in pain relief only in the area of the body involved with pain. At present no such ideal operation exists; however, lesions of the dorsal root entry zone (DREZ) have certain advantages in that they involve a localized neuroanatomic structure (the DREZ) and can result in pain relief in those restricted regions of the body that are painful (one to several dermatomes). The DREZ operation makes it theoretically possible to confine the pain relief to the painful areas involved. A good clinical example of the DREZ localized effect is in the person with postherpetic pain, which usually involves only one or two dermatomes. If these involved roots are surgically treated, pain relief occurs only in a restricted zone.

The DREZ represents the first spinal cord region where initial integration of sensory information takes place in the central nervous system. We believe that in certain pain syndromes (deafferentation) the neural mechanism responsible for the pain originates in the neurons of the damaged dorsal horn. Good examples of this are the dorsal root avulsion injuries paraplegia and post-herpetic pain.

At present the dorsal horn is under intense study by neurophysiologists. The dorsal horn region was first described by Rolando, an Italian anatomist of the 18th century, who identified the region by gross inspection of the spinal cord (3). Later this dorsal spinal region was named the substantia gelatinosa of Rolando. It was Rexed, however, who identified 10 distinctive anatomic layers of the dorsal horn based on its specific cytoarchetectonics (4) (Fig. 7.1). At present neurophysiologists are adding to our knowledge of the neurophysiologic importance of these Rexed zones.

Nociceptive input from small fiber systems are found in Rexed layer I, sometimes designated as the substantia gelatinosa, and Rexed layer V (Fig. 7.2). The DREZ lesions, using special thermal electrodes, are therefore designed to destroy these five superficial layers of the dorsal horn (Rexed layers I–V). In animal experiments, in which deafferentation of the dorsal horn can be experimentally produced, the secondary interneurons in the superficial and deeper Rexed layer (Rexed V) become unstable a few hours after the experimental injury. By monitoring the damaged dorsal horn in these animals with microelectrodes, we have found abnormal electrical activity of the neurons within a few hours of the insult; this electrical abnormality continues for many months. We believe that this abnormal electrical activity (epileptiform) may be the genesis of the pain in both animals and humans. The dorsal horn is rich in a variety of neuropeptides that are altered in the experimental animal model and certainly in humans following injury,

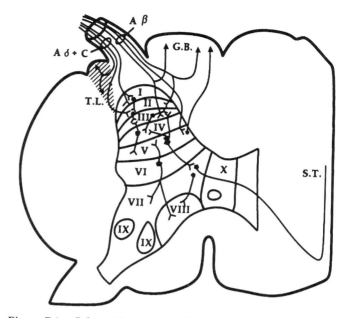

Figure 7.1. **Schematic cross-section of spinal cord showing afferent connections and Rexed layers. DREZ lesions destroy layers I–V.**

but the exact role of these neuropeptides in the pain process is still unknown. We believe that the reduction of pain following lesions of the dorsal horn (DREZ) is the result of destroying the abnormal secondary interneurons and their connections. This was the original theoretical basis for the DREZ operation.

SPINAL ROOT AVULSION

Avulsion of the spinal nerve roots is usually the result of trauma. Years ago it was often due to a fall, with the person striking and depressing the shoulder, causing traction and avulsion of the cervical nerve roots. Today avulsion injuries almost always follow high-speed vehicular accidents, with the motorcycle being the main offender, although we have seen it after automobile, snowmobile, and speedboat accidents, as well as in industrial injuries.

The force of the injury is transmitted to the head and neck along the brachial plexus, avulsing the spinal nerve roots. Both the dorsal and ventral roots can be avulsed with some variation in the number of roots involved, but most of the time in brachial plexus avulsions the dorsal roots from C5 to T1 are involved (Fig. 7.3). Rarely are only one or two roots involved. The person may suffer other serious associated injuries involving the head and neck, so the presence of the avulsion injury may not be evident on the initial examination, particularly if the patient is semiconscious. Intractable pain occurs in about 10% of patients with avulsion, begins very early after the injury, and responds poorly to medical treatment. The DREZ operation has been effective in re-

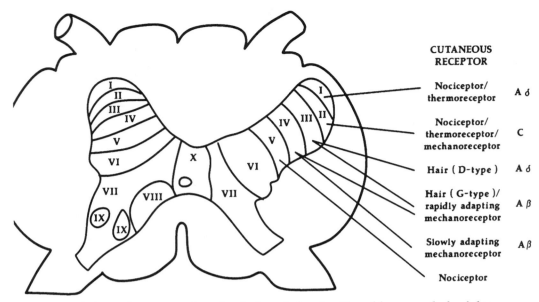

Figure 7.2. Schematic cross-section of spinal cord showing Rexed layers and physiology.

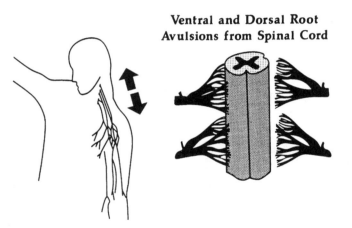

Figure 7.3. Traumatic mechanism of brachial plexus avulsion injury.

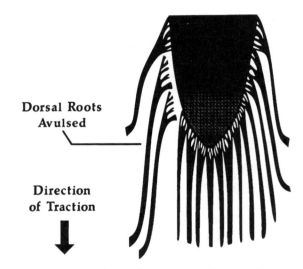

Figure 7.4. Traumatic avulsion of sacral roots from conus medullaris.

lief of the pain in about 70% of patients, with the relief lasting over 5 years (5).

The clinical diagnosis of an avulsion injury is not difficult. The patient complains of severe burning and/or electrical shock–like pains in the paralyzed analgesic arm or leg. In the arm the pain may be referred along the radial aspect into the thumb or index finger, whereas in the leg it may be confined to a specific dermatomal distribution involving the big toe or the lateral aspect of the foot (L4–S1). It should be recognized that the dorsal spinal roots can also be avulsed from injuries involving the conus medullaris that are the result of severe pelvic trauma (Fig. 7.4). The patients complain of the same types of pain, but the pain is localized to the involved lower extremity. After avulsion the involved arm or leg lies immobile and useless, with atrophic changes of the

skin and muscle. Occasionally one finds a patient in whom the paralyzed painful limb has been amputated in order to relieve the pain and unfortunately the patient now has phantom limb pain. Needless to say, this barbaric treatment is not recommended. Amputation is recommended after relieving the pain, because the lifeless limb is now more of a hindrance than a help to the patient.

Along with the neurologic examination, a myelographic study will help confirm the diagnosis of spinal root avulsion (Fig. 7.5). Traumatic myeloceles of varying size and extent can be seen in the spinal region of the avulsion (cervical/lumbosacral). The number of trau-

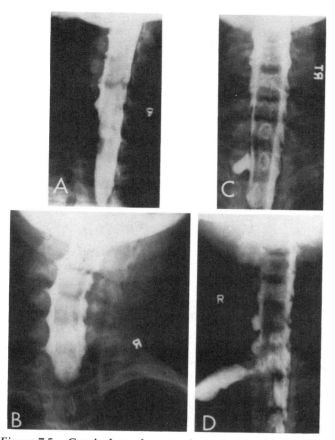

Figure 7.5. **Cervical myelograms in patients with brachial plexus avulsion injury.**

matic myeloceles are not indicative of the extent of the nerve root avulsion, particularly in the cervical region, where it is common for four or five roots to be avulsed with only one or two traumatic myeloceles present (Fig. 7.5). Fewer roots tend to be avulsed in the sacral than in the cervical region, and we have found several paraplegias caused by gunshot wounds with avulsed roots near the site of the spinal cord injury. Additional examination, such as electromyography or the recording of sensory-evoked potentials, is of interest but not diagnostic.

The DREZ operation consists of surgically exposing the region of the spinal cord involved in the avulsion injury and producing small (1–2-mm) thermal lesions in the dorsal horn to destroy the first five Rexed layers of the DREZ (Figs. 7.6 and 7.7). The details of the operation have been reported in the neurosurgical literature and will not be dealt with here. The complications of the DREZ operation are related to the involvement of neighboring spinal cord structures such as the dorsal columns and/or the descending motor pathways or of the ascending spinocerebellar tract, with lesions in the higher cervical cord. No deaths have occurred in over 400 operations, and the morbidity has been about 5% of the patients who have postoperative ipsilateral arm/leg weakness. Transient bladder and motor disorders have occurred in a few paraplegics.

PARAPLEGIA

Traumatic paraplegia is associated with chronic deafferentation pain in about 10% of patients. The onset of pain presents in two ways. In the majority of paraplegics, the pain occurs early after the injury; in another group of paraplegics the pain does not appear until several years after their initial trauma. In these latter paraplegics with a delayed onset of pain, one-third will have an associated spinal cyst at or near the site of spinal cord trauma, visualized either on myelography or at surgery (Fig. 7.8). In our experience, the emptying of the spinal cyst alone may not be sufficient to relieve the patient's pain; in addition, it is necessary to perform the DREZ operation to obtain pain relief. Once the pain syndrome has not responded to medical treatment (6 months), we believe that the DREZ operation should be carried out as early as possible (at 6 months to 1 year). We have had several patients in whom the pain was present for many years; for instance, one man's 30-year pain was finally relieved by the DREZ operation. This suggests that the old idea that the longer the patient suffers pain the more difficult it is to treat may only be partially true, but early treatment is always preferable.

Two main types of pain are described by the paraplegic patient. One is a diffuse burning pain usually involving widespread areas of the legs and sacrum. The DREZ operation will not relieve this type of pain. Another type of pain is that which occurs in those portions of the body near or just above the cutaneous zone of sensory loss. On sensory examination in these patients one finds a zone of cutaneous sensory change for several dermatomes rostral to the upper anesthetic dermatome. Touching or stroking the skin of this area sets off the patient's pain and is described by him as shooting or electrical discomfort referred into the paralyzed limbs. The pain can also be spontaneously triggered by distention of an abdominal viscera, such as the bladder or the lower bowel. Cutaneous trigger spots in distant dermatomes occur in these paraplegics. Stimulation of the skin will trigger the patient's pain, and it is this pain that responds to the DREZ lesions.

The clinical diagnosis of deafferentation pain in the paraplegic is not difficult. It is helpful to carry out a spinal myelogram to define both the upper and lower limits of the spinal cord pathology as well as to look for the presence of one or more spinal cord cysts. The spinal cyst can best be visualized by doing a delayed computed tomography (CT) scan of the spinal cord following the myelogram. After 6 hours, the contrast will have penetrated the cyst cavity sufficiently for good visualization. The use of intraoperative ultrasound studies of the exposed spinal cord at the time of surgery is also very

Figure 7.6. **DREZ electrode (Radionics).**

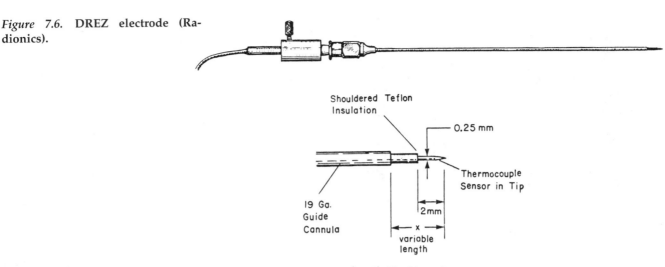

NTCD (0.25) Tip Dimensions

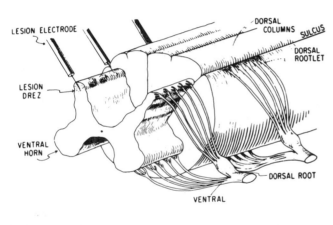

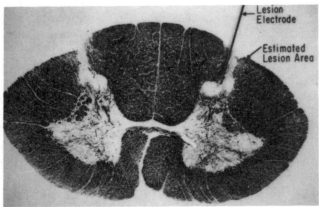

Figure 7.7. **Schematic representation of area of dorsal horn involved in DREZ lesion.**

Figure 7.8. **Intraoperative ultrasound studies in paraplegic with spinal cord cyst and pain.**

useful in defining the extent of the cyst. At times the spinal myelogram with delayed CT scan does not precisely delineate the cyst, and in several patients, using intraoperative ultrasonography, we found two separate spinal cysts that had been missed on the routine myelogram.

The surgical treatment in the paraplegic with deafferentation pain consists of exposing the spinal cord above and below the level of the traumatic lesion (usually two to three vertebral levels). The DREZ lesions are made bilaterally in the DREZ, beginning at the level of the trauma and extending rostrally for at least two to three spinal segments. If a cyst is present, it is drained with a permanent catheter into the subarachnoid space. In paraplegics, good relief of pain can be expected in 50% for at least 5 years (6, 7).

SYRINGOMELIA AND PAIN

In 1827 Ollivier d'Angers coined the term "syringomyelia" from the Greek words for "cavity" and "the spinal marrow" (8). Bastian described one of the earliest reports of traumatic syringomyelia in 1876 in a patient with paraplegia (9). Reports in the literature have shown an incidence of 0.3–2.3% of paraplegics who develop pain post injury and are found to have syringomyelia. Our experience indicates that a higher percentage of paraplegics with pain of delayed onset will also have syringomyelia. As many as 65% of paraplegics who develop pain have traumatic syrinxes (10). The etiology of syringomyelia in paraplegics is still unknown but may result from more than one mechanism including obstruction of the fourth ventricle, arachnoiditis, and increased epidural venous pressure.

By clinical definition, syringomyelia is a slowly progressive disease that can occur at any age but usually begins in the second or third decade of life unless it develops as a result of a traumatic spinal cord injury. In the later case syrinxes may develop within months of an injury or up to a dozen years later. The disease may be congenitally associated in the case of Chiari malformations or may be acquired by traumatic injury to the cord. Syringomyelia has also been reported in a range of clinical settings associated with von Hippel-Lindau's disease, hemangioblastomas, ependymomas, neurofibromas, teratomas, meningiomas, and metastases (11–14).

The classic triad of symptoms are atrophy of the distal upper extremities, hyporeflexia of the arms with hyperreflexia of the legs, and "sensory loss in a cape-like distribution over the cervical dermatones" (15). Cavity formation usually occurs in the lower cervical or upper thoracic region, especially after injuries to this area such as brachial plexus avulsion injuries suffered after motorcycle accidents. Congenital malformations may cause syrinxes to develop in the lumbosacral levels of the cord. The onset of symptoms is usually gradual and intermittent at first as the syrinx impinges on decussating spinothalamic fibers and causes loss of pain sensitivity and the loss of hot and cold discrimination in the distal portions of the upper extremities. Preservation of fine touch and position sense associated with impaired pain and temperature sensations causes the classic picture of dissociated sensory loss as reported by Charcot. Extension of the syrinx causes enlargement of the affected areas in addition to muscle wasting and atrophy in a distal-to-proximal pattern. Expansion into the brainstem may cause symptoms including weakness of the vocal cords, soft palate and pharynx, and unequal pupillary constriction with preservation of the light reflex.

In addition to a thorough history, physical, and neurologic exam, plain radiographs of the spine and skull may indicate other abnormalities associated with syrinxes such as tumors and trauma. Although CT with contrast will delineate extradural and intramedullary lesions accompanying syrinxes, magnetic resonance imaging (MRI) remains the gold standard for detailed axial and saggital imaging of the size and extent of the syrinx and for evaluating the presence of syrinxes with septations, which may complicate proposed surgical treatment of this lesion.

Surgical drainage of the syrinx using either syrinx-to-subarachnoid (SSA) shunting or syringoperitoneal (SP) shunting has been the standard treatment in patients who develop severe pain or exhibit deteriorating motor and sensory deficits. Shannon et al. reported that 10 of 13 paraplegics with syrinxes were relieved of pain by simply opening the cyst to the subarachnoid space or by draining it with an indwelling catheter (16).

Our experience with drainage of cysts indicated that some patients had a return of pain within 6 months to a year postoperatively. When drainage of the cyst was combined with a DREZ operation, pain relief occurred in 77% of these patients with a follow-up of 3.5 years. Cyst drainage was accomplished by either creating an opening between the syrinx and the subarachnoid space or by use of a catheter between the syrinx and the SAS. Patients with paraplegia who develop severe, intractable pain from syringomyelia and who have "failed" multiple medical trials at pain control are suitable candidates for syrinx drainage and the DREZ operation.

POST-HERPETIC PAIN

TRIGEMINAL NUCLEUS CAUDALIS

Chronic facial pain due to post-herpetic infection of the gasserian ganglion has been very difficult to treat. The virus initially affects the gasserian ganglion and the skin, with painful cutaneous lesions involving the three divisions of the trigeminal nerve. If there is involvement of the first trigeminal division (V_1) the pain is referred to the eye and forehead and scarring of the involved skin area may be associated with hyperesthesia and/or hyperalgesia (Fig. 7.9). When the cornea is involved, it becomes anesthetic, with the added problem of corneal scarring and the risk of loss of sight. The second and third trigeminal divisions (V_2 and V_3) are similarly involved in some patients (Fig. 7.10).

The anatomic organization of facial sensation in the trigeminal tract (touch and pain) was determined by Soquist and resulted in his sectioning the descending trigeminal tract in the medulla for relief of certain types of facial pain (Fig. 7.11). The facial sensation via the trigeminal system is organized into three separate nuclei located in the medullocervical junction. The pain afferents end in the trigeminal nucleus caudalis, which lies at the medullospinal junction between the lower end of the obex and the second cervical dorsal root. The trigeminal nucleus caudalis has a neuroanatomic organization similar to that of the spinal dorsal horn (Fig. 7.12). In

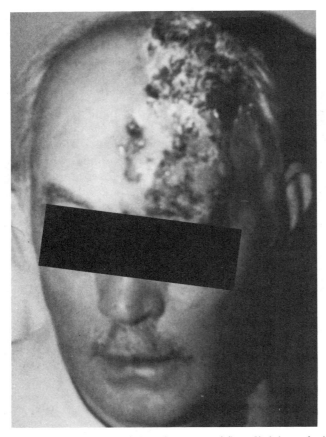

Figure 7.9. Patient with involvement of first division of trigeminal nerve (V₁) during acute phase of herpetic infection.

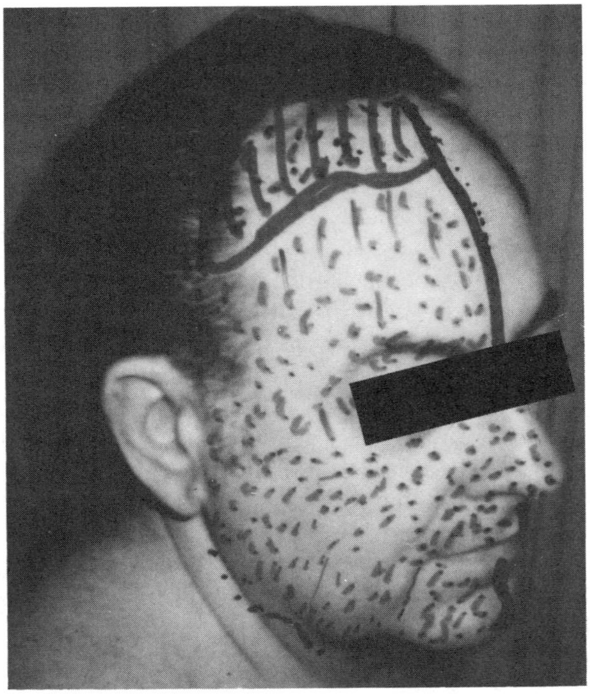

Figure 7.10. Patient with postherpetic pain of the trigeminal nerve, total analgesia over forehead, and remainder of face hyperalgesic to all sensory stimulation. Total relief (3 years pain free) was achieved after caudalis DREZ.

fact, the dorsal horn merges at the level of the cervical cord with the nucleus caudalis. The nucleus caudalis receives the majority of pain afferents and fibers from the face and oral cavity via the descending trigeminal tract. The nucleus has a unique organization in that the three trigeminal divisions are arranged in a laminar fashion beginning at the level of the medullary obex and extending caudally into the upper cervical cord segments. There is also a dorsoventral lamination of the three divisions, with the eye and forehead division (V₁) situated ventrally near the origin of the roots of the spinal accessory nerve while the jaw and lower cheek division (V₃) is dorsally situated with the central facial area division (V₂) interposed between the two. Lying along the lateral length of the nucleus caudalis are the ascending fibers of the spinocerebellar tract, which may be involved by the DREZ lesion, causing a transient ipsilateral ataxia of the arm.

Using a special DREZ caudalis electrode, it is possible to destroy the nucleus caudalis at the cervicomedullary junction and, therefore, interrupt not only the descending trigeminal fibers but the secondary trigeminal neurons and their central connections to the midbrain and thalamus. We have successfully reduced the deafferentation pain associated with post-herpetic infection of the

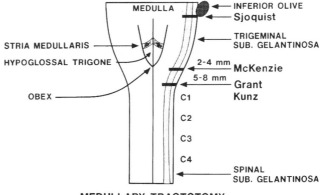

MEDULLA — INFERIOR OLIVE / Sjoquist

STRIA MEDULLARIS — TRIGEMINAL SUB. GELANTINOSA

HYPOGLOSSAL TRIGONE — 2-4 mm McKenzie / 5-8 mm Grant / Kunz

OBEX — C1 / C2 / C3 / C4 — SPINAL SUB. GELANTINOSA

MEDULLARY TRACTOTOMY

Figure 7.11. Schematic drawing of medullary cervical junction showing extent and merging of substantia gelatinosa from trigeminal system and spinal regions. Levels of section of descending trigeminal tract indicated with names of researchers at suggested DREZ lesion points.

gasserian ganglion as well as pain of anesthesia dolorosa by destroying the nucleus caudalis. A therapeutic DREZ lesion of this nucleus results in anesthesia over the entire trigeminal distribution of the face and oral cavity. Relief can be expected in half of the patients (17).

The major postoperative complication of a nucleus caudalis lesion is involvement of the adjacent spinocerebellar tract, which may result in ataxia of the ipsilateral

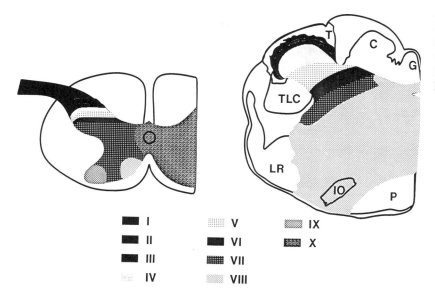

Figure 7.12. **Schematic cross-sections of cervical cord and lower medulla. Shows the similarities of the organization of the Rexed layers in spinal cord and medulla. The DREZ lesions in the cord medulla are produced in the Rexed layers I–V.**

■ I	░ V	▨ IX
■ II	■ VI	▨ X
■ III	▦ VII	
░ IV	▨ VIII	

arm. This complication has occurred in only a few patients and usually clears in a short time. The caudalis DREZ is a good example of DREZ lesions confined to a specific, well-localized anatomic structure such as the trigeminal system, thus relieving pain in a small, specific area of the face and/or oral cavity.

Thoracoabdominal Pain

Herpetic involvement with pain can also occur in the trunk or abdominal region and is more common than facial involvement. The pain of shingles is one of the most difficult to treat medically or surgically. When the pain becomes chronic (10% of patients), most therapy has been unsuccessful (18). In those patients with chronic post-herpetic pain, the DREZ operation has been successful in reducing the pain to manageable levels in 60% of patients.

Shingles is the result of a chicken pox infection, which may lie dormant in the dorsal root ganglion of the elderly, who most often suffer from this painful disorder. The viral infection is often triggered by nonspecific stimuli or stress, such as debilitating diseases, surgical operations, and radiation therapy, and by unknown factors. Shingles occurs three times more frequently in the octogenarian. The dermatomal distribution involves most frequently C3, T5, L1, and L2, as well as the ophthalmic division of the trigeminal nerve (V_1). The ophthalmic branch is affected with 20 times the frequency of the other two divisions of the trigeminal nerve.

Originally it was thought that the pathologic process resulting from the viral infection was localized only to the dorsal root ganglion, but it is now apparent that the virus also invades the spinal cord, especially the DREZ region, and at times even the motor neurons in the ventral horn are involved. We believe that the chronic pain

syndrome of herpes is due to the dorsal horn involvement, because the DREZ lesion of the involved DREZ area results in good pain relief in a significant number of patients.

The onset of the disease is heralded by a deep, lancinating pain appearing several weeks before the skin rash, which is a vesicular eruption occurring in the involved dermatome (thoracic region, 65%; facial region, 20%). When healing of the skin occurs, there are large scarred cutaneous regions that are painful. These cutaneously involved dermatomes outlined by the pathologic skin lesions are found to be grossly abnormal on sensory examination. The scarred areas may be hyperalgesic to light touch and pin prick with zones of complete hypoesthesia. Stroking the skin may activate the patient's pain, and patients often protect these skin areas from stimulation. The patient may also complain of another type of pain other than the lancinating pain. This is described as a deep, aching sensation often unaffected by skin stimulation. This deeper pain may not be involved by the DREZ lesion. It is therefore important for the physician to delineate the kinds of pain the patient is suffering before surgery is advised. If at times the patient experiences both the severe lancinating and the deep type of pain, he still may have partial benefit from the DREZ operation.

The DREZ operation for relief of post-herpetic pain in the thoracic and/or abdominal region requires careful planning by the neurosurgeon since it is essential that the dorsal roots lesioned are only those involved in the painful syndrome (19). The involvement of the thoracic dermatomes is surgically the most difficult since the anatomic localization of the thoracic dorsal roots is variable (Fig. 7.13). Both intraoperative radiographic and physiologic localization using evoked potentials is important for precise placement of the thoracic DREZ le-

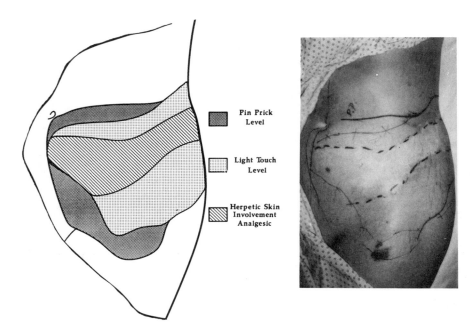

Figure 7.13. **Post-herpetic abdominal involvement with intractable pain. Post-DREZ lesion showing levels of postlesion dermatomes involving dorsal roots T11–L1.**

Pin Prick Level

Light Touch Level

Herpetic Skin Involvement Analgesic

sions. When the appropriate spinal cord segments are surgically exposed, the surgeon inspecting the spinal cord and dorsal roots may find that the involved dorsal roots have an abnormal appearance—atrophied and dullish red in coloration—under the operative microscope. Biopsy of these abnormal dorsal roots reveals specific damage to the larger myelinated sensory fibers with apparent sparing of the smaller (pain) fibers. The entire dorsal root appears to be involved, and we believe this involvement extends into the dorsal horn. For this reason the DREZ lesions are made in the DREZ of the involved painful dermatomes. The thoracic DREZ operation has the greatest potential for postlesion complication because the thoracic cord is sensitive to any type of surgical trauma. The major postoperative risk is weakness in the ipsilateral leg due to encroachment by the DREZ lesions on the pyramidal tract; this occurs in about 5% of patients. The best way to avoid this complication is to carefully control the size of the lesions, which we accomplish by the use of a specially designed thermal DREZ electrode along with the use of steroids in the postoperative period. It is important for the surgeon to warn the patient about this potential complication before the DREZ operation.

THALAMIC SYNDROME

The thalamic syndrome, first described by Dejerine and Roussy in 1906 (20), consists of severe, intractable burning pain with frequent exacerbations, either spon-

taneous or following mild tactile stimuli, as a sequela of an infarction affecting the thalamus. A similar pain may follow brainstem lesions, including tumors, or ablative neurosurgical procedures (21). The patient initially exhibits a "typical stroke" with a hemiparesis. There may be varying degrees of sensory disturbance on the paretic side of the body. As the hemiparesis clears, the patient begins to experience pain that is most often located in the head and arm on the paretic side. The patient often complains of pain centered deep in the eye. The pain is described as burning in nature and can be aggravated by touching the skin of the involved side. Emotional upsets also can often trigger the pain. Fortunately only 10% of stroke patients develop central pain, but when it is present it is difficult to treat. The pain frequently precedes other facets of the syndrome, and is often ill defined. Pain is constant, although paroxysmal, and frequently described as restricting, burning, or coming in waves. Hyperpathia, with varying degrees of stimulation either locally or at distant points being evocative, commonly occurs, with pain rapidly ascending to a crescendo, followed by a slow diminution. This pain is frequently refractory to medical and behavioral modification therapies.

Of the five principal groups of arteries that supply the thalamus (22), the thalamogeniculate stalk (inferior and posterior group) penetrates between the geniculate bodies to supply the nucleus ventralis posterior, anterior pulvinar, and centrum medianum. Involvement of this

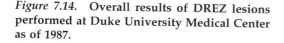

Figure 7.14. **Overall results of DREZ lesions performed at Duke University Medical Center as of 1987.**

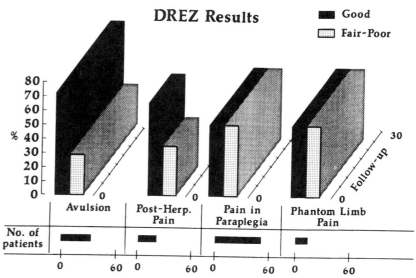

group leads to the classic syndrome of Dejerine and Roussy. The hemiparesis is usually transient, leaving hemianesthesia to light touch with profound loss of deep pressure sensation, the severe paroxysms of pain mentioned above, and mild ataxia and astereognosia on the affected side. Choreotaxic movements on the affected side are routinely seen. Vasomotor symptoms, consisting of cyanosis, hyperthermia, pallor, and diaphoresis, are not uncommon (23).

The nucleus ventralis posterior receives the spinothalamic tracts and the medial lemniscus in its pars lateralis, as opposed to the trigeminothalamic tracts, which terminate in the pars medialis. The head is medial with the body lateral in somatotopic organization within the nucleus. Most afferents from this nucleus are directed to the postcentral gyrus.

The pulvinar is mainly an association nucleus with afferents derived from the auditory pathways and nucleus geniculatus lateralis, although this is still under investigation. It has diffuse efferent pathways to the cerebral cortex and probably plays a role in speech formation.

The centrum medianum is divided into a dorsomedial pars magnocellularis, with efferents to the caudate nucleus, and the pars parvocellularis (ventrolateral), which projects to the putamen (23).

The thalamic pain described above has been reported with thalamic lesions in several locations (lateral formation, alone or with the medial nucleus or ventral posterior nucleus, or in the latter alone) (23). Of note, thousands of stereotaxic thalamic lesions have been made with only extremely rare reports of thalamic pain (24). The surgeon defines this by requiring additional lesions in the internal capsule or parietal lobe to explain the "thalamic" pain.

Several forms of surgical therapy for the thalamic pain syndrome have been reported, with varying degrees of success. Extirpation of the postcentral gyrus (25) as well as cervical cordotomy (26) have reportedly been successful. Partial pain relief was noted in one reported case using posteromedial hypothalamotomy (27). The same author has used thermocoagulation of the posterior internal medullary lamina of the thalamus with excellent results (28). Stereotaxic lesions in the pulvinar were completely successful in 3 of 11 cases (29). Pain perception is unaffected by interrupting pathways to the frontal lobes via prefrontal lobotomy (30) or cingulotomy (31), although the "suffering" component may be diminished. Bilateral amygdalectomies have had similar limitations (32). Electrical stimulation of the central gray matter (33), thalamus (34, 35) mesencephalic medial lemniscus (36), and periventricular gray matter have all been reported with varying degrees of success, limited mainly by adaptation, patient compliance, and expense (37, 38). Stereotaxic mesencephalotomy was first reported by Spiegel and Wycis (39), and its success in several series has supported its continued use in certain settings (40–43).

Sixteen of 24 (67%) patients in our series at Duke University Medical Center had long-term relief of their thalamic pain after mesencephalic tractotomy, with two deaths. None of 12 (75%) of those who had lesions made at the "superior colliculus" site reported significant long-term improvement. Seven of 12 (58%) who had surgery at the "inferior colliculus" site reported good pain relief. Postoperative disorders of ocular movement and difficulties with binocular vision have been reduced with recent improvements in technique (Colin Shieff, unpublished information; 44–48).

CHEMICAL HYPOPHYSECTOMY

Chemical hypophysectomy has been used by Levin and colleagues to treat three patients with thalamic syndrome (49). Two patients were significantly relieved of their pain with a follow-up of 19–58 months. The mechanism of pain relief is unknown. The authors suggested several theoretical possibilities. One is that the relief of pain is due to a humoral effect produced by the hypophysectomy on peripheral receptors. Another theory is that the humoral agent acts centrally to relieve pain. The use of pituitary ablation for cancer pain due to prostate and breast bone metastasis is well known, but more clinical studies are needed before hypophysectomy can be applied for the treatment of thalamic pain.

CONCLUSIONS

Our understanding and treatment of deafferentation pain has improved but is far from complete. The goal of the neurosurgeon is to devise surgical treatments that are localized to the site of pathophysiologic changes responsible for the pain, reducing adverse side effects to a minimum. This goal has been in part achieved with the DREZ lesions (Fig. 7.14), but much work is yet to be done in the laboratory and at the bedside.

REFERENCES

1. Tasker RR, Organ LW, Hawrylyshyn P: Deafferentation and causalgia. In Bonica J (ed): *Pain.* New York, Raven Press, 1980, pp 305–329.
2. Wall P, Devar M: Sensory afferent impulses originate from dorsal root ganglia as well as from the periphery in normal and nerve injured rats. *Pain* 17:321–339, 1983.
3. Rolando L: *Ricerche Anatomiche sulla Struttura del Midollo Spinale.* Torino, Dalla Stamperia Renle, 1824.
4. Rexed B: A cytoarchitectonic atlas of the spinal cord of the cat. *J Comp Neurol* 100:297–380, 1954.
5. Nashold BS, Ostdahl RH: Dorsal root entry zone lesions for pain relief. *J Neurosurg* 51:59–69, 1979.
6. Nashold BS, Bullitt E: Dorsal root entry zone lesions to control pain. *J Neurosurg* 55:414–419, 1981.
7. Friedman AH, Nashold BS: DREZ lesions to relieve pain related to spinal cord injury. *J Neurosurg* 1986, Vol 65, pp 465–469.
8. Olliver CP: *Traite de la Moelle epiniere et de ses maladies,* ed 2, vol 1. Paris & Brussels, Crevot, 1827, p 178.
9. Bastian HC: On a case of concussion lesion with extensive degeneration of the spinal cord. *Proc R Med Chir Soc Lond* 50:499, 1867.
10. Nashold BS, Vierira J, El-Naggar AO: Pain and spinal cysts in paraplegia: Treatment with drainage and DREZ operation. *Br J Neurosurg* 4:327–336, 1990.
11. De Reuck J, Alva HR, vander Eecken H: Relation between syringomyelia and von Hippel-Lindau's Disease. *Eur Neurol* 12:116–127, 1974.
12. Iannotti F, Scaravilli F, Symon L: Spinal haemangioblastoma associated with syringomyelia and multiple lung lesions. *Surg Neurol* 6:373–379, 1981.
13. Enomoto H, Shibata T, Ito A, Harada T, Satake T: Multiple Hemangioblastomas accompanied by syringomyelia in

the cerebellum and the spinal cord. *Surg Neurol* 22:197–203, 1984.
14. Probst A, Lotz M, Heitz P: Von Hippel-Lindau's disease, syringomyelia and multiple endocrine tumors: A complex neuroendocrinopathy. *Virchows Arch [A]* 378:265–272, 1978.
15. Long DM: *Current Therapy in Neurologic Surgery.* Toronto, BC Decker, 1985, p 161.
16. Shannon N, Symon L, Logue V, et al: Clinical features of investigation and treatment of post-traumatic syringomyelia. *J Neurol Neurosurg Psychiatry* 44:35–42, 1981.
17. Bernard EJ, Nashold BS, Caputi F, Moossy J: Nucleus caudalis DREZ lesions for facial pain. *Br J Neurosurg* 1:81–92, 1987.
18. Friedman HH, Nashold BS: Postherpetic neuralgia. In Wilkins RH, Rengachary SS (eds): *Neurosurgery,* vol 3. New York, McGraw-Hill, 1985, pp 2367–2368.
19. Friedman AH, Nashold BS, Ovelmen-Levitt J: Dorsal root entry zone lesions for treatment of post-herpetic neuralgia. *J Neurosurg* 60:1258–1262, 1984.
20. Dejerine J, Roussy G: Le syndrome thalmique. *Rev Neurol (Paris)* 14:521–532, 1906.
21. Currier RD, Giles CL, DeJong RW: Some comments on Wallenberg's lateral medullary syndrome. *Neurology* 11:778–791, 1961.
22. Lazorthes G: *Vascularisation et Circulation Cerebrales.* Paris, Masson & Cie, 1961.
23. Martin JJ: Thalamic syndromes. In Vinken PJ, Bruyn GW (eds): *Handbook of Clinical Neurology,* Vol 2. Amsterdam, North-Holland, 1969, pp 469–496.
24. Cooper IS: Clinical and physiologic implications of thalamic surgery for disorder of sensory communications, parts I and II. *J Neurol Sci* 2:493–553, 1965.
25. Erickson TC, Bleckwenn WJ, Woolsey CN: Observations on the post-central gyrus in relation to pain. *Trans Am Neurol Assoc* 77:57–58, 1952.
26. Frazier CH, Lewy FH, Rowe SN: The origin and mechanism of paroxysmal neuralgic pain and the surgical treatment of central pain. *Brain* 60:44–51, 1937.
27. Sano K, Sekino H, Hashimoto I, et al: Posteromedial hypothalamotomy in the treatment of intractable pain. *Confin Neurol* 37:285–290, 1975.
28. Sano K, Yoshioka M, Ogashiwa M, et al: Thalamolaminotomy. A new operation for relief of intractable pain. *Confin Neurol* 27:63–66, 1966.
29. Yoshii N, Kudo T, Shimuzu S: Clinical and experimental studies of thalamic pulvinotomy. *Confin Neurol* 37:87–97, 1975.
30. Freeman W, Watts JW: Pain mechanisms and the frontal lobes: a study of prefrontal lobotomy for intractable pain. *Ann Intern Med* 28:747–754, 1948.
31. Foltz EL, White LB: Pain "relief" by frontal cingulotomy. *J Neurosurg* 19:89–100, 1962.
32. Jelasio P: Relations of the lateral part of the amygdala to pain. *Confin Neurol* 37:53–55, 1966.
33. Gybels JM: Electrical stimulation of the central grey for pain relief in humans: A critical review. In Bonica JJ, Liebeskind JC, Albe-Fessard DG (eds): *Advances in Pain Research and Therapy,* vol 3. New York, Raven Press, 1979, pp 499–508.

34. Hosobuchi Y, Adams JE, Rutkin B: Chronic thalamic stimulation for the control of facial anesthesia dolorosa. *Arch Neurol* 29:158–162, 1973.
35. Richardson DE, Akil H: Pain reduction by electrical brain stimulation in man. *J Neurosurg* 47:176–194, 1977.
36. Mundinger F, Salamao JF: Deep brain stimulation in mesencephalic lamniscus medialis for chronic pain. *Acta Neurochir Suppl* 30:245–258, 1980.
37. Nashold BS, Wilson WP: Central pain. Observations in man with chronic implanted electrodes in the midbrain tegmentum. *Confin Neurol* 27:30–44, 1966.
38. Nashold BS, Wilson WP, Slaughter DG: Sensations evoked by stimulation in the midbrain of man. *J Neurosurg* 30:14–24, 1969.
39. Spiegel EA, Wycis HT: Mesencephalotomy for relief of pain. In: *Anniversary Volume for O Pitzl.* Vienna, 1948, p 438.
40. Amano K, Iseki H, Notani M, et al: Rostral mesencephalic reticulotomy for pain relief. *Acta Neurochir Suppl* 30:391–393, 1980.
41. Nashold BS, Wilson WP, Slaughter DG: Stereotaxic midbrain lesions for central dysaesthesia and phantom pain. Preliminary report. *J Neurosurg* 30:116–126, 1969.
42. Orthner H, Roeder P: Further clinical and anatomical experiences with stereotactic operations for relief of pain. *Confin Neurol* 27:418–430, 1966.
43. Voris HC, Whisler WW: Results of stereotaxic surgery for intractable pain. *Confin Neurol* 37:86–96, 1975.
44. Nashold BS: Mesencephalotomy. A current appraisal. In Voris HC, Whisler WW (eds): *Treatment of Pain.* Springfield, IL, Charles C Thomas, 1975, pp 121–131.
45. Nashold BS: Brainstem stereotaxic procedure. In Schaltenbrand G, Walker AE (eds): *Stereotaxy of the Human Brain,* ed. 2. Stuttgart, Verlag, 1982, pp 475–483.
46. Nashold BS, Gills JP: Ocular signs from brain stem lesions. *Arch Ophthal* 77:609–618, 1967.
47. Nashold BS, Seaber JH: Defects of ocular motility after stereotactic midbrain lesions in man. *Arch Ophthalmol* 88:245–248, 1972.
48. Nashold BS, Slaughter DG, Wilson WP, et al: Stereotactic mesencephalotomy. In Krayenbuhl H, Sweet WH (eds): *Progress in Neurological Surgery,* vol 8. Basel, Karger, 1977, pp 35–49.
49. Levin AB, Ramirez LF, Katz J: The use of stereotaxic chemical hypophysectomy in the treatment of thalamic pain syndrome. *J Neurosurg* 59:1002–1006, 1983.

CHAPTER **8**

NEURAL STIMULATION TECHNIQUES FOR CHRONIC PAIN

RICHARD B. NORTH

Since the late 1960s, electrical stimulation devices have been employed increasingly in the management of pain. Although the underlying mechanisms remain controversial, thousands of spinal, peripheral nerve, and brain implants, as well as a much larger experience with transcutaneous electrical nerve stimulators, have shown these techniques to be effective empirically in properly selected patients.

The pain-relieving effects of electrical stimulation have been appreciated since antiquity. In the first century BC, Scribonius Largus described the relief of pain by application of a torpedo fish to an injured limb (1). Medical applications were prominent in early investigations of artificially generated electrical current, beginning in the seventeenth century.

The modern era of pain management with electrical stimulation devices began in the late 1960s. Development of compact, solid-state electronics made portable, and even implantable, devices a practical possibility, and techniques for packaging implanted circuitry were already under development for cardiac pacing.

The publication in 1965 of the "gate theory" by Melzack and Wall gave new impetus to this form of treatment (2). According to this theory, the central transmission of neural activity signaling pain is governed by a spinal "gate," which opens in response to an excess of small fiber activity in the peripheral nervous system. Because the large fibers in a mixed population are more susceptible than small fibers to depolarization by typical rectangular stimulation pulses, they may be recruited selectively, closing the central gate. Stimulation to achieve this effect in the dorsal horn may be directed orthodromically, from peripheral nerve, or antidromically, via collateral processes from the dorsal columns of the spinal cord.

The gate theory has always been the subject of controversy (3), but the clinical methods it rationalized have succeeded empirically, to such a degree that their application continues to grow.

PERIPHERAL NERVE STIMULATION

The first clinical application of the gate theory, employing stimulation of large-diameter afferents to manage pain, was reported by Wall and Sweet in 1967 (4). Their initial series included patients with temporary electrodes implanted directly on peripheral nerve. Sweet and Wepsic later reported on selected patients from a larger series (5). At extended follow-up in 1976, with chronically implanted devices, sustained benefit was reported in 19 of 31 patients (61%) (6). Comparable results (45–79%) have been reported by other investigators, at up to 10-year followup (7–12). These series have emphasized the sequelae of peripheral nerve trauma and entrapment, treated with electrodes implanted proximal to the site of injury, as the most consistently successful application of this technique. In general, long-term treatment of pain attributable to lesions proximal to the site of stimulation, in particular lumbosacral radiculopathy, has not been successful (7, 13).

In routine clinical practice, candidates for an implanted peripheral nerve stimulator are screened by transcutaneous electrical nerve stimulation (TENS) trial, electrophysiologic testing (12), and diagnostic peripheral nerve blocks (14). Before a permanent device is implanted, stimulation analgesia is demonstrated in a trial with a temporary percutaneous electrode. For chronic stimulation, electrodes are implanted by open surgical technique, with direct visualization, and under local anesthesia whenever possible, to permit isolation of appropriate sensory fiber populations. Primarily to achieve mechanical stability, electrode arrays backed by cuffs of supporting Silastic and/or Dacron have been used. Although special electrode and cuff geometries and novel stimulation waveforms have been developed to achieve such effects as unidirectional action potential propagation for functional neural prostheses (15), these have not been employed to date in clinical pain management. Multichannel devices have yielded the same advantages as in other applications, by permitting noninvasive alteration of stimulation topography, to isolate the desired sensory effect. Because the threshold for motor effects may be critically close to the sensory thresholds in a mixed peripheral nerve, however, this remains problematic.

TRANSCUTANEOUS ELECTRICAL NERVE STIMULATION (TENS)

Externally applied electrical stimulation devices have been employed in the management of pain, and have been available commercially, for over a century (1), but the modern era of their application began only two decades ago, when they were investigated as screening devices for candidates for spinal and peripheral nerve implants (16). TENS alone proved to be adequate treatment for a substantial number of patients (17). Controlled trials, using placebo stimulation, have demonstrated a rapid decline in placebo effect shortly after institution of therapy, with profiles and incidence comparable to those seen in pharmacologic studies (18, 19). The art and science of electrode placement, and the necessity for extensive, trial-and-error determination of optimal sites in individual patients, are well documented (20). The applications of TENS have expanded to include postoperative pain (21) and acute as well as chronic pain caused by musculoskeletal, neurologic, and even visceral pathology (20). Although a minority of patients with chronic, intractable pain problems such as "failed back syndrome" will achieve adequate analgesia with TENS alone (22, 23), it deserves a routine trial in a program of conservative management, and in patients who are considered for implanted devices. A failure by such a patient to respond to TENS, although sometimes significant, by no means precludes a favorable response to an implant. Like other forms of electrical stimulation for pain, TENS is a reversible, nondestructive, relatively benign form of treatment, with few contraindications or significant adverse effects.

CONTRAINDICATIONS

1. *Implanted cardiac pacemakers.* Such pacemakers in "demand" mode may be inhibited if an artifactual signal is not recognized as such by R-wave sensing circuitry. Any implanted cardiac pacemaker should be considered a relative contraindication to treatment with electrical stimulation, unless special arrangements can be made for cardiac monitoring and/or the pacemaker can be operated at "fixed rate."
2. *Pregnancy.* Only limited data are available regarding the safety of TENS in pregnancy (20), and in labor and delivery; prudence dictates the restriction of its use in these conditions, pending further investigation.
3. *Inability to use the device.*

PRECAUTIONS

1. Application of TENS electrodes over the eyes, or in contact with mucous membranes, may be injurious.
2. Application over or near the carotid sinus, particularly in patients with cardiac or cerebrovascular disease, may provoke hypotension and/or bradycardia.
3. Application over the anterior chest of a cardiac arrhythmia patient, although never reported to have caused a complication, should be avoided, as should cephalic application in epilepsy and stroke patients.
4. Skin reactions, due to chemical and mechanical irritation, and sometimes allergy, are common with TENS electrodes; less commonly, they occur with radiofrequency antennas applied over implanted devices. Careful routine hygiene is essential.

MECHANISMS OF STIMULATION ANALGESIA

The analgesic effects of TENS delivered at conventional "low intensity" (12–20 mA) and "high frequency" (50–100 Hz) are not reversible by the narcotic antagonist naloxone in humans (24–26), but analgesia achieved with "acupuncture-like" low-frequency stimulation (2-Hz pulse repetition rate [27] or burst repetition rate [28]) reportedly is reversed. This implies separate mechanisms of action for these stimulation regimes.

The gate theory is countered by recent evidence that hyperalgesia is signaled by large fibers (29). The analgesic effects of stimulation, accordingly, might be mediated by an effect such as frequency related conduction block, acting on this fiber population (30). Although stimulation parameters employed clinically in peripheral nerve may (31, 32) or may not (33) achieve this effect locally, branch points are particularly vulnerable. The effect of spinal cord stimulation might occur at branch points of primary afferents into dorsal column and dorsal horn fibers. Such a mechanism would not, however, readily explain the prolonged latency and persistence of stimulation analgesia described by many patients with implanted spinal stimulators (34) (Fig. 8.1).

GENERAL CONSIDERATIONS IN PATIENT MANAGEMENT

Concurrently with improvements in hardware and technique, the diagnosis and management of chronic pain syndromes has been refined considerably, and programs specializing in this field have proliferated (35). In particular, the importance of psychological factors in comprehensive management, and in selection for surgical procedures, especially implantation of stimulation devices (36, 37), is widely recognized. Criteria for treatment with an implanted stimulation device have evolved, empirically, as follows.

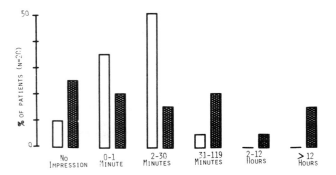

Figure 8.1. **Time lags associated with stimulation analgesia (spinal cord stimulation, 8-year follow-up)** *Open columns,* latency of analgesia after stimulator is turned off; *shaded columns,* persistence of analgesia after stimulator is turned off. **Most patients report that pain relief does not occur instantaneously when stimulation begins, nor does it cease immediately when stimulation ends.**

GENERAL INDICATIONS FOR IMPLANTED STIMULATION DEVICES

1. There is an objective basis for the pain complaint (e.g., myelographically demonstrated arachnoiditis).
2. Alternative therapy has been exhausted or is unacceptable (e.g., decompression, microsurgical lysis of arachnoid adhesions, ablative procedures).
3. Psychiatric clearance has been obtained and demonstrates motivation and long-term commitment (without major psychiatric or personality disorder, issues of secondary gain, serious drug habituation problems, or other abnormal illness behavior).
4. The topography of pain and its underlying pathophysiology are amenable to stimulation coverage (e.g., by spinal cord stimulation for radicular thoracic or lumbosacral pain, or by thalamic nucleus ventralis posteromedialis stimulation for facial anesthesia dolorosa). Periaqueductal gray stimulation will address diffuse, or axial, topographies.

An additional criterion for implantation of a device, required as a condition for reimbursement by some third parties, is that "demonstration of pain relief with a temporarily implanted electrode precedes permanent implantation." This requirement might be met, at least literally, by implantation of a permanent system in a single procedure, if pain relief is reported by the patient intraoperatively; but a high rate of treatment failures (and explants) would be expected. An extended stimulation trial with a temporary electrode has several advantages beyond simple patient selection (except in deep brain stimulation, where the logistics and the morbidity of insertion of new electrodes must be considered):

1. Its placement affords the physician and patient the opportunity to evaluate a greater number of promising stimulation sites more thoroughly.

2. Assessment of analgesic effect can be made under more physiologic conditions of activity and body position, away from the time constraints of the operating room.
3. Assuming the temporary electrode is removed (to minimize the risk of infection) rather than internalized for chronic use, this prior experience on the part of physician and patient expedites implantation of the permanent device, further lowering the risk of infection. Multichannel, programmable devices, permitting noninvasive selection of electrodes from an array even after permanent implantation, make this process easier.
4. Observations relevant to hardware choice for a particular patient can be made: For example, if a fully implanted, primary cell device is under consideration, its adequacy may be inferred from measurements of stimulation current requirements and duty cycle.

During percutaneous testing, and at follow-up assessments following implantation of a device, standard outcome measures should be collected, ideally by an evaluator independent of the surgeon, and blinded to parameters of treatment when feasible. Crossover periods without stimulation clarify the cause-effect relationship of treatment and reported relief of pain. Criteria for placement of a permanent implant (and for long-term assessment of the results of treatment) include direct estimates of analgesic effect, using standard analog rating scales; comparison with effects of prior treatments; and indirect measures such as analgesic use, functional activity levels, and (at long-term follow-up) ongoing health care needs and employment status.

SPINAL CORD STIMULATION (SCS)

The most common application of implanted neural stimulation devices has been spinal cord stimulation (SCS), typically delivered via longitudinally oriented electrode arrays in the dorsal epidural space. The earliest SCS electrodes (38) were fixed, flat arrays that required a laminectomy for implantation under direct vision (39, 40). In the typical patient with "failed back syndrome" or "post-laminectomy syndrome," these electrodes were implanted at upper thoracic levels, so as to provide stimulation coverage of all segments below the array (Fig. 8.2). Experience showed, however, that such broad coverage often was accompanied by uncomfortable thoracic radicular stimulation, and that electrode placement more caudally, which afforded more selective stimulation, was more effective. Optimal placement was facilitated with intraoperative stimulation of an awake patient, under local anesthesia, but this was cumbersome when laminectomy was required, and when the appropriate level of electrode placement for an individual patient was unknown preoperatively.

To determine the proper level of electrode placement

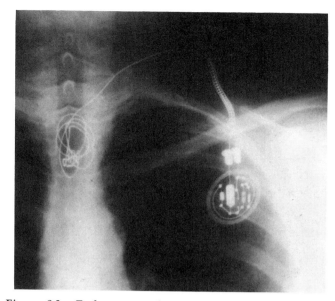

Figure 8.2. Early monopolar spinal stimulation system. High thoracic placement via laminectomy was typical.

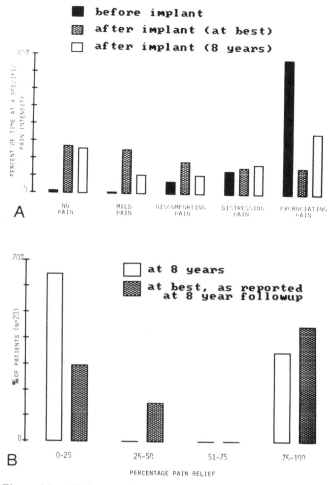

Figure 8.3. Eight-year follow-up on bipolar spinal stimulation systems for pain of lumbar arachnoiditis, expressed as (A) average patient's pain intensity profile, on an analog scale, and (B) direct patient estimates of overall pain relief.

in each patient, and to demonstrate analgesic effect prior to permanent implantation of a stimulation device, techniques were developed for percutaneous temporary electrode placement (41). These evolved into methods for implantation of permanent electrodes, obviating laminectomy in many patients. Multiple, individually inserted electrodes, however, often migrated spontaneously with respect to one another and with respect to the spinal cord, requiring surgical revision (34). The development of multiple electrode arrays that could be inserted via Tuohy needle, and improvements in electrode anchoring techniques, have ameliorated this problem (42, 43). At the same time, programmable implanted pulse generators were developed to take full advantage of these arrays by noninvasively selecting electrode combinations of stimulating anodes and cathodes. The topography of stimulation coverage may thereby be optimized after surgery. Even hardware failures such as electrode migration may be amenable to noninvasive correction with these versatile devices.

Under the general criteria described above for implantation of a stimulation device for pain management, the following have emerged as specific indications for SCS; they are listed in decreasing order of application and reported success rates:

1. Lumbar arachnoiditis (lumbosacral spinal fibrosis), a subset of failed back syndrome with radiculopathic pain, ideally predominating over axial and mechanical pain (43)
2. Peripheral vascular disease, with ischemic pain (44)
3. Peripheral nerve injury, neuralgia, or causalgia (including so-called "reflex sympathetic dystrophy")
4. Phantom limb or stump pain

5. Spinal cord lesions, with well-circumscribed segmental pain
6. Post-herpetic neuralgia

Results of SCS for failed back syndrome, including patients with documented lumbar arachnoiditis, have been reported by a variety of outcome measures, at follow-up periods up to 20 years (45): "Good" or "excellent" results are obtained in approximately half the patients reported in the literature (46). The long-term results (47) in our earliest series of patients treated with percutaneously inserted electrodes, adapted for chronic implantation, are representative. Figure 8.3 presents the largest subgroup of patients, those with intractable low back and leg pain following multiple lumbar spine surgeries, and myelographically documented arachnoiditis. At 8-year follow-up, 35% maintained excellent (75% or better) pain relief. This decline from our early (6-month mean) follow-up (34) reflects, in large measure, hardware problems with early percutaneous electrodes:

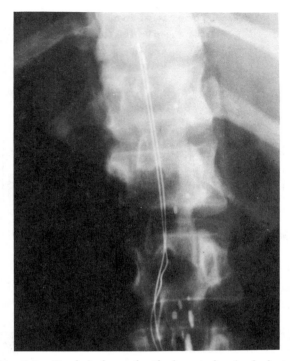

Figure 8.4. Dual, independently inserted spinal electrode systems are vulnerable to migration of either electrode. The result may be a short circuit, as shown.

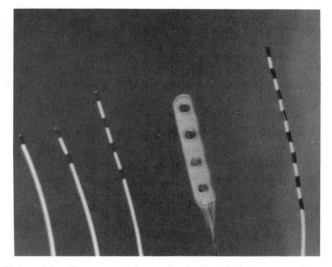

Figure 8.5. Representative spinal stimulation arrays, bearing from one to eight electrodes. Fourth from left is a laminectomy array; the others may be inserted percutaneously, through a Tuohy needle.

In our first 31 patients, followed over 21 months, we recorded 47 instances of electrode migration or malposition, 9 lead wire fractures, 5 lead insulation failures, and 1 receiver failure (47). Although many electrode migrations were radiographically demonstrable (Fig. 8.4), the total of 47 events requiring revision included patients whose topography of stimulation changed follow-

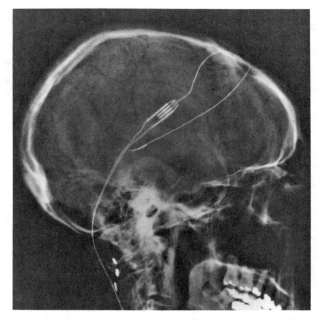

Figure 8.6. A typical deep brain stimulation electrode system, with four available stimulation sites, shown here hardwired in a fixed bipolar configuration.

ing surgery, when they were no longer in the artificial, prone position required for implantation. To an extent, therefore, this figure reflected the inflexibility of single-channel devices.

Because of the high incidence, in our experience, of technical difficulties with percutaneously inserted electrodes placed in tandem for bipolar stimulation, we resumed for some time the implantation of fixed endodural and epidural electrode arrays (Fig. 8.5) via laminectomy. The risk of longitudinal migration of these arrays is inherently minimal, but lateral migration or malpositioning is possible). We continue to employ this technique occasionally in patients with a prior laminectomy or epidural scarring at the level of proposed electrode placement, in whom the technical difficulty of percutaneous electrode insertion has been confirmed at a trial procedure with a temporary electrode. For the typical failed back patient, however, whose postsurgical scarring is caudal to the usual T8–T11 electrode site, percutaneous placement is straightforward. Currently available multiple electrode arrays, designed for insertion via Tuohy needle, are more resistant to migration (and immune, of course, to migration of one electrode with respect to another [Fig. 8.6]). Complemented by multichannel, programmable implants, permitting noninvasive postoperative adjustments of stimulating electrode location, these arrays rarely require surgical revision in our experience (45, 48). By comparison with single-channel devices, these systems have a significantly lower electromechanical failure rate, and significantly better long-term clinical results (45).

Prior to implantation of a permanent device, a trial with a temporary percutaneous electrode is undertaken. This is considered technically adequate when stimulation coverage of most of the patient's topography of pain is maintained for at least 2–3 days, so that its analgesic effects may be assessed fully, and reproducibility may be established. A simple monopolar electrode suffices for this purpose in most patients; its effects may, however, predict imperfectly the results of bipolar stimulation, which has technical advantages as the routine method of chronic implantation (49). Electrode placement away from the dorsal midline, and even ventrally, is more difficult technically, and tends to elicit uncomfortable motor responses at low threshold; it has not been the subject of any recent reports despite encouraging preliminary experiences (50, 51).

DEEP BRAIN STIMULATION (DBS)

The analgesic effects of stimulation via stereotactically implanted brain electrodes (in human supraoptic nuclei and septal area) were first described 30 years ago by Heath and Mickle and by Pool (52, 53). In 1960, Mazars et al. reported successful treatment of deafferentation pain by stimulation of the spinothalamic fasciculus (54); stimulation of specific sensory nuclei (55, 56) and of internal capsule (55, 57, 58) followed.

The antinociceptive effect of periaqueductal gray (PAG) stimulation was reported by Reynolds in 1969 (59), and given new impetus by the discovery in 1973 of specific opiate receptors in the central nervous system (60), found in high concentration in PAG (61). The phenomenon of "stimulus produced analgesia" has been found, in animals, to involve a descending inhibitory pathway, extending through the dorsolateral quadrant of the spinal cord; reversal by the narcotic antagonist naloxone, and the development of tolerance, with crosstolerance to morphine, has been described (62–67). In humans, the analgesic effect has been reported to be naloxone-reversible (68, 69) and to be associated with elevation of cerebrospinal fluid beta-endorphin levels (70, 71), but the latter has been attributed to an artifact produced by contrast ventriculography (72, 73). Mediation of this effect directly by endogenous opiate release, as opposed to other effects of stimulation, remains a matter of controversy; but the method has enjoyed continued clinical success in the management of chronic benign pain as well as cancer pain (74–78). Currently recognized indications for the procedure include the following:

Deafferentation pain syndromes, treated by thalamic electrode placement:

1. Thalamic (Dejerine-Roussy) syndrome, where the anatomic substrate remains for stimulation
2. Anesthesia dolorosa
3. Phantom limb pain
4. Postcordotomy dysesthesia

5. Pain of spinal cord injury
6. Brachial or lumbosacral plexus lesions
7. Chronic lumbosacral radiculopathy
8. Post-herpetic neuralgia

Pain responsive to narcotics, as determined by a morphine infusion test (75), may be an indication for PAG electrode placement (although this may not be a specific test [79]):

1. Chronic low back and leg pain (exclusive of radiculopathic, deafferentation pain)
2. Cancer pain (exclusive of gross infiltration of the peripheral nervous system, causing deafferentation pain)
3. Nonmalignant abdominal and perineal pain

Electrode implantation is performed stereotactically, using standard ventriculographic or computed tomographic techniques, under local anesthesia. In patients with unilateral deafferentation pain, the electrode is placed in contralateral sensory thalamus, in ventral posterolateral (VPL) or ventral posteromedial (VPM) nucleus, as appropriate for the topography of a particular patient's pain. Recording thalamic single unit activity is helpful in defining the target (80). Contralateral PAG or PVG is accessible through the same burr hole. Alternate sites have been reported (e.g., the nuclei of Kolliker-Fuse) (81). Following electrode implantation, stimulation is then delivered via percutaneous test leads to representative electrode combinations. Because analgesia may persist in some patients for 24 hours or more following stimulation, and a new electrode combination may be assessed only when the patient's pain has returned, the number of combinations that may be tested is limited in this (successful) group. If satisfactory stimulation analgesia is achieved, the system is adapted for chronic use: Under general anesthesia, the existing electrodes are connected to subcutaneously implanted electronics. If stimulation is ineffective, the electrode array is easily removed under local anesthesia.

The risks of the procedure, and their frequency of occurrence in the largest published series (75, 77, 82, 83), are as follows: *(1) Intracranial hemorrhage (2–4%),* which is potentially fatal (0–2%). Accordingly, patients should be screened rigorously for clotting abnormalities, particularly if cancer pain is to be treated in this fashion. *(2) Infection (3–6%),* which may require removal of implanted hardware. The use of programmable, multichannel implants minimizes the duration of the test phase with percutaneous leads, reducing this risk. *(3) Eye movement abnormalities (2–4%)* have not occurred when placement of the electrode tip remains rostral to the iter of the aqueduct of Sylvius. *(4) Hardware failures (2–12%)* range from implanted electrode migration to electromechanical and electronic failures, which may require reoperation. Programmable, multichannel devices permit noninvasive adjustments to correct for certain faults, such as electrode migration or malposition, and to optimize therapeutic effects and minimize the side effects of stimulation. Histologic analysis of autopsy material has shown no deleterious effect such as gliosis or parenchymal reaction along the trajectories or at the tips of the electrodes (84).

The results of treatment have been reported using a variety of criteria, among them direct estimates of pain relief, and indirect indicators such as analgesic use, patterns of stimulator use, functional capacity, and employment status. As reviewed by Young et al. (77), "success" was reported in the literature from 13 centers in 57% of 698 chronic pain patients treated with electrical stimulation of the brain: from 50% (83) to 80% (85) for thalamic stimulation, and from 0% (86) to 90% (87) for PAG/PVG stimulation. In the most recent literature on the treatment of cancer pain by these techniques, success is reported in 70–76% of patients (75, 78).

Deep brain stimulation is unique as a reversible, nonablative technique for central deafferentation pain states; and in patients refractory to peripheral nerve or spinal cord stimulation, it represents a worthwhile alternative, although its risks are greater.

IMPLANTED STIMULATION DEVICES

The prototypical neural stimulation device (Fig. 8.7), implanted in a large population of patients over the past two decades, is a passive radiofrequency (RF) receiver. It contains no battery or life-limiting components, and functions only when powered by an external transmitter. The transmitter emits RF (455-kHz–2-MHz) bursts, whose amplitude, duration, and frequency (repetition rate) determine the stimulation waveform delivered to the electrodes by the implanted receiver, which functions as a simple amplitude modulation (AM) demodulator. These stimulation parameters are adjusted by physician and patient to optimize analgesic effect.

The latest generation of devices permits selection of stimulating anode(s) and cathode(s) from an array of four to eight electrodes, thereby varying stimulation in the spatial, as well as the temporal, domain. Formerly, with single-channel devices, this could be accomplished only by surgical revision. This feature is invaluable, because electrode position is the major determinant of the topography of stimulation paresthesias, which for peripheral nerve, spinal cord, and thalamic stimulation should correspond to a patient's painful areas for optimal analgesic effect. In reported clinical applications to date, multichannel systems have been used not only to vary cathodal position to optimize coverage (48), but also to achieve specific configurations of anodes and cathodes more complex than dipoles. "Split anode" or "guarded cathode" configurations are preferred disproportionately by spinal cord stimulation patients (43), presumably because of a favorable current distribution (88, 89).

Because of the flexibility and redundancy of current multichannel implantable stimulation devices, implantation is expedited, technical success and clinical results are enhanced, and the rate of failures requiring surgical revision has fallen dramatically. As the flexibility and number of stimulation channels of these systems increases, however, the task of adjustment and electrode selection for optimal results grows disproportionately, far in excess of the 50 working combinations of anodes and cathodes possible with four electrodes. A general formula for this relationship may be derived as follows:

From an array of (n) electrodes, where $n > 2$, the possible combinations of (m) active and (n-m) inactive electrodes number $C(n,m) = n!/(n-m)!m!$

For each combination of m active electrodes, there are 2^m possible selections of anode(s) and cathode(s). This figure includes two open circuit configurations (all anodes, all cathodes); the number of useful configurations, therefore, is $2m - 2$.

In aggregate, the number of unique electrode combinations numbers

$$\sum_{m=2}^{n} n!(2^m - 2)/(n-m)!m!$$

For example, four electrodes permit:

$$12 + 24 + 14 = 50 \text{ combinations.}$$

Eight electrodes permit:

$$56 + 336 + 980 + 1680 + 1736 + 1008 + 254 = 6050 \text{ combinations.}$$

If "biphasic" stimulation (alternating complementary electrode combinations) is considered, these figures increase by 50%.

Clearly, as the number of available channels increases, the task of thoroughly evaluating potentially useful electrode combinations to optimize effect may grow tremendously, taxing the capabilities and resources of the physician and his staff. As a practical matter, in determining appropriate commercial transmitter settings for routine clinical practice, exhaustive assessment of all possible combinations is rarely necessary. In theory, and in practice, electrode combinations differing in minor ways (addition or deletion of one among multiple anodes, for example) are commonly functionally identical, and therefore redundant.

Like the task of postoperative (and even intraoperative) adjustment of stimulation amplitude and pulse repetition rate, electrode selection generally is managed most efficiently by the patient himself, given appropriate means of control, constraint, supervision, and data collection. For this purpose, we have developed a personal computer interface to standard RF-coupled implants, with supporting user-friendly, expert system software

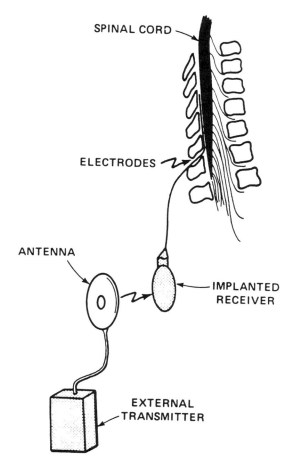

Figure 8.7. **A typical radiofrequency-coupled implant, as employed for spinal stimulation.**

for direct patient interaction (90, 91). The system incorporates commercially available RF transmitters (two four-channel, one single-channel), in routine clinical use for neurologic stimulation. The range of stimulation pulse parameters nominally available from the system is the same as is available from each commercial transmitter in its usual, free-standing mode of operation. The computer and interface simply allow automatic, rapid switching between standard pulse parameters to determine the optimal settings for the patient's standard commercial transmitter. The patient controls the system with simple pushbutton and slide potentiometer controls, designed for greater ease of operation than those of the standard transmitter. Patient responses and impressions are entered through similar controls, and through a simple graphics tablet that conveys topographic data. Comparisons of the perceived location of stimulation paresthesias with a patient's recorded pain topography may be made rapidly, automatically, and systematically, and psychophysical thresholds may be determined reproducibly. Protocols of varying complexity, which present stimulation parameters in random or pseudorandom order, may be implemented as required for each patient, and for each application.

For research purposes, the system is capable of changing stimulation pulse parameters (amplitude, width, interpulse interval) and cathode or anode postitions in as little as 1 msec. This will permit, for example, interleaving pulses delivered from different electrode combinations whose effects are complementary. "Modulation" of pulse parameters in simple, deterministic patterns has been described in the literature on TENS (92); the system allows not only this, but also modulation in a stochastic or even adaptive fashion.

With advances in lithium battery technology that permit a lifespan of a decade for a cardiac pacemaker powered by a primary cell, "totally implanted" neural stimulation devices have been developed. External hardware is still required for control; a permanent magnet commonly is employed for simple adjustments by the patient, and a dedicated programming unit allows full range of adjustment by the physician. Existing devices are limited to fixed menus of stimulation parameters, and lack the flexibility (in accommodating novel stimulation regimes) of passive, RF-powered implants. For spinal or peripheral nerve applications, whose energy requirements often exceed those of cardiac pacing by two orders of magnitude, currently available primary cell devices may not have acceptable longevity in some patients. Periaqueductal gray stimulation, on the other hand, typically requires a small charge per phase, at a low rate, with a duty cycle of minutes per day, well within the design specifications of these devices for a lifespan of several years. Automatic cycling on and off, as permitted by the latency of analgesic effect after the stimulator is turned on, and its persistence after the device is turned off, is among the strategies employed to maximize battery life.

STIMULATION WAVEFORMS

In clinical practice with standard peripheral nerve and spinal stimulation hardware, perception by the patient of stimulation paresthesias corresponding to the topography of pain has proven, empirically, to be a necessary condition for analgesic effect. Achieving specific stimulation coverage, without incurring uncomfortable sensory, reflex, or direct motor effects, requires careful attention to the position of surgically implanted electrodes (49). In a given patient, the final choice of stimulation parameters involves a compromise, and stimulation analgesia is often incomplete. At thoracic spinal cord levels, where electrodes are commonly placed to achieve coverage of multiple caudal segments, radicular thoracic effects may predominate. This relates to anatomic factors: (1) the proximity of entering dorsal root fibers to dorsal epidural stimulating electrodes, (2) the relatively superficial location of these fibers in the dorsal columns, within a few segments of their entry (93), and (3) fiber diameter, in that the mean diameter of fibers in fasciculus gracilis decreases at cephalad levels (94).

The effects of "stimulation" are not necessarily excitatory (95); with appropriate electrode geometries and stimulation waveforms, inhibition, blockade, or even unidirectional action potential propagation (15) may be achieved. Likewise, specific subpopulations of different fiber diameters may be selected (96). These effects have been modeled, and observed experimentally, in idealized peripheral nerve preparations, with directly applied and even circumferential electrodes. These are not, however, directly relevant to the most common clinical situation, spinal cord stimulation, which involves an anisotropic medium and electrodes that are neither directly applied nor circumferential.

Finite element modeling of electrical fields applied to the spinal cord and surrounding structures (88, 89) has yielded voltage and current profiles that correspond well to in-vitro measurements in primate and cadaver spinal cord (97) for electrode configurations currently in clinical use. This model has addressed only the simple case of cathodal excitatory effects, however; anodal blocking and effects of stimulation waveshape have not been considered. By superimposing a modification of the McNeal model of myelinated fiber excitation, the "spatially extended nonlinear nodal" model (98), one might predict the effects of waveform permutations for representative fiber sizes within the spinal cord tracts of interest. Selective activation of deeper structures, while sparing overlying structures, and selective effects on different fiber sizes are possible. With appropriate modifications to existing RF transmitters that compensate for the series capacitance in the output of existing receivers, a limited regime of novel stimulation waveforms might be tested noninvasively in patients with existing implants.

CONCLUSIONS

Neural stimulation techniques are employed with increasing success, in properly selected patients, in the management of chronic, intractable pain. The mechanisms by which they act, as presently applied, at different levels of the central and peripheral nervous system are poorly understood. Simple, monotonic sequences of pulses, of simple rectangular shape, delivered via simple electrode geometries have been applied to complex neural networks with remarkable empiric success. Further basic and clinical research to optimize this form of treatment may take advantage of (or must contend with) a literally infinite number of possible stimulation regimes. We now have the technology to pursue this intriguing research.

REFERENCES

1. Stillings D: A survey of the history of electrical stimulation for pain to 1900. *Med Instrum* 9:255–259, 1975.
2. Melzack P, Wall PD: Pain mechanisms: A new theory. *Science* 150:971–978, 1965.
3. Nathan PW: The gate-control theory of pain: A critical review. *Brain* 99:123–158, 1976.
4. Wall PD, Sweet WH: Temporary abolition of pain in man. *Science* 155:108–109, 1967.
5. Sweet WH, Wepsic JG: Treatment of chronic pain by stimulation of fibers of primary afferent neuron. *Trans Am Neurol Assoc* 93:103–107, 1968.
6. Sweet WH: Control of pain by direct electrical stimulation of peripheral nerves. *Clin Neurosurg* 23:103–111, 1976.
7. Campbell JN, Long DM: Peripheral nerve stimulation in the treatment of intractable pain. *J Neurosurg* 45:692–699, 1976.
8. Law JD, Swett J, Kirsch WM: Retrospective analysis of 22 patients with chronic pain treated by peripheral nerve stimulation. *J Neurosurg* 45:692–699, 1980.
9. Long DM, Erickson D, Campbell J, North R: Electrical stimulation of the spinal cord and peripheral nerves for pain control. *Appl Neurophysiol* 44:207–217, 1981.
10. Picaza JA, Cannon BW, Hunter SE, Boyd AS, Guma J, Maurer D: Pain suppression by peripheral nerve stimulation. *Surg Neurol* 4: 95–114, 1975.
11. Picaza JA, Hunter SE, Cannon BW: Pain suppression by peripheral nerve stimulation. *Appl Neurophysiol* 40:223–234, 1978.
12. Waisbrod H, Panhans C, Hansen D, Gerbershagen HU: Direct nerve stimulation for painful peripheral neuropathies. *J Bone Joint Surg* 67:470–473, 1985.
13. Meyer GA, Fields HLL Causalgia treated by selective large fiber stimulation of peripheral nerve. *Brain* 95:163–168, 1972.
14. Nashold BS, Goldner JL: Electrical stimulation of peripheral nerves for relief of intractable chronic pain. *Med Instrum* 9:224–225, 1975.
15. Van den Honert, Mortimer J: Generation of unidirectionally propagated action potentials in a peripheral nerve by brief stimuli. *Science* 206:1311–1312, 1979.
16. Long DM: Cutaneous afferent stimulation for relief of chronic pain. *Clin Neurosurg* 21:257–268, 1976.
17. Long D, Hagfors N: Electrical stimulation in the nervous system: The current status of electrical stimulation of the nervous system for relief of pain. *Pain* 1:109–123, 1975.
18. Long D: Electrical stimulation for the control of pain. *Arch Surg* 112:884–888, 1977.
20. Thorsteinsson G, et al: The placebo effect of transcutaneous electrical stimulation. *Pain* 5:31–41, 1978.
21. Vanderark G, McGrath KA: Transcutaneous electrical stimulation in treatment of postoperative pain. *Am J Surg* 130:338–340, 1975.
22. Deyo R: A controlled trial of transcutaneous electrical nerve stimulation (TENS) and exercise for chronic low back pain. *N Engl J Med* 322:1405–1411, 1990.
23. Loeser JD, Black RG, Christman A: Relief of pain by transcutaneous stimulation. *J Neurosurg* 42:308–314, 1975.
24. Abram S, Reynolds A, Cusick J: Failure of naloxone to reverse analgesia from transcutaneous electrical stimulation in patients with chronic pain. *Anesth Analg* 60:81–84, 1981.
25. Freeman TB, Campbell JN, Long DM: Naloxone does not affect pain relief induced by electrical stimulation in man. *Pain* 17:189–195, 1983.
28. Woolf CJ, Mitchell D, Myers RA, Barrett GD: Failure of naloxone to reverse peripheral transcutaneous electro-an-

algesia in patients suffering from acute trauma. *SA Med J* 53:179–180, 1978.

27. Chapman C, Benedetti C: Analgesia following transcutaneous electrical stimulation and its partial reversal by a narcotic antagonist. *Life Sci* 21:1645–1648, 1977.

28. Sjolund B, Eriksson M: The influence of naloxone on analgesia produced by peripheral condition stimulation. *Brain Res* 173: 295–301, 1979.

29. Campbell JN, Meyer RA. Primary afferents and hyperalgesia. In Yaksh TL (ed): *Spinal Afferent Processing.* New York, Plenum Publishing Corporation, 1986, pp 59–81.

30. Campbell JN, Davis KD, Meyer RA, North RB: The mechanism by which dorsal column stimulation affects pain: Evidence for a new hypothesis: *Pain Suppl* 5:228, 1990.

31. Campbell J, Taub A: Local analgesia from percutaneous electrical stimulation. *Arch Neurol* 28:347–350, 1973.

32. Ignelzi RJ, Nyquist JK: Excitability changes in peripheral nerve fibers after repetitive electrical stimulation. *J Neurosurg* 45:159–165, 1976.

33. Swett J, Law J: Analgesia with peripheral nerve stimulation: Absence of a peripheral mechanism. *Pain* 15:55–70, 1983.

34. North RB, Fischell TA, Long DM: Chronic stimulation via percutaneously inserted epidural electrodes. *Neurosurgery* 1:215–218, 1977.

35. Bonica JJ: Basic principles in managing chronic pain. *Arch Surg* 112:783–788, 1977.

36. Daniel M, Long C, Hutcherson M, Hunter S: Psychological factors and outcome of electrode implantation for chronic pain. *Neurosurgery* 17:773–777, 1985.

37. Long DM: A review of psychological considerations in the neurosurgical management of chronic pain: A neurosurgeon's perspective. *Neurosurg Q* 1:185–195, 1991.

38. Shealy CN, Mortimer JT, Reswick JB: Electrical inhibition of pain by stimulation of the dorsal columns: Preliminary clinical report. *Anesth Analg* 46:489–491, 1967.

39. Nashold BS Jr, Friedman H: Dorsal column stimulation for control of pain, preliminary report on 30 patients. *J Neurosurg* 36: 590–597, 1972.

40. Sweet W, Wepsic J: Stimulation of the posterior columns of the spinal cord for pain control. *Clin Neurosurg* 21:278–310, 1974.

41. Erickson DL: Percutaneous trial of stimulation for patient selection for implantable stimulating devices. *J Neurosurg* 43:440–444, 1975.

42. Leclercq TA: Electrode migration in epidural stimulation: Comparison between single electrode and four electrode programmable leads. *Pain Suppl 2* 20:78, 1984.

43. North RB, Ewend MG, Lawton MT, Piantadosi S: Spinal cord stimulation for chronic, intractable pain: Superiority of "multichannel" devices. *Pain* 44:119–130, 1991.

44. Broseta J, Barbera J, DeVera J, Barcia-Salorio J, March G, Gonzalez-Darder J, Rovaina F, Joanes V: Spinal cord stimulation in peripheral arterial disease. *J Neurosurg* 64:71–80, 1986.

45. North RB, Kidd DH, Zahurak M, James CS, Long DM: Spinal cord stimulation for chronic, intractable pain: Two decades' experience [Submitted].

46. De la Porte C, Siegfried J: Lumbosacral spinal fibrosis (spinal arachnoiditis): Its diagnosis and treatment by spinal cord stimulation. *Spine* 8:593–603, 1983.

47. North RB, Long DM: Spinal cord stimulation for intractable pain: Eight-year followup. *Pain Suppl 2* 20:79, 1984.

48. North RB, Fowler KF: Computer-controlled, patient-interactive, multichannel, implanted neurological stimulators. *Appl Neurophys* 50:39–41, 1987.

49. Law J: Spinal stimulation: Statistical superiority of monophasic stimulation of narrowly separated, longitudinal bipoles having rostral cathodes. *Appl Neurophys* 46:129–137, 1983.

50. Hoppenstein R: Percutaneous implantation of chronic spinal cord electrodes for control of intractable pain: Preliminary report. *Surg Neurol* 4:195–198, 1975.

51. Larson SJ, Sances A, Cusick JF, Meyer GA, Swiontek T: A comparison between anterior and posterior implant systems. *Surg Neurol* 4:180–186, 1975.

52. Heath R, Mickle WA: Evaluation of seven years' experience with depth electrode studies in human patients. In Ramey ER: *Electrical Studies on the Unanesthetized Brain.* 1960, pp 214–247.

53. Pool JL: Psychosurgery in elderly people. *J Am Geriatr Soc* 2: 456–465, 1956.

54. Mazars GJ: Intermittent stimulation of nucleus ventralis posterolateralis for intractable pain. *Surg Neurol* 4:93–95, 1975.

55. Hosobuchi Y, Adams JE, Rutkin B: Chronic thalamic and internal capsule stimulation for the control of central pain. *Surg Neurol* 4: 91–92, 1975.

56. Mazars GJ: Intermittent stimulation of nucleus ventralis posterolateralis for intractable pain. *Surg Neurol* 4:93–95, 1975.

57. Adams JE, Hosobuchi Y, Fields HL: Stimulation of the internal capsule for relief of chronic pain. *J Neurosurg* 41:740–744, 1974.

58. Fields HL, Adams JE: Pain after cortical injury relieved by electrical stimulation of the internal capsule. *Brain* 97:169–178, 1974.

59. Reynolds DV: Surgery in the rat during electrical analgesia induced by focal brain stimulation. *Science* 164:444–445, 1969.

60. Pert CB, Snyder SH: Opiate receptor: Demonstration in nervous tissue. *Science* 179:405–423, 1973.

61. Kuhar M, Pert C, Snyder S: Regional distribution of opiate receptor binding in monkey and human brain. *Brain* 245:447, 1973.

62. Basbaum AI, Fields HL: Endogenous pain control mechanisms: Review and hypothesis. *Ann Neurol* 4:451–462, 1978.

63. Liebeskind JC, Guilbaud G, Besson JM, et al: Analgesia from electrical stimulation of the periaqueductal gray matter in the cat: Behavioral observations and inhibitory effects on spinal cord interneurons. *Brain Res* 40:441–446, 1973.

64. Mayer DJ, Wolfe TL, Akil H, et al: Analgesia from electrical stimulation in the brainstem of the rat. *Science* 174:1351–1354, 1971.

65. Mayer DJ, Liebeskind JC: Pain reduction by focal electrical stimulation of the brain: An anatomical and behavioral analysis. *Brain Res* 68:73–93, 1974.

66. Mayer DJ, Hayes RL: Stimulation-produced analgesia: Development of tolerance and cross-tolerance to morphine. *Science* 188:941–943, 1975.

67. Mayer DJ, Price DD: Central nervous system mechanisms of analgesia. *Pain* 2:379–404, 1976.
68. Adams JE: Naloxone reversal of analgesia produced by brain stimulation in the human. *Pain* 2:161–166, 1976.
69. Hosobuchi Y, Adams JE, Linchitz R: Pain relief by electrical stimulation of the central gray matter in humans and its reversal by naloxone. *Science* 197:183–186, 1977.
70. Akil, Richardson DE, Hughes J: Enkephalin-like material elevated in ventricular cerebrospinal fluid of pain patients after analgetic focal stimulation. *Science* 201:463–465, 1978.
71. Hosobuchi Y, Rossier J, Bloom FE, Guilleman R: Stimulation of human periaqueductal gray for pain relief increases immunoreactive β-endorphin in ventricular fluid. *Science* 203:279–281, 1979.
72. Dionne RA, Muller GP, Young RF, Greenberg P, Hargreaves KM. Gracely R, Dubner R: Contrast medium causes the apparent increase in β-endorphin levels in human cerebrospinal fluid following brain stimulation. *Pain* 20:313–321, 1980.
73. Fessler RG, Brown FD, Rachlin JR, Mullan S: Elevated β-endorphin in cerebrospinal fluid after electrical brain stimulation: Artifact of contrast infusion. *Science* 224:1017–1019, 1984.
74. Duncan GH, Bushnell MC, Marchand S: Deep brain stimulation: A review of basic research and clinical articles. *Pain* 45:49–59, 1991.
75. Hosobuchi Y: Subcortical electrical stimulation for control of intractable pain in humans. Report of 122 cases (1970–1984). *J Neurosurg* 64:543–553, 1986.
76. Richardson DE, Akil H: Pain reduction by electrical stimulation in man (Part I). *J Neurosurg* 47:178–183, 1977.
77. Young RF, Kroening R, Fulton W, Feldman R, Chambi I: Electrical stimulation of the brain in treatment of chronic pain: Experience over 5 years. *J Neurosurg* 62:389–396, 1985.
78. Young RF, Brechner T: Electrical stimulation of the brain for relief of intractable pain due to cancer. *Cancer* 57:1266–1272, 1986.
79. Young RF, Chambi VI: Pain relief by stimulation of the periaqueductal and periventricular gray matter: Evidence for a non-opioid mechanism. *J Neurosurg* 66:364–371, 1987.
80. Lenz FA, Dostrovsky JO, Tasker RR, Yamashiro I, Kwan HC, Murphy JT: Methods for microstimulation and recording of single neurons and evoked potentials in the human central nervous system. *J Neurosurg* 68:630–634, 1988.
81. Hodge CJ, Apkarian AV, Stevens RT: Inhibition of dorsal-horn cell responses by stimulation of the Kölliker-Fuse nucleus. *J Neurosurg* 65:825–833, 1986.
82. Levy RM, Lamb S, Adams JE: Treatment of chronic pain by deep brain stimulation: Long-term follow-up and review of the literature. *Neurosurgery* 21:885–893, 1987.
83. Plotkin R: Results in 60 cases of deep brain stimulation for chronic intractable pain. *Appl Neurophysiol* 45:173–178, 1982.
84. Baskin DS, Mehler WR, Hosobuchi Y, Richardson D, Adams J, Flitter M: Autopsy analysis of the safety, efficacy and cartography of electrical stimulation of the central gray in humans. *Brain Res* 371:231–236, 1986.
85. Siegfried J: Monopolar electrical stimulation of nucleus ventroposteromedialis thalami for postherpetic facial pain. *Appl Neurophysiol* 45:179–184, 1982.
86. Amano K, Kitamura K, Kawamura H: Alterations of immunoreactive β-endorphin in the third ventricular fluid in response to electrical stimulation of the human periaqueductal gray matter. *Appl Neurophysiol* 43:150–158, 1980.
87. Boivie J, Meyerson BA: A correlative anatomical and clinical study of pain suppression by deep brain stimulation. *Pain* 13:113–126, 1982.
88. Coburn B, Sin W: A theoretical study of epidural electrical stimulation of the spinal cord. Part I: Finite element analysis of stimulus fields. *Biomed Eng* 32:971–977, 1985.
89. Holsheimer J, Strujik JJ, Rijkhoff NJM: Contact combinations in epidural spinal cord stimulation: A comparison by computer modeling. *Stereotact Funct Neurosurg* 56:220–233, 1991.
90. Fowler KR, North RB: Computer-optimized neurostimulation. *APL Tech Dig* 12:192–197, 1991.
91. North RB, Fowler KR, Nigrin DA, Szymanski RE, Piantadosi S: Automated "pain drawing" analysis by computer-controlled, patient-interactive neurological stimulation system. *Pain* [in press].
92. Mannheimer C, Carlsson CA: The analgesic effect of transcutaneous electrical nerve stimulation (TNS) in patients with rheumatoid arthritis: A comparative study of different pulse patterns. *Pain* 6:329–334, 1979.
93. Dyck PJ, Lais A, Karnes J, Sparks M, Dyck PJB: Peripheral axotomy induces neurofilament decrease, atrophy, demyelination and degeneration of root and fasciculus gracilis fibers. *Br Res* 340:19–36, 1985.
94. Ohnishi A, O'Brien PC, Okazaki H, Dyck PJ: Morphometry of myelinated fibers of fasciculus gracilis of man. *J Neurol Sci* 27:163–172, 1976.
95. Ranck J: Which elements are excited in electrical stimulation of mammalian central nervous system: A review. *Brain Res* 98:417–440, 1975.
96. Accornero N, Bini G, Lenzi G, Manfredi M: Selective activation of peripheral nerve fibre groups of different diameter by triangular shaped stimulus pulses. *J Physiol* 273:539–560, 1977.
97. Sances A, Swiontek TJ, Larson SJ, Cusick JF, Meyer GA, Millar EA, Hemmy DC, Myklebust J: Innovations in neurologic implant systems. *Med Instrum* 9:213–216, 1975.
98. Reilly JP, Freeman VT, Larkin WD: Sensory effects of transient electrical stimulation—Evaluation with a neuroelectric model. *IEEE Trans BME* 32:1001–1011, 1985.

CHAPTER **9**

ROLE OF THE PHYSIATRIST IN MANAGEMENT OF MUSCULOSKELETAL PAIN

ANDREW COLE
STANLEY A. HERRING

PHYSIATRISTS (GREEK *physis*, "nature" + *iatrikos*, "healing") are specialists in Physical Medicine and Rehabilitation who have been educated to distinguish pain and disablity (1). They prescribe comprehensive goal-oriented treatment programs that rapidly restore and optimize physical function and performance while relieving pain and minimizing the psychological, social, and vocational effects of disability and the risk of recurrence or residual disability. Physiatrists are committed to the rehabilitation of patients beyond an absence of symptoms. They are committed to the elimination of any residual weaknesses or abnormal biomechanics that could contribute to future recurrence of painful disorders even when the patient might not be symptomatic any longer. Physiatrists have also been specifically trained to assemble, direct, and coordinate a broad spectrum of health care providers who will implement the rehabilitation plan (2, 3).

BACKGROUND

During the infancy of physical medicine in the 1930s, Frank H. Krusen , M.D. introduced the scientific application of physical agents, including heat, cold, water, electricity, and assistive devices, for the rehabilitation of musculoskeletal disorders. Today's physiatrists routinely write prescriptions for the therapeutic application of these modalities by physical and occupational therapists. For example, appreciating that ultrasound, a deep-heating modality, has thermal effects that can increase collagen distensibility, a physiatrist may prescribe it for glenohumeral joint adhesive capsulitis to stretch the contracted joint capsule (4–7).

Dr. Krusen also demonstrated that therapeutic exercise can be scientifically applied in the treatment of mus-

culoskeletal and neurological disorders (2). Current physiatric prescriptions for exercise are as precise as those written for medication. The type of exercise is specified, as well as its frequency and duration. Side effects of the prescribed therapeutic exercises are discussed with patients, and precautions or contraindications are enumerated. A patient with a history of myocardial infarction who has acute low back pain with minimal motor loss due to a herniated nucleus pulposus would initially be referred to a cardiologist for clearance to undergo a therapeutic exercise program. Upon a review with the patient of the potential side effects of isometric exercise on cardiovascular health, the physiatrist would prescribe a program of these exercises to recruit the abdominal, spinal extensor, and associated muscles. Initially, three sets of five contractions for each exercise would be prescribed twice a day. The frequency, duration, and intensity of each set of repetitions would increase as the patient's pain decreased. These exercises should be performed within the available pain-free range of motion. A physical therapist would be asked to monitor any significant cardiac side effects that were listed on the physiatrist's exercise prescription. The therapist would also be asked to monitor increased weakness, a sign of deterioration of the patient's neurologic status (8–10).

The next major advance in physical medicine took place during World War II. Physiatrists, confronted with catastrophic injuries, soon found that physical agents were not enough to meet the condition of their patients. Howard Rusk , M.D. introduced psychological, social, and vocational interventions that helped patients meet the significant physical challenges that their adjustment and reintegration into society demanded. In 1949, as a reflection of the expanded nature of Physical

Medicine, the field was officially renamed Physical Medicine and Rehabilitation (2).

Since becoming a certified medical specialty in 1949, the number of board-certified physiatrists has expanded exponentially to keep pace with the demands of an increasingly active aging population (2). New residency programs have been established and existing programs have been expanded to meet this need. In addition, subspecialty training is flourishing in many areas including electrodiagnostic medicine, sports injury, spine injury, industrial injury, spinal cord injury, stroke, amputation, pediatrics, and traumatic brain injury (2, 11). Finally, an ever-increasing emphasis has been placed on research to further validate rehabilitation techniques already in use and to develop new ones (2, 11–13).

THE MAKING OF A PHYSIATRIST

Physiatrists are trained as experts who distinguish pain, disease, impairment, disability, and handicap so that specific short- and long-term goals can be most efficiently achieved by the health care team that they assemble. Their patient evaluations include all aspects of the traditional general medical history and physical examination. The scope of the exam is more comprehensive, however. Whereas the short-term goals of the physiatrist's team may be to control pain and re-establish function, their long-term goals are to optimize function, improve the quality of life, and minimize disability, thereby enabling patients to assume responsibility for their conditions (2, 3, 14).

The foundation of physiatric training rests on postgraduate training in anatomy, neuroanatomy, neuromuscular physiology, pathology, pain assessment and management, pharmacology, internal medicine, psychology, biomechanics, kinesiology, therapeutic exercise, prosthetics, orthotics, therapeutic modalities, and specific testing techniques and their interpretation (2, 3, 9, 10, 15). This training provides an ability to diagnose, treat, and rehabilitate the many painful and disabling conditions commonly seen in physiatric practice such as *musculoskeletal disorders* (e.g., lumbar pain, cervical pain, sports-related peripheral joint injuries, myofacial pain, reflex sympathetic dystrophy, amputation), *neurological problems* (e.g., cerebrovascular accidents, traumatic brain injuries, multiple sclerosis, spinal cord injury), and *cardiopulmonary conditions* (e.g., myocardial infarction and restrictive lung disease). What sets physiatrists apart from other physicians, however, is their ability not only to correctly identify and treat the immediate and obvious consequences of disease and injury, but also to anticipate potential problems by rehabilitating the less obvious causes of dysfunction (e.g., subtle alterations in strength, flexibility, and biomechanics).

Whether caused by trauma or illness, *disease* is a pathological condition of the body defined by a particular collection of symptoms and signs. Disease may or may not result in functional deficit (1, 14). *Impairment* is "any loss or abnormality of psychological, physical, or anatomical structure or function" (1, 14, 16). When an impairment prevents performance of activities required for personal independence, a patient has a *disability*. The World Health Organization (WHO) states that a disability is "any restriction or lack (resulting from an impairment) of an ability to perform an activity in the manner or within the range considered normal for a human being" (1, 14, 16). When a disability or impairment prevents performance of patients' social roles, they are said to have a *handicap* (1, 14, 16). For example, Cindy, a 20-year-old college student, had an amputation below the knee that she sustained in an automobile accident because of a crush injury to the distal tibia and ankle complex. Because phantom limb pain interferred with her ability to use a prosthesis, she was unable to ambulate independently or participate in college classes or snow ski. Following successful resolution of her phantom limb pain through multidisciplinary treatment that included desensitization techniques, medication, electrical stimulation, ultrasound, and vibration, she received a below-knee prosthesis. She then learned to ambulate independently, was able to manage all self-care activities, and resumed her regular academic schedule. Subsequently, she purchased special adaptive ski equipment that allowed her to resume snow skiing, her favorite sport.

Cindy's *disease* was a traumatic crush injury of her distal tibia and ankle complex. Her *impairment* was the loss of the distal leg below her knee. Once her phantom limb pain was successfully treated, she learned how to use a prosthesis, thus overcoming an initial *disability* (i.e., her inability to walk to the bathroom). Ultimately, she overcame her *handicap*, the inability to walk to her college classes and to ski.

This example illustrates two unique aspects of physiatric care: the team approach and the special role that pain can play in disability. A health care team is a group of health care professionals from different disciplines who share common values and work toward common objectives (17, 18). Initially, the physiatrist was instrumental in orchestrating Cindy's preoperative and postoperative care. In the preoperative phase, the physiatrist prescribed medication for pain control and helped Cindy develop realistic expectations for the postoperative period. In addition, he ordered a physical therapy program designed to anticipate postoperative needs: upper extremity and opposite leg strengthening to help meet the increased energy demands that a below-knee prosthesis requires, and crutch-walking skills to aid in preoperative and postoperative ambulation. Finally, he discussed Cindy's specific functional needs—i.e., her sporting activites and long-distance ambulation with the surgeon and prosthetist. Therefore, arrangements were made for the prosthetist to be in the operating room for immediate postoperative temporary prosthetic fitting, thus shortening the recovery period. The physiatrist's postoperative plan included physical therapy to train Cindy in the use of her temporary prosthesis, one-leg crutch ambulation techniques, residual limb care, limb-wrapping techniques, edema control methods, and massage and desensitization techniques. Cindy was also trained in techniques to control residual limb pain. The physical therapist continued the programs for upper extremity and opposite leg strengthening for maintaining knee range of motion. An occupational therapist was requested to help Cindy with activities of daily living—toileting, bathing, and driving. A psychologist also played a critical role by helping Cindy adjust to the loss of her limb and the resulting changes in her life. Eventually, the prosthetist was asked to construct a permanent prosthesis and the special adaptive equipment that Cindy needed to ski. The physiatrist then followed Cindy on a routine basis to check her residual limb for skin breakdown, infection, neuromas, and edema, and to evaluate her prosthesis for any mechanical problems or wear and tear so that impending problems could be solved before they created further pain and disability.

Howard Fields defines pain in a clinical context as an unpleasant sensation perceived to arise from a specific region of the body and commonly produced by processes that damage or are capable of damaging bodily tissue (19). Cindy's phantom limb pain, due to amputation, created both a disability and a handicap. Fortunately, her situation was resolved relatively quickly. The physiatric management model is effective in managing complex conditions because physiatrists not only recognize and treat pain but also the associated functional changes and disability patients suffer.

Lumbar spine pain is the most common painful musculoskeletal complaint. It also has one of the highest rates of disability. "Low back *disability* syndrome" is the descriptive phrase most often used when discussing lumbar spine pain in patients in the workplace. However, because workers' injuries actually *handicap* them in the workplace (i.e., result in their losing their social/professional role), the syndrome might be more accurately called "low back *handicap* syndrome." Although there might be social and/or political implications in this change of terminology, there are no obvious implications for physiatric treatment. That said, we will continue to use the term "low back disability syndrome" to describe worker handicaps.

As Shelton and Robinson point out, epidemiologic data suggest that disability from back pain is rare in contemporary primitive societies and apparently was rare in the United States prior to this century (20). Beals and Hickman reported the relation between back injury, time off work, and chances of returning to work. Their research showed that the chances of an injured worker returning to work was only 50% for those off work for 6 months, 10% for those off work for 1 year, and virtually 0% for those off work for 2 years or more (20, 21). Vocational factors also play a role in low back disability. Lumbar spine disability is more likely to occur when a job is physically demanding, the worker perceives his work as "too heavy," or when the worker has little control over pacing tasks (20, 22). Shelton and Robinson also discuss the fact that low back pain disability syndrome cannot be fully explained in medical terms. The syndrome is a product of a medical problem and the patient's adaptation to it (20). Therefore, physiatric intervention has as its focus the control or elimination of underlying pain while setting realistic short- and long-term goals to reestablish and optimize function and quality of life. Primary physiatric goals are minimizing any associated musculoskeletal or biomechanical dysfunction, speeding recovery, and avoiding the possible downward spiral in which disabled workers never return to work, thus creating escalating costs to both the worker and society. As Gamburd points out, a physiatrist's base of knowledge allows him to "maintain a broad perspective about painful disorders of the spine, integrating the anatomic and physiologic information with psychosocial factors . . ." to establish a treatment program that will maximize symptom resolution and functional recovery (15).

A PHYSIATRIC MODEL FOR REHABILITATION OF MUSCULOSKELETAL PAIN

Overload injury to the muscle and the muscle-tendon unit is a common problem seen by physiatrists. In sports medicine, a subspecialty of physical medicine and rehabilitation, 30–50% of all injuries are secondary to overload (23–25). If traumatic causes are included in the evaluation, the injury rate increases.

Initial soft tissue injury first triggers an inflammatory response that is soon followed by tissue healing, repair, and remodeling (26–28). As a result of the inflammatory response, some of the symptoms and signs of soft tissue damage (e.g., pain, swelling, discoloration, decreased range of motion) may soon occur. Although the tissue may repair and remodel, changes in muscle function (i.e., strength, strength balance, flexibility, and proprioception) result in new adaptive functional patterns for a specific activity. These functional deficits persist beyond the resolution of the signs and symptoms associated with initial injury. A subclinical soft tissue injury may produce similar functional changes even without obvious pain and swelling. In this instance, the patient may report a change in athletic performance. Subclinical injury causes a decrement in performance due to less-efficient adaptive patterns that develop secondary to the remaining functional deficits. In fact, not only do injured tissues themselves undergo functional change, but dis-

Table 9.1.
Goals of Musculoskeletal Injury Rehabilitation

1. Establish an accurate diagnosis
2. Minimize deleterious local effects of acute injury
3. Allow proper healing
4. Maintain other components of athletic fitness
5. Return to normal athletic function

Table 9.2.
Types of Clinical Injury Presentation

1. Acute injury
2. Chronic injury
3. Acute exacerbation of a chronic injury
4. Subclinical functional alteration

tant supporting structures may undergo functional adaptive changes as well.

The rehabilitation plan must, therefore, address more than the pain of the initial injury. The plan must be oriented toward return of function, not just relief of symptoms. The goals of any musculoskeletal injury rehabilitation program are to (1) establish an accurate diagnosis, (2) minimize the deleterious local effects of acute injury, (3) allow proper healing, (4) maintain other components of fitness, and (5) return the patient to normal function as soon as possible (29) (Table 9.1). In addition, certain critical considerations may influence the rehabilitation plan. Physiatrists recognize that the clinical presentation of an injury will influence a rehabilitation plan. The four general categories of clinical presentation are (1) acute injury, (2) chronic injury, (3) acute exacerbation of a chronic injury, and (4) subclinical functional alteration (Table 9.2). Each of these requires a different approach during the acute and chronic phases of the rehabilitation process. When prescribing a rehabilitation program, physiatrists should be aware that physiological and psychological needs vary among different patient populations. Highly competitive athletes will require alternative training regimes during rehabilitation to help maintain peak flexibility, strength, and aerobic condition. Recreational performers may be more flexible in this regard. Therefore, the aggressiveness of a rehabilitation plan should be geared to the level of athletic demand.

A thorough rehabilitation plan geared to the clinical presentation of an injury and physiological and psychological patient needs requires physiatrists to make accurate diagnoses as soon as possible. Their diagnoses must be anatomically specific (e.g., impingement syndrome secondary to glenohumeral instability), *not* generic (e.g., "shoulder strain") so that the rehabilitation plan is structured to adequately and thoroughly address all aspects of the injury. Accurate histories help form initial differential diagnostic impressions that might explain degrees of pain and disability. Then, well-planned and focused physical examinations are performed. Working diagnoses, based on a history and physical examination, are a further refinement of differential di-

agnoses and will determine what additional testing may be required to arrive at a correct final diagnosis.

THE SCIENCE BEHIND THE GOALS

After a precise diagnosis, initial treatment aims to control pain and inflammation. The injured tissue may need to be rested and occasionally splinted or kept from bearing weight. There may be up to a 20% loss of muscle strength after 1 week of muscle immobilization and another 20% decline in residual strength with every subsequent week. Atrophy will occur even faster if a muscle is immobilized in a shortened position. Therefore, a prescription for absolute rest must be made only after careful consideration (30, 31). Immobilization may also cause significant changes in joint capsule, cartilage, subchondral bone, and bone-ligament interfaces (32). Although a year or more of aggressive rehabilitation may be necessary to reverse these changes, some tissues, such as articular cartilage, may never completely return to normal, even though joint immobilization may have lasted for as little as 8 weeks (31, 33).

Early use of the joint limits unwanted side effects that immobilization may have produced and also promotes proper tissue healing. Collagen fiber growth and realignment is stimulated by early tensile loading of muscle, tendon, and ligament, and the formation of adhesions is minimized (34, 35). Early motion also helps to preserve proprioceptive skills (34, 35). Relative rest and protected motion help meet the goals of rehabilitation by ensuring that the deleterious effects of prolonged immobilization are avoided while tissue repairs.

Physical modalities and medication can help promote healing and minimize the local side effects of muscle injury. Acute injury is best treated by therapeutic cold, which decreases pain and muscle spasm and causes arteriolar and capillary blood flow to diminish. The time required to cool an injured muscle directly depends on the depth of intervening fat and may vary from 10–30 minutes (36, 37). Compression and elevation of the injured soft tissues are also helpful. Therapeutic modalities that heat superficially (e.g., hydrocollator packs) or deeply (e.g., ultrasound) are best reserved for subacute or chronic soft tissue injuries (7). Acute pain is best treated by high-frequency electrical stimulation, which operates via the gate theory, and chronic pain by low-

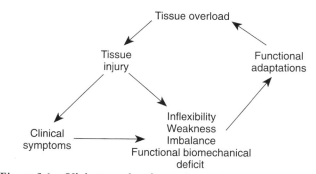

Figure 9.1. **Vicious cycle of muscle overload injury.**

frequency stimulation that causes endorphin release. Electrical stimulation can decrease muscle spasm by inducing post-tetanic relaxation as well as increasing circulation, which helps remove inflammatory waste products (38).

The antiprostaglandin effect of nonsteroidal anti-inflammatory drugs (NSAIDs) can be beneficial during the acute phase of a soft tissue injury. This biochemical effect may control an injury's inflammatory response and provide pain relief. The duration of a NSAID's analgesic effect may be different than its anti-inflammatory effect (39). Some authors have expressed concern that NSAIDs may actually interfere with the later stages of tissue repair and remodeling, where prostaglandins still help mediate debris cleanup (26). The dosage, timing and potential side effects of NSAIDs should be evaluated. Finally, it does not appear possible to predict patient response to a particular NSAID based on its chemical class or pharmacokinetics (40).

In addition to managing the local effects of a soft tissue injury, physiatrists prescribe appropriate alternative exercise programs such as cross-training. Cross-training helps patients maintain their flexibility, strength, and general cardiovascular fitness, and also decreases total rehabilitation time. In the case of athletes, sport-specific retraining is required before they return to play in order to help avoid reinjury. Return-to-play criteria include the resolution of tissue injury, clinical symptoms, and functional adaptation complexes. Patients must have full range of motion and adequate muscle strength, and must be able to perform sports-specific activities safely. Without an adequate and complete rehabilitation program that meets all five rehabilitation goals, the reinjury rate to the same or associated tissue complexes can be remarkably high (41, 42).

The goals of rehabilitation fit nicely into the tissue injury cycle described by Kibler (43) (Fig. 9.1). He identifies *five key components* of a soft-tissue injury complex that may occur with a musculoskeletal injury and that can create and prolong the symptoms and signs of injury. A complete and accurate diagnosis that accounts for the distant adaptations and biomechanical alter-

ations of the injury in addition to the local manifestations of the injury will allow a focused yet comprehensive rehabilitation program to be prescribed. A *tissue overload complex* is that group of tissues subject to tensile or eccentric overloads that may create and prolong symptoms and disability. A *tissue injury complex* is the specific area of tissue damage. A *clinical symptom complex* refers to those symptoms and signs (e.g., pain, swelling, weakness, instability) that were created by the tissue injury complex. A *functional biomechanical deficit* is a combination of specific muscle inflexibilities, weaknesses, and imbalances that cause inefficient performance mechanics. A *functional adaptation complex* represents a set of functional substitutions that the patient employs to maintain performance (43). Using this model to analyze soft tissue injury insures treatment of the obvious painful injury as well as that of any associated subtle biomechanical deficits and functional adaptations that might create further pain and disability. When examining patients who are subject to cumulative trauma (e.g, typists who take longer to type a given length of text or swimmers with an increase in performance times), physiatrists search for historical clues that suggest decreased efficiency and performance drop-off. Changes in efficiency and performance that are not accompanied by pain are the hallmarks of subclinical injury. In these instances, the physiatric task is to uncover all the underlying biomechanical deficits and functional adaptations that decrease patient efficiency and performance. An appropriate rehabilitation program that prevents overt, painful soft tissue failure will then be prescribed (29, 43, 44).

A CASE PRESENTATION OF MUSCULOSKELETAL PAIN

The following presentation will demonstrate how physiatrists manage musculoskeletal pain. A 42-year-old left-handed banker who had been swimming competitively at the Master's level for 15 years presents with a 2-year history of intermittent left anterolateral shoulder pain. The pain is exacerbated during the entry and early pull phases of freestyle, and is felt less during the late pull and early recovery phases. His regular medical doctor has prescribed NSAIDs and rest. Although helping to eliminate his symptoms after each rest period, in the first few days of swimming the patient's pain soon recurred. It got progressively worse with each painful episode. The sports medicine specialist whom he next saw recommended the same treatment plus a brief course of physical therapy using weight machines for rotator cuff strengthening. During his most recent painful flare-up, he sees a physiatrist. The patient's pain is in the same location as in earlier episodes, but is more intense and has forced him to stop swimming. His chronic low back pain would worsen shortly after his shoulder symptoms would flare. Plain radiographs of the left shoulder demonstrated only minimal narrowing of the subacromial interval, and radiographs of the lumbar spine revealed L4-L5 intervertebral disk space narrowing and small vertebral endplate osteophytes both anteriorly and posteriorly at the same level. A recent magnetic resonance imaging (MRI) scan showed minimal dessication of the L4-L5 disk, but no disk herniation.

The physiatrist's physical examination was thorough yet focused and was guided by his understanding of swimming biomechanics. His evaluation was also guided by the way in which repetitive microtrauma can place particular structures in the spine and shoulder complex in jeopardy. The patient had a typical swimmer's posture with rounded shoulders, forward displaced head, increased thoracic kyphosis, and increased lumbar lordosis. He had normal, left shoulder active range of motion with pain in the anterolateral acromial region at roughly 90° of abduction. He also had pain at the end ranges of forward flexion and abduction. Passive range of motion revealed inflexibility of the internal rotators. Anterior glenohumeral instability was present as well as lateral scapular slide. The lateral scapular slide test measures the ability of the posterior shoulder muscles to stabilize and position the scapula. The test is a static measurement of scapular stability in three positions: (1) at relative rest with one's arms by one's side in neutral rotation, (2) with one's hands on one's hips (thumbs pointed posteriorly), thus requiring some shoulder internal rotation and upper trapezius activity, and (3) with one's arm abducted 90° and internally rotated to its extreme, presenting maximum challenge to the shoulder stabilizers and requiring upper and lower trapezius and serratus anterior function. Bilateral measurements in each of these three positions should be made from the spine to the medial border of the scapula. With abnormal scapular stabilization, a difference of greater than 1 cm between sides in positions 2 or 3 is associated with onset of pain and decrease in shoulder function (45).

Evaluation of the patient's lumbar spine revealed normal range of motion, but he had compaints of pain at end-range extension and flexion and hypomobility from L4 to S1 with bilateral lateral bending. There were no signs of dural tension. Manual examination of his lumbar spine revealed decreased spring at L4 with reproduction of his low back pain. Deep palpation over the bilateral L4-L5 and L5-S1 facets also reproduced a component of his pain. Neurologic examination was normal with the following abnormal findings: pain inhibited the testing of the left supraspinatous muscle and there was a 5-/5 weakness of the left external rotators.

The model of the tissue injury cycle helped the physiatrist precisely define the patient's injury. The patient had an acute exacerbation of a chronic shoulder injury. The *tissue overload complex* consisted of tensile loading of the posterior shoulder capsule and muscles as well as the scapular stabilizers. The *tissue injury complex* in-

Table 9.3.
Swimming Stroke Phases (Freestyle)

I. Entry phase
  A. Hand entry
  B. Hand submersion ("ride")
II. Pull phase
  A. Insweep
  B. Outsweep
  C. Finish
III. Recovery phase
  A. Exit
  B. Arm swing

cluded rotator cuff tendon dynamic impingement, anterior glenoid labrum attrition, and anterior capsule stretch and inflammation. The *clinical symptom complex* included dynamic subacromial impingement pain, and anterior-superior glenohumeral instability. In addition, decreased swimming speed resulted from decreased power developed during the pull phase. The *functional biomechanical deficits* were tight internal rotators, rounded shoulders, and strength deficits in the left shoulder scapular stabilizers. When the external and internal rotators were compared, decreased strength in the external rotators was found, a strength differential that created a muscle imbalance. The *substitute activity complex* included a recovery phase using a shortened and lowered left arm, and a shortened and less powerful pull phase using decreased internal rotation of the shoulder. Entry, pull, and recovery phases made with left-arm lateral drift from the midline and continued humeral external rotation of the left arm were also part of this complex (Table 9.3).

The model of the tissue injury cycle helped the physiatrist discern that the patient's recurring shoulder pain was due to extrinsic impingement secondary to glenohumeral instability. His shoulder pain would therefore respond most favorably to conservative management and not to surgical intervention. As discussed by Fu et al., there are extrinsic and intrinsic causes of rotator cuff tendinitis (Fig. 9.2). The extrinsic causes may be either primary or secondary. A primary extrinsic cause of rotator cuff tendinitis is repetitive mechanical impingement of the rotator cuff tendons by structures other than the rotator cuff itself (e.g., by the coracoacromial arch). This mechanical impingement may be a result of alterations on the undersurface of the anterior one-third of the acromion, the coracoacromial ligament, or the acromioclavicular joint. A secondary extrinsic cause of rotator cuff tendinitis is glenohumeral or functional scapular instability, which causes a relative decrease in the volume of the supraspinatus outlet under the coracoacromial arch. Instability is most commonly seen in

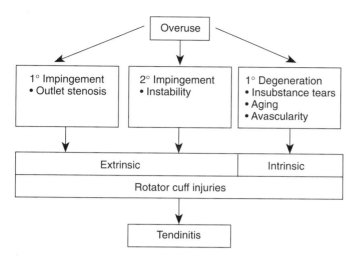

Figure 9.2. **Etiology of rotator cuff tendinitis. Tendinitis is multifactorial and not just due to primary impingement. Extrinsic causes are from outside the rotator cuff. Intrinsic causes are a primary breakdown of the cuff. Extrinsic and intrinsic injuries to the rotator cuff are exacerbated by overuse syndromes. Primary and secondary causes of impingment lead to an indistinguishable tendinitis pattern.**

younger throwing athletes or swimmers. The overhead activities of these athletes cause progressive stretch and damage to the posterior capsular structures, thus allowing anterior-superior glenohumeral instability to occur. In addition, the rounded shoulder posture caused by overdevelopment of the internal rotators (i.e., supraspinatous, pectoralis major and minor, and latissimus dorsi) and by a relative weakness in external rotator muscular strength (i.e., infraspinatous, teres minor) further narrows the supraspinatous outlet. This narrowing magnifies the effect of the instability. Intrinsic causes of rotator cuff tendinitis are due to degeneration of the cuff itself. This degeneration may be the result of overstress impingement of the tendons and diminished blood supply at the hypovascular insertion zone of the supraspinatous tendon into the humeral head. The contribution of this avascularity to inflammation is compounded by aging (46).

Both primary and secondary causes of extrinsic rotator cuff tendinitis can produce similar, and frequently indistinguishable, patterns of tendinitis. The precise cause of tendinitis must be determined in order to provide appropriate treatment. Primary extrinsic impingement responds favorably to surgical treatment if conservative care fails, whereas secondary extrinsic impingement responds well to aggressive conservative management but poorly to surgery (46).

Chronic soft tissue injuries cause functional biomechanical deficits and substitute activity patterns to develop. Therefore, the major focus of this patient's rehabilitation program must extend well beyond symptom relief. He must be rehabilitated beyond an absence of

symptoms. His rotator cuff tissue damage should dissipate with conservative measures that promote healing and minimize side effects. Repair of the tissue injury is only the first goal of his rehabilitation plan. Functional disability will persist until overall strength, proper glenohumeral flexibility, and balance of bilateral shoulder girdle strength occurs. Technique re-training, general conditioning, and a plan for sports-specific return to activity must also be implemented. If his functional biomechanical defects and resultant substitute activity patterns are not addressed, performance dropoff, recurrent injury, or both may occur.

According to Kibler et al., the rehabilitation of soft tissue injuries and their associated deficits can be divided into three parts: (1) an acute phase, (2) a recovery phase, and (3) a maintenance phase (44). Each phase is designed to sequentially address specific aspects of the tissue injury cycle. During the acute phase of rehabilitation, tissue injury and clinical symptom complexes are treated. The goals of this phase are to reduce pain and inflammation, re-establish nonpainful range of motion, improve neuromuscular control of the scapula when in neutral glenohumeral position, and retard the muscle atrophy of the entire upper extremity. Both pain and inflammation can be treated with judicious use of NSAIDs for a short period of time as well as with appropriate choices of modalities. Ultrasound can stimulate tissue regeneration, promote soft tissue repair, increase blood flow to damaged tissue to provide needed nutrients to the healing tissue and aid in the removal of inflammatory byproducts, increase soft tissue distensibility, and decrease muscle spasm and pain (4–7). Electrical stimulation techniques including transcutaneous electrical nerve stimulation (TENS), high-voltage pulsed galvanic stimulation (HVPGS), interferential electrical stimulation, and minimal electrical noninvasive stimulation (MENS) have been reported to promote analgesia, muscle relaxation, resolution of edema, and wound healing, as well as to retard inflammation and muscle atrophy (38). The application of low-energy lasers, electro-acuscope, and neuroprobe, which are newer and less-traditional modalities for the management of pain associated with sports injuries, awaits well-controlled prospective studies to determine their mechanism of action and their efficacy (47).

During the acute phase of rehabilitation, techniques for joint protection are also taught to help prevent the untoward motion and muscle recruitment that could further damage affected tissues. Joint mobilization techniques can also promote healing. Repetitive passive joint oscillations at the limit of the joint's available range can have a mechanical effect on joint mobility by moving the joint tissue into the area of plastic deformation of the stress-strain curve (48). Mechanically controlled passive or active movements of joints improve the rate of tendon repair and the gliding function within tendon sheaths during repair (49). Neurological effects of these passive mobilization techniques include restoration of axonal transport, stimulation of large-fiber joint afferents, and stimulation of clinically effective endorphins (50–52). Passive joint mobilization techniques stretch and lubricate tissues and induce metabolic changes in soft tissue, cartilage, and bone (53, 54). Passive range of motion helps improve the flexibility of tight structures and begins to restore appropriate tissue length and strength to the glenohumeral, sternoclaviclar, acromioclavicular, and scapulothoracic joints and their supporting structures. Manual capsular stretching and cross-friction massage can help to break-up adhesions and improve tendon motion and soft tissue flexibility (55, 56). Active range of motion is produced with Codman's exercises, ropes, and pulleys. When using these devices, care should be taken so as not to increase mobility in structures that are already hypermobile. Muscle atrophy at the site of injury is retarded and neuromuscular control reinstituted by using isometric exercises, scapular control techniques, and closed-chain activities (57). Distant nonpathological structures are also trained through concentric and eccentric open-chain exercises. Criteria for advancement to the recovery phase of rehabilitation include no swelling, the ability to exercise through limited range of motion in pain-free patterns, manual muscle strength at 75% of other muscles, and scapular control in neutral position (44).

The recovery phase of rehabilitation addresses tissue overload and functional biomechanical deficit complexes. The goals of this phase are to help patients regain and improve upper-extremity muscle strength, improve upper-extremity neuromuscular control, normalize shoulder arthrokinematics in single planes of motion, and improve active/passive range of motion and flexibility. Complete resolution of the tissue injury and clinical symptom complexes is necessary in the early recovery phase. Attention should be focused on appropriate loading of the involved tendon and its muscle (58, 59). Physical modalities and NSAIDs are probably unnecessary in this phase. Scapular and glenohumeral proprioceptive neuromuscular facilitation techniques improve general and sport-specific coordination and strength. Independent single-plane motions are emphasized through concentric and eccentric isotonic, isokinetic, tube, pulley, and rotator cuff isolation exercises. The protected range is increased until both passive and active full range of motion and local strength are achieved. Balance between force couples is reached by selectively training specific force couples (e.g., scapular retractors/protractors, glenohumeral elevators/depressors, and glenohumeral internal/external rotators) before extending the program to the entire kinetic chain (60, 61). Criteria for advancement to the maintenance phase include full nonpainful scapulothoracic motion, almost full nonpainful glenohumeral motion, normal scapular stabilizer strength, lat-

eral slide asymmetry less than 0.5 cm, and rotator cuff strength that is 75% of normal.

Maintenance is the final phase of rehabilitation. The goals of this phase are to increase power and endurance in the injured upper extremity, increase normal multiple-plane neuromuscular control by eliminating any functional adaptations and biomechanical deficits, and enable patients to return to unrestricted sport-specific aquatic activities (44). By this phase, patients should have developed sufficient strength and range of motion to begin stroke retraining. Additional patterned motion training using tubing is recommended because it permits enough freedom of movement to mimic swimming patterns. These activities should be performed in front of a wall mirror to further enhance proprioceptive feedback. In addition, specific types of equipment (e.g., the Swim Bench) help to develop strength, endurance, and specific stroke mechanics. Criteria for return to unrestricted competition include normal swimming stroke mechanics, full range of motion, and normal balances of strength and flexibility.

The other musculoskeletal complaint that the patient presented with, an increase in lumbar spine pain, must also be dealt with. Treatment of this complaint should occur simultaneously with the program for shoulder rehabilitation. Simultaneous treatment will insure rapid and complete rehabilitation. Although the details of the tissue injury cycle as it applies to lumbar spine pain are beyond the scope of this chaper, there are certain important points that deserve to be mentioned. Because the entire musculoskeletal system behaves as a functionally linked kinetic chain, a tissue injury and its localized functional biomechanical deficits can produce functional biomechanical adaptations at locations some distance from the primary site of injury. In this patient's case, the instability in his left shoulder and the resulting pain produced subtle yet important changes in his stroke mechanics. These changes had an indirect, yet definite effect on his lumbar spine.

This patient's freestyle stroke underwent many adaptations to avoid further pain due to impingement. He lowered his left arm height above water during the recovery phase and externally rotated his humerus, thus allowing his hand to enter the water palm-down rather than thumb-down. He also allowed his hand to enter the water farther away from the midline. By lowering his arm during the recovery phase, he had to increase the roll of his upper body in order to breathe. The increased roll made it impossible for him to move the lumbar, thoracic, and cervical parts of his spine as a unit (i.e., using "log-roll" or nonsegmental motion). This biomechanical adaptation resulted in an increase in segmental rotation through his lumbar spine. Because he externally rotated his humerus to minimize further loss of supraspinatous outlet space and subacromial impingement, his hand entered the water palm-down. The net effect was to increase the amount of segmental motion (i.e., twist) through his lumbar spine. Widening the entry phase position caused his trunk to rotate away from the entry phase side, which increased the amount of lateral flexion and segmental motion through the lumbar spine. He also adopted a crossover kick to offset the segmental rotation produced through his lumbar spine. Unfortunately, the crossover kick only served to further increase the amount of lateral flexion and segmental motion through his lumbar spine (62–64). The increased forces placed across his dysfunctional L4-L5 motion segment resulted in lumbar spine pain. Torque forces can be particularly damaging to the anular fibers that surround the nucleus (65, 66). Swimming, an activity usually recommended for patients with lumbar spine pain, actually exacerbated an otherwise quiescent lumbar spine syndrome each time the patient returned to aquatic training with his functional biomechanical shoulder adaptations. Most swimmers will experience a myriad of functional adaptations at sites distant from an initial injury because of the effects of the "motion cascade" (64) (Fig. 9.3). Therefore, an initial tissue injury should not be viewed and treated in isolation but should be seen as having the potential to create a cascading effect that can produce or exacerbate other painful musculoskeletal injuries.

CONCLUSION

Physiatrists have been trained to distinguish pain and disability so that they can direct a goal-oriented team to rehabilitate painful musculoskeletal conditions. They prescribe comprehensive treatment programs that rapidly restore and optimize physical function and performance while relieving pain and minimizing the psychological, social, and vocational effects of disability and the risk of recurrence or residual disability. Recognizing the type of clinical presentation of musculoskeletal pain allows physiatrists to develop treatment plans that meet all rehabilitation goals and address each component of the tissue injury cycle rapidly, efficiently and completely.

Acknowledgements The authors wish to thank Marcus G. Calahan and Carolyn A. Cole, M.S. for their editorial assistance and Gregory Mulford, M.D. for reviewing the manuscript.

REFERENCES

1. *Steadman's Medical Dictionary*, ed 23. Baltimore, Williams & Wilkins, 1976, p 1085.
2. Braddom RM, Krebs MA, Meler RH III, Opitz JL: *The Spectrum of a Specialty: Physical Medicine and Rehabilitation 1988. Office of Marketing and Communications of the American Academy of Physical Medicine and Rehabilitation.* Chicago, C.V.B. McMillan. 1988.
3. Herring SA: The physiatrist as the primary spine care specialist. In Herring SA (ed): *Low Back Pain.* Philadelphia, W.B. Saunders, 1991, pp 1–6.
4. Ziskin MC, McDiarmid T, Michlovitz SL: Therapeutic ultrasound. In Michlovitz SL (ed): *Thermal Agents in Rehabilitation.* Philadelphia, F.A. Davis, 1990, pp 134–169.
5. Gann N: Ultrasound: Current concepts. *Clin Mgmt* 11:64–69, 1991.
6. Dyson, M: Therapeutic applications of ultrasound. In Nyberg WL, Ziskin MC (eds): *Biological Effects of Ultrasound: Clinics in Diagnostic Ultrasound.* New York, Churchill Livingston, 1985, pp 121–133.
7. Cole AJ, Eagleston RE: The use of ultrasound, shortwave, and microwave diathermy for rehabilitation of sports injuries. The Physician and Sportsmedicine [In press].
8. Brammel HL: Rehabilitation of the cardiac patient. In DeLisa JA (ed): *Rehabilitation Medicine: Principles and Practice.* Philadelphia, J.B. Lippincott, 1988, pp 671–687.
9. Saal JA, Saal JS: Initial stage management of lumbar spine problems. In Herring SA (ed): *Low Back Pain.* Philadelphia, W.B. Saunders, 1991, pp 187–204.
10. Saal JA, Saal JS: Later stage management of lumber spine problems. In Herring SA (ed): *Low Back Pain.* Philadelphia, W.B. Saunders, 1991, pp 205–221.
11. Ditunno JF: Maturation of a specialty: The early 1980's. *Arch Phys Med Rehabil* 69:35–40, 1988.
12. Granger CV: Breaking new ground: Academy growth from 1975 to 1979. *Arch Phys Med Rehabil* 69:30–34, 1988.
13. deLateur BJ: Fostering research in the physiatrist's future. Or, there is nothing quite so practical as a good sound theory. *Arch Phys Med Rehabil* 71:1–2, 1990.
14. Erickson RP, McPhee MC: Clinical evaluation. In DeLisa JA (ed): *Rehabilitation Medicine: Principles and Practice.* Philadelphia, J.B. Lippincott, 1988, pp 25–65.

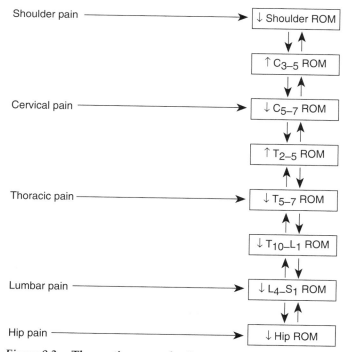

Figure 9.3. **The motion cascade. C = cervical, T = thoracic, L = lumbar, S = sacral, ROM = range of motion. Downward arrows indicate a decrease, upward arrows an increase.**

15. Gamburd, RS: The use of selective injections in the lumbar spine. In Herring SA (ed): *Low Back Pain*. Philadelphia, W.B. Saunders, 1991, pp 79–96.

16. International Classification of Impairments, Disabilities, and Handicaps: *A Manual of Classification Relating to the Consequences of Disease*. Geneva, World Health Organization, 1980.

17. DeLisa JA, Martin GM, Currie DM: Rehabilitation medicine: Past, present, and future. In DeLisa JA (ed): *Rehabilitation Medicine: Principles and Practice*. Philadelphia, J.B. Lippincott, 1988, pp 3–24.

18. Halstead LS: Team care in chronic illnesses: Critical review of literature of past 25 years. *Arch Physical Med Rehab* 61:507–511, 1976.

19. Fields HL: The peripheral pain sensory system. In Fields HL (ed): *Pain*. New York, McGraw-Hill, 1987, pp 13–40.

20. Shelton JL, Robinson JP: Psychological aspects of chronic back pain. In Herring SA (ed): *Low Back Pain*. Philadelphia, W.B. Saunders, 1991, pp 127–144.

21. Beals R, Hickman H: Industrial injuries of the back and extremities: Comprehensive evaluation—An aid in prognosis and management: A study of one hundred and eighty patients. *J Bone Joint Surg* 54:1593–1611, 1972.

22. Bigos S, Crites-Battle M: Acute care to prevent back disability. *Clin Orthop* 221:121–130, 1987.

23. Oravia S: Exertion injuries due to sports and physical exercise. A clinical and statistical study of nontraumatic overuse injuries of the musculoskeletal system of athletes and keep-fit athletes [Ph.D. thesis]. Finland, Ouler University, 1980.

24. Renstrom P, Johnson RJ: Overuse injuries in sports: A review. *Sports Med* 2:316, 1985.

25. Sperryn PN, Williams JGP: Why sports injury clinics? *Br Med J* 5966:364, 1975.

26. Kellett J: Acute soft tissue injuries—A review of the literature. *Med Sci Sports Excerc* 18:489, 1986.

27. Oakes B: Acute soft tissue injuries: Nature and management. *Aust Fam Phys Suppl* 10:3, 1982.

28. Van DerMuelin JHC: Present state of knowledge on processes of healing collagen structures. *Int J Sports Med* 3(Suppl 1):4, 1982.

29. Herring SA: Rehabilitation of muscle injuries. *Med Sci Sports Excerc* 22:453–456, 1990.

30. Hettingger T, Mueller EA: Muskelleistung and muskeltraining. *Arbeitsphysiologie*, 15:111, 1953.

31. Paulos LE, Payne FC, Rosenberg TD: Rehabilitaiton after anterior cruciate ligament surgery. In Jackson D, Drew D (eds): *The Anterior Cruciate Deficient Knee*. St. Louis, CV Mosby, 1987, pp 291–314.

32. Akeson V, Woo S, Amiel D: The connective tissue response to immobility: Biomechanical changes in periarticular connective tissue of the immobilized rabbit knee. *Clin Orthop* 93:356, 1973.

33. Zarins B: Soft tissue injury and repair—Biochemical aspects. *Int J Sports Med* 3(Suppl 1):9, 1982.

34. Leach R: The prevention and rehabilitation of soft tissue injuries. *Int J Sports Med* 3(Suppl 1):18, 1982.

35. Frank G, Woo S, Amiel D, Harwood F, Gomez M, Akeson W: Medial collateral ligament healing. A multidisciplinary assessment in rabbits. *Am J Sports Med* 11:379, 1983.

36. Lehmann J: Therapeutic heat and cold. *Clin Orthop* 99:207, 1974.

37. Lehmann J, deLateur BJ: Diathermy and superficial heat and cold therapy. In Kottke EJ, Stillwell GK, Lehmann JF (eds): *Krusen's Handbook of Physical Medicine and Rehabilitation*. Philadelphia, W.B. Saunders, 1982, pp 275–350.

38. Windsor RE, Lester JP, Herring SA: Electrical stimulation in clinical practice. *Phys Sportsmed* 21:85–96, 1993.

39. Huskisson E: Non-narcotic analgesics. In Wall PD, Melzach R (eds): *Text Book of Pain*. New York, Churchill-Livingstone, 1984, pp 505–513.

40. Dahl S: Nonsteroidal anti-inflammatory agents: Clinical pharmacology/adverse effects/usage guidelines. In Williams RF, Dahl SL (eds): *Therapeutic Controversies in the Rheumatic Diseases*. Orlando, Grune & Stratton, 1987, pp 27–68.

41. Robdy R, Blyth C: Athletic injuries: Application of epidemiologic methods. *JAMA* 217:184, 1971.

42. Lysens R, Steverlynck A, Van Den Auweele Y, et al: The predictability of sports injuries. *Sports Med* 1:6, 1984.

43. Kibler WB: Clinical aspects of muscle injury. *Med Sci Sports Excerc* 22:450–452, 1990.

44. Kibler WB, Chandler TJ, Pace BK: Principles of rehabilitation after chronic tendon injuries. In Renstrom AFH, Leadbetter WB (eds): *Clinics in Sports Medicine: Tendinitis I: Basic Concepts*. Philadelphia, W.B. Saunders, 1992, pp 661–672.

45. Kibler WB: Role of the scapula in the overhead throwing motion. *Contemp Orthop* 22:525–532, 1991.

46. Fu FH, Harner CD, Klein AH: Shoulder impingement syndrome: A critical review. *Clin Orthop Rel Res* 269:162–173, 1991.

47. Dreyfuss P, Stratton S: The use of the low energy laser, electroacuscope, and neuroprobe in sports medicine: A current review. *Phys Sportsmed* [In press].

48. Paris S: Mobilization of the spine. *Phys Ther* 59:988–995, 1979.

49. Woo S, Gomez M, Amiel D, et al: The effects of exercise on the biomechanical and biochemical properties of swine digital flexor tendon. *J Biomech Eng* 103:51–56,1981.

50. Korr IM: Neurochemical and neurotrophic consequences of nerve deformation. In Glasgow EF et al (eds): *Aspects of Manipulative Therapy*. Melbourne, Churchill-Livingstone, 1985, pp 64–71.

51. Wyke B, Polacek P: Articular neurology: The present position. *J Bone Joint Surg* [Br] 57:401, 1975.

52. Ward R: Headache: An osteopathic perspective. *J Am Osteopathic Assoc* 81:458–466, 1982.

53. Frank C, Akeson W, Woo S, et al: Physiology and therapeutic value of passive joint motion. *Clin Orthop Rel Res* 185:113–125, 1984.

54. Farrell JP: Cervical passive mobilization techniques: The Australian approach. In Saal JA (ed): *Neck and Back Pain*. Philadelphia, Hanley and Belfus, 1990, pp 309–334.

55. Wyke BD: Articular neurology and manipulative therapy. In Glasgow EF, Towomey LT, Scull ER, Kleynhans AM, Idczak RM (eds): *Aspects of Manipulative Therapy*. New York, Churchill-Livingstone, 1985, pp 72–77.

56. Kaltenborn FM: *Mobilization of the Extremity Joints: Examination and Basic Treatment Techniques*, ed 3. Oslo, Norway, Olaf Norlis Bokhandel Universitetsgaten, 1980.

57. Eagleston RE: (Unpublished data), 1992.
58. Kibler WB: Concepts in exercise rehabilitation. In Leadbetter W, Buckwalter JA, Gordon SL (eds): *Sports Induced Inflammation.* Chicago, American Academy of Orthopaedic Surgeons, 1990, pp 759–769.
59. Frank CB, Hart DA et al: Cellular response to loading. In Leadbetter W, Buckwalter JA, Gordon SL (eds): *Sports Induced Inflammation.* Chicago, American Academy of Orthopaedic Surgeons, 1990, pp 555–565.
60. Inman V, Sanders J, Abbott L: Observations on the function of the shoulder joint. *J Bone Joint Surg* 26:1–30, 1944.
61. Kadaba MP, Cole AJ, Wooten ME, McCann P, Reid M, Mulford G, April E, Bigliani L: Intramuscular wire electro-

myography of the subscapularis. *J Orthop Res* 10:394–397, 1992.
62. Cole, AJ: Swimming stabilization programs. Presented at the annual meeting of The American College of Sports Medicine, Dallas, TX, 1992.
63. Sanders RH, Stewart AM: Principles relating to reducing resistive forces. *Swim Tech* 29:21–23, 1992.
64. Cole AJ, Moschetti ML, Eagleston RE: Getting backs in the swim. *Rehab Mgmt* August/September:62–71, 1992.
65. Farfan HF: Effects of torsion on the intervertebral joints. *Can J Surg* 12:336–341, 1969.
66. Farfan HF, Cossette JW, Cossette JW, Robertson GH: The effects of torsion on the lumbar intervertebral joints: The role of torsion in the production of disc degeneration. *J Bone Joint Surg* [Am] 52:468–497, 1970.

CHAPTER 10

SPINAL MANIPULATION AND PHYSICAL REHABILITATION

JERRY C. LANGLEY

THROUGHOUT HISTORY, spinal manipulation has been one of the most maligned and controversial modes of treatment for the reduction of back pain. Much of the controversy revolves around the lack of scientific data to demonstrate the efficacy of manipulative therapy. Ultimately, even the results of clinical trials have been overshadowed by the possibility that results occurred by chance because of spontaneous remission or other phenomena.

Confusion and disagreement surround even the basic definition of manipulation. In recent years, spinal manipulation has been broadly defined. Many times the definition has been given to include all procedures in which the hands are used to massage, mobilize, adjust, or manipulate the osseous structures of the body and their surrounding tissue. This broad concept has evolved because most competent manipulators use extensive myofascial and soft tissue techniques along with manipulation in the reduction and control of pain syndromes. Further, many authors have construed the terms *manipulation* and *mobilization* to be synonymous, yet there is a distinct difference between the two. Cassidy et al. have provided a very good clarification of this difference (1). Mobilization involves taking the joint to its limit of passive range of motion, whereas manipulation goes beyond the passive range of motion into the paraphysiologic zone. Of course, extension beyond the paraphysiologic zone causes damage to the articular ligaments.

Further difference of opinion has evolved because of the terminology used to describe the primary manipulative lesion. The chiropractic subluxation has been described by Schafer as the alteration of normal, dynamic anatomic and physiologic relationships of continuous articular structures (2). Schafer indicates that subluxation is always attended to some degree by articular dysfunction, neurologic insult, and stressed muscles, tendons, and ligaments. Once produced, the lesion becomes a focus of sustained pathologic irritation; a bar-

rage of impulses stream into the spinal cord where internuncial neurons receive and relay the impulses to the motor pathways. The subluxation and joint irritation is thereby reinforced, thus perpetuating both the subluxation and the pathologic process engendered.

Neumann refers to the somatic dysfunction as a disturbance of any one of the components of an interrelated system (i.e., joint, intervertebral disk [IVD], muscles, or the nervous system) (3). Johnston cites three cardinal signs of a musculoskeletal dysfunction (4), which is often referred to as a biomechanical fault. The first sign is palpable muscle tension, the second is structural or positional irregularity, and the third is the near-universal presence of altered mobility. Other authors use the terms *fixation* and *blockage,* as well as other broadly described alterations of the spine, to describe a primary manipulable lesion.

In any of the above-mentioned cases, it is readily accepted that the patient has lost clinical stability of the spine. White and Panjabi have defined clinical stability as being the ability of the spine to prevent initial or additional neurologic damage, intractable pain, or gross deformity (5). With this definition of clinical stability in mind, the primary manipulable lesion would include not only positional or postural changes but also any aberrant or restricted motion of the spinal segments. The functional characteristics of this lesion would include, of course, the muscular and soft tissue changes. Other factors that have yet to be established by formal research are the neurogenic and nerve compression abnormalities.

PAIN TOLERANCE

Manipulation can be effective in producing relief in low back pain, neck pain, and headaches. Although scientific data has produced evidence of pain relief and manipulators have claimed clinical success, the exact pathway of pain relief still unknown. Wyke feels that the impact of spinal joint receptor afferentation is a potential component of this pain modulation (6). Denslow and Hassett (7) and Korr (8) projected the role of muscle spindle afferents in both sustaining and abolishing segmental central fasciculation. These authors felt that spinal manipulation produced short-term bursts of proprioceptive sensory bombardment, which could produce secondary effects such as gamma afferent inhibition and inhibition of the pain pathways. This bombardment would occur as a result of an instantaneous stretch of articular and myofascial receptors as their elastic barriers were exceeded in manipulation. Glover found zones of hyperesthesia lateral to the facet joints at painful segments, which he felt were due to fasciculation of cutaneous pain reflexes by nociceptive impulses from the joint receptors (9). He further found that these zones disappeared following rotational manipulation along the involved segment.

Terret and Howard found that a statistically significant elevation of pain tolerance (140%) occurred after manipulation as compared to a control group (10). These authors concluded that the local paraspinal pain tolerance increased following manipulation. Korr's model of spinal fixation focused on the muscle spindle as the coordinator that may increase or decrease muscle contraction according to the direction of motion of the joint (8). The reflex muscle contraction can then produce joint motion by this action or prevent joint motion in the area of spinal fixation. Korr proposed two mechanisms whereby manipulation would be successful in reducing pain associated with spinal fixation. First, stretch of the fibers and muscle against its spindle maintained resistance, which would produce a barrage of afferent impulses of sufficient intensity to signal the central nervous system to reduce the gamma motor neuron discharge (muscle contraction). Second, the Golgi tendon organs could be stimulated by manipulation and forced stretch of the skeletal muscles, causing gamma motor neuron inhibition.

GENERAL SPINAL BIOMECHANICS

Even though there is disagreement on the exact mechanism of how spinal manipulative therapy relieves pain, there are specific biomechanical changes along the spine that demonstrate clinical characteristics of a spinal manipulative lesion. Hildebrandt and Howe (11) have listed the following biomechanical changes in accordance with the static and kinetic aspects of the involved vertebral motor units.

Static Vertebral Motor Distortions

1. *Flexion-subluxation.* This type of malpositioning may force a posterior bulging of the annular fibers with excursion of the nucleus. There is likely to be stretching of the posterior longitudinal, interspinal, and supraspinal ligaments, along with shearing stress to the synovia of the facets.

2. *Extension subluxation.* This type of distortion may force a bulging of the annulus to the anterior with excursion of the nucleus. There is likely to be stretching of the anterior longitudinal ligament and imbrication or overlapping of the facet articulations with stress to the synovia of the facet articulations.

3. *Lateral flexion subluxation.* This spinal distortion may indicate imbrication or overlapping of the facets and stress to the synovia of the facets on the side of flexion, with possible bulging of the annulus with excursion of the nucleus toward the side of extension. There may also be stretching of the anterior longitudinal ligament at the lateral aspect on the side of extension.

4. *Rotational subluxation.* This distortion is indicative of possible torsion binding of the annulus, decreased resiliency of the intervertebral disk due to torsion compression of the annular fibers, and torsion stretching of the anterior and posterior longitudinal ligaments, with rotational overlapping of the facets with reverse shearing stress to the synovia of the facets.

5. *Anterolisthesis subluxation without spondylosis.* This distortion may produce forward shearing stress to the annulus and stretching of the anterior and posterior longitudinal ligaments, with overlapping of the facets with forward shearing stress to the synovia of the facets.

6. *Anterolisthesis subluxation with spondylolysis.* This spinal distortion may produce bulging of the annulus with forced excursion of the nucleus pulposus and forward shearing stress to the annular fibers. There may also be stretching of the anterior longitudinal ligaments.

7. *Retrolisthesis subluxation.* This distortion is characterized by posteroinferior excursion of the vertebral body and facets. With the retrolisthesis, there may be posterior shearing along the annulus with stretching of the anterior and posterior longitudinal ligaments. There may be further overlapping of the facets with posterior stress to the synovia.

8. *Laterolisthesis subluxation.* This distortion may produce lateral and posterior shearing stress to the annulus on the side of deviation and overlapping of the facets with anterior shearing of the synovia of the facets on the side opposite deviation.

9. *Decreased interosseous space subluxation.* Decreased spacing may cause traumatic compression of the intervertebral disk with possible herniation of the nucleus through an endplate and an overlapping of the facets with compression shearing to the synovia. There may be further compression of the contents of the intervertebral foramen.

10. *Increased interosseous space subluxation.* This may be indicative of inflammatory swelling or pathologic enlargement of the intervertebral disk with traction shearing to the annulus and the synovia of the facet articulations. There may also be stretching of the anterior and posterior longitudinal ligaments.

11. *Foraminal encroachment subluxation.* This distortion is characterized by findings of possible osteophytic changes along the intervertebral foramen. These changes may produce compression, irritation, and swelling of the foraminal contents with degenerative changes along the vertebral motor unit.

12. *Costovertebral-costotransverse subluxation.* With this type of distortion, there is misalignment of the costal processes in relation to the vertebral bodies and transverse processes independent of vertebral motion, or misalignment of the costal processes in relation to the vertebral bodies and transverse processes as a result of vertebral subluxation.

13. *Sacroiliac subluxation.* This distortion is characterized by misalignment of the sacrum in relation to the ilia. These distortions classically produce biomechanical improprieties of the pelvis.

KINETIC VERTEBRAL MOTION UNIT SUBLUXATIONS

1. *Hypomobility or fixation.* This type of dysfunction is characterized by fixation of vertebral motion in relation to the supporting structures below. With this classification, there may be stretching along the anterior and posterior longitudinal ligaments and spasticity along the muscles of the involved segment, with possible neurologic involvement of both the neural canal and the intervertebral foramen.

2. *Hypermobility.* This dysfunction is characterized by an increase in the vertebral motion along the motor unit in relation to the normally functioning unit below. Hypermobility produces increased stress to the anterior and posterior longitudinal ligaments with muscular spasticity and possible neurologic insult to the confines of the neural canal and intervertebral foramen.

3. *Aberrant movement subluxation.* The type of distortion is characterized by movement of a vertebra out of the normal phase with the segment above and below the involved unit. This may produce occlusion to the intervertebral foramens above and below the aberrant segment and may also produce shearing stress to the intervertebral disk and synovia of the facets along the involved area.

It is important to note that with the above-mentioned classifications there is alteration in the normal vertebral motion. There are at least two reports wherein increased vertebral movement following manipulation of the cervical spine has been noted on pre- and post-manipulation radiographs (12, 13).

Commonly, a major criterion for manipulation by many clinicians has become the restriction, fixation, and/or blockage of motion at specific joints of the spine (14). The location and characteristics of the fixation must be determined before manipulation can be performed. Motion-palpation of various joints of the spine is an invaluable tool for selecting the site of manipulation, as well as the type of procedure to be used.

In the hands of a skilled clinician, manipulation is both a safe and effective alternative for the correction of many musculoskeletal dysfunctions. As with any critical procedure (e.g., surgery, medication), however, manipulation can have harmful effects if it is incorrectly performed or used for the wrong reasons. Thorough digital examination of the spinal column is important to the evaluation of the joint dysfunction. Static palpation, however, will determine only the probable locations of the subluxation by the variations in muscular tone, texture, and sensitivity. The clinician must understand that there are several types of joint motion. These motions are described as gliding and angular, flexion, extension, abduction, adduction, rotation, and circumduction. Thorough evaluation of these joint movements by motion palpation will allow the clinician to key in on even minor joint dysfunctions. Because manipulation is intended to return joints to a more normal function, it is important for the clinician to fully understand the normal range of motion and the normal limits of the involved joint. Attempts to force joints beyond the normal limits can be harmful to the integrity of the joint and its surrounding soft tissue structures.

Along with motion palpation, it is important to note the surrounding soft tissue tone. Muscle tissue near a joint dysfunction or subluxation will normally present a spastic condition with localized tenderness. Interestingly, muscle tissue near a subluxation is often active as shown by electromyography. Propping the patient in different positions with pillows often increases the electromyographic activity but does not reduce the palpable firmness of the muscles. This indicates that the decreased tone is not necessarily due to muscle contraction from nociceptive input (15). It has been well established that irritation of the posterior joints and ligaments readily leads to reflex spasms of the erector spinae and other extensors (16). This muscle tone evaluation requires a precise knowledge and extensive practice in palpation. Also, because pain from nerve roots or pathways is referred toward the periphery, the entire nerve leading from the area should be explored. Tenderness, masses, temperature changes, and spasm along the areas of the nerve innervation can also give clues to joint dysfunction if the changes remain dermatomal.

During the examination phase, it is essential for the physician to perform numerous neurologic and orthopedic tests. These tests are significant in forming an opinion as to the type of technique to be employed, as well as in detecting contraindications to manipulation. It is important to keep in mind that along the cervical region, the brachial plexus is composed of nerve roots from C5 through T1. Involvements along the nerves radiating from the brachial plexus can be examined through reflex changes, muscle weakness, and sensation along the areas of distribution of the nerves. Nerve root C5 is responsible for the biceps reflex and innervates the deltoid and biceps muscles. This nerve is responsible for sensations over the lateral arm primarily along the deltoid area.

Nerve root C6 is primarily responsible for the brachioradialis reflex with contributing components to the biceps reflex. C6 innervates the wrist extensors and the biceps muscle. C6 is responsible for the lateral forearm and the thumb side of the hand.

Nerve root C7 is responsible for the triceps reflex. The nerve innervates the wrist flexor muscles, finger extension muscles, and the triceps. Primary sensory innervation is of the middle finger.

Nerve root C8 has no reflex component but innervates the finger flexion muscles and the hand intrinsics. Sensory innervation is to the medial forearm.

Nerve root T1 has no reflex component. The muscles innervated by T1 include the hand intrinsics with sensory innervation over the medial upper arm.

In the lumbar spine, nerve root L4 produces the patellar reflex and innervates the anterior tibialis muscle. L4 is responsible for sensory innervation to the medial leg and medial foot.

Nerve root L5 has no reflex component. The muscles innervated by L5 include the extensor hallicus longus with sensory innervation to the lateral leg and dorsum of the foot.

The S1 nerve root is responsible for the Achilles reflex with innervation to the Peronius longus and brevis muscles. S1 gives sensory innervation to the lateral foot. It is important to note that with disk involvement in the lumbar spine, it is typical for the involved nerve to be compressed by the disk one segment below the site of origin.

INDICATIONS FOR MANIPULATION

The determining factor for final selection of the manipulable patient is based on the etiology of the primary pathology. Importance lies in determining possible contraindications for manipulations and determining those patients whose conditions fail to make manipulation the primary treatment of choice. A comprehensive examination allows the clinician to clarify not only the nature but also the extent of the involved lesion. Differential diagnosis, while excluding some patients from the manipulative mode of treatment, also establishes a basis whereby the clinician is able to assess the progress of the patient and the success or failure of the applied treatment.

Difficulty in selecting the manipulable patient is further complicated by the poor understanding of the pathogenesis of back pain. Although a breakdown into numerous differential diagnostic categories is possible, many manipulators have achieved varying results with patients diagnosed with different symptom complexes or specifically diagnosed origins of pain (20).

LOW BACK PAIN

A few of the proposed causes of low back pain that respond to spinal manipulative therapy are discussed below. These causes have been divided into two categories. Category I findings are definite indications for manipulation. With proper techniques and application, excellent results can be expected. Common characteristics found in Category I are (1) absence of radiation and dermatomal pain, (2) little or no alteration in neurologic reflex findings, (3) joint dysfunction, and (4) asymmetric paravertebral muscle spasms. Category II findings, while responding to the proper application of spinal manipulation, yield successful results to a lesser degree.

Category I

Uncomplicated Back Pain

This is a nonspecific category, in which patients present a history of recent onset. There are no sensory changes along the dermatomal tract and no radiation of pain to the extremities. Potter has noted that patients with uncomplicated acute back pain have a high response rate, with 93% of such patients fully recovering or improving greatly following manipulation (16). Hoehler et al. have indicated that 84% of manipulated patients felt reduced pain following first manipulation (17). Fisk used manipulation to obtain complete recovery in 90% of patients suffering from acute low back pain syndrome (18). He found patients to have increased spinal mobility and increased straight leg raising ability following treatment.

Glover et al. used rotational manipulation of the trunk to correct a syndrome that was defined as including back pain, skin hyperesthesia, tenderness, and limitation of the trunk in one or more directions of movement (19). Statistically significant improvement was seen after the first and only manipulation. The patient with uncomplicated back pain is more likely to receive significant relief following the first treatment; the technique favors that of the long lever rotary manipulation.

Uncomplicated Chronic Low Back Pain

Statistically, uncomplicated chronic lower back pain responds to a lesser degree than does acute pain. Potter indicates that 71% of patients in his study who were classified as uncomplicated chronic low back pain sufferers improved following treatment. By the very nature of the pathology, chronic back pain is associated with lower expectations for full recovery than is the case with uncomplicated acute back pain. Further, spontaneous recovery with chronic back pain is rarely seen.

Posterior Facet Syndrome

The pain of the posterior facet joints begins along the midline of the lower back and may be referred to the buttock, thigh, or leg. The referred pain is nondermatomal. The patient may complain of a generalized achiness over the piriformis muscle. As with other Category I pain syndromes, there is no major neurologic deficit. In the majority of cases, these are radiographic signs of reduced lumbar mobility or fixation.

Cassidy et al. have divided the posterior facet syndrome into two divisions, the first being the fixed posterior joint syndrome and the second being the unstable posterior joint syndrome (1). With the fixed posterior joint syndrome, 62% of the patients receiving manipulation had favorable results, whereas only 26% of those patients with unstable posterior joint syndrome showed marked improvement.

Sacroiliac Syndrome

The sacroiliac joint, which is an atypical synovial joint with limited range of motion, is susceptible to mechanical derangements. Pain with the sacroiliac dysfunction may be characterized by local pain to the lateral aspect of the sacrum or referred pain to the buttock area. Many times, the patient will complain of symptoms that are relieved by rest and aggravated by activity. As is characteristic of all Category I pain syndromes, there is little or no alteration of neurologic reflexes. Jarring at the base of the spine causes sharp localized pain over the affected side. There may be either posterior or anterior torsional displacement.

With the posterior displacement, the patient will have a tendency to stand with the hip, knee, and lower back slightly flexed to the involved side. The posterior superior iliac spine and iliac crest will also be lower on the involved side. The pelvis will be shifted away from the involved side. If the patient stands with the leg straight, however, the posterior superior iliac spine and iliac crest will be lower on the involved side, but the anterior superior iliac spine will be higher. In this occurrence, the pelvis will appear to be rotated forward on the involved side.

With the anterior torsional displacement of the sacroiliac joint, the patient will have a tendency to stand with the hip and knee in extension on the involved side. The pelvis will likely be shifted toward or inclined away from the involved side. The posterior superior iliac spine and crest of the ilium will be lower on the uninvolved side. If the patient is able to stand erect with anterior torsional displacement, the posterior superior iliac spine and the iliac crest will be higher on the involved side. Cassidy et al. claim that 71% of patients with fixed sacroiliac syndrome received marked improvement with manipulation of the joint. (1).

Muscles

Manipulators have long recognized the importance of muscle syndromes in the genesis of back pain. Denslow and Hassett studied contracted muscles in individuals shown to have postural abnormalities (7). Good postural alignment of the body consists of bony structures that are in optimal position for weight bearing to allow the weight of the trunk to be balanced, and further consists of muscles that are adequate in length and balanced in strength. When muscles become shortened, the range of motion in the opposite direction is limited and structural misalignment may be produced. This allows the opposite muscle to stretch and weaken.

Muscle groups of the lower extremities and lower spine are significant because they provide a foundation for proper postural alignment. Muscles of particular importance include the abductor muscles, which consist of the gracillis, longus, brevis, and magnus muscles. Other muscles to consider are the gluteal, the piriformis, psoas, quadriceps, and hamstring muscles. Muscles of importance that act in extension and rotation of the vertebral column include the multifidus and rotatory muscles. Specific manipulative techniques have been developed with the aim of stretching or manually massaging these muscles in an attempt to relax them (14).

Category II

Spondylolisthesis

Spondylolisthesis should not be considered a contraindication to nontraumatic specific short lever manipulations. Cox found that the presence of such abnormalities did not produce less favorable treatment results (21). He did, however, note that spondylolisthesis at L4 responded much slower and required more treatments than did L5 spondylolisthesis. Proper manipulative technique will ensure that direct force over the area of slippage is avoided. Manipulation should be directed to the sacroiliac joint or posterior joints above the level of slippage.

Stenosis

Narrowing of the spinal canal secondary to degenerative changes along the joint and/or disk produce multidermatomal and/or bilateral leg pain. The Achilles reflex may be absent after exercise and present when the patient is at rest. Patients may complain of listlessness at night and leg pain that worsens with excessive exercise. A study by Potter found that 70% of patients with stenosis receiving manipulation showed some favorable results (16). Although very few patients become symptom-free, it appears that skilled manipulation may provide at least temporary relief for patients with neurogenic claudication due to spinal stenosis.

Disk

Disk involvement often produces an interesting dilemma for manipulators. The effect of spinal manipulation on the degenerative disk is controversial. Some clinicians feel the primary effect of manipulation is the reduction of the nuclear protrusions of the disk (21, 22). Other authors through clinical trials have found the results of manipulation in patients with disk protrusions to be much poorer than in patients with normal myelograms (23). These studies were unable to present any evidence of reduction in a positive myelogram finding following manipulation. It should be noted that in the event of frank herniation, competent manipulators exclude the use of rotary movement and use alternative methods such as intermittent distraction and/or reflux type techniques, which are less traumatic to the disk.

Hirschberg advocates conservative management in the treatment of patients suffering from symptoms of disk herniation (24). He states that under favorable circumstances, the protruded portion of the nucleus shrinks by dehydration and the symptoms of the nerve root compression are relieved.

CERVICAL PAIN

Flexion, extension, rotation, lateral flexion, and circumduction are the basic movements of the cervical region (25). Mechanical restrictions may occur because of various underlying disorders.

Cervical Strain/Sprain Injuries

Treatment for mild or moderate strain/sprain injuries should include appropriate manipulation to assist in preventing residual joint dysfunction. Manipulation is not the initial treatment of choice in severe strain/sprain injuries, however. These severe cases necessitate immobilization along with physiotherapeutic remedial aid and rest. This regimen of treatment should be followed after several weeks with a series of manipulations to restore the joint function and integrity.

Torticollis

Torticollis can be divided into two types, *viral myalgia* and *acute mechanical*. There is little evidence that manipulation can be effective in the viral myalgia torticollis, although proper maneuvers can provide excellent results in the acute mechanical torticollis. The manipulative technique used in this instance would be more of a stretching technique in a mild and methodic, progressive manner. All maneuvers in this case should be done away from the side of pain.

Acute Cervical Pain

Acute cervical pain may be due to simple mechanical distortions, inflammatory processes, or intervertebral disk lesions. Although the simple mechanical distortions respond excellently to manipulation, inflammatory processes and intervertebral disk lesions do not respond as favorably and should not receive harsh manipulation. Many distraction-type techniques with mild stretching and mild mobilization of the area may be effective. Often, stabilization of the cervical spine with a cervical collar following the treatment is essential.

Headaches of Cervical Origin

Many times headaches will originate in the cervical spine. Normally, these headaches will involve the occipital nerves, which radiate from the posterior branches of C2 and along the anterior branches of C3. Irritation along these nerves can be termed *occipital neuralgia* and may produce headaches along the posterior aspect of the skull or at the base of the skull, and/or radiating pain toward the frontal area. Normally the clinician will find tenderness along the occipital area and at the level of C2 and C3 bilaterally with paravertebral muscle spasms. Many times these headaches are associated with increased stress or tension. Frequently, proper manipulation will produce favorable results with these headaches in three to five treatments. Vernon found evidence of significant decrease in frequency, duration, and severity of headaches in patients treated by chiropractic manipulation (26). It should further be noted that additional symptoms of vertigo, nausea, and tinnitus can be effectively treated with manipulation in many cases (27). Because of the obvious contraindications that are possible in this syndrome, however, the diagnosis of mechanical malfunction along the cervical spine must be established prior to harsh manipulation.

Radicular Pains of Cervical Origin

Many times mechanical dysfunctions along the cervical spine will produce mild irritation along the brachial plexus, which can produce brachial neuralgia. The pain from these dysfunctions can extend across the shoulder and cause irritation to the supraspinous, infraspinous, and bicipital areas. These symptoms, which occur in the absence of frank herniation of disks along the cervical region, will readily respond to manipulation, which will also reduce chronic irritation to the corresponding spinal nerves.

THORACIC PAIN

Acute Thoracic Pain

Thoracic pain may be the result of pain originating along the cervical spine and referred to the thoracic region. This occurrence is typical with a patient who has a cervical dysfunction at the level of C5 through C7. Referred pain will typically appear along T5 and T6. Trigger points will occur along the medial border of the scapulae and along the trapezius or the superior margins of the scapulae. These trigger points can be treated with pressure and can effectively be reduced with stretch techniques if there is absence of frank herniation.

Rib Pain

Painful thoracic conditions can be associated with dysfunctions along the costovertebral or costotransverse articulations. Microtraumas or faulty posture can many times initiate this pain. The patient may complain of intense pain along the thoracic region at the costovertebral joints and may further experience radiating pain along the rib cage toward the sternum. This pain is due to intercostal neuritis and may cause symptoms of intense chest pain. Frequently, these conditions have a dramatic and instantaneous resolution with proper manipulative care.

TYPES OF MANIPULATION

While researchers are continuing to underscore the positive ramifications of spinal manipulation, clinicians have developed numerous methods and techniques of treatment for musculoskeletal dysfunction.

The primary distinguishing factor regarding manipulative methods is the differentiation between general and specific manipulation. General manipulation is a stretch performed to more than one joint and usually more than one spinal segment. Specific manipulation intends to stretch only one segment or one spinal joint (28). Ideally, the use of a specific manipulation tends to reduce increased stress to uninvolved segments.

Further distinguishing characteristics of manipulation involve the direction of motion or line of drive. Direct manipulation involves a line of drive into and past the barrier of restricted motion. Indirect manipulation utilizes line of drive away from the barrier of restricted motion. Generally speaking, indirect manipulation is safer than direct manipulation and exhibits less of a tendency for adverse reaction (14). Usually, manipulators will not attempt direct manipulation until all possibilities of a correction by indirect manipulation have been exhausted. Even so, although direct manipulation may be painful for the patient, there are some specific indications for the use of direct manipulation. In the presence of these indications, its use is both a logical and an effective choice.

The ultimate goal of the manipulator is to correct the musculoskeletal dysfunction and return the patient to a more normal function. The ideal manipulative procedure should take into account the structural relationship of the vertebral segment being manipulated. This consideration would include any abnormalities or structural symmetries. With proper manipulative procedures, it is not necessary to regard all bony or structural malformation as contraindications to manipulation. With manipulation, the areas of restricted and fixated joint movements are mobilized, thereby reducing painful and abnormal joint play and eliminating palpable soft tissue fibers with the ultimate correction of muscle spasms along the imbalanced area. The most important goal of the manipulator is to achieve favorable results without inducing trauma to the spine or soft tissues along the spine and thus allow the patient to receive maximum therapeutic benefit.

A widely used manipulative procedure is the short-lever, high-velocity thrust directed specifically at the manipulable lesion. The proficient clinician must have proper skills to diagnose the clinically significant lesion and must develop the ability to direct the manipulative thrust to one vertebra segment in a specific direction.

As opposed to the specific short-lever, high-velocity adjustment, the long-lever manipulation is an example of a nonspecific manipulation over an entire region of the spine. Without proper care in this type of manipulation, and in the hands of an unskilled manipulator, the most often mobilized segment is the one that is already hypermobile. Nonspecific techniques include what are known as noncontact techniques. These techniques are used when greater force is necessary to achieve joint mobility. The manipulator gains leverage by obtaining contact points away from the manipulable lesion, such as on the chest or the extremity.

Additionally, several authors now propose the use of distraction techniques, specifically for the treatment of intervertebral disk lesions. Cyriax indicates that there are three effects from traction and distraction type techniques (22). First, there is an increase in the spacing between vertebral bodies, thus enlarging the space into which the protrusion must recede. Second, there is a tautening of the joint capsule, which allows the ligaments joining the vertebral bodies to create a centrifugal force around the joint, which squeezes the disk fibers and the nucleus back into place. Third, there is suction created to the joint.

James C. Cox, D.C. uses a specific intermittent distraction technique designed to provide a push, pull, pumping effect on the intervertebral disk space, creating a milking action of the intervertebral disk, thereby allowing resolution (21). Proponents of this distraction manipulation are quick to point out the difference between intermittent distraction and static traction. Whereas the distraction technique is designed to pump the intervertebral disk and the nucleus back to a more normal position, static traction actually opens the intervertebral disk space and can allow the nucleus to imbide fluids, which may increase the intradiskal pressure and cause a worsening of pressure against an already compressed nerve root.

In preparation for manipulation, one must consider a number of general rules. The patient must be relaxed and comfortable. If there are contracted muscles in the general area in which the manipulation is to be applied, a preparatory therapy such as stretching or massage along with a physiotherapeutic modality may be required to assist the patient in obtaining maximum relaxation prior to manipulation.

Additionally, the manipulator must be mentally and physically relaxed. This requires self-assurance and complete confidence in biomechanics, with a concept of how the correction is to be made. Further, it is most helpful if the manipulator wears comfortable clothing, because manipulation often requires close body contact between the clinician and the patient. It is essential to determine the difference between soft tissue stretch and the pain of muscle guarding. Muscle guarding is a significant sign that indicates that the clinician is about to move through the point of pain. It is reiterated here that in general, movement through the point of pain should be avoided. Manipulation through the point of pain requires exact skills and precise techniques that are employed in carefully selected circumstances.

Consideration must be given to the direction in which the thrust is to be made, which is commonly referred to as the *line of drive*. The depth and/or velocity of thrust must also be determined. Additionally, skilled manipulators often use torque during the thrust. This torque is a twisting at the wrist of the contact hand to assist in the correction.

VARIATIONS OF MANIPULATIVE TECHNIQUES

Unquestionably, it is impossible to list all of the techniques and variations that have been developed to reduce spinal dysfunction. Some techniques require the patient to be supine, whereas others require side-lying or seated positions. Many techniques require special types of manipulative tables or traction devices. The following examples will illustrate some of the basic principles of spinal manipulation.

The specific short-lever, high-velocity spinal manipulation requires the patient to be placed in a position that allows movement of the vertebra in the desired position. Normally, contact is made with a small portion of one hand. This could be in the form of a thumb with a pushing action or the pisiform bone of the contact hand. The spinal segment above or below the segment to be manipulated should be stabilized by the clinician's other hand or by moving the spine to the limit of its passive range of motion. The high-velocity thrust is delivered with the contact hand to the short-lever area of the vertebra (i.e., transverse process, spinous process, or mamillary process) in the direction to which the correction should be made (Fig. 10.1).

Lumbar spine manipulations and sacroiliac joint manipulations are frequently performed with the patient in a side-lying position. The point of contact for the clinician is at the segment to be manipulated in the lumbar spine. The patient's upper body is rotated and laterally flexed downward to the lumbar spine at the point of contact. At this point, the superior knee and hip are flexed, which allows the manipulator to rotate the pelvis and localize the point of counter rotation to the spinal segment to be manipulated. With manipulation of the lumbar spine, the clinician is normally contacting the patient with the pisiform section placed across the mamillary process of the lumbar vertebra or is hooking the spinous process with a cupping action of the fingers. With proper placement of the patient, the force of the

manipulation can be localized to higher levels along the lumbar spine; with skilled manipulators, this technique can be delivered to specific levels of the spine (Fig. 10.2).

A similar technique that allows the patient to receive a different effect is the side posture manipulation and rotation with extension. This technique can be effective with patients who have a decrease in the normal lordosis of the lumbar spine. Once again, the patient is on his or her side with the clinician stabilizing the patient along the shoulder. The patient's inferior leg must be placed posteriorly, bringing the patient's lumbar spine into lordosis. From this position, the contact hand is

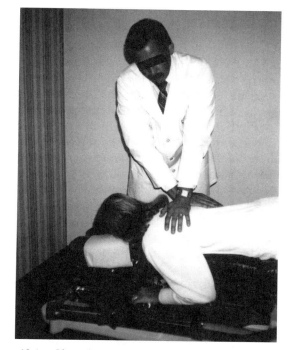

Figure 10.1. **Short lever, high-velocity spinal manipulation.**

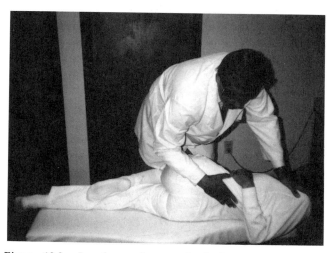

Figure 10.2. **Lumbar spine manipulation with patient in side-lying position.**

placed on the anterior superior portion of the ilium. The specific thrust is injected anteriorly and inferiorly (Fig. 10.3).

Seated positions can be used when manipulating even the lumbar spine. The patient is seated along the end of the adjusting table with the arms across the chest and the hands grasping the opposite shoulders. Normally the clinician will contact the spinous process with a thumb. The stabilizing hand is in front of the patient and grasping the patient's shoulder. The manipulator is then able to flex, extend, rotate, or laterally bend the patient. The thrust is delivered with high velocity to the area to be manipulated (Fig. 10.4). This technique is also effective in the thoracolumbar region.

An effective procedure for the thoracic spine is performed with the patient in a seated position. The patient flexes the neck and grasps his or her hands behind the neck. The manipulator stands behind the patient, placing his forearms under the patient's arms, and grasps the patient's wrists. The contact by the manipulator here is made at the sternum area against the thoracic spine. The patient's shoulders are brought to tension while the manipulator avoids the pressure of the patient's wrists and neck. The thrust is achieved by raising the patients shoulder while delivering simultaneous thrust with the manipulator's sternum (Fig. 10.5).

An excellent manipulation for correction of intercostal pain and distortions along the rib cage is achieved with the patient lying supine. The manipulator stands to the side opposite that of the pain and extends the hand beneath the patient alongside the spine, contacting the patient's costovertebral articulations. The manipulator stabilizes with the anterior hand against the crest of

the opposite ilium. The patient is rotated and the manipulator brings the spine to tension. The thrust is then delivered upward with the contact hand while the stabilizing hand and arm lightly thrust inferiorly (Fig. 10.6).

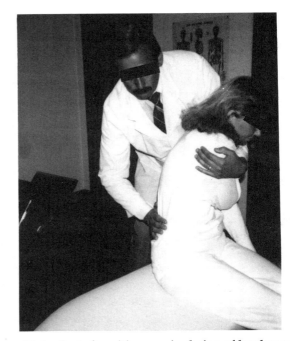

Figure 10.4. **Seated position manipulation of lumbar spine.**

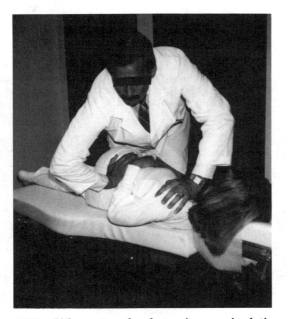

Figure 10.3. **Side posture lumbar spine manipulation and rotation with extension.**

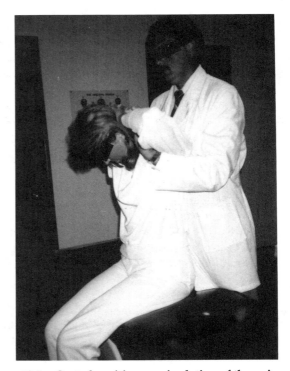

Figure 10.5. **Seated position manipulation of thoracic spine.**

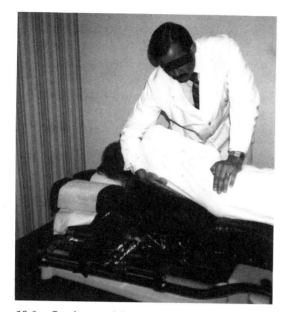

Figure 10.6.   **Supine position manipulation of rib cage.**

CONTRAINDICATIONS FOR MANIPULATION

According to rough estimations based on 50 million manipulations yearly over the past 40 years, the odds of a serious complication due to manipulation is 1/181 million manipulations. It is safe to say that if proper precautions are taken and combined with a full understanding of the case at hand, the frequency of complication is greatly reduced.

The most serious complication to arise is from injury to the cerebral circulation or spinal cord following cervical manipulation. There are predisposing factors that greatly increase the risk of cervical manipulation, however. The most obvious is osteophytic outgrowths, which may obstruct the course of vertebral arteries.

Additionally, degenerative joint disease along the cervical spine may reduce the disk height. This shortens the cervical spine and allows the vertebral arteries to become more tortuous (29).

Yet, the most likely cause of serious injury or complications due to manipulation remains that of an incorrect diagnosis, failure to diagnose, or improper techniques. As with any skilled procedure, the expected results and the resulting complications depend on the skills of the clinician.

REHABILITATION

Interestingly, manipulation should be viewed as only one part of the recovery process. Rehabilitation and exercise are considered vital parts of this process.

Webster defines rehabilitate as "to restore to a former capacity; to restore or bring to a condition of health or useful and constructive activity" (30).

The process of rehabilitation is based on principles of conditioning, but some vital modifications must be made. For example, a patient who has torn or traumatically injured a ligament or tendon should not attempt any strenuous rehabilitation program until the soft tissue is healed. Therefore, any process that assists and enhances healing, such as chiropractic manipulation or physiotherapy, must be considered an important aspect of rehabilitation. Pain must also be taken into consideration, because pain activates neural mechanisms within the body that cause restriction, inhibit normal flexibility, and often cause edema in and around the tissue. Therefore, pain must be reduced before reconditioning can be successful.

There is some misunderstanding, even among professionals, of the term "rehabilitation." Many may confuse it with "exercise," "working with weights," "working with machines," or other erroneous concepts. This is too narrow. Rehabilitation is the entire process of returning an injured patient to health and freedom from pain. Rehabilitation in the treatment of a sports injury occurs when the injured athlete is returned to competition (31).

The process of rehabilitation should progress through a systematic program of physical reconditioning. Kegerreis referred to the "progressive reorientation" and "functional progression" as an ordered sequence of activity (32). He felt that each phase of the physical process is part of the total rehabilitation and should proceed as follows:

1. Intact articulations and muscles
2. Pain-free joints and muscles
3. Joint flexibility
4. Muscular strength
5. Muscular endurance
6. Muscular speed
7. Integrated and coordinated movement
8. Cardiovascular endurance

Obviously, there will be some overlapping, but development of any step of the above sequence will require the successful development of the step that precedes it.

In a well-organized and professionally staffed rehabilitation center, care must be taken to choose the therapeutic modality to be used during a particular phase of rehabilitation. The proper modality must be matched with the therapeutic goal. Modalities should be rated as follows:

1. The modality has a direct effect and is a good choice during a specific phase of rehabilitation
2. The modality can be effective if used in a specific way (e.g., isotonic resistive exercise can be effective only if used with many repetitions)
3. The modality is somewhat effective, but is not the best choice for this particular phase of rehabilitation (33)

Proper rehabilitation requires an accurate professional diagnosis and program of physical reconditioning. Kegerreis referred to the evaluation of the patient to determine the desired response to the program (32).

The goals of a proper rehabilitation program can be listed as follows:

1. Establishment of an accurate diagnosis
2. Minimization of deleterious local effects of the acute injury
3. Allowance for proper healing
4. Maintenance of other areas of physical fitness
5. Return to normal function

Following an injury, the injured area may need to be rested and occasionally kept non–weight bearing or splinted. Never underestimate the significant side effects of immobilization, however. There can be up to a 20% loss of muscle strength after 1 week of immobilization and another 20% decline in residual strength every subsequent week of immobilization. Atrophy may occur rapidly if the muscle is immobilized in shortened position (34).

Side effects due to immobilization extend far beyond the muscle alone. If an associated joint is immobile, significant joint capsule, cartilage, subchondral bone, and bone-ligament changes occur. Some tissues may never completely return to normal after 8 weeks of total immobilization.

Early exercise, guided by a competent professional, is essential to successful rehabilitation. It speeds the healing process, whereas lack of exercise during the early stages of rehabilitation could result in disability. Obviously, caution must be used to prevent exercise that is too vigorous.

Rehabilitation involves functional progression through a systematic program of physical reconditioning. Specific demands must be imposed on the body to bring about redevelopment of each phase. Proper and constant monitoring of the patient's progress during rehabilitation is necessary so that the demands of the therapeutic regimen can be adjusted according to the patient's progress.

A successful rehabilitation evaluation system allows the clinician to determine the initial level of impairment and injury regardless of the symptomatic complaints presented by the patient. This initial level can be used to characterize pain in terms of dysfunction, to develop an individual rehabilitation program, to guide the clinician during the entire rehabilitation process, and to quantify the final result of treatment in terms of restoration. The ultimate goal is to restore the patient to perform his or her tasks at a normal level.

There is growing evidence that back pain disability and other injuries resulting in permanent impairment can be reduced by the application of proper treatment methods in the early stages. We are now aware that overmedicating or immobilizing patients is not the answer. A well-managed and professional rehabilitation program will improve body mechanics and promote cardiovascular conditioning. This decade will very likely endorse the importance of rehabilitation in both preventing and treating traumatic conditions.

REFERENCES

1. Cassidy JD, Kirkaldy-Willis WH, McGregor M: Spinal manipulation for the treatment of chronic low back and leg pain: an observational study. In Buerger AA, Greenman PE (eds): *Empirical Approaches to the Validation of Spinal Manipulation.* Springfield, IL, Charles C Thomas, 1985, pp 199–150.
2. Schafer RC: *Chiropractic Management of Sports and Recreational Injuries.* Baltimore, Williams & Wilkins, 1982, pp 273–274.
3. Neumann H: A concept of manual medicine. In Buerger AA, Greenman PE (eds): *Empirical Approaches to the Validation of Spinal Manipulation.* Springfield; IL, Charles C Thomas, 1985, p 267.
4. Johnston WL: Inter-rater reliability on the selection of manipulable patients. In Buerger AA, Greenman PE (eds): *Empirical Approaches to the Validation of Spinal Manipulation.* Springfield, IL, Charles C Thomas, 1985, p 107.
5. White AA, Panjabi M: The role of stabilization in the treatment of cervical spine injuries. *Spine* 9:229–238, 1984.
6. Wyke BD: Articular neurology. A review. *Physiology* 58:94–100, 1973.
7. Denslow JS, Hassett CC: The central excitatory state associated with postural abnormalities. *J Neurophysiol* 5:393–402, 1942.
8. Korr IM: Proprioceptors and the discussion of mechanisms of manipulative therapy. In Korr IM (ed): *Neurobiologic Mechanisms in Manipulative Therapy.* New York, Plenum, 1978.
9. Glover JR: Back pain and hyperesthesia. *Lancet* 1:1165–1169, 1980.
10. Terrett AC, Howard V: Manipulation and pain tolerance. *Physiol Med J* 63:217–223, 1984.
11. Hildebrant RW, Howe JW: Spinal biomechanics and subluxation classification. Lombard, IL, National College of Chiropractic, 1974.
12. Hviid H: The influence of chiropractic treatment on the rotary mobility of the cervical spine. *Ann Swiss Chirop Assoc* 5:31–44, 1971.
13. Jirout J: The effect of mobilization of the segmental blockage on the sagittal component of the cervical spine. *Neuroradiology* 3:210–215, 1972.
14. Halderman S: Spinal manipulative therapy in the management of low back pain. In Finnesan BE (ed): *Low Back Pain.* Philadelphia, J.B. Lippincott, 1980, pp 245–273.
15. Schafer RC: *Clinical Biomechanics: Musculoskeletal Actions and Reactions.* Baltimore, Williams & Wilkins, 1983.
16. Potter GE: A study of 744 cases of neck and back pain treated with spinal manipulation. *J Can Chirop Assoc* 21:154–156, 1977.

17. Hoehler F, Tobis JS, Buerger AA: Spinal Manipulation for back pain. *JAMA* 245:1835–1838, 1981.

18. Fisk JW: An evaluation of manipulation in the treatment of the acute low back pain syndrome in general practice. In Buerger AA, Greenman PE (eds): *Empirical Approaches to the Validation of Spinal Manipulation.* Springfield, IL, Charles C Thomas, 1985, 228–273.

19. Glover JR, Morris JG, Khosla T: Back pain: A randomized clinical trail of rotational manipulation of the trunk. *Br J Ind Med* 31:59–64, 1974.

20. Dyck P, Pheasant HC, Doyle JB, Rieder JJ: Intermittent cauda equina compression syndrome. *Spine* 261:75, 1977.

21. Cox J: *Low Back Pain: Mechanism, Diagnosis and Treatment,* ed 4. Baltimore, Williams & Wilkins, 1985.

22. Cyriax J: *Textbook of Orthopaedic Medicine,* ed 3. Baltimore, Williams & Wilkins, 1969.

23. Chrisman OD, Mittnacht A, Snook GA: A study of the results of following rotatory manipulation in the lumbar intervertebral disc syndrome. *J Bone Joint Surg [Am]* 46:517–524, 1964.

24. Hirschberg GG: Treating lumbar disc lesions by prolonged continuous reduction of intradiscal pressure. *Tex Med* 70:58–68, 1974.

25. Schafer RC: *Clinical BioMechanics: Musculoskeletal Actions and Reactions.* Baltimore, Williams & Wilkins, 1983.

26. Vernon H: Chiropractic manipulative therapy in the treatment of headaches: A retrospective and prospective study. *J Manipulative Physiol Ther* 5:109–112, 1982.

27. Strange VV: *Essential Principles of Chiropractic.* Davenport, IO, Palmer College of Chiropractic, 1984.

28. Maigne R: Manipulations of the spine. In Basmajian UV (ed): *Mobilization, Traction and Massage,* ed 3. Baltimore, Williams & Wilkins, 1985, pp 71–134.

29. Loach AA: *The Chiropractic Theories,* ed 2. Baltimore, Williams & Wilkins, 1986.

30. *Webster's Ninth New Collegiate Dictionary.* Springfield, MA, Merriam-Webster, 1988, p 993.

31. Knight KL: Total injury rehabilitation. *Phys Sportsmed* 7:111, 1979.

32. Kegerreis S: The construction and implementation of functional progressions as a component of athletic rehabilitation. *J Orthop Sports Phys Ther* 5:14–19, 1983.

33. Knight KL: Cryostretch for muscle spasm. *Phys Sports* 8:129, 1980.

34. Beals RK, Hickman NW: Industrial injuries of the back and extremities. *J Bone Joint Surg [Am]* 54:1593–1611, 1972.

CHAPTER 11

ADJUNCTIVE TREATMENT TECHNIQUES

LARRY A. GAUPP
DON E. FLINN
RICHARD L. WEDDIGE

HYPNOSIS

Hypnoanalgesia and hypnoanesthesia are among the earliest applications of hypnosis, and among the most enduring methods of pain reduction in the clinical setting. The impressive clinical reports of Rejamier (1821), Clouqet (1829), Elliotson (1834), Ward (1842), and Esdaile (1865) of painless surgery under mesmeric sleep fostered a belief in the efficacy of hypnosis in the relief of pain that has prevailed despite an often hostile scientific climate and the discovery of chemical anesthetics. (For a review of current applications of hypnosis in surgery and anesthesia, see references 1, 2.)

Fortunately, the efficacy of hypnosis in the relief of the acute pain of surgery garnered support from the laboratory, where reasonably good laboratory analogues (e.g., cold pressor pain, ischemic pain) permitted the investigation of hypnosis in the reduction of acute pain under controlled conditions. This body of research has repeatedly demonstrated the reality of pain reduction through hypnosis and that the ability to reduce acute pain in the laboratory through hypnosis is related to the level of hypnotic susceptibility (e.g., as measured by the Stanford Hypnotic Susceptibility Scales). The greater the level of hypnotic susceptibility the greater the likelihood of pain reduction (1, 3–6). It has been demonstrated that hypnoanalgesia reduces both the sensory pain and suffering components of acute pain (7). Further, the reduction of acute pain in the laboratory is not attributable to anxiety reduction (1, 3, 8–11), or to hypnotic induction procedures or suggestion alone (1, 5, 9, 12, 13), or to demand characteristics or expectancy (3, 8). Finally, it has been carefully demonstrated that the reduction of acute pain in the laboratory through hypnosis is not attributable to a placebo effect (14, 15) Hypnoanalgesia acts like a placebo for low hypnotic susceptibles only; for high hypnotic susceptibles, the reduction of pain through hypnosis greatly exceeds the reduction via placebo.

The support that these laboratory findings have given to the clinical reports of the successful reduction of acute pain through hypnosis has been bolstered by experimental studies conducted within the clinical setting. These findings have historically mirrored those of laboratory testing. Gottfredson (16), in a well-designed investigation of hypnoanesthesia as the sole anesthetic in the clinical dental context as it relates to hypnotic susceptibility, found that the more hypnotizable the patient, the less pain the patient experienced. Additionally, the effectiveness of hypnoanesthesia in reducing acute dental pain was comparable to that of chemoanesthesia for the high hypnotic susceptibles. The award-winning research of Wakeman and Kaplan (17) and others (18, 19) demonstrated the efficacy of hypnoanalgesia and hypnoanesthesia in the treatment of painful burns (i.e., daily tanking, debridement, and dressing changes) in children, adolescents, and adults.

Although laboratory-induced pain has provided a satisfactory experimental framework for the investigation of hypnosis in the reduction of acute pain, does this body of work apply equally well to chronic clinical pain? Does chronic clinical pain with its attendant biopsychosocial contaminants respond like acute pain insofar as hypnosis is concerned? Extant evidence suggests that it does; the only difference between the reduction of acute pain and chronic pain through hypnosis is that the latter, because of its ongoing and/or recurrent nature, requires that the patient learn self-hypnosis so that self-reliance can be achieved.

As is the case with acute pain, there are abundant clinical reports and methodologically compromised studies attesting to the efficacy of hypnosis in the reduction of chronic clinical pain. Examples of these reports include the successful application of hypnoanalgesia to various types of headache (20–47), back pain (33, 37, 42, 48–55), cancer pain (1, 50, 56–80), phantom pain (50, 81–87), facial pain (42, 88, 89), neck and shoulder pain (90, 91), myofibrositis (92), herpes (93), lupus (94), gastrointestinal pain (34, 95), bruxism (96), tic douloureux (97), vaginismus (98), arthritis (50, 99–101), and peripheral nerve pain (50).

In addition to these reports of the use of hypnosis in the reduction of chronic pain, there are several methodologically satisfactory studies that support the assertion that the findings reported for acute pain in the laboratory are pertinent to chronic pain. For example, in a well-controlled outcome study with 1-year follow-up, Friedman and Taub (102) concluded that hypnosis was a cost-effective treatment for migraine headache, especially for patients exhibiting a high level of hypnotic susceptibility. Similarly, L. A. Gaupp and F. J. Magnavito (unpublished information), using hypnotic dissociation to promote hypnoanalgesia, found that hypnoanalgesia was effective in reducing both the sensory pain and suffering components of chronic pain for patients exhibiting medium and high levels of hypnotic susceptibility. This study was conducted with a group of unselected pain patients with chronic pain of mixed etiology (i.e., low back pain, headache, shoulder pain, neck pain, and chest pain). A significant correlation between standardized measurement of hypnotic susceptibility (e.g., Stanford Hypnotic Clinical Scale) and the reduction of chronic pain through hypnosis has been found for headache (102), facial pain (89), and chronic pain of mixed etiology (L. A. Gaupp and F. J. Magnavito, unpublished information). Thus, although further research is desirable, these systematic investigations of hypnosis in the relief of chronic pain, like those for acute pain in the clinical setting, have mirrored the findings for the relief of laboratory-induced pain through hypnosis.

The well-documented relationship between hypnotic susceptibility and the reduction of pain through hypnosis led Gaupp and Magnavito to suggest that a medium level of hypnotic susceptibility should serve as the minimum criterion for attempting hypnoanalgesia in the clinical setting. The formal assessment of hypnotic susceptibility in the clinical setting has become time-efficient since the development of brief clinically relevant scales such as the Stanford Hypnotic Clinical Scale (1). This allows for an exploration of the kinds of hypnotic experiences the patient may have versus simply the absolute level of hypnotic susceptibility, and brings scientifically validated procedure into the clinical setting. This is not to state that the practitioner, workload permitting, should not attempt hypnoanalgesia with low hypnotic susceptibiles, because some are able to reduce pain. However, given that the single most important determinant of the patient's ability to reduce pain through hypnosis is level of hypnotic susceptibility (1, 103), it would seem prudent to limit such attempts to two to three sessions unless success is clearly evident.

The practitioner's approach to hypnoanalgesia does not differ substantially from hypnotherapy generally. Care must be given to prepare the patient, especially those naive to the experience of hypnosis, by establishing rapport, gaining the patient's trust and cooperation, enhancing and binding the patient's motivation, exploring the patient's expectations and attitudes, and exploring the patient's knowledge of hypnosis so that any misconceptions can be corrected and attendant apprehension alleviated. Specific to the preparation of the chronic pain patient is the correction of the belief that the successful use of hypnosis to alleviate pain means that the pain is psychological or emotional or imaginary, thereby challenging the veracity of the pain complaint and the integrity of the patient. A brief history of hypoanalgesia coupled with a graphic description of the use of hypnosis to control painful burns can readily correct this misconception. Finally, it is important that the patient conceptualize hypnosis as a long-term chronic pain management strategy versus a brief intervention that will completely and forever abolish the pain. The ultimate goal of the hypnotic intervention is to teach the patient self-hypnosis so that the patient may become self-reliant in managing the pain and thereby minimize the pain's adverse impact on daily functioning (104). Additionally, although there is a growing realization that the use of pain medication to manage chronic pain is not without merit, self-hypnosis can be used to effectively modulate reliance on such medications (105).

Hypoanalgesia

Numerous strategies and variations thereof have been used to promote hypnoanalgesia, reflecting the ingenuity and resourcefulness of the practitioner and the patient as they work collaboratively to reduce the pain (106, 107). The approaches described below are neither inclusive nor mutually exclusive, and do not include the almost unlimited variations and combinations the practitioner may realize in adapting to what the patient can do and finds congenial. The practitioner should discuss openly with the patient the rationale for the strategy being used because it may appear unscientific and bizarre to the patient. An explanation that metaphoric and imaginal suggestions mediate neurophysiologic and/or neurochemical processes that alleviate pain will generally be acceptable.

Direct Hypnotic Suggestion

Direct hypnotic suggestion involves giving the patient the direct suggestion that the pain will no longer be experienced. This is not considered a very useful strategy in that it may be perceived by the patient as authoritarian and thus create resistance, or it may limit the effectiveness of other strategies, and is likely to be successful only for high hypnotic susceptibles with extant cognitive coping strategies that can be creatively used to mediate the direct suggestion.

Indirect Hypnotic Suggestion

Indirect hypnotic suggestion is similar to direct suggestion but is worded and offered in a manner conducive to receptiveness and responsiveness, for example: "... As you enjoy ... the comfort of this deeply relaxed state ... you notice that you gradually lose awareness of your body and how it feels ... like the many moments throughout each day when you become so involved in things outside yourself ... you have little or no awareness of your body ... or that it evens exists. ..." This approach is generally considered more effective than direct suggestion, and is applicable to a broader range of hypnotic susceptibility.

Hypnotic Dissociation

Hypnotic dissociation involves transporting the patient away from the present to an imagined pleasing, relaxing, and absorbing place or activity (e.g., walking through a meadow, engaging in some adventure real or imagined), or to an earlier and happier time via age regression. Another approach to this strategy is to suggest a partial or complete out-of-body experience. For example, a patient with a painful foot may be able to imagine disconnecting the painful foot. Or, the patient might be asked to float out of the body and leave the person experiencing the pain behind.

Hypnotic Time Disorientation

Hypnotic time disorientation involves reorientation in time to an earlier stage of the illness or to an earlier time when the pain was of minor consideration. For example, reorientation to a time predating the illness or pain problem can be suggested, along with restoration of normal sensations or of pleasant feelings and sensations and the projection of these into the present to nullify the pain and/or some subjective qualities of the pain experience. Another approach is to suggest reorientation to a time during the course of the illness or pain problem when a medical/surgical intervention successfully relieved the pain (e.g., nerve block), with restoration of attendant sensations or normal sensations and the projection of these into the present.

Hypnotic Replacement or Substitution of Sensations

Hypnotic replacement or substitution of sensations involves the selective, partial, or complete modification of the pain experience through the substitution of or conversion to some other sensation or symptom. Perhaps the most common approach to this strategy is to suggest glove anesthesia, beginning with suggested feeling of coolness or warmth in a hand that gradually develops into a pleasant numbness. The glove anesthesia can then

be demonstrated by pinching or pricking the hand, enhancing the patient's sense of efficacy regarding control over bodily sensations. Then it is suggested that the numbness be "transferred" from the anesthetic hand to the site of pain by having the patient gently rub or message the painful part of the body with the hand as a symbol of the transfer. Another approach to this strategy is to suggest that the patient experience a pleasant sensation (e.g., tingling) at or near the site of the pain to absorb attention along with suggested feelings of warmth, heaviness, or coolness where the pain is experienced. In contrast, an unpleasant and annoying yet bearable sensation (e.g., itching, burning, pain of minor cut) may be suggested to absorb attention along with hypnotic suggestions of warmth and so forth. Or, it may be suggested that the pain be converted to some other annoying yet tolerable symptom (e.g., twitching, cough). One additional approach is to hypnotically promote synesthesia, or the use of sensory images such that pleasure from one sensory modality (e.g., visual, auditory) is shifted to another (e.g., nociceptive perceptions)—for example, "... the pleasant rhythmic sound of the waves rolling gently onto the shore becomes one with the throbbing in your head."

Hypnotic Displacement

Hypnotic displacement involves displacing the pain or selected qualities thereof from one area of the body to another where it does not carry the same threatening significance or does not as readily interfere with daily functioning (e.g., disabling back pain may be displaced to the little finger of the nonpreferred hand), or where it is simply more tolerable, giving the usually painful area a rest. This strategy is also useful for pain that is not well localized and thus seemingly more difficult to manage. It is suggested that the patient consolidate the pain into a smaller area before moving it.

Hypnotic Reinterpretation

Hypnotic reinterpretation and/or dissociation of the meaning attributed to the pain can alleviate pain. This approach requires full awareness of the meaning attributed by the patient to the pain experience, and is especially useful when the pain experience harbors affectual or metaphoric significance. For example, the pain of an old war injury might come to represent the courage and pride of defending Freedom's Frontier. Or, the pain of child abuse fused with traumatic back pain acquired in adulthood can be differentiated and dealt with as separate experiences.

Hypnoplasty

Hypnoplasty involves hypnotically altering the anatomic site of the pain in a manner that counters the pain experience. A patient might imagine installing circuit breakers, switches, or a rheostat that can be readily manipulated to turn off or lower the level of pain. Or, the patient might shore up a structurally compromised vertebral body so as to relieve compressive effects.

Hypnotic Amnesia

Hypnotically suggested amnesia is a useful strategy for pain that is episodic or constant with intermittent exacerbations. Suggestions can be given for partial or complete amnesia of the pain that has been experienced, or for selective subjective qualities and attributes of the pain experience as described by the patient. Forgetting the pain experience can ameliorate the anticipation and dread of future episodes or exacerbations that may increase interepisode discomfort and exacerbate the episode when and if it occurs. Suggestions that any episodes of pain will seem completely transient usually accompany the suggestions for amnesia. Therefore, neither remembered nor anticipated, the experience will seem to have no appreciable duration and thus be more easily tolerated. Hypnotic time distortion can be a useful adjunct to this strategy. Once amnesia is developed for all past episodes of pain, hypnotically developed time distortion can be suggested so that the duration of an episode may be experienced as markedly shortened. For example, it may be suggested that each episode of pain will come as a complete surprise; that when an episode occurs it will cue a hypnotic state during which the patient will experience the enjoyment of a surprise party; that, because time is relative, the time will seem to fly by because of the fun; that the party, during which the entire episode of pain will be experienced, will seem to last only a matter of seconds or minutes; and that on arousal from this hypnotic surprise, amnesia for the entire experience will occur.

Additional Considerations

Regardless of the strategy or strategies the practitioner employs, it is necessary to be sensitive to the patient's experience so that adjustments can be made. For example, for the patient who believes the chronic pain reflects and serves as a marker of occult disease, it can be suggested that the pain be only partially relieved, leaving the patient with a way to monitor health status. Other patients may need to be reassured that the relief of pain through hypnosis will not abolish the ability to experience acute pain indicative of the need for medical attention.

SELF-HYPNOSIS TECHNIQUES

As previously noted, self-hypnosis is generally essential to the long-term management of chronic pain via hypnoanalgesia. Rarely is chronic pain completely abolished through hypnosis; more commonly, partial or complete relief is attained for varying amounts of time. Once a patient has allowed a practitioner to guide him or her into hypnosis, the patient can readily follow the same induction, deepening, hypnoanalgesic strategies,

and termination procedures. For the high susceptibles, a self-induced cue can be used to enter hypnosis. Fortunately, many patients can readily learn to use self-hypnosis with little difficulty following this procedure and with essentially the same results (1). For those who have difficulty, a personalized tape recording of a heterohypnotic session can be made and used by the patient. Many patients can realize effective pain relief within 10 min through self-hypnosis, and should use self-hypnosis at least once daily if not as often as is necessary.

Some patients will report that at times the pain is too severe to concentrate sufficiently to induce self-hypnosis. Two induction techniques that have been useful in effectively dealing with this eventuality are *fractionation* (34) and *pain induction*. With the modified fractionation technique the patient is asked to follow the same induction procedure previously learned, but without any concern as to the depth of hypnosis achieved. Rather, after eye closure, the patient is to simply notice whatever is experienced at the moment of maximal relaxation, no matter how minimal or slight that may be. Next, the patient should rouse up from the hypnosis with readiness to re-experience hypnosis, knowing that with each rehypnotization a deeper state of relaxed hypnosis will be attained. The patient then induces hypnosis again, paying close attention to those relaxing sensations noted during the previous induction. This procedure is repeated again and again until a level of hypnosis is achieved that allows the patient to proceed with the rest of the hypnoanalgesic intervention. This can generally be achieved following four to six inductions.

Utilizing pain to induce hypnosis simply makes use of the fact that the patient is already absorbed (108). The patient is instructed to focus even more intently on the pain and to carefully notice some dimension of the pain (e.g., intensity, quality, temporality)—to notice, for example, how the pain really is not constant but rather fluctuates, albeit ever so slightly, like the ebb and flow of the tides. It is suggested that the patient begin to highlight those fluctuations, first by intensifying the flow of the pain. Implicit is that if the pain can be increased volitionally, it can be decreased in intensity in a similar manner. Then, the patient begins to heighten the ebbing phase. Throughout the exercise the patient notes that with each flow and ebb of the pain a deeper level of relaxed hypnosis is attained. When the patient feels that the tide has subsided sufficiently, he or she can proceed with the hypnoanalgesic intervention.

MECHANISM OF HYPNOANALGESIA

The mechanisms of hypnoanalgesia remain unclear. The failure of naloxone to reduce hypnoanalgesia (109, 110) has led to the assertion that hypnoanalgesia occurs primarily at higher cortical levels (10, 111). It has been reasoned that if hypnoanalgesia is mediated through a neurochemical mechanism involving the release of opioid peptides in the central nervous system (β-endorphins), then naloxone, an opioid antagonist, would reverse it. In contrast to this assertion, Stephenson (112) reported a single case of repeated reversal of hypnoanalgesia by naloxone, and Domangue and colleagues (101) found that mean plasma levels of β-endorphin were significantly higher following successful hypnoanalgesia in a group of arthritic pain patients. These seemingly conflicting results may reflect the fact that naloxone effects may not be comparable between clinical pain and laboratory-induced pain (113), and highlight the methodologic problems that need to be resolved before the mechanism(s) of hypnoanalgesia can be adequately investigated (114, 115).

CONCLUSIONS

Although there remains much to learn about the use of hypnosis in the relief of chronic pain, there clearly is sufficient scientific evidence substantiating its efficacy to warrant its clinical use (116). Equally important, the chronic pain patient is receptive to the use of hypnosis in the relief of pain and finds it very helpful (L. A. Gaupp, unpublished information). Of 145 chronic pain patients who completed a 6-week inpatient comprehensive pain management program, only 1 declined to attempt hypnoanalgesia. Further, when these patients were asked to indicate which of the 14 treatment elements that made up the program were most helpful in learning how to function more actively and productively in spite of pain, and in learning how to control and/or alter the perception of pain, hypnosis/self-hypnosis emerged as the treatment perceived as most helpful for both. This finding also supports the belief that hypnosis has the advantage of creating and promoting beneficial effects beyond the specific effect on pain (1, 109).

It should be noted that although the above information pertains primarily to adults, there is a growing body of literature attesting to the efficacy of hypnosis in the reduction of chronic clinical pain in the pediatric (117–123) and geriatric (124) population.

RELAXATION RESPONSE

The induction of the psychophysiologic state of low arousal that has come to be known as the *relaxation response* (125) has gained widespread use in the management of chronic pain. The relaxation response has been characterized by a generalized decrease in sympathetic nervous system activity and concomitant decreases in respiratory rate, oxygen consumption, heart rate, blood pressure, arterial blood lactate, and muscle tension, as well as increases in skin resistance, skeletal muscle blood flow, and electroencephalographic alpha activity (125). The amelioration of the chronic pain experience is presumed to result in part from the psychophysiologic changes attendant to the induction of the relaxation response (e.g., decreases in muscle tension believed to underlie musculoskeletal pain, such as muscle tension headache, and decreases in cranial vasculature reactivity believed to underlie vascular headache). Although a variety of procedures have been devised to induce the relaxation response in the reduction of chronic pain, only the most commonly used procedures are reviewed here.

Biofeedback

Biofeedback has become a popular procedure for the treatment of chronic pain. This approach assumes that a maladaptive psychophysiologic response is of etiologic significance in chronic pain and that the normalization and/or control of the presumptive maladaptive response will attenuate the pain. These assumptions have led to the development of several frequently used biofeedback methods: (1) electromyographic (EMG) feedback to reduce muscle tension, (2) thermal feedback to increase finger temperature, and (3) cephalic blood volume pulse (BVP) feedback to reduce BVP of the cephalic temporal artery.

Numerous reports attesting to the efficacy of biofeedback in the reduction of chronic pain have appeared. Examples of these include the successful application of biofeedback in treating muscle tension headache (126–167), migraine headache (168–209), cluster headache (210–212), post-traumatic headache (213), low back pain (214–228), arthritis (229–232), temporomandibular joint pain (233–235), myofascial pain (236), phantom pain (237–239), benign chest pain (240), angina (241), dysmenorrhea (242), post-herpetic neuralgia (243), causalgia (244), sickle cell disease (245), burn pain (246), spasticity (247), reflex sympathetic dystrophy syndrome (248), and anal pain (249).

Despite the fact that the support for the use of biofeedback in the reduction of chronic pain appears impressive in its magnitude, consistency, and diversity, the efficacy of application has yet to be firmly and scientifically established (250). Available reports are all too often methodologically weak, making unequivocal conclusions difficult. More troublesome, however, is the fact that the assumptions underlying biofeedback have been seriously questioned. For example, the belief that excessive muscle tension is the primary source of muscle tension headache has been challenged (127, 128, 133, 251–261), as have the belief that excessive cranial vasculature responsivity underlies migraine headache (262–265) and the belief that chronic low back pain reflects abnormal patterns of neuromuscular activity (266–269). Not surprisingly, then, numerous reports and reviews have dampened the enthusiastic claims of the efficacy of biofeedback in the reduction of chronic pain pending clarification of the relative contributions of the physiologic, physiologic self-control, psychological, social, and nonspecific factors involved (234, 270–304). Currently, it is fair to conclude that a scientific basis for the use of biofeedback in the reduction of chronic pain has yet to be established, and that there is only limited and qualified support for its efficacy in this regard, especially when it is used as the sole treatment intervention.

As with hypnosis, there is growing literature pertaining to the application of biofeedback approaches to chronic pain in the pediatric (305–312) and geriatric (313) populations.

RELAXATION TRAINING

As with biofeedback, there are numerous reports attesting to the efficacy of various relaxation training procedures in the reduction of chronic pain. Examples of these reports include the successful application of such procedures to muscle tension headache (153, 159, 314–329), migraine headache (182, 186, 190, 194, 200, 317, 325–335), post-traumatic headache (336), low back pain (337–339), temporomandibular joint pain (340–342), myofascial pain (343–346), arthritis (347, 348), dysmenorrhea (349), cancer pain (350), phantom pain (351), abdominal pain (352–354), chest pain (355), and chronic pain of mixed etiology (225, 226, 356–358).

In contrast to biofeedback, the efficacy of relaxation training is more firmly established (287, 359, 360). In addition, it appears that biofeedback, which requires expensive equipment and technological support, is no more efficacious than relaxation training and, when successful, usually incorporates some form of home-based relaxation training. Finally, relaxation training can be taught more efficiently than biofeedback, and is more amenable to use as an active coping strategy.

Progressive muscle relaxation (361) is the most widely practiced method of relaxation training in the reduction of chronic pain. Although many variations of this approach are currently in practice (e.g., refs. 362, 363), all involve tensing a muscle group for several seconds, passive focusing of attention on how the tensed muscles feel, then releasing the tensed muscles with passive focusing of attention on how the muscles feel as the relaxation takes place. This sequence is systematically applied to the major muscle groups of the body, and highlights two skills that an individual must acquire if relaxation training is to be effective: recognition/discrimination and voluntary induction of the relaxation response. The patient must first learn to recognize the presence of muscle tension. Although this may seem a relatively easy matter, the chronic pain patient may adapt to a state of chronic muscle tension and thus exhibit a blunted awareness of its presence. Additionally, the patient must learn to recognize increasingly low levels of muscle tension because the pain experience may require only partial tightening of muscle fibers

(364). Following this, the patient must first learn to discriminate the presence of muscle tension from the uniquely subjective feelings indicative of the state of relaxation (e.g., heaviness, warmth, calm). Finally, the patient must acquire the ability to induce the relaxation response without using the tension-releasing procedures employed during training.

Several meditative approaches to relaxation training have demonstrated utility. One simple meditative approach calls for the patient to passively focus awareness on the breathing cycle and to silently repeat the word "one" with each exhalation (125). The patient is instructed to sit quietly in a comfortable position with eyes closed and to relax the muscles of the body, beginning with the feet and progressing to the face and head. The patient is then instructed to passively focus awareness on the breathing cycle, to breathe easily and naturally through the nose, and to silently repeat the word "one" with each exhalation; for example, breathe in . . . out ("one"), in . . . out ("one"), and so on. Maintaining a passive attitude and permitting relaxation to occur at its own pace is emphasized. It is recommended that the technique be practiced once or twice daily for 10–20 min.

A more complex meditative approach to relaxation training is that of autogenic training (365). This approach relies on a series of self-directed formulas to induce the relaxation response. The patient is instructed to assume a relaxed position, to close the eyes, and to passively concentrate on a series of six standard autogenic formulas (e.g., "My right arm is heavy"). Standard formula one focuses on promoting the feeling of heaviness in the limbs, and formula two on promoting the sensation of warmth in the limbs. Formulas three and four focus on cardiac and respiratory regulation, respectively. Formula five focuses on promoting the sensation of warmth in the abdomen, and formula six on the feelings of coolness in the forehead. The patient is instructed to practice these formulas daily until such time that a voluntary shift to a state of wakeful low arousal is readily attained. In addition to the six standard formulas that focus on the psychophysiologic aspects of the relaxation response, there are a series of organ-specific formulas, intentional formulas, and meditative formulas.

Integrative Approach

Because a variety of relaxation training procedures and variations thereof have been used in the reduction of chronic pain, it is difficult to draw any conclusions regarding the effectiveness of any one relative to the others. Therefore, the practitioner should consider combining elements of the more commonly employed methods described above to form an integrative approach to relaxation training (e.g., the quieting response [366]). One such approach is described below.

Phase 1: Progressive Muscle Relaxation

This integrative approach begins with training in progressive muscle relaxation. Training is best conducted in a quiet, slightly darkened, and comfortably warm room with the patient in a posture conducive to relaxation. Most patients prefer to assume a supine position on a firm surface or recliner. The legs should be slightly apart and positioned so that the feet are inclined at a V-shaped angle; the heels should not touch each other. The trunk, shoulders, and head should be in a symmetric position. Particular care should be taken to determine the most relaxing position for the head, neck, and shoulders. The arms should lie relaxed and slightly bent beside the trunk. The fingers should remain slightly spread and flexed and not touch the trunk. If the patient presents with chronic low back pain, some support (e.g., folded blanket or pillows) under the knees will help to provide maximum, postural relaxation of the back and both legs. Not everyone finds the supine or knee-raised training postures congenial; a sitting posture can be used (366). It is also advisable that the shoes be removed and clothing loosened, if necessary, to minimize any distracting stimulation. Finally, further reduction in unnecessary stimulation can be achieved by having the patient close the eyes.

Once the optimal relaxation training posture is assumed by the patient, the practitioner, speaking in a calm, melodic voice, instructs the patient to tense and release the gross muscle groups of the body, beginning with the dominant hand and forearm. For example, the practitioner may say: "Inhale slowly and make a fist, tensing the muscles of the right hand and forearm . . . Tense until they slightly tremble . . . hold the tension (for 10 sec) . . . Notice how the tension in these muscles feels . . . become familiar with those sensations of tension so that you can recognize their presence even if they occur when you are not knowingly tensing . . . Now . . . exhale slowly and relax . . . just letting go completely (3–5 sec) . . . allowing all the tension to drain from those muscles . . . just noticing how those muscles feel as the relaxation takes place . . . the comfortable feelings of heaviness . . . of warmth . . . Passively focusing your awareness on these comfortable feelings and associated sense of inner peace and calm that is gradually coming over you . . . As you do . . . allow the phrase, 'my right hand and arm are heavy and warm,' to gently settle into your mind . . ." and so forth, for 20–30 sec before repeating the sequence with the same muscle group for a second time. This sequence of breathing in and tensing, retaining the breath while focusing attention on the tension, breathing out and releasing, and normal breathing while passively focusing awareness on the relaxation is then systematically applied twice to the dominant upper arm, nondominant hand and forearm, nondominant upper arm, forehead, eyes and nose, cheeks and mouth, neck and throat, chest and back, abdomen, dominant upper leg, dominant calf, dominant foot, nondominant upper leg, nondominant calf, and nondominant foot.

The instruction to take a slow deep breath and to retain it until told to "relax" serves to enhance and maintain tension, facilitating its recognition. Conversely, the instruction to exhale slowly while releasing serves to enhance the feelings associated with relaxation, facilitating the discrimination process. When releasing the tensed muscles, the patient should take care not to release too rapidly or too slowly; 3–5 sec is about right for the release process. The 20–30 sec of practitioner-suggested feelings of relaxation (e.g., heaviness, warmth, comfort, calm) and the patient's passive concentration on the appropriate autogenic formula are designed to enhance the relaxation response. The patient is also cautioned to avoid retensing already relaxed muscle groups when tensing each new muscle group. This may take some practice but usually occurs readily.

Once all muscle groups have been relaxed, the patient is instructed to passively listen to the sound of breathing and to silently say the word "relax" with each exhalation. Pairing the word "relax" with the relaxation response allows the patient to develop a conditional cue for the eventual rapid induction of the relaxation response. This association also begins to prepare the patient for the second phase of relaxation training, training in proper breathing.

Training and practice sessions in progressive muscle relaxation usually last 20–30 min, and represent the focus of the first 2 weeks of relaxation training. The patient is instructed to practice at least once daily, twice if possible. Although tape-assisted practice is probably as effective as self-directed practice for inducing the relaxation response, self-directed practice is preferred because it is more likely to foster and/or restore the patient's sense of personal efficacy (367).

The patient is also asked to follow a number of guidelines in daily practice. Practice should take place in a quiet, slightly darkened and comfortably warm room. The relaxing posture employed during the training should be used during practice. Time(s) congenial to the patient's daily activities should be scheduled for practice so that practice becomes an integral part of the patient's daily routine. The patient should adopt a passive attitude while practicing and not be concerned about the level of success; differing levels of perceived success across practice sessions are natural. If the patient experiences the tendency to fall asleep during practice, he or she is instructed to silently repeat the phrase, "I stay free and fresh while practicing." Finally, upon completion of practice, the patient should sit up slowly and remain seated for several minutes while gently moving the limbs before slowly standing up.

Phase 2: Proper Breathing

The next phase of training involves training in proper breathing. Breathing rhythm, the sequence of inhalation and exhalation, is an important determinant of the level of arousal (368). In contrast to the rapid shallow breathing through the mouth indicative and facilitative of tension, proper breathing, characterized by slow and deep rhythmic breathing through the nose, promotes a low level of arousal.

Training in proper breathing begins with the patient assuming the relaxing posture used during the training and practice of progressive muscle relaxation. However, the hands are lightly placed over the abdomen just below the navel, with fingertips touching. The patient is instructed to inhale slowly and deeply through the nose, and at the same time to let the abdomen swell out, making a conscious but relaxed effort to distend the abdomen as if developing a "pot belly." The fingertips should move apart as the abdomen swells out. As the abdomen rises with inhalation, the diaphragm moves downward. As the breath continues, the lower part of the chest and finally the upper chest expands and slightly lifts and the inhalation is completed. The patient is instructed to retain the breath momentarily, and the process is then reversed. The breath is slowly released, the abdomen is drawn in, which lifts the diaphragm, the expanded chest relaxes, and exhalation is completed. The resultant emptiness is momentarily held and then the cycle is repeated.

Thus described, training in proper breathing involves four distinct stages: (1) inhalation, (2) retention of breath, (3) exhalation, and (4) retention of emptiness. However, with practice this becomes one smooth, continuous, and effortless movement. Training in proper breathing may be facilitated by breathing to a count of 3 or 4 (sec), holding for one count, and then exhaling and holding for the same count. In counting, then, a breathing cycle may sound like this: "(inhaling) one. . . . two. . . . three. . . . hold. . . . (exhaling) *relax*. . . . two. . . . three. . . . hold." Beginning the exhalation count with the conditional cue "relax" facilitates the induction of the relaxation response by eliciting the feelings of relaxation previously associated with progressive muscle relaxation. Although the above count is appropriate for most patients, it may have to be shortened early in training for some. Whatever the count, it should be the same for both the inhalation and exhalation phase so that the breathing cycle is smooth and even.

Training and practice sessions in proper breathing usually last 10–20 min, and are the focus of the third week of training. The patient is instructed to practice proper breathing twice daily. The patient is also instructed to practice limited progressive muscle relaxation (i.e., one tensing-releasing sequence per muscle group) on every other day during this week of training.

For relaxation training to be maximally effective, the patient should use the skills acquired as an active coping strategy (279, 359). Thus, once the patient has begun to exhibit mastery of proper breathing, usually after 1 week of practice, he or she is instructed to practice the following applied breathing exercise roughly once every half hour while awake or each time he or she encounters a designated cue (e.g., small piece of tape on the time pieces in the patient's home and work environments). The patient is to first check the breathing rhythm. If it is proper breathing, the patient should smile and silently say, "What a nice thing to do for my body." If the breathing is rapid (shallow mouth breathing), the patient should silently say, "Proper breathing is better for my body." The patient then initiates proper breathing, allows the jaw to slightly lower and the body to relax, and recalls the feelings of deep relaxation (e.g., heaviness, warmth, calm). Once relaxed, usually after several minutes, the patient smiles and silently says, "What a nice thing to do for my body." The patient is also instructed to use the applied breathing exercise when encountering any annoyance or frustration, no matter how minor. On such occasions the patient is instructed to smile and say, "It's silly to get my body uptight and uncomfortable about this," complete the applied breathing exercise, and then smile and silently say, "It's healthier to keep my body relaxed no matter how disturbing things may seem."

Training and practice of the applied breathing exercise becomes the focus of the fourth week of training. The patient is also instructed to practice proper breathing once daily and limited progressive muscle relaxation on every other day during the fourth week.

Phase 3: Dissociative Visualization

The final phase of this integrative approach to relaxation training involves dissociative visualization. Dissociative visualization is designed to induce "mental" relaxation as well as the relaxation response. It calls for the patient to master the ability of passive focusing in some personally meaningful, pleasing, relaxing, and absorbing memory or image. The patient is instructed to assume the relaxing posture used in the previous training phases, close the eyes, and use the applied breathing exercise to induce the relaxation response. Then, the patient is instructed to passively focus attention on the designated imagery and to allow complete absorption by the image and awareness of the sensory information inherent in the image (e.g., colors, sounds). Passive focusing is perhaps the most important element in relaxing at this point because distracting thoughts may occur, at least initially. The patient is informed that such intrusions may occur but that they do not mean the procedure is being performed incorrectly. Ideally, intrusions are best dealt with through the imagery rather than actively resisted. For example, the image may be one of a quiet beautiful lake nestled in a remote mountain valley. It reflects the brilliant warm sun by day and the distant stars by night. By day, distracting thoughts can become birds that fly from this peaceful sanctuary. By night they become shooting stars that quickly disappear from the peaceful sky.

Training and practice sessions in dissociative visualization usually last 15–20 min, and are the focus of the fifth week of training. The patient is also instructed to continue practicing the applied breathing exercise and limited progressive muscle relaxation once every third day.

Week six of the training focuses on the practice of dissociative visualization as an active coping strategy either singly or in combination with the applied breathing exercise. The practice of limited progressive muscle relaxation once every third day is also prescribed. Thereafter, the patient may elect to adhere to the practice schedule of week 6, or focus on using the one or two procedures found to be most helpful. Regardless, periodic practice of each of the training procedures is strongly recommended so that the derived applied coping strategies do not lose their effectiveness.

Handling Adverse Patient Reactions

Relaxation training procedures designed to induce a low level of arousal may be aversive to some patients. When this occurs, care needs to be taken to determine if this is secondary to tension serving to defend against the florid expression of affectively laden material, for example, or if the tension and attendant pain represent internally augmented information that compensates for an extant and aversive state of low arousal (369). The latter is suspected if the patient has a history of seeking high-arousal activities and environments. In the former case, psychotherapy may be necessary before relaxation training can be initiated. If the latter is the case, relaxation procedures should provide more adaptive ways to enhance arousal. High-arousal activities that are within any physical limitation posed by the patient's pain problem (e.g., games, dancing, jogging, bicycling, swimming, rowing) can be substituted for progressive muscle relaxation. Proper breathing can be modified such that the retention of breath is prolonged one count, which will serve to heighten arousal. Finally, dissociative visualization should employ high-arousal imagery (e.g., mountain climbing, sky diving).

Although relaxation training can be considered a benign treatment intervention, untoward reactions may occur (370). Most of these reactions are not cause for alarm (e.g., myoclonic jerks, cramping, muscle soreness, transient respiratory difficulties, dissociation), and usually reflect mild decompressive effects, high levels of tension, disuse effect, increased awareness of tension, or exposure to the unfamiliar state of low arousal. Although such occurrences may be unsettling for the patient, they readily resolve as training progresses or with reassurance that they will subside as the patient becomes familiar and comfortable with states of wakeful low arousal. Two untoward reactions, however, warrant

the special attention of the practitioner and patient. Relaxation training may partially or completely restore physiologic dysfunction as a byproduct of the general homeostasis facilitated by regular induction of the relaxation response. For example, patients taking antihypertensive medication, thyroid medication, and antidiabetic medication should be carefully monitored for possible symptoms of functional overdose. The hypertensive patient should be alert to hypotensive reactions marked by dizziness and/or light-headedness. The patient with hypothyroidism should be alert to heat intolerance, increased appetite, weight loss, increased nervousness or restlessness, increased activity or energy level, decreased need for sleep, and tremor. The diabetic should be alert to tremulousness, tachycardia, mental slowing, confusion, hypoglycemia, excessive thirst, excessive urination, excessive eating, intense itching, and weakness. Relaxation training should be temporarily discontinued with such occurrences and the prescribing physician should be consulted regarding medication adjustments.

Relaxation training may also precipitate an emotional decompression ranging from tearfulness to florid affective expression or abreaction. These expressions, usually of grief or anger or fear, occur when physiologic tension associated with psychological conflict is reduced. Although this is generally not cause for alarm, relaxation training may have to be temporarily discontinued in lieu of psychotherapy and/or continued within the context of psychotherapy.

Conclusions

Whereas conclusions regarding the efficacy of biofeedback in the reduction and/or management of chronic pain remain equivocal, sufficient scientific evidence has emerged substantiating the efficacy of relaxation training to warrant its use in the reduction of chronic pain. In addition, relaxation is cost-effective, found congenial by most chronic pain patients, and perceived by most patients as an effective treatment. In the study of chronic pain patients' perceived effectiveness of various treatment components of a comprehensive pain management program reported earlier (L. A. Gaupp, unpublished information), the integrative approach to relaxation training described above emerged as the second most helpful pain management strategy behind hypnosis/self-hypnosis. This author would hold that for a chronic pain management strategy to be maximally effective it must be congenial to the patient, restore and/or foster the often diminished sense of personal efficacy (367) exhibited by the chronic pain patient, be readily applied in vitro as an active coping strategy, offer a relatively immediate favorable impact on the perception of pain so that long-term in-vitro use thereof is inherently reinforcing, and foster therapeutic benefit beyond the specific effect on pain. It is suggested that hypnosis/self-hypnosis and relaxation training not only meet these requirements but, when combined with operant strategies, which are more efficacious in increasing activity and decreasing medication use than in the reduction of chronic pain (359), offer a reasonably comprehensive, efficacious, and cost-effective chronic pain management program.

Finally, the utility of relaxation training for the management of chronic pain in the pediatric (371–379) and geriatric (380) populations has increasingly been reported.

ACUPUNCTURE

Acupuncture is one of the major therapeutic procedures of traditional Chinese medicine and, along with the use of herbs, has been in use for thousands of years. It had been standardized and was recorded in *The Yellow Emperor's Classic of Internal Medicine* 24 centuries ago (381). Its practice was consistent with *Yin-Yang* theory, the fundamental Chinese philosophy of active and passive complimentary opposites existing as parts of a whole, and inseparable from its relationship to other entities. Health was believed to result from a harmonious relationship of forces within the body and between the individual and nature. The major organs of the body, some of which were Yin and some Yang, were thought to be connected by 12 paired and 2 midline meridians or channels, which were named for the organs with which they were connected. In a state of health, vital energy (*Qi* or *Chi*) and four other fundamental substances flowed along these channels and harmonized the activity of the organs. Disease was believed to be associated with an imbalance of forces. It was corrected by inserting needles at appropriate points along the meridians at sites determined by the complex patterns of disharmony that were diagnosed (382, 383).

Acupuncture was first introduced to Western medicine in a book published in London in the latter part of the 17th century (384). It was used by a French physician in the early 19th century, and was condemned as reckless after an official investigation. There continued to be periodic references to its use in the medical literature, and a translation of a book on acupuncture published in France was available in the United States in 1825. In 1892 William Osler, in the first edition of his *Principles and Practice of Medicine*, recommended it as the most efficient treatment for acute lumbago, and commented that ordinary bonnet needles would do! However, acupuncture attracted little attention in American medicine until the early 1970s. Then, as a result of visits to China by western journalists and physicians, a widespread lay as well as medical interest developed in the phenomenon based on observations of surgery being performed under acupuncture anesthesia (385, 386).

ACUPUNCTURE FOR PAIN TREATMENT

Acupuncture involves inserting needles, usually stainless steel, 28–30 gauge, and approximately 1–10 cm in length, into selected anatomic points (383). Three hundred sixty-five points were recorded in the Yellow Emperor's treatise, but the number has differed subsequently. The depth of penetration varies, and a sensation of "take," described as tingling, numbness, and heaviness, is commonly experienced by the patient if the procedure is to be successful. The needle is twirled to facilitate the sensation of take and, once achieved, electrical stimulation may be applied.

Although acupuncture based on traditional concepts for the treatment of disease is practiced in the United States, particularly in areas with large Chinese populations, its major application has been for pain treatment. Classic acupuncture points as portrayed in ancient charts are commonly used. Recent studies suggest that acupuncture need not be applied precisely at the classical points, however, and that stimulation close to the site of pain is generally more effective than stimulation at distant sites. Acupuncture analgesia has been attributed by some to a placebo effect, particularly after studies showed that stimulation at non-acupuncture points was equally effective. However, it is likely that stimulation is effective within a large area. The production of analgesia in animals also suggests that the effect is not due to placebo alone. Further, it appears that needle puncture is not essential, and that an analgesic effect can be produced by various types of intense sensory stimulation (387). The relationship of acupuncture analgesia to afferent neural transmission is suggested by the demonstration that the analgesic effect is blocked by procaine infiltration of acupuncture points and by the observation that acupuncture points in hemiplegic limbs are ineffective unless sweating is present or there is other evidence that sympathetic nervous innervation is intact (383, 387).

The gate control theory as described by Melzack and Wall provided a possible physiologic mechanism to explain the relief of pain by acupuncture (388, 389). It now appears that this theory alone cannot account for this effect, because it was later shown that electrical stimulation of A fibers did not abolish the pain produced by C fiber stimulation (390). Melzack (389, 391) has subsequently postulated the existence of a central biasing mechanism at higher levels of the central nervous system that inhibits noxious stimulation when activated by intense somatic stimulation. A similar mechanism is thought to account for the pain relief produced by transcutaneous and dorsal column electrical stimulation. The existence of such a mechanism is suggested by the observation that stimulation of midbrain periaqueductal gray by electricity or opiates produces excitation of rostral medulla neurons and inhibits firing of trigeminal and spinal pain transmission neurons. As part of a negative feedback loop, the output of pain transmission neurons is an important factor in activating the pain suppression system (392). Some studies have suggested that the pain suppression mechanism may be mediated in part by endorphins. Pomerantz and Chiu (393) reduced the response to noxious heat stimulation in awake mice 54% by electroacupuncture, as measured by squeak response. Subcutaneous naloxone completely abolished this response. Mayer et al. (394) produced pain by electrostimulation of teeth in volunteers. Analgesia was produced by needling the *Ho-Ku* point on the hand. Significant analgesia was produced by acupuncture, compared to a no-treatment control group and a placebo group given saline injection. In a sample with a 20% increase in pain threshold, naloxone reduced the pain threshold to placebo levels, a significant difference compared to a saline-treated control group. Sjolund et al. (395) found a rise in an endorphin fraction in spinal fluid of patients with chronic pain who were being treated with acupuncture. Kiser et al. (396) studied endorphin levels in 20 patients treated by acupuncture for chronic pain syndromes. They found that symptom relief correlated with higher levels of metenkephalin. However, other studies have not confirmed the reversal of acupuncture analgesia by naloxone. Chapman et al. (397) used acupuncture to reduce pain intensity, as measured by dental dolorimetry and smaller electroencephalograph evoked potential amplitude. Neither of these responses was reversed by naloxone. In a subsequent study Chapman et al. (398) were unable to demonstrate the reversal of dental acupuncture analgesia with a naloxone injection. Thus, the evidence linking endogenous opiates to acupuncture analgesia remains tentative.

Despite the metaphysical classic theory of acupuncture, and the conflicting results of attempts to understand its physiologic mechanisms through scientific studies, a basic question of the clinician dealing with pain problems is—does it work? Although this question has been subject to serious investigation in the past 15 years, the answer is still unclear. Numerous anecdotal reports and the clinical trials in both the Chinese and American literature have reported positive results (399, 400). However, in the absence of no-treatment or placebo control groups, no conclusions can be drawn. Millman (401), after a comprehensive review in 1977, took a rather skeptical stand, and while acknowledging reported pain relief in large, uncontrolled clinical studies in reputable institutions, concluded that suggestion and placebo effect have substantial roles. On the other hand, some early, controlled studies showed increased pain threshold and tolerance (394, 402, 403).

Some of the special problems encountered in research on the effect of acupuncture in pain have been described by Vincent and Richardson (404). Foremost of these is the problem encountered in doing adequately controlled double-blind studies. In psychopharmacologic research, double-blind studies can be done with both the investigator and the patient unaware of whether an active or an inert substance is being given. In acupuncture studies, incorrect acupuncture points have been used as a control, but the acupuncturist is aware of the difference, and might transmit his expectations to the patient. Further, it appears that needle insertion even at incorrect points might produce some pain reduction. If so, the expectation that true acupuncture points should produce a significantly greater effect than bogus points would place an unrealistic expectation on demonstration of the effectiveness of acupuncture. On the other hand, bogus treatments such as taping needles to the skin have less credibility to the subject and presumably less placebo power.

For these and other reasons, the overall quality of much acupuncture research has not been high. Richardson and Vincent (399) have recently done a thorough review of both controlled and uncontrolled studies of the use of acupuncture for the relief of pain. They evaluated a large number of uncontrolled studies that looked at the effects of acupuncture on mixed groups of pain patients. Although acknowledging that uncontrolled studies make a limited contribution to the evaluation of the effectiveness of acupuncture, they noted that most of these studies suggested that 50–70% of patients with chronic pain achieved clinically significant short-term pain relief, compared with the more commonly reported placebo response rate of 30–50%. Among controlled studies, they found headache and back pain to be the two most common pain disorders for which the effectiveness of acupuncture had been studied. In one study comparing acupuncture with a control condition in which needles were inserted 1 cm from the correct point, true acupuncture reportedly had a significantly greater effect on tension headache than placebo acupuncture. In another study, comparing acupuncture with standard medical treatment for chronic headache, 58% of patients improved on acupuncture compared to 25% improvement on medical treatment. Thus, there is evidence that acupuncture is an effective treatment for headache, although Richardson and Vincent believed there were methodologic problems in both studies that limited their validity. A carefully conducted study comparing acupuncture with placebo transcutaneous electrical nerve stimulation (TENS) revealed the commonly reported placebo response rate of 33% for the mock TENS, and at best an incremental response rate of 20% for acupuncture over placebo. Thus, Richardson and Vincent concluded that despite extensive claims for the effectiveness of acupuncture for the treatment of headache, the overall standard of research reports has generally been poor, and the results of the one adequately controlled study were not encouraging.

Richardson and Vincent's review of controlled studies of acupuncture for low back pain (399) included one study in which acupuncture was significantly more effective than spurious TENS, in which the skin electrodes were connected to a dummy electrical apparatus. In four of five studies they reviewed in which acupuncture was compared with needle insertion at incorrect sites, all but one of the studies reported substantial therapeutic effects of acupuncture. Although true acupuncture showed a tendency toward greater effectiveness than placebo, the difference was not significant. The one study that did not show substantial therapeutic effect was a carefully conducted study comparing locally anesthetized irrelevant acupuncture points with classic points. Using multidimensional evaluation and "blind" assessors, the overall success rate for acupuncture was reported to be 28%, compared to 20% for the control condition. Based on their review, Richardson and Vincent concluded that controlled studies suggest that a majority of back pain patients will derive clinically significant short-term benefits from acupuncture, with highly variable response rates ranging from 26 to 79%. Acupuncture shows no significant advantage over TENS, although the data show a trend in favor of acupuncture. Needling theoretically irrelevant sites showed no significant advantage over use of classic acupuncture points, although trends in the data marginally favored the latter.

From their exhaustive review, Richardson and Vincent (399) concluded that there is good evidence from controlled studies for the short-term effectiveness of acupuncture in relieving clinical pain. The reported success rate of 50–80% is greater than might be expected if the effects were mediated entirely by placebo response, which is generally in the 30–35% range. In studies comparing acupuncture with alternative treatment methods such as TENS and physiotherapy, the evidence is mixed, with the majority of studies finding no statistically significant advantage for acupuncture. Five studies comparing acupuncture at classic sites with needle insertion at random or theoretically irrelevant locations have found classic acupuncture to be significantly more effective, whereas six have found no significant difference in favor of acupuncture. Thus, Richardson and Vincent concluded that the significance of point location remains unclear.

In an effort to determine whether compelling evidence from clinical research exists that acupuncture treatment is efficacious in chronic pain, Ter Reit et al. (405) completed a recent review of 51 studies published between 1963 and 1988. The studies included were those in which needles were used for chronic pain, and there was a reference group of either a sham procedure or an existing treatment modality. All studies were scored on a list of 18 predefined methodologic criteria, with a maximum score of 100. The rather poor quality of most publications was indicated by the fact that only 11 studies scored 50 or more points. No studies earned more than 62% of the maximum score, and the results of the better studies were highly contradictory. Although the results differed somewhat, depending on which cut-off point for quality was chosen, it was the authors' opinion that no definitive conclusion on the efficacy of acupuncture in the treatment of chronic pain could be drawn.

ACUPUNCTURE ANALGESIA DURING SURGICAL PROCEDURES

Although many of the diseases treated with traditional acupuncture were associated with pain, it was not until the latter 1950s that the Chinese began using acupuncture anesthesia (or more accurately analgesia) for control of pain during surgical procedures (386). In the early use of acupuncture analgesia, multiple points were stimulated. Initially, for lung resection as many as 80 needles were used, but this was subsequently reduced, and it is said that comparable results can be produced with one needle in the *Nei-kuan* point on the ventral forearm. One author described 29 acupuncture points as sufficient to produce analgesia for surgical procedures in any area of the body (383).

The impression of early visitors that most operations were successfully conducted under acupuncture analgesia was apparently inaccurate. Bonica (386) estimated that less than 10% and perhaps no more than 1–2% of the operations done in China during the 7 years prior to 1973 were conducted under acupuncture analgesia. Although reportedly effective in 90% of patients, the procedures rated as successful included patients who had obvious pain but for whom the operation could still be accomplished, as well as those in whom supplemental opiates and local anesthetic agents were used. The first American medical mission that visited China in 1974 believed that, using their own criteria, only 30–50% of the Chinese patients had pain relief that would be considered acceptable to American patients (386).

Acupuncture analgesia has not received wide acceptance in mainstream anesthesiology. In one standard text on anesthesiology its use in pain treatment is covered in one brief paragraph (406). It is said to apparently produce a relatively weak analgesia, through mechanisms similar to those in TENS, although less satisfactory because of the added expense and patient-therapist commitment. In the chapter on obstetric anesthesia, it is mentioned as an example of various forms of psychological anesthesia such as hypnosis and natural childbirth, and dismissed as rarely used. Although the ability of acupuncture to alter pain perception can be accepted, the effect is not large and apparently cannot alone account for the pain control observed in surgery. Psychological factors, not unlike those observed in natural childbirth, include careful selection of patients, explanations of what the patient can expect during the procedure, expectations that the patient will share responsibility for pain control, and contact with other patients who have undergone the procedure.

Few if any of the American anesthesiologists who have used acupuncture anesthesia on an experimental basis have seen fit to continue its applications, presumably because of the high failure rate and unpredictable results, especially compared with the certainty of regional and general anesthesia (407). The Chinese are apparently more successful with the procedure because of intense preoperative counseling, their willingness to tolerate moderate to severe pain, the intense motivation provoked in the patient and the surgical team by shortage of anesthetic personnel and by political and ideologic factors, and the skill of Chinese surgeons and their willingness to accept less than optimal operating conditions. Other disadvantages of acupuncture include a waiting period of 20–30 min before the onset of analgesia, the frequent need for needle placement close to the surgical field, the need for manipulation of needles by multiple acupuncturists, and the lack of muscle relaxation for abdominal procedures. Most of the patients receiving acupuncture anesthesia require supplemental analgesics or even anesthetic agents. For these reasons it seems unlikely that the use of acupuncture analgesia for surgical procedures will achieve any wide acceptance in the United States.

CONCLUSIONS

Acupuncture is another treatment method that may be useful in some patients with pain complaints. Although sometimes used by inexperienced persons in an unscrupulous manner, it apparently can be useful when used ethically in appropriate settings. Although controlled studies have not yet fully resolved the questions of its efficacy, the preponderance of evidence seems to be that it is more effective than placebo. Like many other procedures such as TENS, hypnosis, and biofeedback, it apparently may provide relief for some patients for whom other methods have been unsuccessful. With the current intense research interest in pain mechanisms, and the increasing sophistication of treatment outcome studies, it can be anticipated that the role of acupuncture in the overall treatment of pain conditions will be further clarified.

PLACEBO ANALGESIA

Placebos may be defined as therapeutic substances or procedures that are deliberately given to have an effect on a system, syndrome, or disease, but that are without specific activity for the condition being treated (408). They can be viewed as medically doing something soothing when nothing curative can be accomplished (409). Substances given as placebos may be classified as to whether they are pharmacologically inert or whether they are pseudomedicaments, which are active medications that are ordinarily prescribed for a different condition or that are given in a subtherapeutic dose. Placebo effect may be defined as any effect attributable to a pill, potion, or procedure, but not to its pharmacodynamic or specific properties (409).

The use of placebos played an integral role in the practice of medicine for centuries, and in fact most of the therapies practitioners had at their disposal were actually placebos. In fact, Weil suggested that the placebo response was the meat of medicine. Brody defines placebo as a form of medical therapy, or as an intervention designed to stimulate medical therapy (409–413). Examples have included unicorn's horn, viper flesh, moss from the skull of a hanged criminal, eunuch fat, dried mummy, and oil of skinned puppy (410, 414). In ancient Egypt, according to the Ebers Papyrus in 1500 B.C., patients were treated with such substances as lizard blood, crocodile dung, the teeth of an ass, putrid meat, and fly specs (410, 415). One scans the pages of Hippocrates in vain for any treatment of specific value (416).

The use of the quinine-containing chinchona bark, the introduction of which into Europe in the 17th century is attributed, perhaps erroneously, to the Countess of Chinchon, vicereine of Peru, is apparently the first example of a drug that was not a placebo. Sydenham, who demonstrated that it was only effective for fever of malarial origin, contributed to the beginning of scientific medicine (417). Even after the introduction of effective drugs, many physicians recognized the limitations of their efforts and the role of factors other than their specific therapies. In 1859, Quimby stated that "Through a great many mistakes and the prescription of a great many useless drugs, I was led to re-examine the question, and came in the end to the position I now hold: the cure does not depend upon any drug, but simply in the patient's belief in the doctor or the medicine" (417). Oliver Wendell Holmes remarked that if all the drugs were sunk to the bottom of the sea it would be all the better for mankind and all the worse for the fish (418).

The use of the term *placebo* dates back to the 116th Psalm of the Hebrew Bible, which begins "I shall walk." Translated into Latin it became *placebo*, used in the 13th century in the sense of "I shall walk before" or "I shall please" (408, 409, 419, 420). The idea of doing something helpful in a difficult situation became associated with the meaning of the word "placebo." In 1787, Quincy's dictionary defined placebo as a "commonplace method or medicine" (408).

In the 1951 *Dorland's Medical Dictionary*, it is defined as "an inactive substance or preparation, formerly given to please or gratify a patient, now also used in control studies to determine the efficacy of medical substance." It is interesting to note that the document detailing the first federal practice guidelines related to pain management was written by a multidisciplinary team that included physicians, a psychologist, an ethicist, and others (421).

STUDIES OF PAIN RELIEF WITH PLACEBOS

Although prior to 1945 the word "placebo" had never appeared in the title of a medical article, there has since that time been an increasing interest, experimentally and clinically, in placebos (411, 417). Comparison of the effects of active analgesic drugs and placebo have been made in a variety of clinical settings. In a review of 15 clinical studies involving 1082 patients, the therapeutic effectiveness of placebo analgesia was determined (422). The patients suffered from a variety of conditions, including postsurgical wound pain, angina pectoris, and headache. About one-third of these patients received significant pain relief after ingesting placebos, a figure that is typical of most clinical studies. Placebo response has been reported for many types of pain, including postsurgical, labor, postpartum, angina pectoris, dental, cancer, arthritic, and peptic ulcer pain (423).

Some clinicians probably underestimate the percentage of patients who will respond to placebo for pain control (411, 424). In general hospitals in the United States, it is estimated that placebos afford 35–40% of patients significant relief from pain, regardless of the lesion responsible. This includes patients with angina of myocardial origin, bone pain from cancer, or severe postoperative pain (423, 425). It is interesting to note that severe pain may be relieved by placebo in 35% of cases and that morphine may relieve pain in about 75% of cases (426). One might then speculate that about one-half of morphine's effectiveness is placebo effect.

The strength of the placebo response is exemplified by the many treatments that were miraculous when introduced, but proved to be no more effective than placebo when subjected to controlled trials. Benson and McCallie reviewed the use of medical and surgical treatments for angina pectoris that have subsequently been found to be ineffective (427). Between the 1930s and the early 1970s, the xanthenes, khellin, and vitamin E were introduced in turn. These were followed in the mid-1950s by internal mammary artery ligation and implantation. Before it was abandoned, 10,000–15,000 of the latter operations were done, with a mortality rate of about 5%. For all of these treatments uncontrolled trials indicated success rates in the 70–90% range, but controlled studies showed them to be no more effective than placebos. Internal mammary artery ligation was no more effective than a skin incision. The pattern was well recognized in the past. Armand Trosseau, an early 19th century physician, stated "you should treat as many patients as possible with the new drugs while they still have the power to heal" (415).

Experimental studies of the placebo effect have shown that placebo relief of pain is much less dramatic in experimental pain induced in the laboratory than in the clinical setting (419, 422). The former have shown an average pain relief of approximately 16%, compared to an average pain relief of 30–35% in the clinical setting. In studies of placebos and hypnosis in experimental pain, it has been found repeatedly that pain relief is related to the presence of anxiety (428). Apparently neither hypnosis nor placebo is as effective in producing pain relief unless some degree of anxiety is present (428, 429). In clinical pain, fear of its physical and economic implications, and its potential effect on important relationships to others introduce variables that increase the emotional suffering experience of pain. It is probably these components of the pain experience, which cannot be duplicated in the laboratory, that account for a significant part of the placebo effect. Gracely et al. studied a group of dental patients postoperatively who might have received fentanyl, but did not. Their pain rating index was lower (430). Pollmann has shown that the effect of the placebo as an analgesic shows circadian variations. This observation might help substantiate vegetative mechanisms as instrumental in placebo analgesic effectiveness (431). However, Stam and Spanos have demonstrated that contextual variables are correlated with the effectiveness of placebo analgesics (432). It appears that both innate mechanisms and circumstances are important in determining a placebo responder.

PLACEBO RESPONSE

Not all studies show relief with placebo analgesia (433). It would be convenient to identify the situational and personality characterists of placebo response. This is a complex area; however there are emerging data (434, 435). The patient's prior treatment experience is influential. Placebos were approximately twice as effective for patients for whom previous analgesics had been effective, compared to these who had had no previous analgesics or for whom they had been ineffective (436). Responsiveness was influenced by the nature of the pain, with pain of osteoarthritis more responsive than that due to rheumatoid arthritis. The classic observations of Beecher during World War II dramatically illustrated the importance of the meaning of the pain to the patient (437). He studied pain reports and the use of morphine in 215 soldiers who suffered major wounds in the European theater during World War II. Only slightly more than 40% reported bad or moderate pain. Three-fourths of the total group of men wanted no morphine, even though they had received none for a matter of hours, and knew it was available for the asking. Beecher attributed the smaller need for morphine, compared to comparable civilian injuries, to the difference in the meaning of the wound. For the soldier it was a ticket to the hospital, and perhaps home, whereas for the civilian an accident is the beginning of a disaster. Other key elements related to predicting response to placebo analgesia seem to be related to the attitudes and expectations of the patient, attitude of the doctor, and the doctor-patient relationship (411).

Patients who are treated by an individual who has a positive conviction about the treatment or drug potency seem to respond better (408). It has also been demonstrated that if the therapist conveys the concept of plausibility about a drug's potency there will be a better response (416, 435). Placebo response is generally thought to be increased when the physician takes time, shows care and concern, listens, elicits the patient's beliefs about the illness, and offers hope (438). Another potential predictor of placebo response is if the placebo is used for a pain syndrome that has previously responded to placebo analgesia in an experimental setting (439). The concomitant presence of distress or anxiety, as is often present in organic pain syndromes, has also correlated with placebo reactivity (409, 440). Two state variables, the perceived pain level and the level of distress, have been correlated with a response to placebo analgesia (441, 442). Levine et al. have suggested that to trigger the intrinsic systems a minimum level of activity in the ascending pain transmission pathway is required (443). Other positive predictors may be the patient's faith in the treatment procedure with the expectation and anticipation of relief, previous positive experience with treatment, and the patient's acquiescence with the treatment (444).

The personality of the patient and his or her cultural attitudes about pain also play a part in the placebo response. Although some individuals are stronger placebo reactors than others, and seem to be characterized by enduring personality traits such as anxiety and social conformity, no typical placebo reactor personality has been consistently identified.

One early study, using Rorschach data, suggested that the reactors were more anxious, dependent, emotionally labile, and preoccupied with their own internal processes (414). However, they were outwardly oriented and able to drain off their tension through talking with others. The placebo reactors were not "whiners" or "nuisances," not typically male or female, not typically young or old, and had the same average intelligence as nonreactors. In a preoperative period of stress, responders may behave in a more dependent yet outwardly responsive fashion and receive relief through attention from nurses and confidence in the effectiveness of drugs. A number of other investigators have analyzed the characteristics of placebo responses, with contradictory results. Some claim there is no predisposition to respond to placebos, whereas others find common denominators in responders. The most reasonable premise appears to be that there is no constellation of traits that will enable one to neatly pigeonhole people into responders and nonresponders. The placebo response will be determined by numerous factors, including the setting, the symptoms being treated, the specific medical features involved, and the personality, past experience, anticipations, and fears of the individual (420).

The profile of nonresponders to placebo analgesia is not well delineated. In the past, nonresponders have been characterized as being vague, nonspecific, rigid, hard to pin down, self-controlled, using denial, and not psychologically oriented (418, 444, 445).

Unfortunately some medical personnel still regard the "placebo test" as a means of separating functional from organic pain (411, 446), and some practitioners have used placebos on "problem patients" about whom nursing staff has complained. In fact, the demanding, undesirable patients are reported to be the least likely to respond to placebos (411, 424).

MECHANISM OF ACTION OF PLACEBOS

The mechanism of action of placebos is not well understood and overlaps with the discussion of placebo responders. Potential mechanisms postulated include psychological, behavioral, and more recently, induction of the endogenous opioid system. From one perspective, placebos can be viewed as another active pharmacologic agent in their own right, whose analgesic effect can be independently evaluated using the same methods that would be used to test any other potent analgesic agent (408). Placebos can mimic certain characteristics of active drugs such as peak effects, cumulative effects, and carry-over effects (447). Individuals receiving placebos have reported side effects such as nausea, thirst, headache, dizziness, insomnia, sleepiness, fatigue, depression, numbness, difficulty in concentrating, hallucinations, feelings of cold or warmth, itching, and angioneurotic edema (410, 428, 448–450). It has also been suggested that tolerance to placebo analgesia may develop, as well as an abstinence-like syndrome when the substance is suddenly withdrawn (411). The above phenomena become particularly fascinating when considering a treatment modality that is not well understood from either a physiologic or psychological basis.

A review of the psychological and behavioral theories of action of placebos encompasses several topics. A regulatory effect produced by placebos has been proposed in that anxious and emotionally unstable individuals may well respond to placebo treatment (451). It has been proposed that such patients have a subjective reaction to illness, that a part of this reaction is anxiety, and that the role of the placebo in pain relief is primarily to relieve that anxiety (422, 452–454). Other authors have suggested the important role and powerful contribution of suggestion and the expectation that relief will be obtained (389, 413, 455–458). The features of psychotherapy noted by Jerome Frank to be common to all psychotherapies, both primitive and contemporary, are similar to the factors that influence the effectiveness of placebos. These include a trusting relationship with a therapist in whom the patient has confidence, a setting that is identified as a sanctuary or place of healing (doctor's office or hospital), a plausible conceptual scheme accepted by the culture that enables the patient to explain and gain a sense of control over subjective distress, and a procedure based on the conceptual scheme that is believed to be effective (459). The effectiveness of the placebo will be influenced by its plausibility, and by the intrinsic character of the treatment. The latter would include such factors as taste, expense, and route of administration.

It has also been proposed that the placebo effect is a conditioned response that can be understood in terms of learning theory (458–461). For example, pills or injections of an active analgesic in the past have become associated with pain relief. Thus a similar stimulus, in this case an inert substance administered by mouth or by injection, will produce a conditioned analgesic response. It has been shown that both behavioral and physiologic responses can be conditioned in animals in this manner (408).

A proposed physiologic mechanism of action of placebos is related to the stimulation of endogenous opioids, although their role is still controversial (462). It has been suggested that placebo responders have increased levels of endorphins and that naloxone can reverse placebo-induced pain reduction (463). There is evidence that enkephalins (and perhaps beta endorphins) inhibit substance P release and may act at the level of the spinal cord or brainstem to block pain transmission. It is thought that substance P may act as a sensory neurotransmitter for relay of pain signals to second-order neurons of the spinothalamic system (425). In some types of postoperative pain naloxone has produced hyperalgesia (441, 464, 465). Also in experimental ischemic pain, placebo analgesia in placebo responders was diminished by naloxone (466). Also the potent analgesia produced by the micro-injection of opiates into several endorphin-containing brainstem sites seems to support the idea that the endorphins in these regions do mediate analgesia (442). It appears that naloxone does not affect the placebo response in the absence of stress, however (462).

ETHICAL CONSIDERATIONS

Although the use of placebos is apparently not uncommon, most physicians would probably agree with the comments made by Richard Cabot, the eminent Harvard physician, 75 years ago (409), who expressed doubt that there "is a physician in this country who has not used them and used them pretty often," and who deplored the fact that so many physicians believed it to be impossible to deal frankly and openly with patients. He argued against placebo use on the basis that the potential loss of trust in the physician by the patient and the community outweighed any short-term benefits. Although the deception might never be discovered, Cabot was of the opinion that it was not good for physicians to have their reputation rest on the expectation of not being found out. He countered the argument that patients will not be satisfied without medicine for every symptom by pointing out that the patient was not born with this expectation, but "learned it from an ignorant doctor."

On the other hand, many who recognize the ethical implications of placebo use believe that it may be justified in some situations, such as in temporary situations to placate the patient until a relationship can be established, in diseases for which placebos have proved efficacious experimentally, or in prolonged diagnostic testing during which the patient, if not placated, might not return for needed treatment. They also point out that there is a placebo component in almost every use of an active medication by a physician and that one should not withhold any remedy that affords some degree of relief (409, 418). The widespread use of placebos that some studies have revealed cannot be responsibly defended, however.

The British Medical Journal editorialized in 1952 that "a bottle of medicine is given as a placebo in about 40% of patients seen in general practice." In a 1952 analysis of 17,000 prescriptions in Great Britain, about one-third were considered placebos. This is close to Cabot's estimate in 1906 that placebos accounted for 44% of prescriptions filled in Boston Back Bay drug stores (417). In a more recent study of placebo use by house staff and nurses, it was found that during a 6-month period nearly two-thirds of house staff had ordered placebos to see if a patient's pain was "real," 9 out of 10 had ordered placebos for patients they thought were asking for more pain medicine than the staff members thought necessary, and three-fourths had ordered placebos for patients the nurses were complaining about (424). Those who believe that placebos present an ethical dilemma would argue that this type of therapy is deceptive and risks the loss of patient trust. The possibility of nurturing unhealthy public attitudes also exists, in that people may become conditioned to expect medication for every symptom (409). Further, the practice does not take patient autonomy into consideration, nor does it honor the doctor-patient relationship or the right of informed consent.

CONCLUSIONS

Despite the remarkable technological advances made in medicine, there are many chronic conditions for which no cure is possible, and the most the physician can offer is symptomatic relief. For this group of patients particularly, the placebo effect can be a significant benefit. This does not imply the intentional use of an ineffective or inert substance, but rather the conscious use of strategies that increase the expectiveness of any treatment.

Foremost of these is the doctor-patient relationship. Whatever increases the quality of this interaction will often facilitate treatment and contribute to the patient's comfort and symptom relief. A personal interest in the patient, demonstrated by a positive regard and nonjudgmental acceptance, is an important ingredient of the relationship. A willingness to work with the patient to achieve the best possible result, to communicate through explanations and the sharing of responsibility for treatment decisions, and to provide plausible rationales for treatment modalities all potentially influence treatment response. One informative study compared the amount of morphine used by patients after undergoing abdominal surgery who had received an explanation of the pain to be expected and instructions in relaxation techniques prior to surgery, with that used by a control group. The experimental group experienced significantly less pain and used significantly less morphine (467).

Maximizing the placebo response to nonspecific therapies does not imply deception or an insincere and exaggerated assurance of benefits. Rather, it implies a manner that stimulates trust and inspires hope. In the context of a positive relationship, the placebo effect of modalities such as relaxation training, therapeutic exercise, diet, mild analgesics, and the like may be magnified, particularly if prescribed with a plausible rationale for their anticipated mental and physiologic effects. Within this type of relationship, placebos may even be openly prescribed. For example, if presented with an explanation as to the manner in which placebos can, through conditioning and the endogenous opioid system, have a genuine psychophysiologic effect, they can be introduced gradually into a patient's analgesic regimen on an unknown schedule with the concurrence of the patient. This strategy is often used in the behavioral component of pain treatment programs to facilitate reduction or discontinuation of narcotic-like analgesics. Used in these ways, within the context of positive doctor-patient relationships, the placebo response, which is actually inherent in and of greater or lesser importance to every therapeutic act, can be maximized and used as an integral part of the physician's healing armamentarium.

REFERENCES

1. Hilgard E, Hilgard JR: *Hypnosis in the Relief of Pain.* Los Altos, CA, William Kaufmann, 1975.
2. Ewin DM: Hypnosis in surgery and anesthesia. In Wester WC III, Smith AH Jr (eds): *Clinical Hypnosis: A Multidisciplinary Approach.* Philadelphia, JB Lippincott, 1984, p 210.
3. Shor RE: Explorations in hypnosis: A theoretical and experimental study. Doctoral dissertation, Brandeis University, 1959.
4. Hilgard ER: A quantitative study of pain and its reduction through hypnotic suggestion. *Proc Nat Acad Sci USA* 57:1581–1986, 1967.
5. Evans MB, Paul GL: Effects of hypnotically suggested analgesia on physiological and subjective responses to cold stress. *J Consult Clin Psychol* 35:362–371, 1970.
6. Hilgard ER, Ruch JC, Lange AF, et al: The psychophysics of cold pressor pain and its modification through hypnotic suggestion. *Am J Psychol* 87:17–31, 1974.
7. Knox VJ, Morgan AH, Hilgard ER: Pain and suffering in ischemia: The paradox of hypnotically suggested anesthesia as contradicted by reports from the "hidden observer." *Arch Gen Psychiatry* 30:840–847, 1974.
8. Shor RE: Physiological effects of painful stimulation during hypnotic analgesia under conditions designed to minimize anxiety. *Int J Clin Exp Hypn* 10:183–202, 1962.
9. Greene RJ, Reyher J: Pain tolerance in hypnotic analgesic and imagination states. *J Abnorm Psychol* 79:29–38, 1972.
10. Miller MF, Barabasz AF, Barabasz M: Effects of active alert and relaxation hypnotic inductions on cold pressor pain. *J Abnorm Psychol* 100:223–226, 1991.
11. DeBenedittis G, Panerai AA, Villamira MA: Effects of hypnotic analgesia and hypnotizability on experimental ischemic pain. *Int J Clin Exp Hyp* 37:55–69, 1989.
12. Hilgard ER: Pain as a puzzle for psychology and physiology. *Am Psychol* 24:103–113, 1969.
13. Hilgard ER: Pain: Its reduction and production under hypnosis. *Proc Am Philos Soc* 115:470–476, 1971.
14. McGlashan TH, Evans FJ, Orne MT: The nature of hypnotic analgesia and the placebo response to experimental pain. *Psychosom Med* 31:227–246, 1969.
15. Moret V, Forster A, Laverriere MC, et al: Mechanism of analgesia induced by hypnosis and acupuncture: Is there a difference? *Pain* 45:135–140, 1991.
16. Gottfredson DK: Hypnosis as an anesthetic in dentistry. *Dissert Abstr Int* 33(7-B):3303, 1973.
17. Wakeman RJ, Kaplan JZ: An experimental study of hypnosis in painful burns. *Am J Clin Hypn* 21:3–10, 1978.
18. Van der Does AJ, Van Dyck R, Spijker RE: Hypnosis and pain in patients with severe burns: A pilot study. *Burns Ind Therm Inj* 14:399–404, 1988.
19. Patterson DR, Questad KA, Boltwood MD: Hypnotherapy as a treatment for pain in patients with burns: Research and clinical considerations. *J Burn Care Rehabil* 8:263–268, 1987.
20. Wolberg LR: *Medical Hypnosis.* New York, Grune & Stratton, 1948.
21. Horan JS: Hypnosis and recorded suggestions in the treatment of migraine. *J Clin Exp Hypn* 1:7, 1953.
22. Blumenthal LS: Hypnotherapy of headaches. *Headache* 2:197, 1963.
23. Hanley FW: Hypnotherapy of migraine. *Can Psychiatr Assoc J* 9:254, 1964.
24. Harding CH: Hypnosis in the treatment of migraine. In Lassner J (ed): *Hypnosis and Psychosomatic Medicine.* New York, Springer-Verlag, 1967.
25. Greenleaf E: Defining hypnosis during hypnotherapy. *Int J Clin Exp Hypn* 22:120, 1974.
26. Anderson JAD, Basker MA, Dalton R: Migraine and hypnotherapy. *Int J Clin Exp Hypn* 23:48–58, 1975.
27. Andreychuk T, Skriver C: Hypnosis and biofeedback in

the treatment of migraine headache. *Int J Clin Exp* 23:172, 1975.

28. Graham GW: Hypnotic treatment of migraine headache. *Int Clin Exp Hypn* 23:165, 1975.

29. Maher LGP: Intensive hypno-autohypnosis in resistant psychosomatic disorders. *J Psychosom Res* 19:361–365, 1975.

30. Cedercreutz C, Lahteenmaki R, Tulikoura J: Hypnotic treatment of headache and vertigo in skull injured patients. *Int J Clin Exp Hypn* 24:195–200, 1976.

31. Daniels LK: The effects of automated hypnosis and hand warming on migraine: A pilot study. *Am J Clin Hypn* 19:91–94, 1976.

32. Daniels LK: Treatment of migraine headache by hypnosis and behavior therapy: A case study. *Am J Clin Hypn* 19:241–244, 1977.

33. Kroger WS, Fezler WD: *Hypnosis and Behavior Modification: Imagery Conditioning.* Philadelphia, JB Lippincott, 1976.

34. Kroger WS: *Clinical and Experimental Hypnosis.* Philadelphia, JB Lippincott, 1977.

35. Stambaugh EE, House AE: Multimodality treatment of migraine headache: A case study utilizing biofeedback, relaxation, autogenic and hypnotic treatments. *Am J Clin Hypn* 19:235–240, 1977.

36. DePiano FA, Salzberg HC: Clinical applications of hypnosis to three psychosomatic disorders. *Psychol Bull* 86:1223–1235, 1979.

37. Wain HJ: Pain control through use of hypnosis. *Am J Clin Hypn* 23:41–46, 1980.

38. Friedman H, Taub HA: An evaluation of hypnotic susceptibility and peripheral temperature elevation in the treatment of migraine. *Am J Clin Hypn* 24:172–182, 1982.

39. Howard L, Reardon JP, Tosi D: Modifying migraine headache through rational stage directed hypnotherapy: A cognitive-experimental perspective. *Int J Clin Exp Hypn* 30:257–269, 1982.

40. Milne G: Hypnobehavioral medicine in a university counselling centre. *Aust J Clin Exp Hypn* 10:13–26, 1982.

41. Milne G: Hypnotherapy with migraine. *Aust J Clin Exp Hypn* 11:23–32, 1983.

42. Toomey TC, Sanders S: Group hypnotherapy as an active control strategy in chronic pain. *Am J Clin Hypn* 26:20–25, 1983.

43. De Shazer S: The imaginary pill technique. *J Strat Syst Ther* 3:30–34, 1984.

44. Friedman H, Taub HA: Brief psychological training procedures in migraine treatment. *Am J Clin Hypn* 26:187–200, 1984.

45. Kapelis L: Hypnosis in a behavior therapy framework for the treatment of migraine in children. *Aust J Clin Exp Hypn* 12:123–126, 1984.

46. Spinhoven P: Similarities and dissimilarities in hypnotic and nonhypnotic procedures for headache control: A review. *Am J Clin Hypn* 30:183–194, 1988.

47. Daly E, Wulff J: Treatment of a post-traumatic headache. *Br J Med Psychol* 60:85–88, 1987.

48. Erickson MH: Special techniques of brief hypnotherapy. *J Clin Exp Hypn* 2:109, 1954.

49. Levit HI: Depression, back pain and hypnosis. *Am J Clin Hypn* 15:266, 1973.

50. Melzack R, Perry C: Self-regulation of pain: The use of alpha-feedback and hypnotic training for the control of chronic pain. *Exp Neurol* 46:452–469, 1975.

51. Crasilneck HB: Hypnosis in the control of chronic low back pain. *Am J Clin Hypn* 22:71–78, 1979.

52. Johnson LS, Wiese KF: Live versus tape-recorded assessments of hypnotic responsiveness in pain-control patients. *Int J Clin Exp Hypn* 27:74–84, 1979.

53. Lemmon KW: Chronic lower back pain differentiation of the real and imagined. *Med Hypnoanal* 4:17–30, 1983.

54. Michels PJ, Adams DB, McBride P: Chronic pain. *J Fam Pract* 17:591–610, 1983.

55. Frank A: Therapies for back pain. *Practitioner* 234:113–115, 1990.

56. Butler B: The use of hypnosis in the care of the cancer patient. *Cancer* 7:1–14, 1954.

57. Butler B: The use of hypnosis in the care of the cancer patient. (Part I). *Br Med Hypn* 6:2–12, 1954.

58. Butler B: The use of hypnosis in the care of the cancer patient. (Part II). *Br J Med Hypn* 6:2–12, 1955.

59. Butler B: The use of hypnosis in the care of the cancer patient. (Part III). *Br J Med Hypn* 6:9–17, 1955.

60. Hedge AR: Hypnosis in cancer. *Br J Med Hypn* 12:2, 1960.

61. Lea P, Ware P, Monroe R: The hypnotic control of intractable pain. *Am J Clin Hypn* 3:3–8, 1960.

62. Cangello VW: The use of the hypnotic suggestion for relief in malignant disease. *Int J Clin Exp Hypn* 9:17–22, 1961.

63. Caricoppa JM: Hypnosis in terminal cancer. *Am J Clin Hypn* 5:205, 1963.

64. Cangello VW: Hypnosis for the patient with cancer. *Am J Clin Hypn* 4:215–226, 1962.

65. Sacerdote P: Additional contributions to the hypnotherapy of the advanced cancer patient. *Am J Clin Hypn* 7:308–319, 1965.

66. Sacerdote P: Theory and practice of pain control in malignancy and other protracted or recurring painful illnesses. *Int J Clin Exp Hypn* 18:160–180, 1970.

67. Saceerdote P: Some individualized psychotherapeutic techniques. *Int J Clin Exp Hypn* 20:1–14, 1972.

68. Sacerdote P: Convergence of expectations: An essential component of successful hypnotherapy. *Int J Clin Exp Hypn* 22:95–115, 1974.

69. Chong TM: The use of hypnosis in the management of patients with cancer. *Singapore Med J* 9:211–214, 1968.

70. LaBaw WL: Terminal hypnosis in lieu of terminal hospitalization: An effective alternative in fortunate cases. *Gerontol Clin* 11:312–320, 1969.

71. Crasilneck HB, Hall JA: Clinical hypnosis in problems of pain. *Am J Clin Hypn* 15:153–161, 1973.

72. Crasilneck HB, Hall JA: *Clinical Hypnosis: Principles and Applications.* New York, Grune & Stratton, 1975.

73. Willard RD: Perpetual trance as a means of controlling pain in the treatment of terminal cancer with hypnosis. *J Am Inst Hypn* 15:111–131, 1974.

74. Clawson TH: The hypnotic control of blood flow and pain and the potential use of hypnosis in the treatment of cancer. *Am J Clin Hypn* 17:160, 1975.

75. Margolis C: Hypnotic imagery with cancer patients. *Am J Clin Hypn* 25:128–134, 1982.

76. Araoz DL: Use of hypnotic techniques with oncology patients. *J Psychosoc Oncol* 1:47–54, 1983.

77. Davidson GP: Hypnotic augmentation of terminal care chemoanalgesia. *Aust J Clin Exp Hypn* 12:133–134, 1984.

78. Jay SM, Elliott C, Varni JW: Acute and chronic pain in adults and children with cancer. *J Consult Clin Psychol* 54:601–607, 1985.

79. Filshie J: The non-drug treatment of neurologic and neuropathic pain of malignancy. *Cancer Surv* 7:161–193, 1988.

80. Wu TJ, Sun WZ, Luu KC, Lin SY: Application of hypnoanalgesia for the treatment of chronic cancer pain—Report of one case. *MA Tsui Hsuch Tsa Chi* 28:361–365, 1990.

81. Bachet M, Weiss C: Treatment of disorders of amputated subjects by hypnotic inhibition. *Br J Med Hypn* 4:15, 1952.

82. Dorcus RM: *Hypnosis and Its Therapeutic Applications.* New York, McGraw-Hill, 1956.

83. Papermaster AA, Doberneck RC, Bonello FJ, et al: Hypnosis in surgery: II. Pain. *Am J Clin Hypn* 2:220–224, 1960.

84. Chappell DT: Hypnosis and spasticity in paraplegic. *Am J Clin Hypn* 7:33, 1964.

85. Cedercreutz C, Uusitalo E: Hypnotic treatment of phantom sensations in 37 amputees. In Lassner J (ed): *Hypnosis and Psychosomatic Medicine.* New York, Springer-Verlag, 1967, pp 65–66.

86. Siegal EF: Control of phantom limb pain by hypnosis. *Am J Clin Hypn* 21:285–286, 1979.

87. Baker SR: Amelioration of phantom-organ pain with hypnosis and behavior modification: Brief case report. *Psychol Rep* 55:847–850, 1984.

88. Swerdlow B: A rapid hypnotic technique in a case of atypical facial neuralgia. *Headache* 24:104–109, 1984.

89. Stam HJ, McGrath PA, Brooke RI, et al: Hypnotizability and the treatment of chronic facial pain. *Int J Clin Exp Hypn* 34:182–191, 1986.

90. Cheek DB: Therapy of persistent pain states: Part 1, neck and shoulder pain of five years' duration. *Am J Clin Hypn* 8:281, 1966.

91. Williams JA: Ericksonian hypnotherapy of intractable shoulder pain. *Am J Clin Hypn* 26:26–29, 1983.

92. Elkins GR: Hypnosis in the treatment of myofibrositis and anxiety: A case report. *Am J Clin Hypn* 27:26–30, 1984.

93. Gould SS, Tissler DM: The use of hypnosis in the treatment of herpes simplex II. *Am J Clin Hypn* 26:171–174, 1984.

94. Smith SJ, Balaban AB: A multidimensional approach to pain relief: Case report of a patient with systemic lupus erythematosus. *Int J Clin Exp Hypn* 31:72–81, 1983.

95. Zane MD: The hypnotic situation and change in ulcer pain. *Int J Clin Exp Hypn* 14:292–304, 1966.

96. Graham G: Hypnoanalysis in dental practice. *Am J Clin Hypn* 16:178–187, 1974.

97. Golan HP: Control of fear reaction in dental patients by hypnosis: Three case reports. *Am J Clin Hypn* 13:279–284, 1971.

98. Schneck JM: Hypnotherapy for vaginismus. *Int J Clin Exp Hypn* 13:92, 1965.

99. Sachs LB, Feuerstein M, Vitale JH: Hypnotic self-regulation of chronic pain. *Am J Clin Hypn* 20:106–113, 1977.

100. Lehew JL: The use of hypnosis in the treatment of musculoskeletal disorders. *Am J Clin Hypn* 13:131–134, 1980.

101. Domangue BB, Margolis CG, Leiberman D, et al: Biochemical correlates of hypnoanalgesia in arthritic pain patients. *J Clin Psychiatr* 46:235–238, 1985.

102. Friedman H, Taub HA: Brief psychological training procedures in migraine treatment. *Am J Clin Hypn* 26:187–200, 1984.

103. Orne MT: Hypnotic control of pain: Toward a clarification of the different psychological processes involved. *Res Publ Assoc Res Nerv Ment Dis* 58:155–172, 1988.

104. Large RG, James FR: Personalized evaluation of self-hypnosis as a treatment of chronic pain: A repertory grid analysis. *Pain* 35:155–169, 1988.

105. Melzack R: The tragedy of needless pain. *Sci Am* 262:27–33, 1990.

106. Carasso RL, Arnon G, Yehuda S, Mastofsky DI: Hypnotic techniques for the management of pain. *J R Soc Health* 108:176–179, 1988.

107. Kleinhauz M: Prolonged hypnosis with individualized therapy. *Int J Clin Exp Hypn* 39:82–92, 1991.

108. Wain HJ, Amen DG: Emergency room use of hypnosis. *Gen Hosp Psychiat* 8:19–22, 1986.

109. Goldstein A, Hilgard ER: Lack of influence of the morphine antagonist naloxone on hypnotic analgesia. *Proc Nat Acad Sci USA* 72:2041–2043, 1975.

110. Barber J, Mayer D: Evaluation of the efficacy and neural mechanism of a hypnotic analgesia procedure in experimental and clinical dental pain. *Pain* 4:41–48, 1977.

111. Hilgard ER: Hypnosis and pain. In Sternbach RA (ed): *The Psychology of Pain.* New York, Raven Press, 1980, p 219.

112. Stephenson JBP: Reversal of hypnosis-induced analgesia by naloxone. *Lancet* 2:991–992, 1978.

113. Terenius L, Wahlstrom A: Endorphins and clinical pain, an overview. *Adv Exp Med Biol* 116:262–277, 1979.

114. Frid M, Singer G: Hypnotic analgesia in conditions of stress is partially reversed by naloxone. *Psychopharmacology* 63:211–215, 1979.

115. Sternbach RA: On strategies for identifying neurochemical correlates of hypnotic analgesia: A brief communication. *Int J Clin Exp Hypn* 30:251–256, 1982.

116. Spiegel D: Uses of hypnosis in managing medical symptoms. *Psychiatr Med* 9:521–533, 1991.

117. Bowers KS, LeBaron S: Hypnosis and hypnotizability: Implications for clinical intervention. *Hosp Commun Psychiatr* 37:457–467, 1986.

118. Olness K, MacDonald JT, Uden DL: Comparison of self-hypnosis and propranolol in the treatment of juvenile classic migraine. *Pediatrics* 79:593–597, 1987.

119. Olness K: Hypnotherapy: A cyberphysiologic strategy in pain management. *Pediatr Clin North Am* 36:873–874, 1989.

120. Lovell DJ, Walco GA: Pain associated with juvenile rheumatoid arthritis. *Pediatr Clin North Am* 36:1015–1027, 1989.

121. Zeltzer LK, Jay SM, Fisher DM: The management of pain associated with pediatric procedures. *Pediatr Clin North Am* 36:941–964, 1989.

122. Caswell LJ, Eland JM: "Don't bump my bed, don't touch my feet!" *J Pediatr Oncol Nurs* 6:111–120, 1989.

123. Valente SM: Using hypnosis with children for pain management. *Oncol Nurs Forum* 18:699–704, 1991.

124. Thomas BL: Pain management for the elderly: Alternative interventions—Part II. *AORN J* 53:126–132, 1991.

125. Benson H: *The Relaxation Response*. New York, William Morrow, 1975.

126. Budzynski TH, Stoyva JM, Adler CS, et al: EMG biofeedback and tension headache: A controlled outcome study. *Psychosom Med* 35:484–496, 1973.

127. Cox DJ, Fveundlich A, Meyer RG: Differential effectiveness of electromyograph feedback, verbal relaxation instructions, and medication placebo with tension headaches. *J Consult Clin Psychol* 43:892–989, 1975.

128. Haynes SN, Griffin P, Mooney D, et al: Electromyographic biofeedback and relaxation instructions in the treatment of muscle contraction headaches. *Behav Ther* 6:672–678, 1975.

129. Chesney MA, Shelton JL: A comparison of muscle relaxation and electromyogram biofeedback treatments for muscle contraction headaches. *J Behav Ther Exp Psychiatr* 7:221–225, 1976.

130. Hutchings DF, Reinkingy RH: Tension headaches: What form of therapy is most effective *Biofeedback Self Regul* 1:183–190, 1976.

131. Reeves JL: EMG biofeedback reduction of tension headache. A cognitive skills training approach. *Biofeedback Self Regul* 1:217–225, 1976.

132. Kondo CY, Canter A: Time and false electromyographic feedback: Effect on tension headache. *J Abnorm Psychol* 86:93–95, 1977.

133. Peck CL, Kraft GH: Electromyographic biofeedback for pain related to muscle tension: A study of tension headache, back, and jaw pain. *Arch Surg* 112:889–895, 1977.

134. Philips C: The modification of tension headache. *Behav Res Ther* 15:119–129, 1977.

135. Budzynski T: Biofeedback in the treatment of muscle-contraction (tension) headache. *Biofeedback Self Regul* 3:409–434, 1978.

136. Tsushima WT, Hawk AB: EMG biofeedback treatment of traumatic headaches: A preliminary outcome study. *Am J Clin Biofeedback* 1:65–67, 1978.

137. Bruhn P, Olesen J, Melgaard B: Controlled trial of EMG feedback in muscle contraction headache. *Ann Neurol* 6:34–36, 1979.

138. Russ KL, Hammer RL, Adderton M: Clinical follow-up treatment and outcome of functional headache patients treated with biofeedback. *J Clin Psychol* 35:148–153, 1979.

139. Gray CL, Lyle RC, McGuire RJ, et al: Electrode placement, EMG feedback, and relaxation for tension headaches. *Behav Res Ther* 18:19–23, 1980.

140. Kumaraiah V: EMG biofeedback and progressive muscular relaxation in treatment of tension headache. *Ind J Clin Psychol* 7:1–5, 1980.

141. Schlutter LC, Golden CJ, Blume HG: A comparison of treatments for prefrontal muscle contraction headache. *Br J Med Psychol* 53:47–52, 1980.

142. Carrobles JA, Cardona A, Santacreu J: Shaping and generalization procedures in the EMG-biofeedback treatment of tension headaches. *Br J Clin Psychol* 20:49–56, 1981.

143. Philips C, Hunter M: The treatment of tension headache: I. Muscular abnormality and biofeedback. *Behav Res Ther* 19:485–498, 1981.

144. Satinsky D, Frerotte A: Biofeedback treatment for headache: A two-year follow-up study. *Am J Clin Biofeedback* 4:62–65, 1981.

145. Blanchard EB, Andrasik F, Neff DF, et al: Sequential comparisons of relaxation training and biofeedback in the treatment of three kinds of chronic headache, or The machines may be necessary some of the time. *Behav Res Ther* 20:469–481, 1982.

146. Blanchard EB, Andrasik F, Neff DF, et al: Biofeedback and relaxation training with three kinds of headache: Treatment effects and their prediction. *J Consult Clin Psychol* 50:562–575, 1982.

147. Andrasik F, Blanchard EB, Edlund SR, et al: EMG biofeedback treatment of a child with muscle contraction headache. *Am J Clin Biofeedback* 6:96–102, 1983.

148. Bell NW, Abramowitz SI, Falkins CH, et al: Biofeedback, brief psychotherapy and tension headache. *Headache* 23:162–173, 1983.

149. Daly EJ, Donn PA, Galliher MJ, et al: Biofeedback applications of migraine and tension headaches: A double-blinded outcome study. *Biofeedback Self Regul* 8:135–152, 1983.

150. Janssen K: Differential effectiveness of EMG-feedback versus combined EMG-feedback and relaxation instructions in the treatment of tension headache. *J Psychosom Res* 27:243–253, 1983.

151. Onorato VA, Tsushima WT: EMG, MMPI, and treatment outcome in the biofeedback therapy of tension headache and posttraumatic pain. *Am J Clin Biofeedback* 6:71–81, 1983.

152. Ahles TA, King A, Martin JE: EMG biofeedback during dynamic movement as a treatment for tension headache. *Headache* 24:41–44, 1984.

153. Gada MT: A comparative study of efficacy of EMG biofeedback and progressive muscular relaxation in tension headache. *Ind J Psychiatr* 26:121–127, 1984.

154. Levine BA: Effects of depression and headache type on biofeedback for muscle-contraction headaches. *Behav Psychother* 12:300–307, 1984.

155. Werder DS, Sargent JD: A study of childhood headache using biofeedback as a treatment alternative. *Headache* 24:122–126, 1984.

156. Abramowitz SI, Bell NW: Biofeedback, self-control and tension headache. *J Psychosom Res* 29:95–99, 1985.

157. Daly EJ, Zimmerman JS, Donn PA, et al: Psychophysiological treatment of migraine and tension headaches: A 12 month follow-up. *Rehabil Psychol* 30:3–10, 1985.

158. Weranch HR, Keenan DM: Behavioral treatment of children with recurrent headaches. *J Behav Ther Exp Psychiatr* 16:31–38, 1985.

159. Lacroix JM, Clarke MA. Bock JC, et al: Muscle-contraction headaches in multiple pain patients: Treatment under worsening baseline conditions. *Arch Phys Med Rehabil* 67:14–18, 1986.

160. Blanchard EB, Andrasik F, Appelbaum KA, et al: Three studies of the psychologic changes in chronic headache patients associated with biofeedback and relaxation therapies. *Psychosom Med* 48:73–83, 1986.

161. Collet L, Cottraux J, Juenet C: GSR feedback and Schultz relaxation in tension headaches: A comparative study. *Pain* 25:205–213, 1986.

162. Diamond S: Treatment of chronic headache. A nonpharmacologic approach. *Postgrad Med* 81:91–93, 1987.

163. Schwartz MS: Biofeedback and stress management in the treatment of headache. *J Craniomandib Disord* 1:41–45, 1987.

164. Blanchard EB, Andrasik F, Guarnieri P, et al: Two-, three-, and four-year follow-up on the self-regulatory treatment of chronic headache with biofeedback and/or relaxation. *J Consult Clin Psychol* 55:257–259, 1987.

165. Blanchard EB, Appelbaum KA, Guarnieri P, et al: Five year prospective follow-up on the treatment of chronic headache with biofeedback and/or relaxation. *Headache* 27:580–583, 1987.

166. Smith WB: Biofeedback and relaxation training: The effect on headache and associated symptoms. *Headache* 27:511–514, 1987.

167. Reich BA: Non-invasive treatment of vascular and muscle contraction headache: A comparative longitudinal clinical study. *Headache* 29:34–41, 1989.

168. Sargent JD, Green EE, Walters ED: The use of autogenic feedback training in a pilot study of migraine and tension headaches. *Headache* 12:120–124, 1972.

169. Sargent JD, Green EE, Walters ED: Preliminary report on the use of autogenic feedback training in the treatment of migraine and tension headaches. *Psychosom Med* 35:129–135, 1973.

170. Johnson WG, Turin A: Biofeedback treatment of migraine headache: A systematic case study. *Behav Ther* 6:394–397, 1975.

171. Adler CS, Adler SM: Biofeedback therapy for the treatment of headaches: A five year follow-up. *Headache* 16:189–191, 1976.

172. Friar LR, Beatty J: Migraine: Management by trained control of vasoconstriction. *J Consult Clin Psychol* 44:46–53, 1976.

173. Medtina JL, Diamond S, Franklin MA: Biofeedback therapy for migraine. *Headache* 16:115–118, 1976.

174. Mitch PS, McGrady A, Iannone A: Autogenic feedback training in migraine: A treatment report. *Headache* 15:267–270, 1976.

175. Reading C, Mohr PD: Biofeedback control of migraine: A pilot study. *Br J Soc Clin Psychol* 15:429–433, 1976.

176. Turin A, Johnson WG: Biofeedback therapy for migraine headaches. *Arch Gen Psychiatr* 33:527–519, 1976.

177. Feuerstein M, Adams HE: Cephalic vasomotor feedback in the modification of migraine headache. *Biofeedback Self Regul* 2:241–254, 1977.

178. Blanchard EB, Theobald DE, Williamson DA, et al: Temperature biofeedback in the treatment of migraine headaches: A controlled evaluation. *Arch Gen Psychiatr* 35:581–588, 1978.

179. Fahrion SL: Autogenic biofeedback for migraine. *Psychiatr Ann* 8:219–234, 1978.

180. Gainer JC: Temperature discrimination training in the biofeedback treatment of migraine headache. *J Behav Ther Exp Psychiatr* 9:185–187, 1978.

181. Sargent JD: Use of biofeedback in the treatment of headache problems. *Int Res Appl Psychol* 27:111–119, 1978.

182. Attfield M, Peck DF: Temperature self-regulation and relaxation with migraine patients and normals. *Behav Res Ther* 17:591–595, 1979.

183. Boller JD, Flom RP: Treatment of common migraine: systematic application of biofeedback and autogenic training. *Am J Clin Biofeedback* 2:63–69, 1979.

184. Drury RL, DeRisi WJ, Liberman RP: Temperature biofeedback treatment for migraine headache: A controlled multiple baseline study. *Headache* 19:278–284, 1979.

185. Lake A, Rainey J, Papsdorf JD: Biofeedback and rational-emotive therapy in the management of migraine headache. *J Appl Behav Anal* 12:127–140, 1979.

186. Silver BV, Blanchard EB, Williamson DA, et al: Temperature biofeedback and relaxation training in the treatment of migraine headaches: One-year follow-up. *Biofeedback Self Regul* 4:359–366, 1979.

187. Bild R, Adams HE: Modification of migraine headaches by cephalic blood volume pulse and EMG biofeedback. *J Consult Clin Psychol* 48:51–57, 1980.

188. Claghorn JL, Mathew RJ, Langen JW, et al: Directional effects of skin temperature self-regulation on regional cerebral blood flow in normal subjects and migraine patients. *Am J Psychiatr* 138:1182–1187, 1981.

189. Allen RA, Mills GK: The effects of unilateral plethysmographic feedback of temporal artery activity during migraine head pain. *J Psychosom Res* 26:133–140, 1982.

190. Houts AC: Relaxation and thermal feedback treatment of child migraine headache: A case study. *Am J Clin Biofeedback* 5:154–157, 1982.

191. Knapp TW: Treating migraine by training in temporal artery vasoconstriction and/or cognitive behavioral coping: A one-year follow-up. *J Psychosom Res* 26:551–557, 1982.

192. Gamble EH, Elder ST: Multimodal biofeedback in the treatment of migraine. *Biofeedback Self Regul* 8:383–392, 1983.

193. Gauthier J, Doyon J, Lacroix R, et al: Blood volume pulse biofeedback in the treatment of migraine headache: A controlled evaluation. *Biofeedback Self Regul* 8:427–442, 1983.

194. Jurish SE, Blanchard EB, Andrasik F, et al: Home versus clinic-based treatment of vascular headache. *J Consult Clin Psychol* 51:743–751, 1983.

195. Lahbe EE, Williamson DA: Temperature biofeedback in the treatment of children with migraine headaches. *J Pediatr Psychol* 8:317–326, 1983.

196. Lacroix JM, Clarke MA, Bock JC, et al: Biofeedback and relaxation in the treatment of migraine headaches: Comparative effectiveness and physiological correlates. *J Neurol Neurosurg Psychiatr* 46:525–532, 1983.

197. Lichstein KL, Hoelscher TJ, Nickel R, et al: An integrated blood volume pulse biofeedback system for migraine treatment. *Biofeedback Self Regul* 8:127–134, 1983.

198. Marrazo MJ, Hickling EJ, Sison GF: The combined use of rational-emotive therapy and biofeedback in the treatment of childhood migraine. *J Rational-Emotive Ther* 2:27–31, 1984.

199. Reading C: Psychophysiological reactivity in migraine following biofeedback. *Headache* 24:70–74, 1984.

200. Fentress DW, Masek BJ, Mehegan JF, et al: Biofeedback and relaxation-response training in the treatment of pediatric migraine. *Dev Med Child Neurol* 28:139–146, 1986.

201. Ellersten B, Nordby H, Hammesborg D, Thorlacius S: Psychophysiologic response patterns in migraine before

and after temperature biofeedback. Prediction of treatment outcome. *Cephalalgia* 7:109–124, 1987.

202. Gauthier J, Fradet C, Roberge C: The differential effects of biofeedback in the treatment of classical and common migraine. *Headache* 28:39–46, 1988.

203. Holroyd KA, Holm JF, Penzien DB, et al: Long-term maintenance of improvements achieved with (abortive) pharmacological and nonpharmacological treatments of migraine: Preliminary findings. *Biofeedback Self Regul* 14:301–308, 1989.

204. Lisspers J, Ost LG: BVP-biofeedback in the treatment of migraine. The effects of constriction and dilatation during different phases of the migraine attack. *Behav Modif* 14:200–221, 1990.

205. Hickling EJ, Silverman DJ, Loos W: A non-pharmacological treatment of vascular headache during pregnancy. *Headache* 30:407–410, 1990.

206. Blanchard EB, Appelbaum KA, Radnitz CL, et al: A controlled evaluation of thermal biofeedback and thermal biofeedback combined with cognitive therapy in the treatment of vascular headache. *J Consult Clin Psychol* 58:216–224, 1990.

207. Blanchard EB, Appelbaum KA, Nicholson NL, et al: A controlled evaluation of the addition of cognitive therapy to a home-based biofeedback and relaxation treatment of vascular headache. *Headache* 30:371–376, 1990.

208. Lisspers DJ, Ost LG: Long-term follow-up of migraine treatment: Do the effects remain up to six years? *Behav Res Ther* 28:313–322, 1990.

209. Blanchard EB, Nicholson NL, Radnitz CL, et al: The role of home practice in thermal biofeedback. *J Consult Clin Psychol* 59:507–512, 1991.

210. Blanchard EB, Andrasik F, Jurish SE, et al: The treatment of cluster headache with relaxation and thermal biofeedback. *Biofeedback Self Regul* 7:185–191, 1982.

211. Hoelscher TJ, Lichstein KL: Blood volume pulse biofeedback treatment of chronic cluster headache. *Biofeedback Self Regul* 8:533–541, 1983.

212. King AC, Arena JG: Behavioral treatment of chronic cluster headache in a geriatric patient. *Biofeedback Self Regul* 9:201–208, 1984.

213. McGrady AV, Bernal GA, Fine T, et al: Post traumatic head and neck pain, a multimodal treatment approach. *J Holist Med* 5:130–138, 1983.

214. Belar CD, Cohen JL: The use of EMG feedback and progressive relaxation in the treatment of a woman with chronic back pain. *Biofeedback Self Regul* 4:345–353, 979.

215. Nouwen A, Solinger JW: The effectiveness of EMG biofeedback training in low back pain. *Biofeedback Self Regul* 4:103–111, 1979.

216. Freeman CW, Calsyn DA, Paige AB, et al: Biofeedback with low back pain patients. *Am J Clin Biofeedback* 3:118–122, 1980.

217. Jones AL, Wolf SL: Treating chronic low back pain: EMG biofeedback training during movement. *Phys Ther* 60:58–63, 1980.

218. Keefe FJ, Schapira B, Brown C, et al: EMG-assisted relaxation training in the management of chronic low back pain. *Am J Clin Biofeedback* 4:93–103, 1981.

219. Keefe FJ, Black AR, Williams RB Jr, et al: Behavioral treatment of chronic low back pain: Clinical outcome and individual differences in pain relief. *Pain* 11:221–231, 1981.

220. Nigl AJ: A comparison of binary and analog EMG feedback techniques in the treatment of low back pain. *Am J Clin Biofeedback* 4:25–31, 1981.

221. Adams J, Pearson SC, Olson N: Innovative cross-modal technique of pain intensity assessment with lower back pain patients given biofeedback training. *Am J Clin Biofeedback* 5:25–30, 1982.

222. Wolf SL, Nacht M, Kelly JL: EMG feedback training during dynamic movement for low back pain patients. *Behav Ther* 13:395–406, 1982.

223. Flor H, Haag G, Turk DC, et al: Efficacy of EMG biofeedback, pseudotherapy, and conventional medical treatment for chronic rheumatic back pain. *Pain* 17:21–31, 1983.

224. Large RG, Lamb AM: Electromyographic (EMG) feedback in chronic musculoskeletal pain: A controlled trial. *Pain* 17:167–177, 1983.

225. Linton SJ, Melin L: Applied relaxation in the management of chronic pain. *Behav Psychother* 11:337–350, 1983.

226. Linton SJ, Gotestam KG: A controlled study of the effects of applied relaxation and applied relaxation plus operant procedures in the regulation of chronic pain. *Br J Clin Psychol* 23:291–299, 1984.

227. Stuckey SJ, Jacobs A, Goldfarb J: EMG biofeedback training, relaxation training, and placebo for the relief of chronic back pain. *Percept Mot Skills* 63:1023–1036, 1986.

228. Biederman HJ, Inglis J, Monga TN, Shanks GL: Differential treatment responses on somatic pain indicators after EMG biofeedback training in back pain patients. *Int J Psychosom* 36:53–57, 1989.

229. Achterberg J, McGraw P, Lawlis GF: Rheumatoid arthritis: A study of relaxation and temperature biofeedback training as an adjunct therapy. *Biofeedback Self Regul* 6:207–223, 1981.

230. Bradley LA, Young LD, Anderson KO, et al: Psychological approaches to the management of arthritis pain. *Soc Sci Med* 19:1353–1360, 1984.

231. King AC, Ahles TA, Martin JE, et al: EMG biofeedback-controlled exercise in chronic arthritic knee pain. *Arch Phys Med Rehabil* 65:341–343, 1984.

232. Flor H, Haag G, Turk DC: Long-term efficacy of EMG biofeedback for chronic rheumatic back pain. *Pain* 27:195–202, 1986.

233. Carlsson SG, Gale EN, Chman A: Treatment of temporomandibular joint syndrome in biofeedback training. *J Am Dent Assoc* 91:602–605, 1975.

234. Carlsson SG, Gale EN: Biofeedback treatment for muscle pain associated with the temporomandibular joint. *J Behav Ther Exp Psychiatr* 7:333–335, 1976.

235. Funch DP, Gale EN: Biofeedback and relaxation therapy for chronic temporomandibular joint pain: Predicting successful outcome. *J Consult Clin Psychol* 52:928–933, 1984.

236. Stenn PG, Mothersill KJ, Brocke RK: Biofeedback and a cognitive behavioral approach to treatment of myofascial pain dysfunction syndrome. *Behav Ther* 10:29–36, 1979.

237. Sherman RA, Gall N, Gormly J: Treatment of phantom limb pain with muscular relaxation training to disrupt the pain-anxiety-tension cycle. *Pain* 6:47–55, 1979.

238. Dougherty J: Relief of phantom limb pain after EMG biofeedback-assisted relaxation: A case report. *Behav Res Ther* 18:355–357, 1980.

239. Tsushima WT: Treatment of phantom limb pain with EMG and temperature biofeedback: A case study. *Am J Clin Biofeedback* 5:150–153, 1982.

240. Schwartz DP, Large HS, DeGood DE, et al: A chronic emergency room visitor with chest pain: Successful treatment by stress management training and biofeedback. *Pain* 18:315–319, 1984.

241. Hartman CH: Response of anginal pain to hand warming: A clinical note. *Biofeedback Self Regul* 4:335–357, 1979.

242. Bennink CD, Hulst LL, Benthem JA: The effects of EMG biofeedback and relaxation training on primary dysmenorrhea. *J Behav Med* 5:329–341, 1982.

243. Barth JT, Downs EJ: Post-herpetic neuralgia: A biofeedback case study. *Am J Clin Biofeedback* 4:104–106, 1981.

244. Blanchard GR: The use of temperature biofeedback in the treatment of chronic pain due to causalgia. *Biofeedback Self Regul* 4:183–188, 1979.

245. Thomas JE, Koshy M, Patterson L, et al: Management of pain in sickle cell disease using biofeedback therapy: A preliminary study. *Biofeedback Self Regul* 9:413–420, 1984.

246. Bird EI, Colborne GR: Rehabilitation of an electrical burn patient through thermal biofeedback. *Biofeedback Self Regul* 5:283–287, 1980.

247. Bodenhamer E, Coleman C, Achterberg J: Self-directed EMG training for the control of pain and spasticity in paraplegia: A case study. *Biofeedback Self Regul* 11:199–205, 1986.

248. Grunert BK, Devine CA, Sanger JR, et al: Thermal self-regulation for pain control in reflex sympathetic dystrophy syndrome. *J Hand Surg Am* 15:615–618, 1990.

249. Grimaud JC, Bouvier M, Naudy B, et al: Monometric and radiologic investigations and biofeedback treatment of chronic idiopathic anal pain. *Dis Colon Rectum* 34:690–695, 1991.

250. Linton SJ: Behavioral remediation of chronic pain: A status report. *Pain* 24:125–141, 1986.

251. Epstein LH, Abel GG: An analysis of biofeedback training effects for tension headache patients. *Behav Ther* 8:37–47, 1977.

252. Epstein LH, Abel GG, Colins F, et al: The relationship between frontal muscle activity and self-reports of headache pain. *Behav Res Ther* 16:153–160, 1978.

253. Beaty ET, Haynes SN: Behavioral intervention with muscle-contraction headache: A review. *Psychosom Med* 41:165–180, 1979.

254. Borgeat F: Some scientific feedback from biofeedback. *Acta Psychiatry Belg* 81:497–505, 1981.

255. Hart JD, Cichanski KA: A comparison of frontal EMG biofeedback and neck EMG biofeedback in the treatment of muscle-contraction headache. *Biofeedback Self Regul* 6:63–74, 1981.

256. Andrasik F, Holroyd KA: Specific and nonspecific effects in the biofeedback treatment of tension headache: 3-year follow-up. *J Consult Clin Psychol* 51:634–636, 1983.

257. Blanchard EB, Andrasik F, Neff DF, et al: Four process studies in behavioral treatment of chronic headache. *Behav Res Ther* 21:209–220, 1983.

258. Borgeat F, Gauthier B, Larouche LM: Muscle tension of patients with tension headaches during and between episodes of pain. *Acta Psychiatry Belg* 84:108–114, 1984.

259. Holroyd KA, Penzien DB, Hursey KG, et al: Change mechanisms in EMG biofeedback training: Cognitive changes underlying improvements in tension headache. *J Consult Clin Psychol* 52:1039–1053, 1984.

260. Lacroix JM, Clarke MA, Beck JC, Doxey NC: Physiological changes after biofeedback and relaxation training for multiple-pain tension headache patients. *Percept Mot Skills* 63:139–153, 1986.

261. Schoenen J, Gerard P, DePasqua V, Juprelle M: EMG activity in pericranial muscles during postural variation and mental activity in healthy volunteers and patients with chronic tension type headache. *Headache* 31:321–324, 1991.

262. Dalessio DJ, Kunzel M, Sternbach R, et al: Conditioned adaptation-relaxation reflex in migraine therapy. *JAMA* 242:2102–2104, 1979.

263. Gauthier J, Bois R, Allaire D, et al: Evaluation of skin temperature biofeedback training at two different sites for migraine. *J Behav Med* 4:407–119, 1981.

264. Gauthier J, Lacroix R, Cote A, et al: Biofeedback control of migraine headaches: A comparison of two approaches. *Biofeedback Self Regul* 10:139–159, 1985.

265. Morrill B, Blanchard EB: Two studies of the potential mechanisms of action in the thermal biofeedback treatment of vascular headache. *Headache* 29:169–176, 1989.

266. Biedermann HJ: Mechanisms of biofeedback in the treatment of chronic back pain: an hypothesis. *Psychol Res* 53:1103–1108, 1983.

267. Nouwevn A: EMG biofeedback used to reduce standing levels of paraspinal muscle tension in chronic low back pain. *Pain* 17:353–360, 1983.

268. Biedermann HJ: Comments on the reliability of muscle activity comparisons in EMG biofeedback research with back pain patients. *Biofeedback Self Regul* 9:451–458, 1984.

269. Bush C, Ditto B, Feuerstein M: A controlled evaluation of paraspinal EMG biofeedback in the treatment of chronic low back pain. *Health Psychol* 4:307–321, 1985.

270. McGeorge CM: Biofeedback and the headache. *N Z Psychol* 5:16–25, 1976.

271. Silver BV, Blanchard EB: Biofeedback and relaxation training in the treatment of psychophysiologic disorders: Or are the machines really necessary? *J Behav Med* 1:217–239, 1978.

272. Belar CD: A comment on Silver and Blanchard's (1978) review of the treatment of tension headaches via EMG feedback and relaxation training. *J Behav Med* 2:215–220, 1979.

273. Blanchard EB, Ahles TA, Shaw ER: Behavioral treatment of headaches. In Eisler RM, Miller PM (eds): *Progress in Behavior Modification.* New York, Academic Press, 1979, vol 8, p 207.

274. Jessup BA, Neufeld RW, Merskey H: Biofeedback therapy for headache and other pain: An evaluative review. *Pain* 7:225–270, 1979.

275. Turk DC, Meichenbaum DH, Berman WH: Application of biofeedback for the regulation of pain: A critical review. *Psychol Bull* 86:1322–1338, 1979.

276. Adams HE, Feuerstein M, Fowler JL: Migraine headache:

Review of parameters, etiology, and intervention. *Psychol Bull* 87:217–237, 1980.

277. Cohen MJ, McArthur DL, Rickles WH: Comparison of four biofeedback treatments for migraine headache: Psychological and headache variables. *Psychosom Med* 42:463–483, 1980.

278. Holroyd KA, Andrasik F, Noble J: A comparison of EMG biofeedback and a creditable pseudotherapy in treating tension headache. *J Behav Med* 3:29–39, 1980.

279. Kewman D, Roberts AH: Skin temperature biofeedback and migraine headaches: A double-blind study. *Biofeedback Self Regul* 5:327–345, 1980.

280. Nuechterlein KH, Holroyd JC: Biofeedback in the treatment of tension headache: Current status. *Arch Gen Psychiatry* 37:866–873, 1980.

281. Sovak M, Dalessio DJ, Kunzel M, et al: Current investigations in headache. *Res Publ Assoc Res Nerv Ment Dis* 58:261–282, 1980.

282. Kremsdorf RB, Kochanowicz NA, Costell S: Cognitive skills training versus EMG biofeedback in the treatment of tension headaches. *Biofeedback Self Regul* 6:93–102, 1981.

283. Steiner SS, Dince WM: Biofeedback efficacy studies: A critique of critiques. *Biofeedback Self Regul* 6:275–288, 1981.

284. Ford MR: Biofeedback treatment for headaches, Raynaud's disease, essential hypertension, and irritable bowel syndrome: A review of the long-term follow-up literature. *Biofeedback Self Regul* 7:521–536, 1982.

285. Johansson J, Ost LG: Self-control procedures in biofeedback: A review of temperature biofeedback in the treatment of migraine. *Biofeedback Self Regul* 7:435–442, 1982.

286. Linton SF: A critical review of behavioral treatments for chronic benign pain other than headache. *Br J Clin Psychol* 2:321–337, 1982.

287. Turner JA, Chapman CR: Psychological interventions for chronic pain: A critical review. I. Relaxation training and biofeedback. *Pain* 12:1–21, 1982.

288. Barrios FX, Karoly P: Treatment expectancy and therapeutic change in treatment of migraine headache: Are they related? *Psychol Rep* 52:59–68, 1983.

289. Haber JD, Thompson JK, Raczynski JM, et al: Physiological self-control and the biofeedback treatment of headache. *Headache* 23:174–178, 1983.

290. Holmes DS, Burish TG: Effectiveness of biofeedback for treating migraine and tension headaches: A review of the evidence. *J Psychosom Res* 27:515–532, 1983.

291. Kerns RD, Turk DC, Helzman AD: Psychological treatment for chronic pain: A selective review. *Clin Psychol Rev* 3:15–26, 1983.

292. Kewman DG, Roberts AH: An alternative perspective on biofeedback efficacy studies: A reply to Steiner and Dince. *Biofeedback Self Regul* 8:487–503, 1983.

293. Libo LM, Arnold GE: Does training to criterion influence improvement? A follow-up study of EMG and thermal biofeedback. *J Behav Med* 6:397–404, 1983.

294. Neff DF, Blanchard EB, Andrasik F: The relationship between capacity for absorption and chronic headache patients' response to relaxation and biofeedback treatment. *Biofeedback Self Regul* 8:177–183, 1983.

295. Thompson JK, Raczynski JM, Sturgis ET: The control issue in biofeedback training. *Biofeedback Self Regul* 8:153–164, 1983.

296. Diamond S, Montrose D: The value of biofeedback in the treatment of chronic headache: A four-year retrospective study. *Headache* 24:5–18, 1984.

297. Sorbi N, Tellegan B: Multimodal migraine treatment: Does thermal feedback add to the outcome? *Headache* 24:249–255, 1984.

298. Spence ND: Relaxation training for chronic pain patients using EMG feedback: An analysis of process and outcome effects. *Aust N Z J Psychiatry* 18:263–272, 1984.

299. Trifiletti RJ: The psychological effectiveness of pain management procedures in the context of behavioral medicine and medical psychology. *Gen Psychol Monogr* 109:251–278, 1984.

300. Passchier J, van der Helm-Hylkema H, Orlekelke JF: Lack of concordance between changes in headache activity and in psychophysiological and personality variables following treatment. *Headache* 25:310–316, 1985.

301. Litt MD: Mediating factors in non-medical treatment for migraine headache: Toward an interactional model. *J Psychosom Res* 30:505–519, 1986.

302. Chapman SL: A review and clinical perspective on the use of EMG and thermal biofeedback for chronic headaches. *Pain* 27:1–43, 1986.

303. Holroyd KA, Penzien DB: Client variables and the behavioral treatment of recurrent tension headache: A meta-analytic review. *J Behav Med* 9:515–536, 1986.

304. Malone MD, Strube MJ, Scogin FR: Meta-analysis of non-medical treatment for chronic pain. *Pain* 34:231–244, 1988.

305. Fentress DW, Masek BJ, Mehegan JE, Benson H: Biofeedback and relaxation-response training in the treatment of pediatric migraine. *Dev Med Child Neurol* 28:139–146, 1986.

306. Womack WM, Smith MS, Chen AC: Behavioral management of childhood headache: A pilot study and case history report. *Pain* 32:279–283, 1988.

307. Smith MS, Glass ST: An adolescent girl with headache and syncope. *J Adolesc Health Care* 10:54–56, 1989.

308. Duckro PN, Cantwell-Simmons E: A review evaluating biofeedback and relaxation training in the management of pediatric headache. *Headache* 29:428–433, 1980.

309. Burke EJ, Andrasik F: Home vs. clinic-based biofeedback treatment for pediatric migraine: Results of treatment through one-year follow-up. *Headache* 29:434–440, 1989.

310. Labbe EE, Ward CH: Electromyographic biofeedback with mental imagery and home practice in the treatment of children with muscle-contraction headache. *J Dev Behav Pediatr* 11:65–68, 1990.

311. Grazzi L, Leone M, Fredicani F, Bussone G: A therapeutic alternative for tension headache in children: Treatment and 1-year follow-up results. *Biofeedback Self Regul* 15:1–6, 1990.

312. Guarnieri P, Blanchard EB: Evaluation of home-based thermal biofeedback treatment of pediatric migraine headache. *Biofeedback Self Regul* 15:179–184, 1990.

313. Kabela E, Blanchard EB, Appelbaum KA, Nicholson N: Self-regulatory treatment of headache in the elderly. *Biofeedback Self Regul* 14:219–228, 1980.

314. Fichtler H, Zimmerman RR: Changes in reported pain from tension headaches. *Percept Mot Skills* 86:712, 1973.

315. Tasto DL, Hinkle JE: Muscle relaxation treatment for tension headaches. *Behav Res Ther* 11:347–349, 1973.

316. Warner G, Lance J: Relaxation therapy in migraine and chronic tension headache. *Med J Aust* 1:298–301, 1975.

317. Sallade JB: Group counseling with children who have migraine headaches. *Elem School Guid Counsel* 15:87–89, 1980.

318. Philips C, Hunter M: The treatment of tension headache: II. EMG "normality" and relaxation. *Behav Res Ther* 19:499–507, 1981.

319. DeBerry S: An evaluation of progressive muscle relaxation on stress related symptoms in a geriatric population. *Int J Aging Hum Dev* 14:255–269, 1981–1982.

320. Sherman RA: Home use of tape recorded relaxation exercises as initial treatment for stress related disorders. *Milit Med* 147:1062–1066, 1982.

321. Bhargava SC: Progressive muscular relaxation and assertive training in case of tension headache. *Ind J Clin Psychol* 10:23–25, 1983.

322. Jacob RG, Turner SM, Szekelv BC, et al: Predicting outcome of relaxation therapy in headaches: The role of "depression." *Behav Ther* 14:457–465, 1983.

323. Hart JD: Predicting differential response to EMG biofeedback and relaxation training: the role of cognitive structure. *J Clin Psychol* 40:453–457, 1984.

324. Richter NC: The efficacy of relaxation training with children. *J Abnorm Child Psychol* 12:319–344, 1984.

325. Williamson DA, Monguillot JE, Jarrell MP, et al: Relaxation for the treatment of headache: controlled evaluation of two group programs. *Behav Mod* 8:407–424, 1984.

326. Blanchard EB, Andrasik F, Appelbaum KA, et al: The efficacy and cost-effectiveness of minimal-therapist-contact, non-drug treatment. *Headache* 24:214–220, 1985.

327. Janssen K, Neutgens J: Autogenic training and progressive relaxation in the treatment of three kinds of headache. *Behav Res Ther* 24:199–208, 1986.

328. Attanasso V, Andrasik F, Blanchard EB: Cognitive therapy and relaxation training in muscle contraction headache: Efficacy and cost-effectiveness. *Headache* 27:254–260, 1987.

329. Blanchard EB, Nicholson NL, Taylor AE, et al: The role of regular home practice in the relaxation treatment of tension headache. *J Consult Clin Psychol* 59:467–470, 1991.

330. Lutker ER: Treatment of migraine headache by conditioned relaxation: A case study. *Behav Ther* 2:592–593, 1971.

331. Hay KM, Maddens J: Migraine treated by relaxation therapy. *J R Coll Gen Pract* 21:664–669, 1971.

332. Andreychuk T, Skriver C: Hypnosis and biofeedback in the treatment of migraine headache. *Int J Clin Exp Hyp* 23:172–183, 1977.

333. Sorbi M, Tellegen B: Differential effects of training in relaxation and stress-coping in patients with migraine. *Headache* 26:473–481, 1986.

334. Sorbi M, Tellegen B: Stress-coping in migraine. *Soc Sci Med* 26:351–358, 1988.

335. Sorbi M, Tellegen B, Dulong A: Long-term effects of training in relaxation and stress-coping in patients with migraine: A 3-year follow-up. *Headache* 29:111–121, 1989.

336. Smith TW, Denney DR: Relaxation training in the reduction of traumatic headaches: A case study. *Behav Psychother* 11:109–115, 1983.

337. Turner, JA: Comparison of group progressive-relaxation training and cognitive-behavioral group therapy for chronic low back pain. *J Consult Clin Psychol* 50:757–765, 1982.

338. Petty NE, Mastria MA: Management of compliance to progressive relaxation and orthopedic exercises in treatment of chronic back pain. *Psychol Rep* 52:35–38, 1983.

339. Sanders SH: Component analysis of a behavioral treatment program for chronic low-back pain. *Behav Ther* 14:697–705, 1983.

340. Newbury CR: Tension and relaxation in the individual. *Int Dent J* 29:173–182, 1979.

341. Stam HJ, McGrath PA, Brooke RI: The effects of a cognitive-behavioral treatment program on temporo-mandibular pain and dysfunction syndrome. *Psychosom Med* 46:534–545, 1984.

342. Stam HJ, McGrath PA, Brooke RI: The treatment of temporo-mandibular joint syndrome through control of anxiety. *J Behav Ther Exp Psychiatry* 15:41–45, 1984.

343. Gessel AH, Alderman M: Management of myofascial pain dysfunction syndrome of the temporomandibular joint by tension control training. *Psychosomatics* 12:302–309, 1971.

344. Raft D, Toomey T, Gregg JM: Behavior modification and haloperidol in chronic facial pain. *South Med J* 72:155–159, 1979.

345. Scott DS: Treatment of the myofascial pain-dysfunction syndrome: Psychological aspects. *J Am Dent Assoc* 101:611–616, 1980.

346. Scott DS: Myofascial pain-dysfunction syndrome: A psycho-biological perspective. *J Behav Med* 4:451–465, 1981.

347. Varni JW: Self-regulation techniques in the management of chronic arthritic pain in hemophilia. *Behav Ther* 12:185–194, 1981.

348. O'Leary A, Shoor S, Lorig K, Helman HR: A cognitive-behavioral treatment for rheumatoid arthritis. *Health Psychol* 7:527–544, 1988.

349. Quillen MA, Denney DR: Self-control of dysmenorrheic symptoms through pain management training. *J Behav Ther Exp Psychiatry* 13:123–130, 1982.

350. Dolan J, Allen H, Sawyer HW: Relaxation techniques in the reduction of pain, nausea and sleep disturbances for oncology patients: A primer for rehabilitation counselors. *J Appl Rehabil Counsel* 13:35–39, 1982.

351. Brena SF, Sammons EE: Phantom urinary bladder pain—Case report. *Pain* 7:197–201, 1979.

352. Taylor CB, Zlutnick SI, Corley MJ, et al: The effects of detoxification, relaxation, and brief supportive therapy on chronic pain. *Pain* 8:319–329, 1980.

353. Shaw L, Ehrlich A: Relaxation training as a treatment for chronic pain caused by ulcerative colitis. *Pain* 29:287–293, 1987.

354. Guthrie E, Creed F, Dawson D, Tomenson B: A controlled trial of psychological treatment for the irritable bowel syndrome. *Gastroenterology* 100:450–457, 1991.

355. Hegel MT, Abel GG, Etscheidt M, et al: Behavioral treatment of angina-like chest pain in patients with hyperventilation syndrome. *J Behav Ther Exp Psychiatry* 20:31–39, 1989.

356. Kabat ZJ: An outpatient program in behavioral medicine for chronic pain patients based on the practice of mind-

fulness meditation: Theoretical considerations and preliminary results. *Gen Hosp Psychiatry* 4:33–47, 1982.

357. Kabat ZJ, Lipworth L, Burney R: The clinical use of mindfulness meditation for the self-regulation of chronic pain. *J Behav Med* 8:163–190, 1985.

358. Linton SJ, Melin L, St Jernlof N: The effects of applied relaxation and operant activity training on chronic pain. *Behav Psychother* 13:87–100, 1985.

359. Linton SJ: Behavioral remediation of chronic pain: a status report. *Pain* 24:125–141, 1986.

360. Hyman RB, Feldman HR, Harris RB, et al: The effects of relaxation training on clinical symptoms: A meta-analysis. *Nurs Res* 38:216–220, 1989.

361. Jacobson E: *Modern Treatment of Tension Patients.* Springfield, IL, Charles C Thomas, 1970.

362. Wolpe J: *The Practice of Behavior Therapy.* Elmsford, NY, Pergamon Press, 1969.

363. Bernstein DA, Borkovec TD: *Progressive Relaxation Training.* Champaign, IL, Research Press, 1973.

364. Brown BB: *Stress and the Art of Biofeedback.* New York, Harper Row, 1977.

365. Schultz JH, Luthe W: *Autogenic Therapy: Autogenic Methods.* New York, Grune & Stratton, 1969, vol I.

366. Ford MR, Stroebel CF, Strong P, et al: Quieting response training: Long-term evaluation of a clinical biofeedback practice. *Biofeedback Self Regul* 8:265–278, 1983.

367. Bandura A: Self-efficacy: Toward a unifying theory of behavioral change. *Psychol Rev* 84:192–215, 1977.

368. Jencks B: Using the patient's breathing rhythm. In Wester WC II, Smith AH Jr (eds): *Clinical Hypnosis: A Multidisciplinary Approach.* Philadelphia, JB Lippincott, 1984, p 29.

369. de la Pena AM: *The Psychobiology of Cancer: Automatization Boredom in Health & Disease.* New York, Praeger, 1983.

370. Carlson CR, Nitz AJ: Negative side effects of self-regulation training: relaxation and the role of the professional in service delivery. *Biofeedback Self Regul* 16:191–197, 1991.

371. Richter IL, McGrath PJ, Humphreys PJ, et al: Cognitive and relaxation treatment of pediatric migraine. *Pain* 25:195–203, 1986.

372. Larsson B, Melin L: Chronic headaches in adolescents: Treatment in a school setting with relaxation training as compared with information-contact and self-registration. *Pain* 25:325–336, 1986.

373. Larsson B, Melin L, Lamminen M, Ullstedt F: A school-based treatment of chronic headaches in adolescents. *J Pediatr Psychol* 12:553–566, 1987.

374. Larsson B, Dalefold B, Hakansson L, Melin L: Therapist-assisted versus self-help relaxation treatment of chronic headaches in adolescents: A school-based intervention. *J Child Psychol Psychiatry* 28:127–136, 1987.

375. Larsson B, Melin L: The psychological treatment of recurrent headache in adolescents—short-term outcome and its prediction. *Headache* 28:187–195, 1988.

376. Larsson B, Melin L: Follow-up on behavioral treatment of recurrent headache in adolescents. *Headache* 29:250–254, 1989.

377. Lascellus MA, Cunningham SJ, McGrath P, Sullivan MJ: "Challenges in pain management." Part 4. Teaching coping strategies to adolescents with migraine. *J Pain Symptom Manage* 4:135–144, 1989.

378. McDonell L, Bowden ML: Breathing management: A simple stress and pain reduction strategy for use on a pediatric service. *Issues Compr Pediatr Nurs* 12:339–344, 1989.

379. Larsson B, Melin L, Doberl A: Recurrent tension headache in adolescents treated with self-help relaxation training and a muscle relaxant drug. *Headache* 30:665–671, 1990.

380. Arena JG, Hightower NE, Chong GC: Relaxation therapy for tension headache in the elderly: A prospective study. *Psychol Aging* 3:96–98, 1988.

381. Veith I: *Huang Ti Nei Ching Su Wen (The Yellow Emperor's Classic of Internal Medicine).* Berkeley, University of California Press, 1966.

382. Kaptchuk T: *The Web That Has No Weaver.* New York, Congdon and Weed, 1983.

383. Lowe W: *Introduction to Acupuncture Anesthesia.* Flushing, NY, Medical Examination Publishing Co., 1973.

384. Quen J: Acupuncture and western medicine. *Bull Hist Med* 49:196–205, 1975.

385. Diamond E: Acupuncture, anesthesia, western medicine and traditional Chinese medicine. *JAMA* 218:1558–1563, 1971.

386. Bonica J: Anesthesiology in the Peoples' Republic of China. *Anesthesiology* 40:175–186, 1974.

387. Melzack R: Acupuncture and related forms of folk medicine. In: Wall PD, Melzak R (eds): *Textbook of Pain.* Edinburgh, Churchill Livingstone, 1984, pp 691–699.

388. Melzack R, Wall P: Pain mechanisms: A new theory. *Science* 150:971–979, 1965.

389. Melzack R: *The Puzzle of Pain.* New York, Basic Books, 1973.

390. Nathan P, Rudge P: Testing the gate control theory of pain in man. *J Neurol Neurosurg Psychiatry* 37:1366–1372, 1974.

391. Melzack R: Prolonged relief of pain by brief intense transcutaneous somatic stimulation. *Pain* 1:357–374, 1975.

392. Basbaum A, Fields H: Endogenous pain control mechanisms: Review and hypothesis. *Ann Neurol* 4:451–462, 1978.

393. Pomerantz B, Chiu D: Naloxone blocks acupuncture analgesia and causes hyperalgesia: Endorphin is implicated. *Life Sci* 19:1757–1762, 1976.

394. Mayer D, Price D, Rafii A: Antagonism of acupuncture analgesia in man by the narcotic antagonist naloxone. *Brain Res* 121:368–372, 1977.

395. Sjolund B, Terenius L, Erikson M: Increased cerebrospinal fluid levels of endorphins after electro acupuncture. *Acta Physiol Scand* 100:382–384, 1977.

396. Kiser R, Khatami M, Gatchel R, et al: Acupuncture relief of chronic pain syndrome correlates with increased plasma metenkephalin concentrations. *Lancet* 2:1394–1396, 1983.

397. Chapman C, Colpitts Y, Benedetti C, et al: Evoked potential assessment of acupunctural analgesia: Attempted reversal with naloxone. *Pain* 9:183–197, 1980.

398. Chapman C, Benedetti C, Colpitts Y, et al: Naloxone fails to reverse pain threshold elevated by acupuncture: Acupuncture analgesia reconsidered. *Pain* 16:13–31, 1983.

399. Richardson P, Vincent C: Acupuncture for the treatment of pain: A review of evaluative research. *Pain* 24:15–40, 1986.

400. Abstracts of the Second National Symposium on Acu-

puncture and Moxibustion and Acupuncture Anesthesia, Beijing, China, August, 1984.

401. Millman B: Acupuncture: Context and critique. *Annu Rev Med* 28:223–234, 1977.

402. Anderson S, Erickson T, Holmgren E, et al: Electro-acupuncture. Effect on pain threshold measured with electrical stimulation of the teeth. *Brain Res* 63:393–396, 1973.

403. Stewart D, Thompson J, Oswald I: Acupuncture analgesia: An experimental investigation. *Br Med J* 1:67–70, 1977.

404. Vincent C, Richardson P: The evaluation of therapeutic acupuncture: Concepts and methods. *Pain* 24:1–13, 1986.

405. Ter Reit G, Kleijnen J, Knipschild P: *J Clin Epidemiol* 43:1191–1199, 1990.

406. Miller R (ed): *Anesthesia*, ed 2. New York, Churchill Livingstone, 1986, vol 3, pp 1692, 2105.

407. Bonica J: Acupuncture analgesia and anesthesia. In Eckenhoff JE (ed): *Controversy in Anesthesiology*. Philadelphia, WB Saunders, 1979, pp 185–200.

408. Jospe M: *The Placebo Effect in Healing*. Lexington, MA, DC Heath, 1978.

409. Brody H: *Placebos and the Philosophy of Medicine*. Chicago, University of Chicago Press, 1980.

410. Shapiro A: The placebo effect in the history of medical treatment: Implications for psychiatry. *Am J Psychiatry* 116:298–304, 1959.

411. Reuler J, Girard D, Nardone D: The chronic pain syndrome: Misconceptions and management. *Ann Intern Med* 93:588–596, 1980.

412. Critelli J, Neumann K: The placebo. *Am Psychol* 39:32–39, 1984.

413. Skelly FJ: The power of suggestion. *Am Med News* Feb. 17:37–38, 1992.

414. Lasanga C, Mosteller F, VonFelsinger J, et al: A study of the placebo response. *Am J Med* 16:770–779, 1954.

415. Findley T: The placebo and the physician. *Med Clin North Am* 37:1821–1826, 1953.

416. Houston W: The doctor himself as therapeutic agent. *Ann Intern Med* 11:1416–1425, 1938.

417. Shapiro A: A contribution to the history of the placebo effect. *Behav Sci* 5:109–135, 1960.

418. Doongaji D, Vahia V, Bharveha M: On placebos, placebo responses and placebo responders (a review of psychological, psychopharmacological and psychophysiological factors). I: Psychological factors. *J Postgrad Med* 24:91, 1978.

419. Evans F: The placebo response. In Bonica J (ed): *Pain (Advances in Neurology 4)*. New York, Raven Press, 1974.

420. Lasanga L: The placebo effect. *J Allergy Clin Immunol* 78:161–165, 1986.

421. Meyer H: First federal practice guideline given; Pain Management. *Am Med News*, 1:48–49, 1992.

422. Beecher H: The powerful placebo. *JAMA* 159:1602–1606, 1955.

423. Blackwell B: Chronic pain. In Kaplan HI, Sadok BJ (eds): *Comprehensive Textbook of Psychiatry*, ed 5. Baltimore, Williams & Wilkins, 1989, pp 1264–1270.

424. Goodwin J, Goodwin J, Vogel A: Knowledge and use of placebos by house officers and nurses. *Ann Intern Med* 91:106–110, 1979.

425. Adams RD, Martin JB: Acute and chronic pain: Patho-

physiology and management. In Petersdorf RG, Adams RD, Braunwold E, Isselbacher KJ, Martin JB, Wilson JD (eds): *Principles of Internal Medicine*, ed 10, New York, McGraw-Hill, 1983, pp 8–9.

426. Beecher H: *Measurement of Subjective Responses: Quantitative Effects of Drugs*. New York, Oxford University Press, 1959.

427. Benson H, McCallie D: Angina pectoris and the placebo effect. *N Engl J Med* 300:1424–1429, 1979.

428. Sternbach R: *Pain: A Psychophysiological Analysis*. New York, Academic Press, 1968.

429. Thorn W: The placebo reactor. *Aust J Pharm* 43:1035–1037, 1962.

430. Gracely RH, Dubner R, Deeter WR, Wolskee PJ: Clinicians expectations influence placebo analgesia [Letter]. *Lance* 1:43, 1985.

431. Pollman L: Circadian variation of potency of placebo as analgesic. *Funct Neurol* 2:99–103, 1987.

432. Stam HJ, Spanos NP: Hypnotic analgesia, placebo analgesia and ischemic pain: The effects of contextual variables. *J Abnorm Psychol* 96:313–320, 1987.

433. Khurmi N, Bowles J, Kohli R, et al: Does placebo improve idexes of effort-induced myocardial ischemia? An objective study in 150 patients with chronic stable angina pectoris. *Am J Cardiol* 57:907–911, 1986.

434. Woodforde J, Merskey H: Personality traits of patients with chronic pain. *J Psychosom Res* 16:167–172, 1972.

435. Liberman R: An analysis of the placebo phenomenon. *J Chronic Dis* 15:761–783, 1962.

436. Batterman R, Lower W: Placebo responsiveness—The influence of previous therapy. *Curr Ther Res* 10:136–143, 1968.

437. Beecher H: Pain in man wounded in battle. *Ann Surg* 123:96–105, 1946.

438. Skelly FJ: Extending the boundaries of healing. *Am Med News*, Feb 24, pp 23–25, 1992.

439. Bourne H: The placebo—A poorly understood and neglected therapeutic agent. *Rational Drug Ther* Nov, pp 1–6, 1971.

440. Merskey H: The status of pain. In Hill O (ed): *Modern Perspectives in World Psychiatry*. London, Oliver & Boyd, 1968, pp 596–613.

441. Gordon NC, Levine JD: Physiological substrates of placebo analgesia. *Pharmacol Bull* 17:76–77, 1981.

442. Fields HL, Levine JD: Biology of placebo analgesia. *Am J Med* 70:45–46, 1981.

443. Levine JD, Gordon NC, Bornstein JC, Fields HL: Role of pain in placebo analgesia. *Proc Natl Acad Sci* 76:3528–3531, 1979.

444. Shapiro A: The placebo response. In Howells J (ed): *Modern Perspectives in World Psychiatry*. London, Oliver & Boyd, 1968, pp 596–613.

445. Fisher H, Olin B: The dynamics of placebo therapy—A clinical study. *Am J Med Sci* 232:504–512, 1956.

446. Hackett T: Chronic pain. In Sederer L (ed): *Inpatient Psychiatry: Diagnosis and Treatment*. Baltimore, Williams & Wilkins, 1983.

447. Lasanga L, Laties G, Dohan L: Further studies on the "pharmacology" of placebo administration. *J Clin Invest* 37:533–537, 1958.

448. Wolf S, Pinsky R: Effects of placebo administration and occurrence of toxic reactions. *JAMA* 155:339–341, 1954.

449. Haegerstam G: Placebo in clinical drug trials—A multidisciplinary review. *Methods Find Exp Clin Pharmacol* 4:261–278, 1982.

450. Lipkin M: Psychiatry in medicine. In Kaplan HI, Sadok BJ (eds): *Comprehensive Textbook of Psychiatry*, ed 5. Baltimore, Williams & Wilkins, 1989, p 1289.

451. Medvedev V, Zavyalova E, Ovchinnikov B, et al: Functional structure of the placebo response. *Hum Physiol* 10:216–221, 1984.

452. Byerly H: Explaining and exploiting placebo effects. *Perspect Biol Med* 19:423–436, 1976.

453. Nash M, Zimring F: Prediction of reaction to placebo. *J Abnorm Psychol* 74:568–573, 1969.

454. Morris L, O'Neal E: Drug-name familiarity and the placebo effect. *J Clin Psychol* 30:280–282, 1974.

455. Wolf S: Effects of suggesting and conditioning on the action of chemical agents in human subjects—The pharmacology of placebos. *J Clin Invest* 29:100–109, 1950.

456. Petrie J, Hazleman B: Credibility of placebo transcutaneous nerve and acupuncture. *Clin Exp Rheumatol* 3:151–153, 1958.

457. Whitehorn J: Comment: Psychiatric implications of the placebo effect. *Am J Psychiatry* 114:662–664, 1958.

458. Ullman L, Kraser F: Cognitions and behavior therapy. *Behav Ther* 1:202–204, 1969.

459. Frank J: General psychotherapy: The restoration of morale. In Arieti S (ed): *American Handbook of Psychiatry*, ed 2. New York, Basic Books, 1975, vol 5, pp 124–125.

460. Voudouris N, Peck C, Coleman G: Conditioned placebo responses. *J Pers Soc Psychol* 148:47–53, 1985.

461. Voudouris N, Peck C, Coleman G: Conditioned response models of placebo phenomena. *Pain* 38:109–116, 1989.

462. Ponser J, Burke A: The effects of naloxone on opiate and placebo analgesia in healthy volunteers. *Psychopharmacology* 87:468–472, 1985.

463. Levine J, Gordon N, Fields H: The mechanisms of placebo analgesia. *Lancet* 2:654–657, 1978.

464. Fields HL, Levine JD: Biology of placebo analgesia. *Am J Med* 70:745–746, 1981.

465. Grevert P, Albert LH, Godstein A: Partial antagonism of placebo analgesia by naloxone. *Pain* 16:129–143, 1983.

466. Egbert L, Battit G, Welch C, et al: Reduction of postoperative pain by management and instruction of patients: A study of doctor-patient rapport. *N Engl J Med* 270:825–827, 1964.

A COGNITIVE-BEHAVIORAL PERSPECTIVE ON CHRONIC PAIN: BEYOND THE SCALPEL AND SYRINGE

DENNIS C. TURK
THOMAS E. RUDY

OVER THE past two decades, numerous books and chapters have been written emphasizing the importance of viewing pain as more than simply a response to tissue damage. Authors have noted that pain is a much more complex perceptual phenomenon that is composed of a multitude of psychosocial factors as well as sensory stimulation. Chronic pain, in particular, extends over lengthy periods and can be augmented, maintained, and even directly initiated by cognitive, affective, and behavioral parameters (1).

Although historically the role of psychological factors was acknowledged, until recently the pendulum had swung to an extreme view of pain as solely a sensory event. The sensory position evolved from advances in sensory psychophysics and sensory physiology during the last half of the nineteenth century. Consideration of pain as a sensory phenomenon resulted in the efforts to measure pain per se, that is, as a pure sensory-physiologic phenomenon ("nociception" [2]) uncontaminated by psychological factors. This perspective also served as the basis for the development of sophisticated surgical procedures designed to ablate the nociceptive pathways from the periphery to the central nervous system and the synthesis of potent analgesic agents to block nociception. Unfortunately, these therapeutic advances have not always had the desired result of complete and permanent elimination of pain, nor is there agreement as to whether "pure" sensory nociception can be isolated and measured (3).

Dissatisfaction with the unidimensional, sensory model was voiced by clinicians, who noted that patients with ostensibly the same degree of tissue damage reacted quite differently to identical therapeutic modalities and that patients with similar diagnoses responded quite dissimilarly to the syndrome or injury. Moreover, despite significant advances in neuroanatomy and physiology, there remained many pain syndromes for which no neurosurgical intervention, no matter how extreme, consistently and permanently eliminated patients' complaints of pain.

The shift away from the perception of pain as a purely sensory phenomenon to pain as a perceptual event was given the greatest impetus by developments in the mid-1960s, most notably by Ronald Melzack and his colleagues (4, 5) and Wilbert Fordyce (6). Melzack and his colleagues presented a multidimensional model of pain—the *gate control model*—designed to deal with the inconsistencies made manifest by different sensory, nociceptive models (5, 7). Melzack and his collaborators postulated that the experience of pain was the result of the neurophysiologic integration of motivational-affective, cognitive-evaluative, and sensory-discriminative contributions. Note that this view differs greatly from sensory views that, when they consider psychological factors at all, relegate them to reactions to "pain" and, consequently, nuisance variables or at best epiphenomena. The gate control model did not give priority to sensory input, nor did it treat the sensory input as isomorphic with pain. Rather, pain was postulated to be the result of the integration and interpretation of sensory and psychological processes and, therefore, a perceptual process. Treatment conceptualizations based on the gate control model lead to an increased emphasis on cognitive and affective components that contribute to the experience of pain and suffering.

Coming from a very different orientation but at approximately the same time, Fordyce and his colleagues, rather than focusing on pain per se, based their model on learning theory, specifically, *operant conditioning* (8). From this perspective, the subjective experience of pain is irrelevant because it cannot be directly observed, and reports and description of it, therefore, are biased by a number of factors. Fordyce's operant conditioning formulation focuses on behavioral expression of pain—"pain behaviors" (9).

According to Fordyce pain behaviors consist of overt sources of communication that convey to an observer that an individual is experiencing pain and suffering (e.g., limping, grimacing, moaning, lying down) (9). Once the focus shifts from the subjective experience to observable behaviors, then the production and maintenance of those behaviors can be viewed as coming under environmental control by means of selective reinforcement. That is, significant others in the patient's environment, whether family, friends, or health care providers, respond to the patient's behavior. Significant others may positively reinforce these behavioral manifestations by providing attention or permitting the patient to avoid the performance of undesirable activities (e.g., physical activity), and thereby unwittingly contribute to the maintenance and frequency of these behaviors. Moreover, the compensation system may positively reinforce displays of pain behaviors when third-party payers provide financial incentives contingent on the continual emission of pain behaviors. Thus, according to the operant conditioning model, pain behaviors may continue after physical pathology has resolved, even in the absence of nociceptive stimulation.

The operant perspective is particularly relevant when we consider chronic pain that extends over long periods. At an acute level, behavioral responses to injury and nociceptive stimulation may be appropriate and serve a protective function, as in the case of immobilization of an injured limb to prevent further injury and promote healing. Continuation of these responses over long periods, however, may be detrimental and can create a new set of problems. For example, frequent performance of pain behaviors may directly influence the experience of pain because they lead to physical deconditioning (reduction in muscle strength and flexibly and increased fatigue). Moreover, the presence of pain behaviors may lead to reduction of previously enjoyed activities and increased affective distress.

In the same way that the unidimensional, sensory model suggests specific interventions (i.e., cutting or blocking nociceptive pathways), the operant conditioning and gate control models each have important implications for treatment. The operant conditioning model emphasizes environmental manipulations whereby pain behaviors that were previously reinforced are eliminated and, conversely, "well behaviors" (e.g., physical activity) are positively reinforced. Moreover,

medications taken on an "as needed" (PRN) basis and exercise on a work-to-tolerance schedule are viewed as inappropriate. Rather, medication is changed to a time-contingent schedule and eventually eliminated, and exercise is performed to quota rather than until pain increases, which previously served as a signal for terminating the activity.

Both the operant and gate control formulations have contributed to a resurgence of interest in chronic pain treatments that extend beyond the traditional approaches of relying on scalpels and syringes to produce pain relief. These two models emphasize psychological factors in chronic pain, not just physical ones.

Although both the operant and gate control models provide important points of departure from sensory models and interventions, each provides a somewhat limited view and is inadequate. The operant model focuses exclusively on the communicative function of observable behaviors and fails to consider the contribution of cognitive appraisals of patients as they affect patients' perceptions and responses to their physical problems (10). The gate control model provides a static view of pain that does not consider the important reinforcing function that environmental factors come to exert as pain persists.

An alternative model that emphasizes both the importance of environmental factors underscored by the operant approach and psychological contributions inherent in the gate control model has been formulated by Turk and his colleagues and labeled a *cognitive-behavioral* perspective (11–13). A comprehensive intervention model based on the cognitive-behavioral conceptualization has been developed and employed with a diversity of pain syndromes. These include headaches (14, 15), temporomandibular pain disorders (16), arthritis (17, 18), and heterogeneous pain syndromes (19, 20). In the remainder of this chapter we will describe the cognitive-behavioral conceptualization and approach to the treatment of chronic pain patients.

A COGNITIVE-BEHAVIORAL CONCEPTUALIZATION OF CHRONIC PAIN

Cognitive-behavioral conceptualizations were originally developed to understand how individuals function in general and not specifically in the area of pain. The impetus for the development of cognitive-behavioral models was the general dissatisfaction with what was perceived as the limited scope and consistent failure of the beneficial effects attributed to interventions based exclusively on operant conditioning to generalize and be maintained following treatment termination (21–23). From the cognitive-behavioral perspective attention to cognitive and affective factors that contribute to the pain experience can be integrated within a comprehensive treatment program that also gives attention to environmental sources of reinforcement and makes use of various behavioral techniques.

According to the cognitive-behavioral perspective, it is the patient's perceptions that interact reciprocally with emotional factors, sensory phenomena, and behavioral responses. Moreover, the patient's behavior will elicit responses from significant others that can reinforce both adaptive and maladaptive modes of thinking, feeling, and behaving. Thus, a transactional perspective is adopted that does not include the linear causation postulated by unidimensional models, such as sensory-physiologic models (7), the purely cognitive model (24), or operant models (9, 25). Rather, the cognitive-behavioral, transactional model views pain as a reciprocal, multidimensional perceptual phenomenon. Pain perception is not the end result of passive transmission and registration of impulses from physically defined stimuli. Instead, it is a dynamic, interpretive process. From the cognitive-behavioral perspective, it is suggested that to better understand and treat pain consideration must be given to the role of cognitions, emotions, and behavior as well as to sensory contributions in the formation of pain perception and as they evolve over time.

Turk and his colleagues hypothesize that a comprehensive, cognitive-behavioral approach has a greater likelihood of fostering maintenance of treatment benefits than focusing exclusively on environmental contingencies of reinforcement, as emphasized by the operant conditioning formulation (11, 12). The use of positive reinforcement for adaptive behaviors would play an important part in this approach, but focus on intrinsic motivation should also play a major role because continued external reinforcement is unlikely to be maintained indefinitely. Some authors have suggested that cognitive and behavioral approaches and philosophies are "antithetical" and cannot be integrated (24, 26). We strongly disagree and will describe how we believe cognitive and behavioral approaches can be integrated within a comprehensive cognitive-behavioral treatment.

ASSUMPTIONS OF THE COGNITIVE-BEHAVIORAL PERSPECTIVE

There are five general assumptions that characterize the cognitive-behavioral perspective. These are summarized in Table 12.1. The first assumption is that individuals are active processors of information rather than passive reactors. That is, individuals attempt to make sense of the stimuli that impinge on them from the external environment by filtering information through organizing templates derived through their prior learning histories and through the use of general strategies that guide the processing of information (27, 28). Individuals' responses (overt as well as covert) are based on these appraisals and subsequent expectations rather than being contingent exclusively on the actual consequences of their behaviors (i.e., positive and neg-

Table 12.1.
Assumptions of Cognitive-Behavioral Treatment

1. Individuals are active processors of information.
2. Thoughts can elicit or modulate affect and physiology and can serve as impetuses for behavior. Conversely, affect, physiology, and behavior can instigate or influence thoughts.
3. Behavior is reciprocally determined by the individual and the environment.
4. Clients or patients can learn more adaptive ways of thinking, feeling, and behaving.
5. Clients or patients are capable of and should be involved as active agents in change of their maladaptive thoughts, feelings, and behaviors.

ative reinforcements and punishments). Thus, from this perspective, the *anticipated* consequences are as important in the governing of behavior as the actual consequences.

A second assumption of the cognitive-behavioral perspective is that individual's thoughts (e.g., appraisals, attributions, expectancies) can elicit or modulate affect and physiologic arousal, both of which may serve as impetuses for behavior. Conversely, affect, physiology, and behavior can instigate or influence the individual's thinking processes. Thus, the causal priority depends on where in the cycle one chooses to begin. Much energy has been devoted toward establishing the priority of thoughts, feelings, and behaviors. This approach seems to be futile and reminds us of a merry-go-around. Each champion has his or her favorite horse and thinks, feels, and behaves as if he or she is leading the pack when in reality all are going around in circles with little progress but perhaps an exhilarating ride all the same. Causal priority may be less of a concern than the view of a transactional process that extends over time with the interaction of thoughts, feelings, physiology, and behavior (29).

Unlike the operant conditioning formulation that emphasizes the influence of the environment on behavior, the cognitive-behavioral perspective focuses on the reciprocal effects of the individual on the environment as well as the influence of the environment on the individual's behavior. That is, individuals elicit environmental responses by their behavior. The individual who acts in a hostile manner toward others is likely to elicit a response in kind. At least to some extent, then, individuals create their own environments. The third assumption of the cognitive-behavioral perspective is that behavior is reciprocally determined by both the environment and the individual (30).

If it is assumed, as it is from the cognitive-behavioral perspective, that individuals have learned maladaptive

Table 12.2.
Objectives of Cognitive-Behavioral Treatment

1. Reconceptualize clients' or patients' views of their problems from overwhelming to manageable (combat demoralization)
2. Convince clients or patients that skills necessary for responding to problems more adaptively will be included in treatment (enhance outcome efficacy)
3. Reconceptualize clients' or patients' views of themselves from passive, reactive, and helpless to active, resourceful, and competent (foster self-efficacy)
4. Ensure that clients or patients learn how to monitor thoughts, feelings, and behaviors and learn the inter-relationship among these (break up automatic, maladaptive patterns)
5. Teach clients or patients how to employ and when to execute the necessary overt and covert behaviors required for adaptive response to problems (skills training)
6. Encourage clients or patients to attribute success to their own efforts
7. Anticipate problems and discuss these as well as ways to deal with them (facilitate maintenance and generalization)

ways of thinking, feeling, and behaving, then successful interventions designed to change behavior should focus on each of these factors and not one to the exclusion of others with the expectancy that changing thoughts, feelings, or behaviors will necessarily result in the others following suit. (For alternative views on this topic see references 24 and 25; the first focuses exclusively on cognition, the second on behavior.) We also believe that environmental contingencies can influence thoughts, feelings, and behaviors. Thus, we suggest employing both cognitive and behavioral techniques to bring about direct changes in behavior that result from environmental contingencies and indirect behavioral changes that follow from changes in cognitive factors, such as attitudes and beliefs.

Behavioral techniques are essential at the beginning of treatment, but unless significant changes in intrinsic motivation occur following behavioral techniques, it is our contention that treatment efficacy will not be obtained when environmental reinforcement is removed. The literature on the relapse following strict operant approaches for a diversity of problems lends support to our reservations regarding the long-term maintenance of treatment effects following exclusively operant approaches in the management of chronic pain (31–33). Research, specifically in the area of chronic pain, needs to address the issue of maintenance.

The final assumption of cognitive-behavioral models is that in the same way as individuals are instrumental in the development and maintenance of maladaptive thoughts, feelings, and behaviors, they can, are, and

should be considered active agents of change of their own maladaptive modes of thinking, feeling, and behaving. Patients, despite their initial conceptualization of their problems, have to accept that they are not helpless pawns of fate. They can and must be instrumental in learning and carrying out more effective modes of responding to their environment.

Most people have learned to adhere to an acute model of illness. That is, there is a specific cause for every symptom, there is an appropriate treatment, there is a specific time course for resolution of the symptoms (usually days or weeks), and there are socially sanctioned healers who are virtually omnipotent and who will provide a cure. In this model, the "good" patient is the one who is passive, permits health care providers to do things to them, asks few questions, complies with the provider's orders, and, consequently, gets better. Most patients with chronic illnesses, especially patients with chronic pain, are confronted with challenges to the acute illness model and, not surprisingly, are frustrating for health care providers who, like their patients, frequently ascribe to the acute illness model. Chronic pain patients often do not have sufficient objective evidence to account for their pain, many therapeutic interventions may have been tried with limited success, their pain extends over long periods, there is little encouraging information that there is an end to their suffering just over the horizon, and, despite the best efforts of providers, their pain problem persists. Thus, it is hardly surprising that chronic pain patients become demoralized and that combating demoralization is the essential ingredient of any treatment for chronic pain (34).

OBJECTIVES OF COGNITIVE-BEHAVIORAL TREATMENT

Given the description of the cognitive-behavioral perspective outlined above, we can now consider what the implications of this perspective are for developing interventions in general and then more specifically for use with chronic pain patients. A number of specific objectives affect any cognitive-behavioral intervention. These are summarized in Table 12.2.

A primary objective, which is addressed repeatedly, is changing patients' views of their problem from overwhelming to manageable. That is, by the time patients are seen for treatment of a chronic illness they have had sufficient time to become demoralized. After all, they have received multiple treatments by various health care providers and they are no better and possibly worse as a result of the potential iatrogenic consequences inherent in any somatic modality. They feel helpless and hopeless and the future appears bleak. A major component of any intervention, then, is to confront and overcome patients' maladaptive conceptualizations because they contribute to and exacerbate the initial problem and facilitate disability.

One way to bring about the change in patients' conceptualizations is to help them to understand and accept that there are ways to address adequately their problems, that the skills required by the patient to respond more effectively are included within the provider's armamentarium, and that these skills can be taught to the patient. Unfortunately, convincing patients that this is the case is not an easy task; even if they believe in the efficacy of the proposed treatment regimen, they may not believe that they are competent to successfully learn and implement these skills as situations demand. Bandura has emphasized the importance of enhancing patients' perceptions of self-control and self-efficacy (35). Convincing patients of their ability is more likely to occur if they are successful and their own behavior then becomes a positive reinforcer than if one relies exclusively on logic and exhortation. Specific goals and paced mastery are primary strategies to use in the fostering of a patient's sense of competence. Only when patients feel a sense of self-efficacy are they likely to try more difficult goals and to persist in their efforts in the face of difficulties.

Patients need evidence that they can exert more control over their situation. It is all too easy to disregard successful behavior and goal attainment and to focus on failures. Moreover, unless individuals specifically attend to the impact of their thoughts, feelings, physiologic responses, and behavior on each other they are likely to see little inter-relationship. To accomplish the levels of awareness of successful goal attainment and of the relationship among thoughts, feelings, physiologic responses, and behaviors requires focused attention. Thus, cognitive-behavioral therapists emphasize self-observation and self-monitoring.

Specific use of charts and diaries of goals and the antecedents and consequences of maladaptive thoughts, feelings, and behaviors are employed. Self-monitoring can serve to bring maladaptive automatic modes of responding into conscious awareness and, consequently, can become the focus of voluntary control. Self-monitoring of overt behavior as well as some covert behaviors is an important component of many behavioral as well as cognitive-behavioral interventions. A difference is that the cognitive-behavioral approach is much more concerned about patients' self-monitoring of their own thinking, especially maladaptive beliefs, because these beliefs relate to patients' appraisals, expectations, and dysfunctional modes of responding.

An additional objective of cognitive-behavioral interventions involves teaching patients specific skills to use that will foster more effective and adaptive modes of responding. A large number of specific skills may be employed but in general some of the most frequently used include problem-solving skills, rationale restructuring, communication skills, and relaxation. Relaxation skills are generic and consist of a variety of different techniques (e.g., biofeedback, autogenic training) geared toward assisting patients in learning how to deal with stress in general and how to reduce general and pain-specific muscular hyperarousal. Cognitive-behavioral therapists do not only focus on the performance of stress-management skills when the patient is aroused but also emphasize the use of problem solving and communication skills to prevent the development of maladaptive stress responses. Problem solving consists of teaching patients to identify sources of distress as problems to be dealt with and then to generate and test various solutions. Rational restructuring focuses on the identification of maladaptive appraisals and expectations and subsequent consideration of more appropriate modes of interpretation. Finally, communication skills relate to the patient's mode of interacting with significant others, including health care providers, and more appropriate means to acquire attention and information.

Teaching patients specific skills is an important component of cognitive-behavioral interventions, but although skills training is viewed as necessary, it is not sufficient in and of itself. Patients need to know not only how to perform specific skills but when to perform them as well. Most people can learn to relax when they are not upset or experiencing aversive symptoms, but it is more difficult to learn how to be aware of stress and automatic, maladaptive responding and how to execute these skills when symptomatic. Moreover, factors that may interfere with the production of these skills need to be addressed. Skills training may lead to a diminution of any skills deficiency but cognitive-behavioral interventions also emphasize and address the importance of production deficiencies—that is, the factors that can inhibit the use of the skills acquired (e.g., insufficient motivation, automaticity of maladaptive responding, affective distress, maladaptive and self-defeating thoughts).

A final important objective of cognitive-behavioral interventions is the fostering of self-attribution of success. Much effort is made toward encouraging patients to view themselves as the agents of change. To the extent that patients attribute improvements to their own skills and efforts there is a greater likelihood that they will feel more competent and thus are more likely to expand greater efforts and to persist in the face of difficulties that evolve (35).

Before implementing any intervention with chronic pain patients, whether cognitive-behavioral or other approaches, it is essential that a comprehensive assessment be conducted. The assessment of the chronic pain patient should evaluate and integrate psychosocial and behavioral information as well as organic and functional pathology (36). The treatment approach undertaken should be guided by the information provided by the thorough assessment of all relevant factors.

COGNITIVE-BEHAVIORAL APPROACH TO THE ASSESSMENT OF CHRONIC PAIN PATIENTS

In thinking about assessment of chronic pain patients, it is helpful to consider the natural history of chronic pain. Initially, an individual with a new set of symptoms attempts to interpret these symptoms—that is, to make sense of them, to try to determine their meaning, and to make decisions regarding the appropriate action to take. If a symptom is severe and persists over time, the individual will usually seek help from a health care provider. The health care provider will typically take a history, perform a physical examination, and refer the patient for a set of diagnostic tests. Once the results of the examination and tests are obtained, the health care provider will attempt to establish the cause of the pain and prescribe a treatment.

Failure to identify an adequate cause is likely to lead to patient frustration and potentially referral to a specialist or set of specialists. The referral process may initiate and lead to "doctor shopping," a search for a health care provider who can provide relief. Referrals to other specialists often will lead to additional costly and invasive diagnostic procedures. The continual failure to identify the cause of the pain complaint will likely contribute to additional frustration and a suggestion, either implicit or explicit, that the patient is malingering or that the pain is psychogenic. Continued patient frustration and anger may lead to increased symptom reporting, displays of pain behavior, and help–seeking. Throughout this downward spiral, the patient and his or her family frequently will become more psychologically distressed.

From a cognitive-behavioral perspective, three central questions guide assessment of pain patients:

1. What is the extent of the patient's injury or disease (physical impairment)?
2. What is the magnitude of the illness? That is, to what extent is the patient suffering, disabled, and unable to enjoy usual activities?
3. Is the illness behavior appropriate to the disease process or is there any evidence of amplification of symptoms for any of a variety of psychological or social reasons or purposes ("abnormal illness behavior")?

We have proposed a model of pain assessment, labeled a *multiaxial assessment of pain (MAP) patients* that incorporates each of these three questions. This MAP approach postulates that three axes, which parallel the questions listed above, are essential to appropriately assess chronic pain patients, namely, medical-physical, psychosocial, and behavioral-functional. From this conceptualization, each of these general domains must be assessed with psychometrically sound instruments and procedures *and* the results of the assessment of each axis must be combined into a meaningful taxonomy or clas-

Table 12.3.
Components of the Multiaxial Assessment of Pain

1. AXIS I: MEDICAL-PHYSICAL, quantification of:
   1.1 Laboratory and other diagnostic procedures
   1.2 Physical examination
   1.3 Functional mobility, strength, and flexibility
2. AXIS II: PSYCHOSOCIAL, including patients' perceptions of:
   2.1 Pain
   2.2 Affective distress
   2.3 Interference of pain with domains of life (e.g., social, vocational, marital, recreational, physical)
3. AXIS III: BEHAVIORAL-FUNCTIONAL, including:
   3.1 Observable communications of pain and distress
   3.2 Pain-related use of health care system
   3.3 Medication
   3.4 Activity levels
   3.5 Responses of significant others

sification system that will guide treatment decision making and planning. Table 12.3 lists the three axes and examples of the constructs that are incorporated within each.

The approach advocated can be contrasted with the taxonomy of chronic pain patients published by the International Association for the Study of Pain, or IASP (37). The IASP taxonomy is based on inference starting with *a-priori* syndromes or diagnoses and, subsequently, rating each diagnosis along each of five axes (i.e., body location, body system, temporal characteristics of pain, intensity and onset, and etiology). The end result of this process is the creation of a unique code for each of over 300 diagnoses. The MAP approach focuses on the empirical derivation of patient groups based on the statistical integration of medical-physical, psychosocial, and behavioral-functional data. The suggested approach attempts to identify groups of patients based on their unique characteristics rather than assigning patients to a hypothesized set of diagnoses, as is the case of the IASP approach.

A cornucopia (or Pandora's box) of assessment instruments and procedures are available to operationalize the three MAP axes; we will not review these here (38). What will be described is our own attempts to operationalize each of these axes and to develop a taxonomy of chronic pain patients that is based on the integration of these results.

QUANTIFICATION OF MEDICAL-PHYSICAL FINDINGS

Difficulties in assessing the physical contributions to chronic pain are well recognized, and there are no universal criteria for scoring the presence, absence, or importance of a particular sign (e.g., abnormal radiograph, distorted gait, limitation of spinal mobility), for establishing the association of these findings to treatment success, or for quantifying the degree of disability (39). Rather, interpretation of medical-physical findings have tended to rely on clinical judgments and medical consensus based on the physician's experience and occasionally quasi-standardized criteria (40, 41). As Brand and Lehmann note, "Most rating schemes provide only general guidelines from which a physician must develop his own standards" (42).

A frequent source of confusion in the medical evaluation of chronic pain patients relates to what clinical and laboratory findings are useful and appropriate for chronic pain patients, how much importance should be given to each test result, and how to reliably assess physical pathology. For example, is determination of the amount of pathology based on radiographic and electromyographic findings equivalent to determining pathology based on physical examination? Should magnetic resonance imaging (MRI) be given more weight than a functionally oriented finding even though the structural finding may be less reliable than the functional one? Does an abnormal radiograph predict a successful surgical outcome? Currently, there are no definitive answers to any of these questions.

Most assessments of physical pathology rely on a simple linear combination or summation of identified abnormalities, resulting in a total score (40, 41). This procedure is predicated on the assumption that the importance of all abnormalities, regardless of how assessed, are equivalent. It is possible, if not probable, however, that some positive (abnormal) findings are more important than others and thus should be weighed more heavily in the total pathology or impairment score. Furthermore, some assessment procedures provide more reliable data than others.

To begin to address these questions, we conducted a study to establish the differential utility of the most commonly employed diagnostic procedures used by physicians specializing in the assessment and treatment of pain (i.e., members of the American Academy of Pain Medicine, or AAPM) (43). One hundred members of the AAPM were surveyed to establish the differential utility of 18 frequently used diagnostic test and examination procedures gleaned from the literature (e.g., electromyography, mobility of weight bearing joints—see Table 12.4). These physicians displayed a high degree of agreement (Kendall's coefficient of concordance = .65, $p < .001$) regarding the relative importance of the different procedures included in the survey. The average individual physician's rank ordering of these procedures, from 1 (most useful) to 18 (least useful) in the evaluation of chronic pain patients is shown in Table 12.4.

The AAPM members surveyed were also requested to list any additional procedures that would be included in medical assessment of chronic pain patients. Al-

Table 12.4.
Rank-Ordering of 18 Medical Procedures Used in Chronic Pain Assessment

Rank Order Average	Medical Procedure
2.97	Neurologic examination
4.14	Observation of gait and posture
4.39	Assessment of spinal mobility
4.55	Examination of muscular function (tone, mass, strength)
5.94	Examination of soft tissues
6.35	Assessment of mobility of weight-bearing joints
7.95	Plain radiography
8.08	Assessment of mobility of joints other than spine or weight bearing
8.34	Computed axial tomography
9.61	Electromyography
10.42	Contrast radiography
11.69	Examination of internal organs (inspection, palpation, auscultation, percussion)
12.68	Nuclear medicine
13.45	Laboratory tests (other than blood count)
13.93	Thermography
14.00	Blood count
16.10	Electroencephalography
16.40	Electrocardiography

though psychological evaluation and testing were frequently listed, there were no consistent medical tests or procedures suggested by those surveyed, and thus it appears that the content validity of the 18 medical tests and examination procedures is acceptable. Thus, if the information gained from these procedures can be reliably scored in the evaluation of chronic pain patients, the results will be useful in developing a weighted scoring procedure for quantifying medical-physical findings.

A second study was conducted to assess the reliability of the medical-physical screening of the 18 procedures included in the survey of AAPM members (43). Two AAPM members performed chart reviews of 30 chronic pain patients using three-point or four-point scales to rate each of the 18 procedures listed in Table 12.4, two AAPM members performed direct assessments on 30 chronic pain patients, and two AAPM members either reviewed the charts or directly examined the same 30 chronic pain patients. Although more complicated rating scales could have been devised, they would likely make it more difficult to establish inter-judge reliability and would be less likely to be used in clinical settings.

Results from this study (43) indicated that only 1 of the 18 procedures could not be reliably judged (i.e., assessment of mobility of joints other than spine or weight bearing); the remaining had an average kappa reliability coefficient of .64, $p < .001$. The broad range in the linear utility weights computed for the 18 medical procedures (e.g., .394 for neurologic examination to .007 for electrocardiography) suggested that the development of assessment procedures that incorporate these medical findings should consider a weighted scoring system. For example, because neurologic examination findings were weighted as over 56 times more useful than electrocardiographic findings in the evaluation of chronic pain patients, a scoring system that does not reflect these types of utility differences will likely lead to a skewed or biased scale that does not accurately reflect medical consensus.

The results of this study (43) have recently been extended in a subsequent study that led to the development and scoring of a standardized biomedical assessment procedure, the Medical Examination and Diagnostic Information Coding System (MEDICS) (44). In addition to demonstrating the inter-rater reliability of the MEDICS for chronic pain patients, Rudy et al. also developed an innovative scoring approach that permits (1) the use of weighted scores that reflect medical consensus and (2) reliable scoring when only a subset of the 18 MEDICS test results is available for a specific patient (44). Thus, comparisons across subjects can be made despite differences in the biomedical data available. These results provide preliminary support for the appropriateness of assessing chronic pain patients using these basic quantification procedures and subsequently integrating the results of this examination with psychosocial and behavioral assessment data.

QUANTIFICATION OF PSYCHOSOCIAL AND BEHAVIORAL DATA

As noted, a central emphasis is of the cognitive-behavioral perspective, individuals and their interpretation and understanding of their problems and their fears, beliefs, and attitudes about their symptoms, treatment, and the health care system. These cognitive variables are important because they will influence how patients present their symptoms to families, friends, and employers (as well as to health care providers), respond to explanations provided, are motivated for treatment, and adhere to recommendations. Thus, it is useful to ask patients about what they think is wrong with them, what worries them, what they have been told about their symptoms, what problems the symptoms have caused them, and how they think their pain should be treated. Once a rationale for the persistent pain is presented, it is helpful to ask patients and their family members if the explanation makes sense to them. Similarly, once a treatment has been prescribed, the therapist should ask how credible the treatment seems and whether they feel that it will be effective for them.

In addition to structured interviews to identify patients' attitudes and beliefs, it is also helpful to use psychometric instruments, especially those designed (and normed) on relevant populations. Kerns, Turk, and Rudy developed a comprehensive assessment inventory, the West Haven–Yale Multidimensional Pain Inventory (MPI), that was designed to assess the impact of pain from the patient's perspective (45). That is, the MPI operationalizes psychological reactions to chronic pain, perceived responses of significant others, and activities interfered with because of pain. This inventory is composed of three sections. The first section was specifically designed to evaluate chronic pain patients' (1) reports of pain severity and suffering, (2) perceptions of how pain interferes with their lives, including interference with family and marital functioning, work, and social-recreational activities, (3) dissatisfaction with present levels of functioning in family, marriage, work, and social life, (4) appraisals of support received from significant others, (5) perceived life control, incorporating perceived ability to solve problems and feelings of mastery and competence, and (6) affective distress, including ratings of depressed mood, irritability, and tension.

The second section of the MPI assesses the patient's perspective as to how significant others within their environment respond when he or she is suffering (i.e., punishing, solicitous, or distracting responses). The last section evaluates the frequency of performing a set of common activities (e.g., cooking a meal). Thus, the first section of the MPI provides an operationalization of the psychosocial axis, and the latter two sections the behavioral axis.

The MPI displays good internal consistency, test-retest reliability, and convergent and discriminant validity (45). Thus, the psychometric properties that are a prerequisite for the development of a classification system suggested by the MAP approach appear to have been met. The next step in the development of the MAP-based taxonomy consists of the integration of the medical-physical findings, based on the procedures described in the preceding section of this chapter, with the results of the psychosocial and behavioral data acquired on the MPI.

INTEGRATION OF ASSESSMENT FINDINGS: TOWARD A TAXONOMY OF CHRONIC PAIN PATIENTS

The MPI (45) and the medical-physical assessment described above were used in the initial phase of taxometric development (36). Using recent statistical advances in clustering techniques that increase the accuracy of these methods (46, 47), cluster analyses and multivariate classification methods were conducted on a heterogeneous group of 100 patients to determine whether there were different response patterns that could reliably classify patients into unique groups (48). The k-means clustering approach was used to discover more about the similarities and differences among chronic pain patients in order to identify subgroups or "homogeneous" samples of pain patients and to guard against the superimposing of an a-priori but potentially invalid structure to the data.

Four distinct chronic pain patient profiles were identified by means of this analysis. These profiles were labeled (1) *Disabled,* patients who had higher than average (for chronic pain patients) medical-physical findings, perceived the severity of their pain to be high, reported that pain interfered with much of their lives, and reported a higher degree of psychological distress and low activity levels; (2) *Dysfunctional,* patients who had less severe medical findings than the disabled group but who had high degrees of psychosocial and behavioral disability; (3) *Interpersonally Distressed,* patients with a common perception that significant others were not very understanding or supportive of their pain problems; and (4) *Adaptive Copers,* patients who reported higher levels of social support, relatively low levels of pain and interference compared to the other three groups, and higher levels of behavioral activity. The percentage of patients falling within each of the four clusters were 24%, 24%, 31%, and 21%, respectively.

In a subsequent study, we examined whether similar subgroups of chronic pain patients would emerge if the medical findings were eliminated (49). We cluster-analyzed patients' MPI scores excluding medical findings. This analysis resulted in the identification of three subgroups of patients. Two of the subgroups identified in the original study, interpersonally distressed and adaptive copers, emerged along with a large cluster of patients with high levels of pain and psychological distress and low levels of activity. This latter subgroup, on a psychosocial and behavioral basis, appeared to be virtually identical to the dysfunctional subgroup identified in the original study. In short, what seems to have occurred with the removal of medical findings is that the disabled and dysfunctional subgroups merge together. The generalizability of the three subgroups, dysfunctional, interpersonally distressed, and adaptive copers, has been demonstrated in a subsequent study (50). We noted that, although the proportions of patients assigned to the subgroup were different, chronic back pain, head pain, and temporomandibular disorder (TMD) patients could be classified as falling within the three subgroups originally identified. There were more back pain patients classified as dysfunctional than was the case with head pain or TMD patients. Despite these proportional differences, patients with two different medical diagnoses might be psychosocially and behaviorally more similar to each other than two patients with the same medical diagnoses.

Additional research is required to examine the incremental validity of behavioral observation of pain behaviors (51), coping resources (52), and idiosyncratic beliefs (53). The goal should be the development of a triarchic, MAP-based taxonomy that will enhance our understanding of pain, assist in evaluation and the prescription of specific therapeutic interventions, and further our ability to predict treatment outcome.

The tendency has been to provide all patients with much the same intervention and to compare the treatment outcome to pretreatment measures or a no-treatment comparison group. The unfortunate results of this type of research is that although patients with certain characteristics may benefit from the intervention, others with a different set of characteristics may be inappropriate for the intervention. Combining both groups together in a single study is likely to lead to results of modest success at best. Classification of patients into more homogeneous subgroups should permit the direct assessment of the relative effectiveness of different treatments for different patient groups on relevant characteristics and not just on the specific diagnosis as suggested by the IASP approach to classification (e.g., reflex sympathetic dystrophy of the arm, IASP classification code 203.91b) or heterogeneous groups composed of generic "chronic pain syndrome" (54).

The differential approach to treating pain patients does not mean necessarily that the philosophy of treatment will change depending on patient characteristics, but rather that specific interventions may be used to supplement treatment approaches that offer much that is consistent across patients. For example, the cognitive-behavioral philosophy may govern the treatment approach we use with all patients, but patients with a profile that we have classified as "interpersonally distressed" might benefit from the inclusion of more active family involvement than will patients who fall within the group we labeled "adaptive copers," who report that their social supports are more adequate.

COGNITIVE-BEHAVIORAL TREATMENT FOR CHRONIC PAIN

To understand the cognitive-behavioral approach to the treatment of chronic pain patients, it is important to understand that the techniques actually employed are viewed as significantly less important than the more general philosophy and orientation described above in general and more specifically with regard to chronic pain in this section. These factors, which are often referred to somewhat disparagingly as the "nonspecifics" of treatment, may actually be the most important component of successful treatment. Thus, we will spend some time discussing these factors to emphasize their importance and to inoculate the reader against focusing on details, such as what method of relaxation to use, what are the specific images used to enhance distraction, where to place the biofeedback electrodes, what physical exercises are best for what types of patients, what should be included in the homework assignments, and so forth. Although these technical details are important, they will only contribute to treatment efficacy *if* they are embedded in a more general comprehensive treatment framework (13, 34).

OVERVIEW

By the time patients come to a treatment program for chronic pain they have received multiple evaluations and a range of treatment modalities, often beginning with suggestions for bed rest and non-narcotic analgesic medication through therapeutic nerve blocks and passive physical therapy (e.g., hot pack, cold packs) and, finally, when all else has failed, large dosages of psychotropic and/or narcotic analgesic medications and multiple surgical procedures. In addition to these conventional medical interventions, many patients have submitted to a host of alternative therapies (e.g., acupuncture, hypnosis, biofeedback). A common feature across all patients regardless of diagnosis is that an array of interventions have failed to adequately alleviate their suffering. Patients treated at pain programs have an average duration of pain of over 7 years (55). Thus, it is not surprising that by the time these patients are seen at a pain center they are quite demoralized, feel frustrated, and feel their situation is hopeless, and yet still are seeking THE cure for their suffering. This, then, is the background against which any therapeutic regimen that will be offered must be viewed.

The strategic goal of a cognitive-behavioral pain treatment program is to help patients to reconceptualize their view of their situation and their pain. Patients frequently come to pain clinics with a view of pain as a totally medical symptom that is all-encompassing and over which they have no control (fostered by the acute illness model described earlier). The cognitive-behavioral approach is designed to be optimistic, emphasizing both the effectiveness of the rehabilitation approach *and* the patient's ability to alleviate much of his or her pain and suffering if he or she is willing to work *with* the treatment team. That is, the treatment methods that we will recommend will only be effective if the patient accepts responsibility for a large part of the treatment with the guidance, supervision, and support of all members of the treatment team. This view can be sharply contrasted with previous approaches that have been geared toward "doing something to the patient," with the patient assuming a passive "sick-role."

Throughout the rehabilitation process, pain is reconceptualized so that the patient comes to view his or her situation as amenable to change by means of combined psychologically based and physically based approaches. The treatment program is designed to teach the patient a range of physical and psychological coping skills and to assist him or her in dealing with maladaptive thoughts and feelings as well as noxious sensations that may initiate or exacerbate suffering. The cognitive-behavioral treatment relies heavily on active patient participation and emphasizes a mutual problem-solving approach among the treatment team, the patient, and the significant others in the patient's environment.

The cognitive-behavioral approach is very much a collaborative endeavor that attempts to foster an increased sense of self-efficacy and intrinsic motivation. Even the most ideal treatment plan has little likelihood of success if the patient does not continue to engage in the prescribed behaviors once he or she is discharged from the treatment program. In one recent study surveying chronic pain patients 18 months to 10 years following treatment at a multidisciplinary pain center, adherence to various self-care behaviors was quite low, ranging from less that 10% for diet management and appropriate use of communication skills to 52% for following the recommended exercise regimen (56).

The likelihood of the continued adherence to the self-care regimen is limited to the extent the patient (1) does not have the necessary skills, (2) does not feel competent to perform the recommended overt and covert behaviors, particularly on an ad-hoc basis, (3) permits other factors to interfere with the performance of the adaptive behaviors, and (4) experiences no external or intrinsic motivation to persevere with the performance of the behaviors (57). Kanfer and Karoly suggest that for self-management to operate there must be a shift in the patient's repertoire from well-established, habitual, and automatic but ineffective responses toward systematic problem-solving and planning, long-term control of affect, and behavioral persistence (58).

Cognitive and behavioral methods are used to teach the patient to recognize and alter the association between thoughts, feelings, behaviors, environmental factors, and pain. From the cognitive-behavioral perspective, therapeutic gain is enhanced and only maintained when the patient is actively involved, accepts responsibility for change, and is intrinsically motivated rather than externally manipulated (59). Improvement is thus a function of the clinic team, the patient, and other significant people in the patient's environment (e.g., family, attorneys, claims adjusters, and members of the health care system).

The cognitive-behavioral approach can be adapted for use with inpatients and outpatients, conducted on an individual or group basis, and used as a total program for treatment of chronic pain patients in a multidisciplinary setting or by a set of solo practitioners from different disciplines. Before describing the outline of treatment, we need to address briefly the composition and function of an interdisciplinary team, the involvement of significant others, and the disability/compensation morass.

INTERDISCIPLINARY TEAM

We believe that the most effective approach to treating chronic pain patients is by means of an interdisciplinary team. We use the term *interdisciplinary* rather than *multidisciplinary* to describe what we feel is the optimal treatment working relationship. Interdisciplinary implies a close working relationship among health care professionals rather than the distal involvement of many consultants with information integrated by the primary health care provider. The core of the team is composed of representatives from medicine, nursing, psychology, and the physical therapy and occupational therapy disciplines. The specialty of the physician member of the team is less important than his or her dedication to working with pain patients and to a non-autocratic approach to participation on rather than command of a team. Each team member has specific areas of expertise and his or her contribution to decision making and planning is of equal importance in formulating the treatment. It is essential that the treatment team share a common philosophy so that patients are treated consistently regardless of the disciplines or techniques used by the various team members (60).

Although we have listed the core professional team, it is important to realize that the patient and significant others are part of the interdisciplinary *team* as well. That is, patients and family members are not passive. They bring with them to the pain clinic thoughts, attitudes, and wishes that are important and must be incorporated or modified if treatment is to be successful. All too often health care providers forget to LISTEN to what patients and families are trying to tell them. We are not just referring to the "facts" of their injury but also to the impact on their lives. We could contrast the unidimensional health care provider as Sergeant Joe Friday (played by Jack Webb) in the 1950s detective show *Dragnet* with the cognitive-behaviorally oriented health care provider, Lieutenant Columbo (played by Peter Falk) in the detective show *Columbo*. Sergeant Friday only wanted to know "the facts, nothing but the facts," whereas, Lieutenant Columbo was probing, acknowledged confusion and lack of understanding, and readily asked for opinions and not "just the facts." (Perhaps that is why Joe Friday never reached the rank of lieutenant, as Columbo did.)

Often there has been a tendency in the treatment of chronic pain patients to forget about the importance of the family (61). Chronic pain, however, by virtue of extending over time, impacts on all aspects of the patient's life, including his or her family life. Failure to include family members is likely to contribute to the problems of maintenance and generalization of treatment gains. At a minimum, families need to be aware of the nature and logic for the treatment goals and modalities employed. Some families may require additional involvement or family counseling if there is to be any hope for success. We might speculate that patients who lie within the interpersonally distressed subgroup described earlier might require extensive family counseling and in-

terpersonal problem solving in addition to the basic family involvement required for all patients.

There are three other groups who are essential to the maintenance of treatment gains, but they have been given much less attention, namely, referring physicians, attorneys, and claims adjusters. Referring physicians provide the background set that patients acquire and carry with them to the clinic. Many patients are unsure why they are being referred ("Is this where I get more pills?"), others are angry ("You're referring me there because you don't believe my pain is real"), and still others have been given misinformation ("I was told to come here so that you could give a deposition indicating that I should receive complete disability from my worker compensation board").

Moreover, patients who are treated for chronic pain are going to return to referring or primary physicians for continued care. We have seen all too many patients who were successfully treated at other pain centers relapse shortly thereafter because, in part, the referring physician was not informed how best to follow through with the chronic pain patient—namely, by positively reinforcing progress and avoiding rewards for abnormal illness behavior, including passivity and medication seeking. Both prior to evaluation and treatment and subsequent to treatment termination, referring physicians play an essential role. Referral agents need to be informed about the nature of the evaluation process and treatment program, what to tell patients who are being referred, and how to continue to care for patients following treatment at the pain center. Additionally, the referring physician should be provided with the evaluation results, a thorough description of the treatment plan including a specific set of objectives, and a report on how successful the patient was in accomplishing the treatment goals. Involvement and information sharing with referral agents is crucial to all phases of treatment and to facilitate maintenance of benefits.

Third-party payers have often had adversarial relationships with chronic pain patients and pain clinics. Part of the problem has been the failure of pain clinics to address the concerns of third-party payers while expecting them to continue to pay for the services provided (62). Health care providers have tended to take a "holier than thou" stance with insurance companies without understanding the needs of claims adjusters and thus have contributed to the adversarial tension. Certain questions are essential from the standpoint of the insurance company, and these need to be addressed even if the answers are not what the insurance company would like to hear. Questions such as "Can this patient return to work?," "Can he or she be rehabilitated?," "Should he or she be awarded total and permanent disability?," "Could the car accident have exacerbated a previous pathologic condition?," "What is this patient's residual function capacity?," and "Is another operation likely to permit us to close out this case?" Although health care providers need to be concerned primarily about the welfare of their patients, answers to these questions can be crucial in treatment planning and are important to address in order to assist third-party payers (62).

Personal injury lawyers and the legal system also can hamper attempts to provide optimal rehabilitation. Often the litigation process extends over years and may make the task of rehabilitation much more difficult because the patient may be much more physically deconditioned and psychologically distressed following prolonged legal wrangling (63, 64). Pain centers have not done a very good job of education and must be aware of these forces as they develop treatment and rehabilitation programs. A recent meta-analysis reported by Flor et al. has demonstrated that pain clinic treatment not only has significantly improved the subjective quality of life of chronic pain patients but also has resulted in important functional benefits, notably high rates of return to work (55).

COMPONENTS OF TREATMENT

With the background provided, we can now consider some of the specific components of the cognitive-behavioral treatment. Following assessment, although it should be noted that assessment is an ongoing process that should continually guide treatment, treatment is composed of four inter-related components: (1) education, (2) skills acquisition, (3) cognitive and behavioral rehearsal, and (4) generalization and maintenance.

Education

The educational component of treatment consists of the presentation of the cognitive-behavioral perspective on pain and the control of pain (i.e., role of cognitions, affect, behavior, environmental factors, and physical factors). At the outset of treatment and continuing throughout, we attempt to discuss pain and the impact on the patient's life in a manner that is most appropriate to each individual patient. We try to use the patient's vocabulary, and start with their understanding of their situation and problems. We continue in a collaborative rather than didactic manner through the treatment (65). That is, we convey to patients that we will not do anything to them but rather that we will work together with them to achieve the best possible outcome given the restraints imposed by any physical impairments. This collaborative approach can be contrasted with the more traditional autocratic medical approach inherent in many settings.

Many patients have unspoken fears about progression of their condition, about injuring themselves by performing certain exercises ("I can't bend over too far or I might break my spinal fusion"), and that people think their pain is not real. In short, we begin by assuming the "Columbo" role and listen to the patient's "story," his or her fears and concerns. Many patients are reluctant to express such concerns or may not even be aware of them even though they influence their behavior. We often use the "imaginary patient" to help discuss sensitive issues. That is, we might say, "Some patients are concerned that they have limits on their physical activity due to their medical problem. Do you have any concerns about what activities might make your condition worse? Let me assure you that we will not recommend any exercises that would be harmful to you. Have any of the other physicians who have treated you suggested that you should not do certain things?" If the answer is yes, we might ask "How long were you told you should not lift heavy objects and how heavy were the objects you were told that you should not lift?" We have found such questions to be important because many patients misunderstand the information provided by previous health care providers. If significant others are present, we may turn to them and ask a similar set of questions to elicit their views, worries, and possible misconceptions. The important point is to not only reassure the patient and significant others but also to identify idiosyncratic beliefs and inaccurate understanding of information.

We then employ a somewhat more didactic approach, using the information obtained from the assessment, to clarify patients' medical conditions and explain to them what we have found and what is going on physically as well as psychosocially in a manner that patients can understand. We prefer to do this with significant others present so that we can determine the level of misinformation they have acquired as well as educate them about any restrictions and provide them with appropriate reassurances. We review psychosocial and behavioral results acquired during the assessment and try to demonstrate to the patient how his or her situation may be influenced by these factors. We use this information to begin the process of reconceptualization. That is, pain interferes with different areas of their lives, people respond to them in different ways. We ask patients to consider how these responses might affect how they think, feel, and behave, as well as influence how others respond to them.

The educational component continues throughout the treatment. All members of the treatment team use information and material that comes up during and between sessions to underscore the important inter-relationships among thoughts, feelings, and behaviors. Specific homework tasks may be prescribed to help patients to identify situations in which thoughts, feelings, and behaviors exacerbated or inhibited their pain. Because homework is such a crucial element in cognitive-behavioral treatment, we will devote a section to this topic later in this chapter.

Skills Acquisition

In all cases, it is important for patients to understand the rationale for the specific skills being taught and the behaviors they are being asked to perform. Again, unless patients understand the rationale for the treatment components and have an opportunity to raise issues and confusions, they are less likely to persevere in their efforts in the face of difficulty, to benefit, or to maintain any therapeutic gains. Cognitive and behavioral treatment techniques consist of a whole range of strategies and procedures designed to bring about alterations in patients' perceptions of their situation and thus their ability to control their condition (12).

Cognitive-behavioral therapists, regardless of specialty or discipline, serve as teachers, coaches, collaborators, and at times "cheerleaders" helping patients learn new ways of behaving, feeling, and thinking. The health care provider should encourage patients to become active contributors to their experiences and not helpless victims. The responsibility for acquiring and maintaining any treatment gains rests ultimately with the patient.

Various strategies and techniques are available to the cognitive-behavioral team. As Holzman and his colleagues note, *"We have found no one treatment technique essential for all patients"* (59). There is a need to individualize the treatment program for the specific patient. Although two patients both participate in a cognitive-behavioral pain management program, the specific details of their treatment and the techniques that are employed may be very different. Therefore, commonalities among treatments may be obscured if only the techniques used are compared (34). Rather, the rationale for the techniques used and the overall plan of treatment are more important in this therapeutic approach. Techniques such as relaxation training, active physical therapy using paced mastery, problem-solving training, stress management, distraction skills training, rational restructuring, and communication skills training, to name only a few, have all been incorporated within the general cognitive-behavioral approach. A number of papers and volumes have described in detail some specific techniques used; the interested reader should consult these (11–13, 59, 66).

More important than the techniques is the goal of enhancing self-control and intrinsic motivation and the manner in which these skills are described, taught, and practiced. Once again, it is essential for health care providers to keep in mind the patient's perspective and how he or she perceives each skill and assignment. The listening and observational skills of the provider become quite important because they will influence subsequent strategies, revisions of goals and methods, and so forth. These clinical skills and the relationship that is established between providers and patients become the oil that keeps the gears of treatment moving forward, and without these treatment will come to a grinding halt (13).

Cognitive and Behavioral Rehearsal

In this component of the cognitive-behavioral treatment, the patient practices and further consolidates the skills that he or she has learned during the skills-acquisition phase and learns to apply them to natural situations. The rehearsal techniques employed include mental *imagery*, during which time the patient imagines using the skills in different situations, difficulties to be encountered, and how these difficulties can be handled and overcome. *Role-playing* is also used. The patient interacts with the provider as if he or she was in a specific situation and needs to use specific skills (e.g., argument with spouse). *Role-reversal* is also employed, in which the patient and provider switch roles and the patient "teaches" skills to the provider, who has assumed the role of a patient. Specific details of these approaches are described in Holzman et al. (59) and Turk et al. (12).

Homework

An essential component of the cognitive-behavioral approach is the active involvement of the patient and significant others outside the therapy sessions. Turk et al. have outlined the purposes of the tasks to be conducted between sessions (12):

1. To assess various areas of the patient's and significant others' lives and how these influence and are affected by the pain problem.
2. To assess the typical responses of significant others and the patient to pain and pain behaviors.
3. To make the patient and significant others more aware of the factors that exacerbate and alleviate suffering.
4. To help the patient and significant others identify maladaptive responses to pain and pain behaviors.
5. To consolidate the use of coping procedures and physical exercises discussed during therapy sessions.
6. To increase physical activity levels.
7. To illustrate to the patient and significant others that progress can be made in living with pain but with less suffering.
8. To serve as reinforcers and as enhancers of self-efficacy as the patient achieves his or her goals.
9. To assist the provider and patient in assessing progress and in modifying goals and treatment strategies.

Homework assignments are established within the same collaborative framework as all of the cognitive-behavioral therapy that we have described is conducted. Each homework assignment is geared toward observable and manageable tasks, starting with those that are most readily achievable and progressing to more difficult ones. The purpose of such graded tasks is to enhance the patient's sense of competence and to reinforce his or her continued efforts. The provider uses the assessment results to establish short-, medium-, and long-term goals, and the accompanying tasks are designed to attain these goals. Goals and assignments are most effective when they are individually customized to the particular condition, lifestyle, and possible wishes of each patient.

When establishing homework assignments, we have found it extremely useful to use several steps. We ask patients to write down what it is that they are to do, when, and how frequently. We also ask them if they can foresee any problems in successfully completing the homework assigned and how they will deal with these problems. Occasionally, it is useful to use the imaginary patient technique that we mentioned earlier. Namely, we might note that "some patients have had difficulties with similar homework tasks and although you might not, let us tell you what we found helpful for these patients."

The emphasis on homework is consistent with operant approaches. This illustrates our point regarding the potential of integrating behavioral techniques within a cognitive-behavioral treatment regimen.

Generalization and Maintenance

In the final stage of treatment, discussion focuses on possible ways of predicting and avoiding or dealing with pain following treatment termination. We have found it useful to help patients to anticipate future stress or pain-eliciting events and to plan coping strategies and response strategies before they occur. Marlatt and Gordon refer to this process as "relapse prevention" (67).

It is important to note that all possible situations cannot be anticipated. Rather, our goal during this phase, as with the rest of the treatment, is to enable patients to develop a problem-solving perspective to coping wherein they believe that they have the skills and competence to respond in an adaptive fashion. In this manner, the patient will learn to try to anticipate future difficulties, develop plans for coping, and adjust his or her behavior accordingly. Successful performance of these strategies should further serve to enhance self-efficacy and may help to form a "virtuous circle" in contrast to the "vicious circle" created and fostered by inactivity, passivity, physical deconditioning, helplessness, and hopelessness that characterizes chronic pain patients.

The relapse prevention phase serves at least two purposes: it permits the patient to anticipate and plan for future events, and it focuses on the necessary conditions for long-term success. More specifically, relapse prevention provides the patient with the expectation that minor setbacks may in fact occur but that these setbacks do not signal total failure and should be viewed as cues to use in a more effective manner the coping skills already learned. It is important for the patient not to think of his or her work as ending at termination of treatment, but rather that he or she is entering into a different phase of maintenance.

During the final session, all aspects of the program are reviewed. A review with patients of what they have learned and how they have changed from the onset of treatment can encourage recognition of how patients' own efforts contributed to the positive changes. The goal is to help patients realize that they have plans, skills, and abilities within their repertoire to cope with their situation without the need of direct contact with therapists. Thus, change has been achieved and can be maintained if the patient continues to take charge of his or her life.

CONCLUSIONS

Obviously in this chapter we have been unable to address all of the nuances of cognitive-behavioral treatments, but we hope we have whetted the appetite of the reader to consider more carefully the nature of his or her treatment and mode of interacting with patients. As is obvious from any scanning of the literature, single-modality interventions imposed on passive patients seem of limited value for the complexity of problems inherent in chronic pain. The history of treatment of chronic pain is replete with technically elegant interventions that have proven to be failures (7, 68, 69). We do not mean to suggest that there is no place for conventional medical and surgical modalities in chronic pain, but it seems apparent that optimal treatment for chronic pain patients must extend beyond the scalpel and syringe. We have attempted to describe one multidimensional approach to this major problem in health care. Research has begun to support the efficacy of this approach for a diversity of chronic pain syndromes (see refs. 13 and 70 for reviews); however, the hackneyed statement "more research is needed" still is relevant.

Acknowledgement Preparation of this manuscript was supported by grant 2R01DE07514 from the National Institute of Dental Research and grant 2R01AR38698 from the National Institute of Arthritis and Musculoskeletal and Skin Diseases.

REFERENCES

1. Turk DC, Rudy TE: Assessment of cognitive factors in chronic pain: A worthwhile enterprise? *J Consult Clin Psychol* 54:760–768, 1986.
2. International Association for the Study of Pain. Pain terms: A list with definitions and notes on usage. *Pain* 6:249–252, 1979.
3. Fernandez E, Turk DC: Sensory and affective components of pain: Separation and synthesis. *Psychol Bull* 112:205–217, 1992.
4. Melzack R, Casey KL: Sensory, motivational and central control determinants of pain: A new conceptual model. In Kenshalo D (ed): *The Skin Senses.* Springfield, IL, Charles C Thomas, 1968.

5. Melzack R, Wall PD: Pain mechanisms: A new theory. *Science* 50:971–979, 1965.

6. Fordyce WE, Fowler RS, DeLateur B: An application of behavior modification technique to a problem of chronic pain. *Behav Res Ther* 6:105–107, 1968.

7. Melzack R, Wall PD: *The Challenge of Pain.* New York, Basic Books, 1983.

8. Fordyce WE, Fowler RS, Lehmann JF, DeLateur BJ, Sand PL, Trieschmann RB: Operant conditioning in the treatment of chronic pain. *Arch Phys Med Rehab* 54:399–408, 1973.

9. Fordyce WE: *Behavioral Methods for Chronic Pain and Illness.* St Louis, CV Mosby, 1976.

10. Turk DC, Matyas T: Pain-related behaviors: Communication of pain. *Am Pain Soc J* 1:109–111, 1992.

11. Turk DC, Meichenbaum D: A cognitive-behavioral approach to pain management. In Wall PD, Melzack R (eds): *Textbook of Pain,* ed 2. London, Churchill Livingstone, 1989.

12. Turk DC, Meichenbaum D, Genest M: *Pain and Behavioral Medicine: A Cognitive-Behavioral Perspective.* New York, Guilford Press, 1983.

13. Turk DC, Holzman AD, Kerns RD: Chronic pain. In Holroyd KA, Creer TL (eds): *Chronic Disease: A Handbook of Self-Management Approaches.* New York, Academic Press, 1985.

14. Holroyd KA, Nash JM, Pingel JD, Cordingley GE, Jerome A: A comparison of pharmacological (Amitriptyline HCL) and nonpharmacological (cognitive-behavioral) therapies for chronic tension headaches. *J Consult Clin Psychol* 59:121–133, 1991.

15. Newton CR, Barbaree HE: Cognitive changes accompanying headache treatment: The use of a thought-sampling procedure. *Cognitive Ther Res* 11:635–652, 1987.

16. Olson RE, Malow RM: Effects of biofeedback and psychotherapy on patients with myofascial pain dysfunction who are nonresponsive to conventional treatments. *Rehabil Psychol* 32:195–205, 1987.

17. Bradley LA, Young LD, Anderson KO, Turner RA, Agudelo CA, McDaniel LK, Pisko EJ, Semble EL, Morgan T: Effects of psychological therapy on pain behavior of rheumatoid arthritis patients. Treatment outcome and six-month follow-up. *Arthritis Rheum* 30:1105–1114, 1987.

18. O'Leary A, Shoor S, Lorig K, Holman HR: A cognitive-behavioral treatment for rheumatoid arthritis. *Health Psychol* 7:527–544, 1988.

19. Kerns RD, Turk DC, Holzman AD, Rudy TE: Efficacy of a cognitive-behavioral approach for the treatment of chronic pain. *Clin J Pain* 1:195–203, 1986.

20. Nicholas MK, Wilson PH, Goyen J: Comparison of cognitive-behavioral group treatment and an alternative nonpsychological treatment for chronic low back pain. *Pain* 48:339–347, 1992.

21. Bandura A: *Principles of Behavior Modification.* New York, Holt, Rinehart & Winston, 1969.

22. Keeley SM, Shemberg KM, Carbonell J: Operant clinical intervention: Behavior management or beyond? Where are the data? *Behav Ther* 7:292–305, 1976.

23. Mahoney MJ: *Cognition and Behavior Modification.* Cambridge, MA, Ballinger, 1974.

24. Ciccone DS, Grzesiak RC: Cognitive dimensions of chronic pain. *Soc Sci Med* 19:1339–1346, 1984.

25. Racklin H: Pain and behavior. *Behav Brain Sci* 8:43–53, 1985.

26. Sternbach RA: Behavior therapy. In Wall PD, Melzack R (eds): *Textbook of Pain.* London, Churchill Livingstone, 1984.

27. Kahneman D, Slovic P, Tversky A: *Judgment Under Uncertainty: Heuristics and Biases.* New York, Cambridge University Press, 1982.

28. Nisbett R, Ross L: *Human Inference: Strategies and Shortcomings of Social Judgment.* Englewood Cliffs, NJ, Prentice Hall, 1980.

29. Lazarus RS, Folkman S: *Stress, Appraisal, and Coping.* New York, Springer, 1984.

30. Bandura A: The self-system in reciprocal determinism. *Am Psychol* 3:344–359, 1978.

31. Cairns D, Pasino J: Comparison of verbal reinforcement and feedback in the operant treatment of disability due to chronic low back pain. *Behav Ther* 8:621–630, 1977.

32. Dolce JJ, Crocker MF, Moletteire C, Doleys DM: Exercise quotas, anticipatory concerns and self-efficacy expectations in chronic pain: A preliminary report. *Pain* 24:365–372, 1986.

33. Doleys DM, Crocker M, Patton D: Responses of patients with chronic pain to exercise quotas. *J Am Phys Ther Assoc* 62:1111–1114, 1982.

34. Turk DC, Holzman AD: Commonalities among psychological approaches in the treatment of chronic pain: Specifying the meta-constructs. In Holzman AD, Turk DC (eds): *Pain Management: A Handbook of Psychological Treatment Approaches.* Elmsford, NY, Pergamon Press, 1986.

35. Bandura A: Self-efficacy: Toward a unifying theory of behavior change. *Psychol Rev* 84:191–215, 1977.

36. Turk DC, Rudy TE: Toward the comprehensive assessment of chronic pain patients. *Behav Res Ther* 25:237–249, 1987.

37. International Association for the Study of Pain: Classification of chronic pain: Descriptions of chronic pain syndromes and definitions of pain terms. *Pain Suppl* 3:1–225, 1986.

38. Turk DC, Melzack R (eds): *Handbook of Pain Assessment.* New York, Guilford Press, 1992.

39. Brena SF, Turk DC: Vocational disability: A challenge to pain rehabilitation programs. In Aronoff G (ed): *Interdisciplinary Pain Clinics.* New York, Raven Press, 1988.

40. Brena SF, Koch DL: A "pain estimate" model for quantification and classification of chronic pain states. *Anesthesiol Rev* 2:8–13, 1975.

41. Waddell G, McCulloch JA, Kummel E, Venner RM: Nonorganic physical signs in low-back pain. *Spine* 5:117–125, 1980.

42. Brand RA, Lehmann TR: Low-back impairment rating practices of orthopedic surgeons. *Spine* 8:75–83, 1983.

43. Rudy TE, Turk DC, Brena SF: Differential utility of medical procedures in the assessment of chronic pain patients. *Pain* 34:53–60, 1988.

44. Rudy TE, Turk DC, Brena SF, Stieg RL, Brody MC: Quantification of biomedical findings of chronic pain patients: Development of an index of pathology. *Pain* 42:167–182, 1990.

45. Kerns RD, Turk DC, Rudy TE: The West Haven-Yale Mul-

tidimensional Pain Inventory (WHYMPI). *Pain* 23:345–356, 1985.

46. Milligan GW, Cooper MC: An examination of procedures for determining the number of clusters in a data set. *Psychometrika* 50:159–179, 1985.

47. Scheibler D, Schneider W: Monte Carlo tests of the accuracy of cluster analysis algorithms: A comparison of hierarchical and nonhierarchical methods. *Multivariate Behav Res* 20:283–304, 1985.

48. Tatsuoka MM: *Multivariate Analysis.* New York, John Wiley & Sons, 1971.

49. Turk DC, Rudy TE: Toward an empirically derived taxonomy of chronic pain patients: Integration of psychological assessment data. *J Consult Clin Psychol* 56:233–258, 1988.

50. Turk DC, Rudy TE: The robustness of an empirically derived taxonomy of chronic pain patients. *Pain* 43:27–36, 1990.

51. Keefe FJ, Block AR: Development of an observation method for assessing pain behavior in chronic low back pain patients. *Behav Ther* 13:363–375, 1982.

52. Rosensteil AK, Keefe FJ: The use of cognitive coping strategies in chronic low back pain patients: Relationship to patient characteristics and current adjustment. *Pain* 17:33–44, 1983.

53. Lefebvre MF: Cognitive distortion and cognitive errors in depressed psychiatric and low back pain patients. *J Consult Clin Psychol* 49:517–525, 1981.

54. Black RG: The chronic pain syndrome. *Surg Clin North Am* 55:999–1011, 1975.

55. Flor H, Fydrich T, Turk DC: Efficacy of multidisciplinary pain treatment centers: A meta-analytic review. *Pain* 49:221–230, 1992.

56. Meilman PW, Skultety FM, Guck TP, Sullivan K: Benign chronic pain: 18 month to ten-year follow-up of a multidisciplinary pain unit treatment program. *Clin J Pain* 1:131–137, 1985.

57. Meichenbaum D, Turk DC: *Facilitating Treatment Adherence: A Practitioner's Guidebook.* New York, Plenum Press, 1987.

58. Kanfer FH, Karoly P: The psychology of self-management: Abiding issues and tentative directions. In Karoly P, Kanfer FH (eds): *Self-Management and Behavior Change.* Elmsford, NY, Pergamon Press, 1982.

59. Holzman AD, Turk DC, Kerns RD: The cognitive-behavioral approach in the management of chronic pain. In Holzman AD, Turk DC (eds): *Pain Management: A Handbook of Psychological Treatment Approaches.* Elmsford, NY, Pergamon Press, 1986, p 40.

60. Turk DC, Stieg RL: Chronic pain: the necessity of interdisciplinary communication. *Clin J Pain,* 3:163–167, 1987.

61. Turk DC, Rudy TE, Flor H: Why a family perspective for pain? *Int J Fam Ther* 7:223–234, 1985.

62. Stieg RL, Turk DC: Chronic pain syndrome: The necessity of demonstrating the cost-benefit of treatment. *J Pain Management* 1:56–63, 1988.

63. Beals RK: Compensation and recovery from injury. *West J Med* 140:232–237, 1984.

64. Brena SF, Turk DC: Chronic pain and disability: An overview for legal professionals. *Insurance Counsel J* 54:122–130, 1987.

65. Hanlon R, Turk DC, Rudy TE: A collaborative approach in the treatment of chronic pain patients. *Br J Counsel Guidance* 15:37–49, 1987.

66. Kanfer FH, Goldstein AP (eds): *Helping People Change: A Textbook of Methods.* Elmsford, NY, Pergamon Press, 1986.

67. Marlatt GA, Gordon JR: Determinants of relapse: Implications for the maintenance of behavior change. In Davidson PO, Davidson SM (eds): *Behavioral Medicine: Changing Health Life Styles.* New York, Brunner/Mazel, 1980.

68. Flor H, Turk DC: Etiological theories and treatments for chronic back pain: I. Somatic factors. *Pain* 19:105–121, 1984.

69. Turk DC, Flor H: Etiological theories and treatments for chronic back pain: II. Psychological factors. *Pain* 19:209–233, 1984.

70. Turner JA, Chapman CR: Psychological interventions for chronic pain: A critical review: II. Operant conditioning, hypnosis, and cognitive-behavior therapy. *Pain* 12:23–46, 1982.

SECTION III
PHARMACOLOGIC INTERVENTIONS

CHAPTER 13

ANALGESIC MEDICATIONS
GLEN D. SOLOMON

THIS CHAPTER presents the pharmacologic properties of the opioids and opioid agonist-antagonists, as well as some novel agents used in pain therapy. The term *opioid* is used to describe substances that have morphine-like actions, as well as receptors that combine with such agents. The term *opiates* is confined to the drugs that have been naturally derived from opium—morphine, codeine, and the semisynthetic cogeners of morphine. The term *narcotic*, from the Greek word for stupor, is a pharmacologically obsolete word that at one time referred to any drug that induced sleep, and for years applied to any morphine-like strong analgesic. Today, "narcotic" has become more of a legal term, describing substances that can cause dependence (1, 2).

HISTORY

Knowledge of the effects of opium dates back at least to 4000 BC to the ancient Sumerians, whose ideograph for the poppy (*Papaver somniferum*) was "joy plants." Undisputed reference to the juice of the poppy is found in the third century BC writing of Theophrastus. The word *opium* comes from the Greek word for juice, because the drug is derived from the juice of the poppy capsule. Arabian physicians were expert in the prescription of opium. Arabian traders introduced the drug to the Orient, where it was used primarily to control dysentery. In the early 16th century, Paracelsus repopularized the use of opium in Europe. By the middle of the 16th century, the use of opium for analgesia was well understood in Europe. In 1680, Sydenham wrote, "Among the remedies which it has pleased Almighty God to give to man to relieve his sufferings, none is so universal and so efficacious as opium." Three centuries later, this statement remains valid.

In 1803, the German pharmacist Serturner isolated the opium alkaloid that he named *morphine*, after Morpheus, the Greek god of dreams. It is morphine that gives opium its analgesic activity. In 1838, Robiquet discovered the opium alkaloid codeine. In 1848, Merck discovered the opium alkaloid papaverine. By the middle of the 19th century, pure alkaloids replaced the use of crude opium extracts throughout the medical world.

Recreational use of opium developed in the 18th century when opium smoking became popular in the Orient. In Europe, the problem of "opium eating" (drinking laudanum) existed, but never became as serious or widespread as alcohol abuse. In the United States, the immigration of opium-smoking Chinese laborers, the widespread use of morphine among wounded Civil War veterans, and the unrestricted availability of opium until the early 1900s led to an increasing problem with opiate use.

The concern over opiate addiction stimulated a search to develop potent analgesics free of the potential for addiction. About the time of World War II, synthetic medications such as meperidine and methadone were introduced, but proved to have the same habituation liability as morphine. By the early 1950s, nalorphine was found to antagonize the effects of morphine, and was used as an antidote for morphine poisoning. The finding by Lasagna and Beecher, that nalorphine had analgesic properties, stimulated research that led to the development of new drugs such as naloxone, an antagonist, and mixed agonist-antagonist drugs such as pentazocine, butorphanol, and buprenorphine.

By the late 1960s and early 1970s, several groups discovered both specific receptor binding sites for opioid drugs within the nervous system and families of endogenous opioid peptides (1, 3). It is hoped that these discoveries will ultimately lead to the development of potent analgesics without significant adverse effects or habituation potential.

OPIOID RECEPTORS

To understand the multiplicity of actions of various opioids, it is valuable to review the subtypes of opioid receptors. There are a variety of opioid receptors differing in ligand specificity and location within the nervous system, each mediating different functions (Table 13.1) (4).

Physiologic effects of mu receptor stimulation include

**Table 13.1.
Receptor Subtypes**

Receptor	Agonist	Antagonist	Physiologic Actions	Pharmacologic Effects
Mu_1	Normorphine	Naloxone	Analgesia, Temperature control	
Mu_2	Morphine Sufentanil	Naloxone	Respiratory depression, constipation, growth-hormone release	Miosis, bradycardia, hypothermia, indifference to environment
Delta	Enkephalins		Euphoria, brain reward	
Kappa	Metenkephalin B-endorphin Dynorphin		Stimulation, ataxia, locomotor activity	Miosis, sedation
Epsilon	B-endorphin		Heat-related anti-nociception	
Sigma	Pentazocine Phencyclidine Ketamine	Haloperidol	Psychomimetic effects	Mydriasis, respiratory stimulation, tachycardia, delirium

miosis of the pupils, bradycardia, hypothermia, indifference to environmental stimuli, and a decrease in spinal and supraspinal nociceptive reflexes (5). Agonists for these receptors include morphine, sufentanil, and dihydromorphine; antagonists include naloxone.

Mu receptors are divided into mu_1 and mu_2 receptors. Mu_1 receptors mediate supraspinal analgesia, prolactin release, free feeding and deprivation-induced feeding, acetylcholine turnover in the brain, and temperature control (6). High concentrations of mu_1 receptors are located in the periaqueductal gray and medial thalamus in the brain (6) and in the substantia gelatinosa of the spinal cord (7). The periaqueductal gray and medial thalamus are regions known to play major roles in opioid analgesia.

In animal models, the density of mu_1 receptors correlates well with the sensitivity of the animal to morphine analgesia. Phylogenetically, higher densities of mu_1 receptors are noted in higher species. Ontogenetically, mu_1 receptors appear at a later developmental stage than either mu_2 or delta receptors, and their presence correlates with sensitivity to opioid analgesia (6).

Mu_2 receptors mediate respiratory depression, gastrointestinal transit (constipation), and growth hormone release (4). Additional effects mediated by these receptors may include dopamine turnover in the brain, feeding, and cardiovascular effects (6), including decreased peripheral resistance and inhibition of baroreceptor reflexes (1).

Localization of mu_2 receptors appears to be similar to that of mu_1 receptors. Mu_2 receptors are also found in the nerve plexus of the ileum, where they help mediate gastrointestinal transit time (6), and in the medullary areas believed to be important in ventilatory control (1).

Delta receptors mediate euphoria and brain reward. Enkephalins appear to be the primary agonists for these receptors (4). Delta agonists act antinociceptively at the spinal level against thermal stimuli (7). Additional proposed actions of delta receptors include dopamine turnover in the brain, growth hormone release, and feeding (6).

Kappa receptors mediate stimulation, ataxia, and locomotor activity (4). Spinal kappa receptors mediate antinociception against nonthermal noxious input, such as pressure (7). Additional proposed actions of kappa receptors include inhibition of antidiuretic hormone release and feeding (6). Agonists of the kappa receptor include dynorphin, met-enkephalin, and beta-endorphin. Physiologic effects of kappa stimulation include miosis of the pupils, sedation, and a decrease in spinal nociceptor reflexes (spinal analgesia) (5).

Epsilon receptors are not well defined, but appear to be stimulated by beta-endorphin. The possible role of epsilon receptors is control of heat-related antinociception (7).

Sigma receptors mediate psychomimetic effects including hallucinations, dysphoria, and excitation (4). It is unlikely that sigma receptors have a major role in nociception. Sigma receptor agonists include pentazocine, phencyclidine (PCP), and possibly ketamine. The receptor antagonist is haloperidol (4). Physiologic effects of sigma stimulation include mydriasis of the pupils, respiratory stimulation, tachycardia, delirium, and a slight effect on nociceptive reflexes (5). Many of the drugs that bind to sigma receptors also interact with D_2-dopaminergic receptors. Sigma receptors likely mediate the naloxone-insensitive psychomimetic effects of certain opioids (1).

While biochemical and pharmacologic evidence indicates that mu, delta, and kappa receptors are distinct, certain characteristics are common to these opioid receptors. These receptors function through coupling to guanine nucleotide-binding regulatory proteins (G proteins). Therefore, it is likely that opioids regulate transmembrane signaling systems through regulation of adenylate cyclase, various ion channels, and phospholipases (1). Mu and delta receptor stimulation produces activation of potassium channels and membrane hyperpolarization. Stimulation of these receptors also can inhibit adenylate cyclase in many regions of the brain. Kappa receptors, in contrast, influence calcium channels (1).

Mu, delta, and kappa receptors all function primarily by inhibition of synaptic transmission in both the central nervous system and the myenteric plexus. They are often found on presynaptic nerve terminals, where their activation results in decreased release of excitatory neurotransmitters (1).

ANATOMY OF OPIOID ACTION

To better understand how opioids act, it is worthwhile to briefly review the anatomy of pain sensation. Pain is generally thought of as having two components—a fast, localized sensation carried by myelinated A-delta fibers that respond to mechanical (i.e., sharp) or thermal stimulation, and a slower, more unpleasant and diffuse sensation carried by unmyelinated C-fibers (8).

Nociceptive fibers enter the spinal cord through the dorsal horn, synapse in laminae I, II, and V of the spinal cord, and ascend as the spinothalamic tract. The spinothalamic tract consists of the neospinothalamic and the paleospinothalamic tracts. The neospinothalamic tract ascends to the thalamus, terminates in the ventral posterolateral nucleus, and projects to the somatosensory cortex. The neospinothalamic tract provides information on the quality, intensity, and location of the painful stimulus. The paleospinothalamic tract is polysynaptic, with many interactions with the reticular system and periaqueductal gray. It terminates in the medial, intralaminar, and posterior thalamic nuclei, and then projects diffusely to limbic and subcortical areas. The paleospinothalamic tract, unlike the neospinothalamic tract, is not topographically organized and does not project to the somatotopically organized cerebral cortex (6). Thus, pain impulses carried by the paleospinothalamic tract are perceived as diffuse, whereas pain impulses carried by the neospinothalamic tract are highly localized.

The first component of pain—the sharp, localized sensation—is initiated by mechanothermal nociceptors, transmitted to the spinal cord via myelinated A-delta fibers, and carried by the neospinothalamic tract to the thalamus and cortex. The second component of pain— the prolonged, burning, poorly localized "hurt"—is initiated by C-polymodal nociceptors, transmitted to the spinal cord via unmyelinated C-fibers, and carried by the paleospinothalamic tract to the reticular system, limbus, and subcortex. Because of these projections to reticular and limbic systems, the second component of pain is associated with the arousal and emotional aspects of pain.

The opioid system is organized such that there are a multiplicity of sites where opioids, either endogenous or exogenous/pharmacologic, potentially modify nociception (7).

First, peripheral nerve endings are accessible to opioids in systemic circulation, such as beta-endorphin and proenkephalin A (7). The primary afferent nociceptor is a bipolar neuron with its centrally directed process innervating the central nervous system and its peripherally directed process innervating tissues such as skin and joints. Opioid receptors, synthesized in the cell body of the neuron, are transported not only centrally but peripherally as well. Stimulation of these peripheral opioid receptors may raise the stimulation (pain) threshold of the nociceptor terminal and inhibit the release of pain-producing inflammatory mediators (i.e., substance P) from the peripheral terminals of the primary afferent nociceptors (9).

Second, the dorsal horn of the spinal cord is the primary processing site of the primary afferent nociceptive information. It is rich in dynorphin and enkephalin.

Third, the midbrain, brainstem, and thalamus are relay stations for nociceptive information ascending to the cerebral cortex. These structures are rich in dynorphin and enkephalin, and receive beta-endorphin innervation from the hypothalamus.

Fourth, the limbic system and the cortex produce the emotional dimension of pain, and are very rich in dynorphin and enkephalin neurons and have beta-endorphin input (7).

CLINICAL USE OF OPIOIDS

The clinical utility of the opioid drugs is in three primary areas: analgesic, antitussive, and antidiarrheal. Many opioids are potent suppressors of the cough reflex, usually at doses lower than that required for analgesia (e.g., 15 mg of codeine orally). This effect is mediated by a direct effect on the cough center in the medulla. There is no relationship between depression of respiration and suppression of coughing (1).

The constipating effect of opioids can be used therapeutically in patients after ileostomy or colostomy, in patients with exhausting diarrhea, or in patients with certain dysenteries. These agents should be avoided (or used with great caution) in patients with inflammatory bowel disease or infectious diarrhea because of the risk of toxic megacolon or systemic bacteremia. Care must be used in prescribing these drugs for long-term treatment of diarrhea because of the risk of physical and psychological dependence. As with the antitussive effect, the dose of opioid required to produce constipation is much lower than is needed for analgesia (3).

The primary use of opioids is for analgesia. The next

section will review the specific medications used for opioid analgesia.

DRUGS

PURE AGONIST ANALGESICS

Morphine

Morphine is the prototypical opioid and produces analgesia, drowsiness, changes in mood, and mental clouding. This analgesic effect occurs without loss of consciousness. The analgesia is selective, occurring without loss of touch and vibration sensation. At therapeutic levels, the painful stimulus may still be recognized but it may not be perceived as painful. Continuous dull pain, described above as the second component of pain and transmitted by C-fibers through the paleospinothalamic tract, is better relieved than intermittent sharp pain, although with high enough doses even severe pain is controlled (1).

Morphine and other opioids, except pentazocine, have no ceiling dose (10). *Ceiling dose* is defined as a dose beyond which additional drug provides no further analgesia. Opioids have no ceiling dose because pain is a natural antagonist of the opioid action. The stronger the painful stimulus, the more opioid required to relieve it (10). Opioid analgesia is limited by adverse effects of the medications (e.g., respiratory depression), rather than by the ability to relieve pain. Non-opioid analgesics, such as nonsteroidal anti-inflammatory drugs, have a ceiling dose for analgesia. Once the maximal analgesic effect of a non-steroidal drug is reached, higher doses provide no additional pain relief.

The analgesic effect of 10 mg of morphine intramuscularly is the standard against which other analgesics are compared (Table 13.2). A single oral dose of 60 mg is required to produce the same analgesic effect of 10 mg intramuscularly, because of first-pass metabolism in the liver. With repeated dosing, the bioavailability of oral morphine is about 25% (1), and the oral dose must be three times larger than the parenteral dose (10). Although the oral dosage is higher than the parenteral dosage, the ultimate quantity of drug reaching the opioid receptors in the central nervous system (CNS) will be the same, and have identical analgesic, respiratory depressant, and addictive effects (3).

Morphine can be administered intravenously for cardiac pain, pulmonary edema, postoperative pain, and minor surgical procedures. The usual dose is 2.5–10 mg. The analgesic effect begins immediately and peaks in 20 min. Maximal respiratory depression occurs within 10 min (1). When used in patient-controlled analgesia, a loading dose of 2–10 mg is titrated to provide initial analgesia, with 1 mg bolus doses given on demand, and a lockout interval of about 10 min between doses (2). Morphine can also be administered epidurally and intrathecally for postoperative analgesia or when conventional routes are ineffective.

Morphine is generally not used for spinal administration. Because morphine is hydrophilic, it remains in the cerebrospinal fluid for long periods and may cause respiratory depression up to 18 hours after administration. This problem does not occur with lipid-soluble drugs such as fentanyl, meperidine, or buprenorphine (2).

The half-life of morphine is 2–4 hours, and the drug must be administered at least every 4 hours. Sustained-release oral morphine products are designed to have a long half-life and produce stable plasma levels with 8- or 12-hour dosing. Patients should initially be titrated to analgesia with short-acting morphine, then changed to an equivalent milligram dosage of the sustained-release preparation, divided into two equal doses at 12-hour intervals (10).

Because of its respiratory depressant effects and blunting of the respiratory response to carbon dioxide, morphine and other opioids should not be used, or be used with great caution, in patients with chronic obstructive pulmonary disease, emphysema, kyphoscoliosis, severe obesity, or cor pulmonale (1). Because morphine increases cerebrospinal fluid pressure, patients with suspected CNS disease, especially acute head injury, should not receive opioids (1).

Metabolism of opioids is by the liver, and these agents should be used with caution in patients with hepatic disease. Renal failure can cause accumulation of metabolites, resulting in overdose. With meperidine, the accumulation of its metabolite, normeperidine, may cause tremor and seizures. With propoxyphene, the accumulation of its metabolite, norpropoxyphene, can cause cardiac toxicity (1).

Morphine and related opioids can produce a number

Table 13.2.
Morphine Equivalent Dose of Opioids

Drug	Dose (mg) i.m.	Dose (mg) p.o.	Duration (hours)
Morphine	10	30	4–5
Hydromorphone	1.5	7.5	4–5
Codeine	130	200	4–6
Hydrocodone	—	5–10	4–8
Methadone	10	20	4–5
Levorphanol	2	4	4–5
Oxycodone	15	30	4–5
Oxymorphone	1	6	4–5
Meperidine	75	300	1–3
Pentazocine	60	180	
Nalbuphine	10	—	
Butorphanol	2	—	
Buprenorphine	0.4	0.3 (s.l.)	

of adverse effects including respiratory depression, nausea, vomiting, dizziness, mental clouding, dysphoria, pruritis, constipation, increased biliary tract pressure, urinary retention, and hypotension (1). Patients with reduced blood volume are particularly prone to the hypotensive effects of opioids (1).

Hydromorphone

Hydromorphone is a congener of morphine with rapid onset of action and a duration of action similar to that of morphine. Because of a short half-life of 2–3 hours, there is less drug accumulation in patients with renal or hepatic insufficiency, and in the elderly. The routes of administration include oral, rectal, and parenteral. An intramuscular dose of 1.5 mg, or an oral dose of 7.5 mg, is equipotent to morphine 10 mg intramuscularly (3).

Levorphanol

Levorphanol is pharmacologically similar to morphine, but with a half-life of 12–16 hours and a duration of action of 4–5 hours. Repeated administration at short intervals may lead to drug accumulation in plasma. An intramuscular dose of 2 mg, or an oral dose of 4 mg, is equipotent to morphine 10 mg intramuscularly (1).

Codeine

Codeine is available orally as codeine sulfate and codeine phosphate; it is available for injection as codeine phosphate. When given parenterally, 120 mg of codeine is equipotent to 10 mg of morphine. By injection, codeine has no advantages over morphine. Given orally, it is 60% as effective as when given parenterally. An oral dose of 30 mg of codeine is equianalgesic with aspirin 325–600 mg. When 30 mg of codeine is combined with aspirin or acetaminophen, the analgesic effect sometimes exceeds that of 60 mg of codeine alone (1). There is considerable variability of analgesic response at this dose level. In prescribed doses large enough to provide prolonged analgesia, codeine has limited utility because of its side effects of nausea, vomiting, constipation, and dizziness (3).

Oxycodone

Oxycodone is about as potent as morphine and nearly 10 times more potent than codeine. Like codeine, it is almost half as potent orally as parenterally. It is available in tablets or solution, or in combination with either aspirin or acetaminophen (1). Because of its morphine-like potency, physical dependence on oxycodone is common in chronic nonmalignant pain states (3).

Meperidine

Meperidine is a synthetic opioid with an onset of action within 10 min of intramuscular injection or 15 min of oral administration, peak analgesia within 60 (intramuscular) to 120 (oral) min, and duration of analgesia

of 2 to 5 hours. The short duration of action requires that meperidine be dosed at frequent intervals (2–4 hours), rather than the customary 4–6 hour dosing (1, 3). Equipotent to 10 mg of morphine is meperidine 75–100 mg parenterally or 200–300 mg orally. The high doses required for analgesia, and the concomitant adverse effects, make oral meperidine a poor choice for long-term therapy. In equianalgesic doses, meperidine produces as much sedation, respiratory depression, and euphoria as does morphine. Because it has less smooth muscle effect than morphine, meperidine is often selected for patients with biliary colic or pancreatitis. Meperidine does not inhibit cough.

Meperidine is metabolized to normeperidine, a product with a half-life four times longer than that of meperidine. Accumulation of normeperidine is associated with CNS excitation, myoclonus, tremulousness, and seizures. This is most likely to occur in patients with renal failure and in those with prolonged use of the oral drug at high doses (10).

In patients taking monamine oxidase inhibitors, meperidine may cause a severe reaction characterized by excitation, delirium, hyperpyrexia, convulsions, severe respiratory depression, and death. This drug interaction does not occur with other opioids. When meperidine is given concurrently with phenothiazines, respiratory depression may be increased. Meperidine-induced respiratory depression may also be enhanced by tricyclic antidepressants (1).

Methadone

Methadone is a synthetic opioid with the longest half-life of any opioid—15–57 hours. The important properties of methadone are its effective analgesic efficacy, its activity by the oral route, its extended duration of action in suppressing withdrawal symptoms in physically dependent individuals, and its tendency to show consistent effects with repeated administration (1). Methadone given orally is about half as potent as the parenteral form; 20 mg orally is equivalent to 10 mg intramuscularly and is equianalgesic to morphine 10 mg intramuscularly. Methadone undergoes extensive biotransformation in the liver. The drugs phenytoin and rifampin can accelerate the metabolism of methadone and precipitate withdrawal symptoms (1).

In a single dose, methadone is comparable to morphine in potency and duration of action; after 4 days of regular dosing at fixed intervals the drug provides long periods of analgesia (3). Because of the long half-life, gradual accumulation of the drug can occur for a week or longer when dosing is instituted or the dosage is increased, resulting in serious toxicity (10). The long half-life and oral formulation make methadone one of the opioids of choice in chronic cancer pain. Its use may avoid periodic abstinence effects, and the prolonged analgesia reduces the anticipation of pain commonly observed with short-duration analgesics (10).

Although the abuse potential of methadone is comparable to that of morphine, withdrawal from methadone develops more slowly and is more prolonged and less intense (1). The abstinence syndrome causes no symptoms until 24–28 hours after the last dose of methadone. At high doses, methadone blocks heroin-induced euphoria. It is frequently used for the treatment of heroin withdrawal.

Propoxyphene

Propoxyphene is a sterioisomer of methadone with limited analgesic potency. It is available only for oral use as capsules and tablets, in combination with aspirin or acetaminophen, or as a suspension.

As an analgesic, propoxyphene is one-half to two-thirds as potent as oral codeine. Ninety to 120 mg of propoxyphene is equianalgesic to 60 mg of codeine or 600 mg of aspirin. Combinations of propoxyphene with aspirin or acetaminophen provide higher levels of analgesia than either agent used alone (1).

The abuse liability of propoxyphene is approximately the same as with codeine (1), with an abstinence syndrome caused by abrupt withdrawal that is generally mild. As with oral codeine preparations, toxicity at high doses may be from the aspirin or acetaminophen used in combination (3).

Fentanyl

Fentanyl is a synthetic opioid that is 80 times as potent an analgesic as morphine. The respiratory depressant effects are of shorter duration than is the case with meperidine. For these reasons, it is primarily used for anesthesia, but it can be used for postoperative analgesia. Fentanyl is often used in combination with the neuroleptic agent droperidol for use as an intravenous anesthetic. Cogeners of fentanyl such as sufentanil citrate and alfentanil hydrochloride are also potent analgesics and can be administered intrathecally, epidurally, and for postoperative analgesia (1).

Fentanyl is also available by a transdermal delivery system for the management of chronic (cancer) pain. The transdermal system delivers fentanyl over a 72-hour period. After application of the patch, stable drug levels occur after 12–24 hours. Peak serum levels occur between 24 and 72 hours. After removal of the patch, serum drug levels fall by 50% over 17 hours because of continued absorption of fentanyl from the skin. Fentanyl transdermal is available in doses ranging from 25 µg/hour to 100 µg/hour. The 25-µg/hour dose is the starting dose for patients who are not opioid-tolerant, and is equivalent to 8–22 mg of intramuscular morphine per day (or 45–134 mg/day oral morphine). The initial dose may be increased after 3 days, but subsequent doses may take up to 6 days to reach equilibrium. Titration should be based on the dose of supplementary opioids, using the ratio of 90 mg/24 hours of oral morphine to a 25 µg/hour increase in transdermal fentanyl.

AGONIST-ANTAGONIST ANALGESICS

The term *agonist-antagonist* has been used generally to describe drugs acting as partial agonists at opioid receptors. An agonist-antagonist binds to the receptor and exerts limited activity (*partial agonist*) or binds to the receptor to prevent the activation by agonist drugs (*competitive antagonists*) (1). Partial agonists have low intrinsic activity, so that there is a ceiling effect at less than the maximal effect produced by a full agonist (11). The term agonist-antagonist also refers to drugs that behave as agonists, partial agonists, or antagonists at different opioid receptors.

These agents were developed in the hope of maintaining effective analgesia without the adverse effects of physical dependence and respiratory depression. The differences between these drugs and the pure agonist opioids have been few, and they have not constituted a major clinical advance in analgesia (11).

Buprenorphine

Buprenorphine is a semisynthetic derivative of thebaine that binds strongly to the mu receptor. It is 25–50 times more potent than morphine. Like morphine, its onset of action is within 15–60 min, but its duration of action averages over 8 hours (12).

Buprenorphine is unique among agonist-antagonists in that it is available for sublingual administration. A 0.4-mg sublingual dose is equianalgesic to 0.2–0.3 mg intramuscularly, with an onset of action within 5 min after injection or 30–120 min after sublingual dosage, and a duration of analgesia of 6–9 hours. This dose is equipotent to morphine 10 mg intramuscularly (11). Oral buprenorphine is a poor analgesic because of extensive presystemic elimination (11).

Buprenorphine has minimal effects on the cardiovascular system. Respiratory depression occurs after 3 hours and lasts for 7 hours after a single dose. The respiratory depression is only partially reversible with naloxone (3). It can induce abstinence syndromes in patients dependent on opioids. It is classified as a drug with low abuse potential because withdrawal signs and symptoms are generally mild and are delayed from 2 days to 2 weeks after discontinuation (1).

The usual dose of buprenorphine is 0.3 mg every 6–8 hours intramuscularly. The primary side effects include sedation, diaphoresis, nausea, constipation, and respiratory depression (3).

Pentazocine

Pentazocine has both weak agonist and weak antagonist activity. A 30–60 mg intramuscular or subcutaneous dose is equianalgesic to morphine 10 mg, with a slightly shorter overall duration of action (11). Given orally, it has relatively weak and unpredictable analgesic activity. In acute myocardial infarction, pentazocine can cause increased left ventricular end diastolic pressure and increased pulmonary artery pressure, and therefore should be avoided (11).

Tolerance and dependence have been reported with pentazocine, but less commonly than with other opioids. Adverse effects include sedation, diaphoresis, and lightheadedness. When high doses are used long-term, hallucinations, euphoria, and depersonalization can occur in up to 20% of people (11).

Nalbuphine

Nalbuphine is an agonist-antagonist structurally related to naloxone. It is equipotent to morphine, but respiratory depression appears to plateau at a 10-mg dose. In single doses, a ceiling effect for analgesia is seen at 20–30 mg. Duration of analgesia is 3–5 hours, with peak effect between 30 and 60 min. The most frequent adverse effect is drowsiness; other adverse effects are similar to those of morphine. Amnesia has been reported in up to 50% of patients receiving nalbuphine postoperatively, even when they were experiencing pain (11).

Butorphanol

Butorphanol is structurally similar to pentazocine and is three to seven times as potent as morphine. Peak effects are seen in 30 min with a duration of analgesic activity of up to 4 hours. The usual dose is 2–4 mg every 3–4 hours. The severity of respiratory depression is not dose-related, with a ceiling effect at 1–2 mg, although the duration of respiratory depression is dose-dependent (11). The major adverse effect with butorphanol is a psychomimetic effect that correlates with the cumulative dose given.

Dezocine

Dezocine has a potency and duration of activity similar to morphine. Increased doses of dezocine are not associated with increasing respiratory depression. Adverse effects are similar to other opioids, but psychomimetic effects and nausea are less common (1, 11).

Maptazinol

Maptazinol is unique for being a specific mu_1 agonist with central anticholinergic activity. It is one-tenth as potent as morphine, with a duration of action of 4 hours. It is a less effective analgesic than morphine with a much higher incidence of adverse effects. It causes less respiratory depression and constipation than morphine, however (11).

GUIDELINES FOR OPIOID DRUG SELECTION

Reasonable guidelines for the selection of opioid drugs in chronic pain management were developed by Portnoy (3, 10). Although these suggestions were designed for patients with cancer pain, the basic concepts are valuable for all chronic uncontrollable pain.

1. *Choose an appropriate drug.*

   The selection of an opioid should be based on analgesic efficacy, additional benefits (e.g., antitussive effects of morphine compared with meperidine), dose-related toxicity (e.g., seizures from meperidine, psychomimetic effects from butorphanol), frequency of adverse effects at appropriate doses, potential toxicities of acetaminophen or aspirin containing combination drugs, or prescribing experience.

   Agonist-antagonist drugs must be initiated as first-line agents, if they are to be used, because they can induce abstinence syndromes in patients physically dependent on opioids. The lack of oral formulations of the agonist-antagonists (except buprenorphine) limit their utility as first-line agents.

   Meperidine is limited by its short duration of analgesia and the accumulation of the long half-life metabolite normeperidine. Normeperidine accumulation can lead to seizures and excitation.

   There is only a loose relationship between plasma half-life and duration of analgesic effect after a given dose. Morphine and hydromorphone should be administered at least every 4 hours, meperidine at least every 3 hours, and methadone every 6 hours. The sustained-release oral morphine formulations can be given every 8–12 hours.

2. *Start with the lowest dose that produces analgesia.*

   A reasonable starting dose for a patient with severe pain is 5–10 mg morphine intramuscularly or its equivalent. Patients who are switched to an alternative opioid after prolonged exposure to an opioid should be started at one-half to two-thirds of the equianalgesic dose of the new medication. Elderly patients, or those with hepatic or renal insufficiency, should be started at lower doses.

3. *Titrate the dose to the relief of pain or to the appearance of intolerable or unmanageable adverse effects.*

   A reasonable approach to dose titration involves the concurrent administration of fixed dosages at a set schedule (usually every 4 hours) and a rescue dose, every 2 hours as needed, for breakthrough pain control. This will guide the need for upward titration of the fixed dose. The rescue drug should be the same as the fixed-dose agent, except when the fixed-dose agent has a prolonged half-life and potential for accumulation (i.e., methadone or levorphanol).

4. *Use as-needed dosing selectively.*

   Routine administration of opioids to chronic pain patients should be on a fixed basis.

5. *Use an appropriate route of administration.*

   The oral route is preferred, when feasible.

6. *Be aware of equianalgesic doses.*

7. *Use a combination of opioid and non-opioid analgesics.*

   The addition of a nonsteriodal anti-inflammatory drug to an opioid may dramatically improve analgesia without significantly increasing adverse effects.

8. *Anticipate and manage side effects.*

   Constipation is so common with chronic opioid use that concurrent treatment should be prescribed for most patients. Nausea can be managed with the addition of an antiemetic. Respiratory depression is rarely a problem because of rapid development of tolerance.

9. *Be aware of tolerance.*

Tolerance usually begins as a reduction in the duration of analgesia after a dose. There is no limit to tolerance, and doses can become enormous in an effort to maintain analgesia.

10. *Understand the distinction between physical and psychological dependence.*

Psychological dependence in a patient with no prior history of substance abuse, who is administered opioid analgesics for the management of intractable pain, is extremely rare.

Although these guidelines are appropriate for patients with cancer pain, or for the short-term management of acute pain states, it is important to note that chronic opioid therapy is inappropriate for patients with chronic, nonmalignant pain. In addition to the concerns of tolerance and physical dependence with prolonged opioid use, opioids will worsen the depression that is typical of patients with chronic nonmalignant pain (13). These chronic pain states are better managed with physical modalities, psychotherapy, antidepressants, and nonsteroidal anti-inflammatory drugs.

NON-OPIOID ANALGESICS

In addition to the opioids and their receptors, various neuropeptides play key roles in pain transmission and the inflammatory response. Modulating the effects of these neuropeptides offers an additional approach to the management of specific pain syndromes.

PROSTAGLANDINS AND NONSTEROIDAL ANTI-INFLAMMATORY DRUGS

Nonsteroidal anti-inflammatory drugs act both centrally and peripherally to induce analgesia and reduce inflammation. This group of drugs constitutes the major non-opioid analgesics used in clinical practice. They will be reviewed in detail in the next chapter.

SUBSTANCE P AND CAPSAICIN

Substance P is a neuropeptide that acts as a potent vasodilator and a powerful spasmogenic agent on nonvascular smooth muscle, triggering the inflammatory process in local tissue (14). It is synthesized in the cell bodies of nociceptive neurons located in the dorsal root ganglia. Substance P is distributed throughout the neuron by axonal transport, and is distributed to skin, joints, and the spinal cord. It is stored in terminal nociceptive endings of type-C nerve fibers. Substance P is released at the central end of the primary nociceptive fibers in response to noxious stimuli, acting as the neurotransmitter to stimulate the secondary neuron of the spinothalamic tract to transmit the pain signal to the brain.

Substance P functions to mediate pain both at the local tissue level and as a neurotransmitter for the pain signal within the CNS. On the local level, substance P is released from distal nerve terminals of nociceptive neurons when activated by painful stimuli. Substance P causes the degranulation of mast cells, with the subsequent release of histamine, vasodilation, and exudation of fluids into the tissues, resulting in inflammation, swelling, and pain. Substance P is also released from proximal nerve terminals of the nociceptive neurons (C-fibers) to activate the spinothalamic tract for transmission of the pain impulse to the CNS.

Capsaicin is a white crystalline material found in minute quantities in red pepper, and is what imparts the pungency to chili and other foods made from hot peppers. When topically applied to peripheral type-C nociceptive nerve fibers, capsaicin induces the initial release of substance P with an excitatory effect. After the initial excitatory effect, substance P is subsequently depleted from the nerve ending and the neuronal membrane is desensitized to noxious stimuli. Capsaicin depletes substance P throughout the length of the neuron, providing both local and central analgesic effects. Because its effect is limited to type-C nociceptive fibers, capsaicin does not alter sensory modalities other than pain.

Capsaicin has been shown to be effective for pain reduction in several pain syndromes including osteoarthritis (15), rheumatoid arthritis (15), diabetic neuropathy (16), post-herpetic neuralgia (17), trigeminal neuralgia (18), and cluster headache (19). It is available as a topical cream containing 0.025% or 0.075% capsaicin. For arthritis and neuralgia, capsaicin is applied topically to the affected area, three to four times daily. For cluster headache, it is applied intranasally to the affected side, once daily.

SEROTONIN AND L-TRYPTOPHAN

Serotonin (5-HT) is a neurotransmitter that plays a role in the endogenous modulation of pain. Decreased central serotonergic function causes increased sensitivity and reactivity to noxious stimuli and partial failure of the analgesic effects of opioids (20). Decreased serotonergic function plays a role in the pathogenesis of depression, and the effects of serotonin on opioid analgesia may explain the increased pain complaints (and decreased efficacy of analgesic medications) in patients with depression. Conversely, increased serotonergic neurotransmission is associated with both analgesia and normalization of the pain threshold.

Pain seems to increase the turnover of serotonin. The cerebral synthesis of serotonin requires the passage of the amino acid tryptophan (unbound to protein) through the blood-brain barrier by carrier-mediated active transport. Increased free-plasma tryptophan is essential to augment central serotonin synthesis.

Intravenous L-tryptophan, 7.5 and 15 mg/kg, has been shown to be effective in the treatment of postoperative (cholecystectomy) pain. Oral L-tryptophan has given good results in patients suffering from deafferentation pain, and oral 5-hydroxytryptophan has benefited patients with acute migraine headache (20). Oral L-tryptophan is no longer available in the United States because of an outbreak of eosinophilic myalgia syndrome attributed to a contaminant produced in the manufacture of the product. The serotonin receptor agonist sumatriptan is effective in treating acute migraine, although it has not been shown to have intrinsic analgesic properties. Antidepressant drugs probably exert their analgesic effects through the modulation of central serotonin (see Chapter 20).

GABA and the GABA-Agonist THIP

Gamma amino butyric acid (GABA) is the major inhibitory neurotransmitter in the central nervous system. Inhibitory neurotransmitters, such as GABA, are thought to have a role in analgesia. THIP (4, 5, 6, 7-tetrahydroisoxazole [5, 4c] pyridine-3-ol) is an analog of the GABA-mimetic drug muscimol. THIP was shown to be an effective analgesic in patients with chronic pain, although side effects of dizziness, sedation, and nausea were commonly observed (21).

Anticonvulsants

Valproic acid (sodium valproate) is an anticonvulsant that is a GABA agonist (1). Valproic acid easily crosses the blood-brain barrier and increases the GABA concentration in various areas of the CNS, including the hypothalamus (22). It has been shown to be effective in the prophylaxis of migraine (22), cluster (23), and chronic daily, or mixed (24), headache syndromes.

Other anticonvulsants, such as carbemazepine and phenytoin, have been used in specific pain states such as trigeminal neuralgia. These drugs are not analgesics, nor do they possess anti-inflammatory properties. These drugs are thought to work by reducing or inhibiting synaptic transmission, interrupting the temporal summation of afferent impulses that set off a painful neuralgia attack (25). Carbemazepine is the treatment of choice in trigeminal neuralgia, and is useful in other neuropathic types of pain, such as glossopharyngeal neuralgia, intercostal neuralgia, herpetic and postherpetic neuralgia, phantom limb states, and central pain states. Pain is frequently controlled at dosages lower than those used for seizure control. The addition of a low dose of a tricyclic antidepressant along with carbemazapine may improve the analgesic effect (26).

CONCLUSIONS

Sir William Osler referred to morphine as "God's own medicine." For patients with severe acute pain or chronic cancer pain, morphine and morphine-like drugs remain the primary hope of respite from suffering.

With every advance in opioid receptor biology and neurotransmitter pharmacology, we move closer to the development of analgesics without the adverse effects and dependency risks of our present drugs. For those who suffer in pain, these advances cannot come quickly enough.

References

1. Jaffe JH, Martin WR: Opioid analgesics and antagonists. In Gilman AG, Rall TW, Nies AS, Taylor P (eds): *Goodman and Gilman's The Pharmacologic Basis of Therapeutics*, ed 8. New York, Pergamon Press, 1990, pp 485–521.

2. Schug SA, Merry AF, Acland RH: Treatment principles for the use of opioids in pain of nonmalignant origin. *Drugs* 42:228–239, 1991.

3. Solomon GD: Analgesic and anti-inflammatory medication. In Tollison CD, Satterthwaite JR (eds): *Painful Cervical Trauma*. Baltimore, Williams & Wilkins, 1992, pp 168–183.

4. Brown RM, Clouet DH, Friedman DP (eds): *Opiate Receptor Subtypes and Brain Function*. NIDA Research Monograph Series. Rockville, MD, NIDA, 1986.

5. Offermeier J, Van Rooyen JM: Opioid drugs and their receptors. *S Afr Med J* 66:299–305, 1984.

6. Pasternak GW: Multiple morphine and enkephalin receptors and their relief of pain. *JAMA* 259:1362–1367, 1988.

7. Milan MJ: Multiple opioid systems and pain. *Pain* 27:303–347, 1986.

8. Fields HL: *Pain* New York, McGraw-Hill, 1987, pp 20–22.

9. Edmeads J: Bringing treatment to a head. *Headache* 31:695, 1991.

10. Portnoy RK: Practical aspects of pain control in the patient with cancer. *CA* 38:327–352, 1988.

11. Hoskin PJ, Hanks GW: Opioid agonist-antagonist drugs in acute and chronic pain states. *Drugs* 41:326–344, 1991.

12. Halpern LM: Analgesic and anti-inflammatory medications. In Tollison CD (ed): *Handbook of Chronic Pain Management*. Baltimore, Williams & Wilkins, 1989, pp 54–68.

13. Gildenberg PL, De Vaul RA: *The Chronic Pain Patient*. Basel, Karger, 1985, p 97.

14. McGregor GP, Bloom SR: Radioimmunoassay of substance P and its stability in tissue. *Life Sci* 32:655–662, 1984.

15. Deal CL, Schnitzer TJ, Lipstein E, Seibold JR, Stevens RM, Levy MD, Albert D, Renold F: Treatment of arthritis with topical capsaicin: A double-blind trial. *Clin Ther* 13:383–395, 1991.

16. Ross DR, Varipapa RJ: Treatment of painful diabetic neuropathy with topical capsaicin. *N Engl J Med* 321:474–475, 1989.

17. Bernstein JE, Bickers DR, Dahl MV, Roshal JY: Treatment of chronic postherpetic neuralgia with topical capsaicin. *J Am Acad Dermatol* 17:93–96, 1987.

18. Fusco BM, Geppetti P, Fanciullacci M, Sicuteri F: Local application of capsaicin for the treatment of cluster headache and idiopathic trigeminal neuralgia. *Cephalalgia* 11(Suppl 11):234–235, 1991.

19. Sicuteri F, Fanciullacci M, Nicolodi M, Geppetti P, Fusco BM, Marabini S, Alessandri M, Campagnolo V: Substance

P theory: A unique focus on the painful and painless phenomena of cluster headache. *Headache* 30:69–79, 1990.

20. Ceccherelli F, Diani MM, Altafini L, Varotto E, Stefecius A, Casale R, Costola A, Gitron GP: Postoperative pain treated by intravenous L-tryptophan. *Pain* 47:163–172, 1991.

21. Jensen LK, Egsmose C, Lund B, Halskov O: Evaluation of the effect of the GABA-agonist THIP in the treatment of chronic pain. *Clin J Pain* 4:51–54, 1988.

22. Hering R, Kuritzky A: Sodium valproate in the prophylactic treatment of migraine: A double-blind study versus placebo. *Cephalalgia* 12:81–84, 1992.

23. Hering R, Kuritzky A: Sodium valproate in the treatment of cluster headache: An open clinical study. *Cephalalgia* 9:195–198, 1989.

24. Mathew NT, Ali S: Valproate in the treatment of persistent chronic daily headache. An open label study. *Headache* 31:71–74, 1991.

25. Dalessio DJ: The major neuralgias, postinfectious neuritis, and atypical facial pain. In Dalessio DJ (ed): *Wolff's Headache*. New York, Oxford University Press, 1987, pp 266–288.

26. Browne TR, Empting L, Lydiard RB, Yerby MS: New uses and old for carbamazepine. *Patient Care* 24:48–81, 1990.

CHAPTER 14

NONSTEROIDAL ANTI-INFLAMMATORY DRUGS

STEPHEN M. HONIG

LANGUAGE IS a powerful tool in the representation of images. In the medical literature, simple words or phrases often dramatically and economically focus the attention of the reader. An example is the now familiar acronym *NSAIDs*, which immediately conjures to mind a group of drugs used in the treatment of a variety of inflammatory disorders, most notably the generic "arthritis." By tradition, nonsteroidal anti-inflammatory drugs (NSAIDs) include both salicylate and nonsalicylated moieties, agents whose clinical utility results from both their anti-inflammatory and analgesic properties, the latter being the focus of this chapter. Historically, the analgesia provided by acetylsalicylic acid (aspirin—first synthesized by Hoffman in 1899), arguably the world's most popular drug, was appreciated almost 50 years before its anti-inflammatory properties were first recognized. The subsequent development of nonsteroidal drugs resulted primarily from a desire to provide physicians and patients with non-aspirin alternatives. Phenylbutazone, the first nonsalicylate NSAID, was introduced in 1949, but its use has been limited by its significant toxicity profile (1). The introduction of indomethacin in 1963 and ibuprofen nearly a decade later marked the beginning of the NSAID era, an era that continues with the marketing of an ever-increasing number of nonsteroidal drugs. The recent observation that indomethacin is useful as a non-narcotic analgesic replicates (in complementary fashion) the aspirin experience of the early to middle 20th century (2, 3). A derivative benefit of the clinical recognition of the analgesic properties of NSAIDs has been the search for the basic mechanism(s) that can explain these effects. A fuller understanding of the mechanisms and events involved in pain production and nociception should aid this effort (4).

The confluence of several important forces has resulted in numerous clinical trials testing the efficacy of one or another NSAID in the treatment of a variety of "pain models." Among the most important of these factors are an increasing understanding of the events involved in pain production and the putative pain pathway, an expanding body of knowledge regarding the mechanisms of actions and sites of activities of nonsteroidal drugs, and the clinical recognition that many patients would benefit from the use of more effective nonnarcotic analgesics as alternatives to opioid compounds.

MECHANISMS OF PAIN PRODUCTION AND THE PAIN PATHWAY

Pain can be defined as the perception of an uncomfortable or disquieting sensation. This perception may or may not be associated with measurable tissue damage. *Nociception* is a term that defines the actual sensation resulting from the activation of specific nerve pathways as a consequence of this tissue damage (5). Current theoretical paradigms suggest that activation of the pain pathway begins with depolarization of specialized receptors (nociceptors) that occurs with tissue injury or inflammation. These specialized receptors are classified by their ability to respond to specific mechanical, thermal, and/or chemical stimuli. The nociceptors have either myelinated axons and respond to mechanical and/or thermal stimuli or unmyelinated axons (polymodal nociceptors) capable of responding to all three types of stimuli (6). Activation of these axons results in the transmission of "pain" from the periphery (site of injury) to the dorsal root ganglion adjacent to the spinal cord and from this site into the dorsal gray matter of the cord itself. During tissue injury, a variety of chemical mediators capable of activating the polymodal nociceptors (electrical depolarization) are released locally at the site of tissue damage. Among these mediators are products of arachidonic acid metabolism, including prosta-

Figure 14.1. Nociceptor and its microenvironment. A, Action poentials of a muscle nociceptor recorded in an animal experiment following administration of bradykinin (upper) or prostaglandin E$_2$ and bradykinin. B, Histologically, the nociceptor is seen as the arbor of free nerve terminals of afferent A-delta and C-fibers. This sensory nerve ending may respond to high-intensity physical stimuli. Endogenous analgesic chemical substances sensitize or excite the nociceptor, affect the local microcirculation, and increase vascular permeability. Substance P, a neuropeptide synthesized in the dorsal root ganglion neurons, is released from the nerve ending and results in mast cell degranulation and neurogenic inflammation. Acetylsalicylic acid and related drugs interfere with the synthesis of prostaglandins and the excitation of the nociceptor. Opioids also can inhibit excitation of nociceptors and release of substance P. (From Zimmerman M: Pain mechanisms and mediators in osteoarthritis. *Semin Arthritis Rheum* 18:24, 1989.)

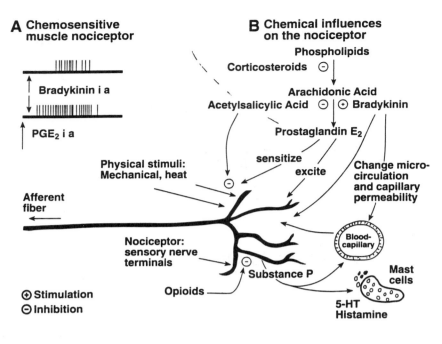

glandins (cyclo-oxygenase dependent) and leukotrienes (lipoxygenase dependent). Prostaglandin E$_2$ (PGE$_2$) sensitizes the polymodal nociceptors, presumably making them more responsive to bradykinin, another compound released locally during tissue injury. Acetylsalicylic acid and the other NSAIDs inhibit the activity of the cyclo-oxygenase enzyme, an effect originally described by Vane over 20 years ago (7). It was this observation that led to the hypothesis that NSAIDs exert their analgesic and anti-inflammatory effects through their inhibition of cyclo-oxygenase at the site of tissue injury. Although this hypothesis is still, in part, felt to be true, recent observations suggest that NSAIDs have other effects independent of cyclo-oxygenase inhibition (8–11). Another chemical mediator thought to be important in the pain pathway is the 11-amino-acid substance P. This neuropeptide is synthesized in the dorsal root ganglion and has effects both at the site of tissue injury and in the spinal cord. At the periphery, it causes mast cell degranulation and contributes to neurogenic inflammation, whereas in the spinal cord, it serves to facilitate activation of spinal interneurons. Figure 14.1 depicts, in schematic fashion, both stimulatory and inhibitory influences on the pain pathway at the receptor level. In the spinal cord, the pain pathway is influenced by a number of neurotransmitters including those released as a result of activation of descending supraspinal pathways. Whether or not a sensory event will be perceived as pain depends on the intensity of the stimulus, the endogenous pain control systems of the brain and spinal cord, and the affective state of the individual under study. Previous chapters in this volume, detailing the anatomy, taxonomy, and classification of pain, are recommended to the reader interested in additional information on pain mechanisms.

NSAIDS, INFLAMMATION, AND ANALGESIA

Since Vane's observations relating the ability of NSAIDs to inhibit prostaglandin production, this "unifying hypothesis" has been held as the explanation for the anti-inflammatory and analgesic properties of this class of drugs. When a tissue is "injured," the cell membrane produces arachidonic acid, de novo, from phospholipid precursors. As noted above, arachidonic acid is a substrate for two major enzyme pathways: cyclo-oxygenase and lipoxygenase. Most NSAIDs inhibit the transformation of arachidonic acid to the stable prostaglandins, and some drugs of this class also interfere with lipoxygenase activity (12). Prostaglandin E$_2$ has been thought only to sensitize and not directly stimulate the nociceptor (Fig. 14.2), a conclusion based on the study of Ferreira 20 years ago (13). More recent work using the rat paw-withdrawal test concluded that both PGE$_2$ and prostaglandin I$_2$ (PGI$_2$) are the main hyperalgesic metabolites of the cyclo-oxygenase pathway of arachidonic acid (14). NSAIDs have been demonstrated to inhibit the production of prostaglandins both in vitro and in vivo. In chronic inflammatory states, NSAIDS (bound to albumin) accumulate in chronically inflamed tissue. The ability of an NSAID to inhibit the microsomal prostaglandin endoperoxide synthetase enzyme system depends in part on the intracellular accumulation of the drug (15). The clinically useful and anti-inflammatory

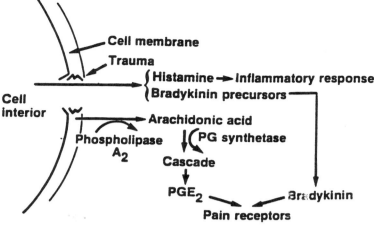

Figure 14.2. **Proposed peripheral mechanism of pain.**

NSAIDs are weak organic acids, a feature of these agents thought to be important in their ability to accumulate intracellularly. The intracellular region is relatively more alkaline than the acidic extracellular space of chronically inflamed tissue, a situation that favors ion trapping of the NSAID inside cells of inflamed tissue (16). Increased concentration of NSAIDs in chronically inflamed tissue favors maximal inhibition of local prostaglandin production, clearly a desirable pharmacodynamic effect. It has become clear, however, that NSAIDs have other, non–prostaglandin-dependent effects that result in a modification of a variety of cellular and inflammatory processes. NSAIDs can intercalate into the lipid bilayer of the plasma membrane of cells and interfere with several nonprostaglandin cell membrane processes including oxidative phosphorylation in mitochondria and the reduced form of nicotinamide-adenine dinucleotide phosphate (NADPH) oxidase (neutrophil) and phospholipase C (macrophage) enzyme activities (8). Inhibition of neutrophil activation and aggregation (11) and suppression of cytokine release from activated monocytes have been reported with several different NSAIDs (10, 17). Whether these effects can help explain clinical differences among drugs of this class remains to be determined.

In addition to the actions of the nonsteroidal drugs at the "periphery," the site(s) of actual tissue injury, there have been a number of studies reporting on the effects of these agents on the central nervous system (CNS). Measurable cerebrospinal fluid levels of oxyphenabutazone have been reported even after short-term use (18). McCormack and Brune have advanced the hypothesis that there is a dissociation between the antinociceptive and anti-inflammatory effects of NSAIDs (19). These authors, however, have not identified the site(s) of such antinociceptive activity, but furthering the work of Gropetti et al. (in the rat model) (20) speculate that NSAIDs may influence serotoninergic and/or dopaminergic mechanisms involved in nociception at the level of the brain. Intrathecal injections of PGE_2 produce dose-

dependent hyperalgesia in rats; a suggested mechanism is the blocking of endogenous opioid mediated activation of the bulbospinal noradrenergic analgesic pathway (21). There is some evidence, based on a mouse ear-inflammation model, that salicylates can act within the brain to inhibit acute inflammation at the periphery in a manner analogous to alpha-melanocyte–stimulating hormone. This effect is non–PG-dependent and not shared by centrally administered indomethacin or dexamethasone (22). The significance of this observation, potentially very important, awaits elucidation. For the present, however, it is reasonable to speculate that NSAIDs will continue to demonstrate effects on a variety of effector cells, enzymes, and neurotransmitters involved in inflammation and pain production. Such knowledge may allow us to better define the analgesic potential of individual agents, but the myriad animal and test models used in the study of basic mechanisms involved in pain production make it unlikely that clinically relevant information will be available in the immediate future.

NSAIDS AS ANALGESICS

An increasing number of NSAIDS are available to the clinician, but there is a paucity of good comparative efficacy data to help distinguish among agents in this class of drugs. Selecting the most efficacious NSAID for an individual often is an exercise in trial and error. NSAIDs have been suggested for most acute and chronic painful conditions. Efficacy determinations are often based on the results of single-dose postoperative pain and post third-molar extraction dental models. Unfortunately, the results of such single-dose studies may not be relevant or reproducible in multiple dose models (22), clouding a clear interpretation of their clinical significance.

The analgesic response to NSAIDs is marked by a ceiling effect, beyond which dosage increments yield no additional analgesia (5). Based on overall data and clinical experience, however, it is reasonable to recommend a trial of an NSAID analgesic for most acute and chronic pain states. Experimental studies confirm the utility of drugs of this class in numerous pain models, selected examples of which include postoperative pain (24), malignancy-related bone pain (25), orthopedic pain (26), post-thoracotomy pain (27), dental pain (28, 29), as intraoperative adjuvants to anesthetic agents (30), headache syndromes (31), dysmenorrhea (32, 33), and diabetic neuropathy (34).

ADVERSE EFFECTS

Prostaglandin inhibition is also responsible for some of the more common adverse effects of these drugs, particularly those involving the gastrointestinal (GI) tract, platelets, and kidney. All NSAIDs can irritate the gastrointestinal tract, leading to gastritis, bleeding, and frank ulceration of the stomach and duodenum. These drugs inhibit gastric mucus and bicarbonate secretion, leading to a reduction in the effectiveness of the gastric mucosal barrier (35). The lower GI tract is less commonly affected, but patients with inflammatory bowel disease may be at risk for NSAID-induced activation of their underlying bowel disorder (36); therefore these agents should be used with caution in patients with ulcerative colitis or Crohn's disease. Use of the synthetic analogue of prostaglandin E_1 (PGE_1), misoprostol, offers some protection against gastric mucosal injury (37), but its additional cost makes long-term concomitant use of this compound and an NSAID economically difficult for many patients.

NSAIDs inhibit platelet aggregation and prolong the bleeding time, an effect that may be important to patients requiring surgery (38). The acetyl group of aspirin irreversibly binds to platelet cyclo-oxygenase, rendering the platelet ineffective (for clotting) for its entire 7–12 day life span. The nonacetylated salicylates do not share this property. The other nonsalicylate NSAIDs reversibly inhibit platelet cyclo-oxygenase, which results in platelets retaining their capacity to generate thromboxane, a potent platelet-aggregating substance. Clinically, this means that once a patient stops using a particular NSAID and the drug has been cleared from the patient's sera (about five half-lives), the patient's platelets can be expected to clot normally (39).

In the kidney, prostaglandins, which are produced near the juxtaglomerular apparatus and the tubular mucosa, are important to renal hemodynamics and kidney handling of salt and water (40).

NSAIDs can cause acute renal failure, an event more common in the elderly and in those with hypovolemic states. Interstitial nephritis, papillary necrosis, chronic renal failure, and hyperkalemia have all been attributed to the use of NSAIDs (41). Concurrent administration of a diuretic with an NSAID increases the likelihood of renal toxicity, particularly acute renal failure (42).

Less common adverse reactions include hepatotoxicity, hypertension, and several CNS syndromes, including aseptic meningitis (particularly in patients with systemic lupus erythematosus) (43).

Relative toxicity data for NSAIDs has been reported in several studies. Patients with rheumatoid arthritis who chronically used a number of different NSAIDs were studied by a computer model that found that indomethacin had the highest toxicity scores and ibuprofen and coated or buffered aspirin the lowest (44). Elderly patients, particularly those requiring other medications, seem at greatest risk for an adverse reaction (45).

It is imperative that physicians monitor patients who require intermediate or chronic use of an NSAID. This monitoring should include periodic renal and liver function tests, hemograms, and urinalysis. Particular attention is needed for older patients and those patients dependent on other drugs for other medical problems. This latter situation predisposes the patient to possible problems from drug interactions.

INTERACTIONS WITH OTHER DRUGS

Interactions between NSAIDs and aspirin and other drugs are being recognized with increasing frequency. Largely a product of an expanding pharmacopeia and an aging population afflicted with multiple clinical problems, drug interactions are a clinical area requiring physician attention. The incidence of peripheral osteoarthritis and cervical/lumbar spondylosis increases with aging, creating circumstances favoring the prescribing of NSAIDS. Unfortunately other chronic diseases requiring medical treatment also increase with aging. The introduction to the market of new agents for many acute and chronic diseases and conditions virtually assures clinicians that drug interactions involving NSAIDs will be an increasingly frequent phenomenon. Many of these interactions result from NSAIDs causing the displacement of other agents from albumin, increasing the free level of the drug, or interfering with renal excretion of either or both drugs. Table 14.1 lists some of the more common interactions and their mechanisms of interaction.

INDIVIDUAL NSAIDS

NSAIDS are often categorized by their chemical class or by their plasma half-life. In general, these agents reach a steady-state plasma level after three to five half-lives, ensuring that those NSAIDs with longer half-lives will require a longer time before reaching plateau concentrations (41). This may be important in determining whether an individual patient is responding to a particular NSAID. The propionic acids are the most common NSAIDs available in the United States. They include ibuprofen, flurbiprofen, ketoprofen, naproxen, carpro-

Table 14.1.
NSAID-Drug Interactions

Drug Implicated	Mechanism	Management
Lithium	Reduces renal excretion Lithium level increases	Reduce dose of lithium
Oral Hypoglycemics	Inhibits metabolism Increases half-life	Monitor blood glucose
Dilantin	Inhibits metabolism Increases blood level	Avoid NSAIDs Monitor closely
Digoxin	Reduces renal excretion	Avoid NSAIDs Monitor digoxin

fen, nabumetone, etodolac, and diclofenac. Piroxicam, an oxicam, is a drug with a long half-life (57 ± 22 hours), and until the introduction of nabumetone was the only once-a-day NSAID currently available in this country with little evidence to suggest that its long half-life leads to clinically significant drug accumulation, as was the case with the ill-fated benoxaprofen.

PROPIONIC ACIDS

Ibuprofen

This agent, as indicated above, heralded the beginning of the NSAID era. It is the only drug of this type available as an over-the-counter drug (200 mg dose). At this dosage, its safety profile is impressive (46). Ibuprofen is rapidly absorbed after oral administration and has an elimination half-life of 2–3 hours. It requires three to four doses per day as a consequence of its short half-life. When first introduced into the United States, the recommended daily dose was 1200–1600 mg. Presently doses twice that high are routinely used, particularly in the treatment of the inflammatory arthropathies (47). Ibuprofen is available in 300-mg, 400-mg, 600-mg, and 800-mg strengths by prescription and in 200-mg doses as an over-the counter drug. As with all NSAIDs, it is prudent to recommend that ibuprofen be taken with or following meals.

Naproxen

Naproxen is the most frequently prescribed NSAID in the United States. It is available in 250-mg, 375-mg, and 500-mg tablets and as a liquid suspension (125 mg/5 ml), a delivery system helpful for pediatric patients as well as adults who have difficulty swallowing tablets. Naproxen's half-life is 12–14 hours, allowing twice-a-day dosing, with peak plasma levels reached 2–4 hours following ingestion. Naproxen is available as a sodium salt (Anaprox). The sodium salt is more rapidly ab-

sorbed from the gastrointestinal tract, an important feature for an analgesic.

Ketoprofen

Ketoprofen is another popular member of this class of drugs. It has compared favorably to indomethacin in the treatment of acute gouty arthritis. It is available in 25-, 50-, and 75-mg capsules, with a recommended dosing schedule of three times a day. The half-life of this drug is about 2–3 hours. There were scattered reports indicating that patients with rheumatoid arthritis receiving methotrexate therapy may be at particular risk for a drug interaction (hepatotoxicity) with ketoprofen. Increased experience suggests that this effect is seen with other NSAIDs and may reflect reduced clearance of methotrexate through yet-unidentified mechanisms.

Diclofenac

Diclofenac is the most frequently used NSAID outside the United States and has become very widely used in this country since its introduction to the market. It is available at strengths of 25 mg, 50 mg, and 75 mg. It has a short half-life of 1–2 hours. Hepatotoxicity has been a clinical concern because transaminase elevations were found when this drug was undergoing clinical testing. No significant liver damage has been reported with this drug, but it remains good practice to periodically monitor liver function tests in patients who are using the drug with a chronic dosing schedule.

Fenoprofen

This drug has been available in the United States by prescription for over 15 years. It has a short half-life of 2.5 hours and is rapidly absorbed. It is available in doses of 200 mg, 300 mg, and 600 mg. It was one of the earliest NSAIDs to be shown to have an analgesic ceiling at a dose level far lower than its maximal anti-inflammatory dose. It has been thought to cause interstitial nephritis, but the mechanism for this adverse effect is not known (48).

NEWER PROPIONIC ACIDS

Flurbiprofen, etodolac, and nabumetone are drugs that have recently been approved by the United States Food and Drug Administration for prescription use. Flurbiprofen has a half-life of 4–5 hours and is available in 50-mg and 100-mg strengths. It is recommended for dosing of twice or three times a day. Etodolac was available outside the United States for some time before earning FDA approval. Early indications are that it seems to be well tolerated with an acceptable incidence of GI toxicity. Whether this will hold true in the long run will require greater clinical experience with the drug. The elimination characteristics of this drug are interesting and indicate a two-phase elimination process. The first phase, which is the clinically more important one, gives the agent an "effective" half-life of about 3 hours (41).

Nabumetone is a recently introduced NSAID with a long half-life (25–30 hours). This half-life allows dosing of once or twice a day. Postmarketing experience with etodolac and nabumetone is not sufficient to know whether these agents afford any particular advantage over agents that have already been approved for use in this country.

INDOLEACETIC ACIDS

Indomethacin

As noted earlier, indomethacin has been available in the United States for more than 25 years, and much experience with this drug has been reported. It remains the drug of choice for acute gouty arthritis and is the preferred NSAID for the treatment of ankylosing spondylitis. It has significant GI toxicity as listed above. Major CNS adverse effects including headache and depression occur with this agent. Indomethacin is available in 25-mg, 50-mg and 75-mg (sustained release) capsules and in a 50-mg suppository. The half-life is about 5 hours, and dosing of three to four times a day is suggested. The recommended daily dose should not exceed 200 mg, a dose beyond which adverse reactions occur with greater frequency.

Sulindac

This pro-drug becomes active after it undergoes hepatic conversion to its sulfide metabolite. The sulfide circulates in equilibrium with the inactive parent drug; some evidence suggests that there is a shift back to the inactive form in the kidney. The renal excretion of inactive drug has been advanced as the explanation for a reportedly lower incidence of nephrotoxicity with this agent. More recent clinical studies do not consistently support a renal-sparing quality to sulindac relative to other NSAIDs. Sulindac has a long half-life (15–20 hours), allowing for twice-a-day dosing schedules. It is available in 150-mg and 200-mg strengths. There is a lower incidence of CNS side effects than with the older indoleacetic acid, indomethacin.

Tolmetin

This drug has a very short half-life (1–1.5 hours), a feature that allows dosing of four times a day. It was the first NSAID approved for the treatment of juvenile rheumatoid arthritis. It is available in 200-mg and 400-mg strengths. There appears to be an increased incidence of anaphylactoid reactions associated with the use of this NSAID when compared to the other presently available drugs of this type.

OXICAMS: PIROXICAM

Piroxicam is the only drug of this class available in the United States. It has a very long half-life of 50–60 hours and therefore can be used in a once-daily dosage schedule. It is available in 10-mg and 20-mg strengths, with the latter most commonly prescribed. Dosage flexibility is limited by a dramatic increase in GI toxicity at doses above 20 mg daily.

FENAMIC ACIDS

Meclofenamate

Meclofenamate is a drug with a short half-life (3–5 hours) and is recommended for a dosing schedule of three to four times a day. It is available in 50-mg and 100-mg strengths. Its extensive enterohepatic recirculation may be responsible for the high incidence of diarrhea seen with this drug, a side effect that should be carefully monitored. Earlier reports ascribing special benefits to this drug in the treatment of psoriatic arthritis have not been confirmed in subsequent studies. Mefenamic acid, the precursor of meclofenamate, is available for 1-week use only as an analgesic.

Ketorolac

This drug is the first injectable NSAID available in the United States. An oral form of this drug has also been released to the market. The injectable drug was extensively evaluated in the postoperative, single-dose pain model. It compared favorably to morphine sulfate in the reported studies and has been suggested as an adjunct to traditional narcotics because of its "narcotic-sparing" potential. Injectable ketorolac is very expensive (hospital cost of approximately $8 per dose), which may limit its inclusion on cost-conscious hospital formularies. There is some evidence to suggest that indomethacin in suppository form can fill the same therapeutic needs as injectable ketorolac at a fraction of the cost. Whether the very impressive pre-marketing clinical studies reported with this drug will be confirmed is important information that is not yet available. If this NSAID can reliably produce narcotic-comparable analgesia with multiple doses in the manner reported with single administrations, it likely will become an important new NSAID.

CONCLUSIONS

The use of NSAIDs as analgesic agents will likely become more common in the years ahead. Their utility in clinical states as diverse as migraine headache and postoperative pain suggests an expanding role for this class of drug. The literature already indicates that unless a contraindication is present, NSAIDs have a role in the treatment of virtually all acute and chronic pain. Research into understanding and explaining the analgesic effects of these agents is proceeding rapidly and holds out the hope for better and more effective therapies. As with all drugs, understanding the potential for toxicity is of extreme importance. Gastrointestinal and renal toxicity are the most common and potentially most serious adverse effects with this whole class of drugs, regardless of structure. This is particularly problematic for the elderly, who often are in chronic pain as a consequence of degenerative arthropathies and are most likely to require other drugs for other medical illness. Polypharmacy problems for the elderly often involve NSAIDs and diuretics, a combination that increases the potential for nephrotoxicity. NSAIDs are analgesic agents with an important place in the treatment of acute and chronic pain. Tailoring the use of particular NSAIDs according to a patient's concomitant medication and underlying medical condition, and physician awareness of drug-specific features such as half-life and cost, will help ensure that these drugs are used in the most effective way.

REFERENCES

1. Flower RJ, Moncada S, Vane JR: Analgesics—antipyretic and anti-inflammatory agents. In Gilman AG, Goodman LS, Rall TH, Murat F (eds): *The Pharmacologic Basis of Therapeutics,* ed 7. New York, MacMillan Publishing Company, 1985, pp 690–704.
2. Segstro R, Morley-Forster PK, Lu G: Indomethacin as a postoperative analgesic for total hip arthroplasty. *Can J Anaesth* 38:578–581, 1991.
3. Twiston-Davies CW, Goodwin MI, Baxter PJ: Rectal indomethacin for postoperative pain in orthopaedic surgery. A double-blind study. *J Bone Joint Surg (Br)* 72:510–511, 1990.
4. Honig S: Pain and rheumatoid arthritis. *Clin Rheumatol* 1:1–5, 1991.
5. Portenoy RK: Drug treatment of pain syndromes. *Semin Neurol* 7:139–149, 1987.
6. Dubner R, Hargreaves KM: Neurobiology of pain and its modulation. *Clin J Pain Suppl* 5:1–6, 1989.
7. Vane JR: Inhibition of prostaglandin synthesis as a mechanism of action for aspirin-like drugs. *Nature* 231:232–235, 1971.
8. Abramson SB, Weissman G: The mechanism of action of nonsteroidal anti-inflammatory drugs. *Arthritis Rheum* 30:1023–1031, 1989.
9. Abramson S: Therapy with and mechanisms of nonsteroidal anti-inflammatory drugs. *Curr Opin Rheum* 3:336–340, 1991.
10. Lozanski G, Ballou SP, Kushner I: Effect of flurbiprofen on cytokine production by human monocytes and U-937 and THP cell lines. *J Rheumatol* 19:921–926, 1992.
11. Abramson S, Korchak, HM, Luddewig, R, Edelson H, Haines K, Levin R, Rider L, Kimmel S, Weissmann G: Modes of action of aspirin-like drugs. *Proc Natl Acad Sci USA* 82:7227–7231, 1985.
12. Siegel MI, McConnell RT, Cuatrecasas P: Aspirin-like drugs interfere with arachidonate metabolism by inhibition of the 12-hydroxy-5,8,10,14-eicosatetraenoic acid peroxidase activity of the lipoxygenase pathway. *Proc Natl Acad Sci USA* 76:3774–3778, 1979.
13. Ferreira SH: Prostaglandins, aspirin-like drugs and analgesia. *Nature New Biol* 240:200–203, 1972.
14. Taiwo YO, Levine JD: Effects of cyclooxygenase products of arachidonic acid metabolism on cutaneous nociceptive threshold in the rat. *Brain Res* 537:372–374, 1990.
15. McCormack K, Brune K: Classical absorption theory and the development of gastric mucosal damage associated with the nonsteroidal anti-inflammatory drugs. *Arch Toxicol* 60:261–269, 1987.
16. Brune K, Graf P: Nonsteroidal anti-inflammatory drugs: Influence of extracellular pH on biodistribution and pharmacological effects. *Biochem Pharmacol* 27:525–530, 1978.
17. Chang DM, Baptiste P, Schur P: The effect of of anti-rheumatic drugs on interleukin-1 beta release from human peripheral blood monocytes. *J Rheumatol* 17:1148–1157, 1990.
18. Gaucher A, Netter P, Faure G, Schoeller JP, Gerardin A: Diffusion of oxyphenbutazone into synovial fluid, synovial tissue, joint cartilage and cerebrospinal fluid. *Eur J Clin Pharmacol* 25:107–112, 1983.
19. McCormack K, Brune K: Dissociation between the antinociceptive and anti-inflammatory effects of the nonsteroidal anti-inflammatory drugs. *Drugs* 41:533–547, 1991.
20. Gropetti A, Braga PC, Biella G, Parenti M, Rusconi L, et al: Effect of aspirin on serotonin and met-enkephalin in brain: Correlation with the antinociceptive activity of the drug. *Neuropharmacology* 27:499–505, 1988.
21. Taiwo YO, Levine JD: Prostaglandins inhibit endogenous pain control mechanisms by blocking transmission at spinal noradrenergic synapses. *J Neurosci* 8:1346–1349, 1988.
22. Catania A, Arnold J, Macaluso A, Hiltz ME, Lipton JM: Inhibition of acute inflammation in the periphery by central action of salicylates. *Proc Natl Acad Sci USA* 88:8544–8547, 1991.
23. Honig S, Murray KA: An appraisal of codeine as an analgesic: Single-dose analysis. *J Clin Pharm* 24:96–102, 1984.
24. Honig S: Nonsteroidal anti-inflammatory drugs as postoperative analgesics. *Orthop Rev Suppl* 18:30–34, 1989.
25. Wycross RG: The management of pain in cancer: A guide to drugs and dosages. *Oncology* 2:35–44, 1988.
26. Fetrow KO: The management of pain in orthopaedics. *Clin J Pain* 5(Suppl 2):26–32, 1989.
27. Rhodes M, Conacher I, Morritt G, Hilton C: Nonsteroidal antiinflammatory drugs for postthoracotomy pain. A prospective controlled trial after lateral thoracotomy. *J Thorac Cardiovasc Surg* 103:17–20, 1992.
28. Cooper SA, Kupperman A: The analgesic efficacy of flurbiprofen compared to acetaminophen with codeine. *J Clin Den* 2:70–74, 1991.
29. Troullos ES, Hargreaves KM, Butler DP, Dionne RA: Comparison of nonsteroidal anti-inflammatory drugs, ibuprofen and furbiprofen, with methylprednisolone and placebo for acute pain, swelling and trismus. *J Oral Maxillofac Surg* 48:945–952, 1990.
30. Watcha MF, Jones MB, Laguerela RG, Schweiger C, White PF: Comparison of ketorolac and morphine as adjuvants during pediatric surgery. Anesthesiology 76:368–372, 1992.
31. Welch KM, Ellis DJ, Keenan PA: Successful migraine prophylaxis with naproxen sodium. *Neurology* 35:1304, 1985.
32. Dingfelder JR: Primary dysmenorrhea treatment with prostaglandin inhibitors: A review. *Am J Obstst Gynecol* 140:874–879, 1981.
33. Dawood MY: Nonsteroidal anti-inflammatory drugs and changing attitudes toward dysmenorrhea. *Am J Med* 84:23–29, 1988.

34. Cohen KL, Harris S: Efficacy and safety of nonsteroidal anti-inflammatory drugs in the therapy of diabetic neuropathy. *Arch Intern Med* 147:1442–1444, 1987.

35. Rainsford KD: The biochemical pathology of aspirin-induced gastric damage. *Agents Actions* 5:326–344, 1975.

36. Rampton DS, McNeil NI, Sarner M: Analgesic ingestion and other factors preceding relapse in ulcerative colitis. *Gut* 24:187–189, 1983.

37. Ryan JR, Vargas R, Clay GA, McMahon FG: Role of misoprostol in reducing aspirin induced gastrointestinal blood loss in arthritic patients. *Am J Med* 83(Suppl 1A):41–46, 1987.

38. Miller LG, Prichard JG: Clinical review: Selecting nonsteroidal anti-inflammatory drugs: Pharmacologic and clinical considerations. *J Am Board Fam Pract* 2:257–271, 1989.

39. Green, Given KM, Tsao C, Ehipple JP, Rossi EC: The effect of a new nonsteroidal anti-inflammatory agent, sulindac, on platelet function. *Thromb Res* 10:283–289, 1977.

40. Lifschitz MD: prostaglandins and renal blood flow: In vivo studies. *Kidney Int* 19:781–85, 1981.

41. Brooks PM, Day RO: Nonsteroidal antiinflammatory drugs—Differences and similarities. N Engl J Med 24: 1716–1725, 1991.

42. Brown J, Dollery C, Valdez G: Interaction on nonsteroidal anti-inflammatory drugs with antihypertensive and diuretic agents. *Am J Med* 81(Suppl 2B):43–57, 1986.

43. Peck MG, Joyner PU: Ibuprofen-associated aseptic meningitis. *Clin Pharm* 1:561–565, 1982.

44. Fries JF, Williams CA, Bloch DA: The relative toxicity of nonsteroidal antinflammatory drugs. *Arthritis Rheum* 34:1353–1360, 1991.

45. Brawn LA, Castleden CM: Adverse drug reactions. An overview of special considerations in the management of elderly patient. *Drug Saf* 5:421–435, 1990.

46. Proceedings of the 22nd Arthritis Advisory Committee of the U.S. Food and Drug Administration. Federal Registry, 5/16/88.

47. Kantor TC: Ibuprofen. *Ann Intern Med* 91:877–883, 1979.

48. Garella S, Matarese RA: Renal effects of prostaglandins and clinical adverse effects of nonsteroidal anti-inflammatory drugs. *Medicine (Baltimore)* 64:165–181, 1984.

CHAPTER **15**

MUSCLE RELAXANT MEDICATIONS

R. MICHAEL GALLAGHER

THE INCLUSION of muscle relaxant medications in the treatment of pain has added another dimension to the clinician's pharmacologic armamentarium. Many pain states are associated with varying degrees of increased muscle spasm. As complex neurologic mechanisms are involved in the maintenance of muscle tone, any malfunction of, or interference with, these mechanisms can result in or contribute to abnormal muscle contraction.

Abnormal muscle contraction can arise from a multitude of sources. The most frequently encountered are injury (often the result of motor vehicle accidents), falls, work accidents, athletics, and overstretching. Others include inflammatory disease states and prolonged or excessive anxiety. In some cases, a pain state in itself can generate anxiety which, in turn, can lead to muscle spasm and more pain. Thus, a potentially frustrating and self-perpetuating "pain–anxiety–muscle spasm" cycle develops (Fig. 15.1).

Pharmacologic agents that interfere with the above-mentioned cycle at one or more stages will often help to reduce pain. Muscle relaxants alone or in combination with analgesics can be effective.

A group of pharmacologic agents used in the treatment of pain associated with muscle contraction are the central-acting skeletal relaxants (Table 15.1). These agents have no direct effect on muscle, the myoneural junction, or motor nerves. Muscle relaxation is produced by a depression of the central nerve pathway and possibly through the effect on higher centers.

It is believed by some clinicians and researchers that the central-acting muscle relaxants have direct analgesic activity without relation to muscle relaxation (1, 2). These medications are sometimes used in pain states not usually thought to be related to abnormal muscle contraction.

The central-acting muscle relaxants exert effects on higher centers of the brain, and because of this are sometimes used as anxiolytics as well as analgesics. The muscular pain is reduced through a modification of central perception without interfering with normal pain reflexes or motor activity. This group of medications is generally well tolerated and has a low toxicity profile. Tolerance can develop after extended use, and dependency is not common.

In general, the muscle relaxants are used for the symptomatic treatment of pain for relatively short periods. Benzodiazepines, carisoprodol, and the tricyclic-like cyclobenzeprine are sometimes used for longer periods. The types of pain states that more commonly respond are neck and back pain, myofascitis, headaches, craniomandibular disorders, and other types of pain associated with muscle spasm or injury. There are reports of their effectiveness for non–muscle-related pain such as dental pain and trigeminal neuralgia (1).

BACLOFEN

Baclofen is a skeletal muscle relaxant related to GABA (gamma-aminobutyric acid). It is believed to act presynaptically to decrease the release of excitatory amino acids (3). It is generally used in the treatment of spasticity associated with multiple sclerosis. It may have limited use in the treatment of head and facial pain such as trigeminal neuralgia or glossopharnyngeal neuralgia and atypical facial pain (4–6).

Baclofen is not well-studied in its use for head and facial pain. Fromm reported a 74% improvement of trigeminal neuralgia symptoms in patients who had previously been unresponsive to carbamazepine (7). In some of the patients, the addition of baclofen to carbamazepine was helpful. Parmar et al. reported improvement in 65% of 20 patients treated for the same condition (8).

Baclofen is rapidly absorbed, with peak serum concentration being reached in 2–3 hours. It is primarily excreted through the kidneys with 70–80% being eliminated in 1 day. The biologic half-life is variable, averaging about 3–4 hours in most patients.

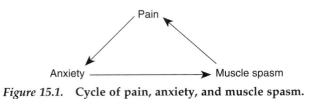

Figure 15.1. **Cycle of pain, anxiety, and muscle spasm.**

DOSAGE

Baclofen is available orally in 10- and 20-mg tablets. The usual maintenance dosage is 50–60 mg/day. It is initiated at 10–15 mg/day in divided doses and slowly increased. It should be withdrawn slowly after prolonged use, because hallucinations, anxiety, and tachycardia can occur.

SIDE EFFECTS

The most common untoward side effects include drowsiness, dizziness, ataxia, mental confusion, and gastrointestinal distress. An acute confusional state after the initiation of treatment is a rare complication, but clears after discontinuation of the drug.

CARISOPRODOL

Carisoprodol is a central nervous system (CNS) depressant and is chemically related to meprobamate and mephenesin. It is reported to have analgesic properties and to reduce local muscle spasm without significantly interfering with muscle or neuromuscular function (1, 9). The exact mechanism of action is not completely understood, but is thought to involve a depression of polysynaptic transmission in interneuronal pools at the supraspinal level in the brainstem reticular formation. It does not produce behavioral changes, and its muscle relaxation effects may be in part due to sedative qualities (10).

Cullen studied 65 patients with a variety of acute musculoskeletal conditions treated with carisoprodol or placebo (11). Carisoprodol was significantly more effective than placebo in the relief of muscle spasm, pain, and stiffness. The conditions treated included sprains and strains of the cervical, thoracic, lumbar, and sacroiliac regions.

Vaeroy et al. studied 58 patients with fibromyalgia who were treated with carisoprodol in combination with acetaminophen and caffeine or placebo (9). Seventy percent of the active treatment group showed significant improvement of pressure pain thresholds at the most tender point sites. In addition, these patients reported a significant improvement in their feeling of sickness.

Various studies have compared carisoprodol to other muscle relaxants, analgesics, and sedatives. Hindle studied 48 patients with back pain who were treated with carisoprodol, butalbital, or placebo (12). Carisoprodol was shown to be significantly more effective. Baratta

Table 15.1.
Central-Acting Skeletal Muscle Relaxants

Drug	Brand Name
Baclofen	Lioresal
Carisoprodol	Soma, Soma Compound
Chlorphenesin carbamate	Maolate
Chlorzoxazone	Parafon Forte DSC, Paraflex, Remular-S
Cyclobenzaprine HCl	Flexeril
Diazepam	Valium, Valrelease
Metaxalone	Skelaxin
Methocarbamol	Robaxin, Robaxisal
Orphenadrine citrate	Norflex, Norgesic, Orphengesic
Tizanidine	Surdalud

reported that carisoprodol was significantly more effective than propoxyphene or placebo in the treatment of low back syndrome in 94 patients (13). In a multicenter study involving 71 patients with thoracic strain or sprain, Boyles et al. showed carisoprodol to be slightly more effective than diazepam in reducing painful muscular spasm (14).

Carisoprodol is a relatively short-acting drug with minimal cumulative effect. Peak blood levels are achieved in 1–2 hours after ingestion, and the duration of effect is about 4–6 hours. It is generally well tolerated, and its potential for organ toxicity is extremely low. Metabolization takes place in the liver with excretion through the kidney. Drug interactions include an additive sedative effect when taken with CNS depressants such as alcohol or antihistamines.

DOSAGE

The adult oral dose of carisoprodol is 350 mg three to four times daily. It is usually recommended for adult use, but its use in the pediatric age groups is not uncommon. Baird and Menta tested 29 children aged 5 months to 14 years with minimal adverse effects (15). The suggested dosage for children above 5 years of age is 25 mg/kg four times daily (16). Because there are only limited studies involving children, carisoprodol should be used with caution in this group.

Carisoprodol is not recommended during pregnancy or in nursing women.

Carisoprodol (200 mg) is combined with aspirin (325 mg) or with both aspirin (325 mg) and codeine (16 mg) for those patients experiencing significant pain. The rationale for this combination is to add an anti-inflammatory and additional analgesic effect. These medications are given in a dose of one or two tablets four times daily. The usual aspirin and codeine prescribing precautions should be followed.

SIDE EFFECTS

Untoward side effects are usually transient and occur within the first several days of use. These include drowsiness, dizziness, vertigo, ataxia, tremor, agitation, irritability, headache, depression, syncope, and insomnia. Side effects that do not resolve within 48–72 hours may do so with a reduction in dose. Allergic or idiosyncratic reactions, although rare, can occur and are usually evident within the first several doses.

CHLORPHENESIN

Chlorphenesin is a central-acting skeletal muscle relaxant structurally and pharmacologically similar to methocarbamol. The precise mechanism of action is not known. Its direct muscle relaxation effects are minimal, and benefit is probably related to its sedative effects. In animals, chlorphenesin appears to modify central pain reception (16).

Investigational studies involving chlorphenesin are limited. It is more commonly used in the treatment of skeletal muscle hyperactivity secondary to neurologic disorders, but is used for painful musculoskeletal conditions. Stanko reports chlorphenesin to be as effective as carisoprodol for craniomandibular disorders (17).

Chlorphenesin is rapidly absorbed, with peak blood levels being attained at 1–3 hours. It is partially metabolized in the liver and excreted in the urine.

DOSAGE

Chlorphenesin is administered orally in 400-mg tablets. The usual adult daily dosage is 1600 mg in divided doses. In more difficult cases, dosage can be begun at 800 mg three times daily and lowered as improvement occurs. Chlorphenesin should not be administered for more than 8 weeks.

Chlorphenesin is not recommended in children under 12 years of age or in pregnant or lactating women. It should be used with caution in patients with hepatic dysfunction.

SIDE EFFECTS

The most commonly reported side effects from chlorphenesin are drowsiness and dizziness. Other side effects include confusion, paradoxical stimulation, insomnia, headache, nausea, and epigastric distress. Rash, pruritis, fever, and anaphylaxis are rare.

CHLORZOXAZONE

Chlorzoxazone is a central-acting skeletal muscle relaxant with sedative qualities. The mode of its action has not been clearly identified. It acts at the spinal cord level and subcortical areas of the brain, inhibiting reflex arcs involved in producing and maintaining muscle spasms. Chlorzoxazone is commonly used in combination with aspirin or acetaminophen for mild to moderate musculoskeletal disorders.

Vernon studied 59 patients with chlorzoxazone or placebo for (painful) musculoskeletal back conditions over 8 days (18). By day 2, those treated with chlorzoxazone reported a reduction in symptoms of spasm, pain, tenderness, and restricted ranges of motion. At completion of the study, 97% of the chlorzoxazone group experienced complete remission of symptoms, as opposed to 39% of the placebo group.

Scheiner reported on 53 patients treated with chlorzoxazone (300 mg) and diazepam (20 mg) for muscular spasm in a controlled double-blind study (19). In this study, chlorzoxazone was shown to be significantly more effective in relieving symptoms and had fewer side effects than diazepam. Gready studied 49 patients treated with chlorzoxazone in combination with acetaminophen, methocarbamol in combination with aspirin, or placebo for various musculoskeletal disorders, including cervical sprains (20). In this study, the chlorzoxazone combination was shown to be the most effective.

Chlorzoxazone is rapidly absorbed, with an onset of action in 1 hour following ingestion. Peak blood levels are attained in 3–4 hours, and its duration of action is approximately 3–4 hours. Chlorzoxazone is rapidly metabolized in the liver and excreted in the urine.

DOSAGE

Chlorzoxazone is administered orally and is available in 250-mg and 500-mg tablets. The usual initial adult dosage is 750–2000 mg daily in three to four divided doses. In unresponsive patients, the daily dosage can be increased to 3000 mg and then lowered as improvement occurs.

Chloroxazone can be administered to children. The daily dosage is 375–1000 mg in three to four divided doses. Dosage should take into account the age and weight of the child. As with many other medications, chlorzoxazone should be administered only when clearly necessary.

The safe use of chlorzoxazone during pregnancy has not been established, and therefore this drug is not recommended in pregnant women. Chlorzoxazone should be used with caution in those patients with liver or renal impairment.

SIDE EFFECTS

Chlorzoxazone is generally well tolerated, and undesirable side effects are not common. Side effects include gastrointestinal disturbances, drowsiness, dizziness, light-headedness, overstimulation, and allergic skin rash. Serious reactions such as angioneurotic edema or anaphylaxis are extremely rare.

CYCLOBENZAPRINE

Cyclobenzaprine is a central-acting skeletal muscle relaxant similar to the tricyclic antidepressants, and is thought by many to have analgesic qualities (21). It is believed to relieve pain via inhibition of endogenous monoamine-dependent pain-modulating systems and to relieve skeletal muscle spasm within the CNS (22, 23). It was initially studied for psychotherapeutic use with limited benefit and is more widely used for the relief of muscle spasm. Cyclobenzaprine can be sedating, but does not appear to interfere with muscle function (24).

Basmajian studied 55 patients treated with 30–50 mg of cyclobenzaprine or placebo for chronic neck spasm (25). The cyclobenzaprine group experienced significantly more reduction in both pain and muscle spasm. Rollings et al. reported on 78 patients treated with cyclobenzaprine or carisoprodol for acute thoracolumbar strain and sprain (26). Cyclobenzaprine and carisoprodol were equally effective in relieving spasm and pain. Brown and Womble studied 49 patients treated with cyclobenzaprine, diazepam, or placebo for long-term cervical and lumbar pain and skeletal muscle spasm (27). Although both active drug groups showed significant improvement, cyclobenzaprine was the most effective. I studied 41 patients treated with cyclobenzaprine for post-traumatic headache, 46% of whom showed significant improvement (28).

Cyclobenzaprine is relatively long-acting as compared to other central-acting skeletal muscle relaxants. The onset of action is within 1 hour of ingestion, with plasma therapeutic levels being attained in 3–8 hours. Its duration of action is 12–24 hours, and its elimination half-life is 1–3 days.

DOSAGE

Cyclobenzaprine is administered orally. The usual daily dosage is 20–40 mg in divided doses. Prescribing information often recommends a treatment period of 2–3 weeks. A postmarket surveillance study of 6311 patients by Nibbelink and Strickland (29), however, showed no unexpected adverse effects after as long as 237 days of therapy. Cyclobenzaprine is excreted in the urine as inactive metabolites and in the feces as unchanged drug. It is extensively metabolized, and its metabolites may undergo enterohepatic recycling.

Cyclobenzaprine is not recommended in children under 15 years of age or in nursing women. Reproductive studies involving rats, mice, and rabbits using comparatively high doses have revealed no fetal abnormalities. Cyclobenzaprine should be used in pregnant women only when absolutely necessary and only with extreme caution, however.

SIDE EFFECTS

Drowsiness is a common side effect and may occur in as many as 40% of treated persons. This symptom often lessens with time. Dry mouth and dizziness also are commonly experienced. Other possible side effects include nausea, constipation, dyspepsia, unpleasant taste, headache, nervousness, confusion, syncope, tachycardia, arrythmia, hypotension, vomiting, anorexia, edema of the tongue, abnormal liver function, jaundice, tremors, depressed mood, sweating, and urinary retention.

Because of its anticholinergic properties, cyclobenzaprine should be used with caution in patients with angle-closure glaucoma or prostatic enlargement.

DIAZEPAM

Diazepam is a benzodiazepine commonly used as a sedative. The effects of the benzodiazepines, as a group, are the result of their action on the CNS. Their most significant clinical effects are sedation, hypnosis, decreased anxiety, anticonvulsant activity, and muscle relaxation. They may exert independent analgesic effects, however. The effects are believed to be from a potentiation of GABA on neurons at all levels (30). In addition, muscle relaxation may in part be due to the interruption of the pain–anxiety–muscle spasm cycle through an anxiolytic effect. Other benzodiazepines, such as clonazepam, chlordiazepoxide, or meprobamate, are sometimes prescribed.

Diazepam has been used for many painful musculoskeletal disorders with varying results. Some researchers believe that its effectiveness is due to its anxiolytic effects. Basmajian studied 40 patients treated with diazepam, phenobarbital, or placebo over 4 days for cervical muscle spasm (31). The muscle symptoms were due to trauma, nervous tension, cold weather, degenerative joint disease, overexertion, and unknown causes. Patients treated with diazepam showed a statistically significant improvement over those treated with phenobarbital or placebo. Boyles et al. showed diazepam to be of benefit in painful skeletal muscle spasm in a comparison study with carisoprodol (14). Fryda-Kaurinsky and Muller-Fassbender reported its effectiveness for pain and tenderness in the treatment of acute paravertebral spasm (32).

Other benzodiazepines with similar pharmacologic properties have also been used for the treatment of painful conditions. The effect of these agents is expected to be similar to that of diazepam. Goldenberg reported temazepam to be effective in fibromyalgia syndrome (33). Swerdlow reported clonazepam to be effective in the treatment of trigeminal neuralgia (34).

Diazepam is rapidly absorbed, with peak blood levels being attained at 1 hour in adults and as soon as 15 min after ingestion in children. Secondary peak blood levels can occur at 6–12 hours, most likely as a result of enterohepatic recirculation. Diazepam is metabolized in the liver and excreted in the urine, and has an elimination half-life of 30–60 hours.

Diazepam and other benzodiazepines should be used with caution because tolerance and dependency can occur. Careful surveillance of the amounts of the drug prescribed is mandatory. In patients who may be prone to addiction, such as those with histories of alcoholism or previous addiction, benzodiazepines should be used only when absolutely necessary.

Dosage

Diazepam can be administered orally or by injection. The oral route is preferred except for the most serious cases of cervical muscle spasm. The usual adult daily dosage of diazepam is 6–40 mg in three to four divided doses. The pediatric daily dosage is 1–2.5 mg in three to four divided doses.

When parenteral diazepam is necessary, 5–10 mg can be injected intramuscularly. The dose can be repeated as necessary at intervals of 4–6 hours and changed to the oral form when improvement begins. Patients should be monitored for possible undesirable effects for 4–6 hours following administration of the injectable form.

Side Effects

The most commonly reported side effect is drowsiness. Ataxia, dizziness, confusion, headache, gastrointestinal disturbances, rash, and chills can occur, but are infrequent. There may be an increased risk of congenital malformations associated with minor tranquilizers during the first trimester of pregnancy. Diazepam is not recommended during pregnancy.

METAXALONE

Metaxalone is a central-acting skeletal muscle relaxant that is chemically similar to mephenoxalone, a mild tranquilizer. Its mode of action is unclear, but its action is thought to act centrally by suppressing polysynaptic spinal cord reflexes. It is used clinically as adjunctive therapy in acute musculoskeletal disorders.

Dent and Ervin reported on a multicenter study involving 228 patients suffering from acute musculoskeletal disorders (35). Those treated with metaxalone showed a significantly greater improvement of spasm and pain symptoms as compared to those treated with placebo. Fathie studied 100 patients with metaxalone or placebo for low back muscular pain and observed a significant improvement in 69% of patients (36). The entire study was repeated and the results corroborated, with a significant improvement in 75% of treated patients. Diamond conducted a similar study involving 100 patients and found a near-equal result with metaxalone and placebo, 52% and 46% respectively (37).

Metaxalone is rapidly absorbed with an onset of action in approximately 1 hour following ingestion. Peak blood levels are attained in approximately 2 hours, and its duration of action is 2–4 hours.

Dosage

Metaxalone is administered orally and is available in 400-mg tablets. The usual adult daily dosage is 2400–3200 mg in divided doses. It should be administered with caution in patients with impaired liver function. Metaxalone is contraindicated in patients with significant renal or liver disease and in those with a history of drug-induced anemias. It is not recommended in children under 12 years of age.

Reproductive studies in rats have revealed no evidence of reduced fertility or fetal injury as a result of metaxalone. Because its safety has not been established, metaxalone is not recommended in pregnancy, however. It is not known whether metaxalone is secreted in human milk, and therefore it is not advised to be taken by nursing mothers.

Side Effects

Metaxalone is generally well tolerated. Side effects include nausea, vomiting, gastrointestinal upset, drowsiness, dizziness, headache, nervousness and irritability, rash, and pruritis. Leukopenia, jaundice, or hemolytic anemia can occur, but these side effects are extremely rare.

METHOCARBAMOL

Methocarbamol is a central-acting skeletal muscle relaxant with a structure similar to that of mephenesin. It has been available in the United States for over 30 years and has been used with success in the treatment of acute musculoskeletal problems. It is commonly recommended for painful craniomandibular, neck, and back conditions. The mechanism of action is yet to be established. It has no apparent direct effect on striated muscle itself or the myoneural junction. In animals, it inhibits nerve transmissions in the internuncial neurons of the spinal cord and blocks polysynaptic reflexes.

Few thorough comparison studies of methocarbamol have been conducted. In a 180-patient double-blind study of methocarbamol and placebo by Tisdale and Ervin (38), methocarbamol was shown to be effective in the treatment of acute musculoskeletal disorders of both traumatic and inflammatory origin. It was significantly more effective (80%) than placebo (45%), with its greatest effect in the first several days of therapy. Preston et al. concluded that methocarbamol was slightly more effective than cyclobenzaprine and significantly more effective than placebo in the treatment of 227 patients with acute musculoskeletal conditions (39). Stearn studied 200 patients treated with methocarbamol, chlorphenesin, carisoprodol, and placebo and concluded that the three active medications were superior to placebo (40).

Other studies establishing the efficacy of methocarbamol for painful musculoskeletal conditions were reported by Feinberg et al. (41), Valtonen (42), and Dent and Ervin (43).

Methocarbamol is a short-acting drug. In the oral form its onset of action is 30 min after ingestion. Peak blood levels are attained in about 2 hours, and its duration of action is approximately 4–6 hours. Its inactive metabolites are predominantly excreted in the urine, with a small amount excreted in the feces.

DOSAGE

Methocarbamol is available in both oral and injectable forms. Oral tablets are available in 500-mg and 750-mg strengths, and in combination with 325 mg of aspirin. The injectable form is usually used in hospitalized patients and contains 100 mg/ml.

The average starting daily oral dosage of methocarbamol is 6 g in four divided doses; this is then decreased to 4.0–4.5 g for maintenance. Two tablets of the combined methocarbamol and aspirin tablets are given four times daily. In severely suffering patients, three tablets can be given four times daily as tolerated for several days. Methocarbamol is not recommended in children under 12 years of age or in pregnant or lactating women.

The injectable form of methocarbamol can be administered intramuscularly, by intravenous push, or by slow intravenous drip. It should not be administered subcutaneously. Intramuscularly 200–500 mg (2–5 ml) can be injected into each gluteal region, and this dose can be repeated at 8-hour intervals as necessary. As soon as improvement occurs, the patient can be switched to the oral form.

As much as 3000 mg (30 ml) of methocarbamol can be given by the intravenous route in divided doses daily for up to 3 days. For intravenous drip, methocarbamol is mixed with up to 240 ml of sodium chloride or 5% dextrose solution. By direct intravenous push it can be administered at a maximum rate of 300 mg (3 ml) over 1–2 min. Patients receiving intravenous methocarbamol should be in the recumbent position during administration and for at least 15 min following treatment.

SIDE EFFECTS

Methocarbamol is generally well tolerated by most patients. Many of the reported side effects occur early in treatment and improve with time. Reported side effects include light-headedness, dizziness, vertigo, headache, mild muscular incoordination, blurred vision, urticaria, rash, flushing, gastrointestinal upset, nasal congestion, fever, and a metallic taste in the mouth (with the injectable form). The most significant adverse effects with parenteral use are syncope and light-headedness.

ORPHENADRINE

Orphenadrine, a derivative of diphenhydramine, is a central-acting skeletal muscle relaxant with anticholinergic properties. It has been used extensively as a muscle relaxant and analgesic, both alone and in combination with other analgesics. Although it is prescribed for numerous conditions, it is more commonly used in the treatment of back, neck, dental, and head pain.

Available data indicate that orphenadrine has antinociceptive and muscle relaxant effects (44). It is presumed to relax skeletal muscle by blocking neuronal circuits whose hyperactivity may be implicated in hypertonia and spasm. The mechanism of its antinociceptive effect is not known. Various actions on the CNS are known and include parasympatholytic, antihistaminic, and serotonergic effects.

Gold studied 40 patients treated with orphenadrine or placebo intravenously for painful muscle spasm (45). The patients treated with orphenadrine showed a statistically significant improvement in overall clinical progress and acute painful muscle spasm. Bakris et al. studied 38 patients treated with orphenadrine, diazepam, or placebo for prolonged headache resulting from continuous muscle spasm (46). Orphenadrine and diazepam were equally effective in relieving muscle spasm and pain as compared to placebo. Winter and Post reported orphenadrine's effectiveness in treating pain of dental origin and pain following oral surgery (47).

Orphenadrine is relatively rapid-acting, with peak blood levels being attained within 2 hours of ingestion. Its duration of action is 4–6 hours. In the sustained-release form, absorption takes place over 8–10 hours, and peak blood levels are attained within 8 hours of ingestion. Orphenadrine is extensively metabolized, and its metabolites are excreted in the urine. A small amount is excreted unchanged in the urine.

DOSAGE

Orphenadrine can be administered in both injectable and oral forms. Parenteral orphenadrine contains 30 mg/ml in aqueous solution. An injection of 2 ml (60 mg) is administered intramuscularly or intravenously twice daily. When improvement occurs, parenteral therapy can be changed to oral tablets.

Orphenadrine is available in three oral tablet forms: 100 mg in a sustained-release formulation, 25 mg in combination with 30 mg caffeine and 385 mg aspirin, and 50 mg in combination with 60 mg caffeine and 770 mg aspirin. The 100-mg tablet is administered twice daily. One or two of the 24-mg combination tablets are administered three to four times daily, and one half or one of the 50-mg combination tablets is administered three to four times daily. The safety of orphenadrine has not been established in children or in pregnant women, and thus it is not recommended in these patients. Because of its anticholinergic effects, it should not be taken by patients with glaucoma, achalasia, prostatic enlargement, or bladder outlet obstruction. The usual aspirin guidelines should be followed when prescribing the orphenadrine combination products.

SIDE EFFECTS

Many of the reported side effects that do occur are related to orphenadrine's anticholinergic effects and are dose-related. Possible side effects include tachycardia, palpitations, urinary retention, dry mouth, blurred vision, increased intraocular pressure, weakness, nausea, vomiting, headache, dizziness, constipation, and drowsiness. Although rare, confusion, excitation, hallucinations, and syncope have been reported.

TIZANIDINE

Tizanidine is a new centrally-acting skeletal muscle relaxant. Its major site of action is the spinal cord. It inhibits polysynaptic mechanisms responsible for excessive muscle tone by affecting the release of excitatory amino acids from interneurons. It has been shown to be effective in the treatment of tension headache and neck and low back pain.

There are limited clinical investigative data available on tizanidine. Shimomura et al. reported that 65% of 78 patients treated for tension-type headache with tizanidine showed excellent to moderate improvement (48). Berry and Hutchinson reported improvement of pain and duration of symptoms in one study of 112 patients for back pain (49), and some advantage to adding tizanidine to ibuprofen in the treatment of acute low back pain in another study (50). Fryda-Kaurinsky and Muller-Fassbender showed a significant analgesic effect on neck and back pain in a 20-patient comparative study with diazepam (32).

Tizanidine is rapidly absorbed, and peak plasma concentrations are reached in 1–2 hours. Metabolism is mostly by the liver, and it and its metabolites are excreted predominantly by the kidney. Its half-life is 3–5 hours.

DOSAGE

Tizanidine is presently not approved for use in the United States, but is available in 2-mg, 4-mg, and 6-mg tablets and in 6-mg and 12-mg modified-release capsules elsewhere. It is administered orally 6–12 mg per day in divided doses. It should be used with caution in patients with hepatic or renal impairment.

SIDE EFFECTS

With usual recommended dosage, untoward effects are minimal. They include drowsiness, fatigue, dizziness, dry mouth, nausea, and reduction in blood pressure. At higher dosage, additional untoward effects

such as bradycardia, hypotension, insomnia, and muscle weakness can occur.

CONCLUSIONS

The central-acting skeletal muscle relaxants are frequently used in the treatment of painful conditions associated with abnormal muscle contraction, and in some cases in painful conditions not thought to be related to muscle. Their use adds to the clinician's array of pharmacologic choices and provides an alternative to nonsteroidal anti-inflammatory drugs and potentially habituating analgesics. The muscle relaxants are generally more useful in those patients who have not reached tolerance and who are not dependent on habituative medications.

REFERENCES

1. Bergen FM, Kletztein M, Ludwig BJ, Margolin S: History, chemistry, and pharmacology of carisoprodol. *Ann N Y Acad Sci* 86:90–107, 1960.
2. LaBelle A, Tislow R: A method of evaluating analgesics of the antiarthralgic type in the laboratory animal. *J Pharmacol Exp Ther* 98:19–21, 1950.
3. Fox S, Krnjevic K, Morris ME, et al: Action of baclofen on mammalian synaptic transmission. *Neuroscience* 3:495, 1978.
4. Fromm GH, Terrence CF, Maroon JC: Baclofen in the treatment of trigeminal neuralgia: Double-blind study and long term follow-up. *Ann Neurol* 15:240–244, 1984.
5. Green MW, Selman JE: Medical management of trigeminal neuralgia. *Headache* 31:588–592, 1991.
6. Martins IP, Ferro JM: Atypical facial pain, ectasia of the basilar artery and baclofen. *Headache* 29:581–583, 1989.
7. Fromm GH: Clinical pharmacology of drugs used to treat head and face pain. *Neurol Clin* 8:143–151, 1990.
8. Parmar BS, Shah KH, Gandhi IC: Baclofen in trigeminal neuralgia—A clinical trial. *JDR* 1:109–113, 1989.
9. Vaeroy H, Abrahamsen A, Forre O, Kass E: Treatment of fibromyalgia (Fibrositis Syndrome): A parallel double blind trial with carisoprodol, paracetamol and caffeine vs placebo. *Clin Rheumatol* 8:245–250, 1989.
10. [Editorial]: Today's drugs. Carisoprodol. *Br Med J* 1:1364, 1964.
11. Cullen AP: Carisoprodol (Soma) in acute back conditions. *Curr Ther Res* 20:556–562, 1976.
12. Hindle TH: Comparison of carisoprodol, butalbital and placebo in treatment of the low back syndrome. *Calif Med* 117:7–11, 1972.
13. Baratta RR: A double blind comparative study of carisoprodol, propoxyphene and placebo in the management of low back syndrome. *Curr Ther Res* 20:233–239, 1976.
14. Boyles WF, Glassman, JM, Soyka MD: Management of acute musculoskeletal condition. *Today Ther Trend* 1:1–16, 1983.
15. Baird HW, Menta DA: Preliminary observations on the use of carisoprodol in infants and children. In Miller EG (ed): *Pharmacology and Clinical Use of Carisoprodol.* Detroit, Wayne State Univ Press, 1959, pp 85–96.

16. McEvoy GK (ed): Autonomic drugs. In *Drugs Info 85*. Bethesda, MD, American Society of Hospital Pharmacists, 1985, pp 417–548.

17. Stanko JR: A review of oral skeletal muscle relaxants for the craniomandibular disorder practitioner. *J Cranioman Pract* 8:234–243, 1990.

18. Vernon WG: A double-blind evaluation of Parafon Forte in the treatment of musculo-skeletal back conditions. *Curr Ther Res* 14:801–806, 1972.

19. Scheiner JJ: Muscle relaxants: Chlorzoxazone compared with diazepam (a double-blind study). *Curr Ther Res* 19:51–57, 1976.

20. Gready DM: Parafon Forte vs Robaxisal in skeletal muscle disorders: A double-blind study. *Curr Ther Res* 20:666–673, 1976.

21. Walsh TD: Antidepressants in chronic pain. *Clin Neuropharm* 6:271–295, 1983.

22. DePalma JR, DeGregorio GJ: Management of low back pain by analgesics and adjuvant drugs. *Mt Sinai J Med (NY)* 58:101–108, 1991.

23. Share NN, McFarlane CS: Cyclobenzaprine: A novel centrally acting skeletal muscle relaxant. *Neuropharmacology* 4:675, 1975.

24. Nibbelink DW: Flexeril (cyclobenzaprine HCl/MSD). Review of clinical double-blind evaluations of efficacy and tolerability. *Postgrad Med Commun* May:19–24, 1978.

25. Basmajian JV: Cyclobenzaprine HCl effect on skeletal muscle spasm in the lumbar region and neck: Two double-blind controlled clinical and laboratory studies. *Arch Phys Med Rehabil* 59:58–63, 1978.

26. Rollings HE, Glassman JM, Soyka JP: Management of acute musculoskeletal conditions—thoracolumbar strain and sprain: A double-blind evaluation comparing the efficacy and safety of carisoprodol with cyclobenzaprine. *Curr Ther Res* 34:917–928, 1983.

27. Brown BR, Womble J: Cyclobenzaprine in intractable pain syndromes with muscle spasm. *JAMA* 240:1151–1152, 1978.

28. Gallagher RM, Gallagher JG: Cyclobenzaprine HCl in the treatment of post-traumatic headache. *Headache* 27:304–305, 1987.

29. Nibbelink DW, Strickland SC: Cyclobenazprine (Flexeril): Report of a post-marketing surveillance program. *Curr Ther Res* 28:894–903, 1980.

30. Harvey CH: Hypnotics and sedatives. In Gilman AG, Goodman IS, Rall TW, Murad (eds): *Pharmacologic Basis of Therapeutics*. New York, MacMillan, 1985, p 345.

31. Basmajian JV: Reflex cervical muscle spasm; Treatment by diazepam, phenobarbital or placebo. *Arch Phys Med Rehabil* 64:121–124, 1983.

32. Fryda-Kaurimsky Z, Muller-Fassbender H: Tizanidine in the treatment of acute paravertebral muscle spasm. *J Int Med Res* 9:501–505, 1981.

33. Goldenberg DL: Management of fibromyalgia syndrome *Rheum Dis Clin North Am* 15:499–512, 1989.

34. Swerdlow M: The treatment of "shooting" pain. *J Postgrad Med* 56:159–161, 1980.

35. Dent RW, Ervin DK: A study of metaxalone (Skelaxin) vs placebo in acute musculoskeletal disorders. *Curr Ther Res* 18:433–440, 1975.

36. Fathie K: Second look at a skeletal muscle relaxant: a double-blind study of metaxalone. *Cur Ther Res* 6:677–683, 1964.

37. Diamond S: Double-blind study of metaxalone *JAMA* 195:479–480, 1966.

38. Tisdale SA, Ervin DK: A controlled study of methocarbamol (Robaxin) in acute painful musculoskeletal conditions. *Curr Ther Res* 17:524–530, 1975.

39. Preston EJ, Miller CB, Herbertson RK: A double-blind multicenter trial of methocarbamol (Robaxin) and cyclobenzaprine (Flexeril) in acute musculoskeletal conditions. *Today Ther Trends* 1:1–11, 1984.

40. Stern TH: A controlled comparison of three muscle relaxant agents. *Clin Med* 68:367–372, 1961.

41. Feinberg I, Carey J, Hussussien J, Arias B: Treatment of painful skeletal muscle disorders: A report of a double-blind study of methocarbamol, aspirin, and placebo. *Am J Orthop* 4:280–282, 1962.

42. Valtonen EJ: A double-blind trial of methocarbamol vs placebo in painful muscle spasm. *Curr Med Res Opin* 3:382–385, 1975.

43. Dent RW, Ervin MS: Relief of acute musculoskeletal symptoms with intravenous methocarbamol (Robaxin injectable): A placebo-controlled study. *Curr Ther Res* 20:661–665, 1976.

44. Hunskaar S, Donnell: Clinical and pharmacological review of the efficacy of orphenadrine and its combination with paracetamol in painful conditions. *J Int Med Res* 19:71–87, 1991.

45. Gold RH: Orphenadrine citrate in low-back pain. *Clin Trial J* 15:145–149, 1978.

46. Bakris GL, Mulopulos GP, Subhash T, Franklin C: Orphenadrine citrate: An effective alternative for muscle contraction headaches. *Ill Med J* 16:106–108, 1982.

47. Winter L, Post A: Analgesic combinations with orphenadrine in oral postsurgical pain. *J Int Med Res* 7:240–246, 1979.

48. Shimomura T, Awake E, Kowa H, Takahashi K: Treatment of tension-type headache with tizanidine HCl. *Headache* 31:601–604, 1991.

49. Berry H, Hutchinson DR: A multicenter placebo-controlled study in general practice to evaluate the efficacy and safety of tizanidine in acute low back pain. *J Int Med Res* 16:75–82, 1988.

50. Berry H, Hutchinson DR: Tizanidine and ibuprofen in acute low back pain. *J Int Med Res* 16:83–91, 1991.

Chapter 16

Psychopharmacologic Agents in the Treatment of Pain Syndromes

JOSEPH H. ATKINSON, JR.
MARK A. SLATER
JASON N. DOCTOR
JOSHUA C. KLAPOW

Psychotropic drugs (the antidepressants, neuroleptics, antianxiety drugs, and psychostimulants) have been used as analgesics, as adjunctive agents to enhance conventional analgesics, and as primary treatment for psychological symptoms or disorders associated with pain. Psychological factors, including anxiety and depression, can profoundly influence pain expression. In addition, the burden of pain itself can produce considerable psychological distress. The use of psychiatric medications for symptomatic treatment of anxiety, depression, and insomnia is widely practiced. This chapter reviews the therapeutic efficacy of psychiatric medications in acute and chronic pain syndromes and provides guidelines for their use.

Despite the importance of the problem of pain, and the abundant literature on psychotropic drugs and pain, few of the available studies can be considered scientifically complete. To rigorously assess the efficacy of an agent in pain management, a clinical trial should meet the following criteria: (1) a reliable method to measure the intensity of pain, functional impairment, and emotional distress, (2) an established and appropriate control or reference standard to compare with the experimental drugs, (3) differentiation between the analgesic, mood-altering, and sedative components of the drug, (4) serum levels of drugs or dose-response curves, and (5) double-blind or crossover design trials.

Two additional points must be noted. First, pain is a multidimensional phenomenon with sensory, affective, and behavioral dimensions. Future research is needed to assess which of these dimensions responds to the particular pharmacologic agent in question. Second, acute pain must be considered separately, because its neuro-physiologic, psychological, and behavioral aspects may well differ from those of chronic pain states.

This chapter is in two parts. The first critically assesses drug therapy outcomes, mainly from controlled studies. It reviews each major class of psychopharmacologic agent. Following the principle that accurate diagnosis is essential, drug efficacy is discussed in relation to specific pain disorders. Experimentally induced and clinical acute pain are differentiated from their chronic pain counterparts. Where psychiatric disorders complicate the pain syndromes, their response to treatment is also discussed. The second section offers some clinical guidelines for using psychoactive drugs. It describes selecting a drug, preparing and evaluating patients for treatment, and conducting initial and longer-term pharmacotherapy. Thus, a clinician considering drug treatment of a particular pain disorder can review selected examples of evidence for efficacy in the text and tables of the first part. The next part provides specifics on treatment.

DRUG THERAPY OUTCOMES OF PSYCHOPHARMACOLOGIC AGENTS

Antidepressants

Cyclic antidepressants (tricyclic antidepressants [TCAs] and newer or "second generation" agents), monoamine oxidase inhibitors (MAOIs), and lithium carbonate have long been used as primary or adjunctive agents in pain management. There are four major clinical questions with regard to antidepressants in acute and chronic pain: (1) Are some antidepressants analgesic, and if so, in which pain disorders? (2) Is this analgesia independent of an antidepressant effect? (3) Do antidepressants potentiate narcotic or non-narcotic analgesics in a clinically relevant manner? and (4) Do antidepressants relieve depression associated with chronic pain syndromes?

Crucial to evaluating the role of antidepressant medication is defining what is meant by the term *depression.* It can be used to describe a mood, a symptom, and a syndrome or disorder. Fluctuations in mood or unhappiness as a reaction to life events or physical limitations is not a disorder. Indeed, the symptom of depressed mood or severe sadness may not be present even in patients diagnosed as having a depressive disorder. A diagnosis of a major depressive disorder, as described by the third revised edition of *The Diagnostic and Statistical Manual of Mental Disorders,* requires either a depressed mood or markedly diminished interest or pleasure in almost all activities. Accompanied by this is a set of at least four of these associated symptoms: sleep disorder, decreased appetite, substantial loss or gain of weight, loss of energy, sense of worthlessness, difficulty concentrating, observable psychomotor agitation or slowing, and thoughts of death or suicide. Major depression differs from depressive symptoms in that the above problems are persistent, interfere with function, and are not explained better by other illness (1). Chronic pain can be associated with intermittent fatigue, withdrawal, insomnia, or other depressive symptoms, and up to 50% of chronic pain patients may suffer a major depressive episode at some point in their pain career.

Tricyclic Antidepressants

Acute Pain

Treatment outcomes for acute and chronic pain in humans are described in Table 16.1. TCAs as a class inhibit the neuronal reuptake of neurotransmitters, chiefly serotonin and noradrenalin, from the synaptic cleft, thereby prolonging and enhancing their biologic activity, and presumably lending to their therapeutic effects as antidepressants. Studies using animal paradigms demonstrate that TCAs provide species-specific analgesia for acute pain (2). The data with regard to analgesia in humans are contradictory. One careful report noted that single doses of doxepin (Sinequan, Adapin) did not alter laboratory-induced dental pain threshold in 18 normal adult males, who were repeatedly tested in a double-blind, placebo-controlled study over a 4-week period (3). There was no effect on acute anxiety or other mood variables measured by standardized inventories. The authors concluded that doxepin did not have straightforward analgesic properties because it did not alter sensory sensitivity or detection thresholds, and that it had no detectable effect on pain-induced anxiety at the dosages studied. Another rigorous study reported that single doses of imipramine (Tofranil) reduced pain ratings in response to an intracutaneous electrical stimulus by 40% (4). This reduction was equivalent to oral meperidine (Demerol) and superior to placebo.

With regard to clinical pain, in a double-blind, placebo-controlled study, Levine et al. observed that neither amitriptyline (Elavil) nor desipramine (Norpramin, Pertofrane), given for 1 week preoperatively at 25–75 mg daily provided analgesia after dental extraction (5).

Chronic Pain

Tricyclic antidepressants and other cyclic antidepressants have been tested in numerous intractable pain syndromes, as summarized in Table 16.1. These data most clearly support the efficacy of TCAs for neurologic (deafferentation) pain and headache syndromes. Their effectiveness in other chronic pain syndromes (e.g., low back pain, arthritis, fibromyalgia, mixed syndromes), which may well represent the conditions for which the drugs are most commonly employed, however, is less certain. Several TCA trials in non-neurologic and non-headache samples have been conducted, and although results are generally favorable, several methodologic and design difficulties exist that serve to reduce the strength of the obtained conclusions. As demonstrated in a recent meta-analysis of 53 heterocyclic antidepressant trials (6), methodologic difficulties, including inadequate blinding conditions, lack of control groups, high attrition rates, and incomplete descriptions of outcome measures are typically present in non-neurologic and non-headache syndrome TCA trials. Despite the prevalence of methodologic problems in TCA trials, a description of some of the more rigorous studies in the field is worthy of note.

Neurologic Disorders. Neuropathic and deafferentation pain are thought to arise from spontaneous neuronal hyperactivity or disturbed inhibition following central nervous system (CNS) or peripheral nerve injury. Disorders reported to respond to TCAs include post-herpetic neuralgia (7, 8), painful peripheral neuropathy from diabetes mellitus (11–14), and persistent postoperative scar pain (9, 10), trigeminal neuralgia, thalamic pain, and neuralgias from lesions of plexus or peripheral nerves (e.g., postamputation stump pain) (15). Treatment is effective in depressed or nondepressed patients.

For example, placebo-controlled studies by Watson et al. (7, 8), demonstrated a therapeutic effect of amitriptyline (25–150 mg daily). In two-thirds of one sample, pain was reduced from "severe" to "mild" within 3 weeks (8). Nine patients with mild depressive symptoms reports good relief of pain, with an accompanying antidepressant effect. Some had pain relief without a change in mood, however. Serum TCA levels were below those associated with antidepressant activity. The authors reported that increases in dosage produced increased pain in some patients, suggesting that there was a "therapeutic window" for dosage. In about half of the

Table 16.1.
Tricyclic Antidepressants: Populations, Experimental Design, Treatment Outcome

Authors	Population	N	Interventions	Design	Control	Dependent Measures	Follow-Up	Results
Chapman & Butler (1978)	Experimentally induced dental pain threshold	18	Compared doxepin 150 mg and placebo	Double-blind, single-dose crossover	Placebo medication	Sensory sensitivity and detection thresholds	4 weeks	Doxepin did not alter sensory sensitivity or detection thresholds or mood variables
Bromm & coworkers (1986)	Experimentally induced cutaneous pain	20	Compared imipramine 100 mg, meperidine, placebo	Randomized, double-blind, crossover	Placebo medication, meperidine	Pain estimates, soma to sensory-evoked cerebral potentials, EEG	Hours	Imipramine reduced pain ratings & somatosensory amplitudes to same extent as meperidine
Levine & coworkers (1985)	Postoperative dental extraction	30	Compared amitriptyline (25–75 mg), desipramine (25–75 mg) and placebo	Double-blind, group outcome	Placebo medication	Visual analog pain scale	None; single dose	Desipramine enhanced prolonged morphine analgesia; amitriptyline did not; neither agent was itself analgesic
Kvinesdal & coworkers (1984)	Diabetic neuropathy	12	Compared imipramine 100 mg and placebo	Crossover, double-blind	Placebo medication	Clinical assessment of neuropathy & global improvement	5 weeks for each arm	Imipramine superior for global improvement
Turkington (1980)	Diabetic neuropathy with depression and depressive symptoms	59	Compared amitriptyline 100 mg, imipramine 100 mg, and diazepam 15 mg	Randomized, double-blind	Diazepam	Kupfer-Detre depression inventory; unspecified pain estimates	3 mos	Antidepressants superior to diazepam for relief of pain and mood disorder
Max & coworkers (1992)	Diabetic neuropathy in depressed and nondepressed subjects	56	Amitriptyline vs. desipramine (38 patients) and fluoxetine vs. placebo (46 patients)	Two randomized, double-blind, crossover	Placebo	Global pain relief with verbal descriptions	Unspecified	No significant differences between fluoxetine & placebo. Both amitriptyline and desipramine superior to placebo. No difference in effect between depressed and nondepressed subjects
Langohr & coworkers (1982)	Mixed Mono- and poly-neuropathy	48	Compared clomipramine 100 mg and aspirin	Open-label, double-blind, crossover	Aspirin	Rated degree of relief and overall function	5 weeks	Clomipramine superior to aspirin; on 14-mo. follow-up 41% maintained good relief
Mathew (1981)	Mixed vascular and muscle contraction headaches	281	Compared amitriptyline 50–75 mg; propranolol; biofeedback; propranolol and biofeedback; amitriptyline and biofeedback; amitriptyline, propranolol, and biofeedback; and ergotamine	Randomized trial	Treatment with ergotamine	Zung depression scores, headache severity & frequency	6 mos	Amitriptyline superior to other agents alone; combination of amitriptyline, propranolol, and biofeedback was most effective therapy
Feinman & coworkers (1983)	Atypical facial pain	93	Compared dothiepin 150 mg and placebo	Double-blind, group outcome	Placebo medication	Rigorous psychiatric diagnosis (ICD-9); Montgomery Asberg depression scale	12 mos	Dothiepin superior to placebo; over 70% had relief of pain at 9 weeks; pain relief independent of relief of depressive symptoms; long-term (>1 yr) treatment needed to prevent relapse
Alcoff & coworkers (1982)	Chronic low back pain	41	Compared imipramine 150 mg and placebo	Double-blind, group outcome	Placebo medication	Beck decompression scores, activity level, work function, pain severity, analgesic use	8 weeks	Imipramine significantly improved activity and work function, but not pain severity, analgesic use, or level of depression
Jenkins & coworkers (1976)	Chronic low back pain	44	Compared imipramine and placebo	Double-blind, group outcome	Placebo medication	Standardized personality inventory, Beck depression inventory, self-reported pain and stiffness	4 weeks	Imipramine no different from placebo

Table 16.1.
(Continued)

Authors	Population	N	Interventions	Design	Control	Dependent Measures	Follow-Up	Results
Sternbach & coworkers (1976)	Chronic low back pain	9	Compared chlorimipramine, amitriptyline, and placebo	Double-blind, counter-balanced	Placebo medication	Self-reported of pain, pain tolerance on tourniquet test	2 weeks	Chlorimipramine reduced pain estimate and increased pain tolerance; amitriptyline ineffective
Goodkin & coworkers (1990)	Chronic low back pain	42	Compared trazodone and placebo	Randomized, double-blind	Placebo medication	Beck depression inventory, Sickness Impact Profile, self-reported and observer pain ratings, Vitalog measure of activity		Trazodone equivalent to placebo
Ward & coworkers (1979)	Low back pain with major depression	16	Doxepin 150 mg	Single-blind, group outcome	None	Rigorous (Research Diagnostic Criteria) diagnosis of depression; retrospective self-report of pain before and after treatment; Hamilton depression score	4 weeks	Pain "diminished" as depression remitted
Ward (1986)	Low back pain with major depression	35	Compared doxepin (3 mg/kg) and desipramine (3 mg/kg)	Double-blind, group outcome	Placebo responders eliminated from study pool	Hamilton depression; Spielberger anxiety; Profile of Moods; McGill Pain Inventory; Illness Behavior; EMG recording; ice-water pain tolerance	4 weeks	Doxepin and desipramine equally reduced pain intensity, frequency, depression, and anxiety; ice-water pain tolerance unaffected
Evans and coworkers (1973)	Mixed arthritic disorders	18	Compared doxepin 150 mg added to analgesic regimen and placebo	Double-blind, group outcome	Placebo medication	Investigator judgement of mood; objective count of analgesic consumption	4 weeks	Doxepin improved mood; analgesic use dramatically decreased in both groups
Gringas (1976)	Mixed arthritic disorders	55	Compared imipramine 75 mg and placebo	Double-blind, counter-balanced, crossover	Placebo medication	Self-reported pain and stiffness; objectively assessed grip strength; observer-assessed function and stiffness	4 weeks	Treatment group showed significantly less subjective pain and stiffness and improved observer ratings of function and stiffness; objective grip strength unchanged
McDonald-Scott (1969)	Mixed arthritic disorders	22	Compared imipramine 75 mg added to anti-inflammatory regimen with placebo	Double-blind, crossover	Placebo medication	Patient "preference" of interventions	3 weeks	Patients "preferred" imipramine to placebo
McNeill (1976)	Mixed arthritic disorders	29	Compared imipramine with placebo	Double-blind, group outcome	Placebo medication	Pain self-report; objectively determined grip strength; Beck depression inventory	10 weeks	No between-group differences in pain report on grip strength; results potentially confounded because imipramine group significantly more depressed at baseline
MacFarlane & coworkers (1986)	Rheumatoid arthritis	36	Trimipramine	Randomized, double-blind	Placebo	Pain ratings	Unspecified	Significant reductions in pain ratings over 12 weeks
Carette & coworkers (1986)	Fibromyalgia	70	Amitriptyline	Randomized, double-blind	Placebo	Visual analogue scale ratings of pain; clinician's global impressions	Unspecified	No significant improvements in pain or clinician global impressions
Goldenberg & coworkers (1986)	Fibromyalgia	62	Amitriptyline	Randomized, double-blind	Placebo	VAS Pain	Unspecified	Significant improvement in pain

**Table 16.1.
(Continued)**

Authors	Population	N	Interventions	Design	Control	Dependent Measures	Follow-Up	Results
Blumer & coworkers (1980)	Mixed chronic pain	129	Compared high-dose (300 mg) and low-dose (unspecified) regimens of amitriptyline, doxepin, imipramine	Open-label, group outcome	None	Investigator assessment of mood, pain intensity, activity, sleep	9–16 mos	Investigators rated 55% of high-dose and 32% of low-dose groups as "improved"; no statistical comparisons
Lindsay & Olsen (1985)	Mixed chronic non-back pain with major depression	25	Maprotiline 75–225 mg	Open-label	None	Self-report of percentage pain reduction	Unspecified	Maprotiline reduced pain by 50% in 72% of sample
Lindsay & Wycoff (1981)	Mixed chronic pain with unipolar depression	116	Sequential trials of amitriptyline, imipramine, or doxepin until antidepressant response	Open-label, group outcome	None	Rigorous (Feighner) clinical assessment of depression; retrospective self-report of pain decrement	8–12 weeks	Significant proportion of those who responded to antidepressant reported pain decrement >50%
Pilowsky & coworkers (1982)	Mixed chronic pain without organic findings	52	Compared amitriptyline and placebo	Double-blind, crossover	Placebo medication	Illness Behavior; questionnaire; Zung and Levine-Pilowsky depression; Spielberger anxiety; Sickness Impact Profile	6 weeks on each arm	Amitriptyline superior to placebo at 2 and 4 weeks; no group differences at 6 weeks; high drop-out (40%) and variability of scores may have obscured treatment effect
Singh & Verma (1971)	Mixed chronic pain	60	Sequential trials of imipramine, amitriptyline, and chlordiazepoxide	Open-label	None	Observer assessment of pain relief and psychiatric symptoms	Unspecified	Imipramine and amitriptyline therapeutically equivalent and superior to chlordiazepoxide for relief of pain and mood disturbance

subjects who responded initially, there was a later decay of efficacy, casting doubts on the long-term benefits of treatment. Nevertheless, several patients were able to discontinue therapy and maintain their improvement beyond 12 months. This development may indicate spontaneous remission (which is prevalent in post-herpetic neuralgia) rather than an effect of treatment itself.

In another study these investigators compared amitriptyline and maprotiline in a 5-week, double-blind, placebo-controlled crossover trial (9). Both amitriptyline (median daily dose 100 mg; median serum concentration 450 nmol/L amitriptyline and nortriptyline) and maprotiline (median daily dose 100 mg; median serum concentration 400 nmol/L) outperformed placebo. Overall, amitriptyline was more likely to be effective than maprotiline, but some patients reported improvement on both agents, some reported improvement on one but not the other, and some reported no benefit on either treatment.

Independently Max and colleagues also reported that amitriptyline (12.5– mg daily) relieved post-herpetic neuralgia. The mean daily dose of amitriptylne was 65 mg daily. Greater pain relief was associated with higher amitriptyline doses (up to 150 mg daily) and higher serum tricyclic concentrations.

Other tricyclics are also effective. In a double-blind, controlled, crossover study of patients with post-herpetic neuralgia, desipramine also was found to be superior to placebo for alleviating pain (9). The mean daily dose was 167 mg. Both nondepressed and depressed patients were equally likely to benefit. For many patients a full response was not evident until 2 weeks after the maximum daily dose was attained, suggesting that analgesia involves longer-term neurologic processes.

Controlled studies indicate that TCAs are effective for the pain of diabetic peripheral neuropathy in patients with and without associated depressive symptoms. Kvinesdal and associates (11) used imipramine (100 mg daily) in insulin-requiring diabetics in good glycemic control with neuropathic symptoms of at least 2 years' duration. None were reported as depressed, although psychometric assessment was not done. Observer ratings of improvement were positively correlated with the plasma concentration of drug. The analgesia did not seem to be mediated by an antidepressant effect because pain relief often occurred within 2 weeks and was achieved at about one-half the drug concentrations usually required for antidepressant activity. Benefit did not appear to be related to changes in glycemic control.

Turkington (12) studied 59 diabetic patients, all with psychometrically documented depressive symptoms, in a trial comparing amitriptyline (100 mg), imipramine (100 mg), and diazepam (Valium) (15 mg) daily. The antidepressants produced equivalent pain relief (and remission of symptoms of depression) within 8–12 weeks. Diazepam produced no improvement in pain or depression scores. Again, level of control of blood glucose did not appear to mediate the improvement. On 2-year follow-up after discontinuation of therapy, pain recurred in 26% of the patients, and remitted with antidepressants.

A very carefully conducted study confirmed that both amitriptyline and desipramine outperformed placebo in alleviating painful diabetic neuropathy (13).

The efficacy of newer generation selective serotonin reuptake inhibitors is unclear. One report indicated that fluoxetine (Prozac) was equivalent to placebo (13). Another study found that paroxetine (Paxil) was effective for painful diabetic neuropathy (14).

Bourhis et al. (16) have reported an uncontrolled trial of trimipramine (Surmotil) (50–200 mg) alone and in combination with a phenothiazine, methotrimeprazine (Levoprome), in cancer pain patients. Although pain diagnoses were not stated, patients with head and neck pain syndromes were particularly benefitted, and it is likely that postsurgical or postirradiation deafferentation pain states were responsible for the head and neck pain. There was no evidence that psychotropics diminished pain caused by metastasis to bone, or by tumor involvement of viscera or other direct effects of neoplasia.

Taken together these data would indicate that cyclic antidepressants can alleviate neuropathic pain and depressive symptoms associated with this disorder. There is some suggestion that selective serotonergic agents may be less effective in neuropathic pain than those with noradrenergic activity. Pain relief occurs in 1–2 weeks, whereas an antidepressant effect may take 8–12 weeks. About 60–75% of cases can be expected to experience meaningful pain relief. There is some formal evidence for a dose-response relationship for pain relief (10), and doses of TCA (e.g., amitriptyline, desipramine) from 75–150 mg or higher appear to be effective.

Migraine Headache Syndromes. Couch and Hassanin reported that amitriptyline (100 mg daily) was superior to placebo in preventing migraine attacks, and in reducing headache severity in attacks that did occur (17). The best response occurred in nondepressed patients with severe migraine and in depressed patients with mild headaches; depressed subjects with severe headaches noted little relief. Correlation between improvement in migraine and change in depression was low but significant.

A subsequent study of 340 patients with classic migraine compared amitriptyline, propranolol, and biofeedback in a randomized trial using treatment with ergotamine and conventional analgesics as a comparison control (18). Amitriptyline (50–75 mg) gave significantly better prophylaxis than control therapy but was inferior to propranolol. The combination of amitriptyline and propranolol offered no advantage. The antimigraine action of amitriptyline was relatively independent of its antidepressant effect because even patients with Zung depression scores within the normal range showed significantly more improvement than did control subjects. Uncontrolled studies also report that amitriptyline prevents migraine attacks (19–21).

With regard to prophylaxis of migraine-contraction headache an intriguing study compared ergotamine to (1) propranolol or amitriptyline (50–75 mg) alone, (2) biofeedback alone, and (3) combinations of drugs and biofeedback (18). Amitriptyline was superior to other single agents, and the combination of biofeedback, amitriptyline, and propranolol was overall the most effective regimen. The beneficial effect of amitriptyline alone was significantly correlated with a high initial self-rating depression score, even though the dosage regimen was "subtherapeutic" for depression.

Tension Headaches. Several studies suggest that low doses of TCAs may be effective for chronic tension headaches, perhaps more effective than the commonly used antianxiety drugs. In controlled, crossover studies Lance and coworkers demonstrated that amitriptyline was superior to placebo (22) and to imipramine (23) for relief of chronic muscle contraction headache. Amitriptyline was most effective in patients over 60 years old. The majority of patients maintained their improvement for at least 6 months. In an open-label study these authors found amitriptyline (30 mg–75 mg daily) and imipramine (30 mg–75 mg daily) superior to barbiturates for overall pain relief (22). Similarly Okasha et al. (24) reported that amitriptyline (50 mg daily) and doxepin (40 mg daily) were superior to diazepam for tension headache. Interestingly, doxepin relieved headache and diminished anxiety and depression, whereas amitriptyline improved mood without concurrent headache relief.

More recently, Langemark and colleagues found clomipramine (Anafranil) to produce significant decreases in chronic tension headaches in a placebo-controlled trial (25).

In addition, the literature consistently reports that depressed psychiatric clinic patients frequently experience muscle contraction headache (26). Two studies reported that TCAs reduce pain complaints in rigorously diagnosed depressed psychiatric patients whose depression also remitted with treatment (27, 28). Whether pain remits before mood improves is not documented.

Other Headache. There are anecdotal reports of successful use of TCAs for cluster headaches (29). Similar reports suggest that the chronic headache syndrome resulting from closed head injury, which is frequently accompanied by compensation claims, depression, and anxiety, does not respond to TCAs (29).

Atypical Facial Pain. This classification contains two conditions. One is the temporomandibular joint syndrome, with pain affecting the temporomandibular joint and its musculature. The other, sometimes collectively termed *atypical facial neuralgia,* includes both atypical odontalgia (pain in the teeth) and oral dysesthesia, which features disturbed taste, dry mouth, and a burning tongue, all in the absence of physical disease (30). These conditions are to be distinguished from the typical facial pain due to trigeminal or post-herpetic neuralgia, in which pain occurs in superficial tissues, as opposed to the deep vague aches found in atypical facial pain.

Feinmann et al. described a controlled study using dothiepin (150 mg), an analog of doxepin (Sinequan) not available in the United States, in patients having temporomandibular joint pain or another atypical facial pain (30). One-third of the sample met rigorous diagnostic criteria for a depressive disorder. By 9 weeks, drug treatment produced significant reduction in pain (71% pain-free) and analgesic use, but not in depression rating scores or overall rating of psychiatric morbidity. Pain diminished equally in depressed and nondepressed patients. Many successfully treated patients who discontinued treatment after 6 months experienced recurrence of pain, which remitted when drug was reinstituted. At 12 months over three-fourths of the sample was pain-free on treatment. This study demonstrates that patients with atypical facial pain respond well to antidepressant therapy, but that continuous drug treatment may be required to maintain improvement.

Low Back Pain. Two basic groups of chronic low back pain (CLBP) patients have been studied. The first includes those with rigorously diagnosed major mood disorders (major depression or dysthymic disorder) that either precedes or is secondary to pain. The second includes patients with depressive symptoms, but who do not meet criteria for a diagnosable depressive disorder. To a large degree, the efficacy of antidepressants depends on the group considered.

Several studies report that CLBP with diagnosable major depression responds well to TCAs. For example, Ward noted that both doxepin and desipramine reduced self-reported and objective ratings of depression and anxiety, pain severity, and percentage of day in pain (31). Clinical pain relief and clinical depression relief were significantly related. The doses achieved were within the usual antidepressant range (3 mg/kg, or at least 150 mg daily for either agent), and the onset of maximum therapeutic response occurred after 3–4

weeks. These factors argued for a primary antidepressant effect. The best clinical predictor of response was a shorter duration of pain complaint; age, number of surgical procedures, employment status, and orthopedic ratings of the amount of physical impairment were not associated with outcome.

Contradictory effects are reported in CLBP patients having depressive *symptoms* not severe enough to qualify as major depression. Alcoff et al. described a group of CLBP patients, 10% of whom had documented depressive symptoms (32). Those treated with imipramine (150 mg daily) showed significantly higher activity levels and work capacity, but did not differ from those on placebo in pain severity, analgesic use, or degree of change in Beck depression scores after 6 weeks of therapy. This study is particularly informative because the groups were well matched for pain chronicity, prior surgery or injury, and depressive symptoms. Plasma antidepressant concentrations did not correlate with change in depression scores or pain intensity in the subgroup of patients with higher depression scores.

In another controlled study of back pain patients with documented depressive symptoms, Hameroff et al. reported that doxepin (2.5 mg/kg daily) was clearly superior to placebo for improving mood and sleep and reducing both muscle tension and the percentage of time patients reported being in pain (33). Pain intensity, level of activity, and analgesic consumption did not respond to the antidepressant.

Pheasant et al. reported a controlled, crossover trial of amitriptyline (50–150 mg daily) in CLBP patients with depressive symptoms (34). Analgesic consumption significantly decreased (by 46%) during treatment with amitriptyline, but mood and activity level were unaltered. A related finding from another controlled trial was that clomipramine (150 mg), an analogue of imipramine, significantly decreased verbal pain estimates in low back pain patients and increased tolerance to experimentally induced pain after 2 weeks of therapy (35). The same study showed, however, that amitriptyline (150 mg) did not differ from placebo. Studies using lower dosages of imipramine (75 mg) reported no significant differences between treatment and control groups in objective or self-reported mood, pain, or stiffness in patients with and without documented depressive symptoms (36).

Finally, in a meticulously conducted controlled investigation, Goodkin and associates reported that trazodone (Desyrel), a nontricyclic antidepressant administered 200 mg daily, was ineffective in altering pain report, activity, mood, or analgesic intake in patients with CLBP who were without major depression (37).

In summary, it would appear that TCAs are especially effective in CLBP with associated major depression, and that full antidepressant dosages are necessary. In patients not having major depression, symptoms such as insomnia or subjective muscle tension may well be improved, but an increase in functional activity and a reduction in analgesic consumption may not occur. Imipramine and desipramine may reduce pain intensity in uncomplicated CLBP, but this is not thoroughly documented.

Arthritic Disorders and Fibromyalgia. Some evidence indicates that TCAs have anti-inflammatory effects in chronic adjuvant-induced arthritis in rats. This effect reduces the physical signs of arthritis itself, increases mobility, and reduces pain-associated behaviors (38).

Four placebo-controlled trials of imipramine have evaluated its use as an adjunct for relief of symptoms of arthritic disorders (rheumatoid arthritis, osteoarthritis, ankylosing spondylitis). In three studies imipramine (75 mg) was added to a nonsteroidal anti-inflammatory drug (NSAID) regimen. One study (39) noted no significant drug effect, whereas another (40) showed significant improvement in pain, stiffness, and activity. In the third study patients "preferred" the antidepressant to placebo, but specific dependent variables (mood, pain, grip strength, and physical function) were not assessed (41). The fourth study examined the efficacy of imipramine alone in a randomized, placebo-controlled trial. Results indicated a significant reduction in pain ratings over a 12-week period. Thus, in humans, imipramine may have therapeutic effects, but more controlled studies are needed to establish its role in arthritic disorders.

More recently, two randomized, placebo-controlled trials of amitriptyline have evaluated its use for relief of symptoms of fibromyalgia. In each study amitriptyline (50 mg) was administered in a 9-week regimen. One study (42) failed to obtain significant improvements in pain or clinicians' global ratings, whereas the other (43) reported significant benefit after a 6-week regimen.

Thus, although amitriptyline may have therapeutic effects in reducing symptoms of fibromyalgia, results from more rigorously controlled trials appear to be mixed. Additional trials examining the differential effectiveness of variations in dose and duration are clearly needed.

Mixed Chronic Pain Syndrome. This term describes a heterogeneous group of patients who do not fit into the diagnostic categories discussed previously. The efficacy of TCAs in these patients again appears to depend on the presence of coexisting major depression.

In a crossover study of amitriptyline, Pilowsky et al. reported that the treated group had significantly less pain than the untreated group at weeks 2 and 4, but that pain ratings became equivalent to placebo after 6 weeks of drug treatment (44). Although amitriptyline generally did not improve daily functioning or symptoms of anxiety and depression, the authors concluded that patients showing clear-cut endogenous depression were the most responsive.

Among the open-label investigations, Blumer et al.

addressed the differential effect of high-dose (antidepressant) versus low-dose (analgesic) regimens of amitriptyline, imipramine, or doxepin in a pain clinic population (45). The high-dose groups had a more favorable outcome (50% versus 30% "improved"), but the clinical and statistical significance of these results is difficult to evaluate.

Singh and Verma reported that imipramine and amitriptyline were superior to chlordiazepoxide for relief of both pain and associated anxiety and depressive symptoms in a sample of patients with pain referred for psychiatric assessment (46).

In another uncontrolled study Lindsay and Olsen treated 25 non–back pain patients with rigorously diagnosed major depression using maprotiline (Ludiomil) at doses of 150–300 mg daily (47). Pain estimates diminished by at least one-half in 72% of patients. Among patients who had received previous unsuccessful antidepressant treatment, 62% had pain reduced by half or more. This finding probably reflects the known antidepressant action of maprotiline.

Novel Agents. New antidepressants are being introduced that have in common a more selective ability to inhibit neuronal reuptake of either serotonin (*selective serotonin reuptake inhibitors,* or *SSRIs*) or noradrenalin than do standard TCAs. Examples of SSRIs include fluoxetine, paroxetine, and sertraline (Zoloft). A more specific noradrenalin reuptake inhibitor is maprotiline. Two of the most notable features of these newer SSRI agents are an absence of anticholinergic properties, and with this a remarkably low incidence of side effects, and antidepressant efficacy in the range expected for first-generation agents (e.g., amitriptyline and imipramine). The low rates of CNS, cardiac, and other side effects of SSRIs are particularly important because many patients with pain have concurrent medical illness that complicates the use of standard agents. Studies exploring the efficacy and indications for these novel agents need to examine homogeneous groups of pain syndromes.

In summary there appears to be strong support for the efficacy of TCAs in reducing reports of pain for individuals suffering from neurologic and headache syndromes. The efficacy of TCAs for other chronic pain syndromes, however, remains largely unproven because of methodologic flaws in the majority of trials. The efficacy of newer, more selective serotonergic and noradrenergic reuptake inhibitors is just now being assessed. Further, in general, a greater emphasis on a multidimensional assessment of treatment outcome (e.g., on pain, mood, and activity) is strongly needed to bolster confidence in the efficacy of TCAs and other cyclic antidepressant interventions for pain syndromes.

Tricyclic Antidepressants as Adjuncts to Analgesics

Amitriptyline (47), nortriptyline (Aventyl, Pamelor) (48), desipramine (49), nomifensine (Merital) (50), and doxepin (50) have long been reported to potentiate opiate analgesia in animal models, perhaps by increasing opiate receptor sensitivity (47). In human acute clinical pain, chronic administration of desipramine (25–75 mg), but not amitriptyline, potentiates and prolongs morphine analgesia, resulting in 10–20% lower verbal estimates of pain intensity (5).

In chronic pain France et al. and Urban et al. report that the combination of either doxepin or amitriptyline with a narcotic analgesic reduced pain intensity more than either an antidepressant or a narcotic agent alone in patients with low back (51) and phantom limb pain (52). Narcotic dose escalation and narcotic abuse did not occur, and no patient required more than the equivalent of methadone (Dolophin) 20 mg daily. Because these patients also were enrolled in a comprehensive pain management program, the authors speculate that both the program itself and the TCAs may have contributed to the low maintenance dosages of narcotic. Of particular interest is that narcotics generally are ineffective in central pain states such as phantom limb (53), and that TCAs may promote narcotic efficacy in these disorders. Controlled trials assessing combination versus single drug on pain intensity, side effects, functional status (e.g., employment, exercise tolerance) and emotional state are needed.

Mechanisms of Action

Tricyclic antidepressants have several putative actions that may affect pain or its associated disability, including (1) antidepressant effects, (2) "anticonvulsant" effects, (3) serotonergic or noradrenergic effects with augmentation of endogenous pain inhibitory mechanisms, (4) anti-inflammatory properties, and (5) central skeletal muscle relaxation. It is possible to speculate that the major therapeutic action depends on the etiology of the pain syndrome. An antidepressant effect would be paramount in pain patients with coexisting major depressive illness. In migraine headache and other neurologic pain from deafferentation disorders, stabilizing aberrantly conducting neurons or inhibiting their afferent transmission at the level of the spinal cord may be crucial. An anticonvulsant mechanism (54, 55) is possible, given the evidence of epileptiform activity in deafferentated neurons, the structural similarity of TCAs to traditional anticonvulsants like carbamazeine, and their ability to suppress firing in polysynaptic neurons (10, 54, 55). Peripheral anti-inflammatory properties may be therapeutic in other pathologic states. Possible sites of action include (1) altering the transport or activity of substances involved in inflammation at the tissue level, such as serotonin, (2) inhibiting prostaglandin synthetase, an enzyme crucial to inflammation, and (3) modifying of blood-protein binding capacity, another property shared with conventional anti-inflammatory drugs (37). Finally, amitriptyline has a chemical structure almost identical to that of cyclobenzaprine (Flexeril), a centrally acting skeletal muscle relaxant. The centrally acting skeletal muscle relaxants are sedatives and preferentially depress polysynaptic reflexes without directly relaxing skeletal muscle or depressing neuronal conduction or muscle excitability. Amitriptyline may act by sedative or neuronal mechanisms to reduce muscle tension in selected headache or low back disorders. Of course, an augmentation of serotonergic or other endogenous pain-inhibitory neurotransmitter systems may be fundamental to any therapeutic effect.

Monoamine Oxidase Inhibitors

Acute and Chronic Pain

Monoamine oxidase (MAO) is a term for intramitochondrial enzymes widely distributed throughout the body. An intraneuronal MAO deactivates biologically active amines potentially important in pain perception, including norepinephrine, 5-hydroxytryptamine (serotonin), and dopamine. Monoamine oxidase inhibitors (MAOIs) increase intraneuronal pools of these neurotransmitters by inhibiting their degradation. Phenelzine (Nardil) and tranylcypromine (Parnate) are the most commonly prescribed MAOIs.

Monamine oxidase inhibitors do not appear to have analgesic properties in acute pain. With regard to chronic pain syndromes, the MAOIs show promise for migraine headache, atypical facial pain, and major depression with secondary pain, as noted in Table 16.2. One uncontrolled study using phenelzine for treatment-resistant migraine headache reported that 20 of 25 patients had a reduction in frequency of headache to less than one-half that of the preceding 12-month control period, and that 7 of these patients became headache-free (56). Although serotonin is thought to be important to the pathogenesis of migraine, no correlation was observed between changes in pain and in platelet serotonin concentrations.

Cyclic migraine, consisting of daily headaches in recurrent episodes lasting 2 weeks or more, also may be a phenelzine-responsive disorder. Uncontrolled studies noted complete remission in 20% of patients, and reduced duration of attacks in the remaining patients (57, 58).

Lascelles described a controlled trial of phenelzine (45 mg) in patients with prolonged atypical facial pain, without detectable organic pathology (59). This group suffered deep, aching pain in the soft tissues and bone, and diagnostically embraced temporomandibular joint syndrome and atypical facial neuralgias (described earlier). Phenelzine significantly outperformed placebo at 4 weeks in relieving both objectively rated depressive symptoms and facial pain. Three-fourths of the treated patients showed improvement of pain and depression. Pain relief was associated with improve-

Table 16.2.
Lithium and Monoamine Oxidase Inhibitors: Populations, Experimental Design, and Treatment Outcome

Authors	Population	N	Interventions	Design	Control	Dependent Measures	Follow-Up	Results
Anthony & Lance (1969)	Migraine headache	25	Phenelzine	Case studies, open-label	None	Self-reported headache frequency	5–24 mos	Phenelzine reduced headache frequency by >50% in 20/25; 7/25 headache-free
Lascelles (1966)	Atypical facial pain	20	Compared phenelzine 45 mg and placebo	Double-blind, group outcome	Placebo medication	Clinical psychiatric diagnosis; Hamilton depression scale; self-report of pain	1 mo	Phenelzine superior to placebo; pain relief in 15/20; relief of depression associated with pain relief
Raft & coworkers (1981)	Primary unipolar depression; pain secondary to depression	23	Compared phenelziine, amitriptyline, & placebo	Double-blind, group outcome	Placebo medication	Beck depression inventory; Hamilton Rating Scale for Depression	6 weeks	Phenelzine (1.5 mg/kg) superior to placebo for relieving depression at 6 weeks
Chazot (1979)	Migraine headache	25	Lithium	Case studies, open-label	None	Self-reported headache frequency		Lithium decreased number of headache attacks in 50% of patients.
Medina & Diamond (1981)	Cyclical migraine	22	Lithium	Case studies, open-label	None	Self-reported headache frequency & duration	3–4 mos	19/22 patients had decreased duration, frequency of attacks
Peatfield & Rose (1981)	Migraine headache	5	Lithium	Case studies, open-label	None	Self-reported headache frequency, intensity	2 weeks	All had more severe, more frequent headache
Damasio & Lyon (1980)	Acute cluster headache	8	Lithium	Case studies, open-label	None	Self-reported headache frequency, severity	1–5 mos	Headache remitted in 3/8 patients at 2 weeks; lithium prophylactic if initiated during remission.
Ekbom (1977)	Acute cluster headache	7	Lithium	Case studies, open-label	None	Self-reported headache frequency, intensity	1–36 mos	No response in 3/7 patients; headache intensity decreased by 20–33% in others; lithium prophylactic if initiated during remission
Kudrow (1978)	Cluster headache	15	Compared lithium, prednisone, & methylsergide	Group outcome, open-label	Reference medication	Self-reported headache improvement	1–12 mos	87% had >75% improvement with lithium, 50% and 41% improved with prednisone and methylsergide, respectively
Damasio & Lyon (1980)	Chronic cluster headache	12	Lithium	Case studies, open-label	None	Self-reported headache improvement	1–24 mos	Complete remission in 6/12 patients on follow-up
Ekbom (1981)	Chronic cluster headache	8	Lithium	Case studies, open-label	None	Self-reported headache improvement	1–24 mos	All reported pain decreased 75–100% at 2 weeks; 11/12 had return of headache to baseline by 8 mos
Lieb & Zeff (1978)	Chronic cluster headache	2	Lithium	Case studies, open-label	None	Self-reported headache frequency	12–27 mos	Markedly reduced frequency of headache
Medina & coworkers (1978)	Chronic cluster headache	12	Lithium	Case studies, open-label	None	Self-reported headache improvement	3 mos	Complete remission in all 12 patients

ment in depression, and was ascribed to an antidepressant effect.

Raft et al. reported a significant antidepressant effect of phenelzine (1.5 mg/kg) in a controlled study of psychiatric patients with definite primary depression in whom pain was symptomatic of depression and did not precede it (60). The effect of phenelzine on pain was not reported, but the patients' daily functioning improved. Interestingly, the authors posit that pain clinic populations may contain a high proportion of patients with "atypical" depression. Such patients exhibit reverse vegetative symptoms of depression (e.g., increased sleep, appetite, and libido) and may be specifically responsive to MAOI agents.

Relatively few outcome studies of MAOIs have been conducted, and only two drug trials employed rigorous research methods (59, 60). Thus, strong evidence for the effectiveness of MAOIs is lacking. More studies need to be conducted to provide conclusive evidence with regard to the effectiveness of MAOIs.

Lithium Carbonate

Acute and Chronic Pain

Lithium is widely used in psychiatric disorders and has been employed for numerous medical and neurologic conditions (61). The rationale for its use in pain syndromes derives from its postulated effects on CNS dopaminergic and serotonergic systems, and its demonstrated efficacy in treating cyclic or recurrent disorders (e.g., bipolar mood disorder). Lithium has been used to treat common migraine, cyclic migraine, and cluster headaches, but its efficacy in these syndromes is not established (see Table 16.2). Open-label reports (52, 58, 63) suggest that lithium diminishes the frequency and severity of common migraine attacks, but there are also indications that the drug precipitates more frequent and severe migraine headaches (64). Lithium has been used to abolish acute attacks of cluster headache but has not been consistently beneficial (65, 66). Several studies (65–70) noted that lithium relieves chronic cluster headache, although in many patients headaches returned to pretreatment levels within 18 months, despite continued lithium therapy (66).

There have been no known controlled trials examining the efficacy of lithium in treating chronic pain conditions, and experimental investigations need to be conducted if the role of this agent is to be understood. Although some reports are encouraging, there presently is no definitive indication that this drug is effective with chronic pain populations.

Mechanism of Action of MAOIs and Lithium Carbonate

The therapeutic mechanism of action of MAOIs and lithium in headache syndromes is unknown, but probably is not simply a primary antidepressant effect. Their widespread effects on serotonergic and noradrenergic neurotransmission may activate endogenous pain-modulating systems.

Summary

In summary, these studies identify promising treatments and illuminate deficits in our current approach to using antidepressants in the treatment of these patients. First, there are no clinical or biologic markers to predict drug responders from nonresponders. Second, the high dropout rate in many studies indicates that antidepressants alone are insufficient to treat these patients and that a more comprehensive approach is required. Finally, improved laboratory methods for detecting major depression may permit the more specific application of these drugs.

NEUROLEPTIC DRUGS

Neuroleptics include the various classes of phenothiazines, butyrophenones, and other compounds used primarily as antipsychotics or "major tranquilizers." Like opiates they inhibit gross motor activity and act at higher centers to produce affective indifference and emotional quieting. Neuroleptics are used widely in combination with narcotics to treat postoperative pain and have been employed for chronic pain syndromes. Recently, however, it has been recognized that there is very little evidence that neuroleptics have analgesic effects or that they potentiate opiate analgesia, and a reassessment of their use is in order. Details of these studies are presented in Table 16.3.

Phenothiazines and Related Drugs

Acute Pain

Experimentally Induced Pain. The extensive work of Dundee et al. assessed the effect of 14 different phenothiazines on pain experimentally induced by pressure on the anterior surface of the tibia, using healthy patients admitted to a gynecologic service for minor surgical procedures (71–74). All phenothiazines tested increased sensitivity to pain at 20 min after injection. By 60 min, however, two distinct response patterns emerged. First, some agents showed mild analgesic activity: chlorpromazine (Thorazine), promazine (Sparine), propiomazine (Largon), and methotrimeprazine (Levoprome) (72). Next, some agents moderately amplified pain reports: prochlorpromazine (Compazine), perphenazine (Trilafon), and trifluoperazine (Stelazine). And one agent markedly increased pain report over baseline: promethazine (Phenergan) (72). Further observations suggested that the action of certain phenothiazines was biphasic—first anti-analgesic and later analgesic. Promethazine, trifluorperazine, and perphenazine, for example, enhanced pain sensitivity at 20 and 60 min post injection but demonstrated some slight analgesic activity by 180 min after administration (71–74).

The Dundee group (72) also explored the ability of phenothiazines to potentiate a narcotic analgesic, meperidine (Demerol). Promazine slightly but significantly increased the analgesic activity of meperidine at 60–90 min after injection. Other phenothiazine derivatives (propiomazine, trifluopromazine) had no effect on meperidine analgesia. An important finding was that perphenazine and promethazine were strongly anti-analgesic and diminished the therapeutic effect of meperidine when given in combination with the narcotic.

A later placebo-controlled crossover trial reported that promethazine, promazine, and propiomazine were not of themselves significantly analgesic and did not enhance meperidine analgesia (75). This report replicated the finding that promethazine strongly antagonized meperidine analgesia.

Postsurgical Pain. Many clinical studies of the analgesic and narcotic-potentiating properties of neuroleptics consist of single-dose trials with limited follow-up. Methotrimeprazine (Levoprome), a congener of chlorpromazine, is the only phenothiazine with replicable an-

Table 16.3.
Antipsychotic Drugs: Populations, Experimental Design, Treatment Outcome

Authors	Population	N	Interventions	Design	Control	Dependent Measures	Follow-Up	Results
	Acute Pain							
Dundee & coworkers (1960, 1961, 1963)	Patients awaiting minor surgery; experimentally induced pain sensitivity	20–140	Compared effect of 14 different phenothiazines on sensitivity to experimentally induced pain	Group outcome, open-label	No treatment	Self-report of sensitivity to experimentally induced pain	3 hours	All phenothiazines increased sensitivity to pain at 20 min; methotrimeprazine, chlorpromazine, promazine, & propiomazine slightly analgesic 60 min after injection
Moore & Dundee (1961)	Patients awaiting minor surgery; experimentally induced pain sensitivity	42–60	Compared ability of 5 phenothiazines to enhance meperidine	Group outcome, open-label	No treatment	Self-report of sensitivity to experimentally induced pain	3 hours	Promethazine & perphenazine antagonized meperidine analgesia; promazine slightly enhanced meperidine; propiomazine, trifluoperazine ineffective
Siker & coworkers (1966)	Healthy volunteers; experimentally induced pain threshold	16	Compared promethazine and placebo	Double-blind, group outcome	Placebo medication	Self-report, scale unspecified	Hours	Promethazine antagonized meperidine analgesia
Keats & coworkers (1966)	Postoperative patients	13	Compared promethazine and placebo; meperidine with and without promethazine	Double-blind, group outcome	Placebo medication	Self-report, pain improvement	Hours	Promethazine equivalent to placebo; promethazine did not enhance meperidine
Lasagna & DeKornfeld (1961)	Postoperative, postpartum pain	37–66	Compared methotrimeprazine and morphine; methotrimeprazine and placebo	Double-blind, case control	Placebo, reference analgesic (morphine)	Self-report, pain improvement	Hours	Methotrimeprazine 15 mg equivalent to morphine 10 mg
McZuitty (1967)	Labor pain	525	Compared promethazine, promazine, or propiomazine with & without meperidine	Double-blind	Placebo medication	Observer rating of pain intensity	Hours	Promazine, promethazine & propiomazine not analgesic and did not enhance analgesia obtained from meperidine 100 mg
Minuck (1972)	Postoperative pain	197	Compared methotrimeprazine, meperidine, & placebo	Double-blind, group outcome	Placebo medication	Observer rating of analgesia as excellent, good, fair, poor	Hours	Methotrimeprazine 5–10 mg equal to meperidine 25–50 mg; both superior to placebo for analgesia
Powe & coworkers (1962)	Labor pain	520	Compared (1) meperidine, (2) meperidine with propromazine, (3) meperidine with propromazine	Group outcome	Reference analgesic (meperidine)	Observer ratings of pain	Hours	Promethazine and propiomazine combined with meperidine produced "calmer" course of labor; outcome criteria confounded by sedative effects of phenothiazines
	Chronic Pain							
Bloomfield & coworkers (1964)	Mixed chronic pain	18	Compared methotrimeprazine with morphine	Group outcome	Placebo medication	Self & observer ratings	4 hours	Methotrimeprazine 15 mg equivalent to morphine for analgesia
Caviness & O'Brien (1980)	Cluster headache	13	Chlorpromazine given to patients who had not responded to conventional therapy	Case study, open-label	None	Self-report of headache frequency, intensity	Up to 8 mos	Chlorpromazine associated with headache suppression within 2 weeks in 13 patients
Hakkarairen (1977)	Tension headache	48	Compared fluphenazine and placebo	Group outcome, double-blind	Placebo medication	Self-report of headache duration, intensity, frequency	2 mos	Fluphenazine 1 mg produced significant decreases in headache duration, intensity, frequency

Table 16.3.
(Continued)

Authors	Population	N	Interventions	Design	Control	Dependent Measures	Follow-Up	Results
Montilla & coworkers (1963)	Mixed chronic pain	105	Compared methotrimeprazine and morphine	Group outcome, double-blind	Reference analgesic (morphine)	Self and observer pain ratings	4 hours	Methotrimeprazine 15 mg equivalent to morphine 10 mg
Beaver & coworkers (1978)	Chronic cancer pain	40	Compared single dose of methotrimeprazine and morphine	Case control, single-blind	Reference analgesic (morphine)	Observer-rated pain hourly for 6 hours	6 hours	Methotrimeprazine about half as potent as morphine on a milligram basis
Bourhis & coworkers (1978)	Chronic cancer pain	100	Methotrimeprazine added to ongoing treatment	Case studies, open-label	None	Observer rating of invalidism and of unsolicited pain reports during interview	15 days	Methotrimeprazine contributed to reduced pain disability
Houde & Wallenstein (1955)	Severe cancer pain	34	Compared chlorpromazine, morphine, and their combination	Case control, double-blind	Placebo medication, reference analgesic (morphine)	Self-report of pain intensity	Hours	Chlorpromazine had no analgesic effect and did not potentiate morphine analgesia
Moertl & coworkers (1972)	Cancer pain	100	Compared promazine 50 mg, aspirin, and other non-narcotic oral analgesics	Case control, double-blind	Placebo medication	Self-rated percentage pain relief for 6 hours after each drug	6 hours	Promazine 50 mg orally had no analgesic activity and did not potentiate aspirin
Cavenar & Meltabie (1976)	Cancer pain	2	Haloperidol added to clinical treatment regimen	Open-label, case studies	None	Self & observer report of pain, activity	1 mo	Haloperidol associated with decreased pain report, increased activity
Daw & Cohen-Cole (1981)	Cancer pain	1	Haloperidol added to clinical treatment regimen	Open-label, case study	None	Self & observer report of pain, function	6 mos	Haloperidol associated with decreased pain report, improved function

algesic properties in postoperative pain. One double-blind multiple-dose study of 66 postoperative and postpartum patients concluded that methotrimeprazine, 15 mg subcutaneously, was equivalent to morphine sulfate, 10 mg (76). A similar controlled study of 197 postoperative patients yielded equivalent results (77).

The balance of the controlled investigations on other antipsychotic drugs indicates that promethazine, promazine, and propiomazine have no analgesic activity and do not enhance narcotic analgesia in the clinical setting (78, 79). The one study reporting a therapeutic effect of these agents confounded analgesia and sedation, making it difficult to assess the results (80). The one placebo-controlled double-blind study of chlorpromazine for postoperative pain is uninterpretable because of the likelihood of a carryover effect from previously administered analgesics and the lack of statistical analysis (81).

It is important to note that even analgesics of proven efficacy may decrease laboratory-induced pain threshold by no more than 30% over placebo (82, 83). Nevertheless, the data from studies of both experimentally induced and acute clinical pain demonstrate that most neuroleptic drugs do not provide clinically relevant analgesia. In addition, some of these agents, such as promethazine, which is used commonly in postoperative patients to "potentiate" narcotic analgesia, lack analgesic properties and may antagonize narcotic analgesia. Methotrimeprazine is an exception to this rule. Methotrimeprazine apparently alone among the phenothiazines assessed is analgesic, but it confers no advantage over narcotics in acute pain and has not had widespread clinical acceptance.

Chronic Pain

The risk of tardive dyskinesia must be considered before employing antipsychotic agents to treat chronic pain. Although the daily dosages of antipsychotic medications indicated in chronic pain used are small, the cumulative amounts pose some risk, and lasting dyskinesias may appear even after brief treatment (84). This problem is discussed in detail later (see "Treatment Approaches"). Investigations of neuroleptic medications for chronic pain syndromes focus on chronic headaches, neuropathic disorders, and cancer-related pain.

Headaches. Hakkarainen reported a placebo-controlled trial of fluphenazine (Prolixin) (1 mg daily) for chronic tension headache (85). Fluphenazine produced significant decreases in self-reports of headache duration, intensity, and frequency.

An open-label study (86) of chlorpromazine in the treatment-resistant cluster headache patients reported that oral doses of 75–700 mg daily uniformly induced a remission, and that suppression of headache continued for at least 8 months in some patients. Although the lack of placebo control and the possibility of spontaneous remission diminish confidence in these results, the persistent benefit in some patients indicates that more rigorous trials should be considered. Similarly an uncontrolled trial of intramuscular chlorpromazine (1 mg/kg) for acute migraine attacks demonstrated complete relief of pain, nausea, and emesis within 1 hour in the vast majority of patients (87). A sizable percentage of patients experienced orthostatic hypotension. There is no evidence that chlorpromazine is effective for migraine prophylaxis.

Neurologic Disorders. Several anecdotal reports suggest that phenothiazine or butyrophenone neuroleptic agents, when used in combination with TCAs, are effective for deafferentation syndromes (88, 89). In selected cases, diabetic peripheral neuropathy, post-herpetic neuralgia, and similar conditions were reported to respond to combination therapy, whereas treatment with a tricyclic agent alone was ineffective (88). Suggested combinations include amitriptyline (25–75 mg) plus fluphenazine (1–3 mg) (9, 88) or imipramine (25–75 mg) with haloperidol (Haldol) (1–3 mg) (11). It is possible that the therapeutic effect of the neuroleptic is attributable to its increasing TCA serum concentrations, rather than to an independent effect. The use of an antipsychotic agent alone is less likely to be helpful in these conditions.

Cancer Pain. Pain in cancer arises from direct effects of tumor (e.g., compression, infiltration) or as a side effect of treatment (e.g., postirradiation neuropathy). Neuroleptics, with the exception of methotrimeprazine (76), lack analgesic properties in pain secondary to direct effects of tumor (16, 90–95). For example, Moertel et al. rigorously compared single doses of promazine, aspirin, acetaminophen, and other non-narcotic oral analgesics in ambulatory patients suffering mild to moderate cancer-related pain (90). Promazine was chosen as the reference antipsychotic because it was one of the few phenothiazines to show promise in studies using experimentally induced pain (71). Aspirin was superior to all other tested agents for relief of cancer pain. Oral promazine has no analgesic activity (95), and did not potentiate the effect of aspirin (90).

In addition, the controlled studies by Houde and Wallenstein of hospitalized cancer patients in severe pain demonstrated that chlorpromazine alone had no significant analgesic effect and did not promote the analgesic activity of morphine (91).

The butyrophenones are neuroleptic drugs structurally related to meperidine. Haloperidol in preliminary animal models augments opiate analgesia (96). Anecdotal reports indicate that haloperidol can reduce or eliminate narcotic requirements and reverse clinical depression in cancer pain patients (97–100), but controlled trials are not available.

In summary, most neuroleptic drugs have limited efficacy as primary analgesics or as adjuncts to narcotic analgesia. Many studies supporting the use of neuroleptics to potentiate or replace opiate analgesia neither exploit a crossover design (77, 79, 80, 102) nor have a placebo control (75, 79, 80, 102–104), and use low or inadequate doses of a reference analgesic (78, 81) or confound sedation and analgesia (103).

Some of the rationale for using neuroleptics derived from hopes that troublesome aspects of narcotic use (tolerance, addiction, emesis, and respiratory depression) would be avoided. Data suggest, however, that addictive behavior initiated by prescription narcotics is rare (104) and that escalation of narcotic requirements by a cancer patient more often indicates progression of the malignancy rather than drug tolerance. Acute adverse reactions (sedation, restlessness, hypotension) to phenothiazines are more common and severe than those attributed to narcotics, and phenothiazines amplify these side effects of narcotics. Although some chronic headache and deafferentation syndromes may respond to antipsychotics, clinical trials with homogenous populations would be needed to clarify the efficacy of these drugs, and the risk of tardive dyskinesia argue against their prolonged use.

Mechanism of Action

The therapeutic mechanism of action of neuroleptic medications for pain syndromes is unclear. Antidopaminergic activity may explain the analgesic effects of methotrimeprazine in acute pain, although other neuroleptic agents with similar ability to block dopamine neurotransmission are not analgesics. The membrane-stabilizing properties of antipsychotic drugs may account for their therapeutic effects in some deafferentation syndromes (54, 55). When a TCA is being coadministered, the neuroleptic may simply increase serum concentrations of the TCA, or may provide an independent or synergistic effect. Obviously the ability of neuroleptics to reduce extreme anxiety may be therapeutic when anxiety amplifies their pain complaints.

ANTIANXIETY AND SEDATIVE AGENTS

Three classes of antianxiety drugs are used in pain syndromes. These are the benzodiazepines, chlordiazepoxide (Librium), diazepam (Valium), clonazepam (Clonopin), and others; the diphenylmethane derivatives, such as hydroxyzine (Vistaril); and the barbiturates, phenobarbital, secobarbital, and others. The benzodiazepines have generally replaced the barbiturates in routine clinical care. The rationale for antianxiety agents is to treat anxiety secondary to pain, or to alleviate the painful muscular spasm and muscular contraction in low back pain and tension headache presumed to be a response to anxiety. These medications also show promise in the treatment neuralgias, perhaps by reducing neuron firing rates. An overview of outcome studies is described in Table 16.4.

Benzodiazepines and Hydroxyzine

Acute Pain

Diazepam decreases the affective response to pain and potentiates this property of opiates in experimentally induced pain in humans (105, 106). Chapman and Feather noted that diazepam (10 mg orally) prolonged tolerance to experimentally induced pain significantly more than did placebo and aspirin, and diminished pain-associated anxiety better than did placebo (105). Graceley and colleagues confirmed that diazepam reduced the affective response to experimentally induced pain without altering sensory sensitivity (106). The use of benzodiazepines as adjuvants for reducing the affective response to acute clinical (e.g., postoperative) pain, however, has not been widely investigated. Clinical experience indicates that benzodiazepines are often useful in anxious postoperative patients, and that reduction of anxiety helps diminish pain complaints.

Hydroxyzine is a diphenylmethane derivative having antihistaminic, antiemetic, spasmolytic, and anxiolytic activity. In animals hydroxyzine, like the benzodiazapines, has minimal analgesic activity and an inconsistent ability to enhance opiate analgesia, but it potentiates opiate reduction of the affective component of pain (107).

Results of studies in clinical pain are equivocal. Hydroxyzine (100 mg orally) is equivalent to placebo in relieving postoperative pain, and does not potentiate oral meperidine (107) or alter meperidine pharmacokinetics or metabolism (108). Hydroxyzine (100 mg parenterally) is reported to be superior to placebo and equivalent to very-low-dose morphine (8 mg) in patients suffering severe pain (109). Two studies indicate that hydroxyzine (100 mg intramuscularly) combined with morphine produce greater pain relief than does morphine alone (109, 110). Nevertheless, in these studies the addition of hydroxyzine to morphine did not increase the percentage of patients who reported better than 50% reduction in pain. The combination did, however, produce significantly greater drowsiness, which may have confounded pain reports.

Thus, hydroxyzine (75–100 mg parenterally) may have an analgesic effect equivalent to 8–10 mg of morphine. Hydroxyzine administration causes sedation and marked discomfort at the injection sites, and subcutaneous administration can produce severe tissue damage. Because of these liabilities and the limited data for therapeutic efficacy, the routine use of hydroxyzine to potentiate opiate analgesia in acute pain cannot be recommended.

Chronic Pain

Headache Syndromes. In controlled studies Lance and Curran concluded that both oral diazepam and chloridazepoxide were superior to placebo (but inferior to TCAs) for relief of chronic tension headache (22, 23). A controlled trial has indicated that diazepam (10–15 mg orally) is superior to placebo for relief of chronic tension headache (111). By comparison one carefully controlled study of a small, heterogeneous sample of chronic pain patients found neither chlordiazepoxide nor hydroxyzine to be superior to placebo for relieving nonheadache pain or improving mood (112).

Other Neurologic Disorders. A substantial number of uncontrolled trials support the effectiveness of oral clonazepam for treatment of chronic neuropathic pain, particularly cranial neuralgias (113–116). Responsive syndromes include trigeminal neuralgia, sphenopalatine ganglion neuralgia (113–115), and diverse neuropathies (116). These preliminary reports are encouraging, but limitations of the data include their open design, the difficulty in assessing the magnitude of functional improvement, and the limited follow-up (117).

Chronic Back Pain. Hollister and coworkers suggested that oral diazepam produces extended relief in chronic pain from musculoskeletal disorders (e.g., back pain) (118). Intrathecal administration of benzodiazepines is also being investigated in pilot studies of chronic back pain. One double-blind, placebo-controlled study examined the efficacy of midazolam (Versed) in 28 patients with chronic "mechanical" low back pain unresponsive to prior therapy. Intrathecal midazolam (2 mg) produced improvement in pain, sleep, and activity in over 50% of the sample, which was sustained on follow-up at 2 months (119). The overall benefit was said to be comparable to epidural steroid (methyl prednisolone). Because only limited toxicity data is available for intrathecal administration of benzodiazepines, widespread investigation of this approach must await appropriate dose-toxicity studies in animal models.

The relative efficacy of benzodiazepines compared to other drugs for treatment of selected neuropathic pain syndromes is an important therapeutic issue. Controlled reports indicate that both imipramine and amitriptyline (100 mg) outperform diazepam (15 mg) (11) and lorazepam (9) in relieving painful diabetic peripheral neuropathy. Given the extensive use of benzodiazopines it is surprising that there are so few rigorous studies of their efficacy, indications, interactions with other treat-

Table 16.4.
Anti-Anxiety Agents: Populations, Experimental Design, Treatment Outcome

Authors	Population	N	Interventions	Design	Control	Dependent Measures	Follow-Up	Results
	Acute Pain							
Chapman & Feather (1973)	Experimentally induced pain in non-patients	30	Diazepam compared to aspirin & placebo	Double-blind, group outcome	Placebo and reference analgesic	Self-report of pain (0–4 scale); pain tolerance	Hours	Diazepam 10 mg orally prolongs tolerance to pain, diminishes pain-associated anxiety; does not alter sensory sensitivity
Gracely & coworkers (1978)	Experimentally induced pain in dental patients	16	Compared pain intensity and quality before and after diazepam	Group outcome within subject	Within subject, no treatment	Verbal descriptions of affective & sensory quality of pain; match hand-grip force to pain intensity	Hours	Diazepam reduced affective response to pain without altering sensory perception
Beaver & coworkers (1976)	Postoperative patients	96	Single dose of hydroxyzine alone and in combination with morphine	Double-blind, group outcome	Placebo medication	Self-reported & observer ratings of pain	Hours	Hydroxyzine 100 mg intramuscularly was superior to placebo and equivalent to morphine 8 mg; hydroxyzine analgesia additive to morphine analgesia
Hupert & coworkers (1980)	Postoperative patients	82	Compared hydroxyzine 100 mg in combination with morphine to morphine alone	Double-blind, group outcome	Morphine	Self-reported pain intensity (0–3) and pain relief (0–4)	Hours	Hydroxyzine 100 mg intramuscularly with morphine gave significantly greater analgesia than morphine alone; combination did not increase percentage of patients reporting >50% pain reduction; increased drowsiness with hydroxyzine confounded analgesia
Kantor & Steinberg (1976)	Postoperative patients		Compared oral hydroxyzine 100 mg with meperidine and placebo	Double-blind, group outcome	Placebo medication	Self-reported pain intensity	Hours	Hydroxyzine 100 mg orally equivalent to placebo
	Chronic Pain							
Lance & coworkers (1964, 1965)	Tension headache	280	Compared chlordiazepoxide, diazepam, amitriptyline, imipramine, placebo	Double-blind, group outcome	Placebo medication	Self-report of improvement	Up to 12 mos	Chlordiazepoxide and diazepam superior to placebo
Weber (1983)	Tension headache	19	Compared diazepam and placebo	Double-blind, group outcome	Placebo medication	Self-report of improvement	3 weeks	Diazepam superior to placebo in producing improvement
Yosselson-Superstine & coworkers (1985)	Mixed chronic cancer & non-cancer	9	Compared chlordiazepoxide, hydroxyzine, prochlorperazine	Double-blind, group outcome	Placebo	Self-report of pain (0–5); Multiple Adjective Affect Checklist (MAACL)	8 weeks	No overall differences between study drugs and placebo on any dependent measure; individual comparisons reveal anxiety and depression lower with chlordiazepoxide vs. placebo
Serro & coworkers (1992)	Chronic back pain	28	Compared inthrathecal midazolam to epidural steroid	Double-blind, randomized, group outcome	Epidural Prednisolone (80 mg)	Self-report of pain, sleep, activity, analgesic intake	8 weeks	Midazolam equivalent to prednisolone for pain relief, sleep, activity

ments, therapeutic mechanisms, and liabilities. Hollister suggests that benzodiazepines are rarely associated with abuse in chronic pain (118). Others argue that conventional measures such as heat, rest, and non-narcotic analgesics are as effective as diazepam, and that even high doses of this drug do not produce clinically de-tectable skeletal muscle relaxation (120). Furthermore, Hendler et al. reported significantly more evidence of cognitive impairment in chronic pain patients receiving diazepam than in those receiving narcotic analgesics (121). The clinical impact and reversibility of benzodiazepine-associated deficits in cognitive functioning, memory, and motor-perceptual performance deserve much further investigation. This is especially important because many chronic pain management programs emphasize behavioral approaches that require intact cognitive skills.

Mechanism of Action

Benzodiazepines increase the ability of gamma-aminobutyric acid (GABA) to inhibit brain and spinal cord neurotransmission; they also inhibit cholinergic and monoaminergic pathways (121). Because GABA is thought to mediate presynaptic and postsynaptic inhibition and to facilitate recurrent inhibition (121), benzodiazepines might decrease the central transmission of ascending noxious stimuli, or inhibit firing peripherally in aberrant neurons. The anxiolytic effects are mediated by poorly understood mechanisms, perhaps by inhibitory effects on the limbic system.

CENTRAL NERVOUS SYSTEM STIMULANTS

The most common stimulants now in medical use are the amphetamines (d,1 amphetamine [Benzedrine], d-amphetamine [Dexedrine], and methamphetamine [Methedrine]) and the related compound, methylphenidate (Ritalin). The amphetamines and methylphenidate are used primarily for attention-deficit disorders and hyperactivity associated with minimal brain dysfunction in children, and in narcolepsy. Cocaine has traditional use as a local anesthetic, and caffeine appears in numerous combinations with analgesics. Evidence with regard to efficacy is described in Table 16.5.

Acute Pain

Psychostimulants lack primary analgesic properties (123). Amphetamines potentiate narcotic and non-narcotic analgesia in animals (124, 125) and in man (126–128), presumably by catecholaminergic mechanisms (124). Several laboratories have demonstrated that dextroamphetamine enhances the analgesic effect of morphine in experimentally induced pain in humans (126, 127). With regard to clinical pain, a single-dose study of postoperative patients concluded that the combination of dextroamphetamine (10 mg parenterally) and morphine (10 mg) was twice as potent as morphine alone, and a combination with dextroamphetamine (5 mg) was one-and-a-half times as potent as a given dosage of morphine (128). There were minimal effects on blood pressure, pulse, and respiratory rate. Because of the study design, the effects of longer-term use of amphetamine on mood, appetite, sensorium, and other aspects of postoperative convalescence could not be addressed.

Cocaine has a long history of use as a primary abortive agent for acute cluster headache, via topical cocainization of the sphenopalatine fossa. Because the therapeutic mechanism depends on local anesthesia, conventional

topical anesthetics such as lidocaine (Xylocaine) are now preferred (129).

Caffeine may be a useful addition to NSAID analgesics. A review of the results of single-dose trials in over 10,000 patients suffering from episiotomy pain indicated that caffeine (100–200 mg orally) increased the analgesic potency of aspirin and acetaminophen by 40% (130). Oral dosages up to 600 mg/day of caffeine cause few side effects. Thus caffeine may be a useful adjunct to mild analgesics in acute pain. The basic pharmacology and clinical effects of caffeine and its relationship to pain have been recently and comprehensively reviewed by Sawynok and Yaksh (131).

Chronic Pain

Brompton's mixture, a variable combination of cocaine with morphine and a phenothiazine, has been advocated for chronic cancer pain (132). There is no systematic evidence that this combination is superior to morphine alone (133). Cocaine retards the gastrointestinal absorption of morphine; because tolerance to the sedating effects of opiates usually develops rapidly, cocaine is not required for its alerting properties.

More recently Bruera and associates conducted a placebo-controlled study in cancer patients with persistent pain and demonstrated that methylphenidate (15 mg daily) added to a regimen of narcotic analgesia decreased pain intensity by an additional 20% (134). This study evaluated patients only during a 3-day trial. Another open-label study has suggested that methylphenidate (20 mg daily) may be an effective adjunct to narcotic analgesia in cancer pain by antagonizing sedation (a frequent dose-limiting side effect) and permitting higher doses of the narcotic (135). A recommendation for general use of these adjuvants must await longer-term outcome studies assessing their effects and benefits.

There is some evidence that psychostimulants are effective antidepressants in depressed medically ill subjects. Recent anecdotal reports (136–138) indicate that dextroamphetamine (2–20 mg/day) and methylphenidate (20 mg/day) are effective antidepressants in hospitalized medically ill patients both with depressive symptoms and with major depression related to medical illness (135). Improved mood, reduced focus on pain, and renewed interest in rehabilitation occurred in about 50% of patients in 2–7 days. The major side effect was confusion, which developed in demented patients. Most patients were treated for about 1 week, although some required longer therapy.

Mechanism of Action

The mechanism of action is unclear. The therapeutic effects probably result from activation of monoamine systems important in pain suppression. Amphetamines exert their effects directly by stimulating adrenergic re-

Table 16.5.
Psychostimulants: Populations, Experimental Design, Treatment Outcome

Authors	Population	N	Interventions	Design	Control	Dependant Measures	Follow-Up	Results
	Acute Pain							
Ivy & coworkers (1944)	Experimentally induced pain in non-patients	30	Dextroamphetamine added to morphine	Double-blind, group outcome	Morphine	Self-reported pain intensity	Hours	Dextroamphetamine improved morphine analgesia
Evans (1962)	Experimentally induced pain in non-patients	24	Dextroamphetamine 10 mg added to morphine	Double-blind,	Morphine	Self-reported pain intensity	Hours	Dextroamphetamine improved morphine analgesia
Forest & coworkers (1977)	Postoperative patients	450	Single dose of dextroamphetamine 5–10 mg added to morphine	Double-blind, group outcome	Morphine	Observer- and self-rated pain intensity	Hours	Dextroamphetamine 10 mg doubled analgesic activity of morphine 10 mg
Johnstone (1974)	Postoperative patients	60	Single dose of methylphenidate	Open-label, anecdotal case studies	None	Self-reported pain intensity	Hours	Methylphenidate produced analgesia
Dodson & Fryer (1980)	Postoperative patients	63	Single dose of methylphenidate (0.4 mg/kg parenterally)	Double-blind	Placebo medication	Self-report of pain; observer-related alertness	Hours	Methylphenidate did not produce analgesia at 30 or 180 min postoperatively. Alertness improved at 30 min only
Laska & coworkers (1984)	Post-partum pain	>10,000	Caffeine added to aspirin, acetaminophen, or salicylamide	Double-blind, group outcome	Aspirin, acetaminophen, salicylamide	Self-rated pain (0–3 scale)	Hours	Caffeine 100–200 mg orally increased relative potency of analgesic by 40%
Kaufman & coworkers (1982)	Hospitalized medically ill patients with major depression secondary to illness, with and without pain	5	Dextroamphetamine or methylphenidate given daily	Open-label, case studies	None	Unspecified assessment of mood, activity, pain	4 weeks	Dextroamphetamine 2–20 mg/daily and methylphenidate 10–20 mg/daily improved mood, increased activity, and reduced pain report
Woods & coworkers (1986)	Hospitalized medically ill patients with major depression secondary to illness, with and without pain	66	Dextroamphetamine or methylphenidate given daily	Retrospective chart review	None	Clinical response of depression	1–87 days	Dextroamphetamine 2–20 mg/daily and methylphenidate improved mood, increased activity, and reduced pain report
	Chronic Pain							
Bruera & coworkers (1987)	Outpatients and inpatients with advanced cancer and chronic cancer pain	32	Methylphenidate added to narcotic analgesics	Randomized, double-blind, crossover	Placebo medication	Self-rated pain intensity; narcotic intake; self-estimate of anxiety, depression, activity	3 days	Methylphenidate 15 mg daily significantly improved analgesia and activity, decreased extra doses of narcotic, decreased sedation
Bruera & coworkers (1992)	Inpatients with Cancer pain	14	Methylphenidate added to narcotic analgesic	Open-label	None	Pain, sedation, narcotic dose		Methylphendate 20 mg reduced sedation, allowed higher dose of narcotic

ceptors, and indirectly by releasing catecholamines and inhibiting their degradation by the enzyme monoamine oxidase. Cocaine appears to inhibit the neuronal reuptake of norepinephrine, thereby potentiating the activity of this neurotransmitter. Caffeine has peripheral and CNS effects that may explain its augmentation of NSAIDs. At the periphery, extracellular levels of adenosine may be elevated following injury or local ischemia, and this may stimulate small-diameter afferents.

Caffeine is an adenosine antagonist and may attenuate such nociceptive activity. Centrally, its stimulating effects on mood may influence the perception or report of pain.

In summary, it is important to realize that this review has been conservative. It may well underestimate therapeutic effects of psychotropic agents in many pain syndromes. Several experimental factors may mask actual therapeutic effects. First, given the limits of present diagnostic methods, drug-responsive and nonresponsive subtypes of disorders may be lumped under a common name (e.g., low back pain). Benefits for responsive subtypes could be lost when overall group outcome is determined. Secondly, problems such as extreme variability of outcome scores, small sample size, or pretreatment between-group differences may obscure significant results. In addition, some drugs produce a therapeutic effect only after 6 weeks or more of treatment. Patients not followed longitudinally may appear to be treatment failures. Also, these agents may improve a variable that is not being assessed (e.g., activity level) while not altering a measured variable (e.g., mood or pain report).

In the next section, we emphasize psychopharmacologic treatments that have solid support in controlled studies, but also indicate less-proven alternatives worth exploring.

TREATMENT APPROACHES

TRICYCLIC ANTIDEPRESSANT AGENTS

The indications for tricyclic antidepressants are described in Table 16.6, and the compounds and dosages in Table 16.7.

Properties and Side Effects

Tricyclic antidepressants (TCAs) were derived from neuroleptics; imipramine, the first TCA, was a modification of chlorpromazine, and amitriptyline was derived from imipramine. These agents increase serotonergic and/or noradrenergic tone by blockade of serotonin and norepinephrine reuptake at presynaptic nerve endings, may increase norepinephrine or serotonin receptor density or sensitivity, and may reduce beta-adrenergic receptor sensitivity (139). The TCAs also have strong anticholinergic properties, producing autonomic, cardiac, and CNS side effects. Autonomic effects include dry mouth, blurred vision, constipation, ileus, and urinary retention. Cardiovascular effects include orthostatic hypotension, increased heart rate, and repolarization abnormalities on the electrocardiogram, or ECG (Q-T interval prolongation and T-wave inversion or flattening). Atrial and ventricular arrhythmias, as well as conduction delay with bundle branch block, may occur. This results from prolongation of the H-V interval, the time from activation of the bundle of His to activation of ventricular myocardium. These effects resemble the properties of Type I cardiac antiarrhythmics, such as quinidine and procainamide (140). The TCAs also can depress myocardial contractility. Central nervous system effects can include agitated states (not uncommon in elderly patients, perhaps because there is less plasma protein binding of the drug in the elderly and higher plasma concentration) and deliria caused by an anticholinergic brain syndrome. Other common side effects are

weight gain, delayed ejaculation, and impotence. Extrapyramidal symptoms are rare.

Selected Drug Interactions

Sympathomimetic Amines

Tricyclic antidepressants potentiate the pressor response of direct-acting amines such as norepinephrine, epinephrine, and phenylephrine (141), with possible hypertensive crisis characterized by hypothermia, sweating, severe headache, and cerebrovascular accident.

Neuroleptics

Because TCAs and neuroleptics compete for the same hepatic metabolic pathways, their anticholinergic and hypotensive properties may be additive or potentiated (142).

Sedative-Hypnotics

Tricyclic antidepressants increase the CNS and respiratory depressant activity of barbiturates and related sedatives (142, 143) and increase the toxicity and potential lethality of these agents.

Propranolol

Tricyclic antidepressants may potentiate propranolol-induced depression of myocardial contractility and hypotension from central vasomotor regulatory centers (143), and patients with migraine headaches treated with these combinations should be monitored closely.

Opiates

Tricyclic antidepressants potentiate meperidine-induced respiratory depression in animals (143) and increase anticholinergic activity of opiates.

Pretreatment Evaluation

Patients over the age of 50 or who have a history of cardiovascular disease (stroke, myocardial infarction, angina, congestive heart failure, syncope, or arrhythmias) should have an ECG and standing and supine blood pressure measurements before treatment. Careful assessment of the risk/benefit ratio and cardiology consultation are indicated in the presence of bradyarrhythmias, heart block, or very long Q-T intervals. Orthostatic blood pressure changes of over 10 mm Hg before drug treatment are associated with pronounced postural changes during treatment, and these patients should be carefully observed. A careful drug history should be obtained, not only to assess possible drug interactions, but to determine past response and reactions to TCAs. Additional laboratory investigation should include a complete blood count with differential and liver function tests.

Drug Selection

Amitriptyline, nortriptyline, imipramine, desipramine, and doxepin are probably equally effective in the

Table 16.6.
Diagnostic Indications for Psychotropic Drug Treatment in Acute and Chronic Pain

Treatment	Diagnosis and Clinical Efficacy	
	Relatively Well-Established Clinical Efficacy[a]	Possible Clinical Efficacy[b]
Tricyclic antidepressants	*Chronic Pain* Atypical facial pain Diabetic neuropathy Post-herpetic neuralgia Migraine headache Tension headache Mixed migraine-tension Primary major depression with secondary pain Major depression secondary to chronic pain	*Acute Pain* Augment narcotics *Chronic Pain* Thalamic pain Other neuropathic pain Augment narcotics
MAO Inhibitors	*Chronic Pain* Atypical facial pain Primary major depression with secondary pain Major depression secondary pain to chronic pain	*Chronic Pain* Migraine headache
Lithium carbonate		*Chronic Pain* Chronic cluster headache
Neuroleptics	*Acute Pain* Severe anxiety or delirium post-surgery *Chronic Pain* Psychosis with delusional pain Tension headache[c]	*Acute Pain* Acute migraine *Chronic Pain* Neuralgia-neuropathy Thalamic pain
Antianxiety agents	*Acute Pain* Acute anxiety *Chronic Pain* Tension headache	*Acute Pain* Muscular-skeletal strain *Chronic Pain* Chronic anxiety
Stimulants	*Acute Pain* Augment narcotics[c]	*Chronic Pain* Depression-pain syndromes

[a]Effectiveness established in controlled trials
[b]Effectiveness reported in open-label studies
[c]Effective but not recommended for use because of toxicity

pain syndromes for which they are indicated. Additionally, these agents all have approximately equivalent antidepressant efficacy. Drug selection therefore depends on side effects. In general, anticholinergic, cardiac, and CNS side effects are more common with tertiary amines (amitriptyline, imipramine, and doxepin) than with demethylated secondary amines (nortriptyline, desipramine, and others). Thus desipramine is the least anticholinergic and sedating of the tricyclic drugs. Patients with agitation or insomnia may benefit more from sedating drugs. There is some evidence that nortriptyline is less likely to depress H-V conduction and less likely to produce orthostatic hypotension (at the serum concentrations usually employed to treat depression) than other TCAs (144, 145). Nortriptyline may thus be preferred in patients with bradyarrhythmias, heart block, or prolonged Q-T interval. Doxepin is also thought to be relatively noncardiotoxic, but that is not

well documented. All TCAs will increase heart rate secondary to adrenergic and anticholinergic effects. Furthermore, imipramine suppresses ventricular arrhythmias (ectopy), and patients on quinidine may need their dosage of that agent revised. Newer antidepressants (e.g., the selective serotonin reuptake inhibitors) have far fewer side effects than the TCAs. The efficacy of these agents for chronic pain syndromes has not been adequately assessed. Although their antidepressant efficacy approaches that of the first-generation agents (amitriptyline and imipramine), most patients with responsive pain syndromes probably should be treated initially with a first-line drug, unless side effects preclude its use.

Treatment Technique for Acute Pain

Although desipramine may potentiate opiate analgesia in acute pain, the practical clinical significance of this is undetermined, and there is no present indication to use TCAs in acute pain.

Treatment Technique for Chronic Pain

Nondepressed Pain Patients

Initial Treatment. Patients without evidence of complicating medical or psychiatric disorders are generally started on a dose of amitriptyline or imipramine at 10–25 mg at night, with increases of 10–25 mg every 3 days to a maximum of 75 mg daily. The drug is usually given at bedtime to take advantage of any sedating effects, although doses initially may be divided if a single dose produces excessive side effects. Elderly patients or those with cardiovascular disease should receive a test dose of 10–25 mg and have orthostatic blood pressure determinations taken 1 hour later.

A therapeutic response usually ensues within 2 weeks, often within 5–7 days. Follow-up appointments are at least every week during the initial month of treatment, with orthostatic blood pressure determinations or ECGs as warranted. Every-other-week appointments are useful in the next month of therapy.

If no benefit appears within 3–4 weeks, or if side effects are unusually severe, a determination of the plasma concentration of the antidepressant is warranted. Plasma concentrations may be used to check compliance, improve efficacy, diminish toxicity, and detect unsuspected drug interactions (146). This allows the clinician to assess whether an alternative therapy is indicated, or if an increase or decrease in dose is necessary. The practitioner should use an experienced laboratory and have his own history of interpreting results from this laboratory.

The most effective plasma concentrations of antidepressants for pain syndromes generally are thought to be below those usually therapeutic for depression. Therapeutic levels for treating depression with amitriptyline are 200 ng/ml total TCA (amitriptyline plus nortriptyline); for nortriptyline there may be a therapeutic window of efficacy between 50 and 150 ng/ml. Concentrations below or above this interval may be ineffective for an antidepressant response. With imipramine, concentrations exceeding 225 ng/ml are therapeutic in depression; doxepin therapeutic concentrations are uncertain, but perhaps in the range of 150–250 ng/ml.

Blood samples drawn for plasma concentrations of antidepressants should reflect steady-state levels, and a patient's dosage should have been stabilized for at least 1 week. Samples are obtained 10–16 hours after a single dose, or 2–5 hours after the morning dose if a divided dosage regimen is employed.

Other indications for a plasma concentration include patients with cardiovascular disease, who may warrant routine plasma monitoring because of being at increased risk for toxicity.

**Table 16.7.
Commonly Used Antidepressants**

Tricyclics	Usual Daily Oral Dose in Pain Treatment (mg)	Usual Daily Antidepressant Dose (mg)
Tertiary amines		
Imipramine (Tofranil)	10–75	150–250
Amitriptyline (Elavil)	10–75	150–250
Doxepin (Sinequan)	10–75	150–250
Secondary amines		
Desipramine (Norpramin)	10–75	100–250
Nortriptyline (Aventyl)	10–75	100–150
Other		
Trazodone (Desyrel)	[NA][a]	
Monoamine oxidase inhibitors		
Tranylcypromine (Parnate)	10–30	10–30
Phenelzine (Nardil)	15–90	45–90
Lithium carbonate	300–1200	900–2400

[a]Experience insufficient to determine usage. Probably below usual antidepressant dose.

Maintenance Treatment. A positive response warrants treatment for about 5–6 months. The maintenance dose should be the minimum effective level after control is established. Attempts to discontinue the TCA should be made at 6-month intervals thereafter, because some neuropathic syndromes spontaneously remit or no longer require treatment. One important exception may be atypical facial pain, which appears to require prolonged treatment (over 1 year) to maintain relief (30). The TCA should be discontinued over a 2- to 3-week period to avoid an abstinence syndrome.

Treatment Nonresponse. An inadequate response is defined as less than 50% reduction in pain, providing there is clinical or laboratory evidence of adequate dosage, after a trial of 3–4 weeks. The antidepressant should be changed to a drug of different class (i.e., if a serotonergic agent is used first, then the switch would be a noradrenergic drug) for another trial of 3–4 weeks. Alternatively, an adjunctive neuroleptic drug may be added to the TCA regimen. (This technique is described in the section on "Neuroleptics," below.) The usual neuroleptics used are haloperidol (0.5–3 mg daily) and fluphenazine (0.5–3 mg daily). Results of adjunctive therapy should be evident within 2 weeks. If this combination therapy is unacceptable because of side effects or concerns about tardive dyskinesia, and if TCAs have not been helpful, a trial of clonazepam (usually 1–3 mg daily) may be indicated. Conventional anticonvulsants (diphenylhydantoin [Dilantin], carbamazepine [Tegretol]) are an alternative choice but require closer monitoring for plasma drug concentrations and toxicity (e.g., blood dyscrasias with carbamazepine).

Depressed Pain Patients

Initial Treatment. All depressed patients should be evaluated for suicidality and the need for hospitalization. Prescriptions for TCAs should be monitored closely according to the concern about suicide, and hospitalization may be indicated. Tricyclic antidepressant overdoses amounting to 1000 mg produce serious side effects, and overdoses of 2000 mg commonly are lethal. If the symptoms do not meet criteria for major depression, the clinician may decide to treat a TCA-responsive pain syndrome at the usual low dosages of TCA recommended for that disorder, with the view that if the patient's pain remits, so might the depressive symptoms. If the patient has major depression then full antidepressant dosages should be commenced. We usually still begin at a lower initial dosage of, say, 25 mg of imipramine and increase by 25–50 mg every 3 days to a final dose of 150–300 mg daily. Hospitalized patients may receive higher initial dosage with 50-mg increases daily up to the full amount.

An antidepressant effect is evidenced by improved activity, energy, and mood, and should appear within 3–6 weeks. Reduction of pain intensity may lag behind improvement in activity and mood by several weeks, and is not a target symptom in this instance. As above, plasma antidepressant concentrations would be indicated for a poor response after 6 weeks or if severe side effects intervene.

Maintenance Treatment. A maintenance dosage of a TCA is usually at the same dose or slightly (about 25%) lower than the acute antidepressant dosage (139). Treatment is maintained for at least 6 months (the usual length of an affective episode). The antidepressant may then be discontinued but there is evidence that extended maintenance treatment for an indefinite period is warranted, given the risk of recurrence (147). Again, tapering off a TCA regimen over several weeks is indicated to avoid an abstinence syndrome.

Treatment Nonresponse. Further treatment of the depressed pain patient who does not respond to initial therapy is a complex topic beyond the scope of this handbook. An experienced psychiatric consultation to reevaluate the diagnosis and treatment regimen is indicated. If the treatment of depression is still indicated, the choices include adding L-thyronine (Cytomel) (25–50 μg) to the TCA or switching to another antidepressant of a different class, with or without adding L-thyronine; considering electroconvulsive therapy; switching to an MAOI; or attempting combination therapy using lithium or an MAOI with a TCA (139).

Monoamine Oxidase Inhibitors

The indications for MAOIs are described in Table 16.6, and the compounds and doses in Table 16.7.

Properties and Side Effects

Monoamine oxidase inhibitors, like the TCAs, enhance the availability of norepinephrine and serotonin in the brain by inhibiting their catabolism. Antidepressant activity may also be related to effects on norepinephrine and serotonin postsynaptic receptor function or sensitivity.

Psychiatric disorders with major indications for MAOIs are agoraphobia with or without panic attacks, the so-called atypical depressive disorders with "reversed" vegetative symptoms (increased sleep, weight gain, reactive mood), and depression that has not responded to trials of TCAs. The MAOI side effect profile is similar to that of the TCAs but to a lesser degree, and includes postural hypotension, agitation, confusion, and mild anticholinergic symptoms: blurred vision, dry mouth, constipation, ileus, and urinary retention. The major issue in using these agents is the need to instruct patients to avoid foods or medications containing pressor amines. Because the MAOIs block metabolism of tyramine and other pressor amines, a hypertensive crisis may ensue after their ingestion, manifested by abrupt and severe hypertension and possible subarachnoid hemorrhage. Proscribed foods include cheese (except cottage cheese and cream cheese), pickled foods, beer and red wines, and fava beans (148).

Selected Drug Interactions

Sympathomimetic Agents

All medication with sympathomimetic activity, including phenylephrine and ephedrine (found in cold tablets), can produce a hypertensive crisis.

Narcotic Analgesics

This so-called type-I interaction is a potentiation of primary narcotic effects (including analgesia, hypotension, respiratory depression, and coma) as a result of MAOI inhibition of hepatic metabolism of narcotics (140). Naloxone (Narcan) reverses this response. Phenelzine may be safer in this regard than other MAOIs.

The type-II interaction is similar to that resulting from administration of sympathomimetic amines or tyramine to patients on MAOIs. The concurrent use of MAOIs and meperidine (149, 150) or dextromethorphan (151) produces agitation, excitement, restlessness, hypertension, headache, rigidity, and convulsions. The mechanism of this response is unknown but it may be mediated by increased brain serotonin release (152).

Codeine usually may be used safely in patients on MAOIs who require low-dose moderate analgesia (148). If other narcotics are mandatory only 20–25% of the usual therapeutic narcotic dose should be used, and vital signs and level of consciousness should be observed carefully (148). Meperidine should never be used because its interaction with MAOIs is too unpredictable and life-threatening complications can occur rapidly.

Sedative-Hypnotics

Monoamine oxidase inhibitor inhibition of microsomal enzymes prolongs the effects of sedative hypnotics, including barbiturates and chloral hydrate (153). Lower doses of sedative hypnotics and close monitoring are advised.

Pretreatment Evaluation

The physical and laboratory evaluation is similar to that used for TCAs, with a special emphasis on drug and dietary history, the patient's ability to comply with the complex dietary restrictions, and cardiovascular status.

Drug Selection

Phenelzine and tranylcypromine are the most commonly prescribed agents. Tranylcypromine is sometimes preferred because it is much shorter acting and will be out of a patient's system within a day. Phenelzine continues to inhibit MAO for over a week after it is discontinued.

Treatment Technique for Chronic Pain

Initial Treatment

Monoamine oxidase inhibitors are not the drug of first choice for any chronic pain syndrome. They are most often used in complex cases that have failed alternative treatments. It is recommended that appropriate consultations be obtained to reevaluate the patient's diagnosis at the start. Thus, neurologic consultation is indicated to confirm a diagnosis of a facial pain or migraine syndrome, and a psychiatric consultation is useful if a depressive or anxiety syndrome complicates the picture. Serious side effects from use of MAOIs are relatively rare, and their danger has probably been overstated.

Most treatment failures are secondary to inadequate dosage. The clinical end point for correct dosage is mild postural hypotension and muscle fasciculation after the second week of treatment. The usual dosage of phenelzine for initial treatment is up to 90 mg/day. Treatment begins with 15 mg on day 1, 30 mg on day 2, and 15 mg in the morning and 30 mg in the evening on day 3, if the patient is asymptomatic. A dose of 45 mg daily is maintained until day 14 if there are no side effects, and then the dosage is increased to 30 mg each morning and 30 mg in the evening. On day 21 the dosage can be increased to 30 mg in the morning, 15 mg in the afternoon, and 30 mg in the evening; on day 28 the dosage can be increased to 30 mg three times daily if there are no side effects. After adequate or maximum dosage is achieved, the patient should be monitored weekly for another 4–6 weeks (148).

Maintenance Treatment

There are few data regarding proper maintenance dosages for pain syndromes. Psychiatric patients with responsive syndromes often experience a relapse of symptoms at dosages below the initial optimal regimen (148). As with other treatments, an attempt should be made every 6 months to discontinue the medication, cutting back by 15 mg every 1–3 weeks until the patient is off the drug.

Treatment Nonresponse

Another MAOI may be used. Monoamine oxidase inhibitors have been combined with various medications, including TCAs and L-tryptophan. It is difficult to evaluate the efficacy of these combinations, and both TCAs and tryptophan may provoke a hypertensive crisis. There are no data that such combinations are useful in chronic pain syndromes. The primary indication for combination therapy would be a nonresponsive depressive disorder. A TCA is usually added cautiously to ongoing MAOI therapy.

LITHIUM

The indications for lithium treatment are described in Table 16.6, and the dosages in Table 16.7.

Properties and Side Effects

Lithium is a monovalent cation in the same group in the periodic table of elements as sodium and potassium are in. It is excreted by the kidney. The lithium ion has no known physiologic role. It has widespread effects on brain amine metabolism: it inhibits synaptic release of dopamine and norepinephrine, increases the synaptic reuptake and turnover of norepinephrine and serotonin, and inhibits CNS adenylate cyclase. It is not known whether any of these actions is associated with its therapeutic effect (139).

The major indication for the use of lithium is in psychiatric patients with bipolar affective disorder, in whom it decreases the severity and frequency of episodes.

Initial treatment is associated with transient and mild gastrointestinal side effects, including diarrhea and nausea, fine motor tremor, and somnolence. Other side effects include polyuria and polydipsia, weight gain, hypothyroidism, edema, and leukocytosis.

Central nervous system effects may include extrapyramidal symptoms, including rigidity and tremor. Cardiovascular effects are repolarization abnormalities (T-wave flattening and inversion) and inhibition of conduction at the sinoatrial node. The only cardiac contraindication is the sick sinus syndrome, wherein lithium is associated with severe bradycardia. Concern about irreversible nephrotoxic effects of lithium (interstitial fibrosis, tubular atrophy, glomerulosclerosis) appears to have been largely unwarranted.

Selected Drug Interactions

Analgesics

Phenylbutazone (Butazolidin) and indomethacin increase serum lithium levels and can provoke frank lithium toxicity. Changes in plasma lithium levels with ibuprofen (Motrin) are inconsistent and relatively minor (154). There is no reported lithium interaction with opiates, although both agents can diminish thyroid function and antagonize antidiuretic hormone.

Sedative-Hypnotics

Hydroxyzine potentiates lithium's effect on cardiac repolarization and can precipitate cardiovascular toxicity. It is recommended that this combination be avoided (155). At therapeutic lithium levels there are no reported interactions with other sedative-hypnotics.

This describes but a few of the drug interactions pertinent to lithium. More comprehensive sources should be reviewed before prescribing this agent, particularly in the medically ill pain patient (e.g., see ref. 139).

Pretreatment Evaluation

The patient's cardiovascular history should be evaluated and an ECG should be obtained. A complete blood count and measurements of electrolytes and creatinine should be obtained because lithium is fully excreted by the kidneys. Lithium toxicity most often is a result of sodium depletion, because lithium and sodium are absorbed at the same site in the proximal renal tubule. Sodium loss secondary to diarrhea, diuretics, excessive perspiration, or dehydration may produce lithium toxicity. Thyroid function tests (tri-iodothyronine, thyroxine, thyroid-stimulating hormone) should be obtained every 3–6 months. Lithium should not be prescribed to pregnant patients, especially in the first trimester, because it is associated with fetal cardiovascular abnormalities. Lithium is excreted in the breast milk in clinically significant amounts, and is a hazard to nursing infants.

Treatment Technique

Lithium is clearly a second-line agent. Its use with recurrent cluster and perhaps migraine headache syndromes have yielded the only convincing reports of its effectiveness. The patient should be instructed that close monitoring of blood levels of lithium is necessary and that therapeutic effects may not be apparent for several weeks. For headache syndromes, the dosage indicated is that needed to keep blood levels within a range of 0.4–0.8 mEq/l. The customary starting dose is 300 mg twice or three times daily. The usual total daily dosage ranges from 600–2400 mg/day, usually given in two equal divided doses. Blood samples for lithium concentration should be taken 12 hours after the last dose. At the beginning of treatment, blood levels are monitored twice weekly for several weeks, then once monthly. Af-

Table 16.8. Commonly Used Neuroleptics

Class	Relative Potency	Usual Daily Oral Dose in Pain Treatment (mg)
Phenothiazines		
Chlorpromazine (Thorazine)	Low	10–50
Methotrimeprazine (Levoprome)	Low	10–50
Thioridazine (Mellaril)	Low	10–75
Perphenazine (Trilafon)	High	1–5
Trifluoperazine (Stelazine)	High	1–5
Fluphenazine (Prolixin)	High	1–3
Butyrophenones		
Haloperidol (Haldol)	High	1–3

ter the patient has been stable for 6–12 months lithium levels may be obtained as is clinically indicated. Symptoms of lithium toxicity include emesis, diarrhea, tremor, muscle weakness, dysarthria, vertigo, ataxia, and hyper-reflexia. The elderly are particularly susceptible to toxicity, and lithium should be kept in the low therapeutic range for older patients. Lithium does not have proven effectiveness in the treatment of unipolar depression and is not indicated as an antidepressant in chronic pain patients with depressive symptoms complicating their illness.

Maintenance Treatment. In psychiatric patients treatment with lithium has been maintained for years without loss of efficacy. However, there is evidence that therapeutic efficacy decays after 1–2 years in headache syndromes. The lowest possible dose consistent with a therapeutic effect is indicated. The patient's thyroid and renal status should be monitored every 3–6 months.

Nonresponse to Treatment. Carbamazepine has been used in psychiatric patients who have not responded to lithium for bipolar disorder, and in treatment of diverse neuropathic pain disorders (156). It is unknown whether this agent is therapeutic in cyclical headache syndromes nonresponsive to lithium. Some psychiatric patients who do not benefit from lithium alone improve when a TCA, or carbidopa-levodopa (Sinemet), or bromcriptine (Parlodel) is added to lithium to augment the noradrenergic system.

NEUROLEPTIC AGENTS

The indications for neuroleptic drugs are described in Table 16.6, and the compounds and dosages in Table 16.8.

Properties and Side Effects

Neuroleptics increase the central arousal threshold by suppressing afferent sensory transmission from the periphery. The most important pharmacologic effect is widespread inhibition of dopaminergic transmission in the CNS. Blockade of the nigrostriatal system produces extrapyramidal symptoms (tremor, rigidity, bradykinesia, akathisia, and dystonia). Blockade of the tuberoinfundibular system produces hyperprolactinemia with gynecomastia and lactation, and inhibition of pituitary gonadotropins. Blockade at the chemoreceptor trigger zone of the hypothalamus produces antiemetic properties. Blockade in the limbic system and associated cortex produces antianxiety and antipsychotic effects (157).

Neuroleptics also have anti–alpha-adrenergic and anticholinergic effects. These properties are most prominent with the aliphatic agents (e.g., chlorpromazine) and less so with piperazine and piperazine agents and the butyrophenones. Cardiovascular effects include increased heart rate and dose-related postural hypotension. Repolarization abnormalities of the electrocardiogram include T-wave abnormalities, prolonged PQ-T intervals, and S-T segment depression. Direct myocardial depressant effects result in diminished myocardial contractility in patients with pre-existing cardiovascular disease. Neuroleptic agents may alter conduction times and induce potentially fatal ventricular arrhythmias. Cognitive defects on time tasks include diminished performance on tests of speed, reaction time, and accuracy.

Idiosyncratic allergic responses can occur, with suppression of the hematopoietic system (leukopenia, anemia, or thrombocytopenia). These reactions usually occur within the first 6 weeks of treatment; their clinical hallmark is the sudden onset of painful pharyngitis and fever. Similarly, an allergic hepatotoxicity with mild increases in liver function tests can occur, and cholestatic jaundice is reported.

The most commonly encountered clinical side effects are the extrapyramidal symptoms, dystonias, and tardive dyskinesia. Extrapyramidal symptoms can be managed with antiparkinsonism agents (benztropine mesylate [Cogentin], trihexphenidyl [Artane], diphenhydramine [Benadryl], or amantadine [Symmetrel]). The antiparkinsonism drug should not be given prophylactically. Extrapyramidal symptoms often do not occur, especially at the low doses of neuroleptics prescribed to pain patients, and the antiparkinsonism agent can produce adverse anticholinergic effects (toxic megacolon, toxic psychosis). If these agents are used, the usual daily dose is 1–6 mg benztropine mesylate daily or 2–10 mg trihexphenidyl daily. Because of anticholinergic toxicity, some clinicians prefer treating extrapyramidal symptoms with diphenhydramine (10–25 mg three times daily), reserving the antiparkinsonism drugs for symptoms not responsive to less-toxic agents (157). If such symptoms are treated, it is recommended that these drugs be tapered off or discontinued after 3 months.

Dystonia (tonic contraction of muscles, especially involving the head and neck, grimaces, posturing, and torticollis) rarely occurs in the low dosages used in pain patients. It can be treated with diphenhydramine (25–50 mg intramuscularly). Akathisia, the sensation of an inability to sit still, responds best to dose reduction of the offending drug (157).

Tardive dyskinesia is a syndrome of involuntary choreiform movements that commence after prolonged treatment with neuroleptics and persist for up to years after the neuroleptics are withdrawn. Symptoms can include periodic tongue protrusions, lip smacking, chewing movements of the mouth, athetoid movements of the fingers, and restless shifting from leg to leg. In their severe form such movements can be disabling. The mechanism is unknown but may involve (sometimes excessive) dopaminergic receptor supersensitivity or excessive dopaminergic activity in the basal ganglia. Treatment with various agents has been only sporadically effective. The best approach is prevention (158). Elderly patients appear to be at higher risk for this disorder. Dosages for the neuroleptics should be kept below 5 mg daily of the high-potency agents or the equivalent in the low-potency agents. Treatment should be limited to months and not years.

Selected Drug Interactions

Non-Narcotic Analgesics

There are no apparent adverse drug interactions between non-narcotic analgesics and neuroleptics, although acetaminophen inhibits chlorpromazine metabolism and therefore augments its effects.

Narcotic Analgesics

Phenothiazines enhance and prolong the hypotensive and respiratory depressant effect of narcotics. Chlorpromazine also increases serum levels of the neurotoxic and cardiotoxic N-demethylated metabolites of meperidine, which are associated with neuromuscular irritability, seizures, bradycardia, and hypotension.

Pretreatment Evaluation

The medical evaluation is the same as that for candidates for TCAs, including ECG for patients over age 50 or for those with pre-existing heart disease, and genitourinary assessment for benign prostatic hypertrophy. These drugs are metabolized by the liver, and patients with hepatic disease will need lower dosages. Laboratory assessment should include baseline complete blood count with differential, and liver function tests.

Drug Selection

Drug selection depends on the side effect profile, because these agents are generally equivalent for major therapeutic effects. The clinician need select only one neuroleptic in each classification and become thoroughly familiar with its properties and use. There is some concern that thioridazine (Mellaril) is especially cardiotoxic (159).

Treatment Techniques for Acute Pain

Generally, these agents are used only to manage severe postoperative agitation or anxiety, or disruptive behavior. In a patient with acute pain, the first task should be to assess the analgesic regimen, because agitation may be related to inadequate analgesia. Postoperative delirium must also be considered. Because of their low incidence of autonomic and cardiovascular complications, the high-potency neuroleptics (e.g., haloperidol) are generally preferred. Customary doses are 0.5–2.5 mg haloperidol orally, administered every 30 min to 1 hour until adequate sedation is achieved. As a guide to further dosage, the total dosage needed to sedate the patient is calculated. The next dose should be about one-half this total amount, given 12 hours after sedation is achieved. If severe anxiety or agitation re-emerges then this amount is given at that point. After sedation is achieved dosages can be rapidly tapered to 1–3 mg daily (160). Treatment rarely extends beyond 2 or 3 days.

Another acute indication for neuroleptics is the acute management of severe migraine attacks. Because of its sedative effects the usual agent is chlorpromazine (50–100 mg orally or intramuscularly). An acute attack is usually aborted with 1 hour.

Treatment Techniques for Chronic Pain

Initial and Maintenance Treatment

There is evidence that neuroleptics are effective for primary treatment of tension headaches, or for adjunctive treatment of neuropathic pain (e.g., post-herpetic neuralgia, diabetic neuropathy). Because of the risks of tardive dyskinesia, we avoid their use in headache syndromes and use neuroleptics only for treatment-resistant neuropathic pain. We prefer to employ neuroleptics only after a trial of two different classes of TCAs (e.g., desipramine and nortriptyline) has produced unsatisfactory relief. We add a high-potency neuroleptic to the chosen TCA. Generally we use fluphenazine or haloperidol; the starting dose is 0.5–1 mg at night, with an increase to 1 mg twice daily after 3–5 days, or to 1 mg three times daily if there is no improvement after 10 days. Once the maximum dose of 3 mg daily is reached, this is given as a one-time dose at bedtime. There should be a response within 2–3 weeks. If there is no response with a neuroleptic from one drug class (e.g., fluphenazine) the clinician may switch to an agent from a different class (e.g., haloperidol). Some authorities employ low-potency/high-dose aliphatic agents such as methotrimeprazine, a congener of chlorpromazine. The usual dosage is 50 mg or less, given once daily at bedtime (161). At present, assessing neuroleptic plasma drug concentration is not clinically useful.

The patient should be carefully monitored for symptoms of tardive dyskinesia. After 3 months, the dosage should be tapered to the lowest therapeutic amount. At no more than 6 months we taper the patient off the neuroleptic and observe for an increase in pain. If continued treatment is needed the maintenance dosage should be the lowest possible amounts, with periodic attempts to discontinue the neuroleptic.

Neuroleptics are indicated for psychiatric patients with chronic pain on a delusional basis, such as patients with paranoid schizophrenia, whose pain has been fully evaluated and is thought to represent a hallucinatory experience. The complaint is often phrased in bizarre terms (e.g., originating from electrodes implanted by the FBI, or other similar persecutory ideas). The patient with schizophrenia should be treated with a neuroleptic dosage adequate to control the major features of his psychosis. The delusion of pain may persist, but the patient's emotional distress as evidenced by this discomfort should diminish. Eradication of the delusion itself should not be the goal of therapy. Additionally, patients with multiple infarct dementia or other dementing illnesses occasionally develop complaints of pain as symptoms of depression, as psychotic delusions, or as fixed ideas upon which they persevere (162). Neuroleptics may be used in low dosages (e.g., haloperidol, 2–3 mg daily) to reduce the agitation and anxiety associated with pain complaints in demented patients. It goes without saying that physical illness is often silent and undetected in patients with schizophrenia and dementia, and all efforts should be made to determine the etiology of the patient's complaint (162).

Treatment Nonresponse

Some clinicians would prefer to use clonazepam if TCAs fail, and to avoid TCA-neuroleptic combinations. The usual dosage range is 1–3 mg daily. A response should occur within 3 weeks. If no response occurs, then a trial of a conventional anticonvulsant (e.g., diphenylhydantoin or carbamazepine) is indicated.

ANTIANXIETY DRUGS

The indications for anxiolytic drugs are described in Table 16.6, and the compounds and dosages in Table 16.9.

Benzodiazepines

Properties and Side Effects

The benzodiazepines have a broad spectrum of pharmacologic activity. Their primary effect is to enhance GABA-mediated presynaptic and postsynaptic inhibition. This action occurs in spinal cord, brainstem, cerebellar cortex, cerebral cortex, and other structures. The major properties of these drugs are their antianxiety, anticonvulsant, and sedative effects, along with an ability to produce centrally induced muscle relaxation. Like other sedatives, all benzodiazepines have the potential

Table 16.9.
Commonly Used Antianxiety Agents

Class	Usual Daily Oral Antianxiety Dose in Pain Treatment (mg)	Usual Oral Hypnotic Dose (mg)
Benzodiazepines		
Long Half-Life		
Clorazepate (Tranxene)	3–15	15–30
Flurazepam (Dalmane)	—	15–30
Intermediate Half-Life		
Chlordiazepoxide (Librium)	15–30	50
Diazepam (Valium)	2.5–15	15–30
Short Half-Life		
Alprazolam (Xanax)	0.5–3.0	—
Lorazepam (Ativan)[a]	2–5	—
Oxazepam (Serax)[a]	10–50	30–60
Other		
Hydroxyzine	100–400	—

[a]No active metabolites

to produce tolerance, psychological as well as physical dependence, and an abstinence syndrome upon withdrawal. Their effects are additive with those of other CNS depressants, and cross-tolerance and cross-dependence develop.

Sudden discontinuation of benzodiazepines after prolonged, uninterrupted use can produce an abstinence syndrome. The syndrome consist of insomnia, nausea, myalgia, muscle twitching, diaphoresis, and potentially major motor seizures. The probability of developing a withdrawal syndrome appears to vary with the length of treatment: patients treated for less than 4 months at the usual therapeutic dosage are unlikely to develop symptoms; about 5% of those treated for up to 1 year may develop symptoms; and those treated for over 1 year run a much higher risk (163).

The most common side effects are sedation, ataxia, and dysarthria. In the elderly these agents may produce confusion and paradoxical excitement. Teratogenic effects (i.e., cleft palate) during pregnancy are postulated but are not thoroughly documented. There are few autonomic side effects, although bradycardia and hypotension can occur. Allergic phenomena are also reported, and include neutropenia and jaundice.

Drug Interactions

The most important interactions involve additive effects with other CNS depressants. Cimetidine (Tagamet), disulfiram (Antabuse), and oral contraceptives can increase the half-life of benzodiazepines.

Pretreatment Evaluation

In patients for whom benzodiazepines are acutely indicated the major concern is for the patient's ability to tolerate the CNS depressive effects of the drug. The major concern in candidates for prolonged treatment is misuse or abuse. Elderly patients are particularly at risk for falls but also for intoxication and ataxia as well as for acute confusional episodes. Such side effects may occur at relatively low dosages because of the elderly patient's reduced rate of drug metabolism and reduced protein binding. A cardiovascular history and ECG should be obtained as indicated: benzodiazepine withdrawal can precipitate angina, elevated blood pressure, or cardiac arrhythmias. Liver function tests should be obtained; patients with liver disease may require a diminished dose.

Drug Selection

All benzodiazepines have similar anxiolytic properties, side effect profiles, and potential for dependency and abuse. They differ mainly in their elimination half-life and presence of active metabolites. Those with the longest half-lives are clorazepate (Tranxene), parzepam (Centrax), and halazepam (Paxipam). Moderately long-acting agents are diazepam and chlordiazepoxide. The shortest-acting are oxazepam (Serax), lorazepam (Ativan), and alprazolam (Xanax). All these drugs have clinically important active metabolites except for oxazepam and lorazepam. The duration of action reflects the presence of active metabolites. Cumulative clinical effects occur with repeated dosage. If drug accumulation or prolonged effects are problems (as in elderly patients or those with hepatic disease), short-acting agents with no active metabolites may be preferred. The problems of drug accumulation also can be met by reducing the dosage of longer-acting drugs. Again, the best clinical practice is to choose one or two agents and learn to employ them effectively. Overall the benzodiazepines have a good margin of safety. By themselves they are unlikely to be lethal in overdoses. Nevertheless their depressant effects are dangerous if they are taken with alcohol, barbiturates, or other drugs that depress the CNS.

Treatment Technique for Acute Pain

In acute pain the indication is for severe postoperative anxiety or acute musculoskeletal strain.

Acute postoperative anxiety often indicates insufficient analgesia. Assuming analgesia is adequate, situational acute fearfulness usually responds to lorazepam (0.5–1.0 mg orally) or diazepam (5–20 mg orally). This will usually produce an anxiolytic effect within 1 hour. If repeated dosage is necessary, the physician can follow the regimen described earlier for titration of antipsychotic drugs in the surgical patient. Diazepam is given each hour; the total dosage needed to produce sedation is calculated; then one-half that dosage is given approximately 12 hours later, or at the time anxiety returns. The drug is then tapered rapidly over the next few days. Most patients will do well on lorazepam (0.5–1 mg three times daily) or diazepam (5 mg two or three times daily). If treatment is needed beyond several days, the dosage required can usually be given once at bedtime: there will be an initial sedative effect, and because of the drug's prolonged half-life, an extended anxiolytic effect will persist throughout the following day. For the acute medical setting some authorities prefer a short-acting agent with no active metabolites, such as oxazepam (15 mg four times daily). Diazepam and chlordiazepoxide should be given orally or intravenously because intramuscular absorption is erratic and incomplete.

For the pain associated with muscle spasm, sedation with attendant muscle-relaxing effects can usually be achieved with diazepam (5–10 mg twice to three times daily). Treatment rarely extends beyond 2 weeks.

Treatment Techniques for Chronic Pain

Initial and Maintenance Treatment. Trigeminal neuralgia may be responsive to clonazepam. The usual dosage is 1–3 mg daily; a therapeutic effect is usually evident within 2 weeks. A major problem for many patients, particularly the elderly, has been oversedation on the dosage required for a therapeutic effect (117). Maintenance treatment is not well described, but probably should follow guidelines offered for other therapy of neuropathic pain. The lowest therapeutic dose should be maintained for 3–6 months; then an attempt to slowly discontinue the drug may be entertained.

Anxiety as a Special Problem. Many patients with chronic pain appear to be acutely or chronically anxious as well. Chronic tension headaches and chronic back or neck pain, presumably related to painful muscular contraction, are two common clinical examples. We rarely employ antianxiety agents for these patients. Yet if anxiety is believed to be the major etiology of functional disability or of pain, and the clinician decides to institute treatment, then therapy should follow the principles outlined by Hollister (164) and others (165) for the proper use of benzodiazepines. Seven guidelines have been described (164): (1) use benzodiazepines only when indicated; (2) use nondrug methods when possible; (3) drug treatment should be brief and intermittent; (4) doses should be titrated individually; (5) efficacy should be assessed early; (6) avoid benzodiazepines if a history of drug abuse is known; and (7) gradually discontinue the drug after chronic treatment. This approach allows the physician to avoid the pitfalls of overprescribing.

Treatment with benzodiazepines is indicated when anxiety interferes with the patient's performing his usual activities. Nonpharmacologic measures for managing anxiety include psychotherapy, exercise programs, relaxation training, and biofeedback. These methods are often components of a comprehensive pain management program, and can help reduce reliance on anxiolytics.

Ideal drug treatment is intermittent and brief. Most anxiety related to life stress is resolved within 1 month. Chronic anxiety, like chronic pain, waxes and wanes in intensity. Anxiolytics would be used only during exacerbations of the patient's chronic disorder. In any event, chronically anxious patients should not be treated indefinitely without assessing the need for continuous treatment. If prolonged therapy is needed, the lowest possible dosage consistent with efficacy should be used. In both acutely or chronically anxious individuals, a drug response generally occurs within the first 2–3 weeks of treatment, because state anxiety is usually more responsive then trait anxiety (165). Therefore if there is no improvement after several weeks on the proper regimen, then benefit is unlikely with prolonged therapy, and other avenues should be explored. If anxiety is relieved the physician can propose that the drug be discontinued, and reinstituted if symptoms return. Thus tolerance and dependence are avoided (164).

Dose titration involves determining the minimum amount of drug necessary to produce mild sedation. Hollister recommended initiating treatment at night, 2–3 hours before normal bedtime (164). The minimum effective dose is determined as the amount required to produce restful sleep when taken 2–3 hours before bedtime. If the initial dose does not produce effective hypnosis the first night, twice the dose is given the second night, four times the dose is given the third night, and eight times the dose is given the fourth night. The patient can commence with 2.5 mg diazepam and then increase to 5 mg, or 10 mg, or 20 mg. The usual minimum effective hypnotic dose is 10 mg or less. As a result, the patient achieves a good night's rest, unwanted oversedation is avoided during the daytime, and the anxiolytic effect is retained. If additional amounts are required during the day, usually one-half or one-third of the night-time dose will suffice. This approach works best for long-acting benzodiazepines and is not suited for short-acting agents.

Treatment efficacy should be assessed within 3 weeks. Failure to respond may indicate an inadequate dosage regimen, or a misdiagnosis. For example, anxiety frequently accompanies depressive syndromes, and an antidepressant would be required to successfully treat this disorder. Alcohol abuse may also be present, and treatment may be undermined by the patient's tolerance to CNS depressants (164).

Patients with a past history of abuse of alcohol or other CNS depressants generally are not good candidates for benzodiazepines. Some authorities recommend short-term treatment with agents less likely to be abused, such as hydroxyzine.

Maintenance Treatment for Anxiety. Some chronically anxious patients may benefit from long-term treatment. Again the minimum effective dose should be used; reevaluation of the regimen should occur at least every 6

Table 16.10.
Commonly Used Psychostimulants

Agent	Usual Daily Antidepressant and Pain-Management Dose (mg)
d-Amphetamine (Dexedrine)	10–20
Methylphenidate (Ritalin)	15–20

months. Tolerance to anxiolytic effects may not occur. The clinician should be alert to requests for escalating the dose.

Patients who have been treated for more than 4 months with diazepam (20–40 mg daily) (or the equivalent) should have the drug withdrawn slowly, usually over 4–6 weeks.

Buspirone (BuSpar) is a new anxiolytic chemically and pharmacologically unrelated to the benzodiazepines. Because maximum benefit emerges only after 3–4 weeks of treatment, it is advocated for chronic anxiety. Preliminary data indicate it has few CNS side effects. Its abuse potential is unknown.

CENTRAL NERVOUS SYSTEM STIMULANTS

Indications for psychostimulants are described in Table 16.6, and the compounds and dosages in Table 16.10.

Properties and Side Effects

Central nervous system stimulants include d,l-amphetamine (Dexedrine), methylphenidate (Ritalin), and pemoline (Cylert). They are rapidly absorbed orally. Methylphenidate has a half-life of 2–7 hours; dextroamphetamine's is 4–21 hours. They are metabolized by hepatic oxidation and conjugating enzyme systems and also are excreted unchanged in the urine. They produce cerebral stimulation and arousal by decreasing neuronal reuptake and deactivation of norepinephrine and dopamine. Physiologic dependence does not seem to occur in the same sense as with CNS depressants, although a withdrawal syndrome of inertia and depressed mood appears upon sudden withdrawal after high intake. Tolerance to euphoriant effects occurs rapidly (139). Side effects are those of anorexia, plus sympathomimetic actions. Other untoward effects include catatonia (mute and bizarre behavior), paranoid reactions, and confusion (166). These agents generally are thought to have fewer cardiovascular side effects (e.g., bundle branch block) than TCAs.

Drug Interactions

The ability of psychostimulants to compete for hepatic enzymes reduces the metabolization of TCAs, neuroleptics, antianxiety agents, and many other drugs. There are additive effects with other sympathomimetic drugs.

Pretreatment Evaluation

Patients over age 50 years and those with a history of hypertension or cardiovascular disease are at increased risk for the drug's sympathomimetic effects, and risk/benefit ratios must be carefully appraised. The elderly are particularly vulnerable to acute agitation or confusion. History of substance abuse must be elicited.

Drug Selection

There are few data available to help distinguish among the psychostimulants. Methylphenidate and pemoline may be less subject to abuse than are amphetamines (139). Because of its short half-life methylphenidate may be preferred in the elderly, to reduce duration of any toxic effects.

Initial and Maintenance Treatment for Acute and Chronic Pain

The CNS stimulants have limited use in management of acute or chronic pain. Although they augment narcotic analgesia acutely, there really seems to be little advantage to these drugs because simply increasing the dose of analgesic accomplishes the desired goal.

These agents are not recommended for first-line routine use in depressed pain patients because of their limited efficacy and risk of increasing agitation (139). If a TCA is contraindicated in a pain patient with major depression, then a CNS stimulant may be employed. For pain control or depression the initial dose of dextroamphetamine or methylphenidate is usually 5–10 mg each morning. With its longer half-life dextroamphetamine may be given once daily, whereas methylphenidate is administered in two divided doses at 8 AM and at noon. If no response occurs after 2 days, the dose is increased, but more than 20 mg daily is rarely required (138). A response should ensue by 7–10 days.

Maintenance treatment is not well described, and rarely extends beyond several weeks. Reports usually indicate that the agent is discontinued a few days after the patient becomes asymptomatic (138). Given the controversial nature of treatment with CNS stimulants the physician should carefully document his reasons for employing these drugs and his explanation to the patient of side effects and the risk/benefit ratio. Treatment should be brief, prescription quantities limited in size, and follow-up frequent.

CONCLUSIONS

Pain is a multidimensional phenomenon. We know little about the basic mechanisms that produce or perpetuate the sensory component of pain following tissue damage, or of mechanisms relevant to the affective or behavioral response to the pain experience. A better understanding of these mechanisms is necessary to design specific and more effective psychopharmacologic treatments.

Four issues must be addressed to ensure appropriate use of psychotropic agents. First, as clear an understanding as is possible of the etiology of pain must be established to identify drug-responsive pain syndromes. Psychiatric disorders contributing to pain or disability must also be accurately diagnosed so that appropriate psychiatric target symptoms can be selected for treatment. Second, detoxification from excessive regimens of analgesics or sedative-hypnotic medications is essential for evaluating perceived pain, functional capacity, and treatment outcome. Third, psychopharmacologic medications are adjunctive treatment, and are not a substitute for a comprehensive treatment plan agreed upon with the patient, involving education, physical reconditioning, behavioral assessment, and evaluation of family and occupational roles. Fourth, few studies reporting initial therapeutic gains follow patients beyond the first weeks of treatment. This means that meticulous follow-up is necessary to detect recurrent symptoms or discontinue ineffective treatments. Psychopharmacologic treatment is effective if it leads to observable improvement in daily function or psychological symptoms, or to diminished use of analgesics or other medical resources.

ACKNOWLEDGEMENT Supported in part by the Department of Veterans Affairs, and by the National Institutes of Health General Clinical Research Centers Program (M01RR00827).

REFERENCES

1. American Psychiatric Association: *Diagnostic and Statistical Manual,* ed 3 revised. Washington, D.C., American Psychiatric Association Press, 1987.
2. Saarnivaara L, Mattila MJ: Comparison of tricyclic antidepressants in rabbits: Antinociception and potentiation of the noradrenaline pressor responses. *Psychopharmacology* 35:221–236, 1974.
3. Chapman CR, Butler SH: Effects of doxepin on perception of laboratory-induced pain in man. *Pain* 5:253–262, 1978.
4. Bromm B, Meier W, Scharein E: Imipramine reduces experimental pain. *Pain* 25:245–257, 1986.
5. Levine JD, Gordon NC, Smith R, McBryde R: Desipramine enhances opiate postoperative analgesia. *Pain* 27:45–49, 1986.
6. Goodkin K, Gullion C: Antidepressants for the relief of chronic pain: Do they work? *Ann Behav Med* 11:83–101, 1989.
7. Watson CP, Evans RJ, Reed K, Merskey H, Goldsmith L, Warsh J: Amitriptyline versus placebo in postherpetic neuralgia. *Neurology* 32:671–673, 1982.
8. Watson CPN, Chipman M, Reed K, Evans RJ, Burkett N: Amitriptyline versus maprotiline in postherpetic neuralgia: a randomized, double-blind, crossover trial. *Pain* 48:29–36, 1992.
9. Max MB, Schafer RNC, Culhane M, Smoller B, Dubner R,

Gracely RH: Amitriptyline, but not lorazepam, relieves post herpetic neuralgia. *Neurology* 38:1427–1432, 1988.
10. Kishore-Kumar R, Max, MB, Schafer SC, Gaughan AM, Smoller B, Gracely RM, Dubner R: Desipramine relieves postherpetic neuralgia. *Clin Pharmacol Ther* 47:305–12, 1990.
11. Kvinesdal B, Molin J, Froland A, Gram LF: Imipramine treatment of painful diabetic neuropathy. *JAMA* 251: 1727–1730, 1984.
12. Turkington RW: Depression masquerading as diabetic neuropathy. *JAMA* 243:1147–1150, 1980.
13. Max MB, Lynch SA, Muir J, Shoaf SE, Smoller B, Dubner R: Effects of desipramine, amitriptyline and fluoxetine on pain in diabetic neruopathy. *N Engl J Med* 326:1250–1256, 1992.
14. Sindrup SH, Gram LF, Brosen K, Eshoj O, Mogensen EF: The selective serotonin reuptake inhibitor paroxetine is effective in the treatment of diabetic neuropathy symptoms. *Pain* 42:135–144, 1990.
15. Kocher R: Use of psychotropic drugs for treatment of chronic severe pain. In Bonica, JJ, Albe-Fessard D (eds): *Advances in Pain Research and Therapy,* vol. 1. New York, Raven Press, 1976, pp 579–582.
16. Bourhis A, Boudouresque G, Pellet W: Pain infirmity and psychotropic drugs in oncology. *Pain* 5:263–274, 1978.
17. Couch JR, Hassanein RS: Amitriptyline in migraine prophylaxis. *Arch Neurol* 36:695–699, 1979.
18. Mathew NT: Prophylaxis of migraine and mixed headache. A randomized controlled study. *Headache* 21:105–109, 1981.
19. Friedman AP: The migraine syndrome. *Bull N Y Acad Med* 44:45–62, 1968.
20. Mahloudji M: Prevention of migraine. *Br Med J* 1:182–183, 1969.
21. Gomersall JD, Stuard A: Amitriptyline in migraine prophylaxis. *J Neurol Neurosurg Psychiatry* 36:648–690, 1973.
22. Lance JW, Curran DA: Treatment of chronic tension headache. *Lancet* 1:1236–1239, 1964.
23. Lance JW, Curran DA, Anthony M: Investigations into the mechanism and treatment of chronic headache. *Med J Aust* 2:909–914, 1965.
24. Okasha A, Ghaleb HA, Sadek A: A double-blind trial for the clinical management of psychogenic headache. *Br J Psychiatry* 122:181–183, 1973.
25. Langemark M, Loldrup D, Bech P, Olesen J: Clomipramine and mianserin in the treatment of chronic tension headache. A doubleblind controlled study. *Headache* 30:118–121, 1990.
26. Sternbach RA: *Pain patients: Traits and treatment.* New York, Academic Press, 1974.
27. Ward NG, Bloom VL, Friedel RC: The effectiveness of tricyclic antidepressants in the treatment of coexisting pain and depression. *Pain* 7:331–341, 1979.
28. Lindsay PG, Wyckoff M: The depression-pain syndrome and its response to antidepressants. *Psychosomatics* 22:571–577, 1981.
29. Raskin NH, Appenzeller C (eds): *Headache.* Philadelphia, WB Saunders, 1980.
30. Feinmann C, Harris M, Cawley R: Psychogenic pain: Presentation and treatment. *Br Med J* 28:436–438, 1984.

31. Ward NG: Tricyclic antidepressants for chronic low back pain. *Spine* 11:661–665, 1986.
32. Alcoff J, Jones E, Rust P, Newman R: Controlled trial of imipramine for chronic low back pain. *J Fam Pract* 14:841–846, 1982.
33. Hameroff SR, Cork RC, Scherer K, Crago BR, Neuman C, Womble JK, Davis TP: Doxepin effects on chronic pain, depression and plasma opioids. *J Clin Psychiatry* 43:22–27, 1982.
34. Pheasant H, Bursk A, Goldfarb J, Azen SP, Weiss JN, Borelli L: Amitriptyline and chronic low back pain. *Spine* 8:552–557, 1983.
35. Sternbach RA, Janowsky DS, Huey LY, Segal DS: Effects of altering brain serotonin activity on human chronic pain. In Bonica, JJ, Albe-Fessard D (eds): *Advances in Pain Research and Therapy,* vol. 1. New York, Raven Press, 1976, pp 601–606.
36. Jenkins DG, Ebbutt AF, Evans CD: Tofranil in the treatment of low back pain. *J Int Med Res* 4(Suppl 2):28–40, 1976.
37. Goodkin K, Gullion CM, Agras WS: A randomized, doubleblind, placebo-controlled trial of trazodone hydrochloride in chronic low back pain. *J Clin Psychopharmacol* 10: 269–278, 1990.
38. Butler SH, Weil-Fugazza J, Godefoy F, Besson J-M: Reduction of arthritis and pain behavior following chronic administration of amitriptyline or imipramine in rats with adjuvant-induced arthritis. *Pain* 23:159–175, 1985.
39. MacNeill AL, Dick WC: Imipramine and rheumatoid factor. *J Int Med Res* 4(Suppl 2):23–27, 1976.
40. Gringas M: A clinical trial of Tofranil in rheumatic pain in general practice. *J Int Med Res* 4 (Suppl 2):41–45, 1976.
41. McDonald Scott WA: The relief of pain with an antidepressant in arthritis. *Practitioner* 202:802–805, 1969.
42. Cardette S, McCain GA, Bell DA, Fam AL: Evaluation of amitriptyline in primary fibrositis. A double blind, placebo-enrolled study. *Arthritis Rheum* 29:(5) 655–659, 1986.
43. Goldenberg DL, Felson DT, Dinerman H: A randomized controlled trial of amitriptyline and naproxen in the treatment of patients with fibromyaisia. *Arthritis Rheum* 29:(11) 1371–1377, 1986.
44. Pilowsky I, Hallett EC, Bassett DL, Thomas PG, Penhall RK: A controlled study of amitriptyline in the treatment of chronic pain. *Pain* 14:169–179, 1982.
45. Blumer D, Heilbronn M, Pedraza E, Pope G: Systematic treatment of chronic pain with antidepressants. *Henry Ford Hosp Med J* 28:15–21, 1980.
46. Singh G, Verma HC: Drug treatment of chronic intractable pain in patients referred to a psychiatry clinic. *J Ind Med Assoc* 56:341–345, 1971.
47. Lindsay PG, Olsen RB: Maprotiline in pain-depression. *J Clin Psychiatry* 46:226–228, 1985.
48. Malseed R, Goldstein FJ: Enhancement of morphine analgesia by tricyclic antidepressants. *Neuropharmacology* 18:827–829, 1979.
49. Liu SJ, Wang RIH: Increased analgesia and alterations in distribution and metabolism of methadone by desipramine in rats. *J Pharmacol Exp Ther* 195:94–104, 1975.
50. Gonzalez JP, Sewell RDE, Spencer PSJ: Antiociceptive activity of opiates in the presence of the antidepressant agent nomifensine. *Neuropharmacology* 19:613–618, 1980.
51. France RD, Urban BJ, Keefe FJ: Long-term use of narcotic analgesics in chronic pain. *Soc Sci Med* 19:1379–1382, 1984.
52. Urban BJ, France RD, Steinberger EK, Scott DL, Maltbie AA: Long-term use of narcotic/antidepressant medication in the management of phantom limb pain. *Pain* 24:191–196, 1986.
53. Pagni CA. Central pain due to spinal cord and brain stem damage. In Wall, PD, Melzack, R, eds. *Textbook of Pain.* London, Churchill Livingstone, 1984, pp 481–495.
54. Anderson LS, Black RG, Abraham J, Ward AA: Neuronal hyperactivity in experimental trigeminal deafferentation. *J Neurosurg* 35:444–452, 1971.
55. Loeser JD, Ward AA, White LE: Chronic deafferentation of human spinal cord neurons. *J Neurosurg* 29:48–50.1968.
56. Anthony M, Lance JW: Monoamine oxidase inhibitors in the treatment of migraine. *Arch Neurol* 21:263–268, 1969.
57. Medina JL: Cyclic migraine: A disorder responsive to lithium carbonate. *Psychosomatics* 23:625–637, 1982.
58. Medina JL, Diamond S: Cyclical migraine. *Arch Neurol* 38:343–344, 1981.
59. Lascelles RG: Atypical facial pain and depression. *Br J Psychiatry* 112:651–659, 1966.
60. Raft D, Davidson J, Wasik J, Mattox A: Relationship between response to phenelzine and MAO inhibition in a clinical trial of phenelzine, amitriptyline and placebo. *Neuropsychobiology* 7:122–126, 1981.
61. Yung CY: A review of clinical trials of lithium in neurology. *Pharmacol Biochem Behav* 21(Suppl 1):57–64, 1984.
62. Nieper HA: The clinical applications of lithium orotate. A two year study. *Agressologie* 14:407–411, 1973.
63. Chazot G, Chauplannaz G, Biron A, Schott B: Migraines: Treatment per lithium. *Nouv Presse Med* 8:2836–2837, 1979.
64. Peatfield RC, Rose FC: Exacerbation of migraine by treatment with lithium. *Headache* 21:140–142, 1981.
65. Damasio H, Lyon L: Lithium carbonate in the treatment of cluster headaches. *J Neurol* 224:1–8, 1980.
66. Ekbom K: Lithium for cluster headache: Review of the literature and preliminary results of long-term treatment. *Headache* 21:132–139, 1981.
67. Medina JL, Fareed J, Diamond S: Blood amines and platelet changes during treatment of cluster headache with lithium and other drugs. *Headache* 18:112, 1978.
68. Kudrow L: Lithium prophylaxis for chronic cluster headache. *Headache* 17:15–18, 1977.
69. Mathew NT: Clinical subtypes of cluster headaches and response to lithium therapy. *Headache* 18:26–30, 1978.
70. Peatfield RC: Lithium in migraine and cluster headache: A review. *J R Soc Med* 74:432–436, 1981.
71. Moore J, Dundee JW: Alterations in response to somatic pain associated with anaesthesia, Part VII: The effects of nine phenothiazine derivatives. *Br J Anaesth* 33:422–431, 1961.
72. Dundee JW, Love WJ, Moore J: Alterations in response to somatic pain associated with anaesthesia, Part XV: Further studies with phenothiazine derivatives and similar drugs. *Br J Anaesth* 35:597–609, 1963.
73. Moore J, Dundee JW: Alterations in response to somatic pain associated with anaesthesia, Part V: The effect of promethazine. *Br J Anaesth* 33:3–8, 1961.

74. Dundee JW, Moore J: Alterations in response to somatic pain associated with anaesthesia, I: An evaluation of a method of analgesimetry. *Br J Anaesth* 32:396–406, 1960.

75. Siker ES, Wolfson B, Stewart WD, Schaner PJ: The earlobe algesimeter, Part 2: The effect on pain threshold of certain phenothiazine derivatives alone or combined with meperidine. *Anesthesiology* 27:497–500, 1966.

76. Lasagna L, DeKornfeld TJ: Methotrimeprazine—A new phenothiazine derivative with analgesic properties. *JAMA* 178:887–890, 1961.

77. Minuck R: Postoperative analgesia—Comparison of methotrimeprazine and meperidine as postoperative analgesia agents. *Can Anaesth Soc J* 19:87–96, 1972.

78. Keats AS, Telford J, Kurosu Y: "Potentiation" of meperidine by promethazine. *Anesthesiology* 22:34–41, 1966.

79. McZuitty FM: Relief of pain in labour. *J Obstet Gynaecol Br Commonw* 74:925–928, 1967.

80. Powe CE, Kiem IM, Fromhagen C, Cavanagh D: Propiomazine hydrochloride in obstetrical analgesia. *JAMA* 181:290–294, 1962.

81. Jackson GL, Smith DA: Analgesia properties of mixtures of chlorpromazine with morphine and meperidine. *Ann Intern Med* 45:640–652, 1956.

82. Bromm B, Seide K: The influence of tilidine and prazepam on withdrawal reflex, skin resistance reaction and pain rating in man. *Pain* 12:247–258, 1982.

83. Wolff BB, Kantor TG, Jarvik ME, et al: Response of experimental pain to analgesic drugs. I. Morphine, aspirin, and placebo. *Clin Pharmacol Ther* 1:224–238, 1966.

84. Baldessarini RJ: Drugs in the treatment of psychiatric disorders. In Gilman, AG, Goodman, LS, eds. *The Pharmacological Basis of Therapeutics,* ed 7. New York, Macmillan, 1985, pp 387–445,.

85. Hakkarainen H. Fluphenazine for tension headache: A double-blind study. *Headache* 17:216–218, 1977.

86. Caviness VS, O'Brien P: Cluster headache: Response to chlorpromazine. *Headache* 22:128–131, 1980.

87. Iserson KV: Parenteral chlorpromazine treatment of migraine. *Ann Emerg Med* 12:756–758, 1983.

88. Taub A: Relief of post-herpetic neuralgia with psychotropic drugs. *J Neurosurg* 39:235–239, 1973.

89. Merskey H, Hester RA: The treatment of chronic pain with psychotropic drugs. *Postgrad Med J* 48:594–598, 1972.

90. Moertel CG, Ahmann DL, Taylor WF, Schwartau N: Relief of pain by oral medications. *JAMA* 229:55–59, 1974.

91. Houde RW, Wallenstein SL: Analgetic power of chlorpromazine alone and in combination with morphine. *Fed Proc* 14:353, 1955.

92. Sadove MS, Levin MJ, Rose RF: Chlorpromazine and narcotics in the management of pain of malignant lesions. *JAMA* 155:626, 1954.

93. Beaver WT, Wallenstein SL, Houde RW, Schwartau N: A comparison of the analgesic effect of methotrimeprazine and morphine in patients with cancer. *Clin Pharmacol Ther* 7:436–446, 1966.

94. Sigwald J, Bouther D, Solignal P: L'action antalguque des phenothiazines. *Therapie* 14:978–984, 1958.

95. Moertel CG, Ahmann DL, Taylor WF: A comparative evaluation of marketed analgesic drugs. *N Engl J Med* 286:813–815, 1972.

96. Head M, Lal H, Puri S: Enhancement of morphine anal-

gesia after acute and chronic haloperidol. *Life Sci* 24:2037–2043, 1979.

97. Cavenar JO Jr, Maltbie AA: Another indication for haloperidol. *Psychosomatics* 17:128, 1976.

98. Daw JL, Cohen-Cole S: Haloperidol analgesia. *South Med J* 74:364–365, 1981.

99. Maltbie AA, Cavenar JO Jr: Haloperidol and analgesia. *Milt Med* 142:946–948, 1977.

100. Maltbie AA, Cavenar JO Jr, Sullivan JL, et al: Analgesia and haloperidol: A hypothesis. *J Clin Psychiatry* 40:323–326, 1979.

101. Maltbie AA, Cavenar JO Jr, Hammett EB: Treatment of pain syndromes with haloperidol. *North Carolina J Ment Health* 8: 50, 1977.

102. Montilla E, Frederik WS, Cass IJ: Analgesic effects of methotrimeprazine and morphine. *Arch Intern Med* 111:725–728, 1963.

103. McGee JL, Alexander MR: Phenothiazine analgesia—Fact or fantasy. *Am J Hosp Pharm* 36:633–640, 1979.

104. Porter J, Jick H: Addiction rare in patients treated with narcotics. *N Engl J Med* 302:123, 1980.

105. Chapman CR, Feather BW: Effects of diazepam on human pain tolerance and pain sensitivity. *Psychosom Med* 35:330–340, 1973.

106. Gracely RH, McGrath P, Dubner R: Validity and sensitivity of sensory and affective verbal pain descriptors: Manipulation of affect by diazepam. *Pain* 5:19–29, 1978.

107. Kantor TG, Steinburg FP: Studies of tranquillizing agents (hydroxyzine and meprobamate) and meperidine in clinical pain. In Bonica JJ, Alge-Fessard D (eds): *Advances in Pain Research and Therapy,* vol 1. New York, Raven Press, 1976, pp 507–572.

108. Stambaugh JE, Wainer IW: Metabolic studies of the interaction of meperidine and hydroxyzine in human subjects. In Bonica JJ, Alge-Fessard D (eds): *Advances in Pain Research and Therapy,* vol 1. New York, Raven Press, 1976, pp 559–565.

109. Beaver WT, Feise G: A comparison of the analgesic effects of morphine, hydroxyzine and their combination in patients with post-operative pain. In Bonica JJ, Alge-Fessard D (eds): *Advances in Pain Research and Therapy,* vol 1. New York, Raven Press, 1976, pp 553–557.

110. Hupert C, Yacoub M, Turgeon LR: Effect of hydroxyzine on morphine analgesia for the treatment of postoperative pain. *Anesth Analg* 59:690–696, 1980.

111. Weber MB: The treatment of muscle contraction headaches with diazepam. *Curr Ther Res* 15:210–216, 1973.

112. Yosselson-Superstine S, Lipman AG, Sanders SH: Adjunctive anti-anxiety agents in the management of chronic pain. *Israeli J Med Sci* 21:113–117, 1985.

113. Caccia MR: Clonazepam in facial neuralgia and cluster headache. Clinical and electrophysiological study. *Eur Neurol* 13:560–563, 1975.

114. Smirne S, Scarlato G: Clonazepam in cranial neuralgias. *Med J Aust* 1:93–94, 1977.

115. Swerdlow M, Cundill JG: Anticonvulsant drugs used in the treatment of lancinating pain. A comparison. *Anesthesia* 36:1129–1132, 1981.

116. Martin G: Recurrent pain of a pseudotabetic variety after laminectomy for lumbar disc lesion. *J Neurol Neurosurg Psychiatry* 43:283–286, 1980.

117. Maciewicz R, Bouckoms A, Martin JB: Drug therapy of neuropathic pain. *Clin J Pain* 1:39–49, 1985.

118. Hollister LE, Conley FK, Britt RH, Shuer L: Long-term use of diazepam. *JAMA* 246:1568–1570, 1981.

119. Serrao JM, Marks RL, Morley SJ, Goodchild CS: Intrathecal midazolam for the treatment of chronic mechanical low back pain: A controlled comparison with epidural steroid in a pilot study. *Pain* 48:5–12, 1992.

120. Greenblatt DJ, Shader RI, Abernathy DR: Current status of benzodiazepines. *N Engl J Med* 309:410–416, 1983.

121. Hendler N, Cimi C, Terence MA, Long D: A comparison of cognitive impairment due to benzodiazepines and to narcotics. *Am J Psychiatry* 137:828–830, 1980.

122. Haefely WE: Behavioral and neuropharmacological aspects of drugs used in anxiety and related states. In Lipton, MA, DiMascio A, Killam KF (eds): *Psychopharmacology: A Generation of Progress.* New York, Raven Press, 1978, pp 1359–1374.

123. Goetzl FR, Burrill DY, Ivy AC: The analgesic effect of morphine alone and in combination with dextroamphetamines. *Proc Soc Exp Biol Med* 55:248–250, 1944.

124. Notl MW: Potentiation of morphine analgesia by cocaine in mice. *Eur J Pharmacol* 5:93–99. 1968.

125. Sigg EB, Capriob A, Schneider JA: Synergism of amines and antagonism of reserpine to morphine analgesia. *Proc Soc Exp Biol Med* 97:97–100, 1958.

126. Ivy AC, Goetzl FR, Burril DY: Morphine-dextroamphetamine analgesia. *War Med* 6:67–71, 1944.

127. Evans WO: The synergism of autonomic drugs on opiate or opioid-induced analgesia: A discussion of its potential utility. *Milt Med* 127:1000–1003, 1962.

128. Forest WH, Brown BW, Brown CR, Defalque R, Gold M, Gordon HE, James KE, Katz J, Mahler DL, Schraff P, Teutsch G: Dextroamphetamine with morphine for the treatment of post-operative pain. *N Engl J Med* 296:712–715, 1977.

129. Kittrelle JP, Grouse DS, Seybold ME: Cluster headache. Local abortive agents. *Arch Neurol* 42:496–498, 1985.

130. Laska EM, Sunshine A, Mueller F, Elvers WB, Siegel C, Rubin A: Caffeine as an analgesic adjuvant. *JAMA* 251:1711–1718, 1984

131. Sawynok J, Yaksh TL: Caffeine as an analgesic adjuvant: A review of pharmacology and mechanisms of action. To be published in Pharmacological Reviews, 1993.

132. Saunders CM: *The Management of Terminal Disease.* Chicago, Year Book, 1979.

133. Melzack R: The Brompton mixture versus morphine solutions given orally: Effect on pain. *Can Med Assoc J* 120:435–438, 1979.

134. Bruera E, Chadwick S, Brenneis C, Hanson J, MacDonald RN: Methylphenidate associated with narcotics for the treatment of cancer pain. *Cancer Treat Rep* 71:67–70, 1987.

135. Bruera E, Fainsinger R, MacEachern JH: The use of methylphenidate in patients with incident cancer pain receiving regular opiates. A preliminary report. *Pain* 50:75–77, 1992.

136. Katon W, Raskind M: Treatment of depression in the medically ill elderly with methylphenidate. *Am J Psychiatry* 137:963–965, 1980.

137. Kaufman MW, Murray GB, Cassem NH: Use of psycho-

stimulants in medically ill depressed patients. *Psychosomatics* 23:817–819, 1982.

138. Woods SW, Tesar GE, Murray GB, Cassem NH: Psychostimulant treatment of depressive disorders secondary to medical illness. *J Clin Psychiatry* 47:12–15, 1986.

139. Baldessarini RJ: *Chemotherapy in Psychiatry: Principles and Practice.* Cambridge, MA, Harvard University Press, 1985.

140. Risch SC, Groom GP, Janowsky DS: Interfaces of psychoparmacology and cardiology, Parts I and II. *J Clin Psychiatry* 42:23–34, 47–59, 1981.

141. Boakes AJ, Laurence DR, Teoh PC, Barar FSK, Benedikter LT, Prichard BNC: Interactions between sympathomimetic amines and antidepressant agents in man. *Br Med J* 1:311–315, 1973.

142. Thornton WE, Pray RJ: Combination drug therapy in psychopharmacology. *J Clin Pharmacol* 15:511–517, 1975.

143. Griffin JP, O'Arcy PF (eds): *A Manual of Adverse Drug Interactions.* Bristol, John Wright & Sons, 1975.

144. Bigger JT, Kantor SJ, Glassman AH, Perel JM: Cardiovascular effects of tricyclic antidepressant drugs. In Lipton MA, DeMascio A, Killam KF (eds): *Psychopharmacology: A Generation of Progress.* New York, Raven Press, 1978.

145. Roose SP, Glassman AH, Giardina EG, Walsh TB, Woodring S, Bigger JT: Tricyclic antidepressants in depressed patients with cardiac conducion disease. *Arch Gen Psychiatry* 44:273–275, 1987.

146. Risch SC, Kalin NH, Janowsky DS, Huey LY: Indications and guidelines for plasma tricyclic antidepressant concentration monitoring. *J Clin Psychopharmacol* 1:59–63, 1981.

147. Prien RF, Kupfer DJ: Continuation drug therapy for major depressive episode: How long should it be maintained? *Am J Psychiatry* 143:18–23, 1986.

148. Sheehan DV, Claycomb JB, Kouretas N: Monoamine oxidase inhibitors: Prescription and patient management. *Int J Psychiatr Med* 10:99–121, 1981.

149. Palmer H: Potentiation of pethidine. *Br Med J* 2:944, 1960.

150. Shee JC: Dangerous potentiation of pethidine by iproniazid and its treatment. *Br Med J* 2:507–509, 1960.

151. Rivers N, Hornes P: Possible lethal reaction between nardil and dextromorphan. *Can Med Assoc J* 103:85, 1970.

152. Roger KJ: Role of brain monoamines in the interaction between pethidine and tranylcypromine. *Eur J Pharmacol* 14:86–88, 1971.

153. Domino E, Sullivan TS, Luby ED: Barbiturate intoxication in a patient treated with a MAO inhibitor. *Am J Psychiatry* 118:941–943, 1962.

154. Frolich JC, Leftwich R, Ragheb M, Oates JA, Reimann I, Buchanan D: Indomethacin increases plasma lithium. *Br Med J* 1:1115–1116, 1979.

155. Hollister LE: Hydroxyzine hydrochloride: Possible adverse cardiac interactions. *Psychopharmacol Commun* 1:61–65, 1975.

156. Killian JM, Fromm GH: Carbamazepine in the treatment of neuralgia. Use and side effects. Arch Neurol 19:129–136, 1968.

157. Taylor MA, Sierles FS, Abrams R: *General Hospital Psychiatry.* New York, The Free Press, 1985.

158. Lohr JB, Jeste DV: Neuroleptic-induced movement dis-

orders: Tardive dyskinesia and other tardive syndromes. In Michels R, Cavenar JO, Cooper AM, Guze SB, Judd LL, Klerman GL, Solnit AJ, (eds): *Psychiatry: Psychobiological Foundations of Clinical Psychiatry*, vol 3. Philadelphia, JB Lippincott, 1988, pp 1–17.

159. Giles TO, Modlin RK: Death associated with ventricular arrhythmias and thioridazine hydrochloride. *JAMA* 205:108–110, 1968.

160. Cassem NH: The setting of intensive care. In Hackett TP, Cassem NH (eds): *MGH Handbook of General Hospital Psychiatry*. St. Louis, CV Mosby, 1978, pp 319–341.

161. Monks R, Merskey H: Psychotropic drugs. In Wall PD, Melzack RD (eds): *Textbook of Pain*. London, Churchill-Livingstone, 1984, pp 526–537.

162. Hackett TP: The pain patient: Evaluation and treatment. In Hackett TP, Cassem NH (eds): *MGH Handbook of General Hospital Psychiatry*. St. Louis, CV Mosby, 1978, pp 41–63.

163. Marks J: Benzodiazepines—For good or evil. *Neuropsychobiology* 10:115–126, 1983.

164. Hollister LE: Principles of therapeutic applications of benzodiazepines. In Smith DE, Wesson DR (eds): *The Benzodiazepines. Current Standards for Medical Practice*. Lancaster, England, MTP Press Limited, 1985, pp 87–96.

165. Rickels K, Case WG, Diamond L: Issues in long-term treatment with diazepam therapy. *Psychopharmacol Bull* 18:38–41, 1982.

166. Johnstone M: The effects of methylphenidate on postoperative pain and vasoconstriction. *Br J Anaesth* 46:778–783, 1974.

CHAPTER 17
SPECIAL CONSIDERATIONS IN PHARMACOLOGIC PAIN MANAGEMENT

JOSEPH W. TOLLISON

Nowhere in the broad area of chronic pain management are the proper selection, dosage, and frequency of administration of medication more critical than in those two very special patient populations, children and the elderly. Previous chapters emphasizing the adult from youth to middle age have carefully defined the pharmacologic actions and administration of various medications for control of chronic pain. However, in cases involving elderly patients and children, where the safety margin is often reduced, special pharmacologic, physiologic, and developmental factors must be very carefully considered. For example, among the elderly, who often are on multiple medications, increasingly frequent manifestations of adverse drug reactions and interactions are commonplace. Another area that is particularly troublesome with these two groups is that of compliance (1–3). Although this is somewhat understandable when considering the unique characteristics of these patients, it nonetheless compounds the prescribing difficulties and decisions. Underprescribing by physicians, as well as variable compliance, is especially common among children, although chronic pain as a motivating force may enhance responsiveness to the latter (4). Overprescribing is equally common among the elderly, especially in light of their propensity for drug accumulation at standard younger adult dosages.

As discussed earlier, pain is often the sentinel manifestation of many diseases or disorders and may thus be the triggering motivation for a patient to seek medical assistance. Altered perception of pain, which frequently occurs in elderly patients, may present some difficulty for the patient both in characterizing and describing the location of the pain. It may also be the only presenting complaint a child is able to express or define clearly. With young children, the inability to describe their symptoms is complicated by the fact that chronic pain of the non-neoplastic type is infrequently seen in this patient population; only in recent years has much study been done on its management. Therefore, well-designed therapeutic responses that would aid the physician in managing the patient effectively over time are relatively new or are still being developed.

The remainder of this chapter examines a number of those factors which make these patients unique, and which make their management complex. Factors ranging from the size and body surface area of the younger patient to the absorption, metabolism, and excretion differences of the older patient will be addressed. Various pain medications and their applicability to these patients will also be discussed.

CHILDREN

Because children are still developing physically and because of the potential deleterious psychological effects that may result, the management of chronic pain in this patient population is a particularly difficult and complex task. The amount of attention health care providers have given to chronic pain in children has been relatively scant, and much still remains to be learned about appropriate care for these patients. Drug therapy in children has in general been studied infrequently, leading to the term *therapeutic orphan* by Shirkey (5). The key to the approach to the care of the child with chronic pain is individualization of therapy based on an understanding of the expected physiologic and pharmacologic parameters, and a special awareness that these patients are not just smaller adults when it comes to prescribing. The final arbiter remains the individual patient's response to the drug and to his disease (6). An excellent review of chronic pain in children was presented by Lacouture, Gaudreault, and Lovejoy in 1984 in *Pediatrics Clinics of North America* (7).

Non-neoplastically generated chronic pain in children is uncommon. This adds to the complexity of management for this patient population group, especially when one considers that many of the drugs released on the market have undergone limited study for use in children, having been primarily investigated for use in the adult population.

The variables of total body water, as well as percentage of intracellular and extracellular water, are prime determinants of dose selection. In concert with factors of metabolism and excretion, selecting appropriate dosing patterns becomes even more difficult. Fig. 17.1 as adapted by Rane and Wilson from the work of Friis-Hansen provides an overview of the body water factor (4, 8).

Dosing regimens in children have historically been based on either the patient's age, weight, or body surface area. Though no system of dose selection is fail-safe, the body surface area and body weight approaches have the most general acceptance. Nomograms have been made available for the health care provider to assist in dosing selections. Table 17.1, a modification of the earlier work of Catzel (9), was developed as a simplified aid by Leach and Wood (6).

Even greater care should be taken with those drugs which have a narrow therapeutic/safety index. Precision is difficult at best, and in the final analysis the individual response to the drugs and the disease is vital (6). Therapeutic serum dose-level monitoring, as it becomes available, would be of increasing assistance.

Because of their pharmacologic properties, aspirin and nonsteroidal anti-inflammatory agents are often selected for adults who are experiencing mild to moderate pain, especially if accompanied by an inflammatory

Table 17.1.
Dose as Proportion of Adult Dose and in mg per kg for Different Age Groups

		Weight		(A) Dose as proportion of adult dose	(B) Dose in mg per kg if adult dose is 1 mg/kg
	Age	lbs	kg		
Adult	·· ··	145	66	1	1.0
12 yr	·· ··	82	37	3/4	1.25
7 yr	·· ··	51	23	1/2	
3 yr	·· ··	33	15	1/3	1.5
1 yr	·· ··	22	10	1/4	
4 mo	·· ··	14	6.5	1/5	2.0
2 wk	·· ··	7	3.2	1/8	

After Catzel: Modified by Leach RH, Wood BSB: Drug dosage for children. *Lancet* 23:1350–1351, 1967.

component. Only a small percentage of physicians continue to use aspirin for chronic disorders in children, however. Based on the initial findings of Starko in 1979, and on subsequent studies, there was an official announcement in 1985 of an association of aspirin with Reye's syndrome (10–13). Because the incidence of viral illness is so common among children, concurrent disease during long-term chronic pain therapy is very likely. In response to this concern the chronic use of aspirin with its proven analgesic, anti-inflammatory, and anti-pyretic properties is uncommon. Other potential problems with aspirin, even when given at much lower dosages, include adverse effects ranging from gastrointestinal effects to hematologic effects (e.g., delayed clotting time), as well as occasional hypersensitivity. If the decision is made to use aspirin, the dosage is calculated from a base dosage of 65 mg/kg/day in 4–6 divided doses, and routine drug level monitoring is strongly recommended to avoid common toxic effects, including salicylism. Dosage forms include tablets, enteric-coated tablets, and suppositories.

The nonsteroidal agents as a group share the analgesic, anti-flammatory, and to a degree the anti-pyretic potential of the aspirin family. Like aspirin, however, nonsteroidal drugs are occasionally recommended for use for chronic pain in children. Unlike aspirin, such drugs are expensive. The primary problem is that various metabolic concerns, including renal, continue to be studied, and are among the most overlooked (14). Therefore the agents have not been *FDA* approved for use in children. Currently *ibuprofen* (short half-life) *tolemetin* (medium half-life), and *naproxen* (longer half life) are the only exceptions to this rule.

It is important to choose an agent that has proven safe and effective for chronic treatment of mild pain in younger patients while maintaining the essentially sim-

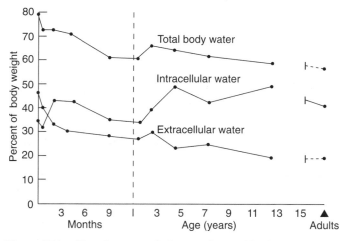

Figure 17.1. **Developmental changes in total body water, intracellular water, and extracellular water in infants and children. The changes are expressed as percentages of body weight. (Data from Friis-Hansen B: Body water components in children: Changes during growth and related changes in body composition. *Pediatrics* 28:169–181, 1961.**

Table 17.2.
Recommended Pediatric Dosing of Acetaminophen by Age and Weight[a]

Age	Weight		Dosing Schedule	
	lb	kg	Single Dose	Frequency
Under 4 months	6–11	2.5– 5.4	40 mg	every 4–6 hours
4 to under 12 months	12–17	5.5– 7.9	80 mg	every 4–6 hours
12 months to under 2 years	18–23	8.0–10.9	120 mg	every 4–6 hours
2 and 3 years	24–35	11.0–15.9	160 mg	every 4–6 hours
4 and 5 years	36–47	16.0–21.9	240 mg	every 4–6 hours
6. 7 and 8 years	48–59	22.0–26.9	320 mg	every 4–6 hours
9 and 10 years	60–71	27.0–31.9	400 mg	every 4–6 hours
11 and 12 years	72–95	32.0–43.9	480 mg	every 4–6 hours
	>96	>44	640 mg	every 4–6 hours

[a]Not to exceed five doses in a 24-hour period (16, 17).

ilar analgesic effects of aspirin. Acetaminophen meets this criterion and does not appear to have an association with Reye's syndrome. Therefore, there has been a dramatic shift from aspirin by most health care providers in recent years to almost exclusive use of this agent for mild pain (14). Expected side effects and adverse reactions are uncommon with acetaminophen, unless used to excess, at which time this agent becomes very problematic. Any residual previous or concurrent hepatic disease could reduce the rate of clearance because of hepatic metabolism and could require one to choose an increased dosing interval. Overdosage with acetaminophen is potentially life-threatening and in any case may result in hepatic damage. Acute renal failure also has been reported when acetaminophen has been taken in excessive dosages. The manifestation of renal damage follows that of hepatic damage by a matter of days, requiring careful follow-up (15). To this point all cases of acute renal failure have been reversible. Acetaminophen comes in various over-the-counter products including chewable tablets, elixir, drops, and suppositories with a dosing formula by age as shown in Table 17.2.

Codeine alone produces excellent analgesia for most patients with moderate pain and is generally the next step in children if acetaminophen therapy alone is insufficient. Dosing levels and frequency for codeine center on a base dosage of 3 mg/kg/day administered in six divided doses. In combination with acetaminophen, it has an additive and perhaps even a synergistic effect, offering improved analgesia to the younger patient in chronic pain.

The opiates and other associated opioid compounds are all commonly used for chronic severe pain, with primary metabolism through the liver. There is a significant "first pass" effect as the agent passes through the liver; therefore, oral doses often range up to 2–6 times that of doses administered parenterally. The oral/parenteral dosage ratios are methadone, 2:1, me-

peridine, 4:1, and morphine, 6:1 (18). Meperidine is representative of this class of narcotics, and through its action on the central nervous system (CNS) creates a level of euphoria and an increase in the pain threshold of as much as 65% (19). Used parenterally, meperidine requires an analgesic ratio of 10:1 to morphine (20). It is notably less effective when given orally. Though it has minimal effect on the cardiovascular system, as with morphine respiratory depression can be a factor (21). Also, because of its propensity for inducing nausea and vomiting, meperidine is often combined with an antihistamine such as promethazine or hydroxyzine, which tends to potentiate the sedative aspects of the drug (20).

A potentially helpful property of these agents is sedation, whereas respiratory depression also becomes an increasing concern with the addition of additive or synergistic medications. The increase in the incidence of seizure disorders in patients who have undergone long-term treatment with meperidine is a possible side effect of which health care providers should be cautious (22). However, the over-riding disadvantage with these agents is the association of potential tolerance and drug dependence (7). These agents appear to work centrally as contrasted with the agents described earlier, which largely act peripherally. Another possible side effect in children may be the development of dysphoria rather than the euphoria commonly seen in adults (7). This concern alone, aside from the dependence concerns, should lead the health care provider to initially choose non-narcotic agents when possible. If narcotic agents are required, a longer-acting agent such as methadone may be selected. Table 17.3 is a catalog of narcotic agents and their side effects as developed by Lacouture, Gaudreault, and Lovejoy (7).

The tricyclic antidepressants, which are frequently used in adults as outlined in the previous chapter, may also be chosen for use in children. The side effect profile often is great, however; and the therapeutic risk/benefit

Table 17.3.
Narcotic Analgesics

Agent	Dosage (Oral)	Indication	Side Effects	Comments
Codeine	.5 mg/kg/dose to 60 mg/dose q 4 hrs	Mild to moderate pain	Metabolic (*see morphine*)	Converted to morphine: elevated level of tolerance
Acetaminophen w/codeine elixir 12 mg/5 ml (Tylenol with Codeine Elixir)	Under 3 yrs—Not indicated 3–6 yrs—5 ml q 3–4 hr 7–12 yrs—10 ml q 3–4 hr			
Hydromorphone (Dilaudid)	.05–.1 mg/kg/dose to 5 mg/dose q 6 hrs	Moderate to severe pain	*See morphine*	Well absorbed: commonly used in terminal pain
Meperidine (Demerol)	1 mg/kg/dose to 100 mg/dose q 4 hrs	Moderate to severe pain	*See morphine*	Caution in renal failure: less sedation: may trigger bronchial asthma: may lead to CNS exitation
Methadone (Dolophine)	.2 mg/kg/dose to 10 mg/dose q 6 hrs	Severe pain	*See morphine*	Long half-life: minimal euphoria
Morphine	.5 mg/kg/q 6 hrs	Severe pain	CNS depression; orthostatic hypotension; decreased GI motility; mental clouding	Tolerance or dependence may develop
Oxycodone	.05–.15 mg/kg/dose to 10 mg/dose q 4–5 hrs	Moderate pain	*See morphine*	Short half-life: excellent short-term effects; commonly combined with aspirin (Percodan or acetaminophen [Percocet])

Adapted from Lacouture PG, Gaudreault P, Lovejoy FH: Chronic pain of childhood: A pharmacologic approach. *Pediatr Clin North Am* 31:1133–1151, 1984.

ratio may therefore be unacceptable. Again, if such agents are used, individualization of therapy is in order, as well as adherence to specific indications that tend to be uncommon in childhood chronic pain (7). Potentiation of analgesia is an expected effect. Occasional use of other agents has also been reported with younger patients but these should be very carefully selected and even more carefully monitored. An example is the use of phenytoin in carefully selected patients (lancinating pain) with mild facial pain, and skeletal muscle relaxants in patients with pain of skeletal muscle origin (7). Significant side effects such as CNS depression (relaxants) in the short and long term, and CNS depression and hyperplastic changes of the gingiva (phenytoin) over the long term are possible with these medications.

Of special note is the potential for drug interactions in this age group. Any other medications that are being taken should be carefully considered, and the potential of the drug for interaction with the medication chosen for treatment of the chronic pain should be carefully studied.

Another key management approach would be to attempt to maintain these patients on a set, yet reasonable, schedule other than PRN scheduling, which has been shown to adversely affect pain behavior. Also, the possibility of the child returning to an environment in which his learned pain behavior elicits a predictable response may be determined and appropriate adjustments may be made (7). Another principle is that the pain process should be closely monitored. For example, a child should not be permitted to remain in pain during the latter portion of a "q4h" regimen. This requires a careful review of all the variables involved in setting appropriate dosage levels and frequency. A caring response while avoiding the pitfalls of chronic narcotic use should be the goal in order to avoid distrust, anger, and other negative emotions. Undertreatment will engender these emotions on the part of the patient, and must be avoided (7).

There are numerous other factors for consideration when selecting an appropriate medication for a child suffering with chronic pain, due in part to the expected differences in psychological impact. For example, in a child who is in the process of developing his or her self-concept and sense of identity, the health care provider has a challenge of significant magnitude in attempting to select a plan of therapy that will be effective while not impacting adversely on this critical stage of development. Another challenge is to use the selected therapy in the optimal manner. This makes the diagnostic evaluation of critical importance, because abbreviating the pain process is the ultimate goal, and arriving at a specific diagnosis may predetermine the family of specific agents that can be used. Patterns of chronic pain behavior develop variably. In certain patients relatively healthy coping patterns emerge. However, those patterns of chronic pain behavior expected to develop over time in response to chronic pain have the potential to impact adversely on the child's development.

The tragedy of chronic pain in children is no more evident than when attempting to deal constructively with the families of these children. Assessment of the parents' nonverbal as well as verbal communication with the child and with you as the health care provider is critical. The response of the family members to the pain itself is important. Do they attempt to overcompensate? Do they overact in other ways? How does this appear to affect the child? Does it enhance or promote his response to the pain? The highly complex and yet foundational impact of the interaction with the parents and other family members plays a vital role in the long-term care of these patients. All of this would lead one to study family relationships and interactions and other environmental aspects carefully and to address as many of these as possible prior to selection of medication.

As stated earlier in this chapter, at this juncture in the history of health care, appropriate treatment of children with chronic non-neoplastic pain has drawn precious little attention and emphasis. Most multidisciplinary pain clinics have understandably emphasized care of the adult with chronic pain because of its resultant impact on the work force and economic factors. There are unique aspects in the care of children, however, including the impact of pain on their development and the different physiologic and pharmacologic aspects of selected therapy, both of which require much more attention than has previously been channeled in that direction. Modification of surrounding factors may alter the pain to some degree, as is all so often the case when specific causes of the pain are identified and are addressed rather than treating the resulting pain alone. Again, individualization of care in this age group is paramount. The simplest regimen possible to achieve the desired effect should be undertaken; when this involves medication it should be with the lowest dosage, the least frequent dosing interval, and the lowest toxicity. If possible, the patient should be administered only one medication (7).

Finally, when one is dealing with children, their trust in the health care provider needs to be honored at all times, and nowhere is this more important than in the relief of pain. A child who presents with chronic pain should be approached with professional concern and constant reassurance. Ambiguity of effort in this regard, albeit unintentional, has deleterious results. Careful and frequent reassessment of children with chronic pain is in order. Under all circumstances, keep in mind that the patient's possible misunderstanding of the health care provider's failure to bring relief may create an environment that makes quality long-term care virtually impossible.

THE ELDERLY

Many perceive pain to be an inevitable by-product of aging (23), occurring with increasing frequency during the aging process. With appropriate care, however, chronic pain in the elderly can be managed effectively over the long term. By almost every diagnostic and therapeutic unit of measurement including psychosocial, physiologic, and pharmacokinetic indexes, the elderly are the most complex patient group in our society. Those over age 65 are an increasing segment of our population and will account for over 20% of the population shortly after the turn of the century, including an expanding percentage of the "older old" (85+). The elderly often present with multiple problems, are seen more frequently in the office setting than are younger patients, and generally require longer hospitalizations. Also, the diagnosis and treatment process may be compounded by communication disorders involving reduced vision and/or hearing. With the older old, increased fragility will also need to be addressed.

The team approach has been helpful in the care of the elderly because it focuses the efforts of all of the health care professionals involved in the patient's total care (*whole patient* concept) and is keyed to the various problems of function the patient encounters. Unquestionably, care of the elderly has been greatly improved through the team approach, which is being increasingly used in many areas. Enhanced commitment and involvement are the potential benefits to the patient when the various health care professionals sense joint responsibility in the care of the whole patient and not just in their area of expertise. Properly developed, this impacts favorably on the role of the individual physician, broadening the professional involvement and time commitment to the patient. Improved care will naturally result.

Also, the once infrequently addressed area of preventive health care for the elderly has come into prominence in recent years. The sense of "inevitability" that was once a permanent and commonly encountered attitude among patients as well as among many health care professionals has been modified and has given way to a new emphasis on preventive health care. Proper exercise, good nutrition, and activities contributing to emotional health are heavily prescribed, as are routine maintenance and preventive health measures, all of which lead to greater longevity and enhanced health and function during the latter years.

Homeostasis is the goal in caring for the elderly patient with chronic pain. It remains a major goal for the health care provider not to disrupt the delicate physiologic balance in which the patient quite often is maintained. The loss of adaptability becomes the critical factor, followed by a loss of homeostasis with resulting disease in the patient. The body systems become progressively less adaptable over the years and eventually a system failure occurs. Pain syndromes in the elderly frequently present in an atypical manner. A high index of suspicion concerning the presenting problem as well as the pattern of presentation is required. Each of us has encountered in our elderly patient population those with silent or painless myocardial infarctions, afebrile pneumonia, or other processes that do not present in the classic manner more commonly seen in younger adults. One factor at work is thought to be an elevation in pain threshold due to a degeneration of dorsal column neurons with a resultant reduced sensory awareness (27, 28). Therefore, a perception of pain by the elderly patient may have a heightened significance over that of a younger patient, and indeed may signal a more involved disorder. Proper diagnosis is compounded further by the fact that depression, often resulting in part from the multiple and accelerating emotional losses experienced by the patient, is more common among the elderly, and yet is usually not diagnosed and, therefore, not treated at the suspected rate of prevalence. Depression must be searched for, with a high level of awareness. Is this isolated elderly lady depressed because she is lonely or lonely because she is depressed? Pain, of course, greatly compounds this presentation.

Pharmacokinetics are of special significance in this age group. There remains much discussion on the effect the aging process has on absorption, with most currently believing that the absorptive process is mildly reduced. Certainly, the rate of absorption is reduced as a patient ages. This is due to various causes ranging from a delayed gastric emptying time to cardiovascular and blood flow determinants, all of which is rather alarming when considering long-term therapy with agents such as aspirin and nonsteroidals, which have the potential of inducing gastric bleeding and adverse kidney effects. The expected reduction in intracellular body water and serum albumin as the patient ages occurs in concert with the previously addressed increase in body fat and reduction of lean muscle mass. This markedly affects drug distribution, and these normal and predictable aspects of biological aging must be appropriately considered when prescribing medications that have their distribution in various body components. Table 17.4 defines the normal expected physiologic changes and resulting pharmacokinetic effects of the various aging body systems.

Major alterations in percentage of body components occur during aging and major changes in total body lipid content (approximate doubling by age 70 from 14% to approximately 30%) take place (Fig. 17.2). Soft tissue and muscle decrease in the range of 25–30%, whereas body water declines approximately 18% (23).

Understanding the expected specific pharmacologic activity of the medication selected is essential. As an example, the medication's lipid solubility is greatly affected. A medication that is highly lipid-soluble has increased distribution in body fat, with an expected decrease in the serum level and resultant availability. Correspondingly, those medications which depend on protein binding will have an increased concentration of unbound drug in the serum as a result of reduced serum albumin in the elderly patient. Prolongation of activity of the medication and the risk of toxicity or adverse reactions is an increasingly frequent result among elderly patients.

Excretion of various pain medications is another area in which the elderly generally differ from the younger population. The liver is reduced in size and weight, and there is a decrease in activity of the hepatic microsomal enzyme system. There is a tremendous reserve in the human liver, however, and it is debatable whether this in itself will result in clinically apparent biochemical changes (24). However, normal physiologic factors in aging such as the gradual decrease in cardiac output by approximately 1% per year following age 35–40, and the decrease in the glomerular filtration rate by 40% by age 80, along with many other changes in organ systems, are the norm, and these cellular changes as yet cannot be prevented (29). These expected reductions in the glomerular filtration rate and tubular reabsorption in the aging patient are accompanied by reduced renal blood flow. This reduces the excretion rate and further increases the likelihood of *pharmacokinetic interaction and/or toxicity.* In general, we should expect accumulation, so prevention of the accompanying toxicity while seeking effective therapy often becomes an elusive goal.

Choosing appropriate dosage levels and dosage frequency is extremely important when prescribing medication for elderly patients. As noted above, the elderly are often acutely sensitive both to medication and procedures. This was very clearly illustrated by the study by Reichel at Franklin Square Hospital. The study involved 500 consecutive admissions of elderly patients to the hospital. Of these, 146 patients had 193 reactions, with 54 reactions being to medications, 42 to falls, and 31 to procedures (30). Admitting elderly patients to the hospital is frequently necessary, but it should be recognized that it puts them in an unfamiliar environment

Table 17.4.
Physiologic and Pharmacokinetic Changes Associated with Aging

Physiologic Changes	Pharmacokinetic Effects
Cardiovascular	
Decrease in cardiac output	Redistribution of blood flow from liver and kidneys, resulting in prolonged plasma
Decrease in arterial flow	half-life and diminished biotransformation[a]
Alteration of circulation to organ systems	
Gastrointestinal	
Decrease in gastric acidity	Alteration of ionization and solubility
Prolonged gastric emptying	
Decrease in absorptive surface	Decrease in drug absorption
Decrease in liver size and in activity	Decrease in rate of biotransformation[a]
of hepatic microsomal system	Increase in plasma half-life[a]
Increase in incidence of	Increases the potential for malabsorption
duodenal diverticula	
Metabolic	
Decrease in intracellular fluid	
Decrease in body weight	Increased effects with standard dosage[a]
Decrease in serum albumen	Increase in free to bound drug ratio[a]
Increase in serum globulin	
Increase in proportion of	Increase in storage of lipid soluble drugs[a]
fatty tissue to muscle mass	Increase in plasma half-life[a]
	Increase in volume of distribution[a]
Neuronal	
Increase in rate of neuron loss	Increased susceptibility to hypoxia[a]
	Increased sensitivity to central depressants[a]
	Potential for confusion about drug depressants[a]
Renal	
Decrease in renal clearance	Increase in plasma half-life[a]

[a]Enchances potential for drug toxicity.
From Lamy PP: *Prescribing for the Elderly.* Littleton, MA, PSG Publishing, 1980.

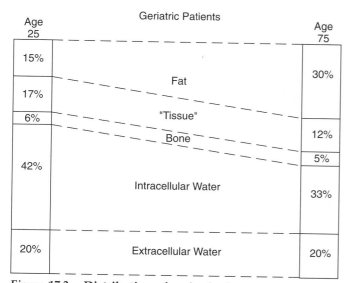

Figure 17.2. **Distribution of major body components with age (25, 26).**

and subjects them to secondary and perhaps even greater pathology (31). Admission of an elderly patient should be carefully weighed. This is especially true with pain patients, because the occurrence of pain in an unfamiliar environment may increase the patient's inability to function effectively.

In the elderly, who are often on multiple medications and have poorly defined absorptive capability, distribution, and excretion differences, drug interactions become an even greater potential hazard. Certain prescribing guidelines for the elderly must be undertaken: (1) Assess very carefully the etiology of the patient's pain and prescribe appropriately. (2) With each visit, reassess the patient's total list of medications (include all OTC medications). (3) Choose the mildest pain medication and simplest regimen possible to achieve the desired effect. (4) Choose the smallest dose possible for initial therapy (a "start low . . . go slow" technique is advised). In general, the elderly often require only one-third to one-half of the initial dose level of younger adults, with a preference for approximately one-third. (5) Because of the above, frequency of dosage should be reduced to avoid the expected accumulation, particularly if the drugs prescribed have extended half-lives of their own that would compound the patient's excretion difficulties. (6) Be alert to various adverse reactions and drug interactions that are major deterrents to medication compliance. An example is the constipating effect of codeine. Consider strongly other factors impacting on compliance as well, including the cost of medications.

Well-intentioned physicians may occasionally compound a patient's medical problem by prescribing dosages, frequencies, or specific medications which are inappropriate. A classic example is the elderly patient who suffers increased orthostatic hypotension from a medication, and, on rising, falls and fractures her hip. Cumulative anticholinergic effects are of major concern and may be additive effects of multiple medications or sufficient dosage of a single medication with this property (32). Antispasmodics or tricyclic antidepressants along with other medications, including some available over the counter, have this potential. When choosing a tricyclic for an elderly patient one may well consider a medication from the lower end of the anticholinergic scale such as desipramine (33). Orthostatic hypotension is a leading manifestation of the anticholinergic effect and has the major potential for causing falls that result in fractures or other injuries. Urinary retention is another frequent result of anticholinergic effects from one or a combination of agents. A "start low . . . go slow" approach to dosage selection is almost always indicated in the elderly except in an emergency situation. A broad review of specific medications and factors affecting selection in the elderly was presented by Rhodes et al. in 1985 (35).

Certainly, drug-induced dementia is among the most common of the reversible forms of dementia and, therefore, along with depression should be high on the list of considered causes. Narcotics, for example, manifest a significantly increased central depressant effect among elderly patients. The decreased respiratory reserve potentially compounds this problem (24). Those experienced in caring for large populations of nursing home patients have long had the impression that physicians have, in general, been more inclined to add medications than to subtract. The less adaptable physiologic systems of the elderly, especially of those most advanced in age, have only compounded the potential of drug-induced dementia. With the increasing attention being given to avoiding adverse reactions and drug interactions, one hopes this is becoming less common of an occurrence. All of these factors, plus others, potentially interact to produce unpredictable results (Fig. 17.3).

This unpredictability of drug effects in the aged is heavily compounded not only by wide variation in re-

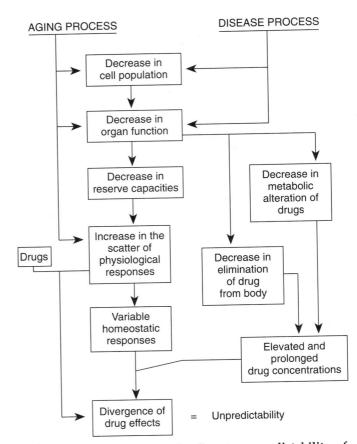

Figure 17.3. **Flow diagram leading to unpredictability of drug effects in the aged. (From Barania JT, et al:** *Management of Dental Behavior in Children.* **Littleton, MA, PSG Publishing, 1979.)**

sponsiveness but by the number of medications taken, which tends to average much higher in the elderly. The term *polypharmacy* to describe the use of multiple medications in the elderly refers both to the number of OTC medications the patient is using and to those medications prescribed by physicians. The additive and even synergistic effects of many of these medications result in compounding problems, and the potency of medications used for pain add significantly to the resulting effects. Drug interactions become an increasing problem.

Seldom should medications for the elderly be ordered or prescribed in isolation, and the prescribing physician must maintain a constant awareness of the cumulative effect and the potential contained therein.

Decreased mobility is another frequently expected problem, often limiting patient visits. Because of this and other factors associated with aging, the management of medications at home is critical. Howard-Ruben discussed this approach well and in depth in 1985 (36).

CONCLUSIONS

The challenge presented by both the very old and the very young in the area of chronic pain management is truly unique, and requires our most thoughtful and carefully selected approach to achieve an optimal effect with a minimum of problems. Although immensely challenging and difficult to achieve, effective pain management for patients of these two groups remains among our most complex responsibilities and should merit our full professional attention as well as ongoing research.

REFERENCES

1. Wilson JT: Compliance with instructions in the evaluation of therapeutic efficacy: A common but frequently unrecognized major variable. *Clin Pediatr* 12:333–340, 1973.
2. Becker MH, Drachman RH, Kirscht JP: Predicting mothers' compliance with pediatric medical regimens. *J Pediatr* 81:843–854, 1972.
3. Wilson JT: Drug compliance problems for hospitalized children. In McMahon (ed): *Principles and Techniques of Human Research and Therapeutics.* New York, Futura, 1976.
4. Rane A, Wilson JT: Clinical pharmacokinetics in infants and children. *Clin Pharmacokinet* 1:2–24, 1976.
5. Shirkey H: Therapeutic orphans. *J Pediatr* 72:119–120, 1968.
6. Leach RH, Wood BSB: Drug dosage for children. *Lancet* 23:1350–1351, 1967.
7. Lacouture PG, Gaudreault P, Lovejoy FH: Chronic pain of childhood: pharmacologic approach. *Pediatr Clin North Am* 31:1133–1151, 1984.
8. Friis-Hansen B: Body water compartments in children: Changes during growth and related changes in body composition. *Pediatrics* 28:169–181, 1961.
9. Catzel P: *Pediatric Prescriber.* Oxford, England, Oxford University Press, 1963, and 1966.
10. Starko KM et al: Reye's syndrome and salicylate use. *Pediatrics* 66:859–864, 1980.
11. Waldman RJ et al: Aspirin as a risk factor in Reye's syndrome. *JAMA* 247:3089–3094, 1982.
12. *Morbidity and Mortality Weekly Report* 34:13–16, 1985.
13. United States Food and Drug Administration, Department of Health and Human Services. *Health and Human Services Release.* 10 January 1988.
14. Brooks PM, Day RO: Nonsteroidal antiinflammatory drugs—Differences and similarities. *N Engl J Med* 324:1716–1725, 1991.
15. Rahwan GL, Rahwan FG: Aspirin and Reye's syndrome.

16. Curry RW et al: Acute renal failure after acetaminophen ingestion. *JAMA* 247:1012, 1982.
17. Korberly BH: Pharmacologic Treatment of Children's Pain. *Pediatr Nurs* July/August:292–294, 1986.
18. Temple AR: Pediatric dosing of acetaminophen. *Pediatr Pharmacol* 3:321–327, 1983.
19. Newburger PE, Sailan SE: Chronic pain: Principles of management. *J Pediatr* 59:429–432, 1982.
20. Bennett CR: The pharmacology of conscious-sedative agents. In Bennett CR (ed): *Conscious-Sedation in Dental Practice,* ed 2. St. Louis, CV Mosby, 1978.
21. Brandt SK, Bugg JL: Problems of medication with the pediatric patient. *Dent Clin North Am* 28:563–579, 1984.
22. Goodman LS, Gilman A: *The Pharmacological Basis of Therapeutics,* ed 6. New York, Macmillan, 1980.
23. Barania JT et al: *Management of Dental Behavior in Children.* Littleton, MA, PSG Publishing, 1979.
24. Lamy PP: *Prescribing for the Elderly.* Littleton, MA, PSG Publishing, 1980.
25. Stimmel B: *Pain, Analgesia, and Addiction: The Pharmacologic Treatment of Pain.* New York, Raven Press, 1983.
26. Benet LZ et al: Pharmacokinetic considerations in geriatric patients. In Benet LZ et al (eds): *Pharmacokinetic Basis for Drug Treatment.* New York, Raven Press, 1984.
27. Rossman I: *Clinical Geriatrics,* ed 2. Philadelphia, JB Lippincott, 1979.
28. Procacci P et al: The cutaneous pain pricking threshold in old age. *Gerontol Clin* 12:213–218, 1970.
29. Andrew W: *The Anatomy of Aging in Man.* New York, Grune & Stratton, 1971.
30. Bender AD: The effect of increasing age on the distribution of peripheral blood flow in man. *J Am Geriatr Soc* 13:192–198, 1965.
31. Reichel W: Complications in the care of 500 elderly hospitalized patients. *J Am Geriatr Soc* 13:973–980, 1965.
32. Vestal RE: Drug use in the elderly: A review of problems and special considerations. *Drugs* 16:358–382, 1978.
33. Muller OF et al: The hypotensive effect of imipramine hydrochloride in patients with cardiovascular disease. *Clin Pharmacol Ther* 2:300–307, 1961.
34. Thompson TL et al: Drug therapy: Psychotropic drug use in the elderly. *N Engl J Med* 308:134–138, 1983.
35. Rhodes RS et al: Management of dental pain in the elderly. *Gerodontics* 1:264–273, 1985.
36. Howard-Ruben J: Managing pain medication at home. *Oncol Nurs Forum* 12:78–82.

CHAPTER 18

DRUG DETOXIFICATION PROTOCOLS

DAVID A. FISHBAIN

OPIATE DETOXIFICATION

Following long-term use of opiates, psychological dependence, physical dependence, and tolerance can develop. It is estimated that of those who use opiates sporadically (nondaily), 25% will become dependent or addicted (1). Physical dependence is a function of the dosage schedule of the opiate, but can be produced by very little opiate exposure, can persist for a long period after drug cessation, and will develop in every patient so exposed. In general, of those who advance to twice-daily use, the majority will become physically dependent within 6–8 weeks (1). Each opiate apparently has its own capacity for inducing physical dependence (2).

In a patient who is opiate physically dependent, abrupt opiate discontinuation leads to the development of the opiate withdrawal syndrome (*distressing physical reaction*) (3). The signs and symptoms of this syndrome are well described (3–6) and will not be delineated here. Some of these signs and symptoms have been incorporated into the DSM-III-R Criteria for Opiate Withdrawal (7).

The elimination half-life of the opiate drug will determine when withdrawal will begin because this syndrome usually begins two to three half-lives after the last opiate dose (3). Thus for short–half-life opiates such as morphine, withdrawal begins in 6–12 hours, whereas for long–half-life opiates such as methadone, withdrawal begins in 36–48 hours. Opiate plasma half-lives are well documented in most reference works (2). In terms of time, the opiate withdrawal syndrome will begin within 6–8 hours after the last opiate dose, peak in 48–72 hours, and last for 7–14 days. However, lingering physical effects of opiate withdrawal can appear for up to 6 months after resolution of acute symptoms (3). The severity of the withdrawal is a function of which opiate was being taken, at what dose, and for how long (3). Generally the severity of opiate withdrawal will reflect the degree of physical dependence.

It is to be noted that there is significant confusion over the use of such terms as drug/alcohol abuse, dependence, and addiction (8). As a result, data on the percentages of chronic pain patients who abuse opiates, or are dependent or addicted to this group of drugs, appear to be limited (8). For chronic pain patients, opiate abuse, dependence, or addiction, in most cases, may not be an adequate reason for opiate detoxification. There are, however, other reasons for detoxifying chronic pain patients from opiates, and these have been reviewed by myself (8).

Until quite recently, opiate detoxification had been a relatively standard procedure whose primary purpose was to *minimize* or *eliminate* the signs and symptoms associated with opiate withdrawal via a slow taper. However, because of the development of new medications such as clonidine for opiate withdrawal, there has been an explosion in the variety of opiate detoxification protocols used. This chapter presents a review of some of the opiate detoxification protocols advocated in the literature.

PRINCIPLES

A number of major principles have been outlined for the management of opiate withdrawal (2–4, 9, 10):

1. Opiate withdrawal can be associated with major patient discomfort, both psychological and physiological, but has no serious medical consequence, such as death, if untreated. Thus opiate physical dependence should not impede rapid tapering. This is not the case for sedative/hypnotic withdrawal.
2. Opiate withdrawal can be treated with any opiate, but if a long-acting opiate is used (long half-life), withdrawal symptoms are milder and there is less patient distress.
3. Opiate dosage equivalencies can be utilized to withdraw patients from methadone or any opiate. Generally, in all detoxification procedures the total amount of opiate that the patient takes over 24 hours is translated via dosage equivalences into the equiv-

Table 18.1.
Methadone Opiate Substitution/Detoxification Protocol[a]

1. Patients given any and as much medication as they need for 24–48 hours.
2. From the amount of drug taken in no. 1 (above), calculate equivalent daily dose of methadone (Table 18.11) required.
3. If unable to determine above, give methadone 15 mg q4h until respiratory rate decreases to 16 breaths/min.
4. The total daily substitution dose of methadone is the total dose given to reduce the respiratory rate to 16 breaths/min.
5. This dose is given in four divided doses for 24 hours.
6. Methadone dose is reduced daily by 15–20% in a "pain cocktail" (drug plus masking vehicle to blind patient to detoxification).
7. Doxepin 50–100 mg is added to cocktail if sleep is a problem.
8. Hydroxyzine 50 mg t.i.d. added to cocktail if patient is anxious.

[a]Compiled from Halpern L: Substitution-detoxification and its role in the management of chronic benign pain. *J Clin Psychiatry* 43:10–14, 1982.

Table 18.2.
Alternative Methadone Substitution/Detoxification Protocols[a]

A. As in Table 18.5, except decrease methadone at 7 mg/day over 20 days.
B. As in Table 18.5, but as follows:
  1. If taking greater than 30 mg/day, drop at 10 mg/day to 30 mg/day, then
  2. Drop at 5 mg/day to 20 mg/day; then
  3. Drop at 2.5 mg/day to zero.
  4. If taking less than 30 mg/day, start at step 2.

[a]From Frances RJ, Franklin JE: Alcohol and other psychoactive substance use disorders. In Talbott JA, Hales RE, Yudofsky SC (eds): *American Psychiatric Press Textbook of Psychiatry.* Washington, D.C., American Psychiatry Press, 1988.

alent amount of opiate with which detoxification will proceed. This is why dosage equivalencies are so important to detoxification protocols. Dosage equivalencies are well documented in most reference works (2) and will not be presented here. However, in order for detoxification to proceed in a correct fashion, the treating physician should have a dosage equivalencies chart. He or she should be prepared to use such a chart especially when a patient is found to use more than one opiate.

4. Titration of methadone, or any opiate, for control of opiate withdrawal should be based on objective withdrawal signs (e.g., dilation of pupils, stuffy nose, gooseflesh). However, there appears to be little correlation between patients' subjective ratings, objective nurse ratings, and physical parameters of severity of withdrawal (9). Thus, clinicians should not base their decision as to the severity of opiate withdrawal syndrome solely on physical parameters. There are opiate withdrawal symptoms rating scales available (10). These should be used if the amount of opiate that the patient will receive is to be determined by the presence or absence of withdrawal symptoms and signs.

5. Some patient discomfort is inevitable; the signs and symptoms of withdrawal can rarely be entirely abol-

ished, unless the detoxification process is much prolonged.
6. Detoxification can be blind (cocktail) or open (pills), depending on patient and physician preference.
7. Usual daily dose *required to prevent withdrawal is equal to 25% of the previous daily dose.* Therefore, daily tapers can be from 75% to 5%, depending on preference. However, the usual figure is 50%.
8. At higher dose levels, the daily dose reduction can be greater because it represents a smaller percentage of the total. As daily dose falls, reduction should be more gradual.

PROTOCOLS

All opiate detoxification protocols generally adhere to the principles outlined above. These protocols can be characterized by the type of opiate that is used in the detoxification process and the time required to complete detoxification. Time is an important element because it is thought that short–half-life opiates require 5–7 days to complete detoxification and that intermediate–half-life and long–half-life opiates require 10–14 days and 14–21 days, respectively (2). Many protocols are designed to decrease the time required for detoxification even further. This is because drug treatment programs usually wish to taper opiates as quickly as possible. To date, the protocols that have appeared in the literature can be classified as follows: methadone substitution/detoxification, nonmethadone substitution/detoxification, nonmethadone opiate detoxification, nonmethadone detoxification, buprenorphine substitution/detoxification, and opiate antagonist precipitated withdrawal/detoxification.

Methadone is an opiate with an extremely long half-life (2). It has negligible euphoria, it plateaus in 2 hours, and its onset of action is in 1/2 hour. It cannot be used to detoxify patients dependent on mixed agonist/antagonist opiates. Additionally, it may accumulate between the 24th and 48th hours, and therefore patients on this drug must be assessed for toxicity (4). Because of its long half-life, methadone has been used in a number of opiate detoxification protocols. The best example

Table 18.3.
Nonmethadone Substitution/Detoxification Protocol[a]

1. Patient given as much opiate of choice as he or she requires for 24–48 hours.
2. Total intake of opiate over the 48 hours is calculated and translated into opiate of doctor's choice (e.g., codeine).
3. This total dose of codeine is divided into four doses and given over 24 hours (q6h).
4. This dose is given for 2 days.
5. Then this dose is decreased by 50% every 2 days.
6. When a dose equivalent to 10 mg methadone is reached, that dose is given for 2 days.

[a]From Inturrisi CE: Role of opioid analgesics. *Am J Med* 10:27–36, 1984.

of this is a protocol presented by Halpern (Table 18.1) (11). This protocol is notable for the following: There is an initial 48-hour time span during which the patient is on an opiate PRN demand schedule; a pain cocktail is used, adjunct medications are used in the cocktail, and the time required to complete this protocol from 50 mg of methadone at 20% reduction is 17 days. Two alternatives to this protocol are presented in Table 18.2. Alternative *A* takes 20 days, whereas alternative *B* requires 11 days to complete from 50 mg of methadone.

An example of a nonmethadone opiate substitution/detoxification protocol is presented in Table 18.3. This protocol will take 8–9 days to complete from an equivalent dose of 50 mg of methadone. There are two reasons for considering this protocol over a methadone substitution/detoxification protocol. Firstly, the longer the half-life of the opiate, the longer the detoxification protocol required. It does not make any sense to transfer patients taking short– and intermediate–half-life drugs to long–half-life drugs and then, by necessity, prolonging detoxification if the goal is rapid detoxification. Secondly, many drug addicts believe, although there is little evidence for this, that methadone may be more difficult to detoxify from than other opiates. In support of this, methadone detoxification protocol with true opiate addicts can be extremely prolonged.

An example of a nonmethadone detoxification protocol is presented in Table 18.4. This protocol has a number of advantages over others: it is simple; it does not use methadone; it does not use cocktails; it can be very rapid, with most patients being detoxified in 10 days; the patient is detoxified with the opiate of his choice and preference (i.e., the one he is most familiar with); and for patients taking one opiate only, there is no need for conversions to other opiates. The major disadvantage to this protocol is that, in most cases, detoxification proceeds with an opiate that has a short or intermediate half-life, thereby potentially permitting more patient discomfort than with methadone. However, this is minimized by *dose* detoxification first, followed by *time* detoxification. This distinction between time and dose detoxification is very important because patients using short–half-life opiates will be taking these at frequent

intervals. There is one literature report of the successful use of this protocol (13). At our center, we have used this protocol for about 10 years without major problems.

Buprenorphine is an opiate with mixed agonist/ antagonist properties, and has a long duration of action, which may be a function of slow disassociation from opioid receptors and not a long half-life, as for methadone (14, 15). Buprenorphine can also block the effects of exogenously used opiates and therefore reduce heroin self-administration (14). The drug is also associated with a very mild withdrawal syndrome which, however, can be prolonged (14, 15). These properties suggested that this drug could be used in an opiate detoxification protocol. Buprenorphine was demonstrated to be as effective as methadone using such a protocol (14). This protocol is presented in Table 18.5.

When working with opiate addicts, it is important to determine if the addict in alleged opiate withdrawal is indeed physically opiate-dependent. To make this determination, a test using naloxone, an opiate antagonist, has been developed. This test is presented in Table 18.6. The naloxone challenge test appears to predict treatment outcome in opiate addicts (16). High naloxone challenge test scores at intake (high levels of opiate dependence) predict poor program retention (16).

In addition to determining if the patient is physically opiate-dependent, opiate antagonists such as naloxone can be used to reduce the time required for opiate detoxification (17). This is called "opiate antagonist precipitated withdrawal." The opiate withdrawal is compressed into as short a time as possible, with the hope that a short period of severe symptoms may be easier to cope with than a prolonged period of milder symptoms. This technique is demonstrated below for opiate detoxification with clonidine.

Clonidine Opiate Protocols

Opiate withdrawal is a state of adrenergic hyperactivity in which neurons of the locus ceruleus become markedly activated. Clonidine is an alpha-2 adrenergic agonist, which suppresses the acute dysphoric state associated with opiate withdrawal and appears to act by inhibiting the firing of the locus ceruleus via opening

Table 18.4.
Nonmethadone Detoxification Protocol

1. Patient given as much opiate of choice as he or she requires for 3 days (i.e., a PRN demand schedule).
2. No intramuscular or intravenous opiates are allowed, and these routes are immediately switched to p.o.
3. At the end of 3 days, total dose of opiate is calculated and is translated into a daily opiate dose.
4. If the patient is taking two or three opiates, as is often the case, the opiates taken less frequently are translated into the opiate taken most frequently, and the daily opiate dose is calculated.
5. Detoxification will proceed with the opiate taken most frequently.
6. The daily opiate dose is split over the day according to the original demand schedule of the patient. For example, if the patient was taking Percodan at q2h intervals, the daily opiate dose will be split at q2h intervals.
7. Patient will be maintained on the q2h schedule for 2 days. This is not a demand schedule, and the patient is brought his medications.
8. Detoxification then proceeds by decreasing the dosage by 25–50% per day. For example, if patient is taking three Percodans every 2 hours, he or she would be detoxified to two every 2 hours, then one every 2 hours.
9. Once dosage detoxification is complete, i.e., patient is taking *one* pill at the time interval, then *time detoxification* begins. An example of this would be:
    (a) one tab q4h × 1 day, then
    (b) one tab q6h × 1 day, then
    (c) one tab q8h × 1 day, then
    (d) one tab q12h × 1 day, then
    (e) one tab q.h.s. × 1 day, then
    (f) D/C
10. No adjunct medications (doxepin, hydroxyzine) are given unless indicated (i.e., reasons other than detoxification problems).
11. Clonidine is given only if the patient has major withdrawal difficulties.
12. This protocol requires the cooperation of the patient. He or she is therefore advised of the following:
    (a) During the first 3 days, he or she should take as much medication as he or she requires; if he or she takes less, detoxification may be more difficult than necessary.
    (b) Total minimization of discomfort is not possible.
    (c) Once the detoxification schedule is written, it will not be changed, no matter how much discomfort the patient experiences.
    (d) During the detoxification, no PRN opiates will be administered.
    (e) The patient is advised not to worry about his schedule during detoxification, because it is now Nursing's responsibility to bring the medications to the patient.
    (f) The patient may refuse a dosage; however, this is not advisable and he or she will not be able to have any medication until the next scheduled dosage.
    (g) If a patient is asleep during the time that he or she should receive an opiate dose, he or she will not be awakened.

Table 18.5.
Buprenorphine Substitution/Detoxification Protocol[a]

1. 2 mg of buprenorphine equivalent to 30 mg methadone.
2. Determine the patient's opiate stabilization dose in milligrams of methadone.
3. Buprenorphine is prepared in 20% aqueous alcohol and given once daily sublingually.
4. Buprenorphine detoxification is to proceed for 4 weeks with cuts of 25% in the first week and of 50% thereafter.

[a]From Bickel WK, Stitzer ML, Bigelow GE, Liebson IA, Jasinski DR, Johnson RE: A clinical trial of buprenorphine: Comparison with methadone in the detoxification of heroin addicts. *Clin Pharmacol Ther* 43:72–78, 1988.

Table 18.6.
Naloxone Opiate Physical Dependence Test[a]

1. Administer naloxone 0.4–0.6 mg IM.
2. Watch for signs of opiate withdrawal syndrome.
3. If no effect, subject is not physically dependent.
4. To relieve withdrawal syndrome, give morphine 15–30 mg.

[a]From Kosten TR, Krystal JH, Charney DS, et al: Rapid detoxification from opioid dependence. *Am J Psychiatry* 146:1349, 1989.

potassium channels (18). The ability of clonidine to suppress the symptoms and signs of opiate withdrawal has made the use of this drug popular for this purpose (19). Clonidine has some opiate-like properties, but does not bind to the opiate receptor and does not produce euphoria. Most signs and symptoms of withdrawal are reversed or prevented by 5–30 μg/kg oral clonidine (19).

Clonidine is not the ideal agent for opiate withdrawal. It cannot be precisely titrated and higher doses may be limited by side effects such as hypotension. As a result, clonidine has limitations in its ability to suppress withdrawal manifestations as compared with methadone (20), and opiate addicts being detoxified with clonidine are more likely to fail at detoxification (21).

As an adjunct to methadone opiate detoxification, clonidine has many assets. With the addition of clonidine, the percentage of narcotic addicts who achieve a symptom-free state in inpatient studies is greater than

Table 18.7.
Clonidine Alone Detoxification Protocol[a]

1. At the first sign of withdrawal, 0.3–0.4 mg p.o. (5 μg/kg body wt.) stat clonidine.
2. Then 0.1–0.25 mg q4h for a total of 0.9–1.6 mg (or 15–20 μg/kg) on the first day.
3. Vital signs are taken hourly the first day, every 2 hours on the second, and every 4 hours thereafter.
4. Hold clonidine if blood pressure is less than 90/50 combined with a bradycardia of 50 beats or less per min. Hold until vital signs acceptable.
5. When vital signs are acceptable, reinstate clonidine q4h.
6. On the second day, and each day thereafter, reduce clonidine dosage by 50%.

[a]From Cuthill JD, Beroniade V, Salvatori VA, Viguie F: Evaluation of clonidine suppression of opiate withdrawal reactions: A multidisciplinary approach. *Can J Psychiatry* 35:377–382, 1989.

Table 18.8.
Variant of Clonidine Alone Detoxification Protocol[a]

1. Calculate the amount of daily opiate required from the history or observe intake.
2. Translate into methadone equivalents.
3. If the required equivalent is 25 mg methadone or less, begin at 0.05 mg clonidine b.i.d.
4. If the required equivalent is greater than 25 mg methadone, use 0.1 mg clonidine b.i.d.
5. Maintain on this dose for 3 days.
6. Then decrease clonidine by 25% per day.

From Ghodse H: *Drugs and Addictive Behavior: A Guide to Treatment.* Oxford, Blackwell Scientific Publications, 1990.

with methadone alone, and the same in outpatients (19). It is also claimed that clonidine can decrease the time required for opiate detoxification to 3–5 days for short-acting opiates, 5–7 days for intermediate-acting opiates, and 7–10 days for long-acting ones (4). Clonidine can be used to detoxify from mixed agonist/antagonist opiates, which is a major plus. Clonidine, therefore, appears to offer additional options in the amelioration of the opiate withdrawal syndrome. Physicians must remember that abrupt discontinuation of clonidine can result in a withdrawal syndrome, however. Therefore, patients placed on clonidine detoxification protocols should then be tapered off this drug (4).

Clonidine opiate detoxification protocols can be classified as follows: clonidine alone, clonidine plus opiate antagonist (naloxone or naltrexone), methadone followed by clonidine, clonidine alone–transdermal patch, and adjunct clonidine. These detoxification protocols are presented in Tables 18.7 through 18.12. The following observations apply to these protocols:

1. There is major variability on how much clonidine is given initially. The doses vary from 0.1–1.6 mg per day.
2. With the clonidine/antagonist protocol, one can detoxify a patient in 3 days.
3. The methadone/clonidine protocol does not contain

a clonidine detoxification step. I believe this is necessary.
4. Transdermal clonidine offers the advantage of weekly application and stable blood levels of clonidine (22). This protocol requires 2 days of oral clonidine and continues for 21 days, however.
5. The adjunct clonidine protocol is only used if there are difficulties in detoxification, and is the protocol used by our pain center. The patient is placed on clonidine until the opiate detoxification is complete, at which point he or she is detoxified from clonidine.

In using clonidine for opiate detoxification, the physician will need to monitor blood pressure and should try to use the lowest possible dose of clonidine necessary. I believe that patients should be carefully selected for adjunct clonidine opiate detoxification using two criteria: difficulties in the detoxification process and presence of addictive behaviors. This selection is necessary because clonidine use will prolong detoxification, because clonidine itself requires a taper.

Protocols Using Other Medications

Detoxification protocols using medications other than opiates and clonidine are presented in Table 18.13. These protocols will ameliorate opiate withdrawal syndrome, but less successfully than opiates or clonidine will. The protocols mainly affect anxiety generated by the syndrome.

The medications used in these protocols are used as *adjuncts* in the detoxification process. Propranolol is one such medication. Often, in opiate withdrawal syndrome, the patients complain of restlessness that presents like anxiety. Propranolol, at doses of 20–40 mg/day, has been used successfully for this problem during detoxification (24).

Doxepin is another adjunct medication used successfully during opiate detoxification. Doxepin appears to augment methadone opiate withdrawal (25). It is administered in doses of 50–100 mg p.o. h.s. during detoxification and is maintained for 6 weeks. It is not clear by what mechanism doxepin augments opiate withdrawal. Doxepin may act by simply increasing the levels of

Table 18.9.
Clonidine Plus Opiate Antagonist (Naloxone) Detoxification Protocol[a]

1. Clonidine 0.1 mg t.i.d. first day.
2. Clonidine 0.2–0.3 mg t.i.d. (monitor blood pressure) and naloxone 0.2 mg IM, then 0.4 mg IM q2h for four doses on the second day.
3. Clonidine (same dose as on day 2), naloxone 0.8 mg IM, five doses at 2-hour intervals on third day.
4. Demonstrate completeness of detoxification by a naloxone challenge: 0.4 mg IM should cause no withdrawal; then follow with 0.8 mg IM 1 hour later (no withdrawal should be noted); this is day 4.

[a]From Ghodse H: *Drugs and Addictive Behavior: A Guide to Treatment.* Oxford, Blackwell Scientific Publications, 1990.

Table 18.10.
Methadone Followed by Clonidine Detoxification Protocol[a]

1. Stabilize the patient on methadone.
2. Taper methadone to 20 mg/day.
3. Then switch to clonidine 0.1–0.3 mg t.i.d. for 2 days.
4. Then clonidine 0.2–0.7 mg t.i.d. for 8–14 days.
5. Then D/C.

[a]From Frances RJ, Franklin JE: Alcohol and other psychoactive substance use disorders. In Talbott JA, Hales RE, Yudofsky SC (eds): *American Psychiatric Press Textbook of Psychiatry.* Washington, D.C., American Psychiatry Press, 1988.

methadone or by combating anxiety and/or depression. Doxepin may therefore be the ideal adjunct for opiate detoxification.

Naloxone-precipitated opiate detoxification is often uncomfortable. Therefore, researchers have concentrated on adjunct medications to make this process more tolerable. Methohextone, a barbiturate (26), and midazolam, a short-acting benzodiazepine (27), appear to be such agents. Both of these agents appear to block objective signs of withdrawal precipitated by naloxone.

Naltrexone is an opiate antagonist that is claimed to be non-addicting. It is administered in the morning three times per week, and will block all euphoriant effects of additional opiates (28). Naltrexone administration is based on the theory that if the opiate addict no longer experiences the opiate euphoria, then drug-seeking behavior will diminish and eventually stop. Data indicate that opiate addicts who receive naltrexone are more likely to complete detoxification and less likely to relapse (28). Thus, naltrexone has been added to some opiate detoxification protocols. An example of the combined use of midazolam (short-acting benzodiazepine), naloxone, flumazenil, and naltrexone in a detoxification protocol is presented in Table 18.14. This recently developed protocol is claimed to be easy, quick, and safe, with the addict being able to tolerate the full dose of naltrexone quickly and to experience little withdrawal because of the midazolam (28).

Lastly, there have been reports of the use of auricular acupuncture to augment opiate detoxification (29). In this study, auricular electrical stimulation acupuncture was provided to the Shen Men and lung points. The current was in pulses of 1–3 Hz alternated with pulses of 600–1000 Hz. Patients received acupuncture for a mean of 3–9 hours per day during detoxification. Acupuncture appears to speed opiate detoxification with few side effects from naloxone-precipitated withdrawal.

CONCLUSIONS

There is no good evidence of the superiority of one opiate protocol over another. Therefore this review cannot recommend the use of a particular opiate detoxification protocol. I believe that the choice of a particular detoxification protocol should be dictated by such clinical factors as the need for rapid detoxification and/or the severity of detoxification symptoms encountered.

HYPNOSEDATIVE DETOXIFICATION

Of the hypnosedatives, the barbiturates and nonbarbiturates are rarely administered. The benzodiazepines are now the most important hypnosedative group to the pain physician. This group is widely used for the treatment of anxiety and insomnia within the general population (30) and with chronic pain patients (31). There is much controversy over abuse/dependence/addiction to benzodiazepines in the chronic pain population (32). This issue and the reasons for benzodiazepine detoxification in chronic pain patients have been reviewed in detail (32).

Benzodiazepines differ in abuse liability (i.e., attractiveness as drugs of abuse). This abuse liability is rated as follows (highest to lowest): diazepam, lorazepam, alprazolam, chlorazepate, oxazepam, and chlordiazepoxide (33). Abuse potential does not appear to depend on the half-life of the drug.

Physical dependence to the benzodiazepines can occur even with doses in the clinical range, but requires 6–8 months to develop (34). The short-acting benzodiazepines may have a stronger potential for physical dependence (34). Interestingly, tolerance to the therapeutic effect *does not* develop (30). Three types of benzodiazepine dependence syndromes have been described (35). The

Table 18.11.
Clonidine-Alone Transdermal Patch Detoxification Protocol[a]

1. Test dose oral clonidine 0.1 mg administered and blood pressure measured 1 hour later. If blood pressure systolic less than 90, patient not to get patch.
2. Place two no. 2 transdermal clonidine patches or three patches (if patient weighs more than 150 lbs.) on a hairless area of the upper body.
3. For first 24 hours after patch application, give oral clonidine 0.2 mg q6h.
4. For the next 24 hours, give oral clonidine 0.1 mg q6h.
5. Change patches weekly.
6. After 2 weeks of two patches, switch to 1 no. 2 patch (or two no. 2 patches if the patient weighs more than 150 lbs.).
7. After 1 week of no. 6 (above), D/C patches.

[a]From Spencer L, Gregory M: Clonidine transdermal patches for use in outpatient opiate withdrawal. *J Substance Abuse Treatment* 6:113–117, 1989.

Table 18.12.
Adjunct Clonidine Detoxification Protocol

1. Only start clonidine if the patient demonstrates signs of withdrawal syndrome and/or exhibits major behavioral problems with detoxification.
2. Clonidine 0.1–0.4 mg per day in divided doses to start.
3. Increase gradually to a maximum of 1.2 mg/per day (divided into three doses) according to symptoms.
4. Blood pressure taken lying and standing q.i.d. If less than 90 systolic, clonidine is held for the next dose.
5. Stop increases as soon as symptoms decrease.
6. Maintain on this dose until completion of opiate detoxification.
7. Then begin clonidine detoxification at 25–50% decrease per day.
8. Space clonidine detoxification over 1 week.

patient takes several times the normal therapeutic dose: primary high-dose dependency. The patient takes therapeutic doses: primary low-dose dependency. The patient takes benzodiazepines to treat alcohol or opiate withdrawal: secondary dependency. Patients who manifest primary high-dose dependence are most likely to display addictive behaviors.

Although the hypnosedatives generally cause the same type of withdrawal syndrome, the different classes of hypnosedatives can vary in some signs and symptoms of withdrawal. Barbiturate withdrawal can result in a classic severe withdrawal syndrome that is much like that of alcohol. The signs and symptoms of this withdrawal syndrome are described in most reference texts (36). In general, the hypnosedative withdrawal syndrome will occur from the 2nd to the 14th day after drug cessation (37), and the withdrawal reaction can last 5–20 days (34). It is claimed that unless a hypnosedative has been administered daily for more than 1 month in amounts equivalent to 400–600 mg of a short-acting barbiturate, a severe withdrawal syndrome will not develop (37). To determine if the patient may or may not develop a severe hypnosedative withdrawal syndrome the treating physician should add the total amount of the hypnosedative taken by the patient per day and translate that total amount into a short-acting barbiturate dosage. This conversion can be made with a hypnosedative dosage equivalence chart (38).

Table 18.13.
Detoxification Protocols Using Other Medications[a]

I. *Neuroleptics*
  (1) Thioridazine 25 mg p.o., b.i.d. and 75 mg h.s. for 2 weeks
  (2) Then tapered for 1 week
II. *Diphenoxylate (Lomotil)*
  (1) Two tabs q.i.d. for 4 days
  (2) Then slowly tapered
  (3) Can be combined with thioridazine
III. *Beta-Adrenoreceptor Blocking Drugs*
  (1) Reduces craving after heroin withdrawal
  (2) May be helpful in high somatic anxiety, as indicated by raised pulse rate and high blood pressure
  (3) Propranolol, 80–160 mg in divided doses for 2–3 weeks
  (4) Then slowly tapered
IV. *Sedative Protocol for Opiate Detoxification*
  (1) Does not relieve opiate withdrawal syndrome, only the anxiety
  (2) Not the treatment of choice
  (3) Use diazepam as follows:
    (a) 10 mg q.i.d. × 3 days; then
    (b) 10 mg t.i.d. × 1 day; then
    (c) 10 mg b.i.d. × 1 day; then
    (d) 5 mg b.i.d. × 1 day; then
    (e) 5 mg h.s. × 1 day; then
    (f) D/C

[a]Compiled from Ghodse H: *Drugs and Addictive Behavior: A Guide to Treatment.* Oxford, Blackwell Scientific Publications, 1990.

Table 18.14.
Protocol Using Naltrexone[a]

1. 24 hours after last oral dose of methadone give bolus of 30 mg midazolam IV.
2. Dilute 4 mg of naloxone in 200 ml of 0.9% saline and inject IV via infusion pump. This step is performed 10 min after step 1 above.
3. Maintain sedation with repeated midazolam injections of 50–75 mg.
4. After completion of naloxone infusion give repeated doses of flumazenil 2–6 mg until fully awake.
5. Then continue with oral naltrexone treatment at 50 mg/day.
6. During the procedure record heart rate continuously by EKG and blood pressure by automatic cuff manometer.

[a]Compiled from Rawson RA, Washton AM, Resnick RB, Tennant FS Jr: Clonidine hydrochloride detoxification from methadone treatment—The value of naltrexone aftercare. *Adv Alcohol Subst Abuse* 3:41–49, 1984.

Hypnosedative withdrawal has been divided into two types: with delirium and uncomplicated withdrawal. The DSM-III-R has developed diagnostic criteria for uncomplicated withdrawal (7). Barbiturates and alcohol use are more likely to be associated with withdrawal delirium, whereas benzodiazepine withdrawal is more likely to be of the uncomplicated type (39).

Benzodiazepine withdrawal has also been divided into major and minor types. Owen (34) has described the signs and symptoms of these two types of withdrawal. These signs and symptoms will also differ between abrupt withdrawal and gradual benzodiazepine discontinuation (39, 40). Even a gradual discontinuation, however, appears not to suppress all the signs and symptoms of benzodiazepine withdrawal. Thus, a benzodiazepine withdrawal syndrome will develop even when a gradual taper of 25% *per week* is undertaken (40). It is not clear if these symptoms are withdrawal, rebound, or simply the return of anxiety in a patient being treated for anxiety (34). It is now clear that some form of withdrawal syndrome can be observed in about half the patients discontinuing benzodiazepines (37).

The tendency to experience the benzodiazepine withdrawal syndrome is a function of dosage and duration of treatment and occurs more rapidly in patients taking short–half-life benzodiazepines (34). In addition, the more rapid the fall in benzodiazepine blood level the more likely a withdrawal will occur (34). Severity of withdrawal may be related to benzodiazepine potency, with high-potency drugs such as lorazepam producing more severe withdrawal than medium-potency drugs such as diazepam and low-potency drugs such as chlordiazepoxide (35). In addition, individuals with a psychobiologic predisposition to addiction (often with a past history or family history of alcoholism) may manifest severe benzodiazepine withdrawal symptoms on abrupt benzodiazepine cessation.

Rebound is the return of a symptom for which the drug was originally prescribed, to a degree that is worse than before the drug (35). The benzodiazepine drugs are associated with rebound, especially the short-acting hypnotic benzodiazepine triazolam, which produces prompt and severe rebound. Because of rebound and re-emerging anxiety symptoms even in a gradual benzodiazepine taper (25% per week), a large percentage (approximately 36%) of patients treated for anxiety syndromes will not complete detoxification. Patients on long–half-life benzodiazepines may achieve detoxification in greater numbers, however (40).

In summary, after benzodiazepine drug reduction or cessation, the patient could experience the following syndromes: none, return of pre-existing disorder, rebound, major withdrawal symptoms, minor withdrawal symptoms, combination of rebound and withdrawal, disturbed social/behavioral problems, mood disturbance (major depression), and new anxiety symptoms not before exhibited, such as panic and emotional reaction to anticipated drug withdrawal (41). It is difficult to make a distinction among these syndromes. The pain physician detoxifying a patient from benzodiazepines should be aware of the possibility of the development of these syndromes, however.

Chronic pain patients taking benzodiazepines for anxiety present a special problem. These patients should have a psychiatric examination to determine the type of anxiety syndrome, and whether this syndrome existed before the onset of chronic pain. If the syndrome existed before the pain condition, that patient is less likely to be successfully detoxified, and may not be a candidate for detoxification. Efforts should be made, however, according to the anxiety syndrome diagnosed, to place the patient on other agents that may control his or her anxiety syndrome (e.g., buspirone, MAO inhibitors, tricyclics, beta-blockers). Patients who do not have pre-existing anxiety syndromes but who have current anxiety problems may also have difficulties during detoxification for reasons described above. These difficulties may complicate pain treatment and may occur no matter how slow the taper.

Benzodiazepine Detoxification Protocols

Drugs within the hypnosedative group are mutually cross-tolerant. Thus, as long as dosage equivalencies are calculated correctly (38), any drug within this group can

Table 18.15.
Acute Benzodiazepine Detoxification Methods[a]

Detoxification Method	Indications	Drugs Used
Graded reduction of the benzodiazepine of dependence	Primarily used in medical setting for therapeutic range dependency	Drug used
Substitution of long-acting benzodiazepine	Primarily used for alcohol and/or alcohol-benzodiazepine combination dependency Also now used for therapeutic range dependency	Chlordiazepoxide Diazepam Clonazepam
Phenobarbital substitution	Primarily used for benzodiazepine-polydrug use. Also useful for high-dose benzodiazepine dependency. This method has the broadest utility for all sedative-hypnotics	Phenobarbital

[a]Adapted from Smith DE, Wesson DR: Phenobarbitol technique for the treatment of barbituate dependence. *Arch Gen Psychiatry* 24:56–60, 1971; and Smith DE, Landry MJ: Benzodiazepine dependence discontinuation: Focus on the chemical dependency detoxification setting and benzodiazepine-poly-drug abuse *J Psychiatric Res* 24(Suppl 2):145–156, 1990.

Table 18.16.
Factors Involved in Benzodiazepine Detoxification Problems[a]

1. Taper too rapid
2. Dosage decrease too large
3. Fear of tapering, patient was not sufficiently prepared
4. Caffeine use
5. Alcohol use
6. Illicit drug use
7. Menstrual syndrome (PMS) symptoms
8. Medical condition problem (e.g., increased pain)
9. Life stressors
10. Difficulties in handling tapering problems in a flexible manner
11. Return of pre-existing disorder
12. Rebound
13. Major and minor withdrawal symptoms
14. Mood disorder
15. New anxiety symptoms

[a]Adapted from Dupont RL: A practical approach to benzodiazepine discontinuation. *J Psychiatric Res* 24(Suppl 2):81–90, 1990.

be detoxified by using any other drug within the group (3). There are three major types of benzodiazepine detoxification protocols: graded reduction of the benzodiazepine of dependence, substitution of long-acting benzodiazepine, and phenobarbital substitution. All three, together with their indications, are presented in Table 18.15. Selection of the technique depends on a variety of factors, including severity of dependency, interaction with other drugs, setting for detoxification, and physician expertise (44).

There is disagreement regarding the speed of detoxification for graded reduction. Some authors advocate a 25% reduction every 3 days, which should be titrated according to the severity of withdrawal symptoms (44).

Other authors advocate a detoxification schedule of 6–12 weeks in which dose reduction is no greater than 5 mg of diazepam per week (45). The manufacturer of alprazolam has recommended that for this drug, dosage should be reduced *weekly*. If taking over 3 mg/day of alprazolam, the dosage reduction should be 0.5 mg/week, whereas for patients taking less than 3 mg the reduction should be 0.25 mg/week. Some authors, however, allege that alprazolam can be detoxified much faster, and advocate a reduction of 1 mg every 3 days, or 0.5 mg every 3 days, with a gradual reduction over 3–12 weeks (46). Again, the pain physician will need to decide between a slow taper and an expeditious taper on clinical grounds.

According to my experience if problems or difficulties appear during benzodiazepine detoxification they can be attributed to one or more of the factors listed in Table 18.16. Difficulties in the detoxification process are best avoided by a high index of suspicion for the presence of these factors and by a patient education approach (45). Because of the great likelihood for the development of detoxification problems, patients characterized by the following problems should have a slow taper: pre-existent anxiety syndromes (pre-pain), intense anxiety, trouble coping with current anxiety, increased anxiety with increased pain, and dependent personality features (45).

Substitution of a long-acting benzodiazepine as a detoxification protocol has been advocated for withdrawal from short-acting benzodiazepines. This is because short-acting benzodiazepines, such as alprazolam, may be associated with more withdrawal symptoms than the longer-acting agents, such as clonazepam (47). Thus, in order to make detoxification more tolerable, four long-acting agents have been used in substitution detoxification: chlordiazepoxide, diazepam, clonazepam, and

Table 18.17.
Benzodiazepine Detoxification Protocol Using Substitution of Long-Acting Benzodiazepine

(A) *Using Diazepam*[a]

The dosage of diazepam equivalent to the patient's total benzodiazepine daily dose is calculated (38) for high-dose benzodiazepine abuse, and a loading dose of diazepam of 40% of the patient's total benzodiazepine daily dose is given. Diazepam is then reduced 10% per day for a probable 14-day taper. A slower variant of this technique is to estimate total daily dose by history. Divide this dose into four equivalent doses and administer for 2 days. Then, decrease by 10% per day. If required, give 5 mg Valium PRN for signs of withdrawal syndrome. When remaining diazepam dose reaches 10%, reduce over 4 days. Although slower, the authors recommend this latter method.

(B) *Using Clonazepam to Substitute for Alprazolam*[b]

   a. First day, transfer to clonazepam at a milligram-to-milligram equivalency.
   b. Divide clonazepam into b.i.d. dosage.
   c. Taper clonazepam at 1–1.5 mg every 2 days.
   d. Taper completed in 7–10 days.

[a]From Harrison M, Busto U, Navanjo CA, Kaplan HL, Sellers EM: Diazepam tapering in detoxification for high-dose benzodiazepine abuse. *Clin Pharmacol Ther* 36:527–533, 1984.
[b]Patterson JF: Withdrawal from alprazolam dependency using clonazepam: Clinical observations. *J Clin Psychiatry* 51(Suppl 5):47–49, 1990.

Table 18.18.
Benzodiazepine Detoxification Protocol using Phenobarbital Substitution[a]

A. To calculate the amount of hypnosedative that the patient requires per day, he or she is given the phenobarbital challenge test (43).
B. The amount of pentobarbital (in milligrams) required for 24 hours is calculated from the test.
C. This dose is translated into phenobarbital equivalency (38).
D. Phenobarbital is divided in q8h doses.
E. Detoxification proceeds at one-tenth the starting dose per day.

[a]From Shader RI, Caine ED, Meyer RE: Treatment of dependence on barbituates and sedative-hypnotics. In Shader RI (ed): *Manual of Psychiatric Therapeutics.* Boston, Little Brown, 1989; and from Smith DE, Wesson DR: Phenobarbital technique for the treatment of barbituate dependence. *Arch Gen Psychiatry* 24:56–60, 1971.

phenobarbital. Examples of long-acting benzodiazepine substitution protocols are presented in Table 18.17. An example of phenobarbital substitution protocol is presented in Table 18.18. It is to be noted that for some patients, substitution to long-acting benzodiazepines for alprazolam withdrawal has not been effective, but phenobarbital has been (44).

Adjunct Medications

To assist hypnosedative detoxification adjunct medications have been used. Research for opiate and alcohol withdrawal syndrome has recommended clonidine for benzodiazepine withdrawal. Unfortunately, it is only partially effective at a dose of 0.1–1.2 mg/day (50). Propranolol in doses of 20 mg q.i.d. is also only partially effective, but should be used for rebound and symptom re-emergence (44, 50). Because carbamazepine demonstrated efficacy in alcohol withdrawal, it was used in benzodiazepine withdrawal. Carbamazepine was initiated at 200 mg p.o. b.i.d. at the onset of detoxification, and increased to 800 mg/day, depending on symptoms. It was then discontinued in 3–14 days after completion of benzodiazepine detoxification (51). Of these three agents, carbamazepine may have the greatest effective-

ness as an adjunct medication for benzodiazepine withdrawal.

Recently, a new nonbenzodiazepine anxiolytic has been developed: buspirone. This drug was used in one study of alprazolam detoxification, and has demonstrated that it can decrease the manifestations of withdrawal (52). Buspirone was initiated 2 weeks before beginning the taper at a dosage of 5 mg t.i.d. Because buspirone appears not to have any abuse liability, it could be very useful. A final approach could be the addition of an anti-panic agent, such as imipramine (TCA) or phenelzine (MAO), before beginning detoxification. Such an approach could minimize rebound and symptom re-emergence problems.

Alcohol Abuse/Dependence/Withdrawal and Psychiatric Dual Diagnosis

Alcohol or ethanol is a depressant drug and is classified under the hypnosedative group. Current alcohol abuse/dependence has been reported to be present in 4.3% of a large sample of chronic pain patients (42). Alcohol abuse/dependence in remission has been reported to be present in 7.4% of chronic pain patients

Table 18.19.
Alcohol Withdrawal Detoxification Protocol[a]

(1) Because of severe medical consequences of alcohol abuse and potential for dehydration/seizure/death, all patients should have adequate medical evaluation for concomitant medical/surgical/psychiatric conditions, including full-range laboratory work-up.

(2) *Minimal syndrome*—Drug-free, reassurance given, adequate but appropriate stimulation, millieu support (social setting detoxification).

(3) *Mild syndrome*—Chlordiazepoxide 10–25 mg p.o. q.i.d. for 2–5 days, regular contact with clinician, titrate dosage as needed.

(4) *Moderate syndrome*—Chlordiazepoxide 50–100 mg p.o. initially, then 25 mg. q. 3–4 h. for first 24 hours, then taper total dose by 25–33%/day.

(5) *Severe syndrome*—Chlordiazepoxide 50–100 mg p.o. initially, then 50–100 mg q1–2h until adequately sedated, then D/C and observe for at least 48 hours.

(6) *Emergency management*—If very severe, diazepam 5–10 mg IV slow push (2–5 mg/min), may be repeated PRN or lorazepam 2–5 mg IM or IV may be given and repeated. When stable, use p.o. regimen as above.

(7) Thiamine 100 mg orally four times daily.

(8) Folic acid 1 mg orally four times daily.

(9) Multivitamin, one per day.

(10) Magnesium sulfate 1 g IM every 6 hours for 2 days (if status following withdrawal invol. seizures).

(11) Use lorazepam or oxazepam in debilitated patients and those with COPD or severe liver disease.

(12) If benzodiazepine must be taken IM, do not administer clordiazepoxide or diazepam, because they are poorly absorbed by IM route; use lorazepam.

(13) Patients must be carefully monitored. Signs of oversedation should lead to withholding doses and decreasing subsequent doses. Continued withdrawal should prompt increased dose or re-evaluation of choice of drug, increased dosing interval and/or route of administration, checking for presence of hypoglycemia or hypomagnesemia.

(14) Phenytoin 100 mg p.o. q.i.d., if history of seizure disorder and/or previous withdrawal seizures.

[a]Adapted from Wartenberg AA: Detoxification of the chemically dependent patient. *Rhode Island Med J* 72:451–456, 1989.

(42). Thus, approximately 12% of chronic pain patients appear to have had a problem with alcohol at one point. As with other drugs of abuse, patients who abuse and/or are dependent on alcohol suffer from other psychiatric disorders (dual diagnosis) (51). The pain physician should therefore maintain a high index of suspicion for potential dual diagnosis in alcoholic patients because the dual diagnosis problem can interfere with alcohol detoxification and the concomitant treatment of chronic pain.

Alcohol withdrawal signs and symptoms have been well described and subdivided into mild, moderate, and severe forms (53). The DSM-III-R divides alcohol withdrawal syndrome into *uncomplicated alcohol withdrawal* and *alcohol withdrawal delirium* (7). This classification is simpler and therefore less confusing. In the mild, moderate, and severe classification, both the moderate and severe forms contain some signs and symptoms of delirium, and this is confusing. The mild, moderate, and severe classification, however, lends itself more to the alcohol withdrawal detoxification protocol to be described below. The most effective treatment of alcohol withdrawal, however, is a preventive approach. The pain physician should be alert to the development of alcohol withdrawal in any patient he or she suspects of alcohol abuse/dependence. These patients should be closely monitored; if they demonstrate symptoms of withdrawal, prophylactic aggressive treatment to prevent delirium should be initiated.

Alcohol Withdrawal Detoxification Protocols

Benzodiazepines are clearly the drugs of choice for the treatment of alcohol withdrawal. This group has consistently demonstrated superiority to placebo in controlled trials for the treatment of alcohol withdrawal (38). Of the benzodiazepines, two drugs—chlordiazepoxide and diazepam—have emerged as the drugs of choice. Chlordiazepoxide may be preferable over diazepam because of its lower abuse potential (33). The use of these benzodiazepines for the treatment of various types of alcohol withdrawal is demonstrated in Table 18.19. This alcohol withdrawal detoxification protocol demonstrates the treatment of alcohol withdrawal according to the type of syndrome. In addition it advises on the use of other benzodiazepines (e.g., lorazepam) in other specific situations. This protocol also lists adjunct treatments such as magnesium. According to my experience this protocol can be extremely effective. Often, however, the mistake is made of placing the patient on a PRN chlordiazepoxide schedule after the initial dosage. This is not correct, because generally the nursing staff withholds the PRN benzodiazepine and the patient continues in withdrawal, especially if the routine dosage has not been calculated correctly. Thus, if a PRN order is written, it should specify the symptom for which the medication should be given (e.g., agitation, tremor). A better way to give the benzodiazepine is as in numbers 4 and 5 of Table 18.19, but at the interval specified *unless the patient is asleep*. This type of order will ensure that the patient will get enough benzodiazepine over a short period in order to terminate the alcohol withdrawal syndrome and prevent delirium. The prevention of delirium in an alcohol withdrawal syndrome should be of primary concern.

In addition to the benzodiazepines, other drugs also appear to control the autonomic dysfunction in alcohol withdrawal. Clonidine is claimed to be as useful as the benzodiazepines, but will not prevent seizures or delirium (54). Atenolol (a beta-blocker) appears to decrease the symptoms of tremor, rapid heart rate, and hypertension in this syndrome (54). In addition, the anticonvulsants carbamazepine and valproic acid have been tried. These drugs retard the development of kindling foci in the limbic system, thereby controlling seizure development (54). Carbamazepine in doses of 800 mg/day has been found to be as efficacious as oxazepam (54).

DRUGS OTHER THAN OPIATES AND HYPNOSEDATIVES

DETOXIFICATION PROTOCOLS FOR PSYCHOMIMETICS, NICOTINE, STIMULANTS, ALPHA-ADRENERGIC BLOCKING AGENTS, ANTIDEPRESSANTS, BETA-ADRENERGIC BLOCKING AGENTS, AND MUSCLE RELAXANTS

The psychomimetics do not require a detoxification protocol. The other groups of drugs (above) may or may not be associated with a withdrawal syndrome, however. Thus, in some situations these drug groups may require a detoxification protocol. For some of these groups (e.g., stimulants) protocols have been developed. For details of these protocols, the reader is referred to a recent review (32).

REFERENCES

1. Newman RG: The need to redefine "addiction". *N Engl J Med* 18:1096–1098, 1983.
2. Inturrisi CE: Role of opioid analgesics *Am J Med* 10:27–36, 1984.
3. Ludwig AM: *Principles of Clinical Psychiatry.* New York, Free Press, 1980.
4. Ghodse H: *Drugs and Addictive Behavior, A Guide to Treatment.* Oxford, Blackwell Scientific Publications, 1990.
5. Madden C, Ong B, Singer G: Mood state of heroin-dependent persons undergoing methadone detoxification. *Int J Addict* 22:93–102, 1989.
6. Haertzen CA, Hooks NT: Changes in personality and subjective experience associated with chronic administration and withdrawal of opiates. *J Nervous Mental Dis* 148:606–614, 1969.
7. *American Psychiatric Association Diagnostic and Statistical Manual of Mental Disorders,* ed 3. Washington, D.C., 1987.
8. Fishbain DA, Rosomoff HL, Steele-Rosomoff R: Chronic pain patients opiate and other drug dependence/addiction. A Review of the evidence. *Clin J Pain* 8:77–85, 1992.
9. Turkington D, Drummon DC: How should opiate withdrawal be measured? *Drug-Alcohol Depend* 24:151–153, 1989.
10. Cuthill JD, Beroniade V, Salvatori VA, Viguie F: Evaluation of clonidine suppression of opiate withdrawal reactions: A multidisciplinary approach. *Can J Psychiatry* 35:377–382, 1989.
11. Halpern L: Substitution-detoxification and its role in the management of chronic benign pain. *J Clin Psychiatry* 43:10–14, 1982.
12. Frances RJ, Franklin JE: Alcohol and other psychoactive substance use disorders. In Talbott JA, Hales RE, Yudofsky SC (eds): *American Psychiatric Press Textbook of Psychiatry.* Washington, D.C., American Psychiatry Press, 1988.
13. Goldstein E, Pollack R, Weiner B, Lazoritz R: Rapid treatment of percodan addiction: A case report. *Int J Addiction* 13:1003–1007, 1978.
14. Bickel WK, Stitzer ML, Bigelow GE, Liebson IA, Jasinski DR, Johnson RE: A clinical trial of buprenorphine: Comparison with methadone in the detoxification of heroin addicts. *Clin Pharmacol Ther* 43:72–78, 1988.
15. Kosten TR, Krystal JH, Charney DS, et al: Rapid detoxification from opioid dependence. *Am J Psychiatry* 146:1349, 1989.
16. Jacobsen LK, Kosten TR: Naloxone challenge as biological predictor of treatment outcome in opiate addicts. *Am J Drug Alcohol Abuse* 15:355–366, 1989.
17. Clarney DS, Riordan CE, Kleber MD, et al: Clonidine and naltrexone: A safe, effective, and rapid treatment of abrupt withdrawal from methadone therapy. *Arch Gen Psychiatry* 39:1327–1332, 1982.
18. Aghajanian GK, Vander Mallen CP: Alpha-2-adreno-receptor-induced hyperpolarization of locus ceruleus neurons: Intracellular studies in vivo. *Science* 215:1394–1396, 1982.
19. Kleber HD, Riordqan CE, Rounsaville B, Kosten T, Charney D, Gaspari J, Hogan I, O'Connor C: Clonidine in outpatient detoxification from methadone maintenance. *Arch Gen Psychiatry* 42:391–394.
20. San L, Cami J, Peri JM, Mata R, Porta M: Efficacy of clonidine quanfacine and methadone in the rapid detoxification of heroin addicts: A controlled clinical trial. *Br J Addict* 85:141–147, 1990.
21. Kosten TR, Rounsaville BJ, Kleber HD: Comparison of clinician ratings to self reports of withdrawal during clonidine detoxification of opiate addicts *Am J Drug Alcohol Abuse* 11:1–10, 1985.
22. Fertig JB, Pomerleau OF, Sanders B: I Nicotine-produced antinociception in minimally deprived smokers and ex-smokers. *Addict Behav* 11:239–248, 1986.
23. Spencer L, Gregory M: Clonidine transdermal patches for use in outpatient opiate withdrawal. *J Substance Abuse Treatment* 6:113–117, 1989.
24. Roehrich HJ, Gold MS: Propranolol as adjunct to clonidine

in opiate detoxification. *Am J Psychiatry* 144:1099–1100, 1987.

25. Dufficy RG: Use of psychotherapeutic drugs in the acute detoxification of heroin addicts. *Milit Med* 138:748, 1973.

26. Loimer N, Schmid R, Lencz K, et al: Acute blocking of naloxone precipitated opiate withdrawal symptoms by methohexitone. *Br J Psychiatry* 157:748–752, 1990.

27. Loimer N, Lencz K, Schmid R, Presslich O: Technique for greatly shortening the transition from methadone to naltrexone maintenance of patients addicted to opiates. *Am J Psychiatry* 148:933–935, 1991.

28. Rawson RA, Washton AM, Resnick RB, Tennant FS Jr: Clonidine hydrochloride detoxification from methadone treatment—The value of naltrexone aftercare. *Adv Alcohol Subst Abuse* 3:41–49, 1984.

29. Kroening RJ, Oleson TD: Rapid narcotic detoxification in chronic pain patients treated with auricular electroacupuncture and naloxone. *Int J Addict* 20:1347–1360, 1985.

30. Uhlenhuth E, DeWit H, Balter MB: Risks and benefits of long-term benzodiazepine use. *J Clin Psychopharmacol* 8:161–167, 1988.

31. King SA, Strain JJ: Benzodiazepine use by chronic pain patients. *Clin J Pain* 6:143–147, 1990.

32. Fishbain DA, Rosomoff HL, Steele-Rosomoff R: The detoxification of non opiate drugs in the chronic pain setting and clonidine opiate detoxification: A review. *Clin J Pain,* 8:191–203, 1992.

33. Griffiths RR, Wolf B: Relative abuse liability of different benzodiazepines in drug abusers. *J Clin Psychopharmacol* 10:237–243, 1990.

34. Owen RT, Tyrel P: Benzodiazepine. A review of the evidence. *Drugs* 25:385–398, 1983.

35. Lader M: Long-term anxiolytic therapy: The issue of drug withdrawal. *J Clin Psychiatry* 48(Suppl 12):12–16, 1987.

36. Shader RI, Caine ED, Meyer RE: Treatment of dependence on barbiturates and sedative-hypnotics. In Shader RI (ed): *Manual of Psychiatric Therapeutics*. Boston, Little Brown, 1989.

37. Noyes R, Garvey MN, Cook BL, et al: Benzodiazepine withdrawal: A review of the evidence *J Clin Psychiatry* 49:382–389, 1988.

38. Wartenberg AA: Detoxification of the chemically dependent patient. *Rhode Island Med J* 72:451–456, 1989.

39. Rickels K, Schwerzer E, Case WG, Greenblatt DJ: Long-term therapeutic use of benzodiazepines. I: Effects of abrupt discontinuation. *Arch Gen Psychiatry* 47:899–907, 1990.

40. Schwerzer E, Rickels K, Case WG, Greenblatt DJ: Long-term therapeutic use of benzodiazepines. II: Effects of gradual taper. *Arch Gen Psychiatry* 47:908–915, 1990.

41. Burrows GD, Norman TR, Judd FK, et al: Short-acting versus long-acting benzodiazepines: Discontinuation effects in panic disorders. *J Psychiatric Res* 24(Suppl 2):65–72, 1990.

42. Fishbain DA, Goldberg M, Meagher BR, Steele R, Rosomoff H: Male and female chronic pain patients categorized by DSM-III psychiatric diagnostic criteria. *Pain* 26:181–197, 1986.

43. Smith DE, Wesson DR: Phenobarbital technique for the treatment of barbiturate dependence. *Arch Gen Psychiatry* 24:56–60, 1971.

44. Smith DE, Landry MJ: Benzodiazepine dependence discontinuation: Focus on the chemical dependency detoxification setting and benzodiazepine-poly-drug abuse. *J Psychiatric Res* 24(Suppl 2):145–156, 1990.

45. DuPont RL: A practical approach to benzodiazepine discontinuation. *J Psychiatric Res* 24(Suppl 2):81–90, 1990.

46. Burrows GD: Managing long-term therapy for panic disorder. *J Clin Psychiatry* 51(Suppl 11):9–12, 1990.

47. Herman JB, Rosenbaum JF, Brotman AW: The alprazolam to clonazepam switch for the treatment of panic disorder. *J Clin Psychopharmacol* 7:175–178, 1987.

48. Harrison M, Busto U, Naranjo CA, Kaplan HL, Sellers EM: Diazepam tapering in detoxification for high-dose benzodiazepine abuse. *Clin Pharmacol Ther* 36:527–533, 1984.

49. Patterson JF: Withdrawal from alprazolam dependency using clonazepam: Clinical observations. *J Clin Psychiatry* 51(Suppl 5):47–49, 1990.

50. Lader M: Long-term anxiolytic therapy: The issue of drug withdrawal. *J Clin Psychiatry* 48(Suppl 12):12–16, 1987.

51. Ries RK, Roy-Byrne PP, Warang, et al: Carbamazepine treatment for benzodiazepine withdrawal. *Am J Psychiatry* 146:536–537, 1989.

52. Udelman HD, Udelman DL: Concurrent use of buspirone in anxious patients during withdrawal from alprazolam therapy. *J Clin Psychiatry* 51(Suppl 9):46–54, 1990.

53. Miller GW Jr: Principles of alcohol detoxification. *Am Fam Physician* 30:145–148, 1984.

54. Castaneda R, Cushman P: Alcohol withdrawal: A review of clinical management. *J Clin Psychiatry* 50:278–284, 1989.

SECTION IV

PAIN MANAGEMENT IN SELECTIVE DISORDERS

CHAPTER 19

DIFFERENTIAL DIAGNOSIS OF HEADACHE PAIN

SEYMOUR DIAMOND
MERLE L. DIAMOND

HEADACHE HAS been termed the most common medical complaint of civilized people, and is the fifth most common reason for outpatient medical care (1). Headache may be intense whether its source is benign or malignant. Although the vast majority of headaches are unrelated to structural neurologic disease, headache can also be the presenting complaint in potentially life-threatening disorders such as meningitis, cerebral hemorrhage, and brain tumor.

In evaluating the diagnosis of headache, it is important to review the pain-sensitive structures of the head and their innervation (Table 19.1). These are the skin of the scalp and its blood supply and appendages, the head and neck muscles, aponeuroses, periosteum, spinal roots, joints, the great venous sinuses and their tributaries, parts of the dura mater at the base of the brain, the dural arteries, the intracerebral arteries, the fifth, sixth, and seventh cranial nerves, and the cervical nerves. The brain, the cranium, the majority of the dura and the pia mater, the ependymal lining of the ventricles, and the choroid plexus are not pain-sensitive (2).

Pain pathways for structures of the anterior and middle fossae are contained in the ipsilateral trigeminal nerve. Pain from these structures is usually felt in the frontal, temporal, and parietal regions of the head. The posterior fossa is innervated by the ipsilateral upper three cervical roots with contributions from the glossopharyngeal and vagus nerves. Pain from these structures is usually felt in the occipital region (2).

HISTORY

Proper evaluation of a complete and detailed history will establish the diagnosis in most cases of chronic recurrent headache. A careful history is particularly important in the diagnosis of headache, because the majority of patients with headache will have normal neurologic and physical examinations.

The first inquiry in a headache history is a precise description of the headache. It is very common for patients to have two or more different types of head pain. For each separate type of head pain, the following data should be obtained.

AGE AT ONSET, LENGTH OF ILLNESS, ASSOCIATED LIFE EVENTS AT TIME OF ONSET

The length of time that a patient has suffered from headache is the first guide to whether the symptom represents a malignant or progressive neurologic disorder that requires further evaluation. The sudden onset of severe headache, possibly with focal neurologic disorder, requires further evaluation. The sudden onset of severe headache, possibly with focal neurologic signs or decreased consciousness, suggests a serious illness such as subarachnoid hemmorrhage or meningitis, whereas a recurrent course of headache over 30–40 years is likely to represent a form of vascular headache. The first attack of migraine may prove confusing to the physician, unless it is preceded by a characteristic prodrome, and may suggest meningitis or intracerebral hemorrhage.

Headaches that have developed over weeks to months may be the most difficult to interpret. In these cases, the physician must consider sinusitis, ocular disease, subdural hematoma, mass lesion, hydrocephalus and, in the patient over 45 years old, temporal arteritis.

TIME, COURSE, AND FREQUENCY OF HEADACHE

The information should include the time of day when the headache begins, duration of headache, and relationship to menses, puberty, pregnancy, and menopause. Frequency and duration establish the temporal pattern that can be the key to diagnosis of recurrent headache. Often, migraine will initially occur during puberty and may resolve after menopause. Migraine may recur irregularly for months or years, or may fol-

Table 19.1.
Pain Sensitivity of Cranial Tissues

Tissue	Pain-Sensitive	Insensitive to Pain
Intracranial	Cranial sinuses and afferent veins Arteries of the dura mater Arteries of the base of the brain and their major branches Parts of the dura mater (in the vicinity of large vessels)	Parenchyma of the brain Ependyma, choroid plexus Pia mater, arachnoid membrane, parts of the dura mater
Extracranial	Skin, scalp, fascia, muscles Mucosa Arteries (veins: less sensitive)	Skull (periosteum: slightly sensitive)
Nerves	Trigeminal, facial, vagal, glossopharyngeal Second and third cervical nerves	

Table 19.2.
Ocular Prodromata of Migraine

Positive	Teichopsia, or fortification spectra Zigzags Flashing lights and colors
Negative	Scotomata Hemianopsia
Metamorphopsia	Illusions of distorted size, shape, and location of fixed objects

low a pattern of occurring at the time of menses or 1–10 times per month. During the later months of pregnancy, migraines frequently improve. The duration of an acute migraine is usually from several hours to several days. It is usually preceded and followed by a headache-free interval.

Episodic cluster headache occurs in bouts lasting from 2 weeks to 3 months followed by episodes of quiescence ranging from months to years. The cluster periods tend to occur in the spring and fall months. During a cluster period, headaches occur one or more times per day, often at night, thus awakening the patient. The pain characteristally lasts from 10 min to 2 hours. This duration differentiates cluster headache from trigeminal neuralgia, which presents with transient, recurrent jabs of pain lasting less than a second. Cluster variant headaches, such as chronic paroxysmal hemicrania, have pain patterns similar to those of cluster headache, although the attacks occur predominantly during the day.

Tension-type (muscle contraction) headache is characterized by the absence of periodicity or a headache-free interval. Most of these patients report a continuous, daily headache. The mixed headache syndrome is marked by intermittent paroxysms of severe, throbbing, sick headache superimposed on a background of constant, daily headache.

LOCATION OF HEAD PAIN

Tension-type headache is commonly bilateral, however, migraine occurs unilaterally in two-thirds of patients. Cluster headache and trigeminal neuralgia are always unilateral, as are headaches associated with local disease of the eye, nose, sinuses, or scalp. Headache due to subarachnoid hemorrhage and space-occupying masses may start as localized or unilateral pain, but will usually become bilateral. Migraine headache may alternate sides with different attacks but may be localized to one side during an entire lifetime. Cluster headache invariably remains on one side during a series of attacks.

SEVERITY AND PAIN CHARACTERISTICS OF HEADACHE

In differentiating migraine, the headache is either throbbing or pulsatile. A constant ache will suggest tension-type headache, whereas deep, boring, intense pain is descriptive of cluster headache. Shock-like intense jabs are typical of trigeminal neuralgia. Because the severity of pain is very subjective, its diagnostic value is limited. Cluster headache and trigeminal neuralgia are consistently described as severe, however. The pain of cluster headache will generally make the patient unable to remain still. In contrast, the common response to migraine is to remain in a darkened, quiet room and to limit activity.

PRODROMAL OR WARNING SYMPTOMS AND SIGNS

The only type of headache with a recognizable prodrome is migraine with aura (formerly known as classic migraine). Visual (Table 19.2) or neurologic symptoms precede the onset of headache by 10–60 min. Premonitory symptoms commonly precede migraine by 12–24 hours and may include euphoria, fatigue, a craving for sweets, or yawning.

ASSOCIATED SYMPTOMS

Associated symptoms of migraine can include photophobia, gastrointestinal disturbance, fluid retention, and focal neurologic signs. Cluster headache can be marked by partial Horner's syndrome, constricted pupils, injected conjunctiva, lacrimation, and rhinorrhea. Nasal congestion and rhinorrhea are also common in sinusitis. Stiff neck and other meningeal irritation signs can be seen with meningitis, encephalitis, and subarachnoid hemorrhage. Decreased level of consciousness can be observed in patients with mass lesions, hydrocephalus, or encephalitis. A colloid cyst blocking the flow of cerebrospinal fluid (CSF) in the third ventricle can cause positional headache and drop attacks. Seizures may reflect cortical irritation associated with mass lesions, or arteriovenous malformation. Fever and sweats may signal an acute infection.

Precipitating Factors

Fatigue, specifically lack of sleep, can precipitate both migraine and tension-type headache. Stress is also a frequent trigger of tension-type headache, whereas migraine often occurs after a stressful period, weekends, or vacations. Patients with migraine often relate their headaches to menses, missing meals, and/or dietary indiscretion, particularly consumption of foods rich in tyramine (Table 19.3). Alcohol usually triggers an attack during a cluster series, but will have no effect during remission. Migraine can also be precipitated by alcohol, such as red wine. Weather changes can exacerbate sinusitis pain and can also trigger migraine.

Emotional Factors and Other Evidence of Psychological Illness

Signs and symptoms of depression, including sleep and appetite disturbances, are frequent markers for tension-type headache and depression (Table 19.4).

Relationship to Work and Occupational Exposure to Toxins, Chemicals, and Infectious Agents

Carbon monoxide poisoning will frequently be manifested by headache. Certain chemicals and toxins, such as nitrites, will induce withdrawal or reintroduction headache. It should be noted that exposure to infectious agents or acquired immunodeficiency syndrome (AIDS) may lead to encephalitis caused by fungi or microbacteria that may not produce fever or stiff neck (3).

Family History of Migraine, Depression, Mental Illness, or Alcoholism

Migraine is a familial disorder, with positive family history noted in up to three-fourths of patients. Cluster headache is familial in only about 2% of patients.

Medical and Surgical History

Head trauma suggests subdural hematoma or skull fractures. Lumbar puncture can be followed by a prolonged headache associated with CSF leakage. The headache is worse on arising and decreases with recumbency. Immunocompromised patients (chemotherapy, cancer, steroids, AIDS) may be at risk for unusual types of meningitis and encephalitis, often without the sentinel signs of fever or still neck. Infectious disease, including syphilis or tuberculosis, may be manifested by headache. It is well to remember that fever, regardless of etiology, is the most common cause of infectious headache.

Systems Review, Including Allergies

It has not been demonstrated that migraine and other types of headache result from allergy (antibody-antigen reaction). The patient may confuse dietary triggers of headache for an allergic reaction. Patients with "triad asthma" (asthma, nasal polyps, and aspirin sensitivity) have a high incidence of migraine (4).

Previous Diagnostic Tests and Work-Up for Headache

If a patient has recently had an adequate work-up, and there are no neurologic or historic reasons to indicate further testing, it is prudent to not repeat tests.

Previous Treatments

A past history of therapeutic successes and failures can serve as both a diagnostic aid and a guide to therapy. The dose and duration should be included if possible. Previous good response to ergotamine tartrate suggests the diagnosis of migraine, whereas acute cluster headache may respond well to oxygen inhalation as well as ergotamine.

Current Medications

Migraine can be exacerbated by oral contraceptives, postmenopausal hormones, and vasodilators. Reserpine can promote both depression and migraine. Although indomethacin can be used in headache prophylaxis, it may trigger headache. The daily use of analgesics, especially narcotics and those analgesics containing butalbital or caffeine, can eventually lead to rebound/withdrawal headaches, thus exacerbating a daily headache pattern. Overuse of ergot preparations can also cause rebound headaches.

The information obtained by each item in the headache history should contribute to the overall differential diagnosis of headache.

PHYSICAL AND NEUROLOGIC EXAMINATION

Every headache patient deserves a thorough physical and neurologic examination. The evaluation should include mental status, examination of the head and skull, and palpation of both the temporomandibular joints and cervical spine to rule out tenderness and mobility. Neurologic examination should include tests of cerebel-

Table 19.3.
Tyramine-Free Diet

Class of Food	Foods Allowed	Foods to Avoid
Beverages	Decaffeinated coffee, fruit juice, club soda, noncola soda (7-UP, ginger ale); Limit caffeine sources to 2 cups/day (coffee, tea, cola)	Chocolate, cocoa, alcoholic beverages
Meat, fish, poultry	Fresh or frozen: turkey, chicken, fish, beef, lamb, veal pork Egg as meat substitute (limit 3 eggs/week) Tuna or tuna salad	Aged, canned, cured, or processed meat, including ham or game; pickled herring, salad and dried fish; chick livers; bologna; fermented sausage; any food prepared with meat tenderizer, soy sauce, or brewer's yeast; any food containing nitrates, nitrites, or tyramine
Dairy products	Milk: homogenized, 2%, or skim Cheese: American, cottage, farmer, ricotta, cream, Velveeta; Yogurt (limit 1/2 cup per day)	Cultured dairy products (buttermilk, sour cream); Chocolate milk; Cheese: bleu, Boursault, brick, Brie types, Camembert types, cheddar, Gouda, Stilton, Swiss (Emmentaler), Roquefort, mozzarella, Parmesan, provolone, Romano
Breads, cereals	Commercial bread, English muffins, melba toast, crackers, RyKrisp, bagel All hot and dry cereals	Hot fresh homemade yeast bread, bread or crackers containing cheese; Fresh yeast coffee cake, doughnuts, sourdough bread; any product containing chocolate or nuts
Potatoes or substitutes	White potato, sweet potato, rice, macaroni, spaghetti, noodles	None
Vegetables	Any except those to avoid	Beans such as pole, broad, lima, Italian, fava, navy, pinto, garbanzo; Snow peas, pea pods, sauerkraut, onions (except for flavoring), olives, pickles
Fruits	Any except those to avoid; Limit citrus fruits to 1/2 cup per day; Limit banana to 1/2 per day	Avocados, figs, raisins, papaya, passion fruit, red plums
Soups	Cream soups made from foods allowed in diet, homemade broths	Canned soup, soup or bouillon cubes, soup base with autolytic yeast or MSG (**read labels**)
Desserts	Fruit allowed in diet, any cake, pudding, cookies, or ice cream without chocolate or nuts, no yeast items, JELL-O	Chocolate ice cream, pudding, cookies, cake, or pies Mincemeat pie
Sweets	Sugar, jelly, jam, honey, hard candy	Chocolate candy or syrup, carob
Miscellaneous	Salt in moderation, lemon juice, butter or margarine, cooking oil, whipped cream, white vinegar and commercial salad dressings in small amounts	Pizza, cheese sauce, MSG in excessive amounts, yeast, yeast extract, meat tenderizer, Accent, seasoned salt; Mixed dishes (macaroni & cheese, beef stroganoff, cheese blintzes, lasagna, frozen TV dinners) Nuts (peanuts, peanut butter); Seeds (pumpkin, sesame, sunflower); **Read labels** on snack items; any pickled, preserved, or marinated food

lar, motor, and sensory function, testing of the cranial nerves, and careful inspection of the optic disks. Cardiopulmonary status should be evaluated, with measurement of vital signs. In most patients, the physical and neurologic examinations will reveal no abnormalities.

LABORATORY AND IMAGING STUDIES

As part of the initial evaluation of most headache patients, routine laboratory studies should be obtained in order to identify systemic causes of chronic recurrent headache, and to indicate potential hazards of certain medical therapies.

LABORATORY STUDIES

Laboratory studies should include complete blood count, chemistries, urinalysis and, if clinically indicated, thyroid studies, serology, and prolactin measurement. In patients above the age of 45, erythrocyte sedimenta-

Table 19.4.
Patterns of Depression

Complaint	Incidence (%)
Physical complaints	
Sleep disturbances	97
Early awakening	87
Headache	84
Dyspnea	76
Constipation	76
Loss of weight	74
Trouble getting to sleep	73
Weakness and fatigue	70
Urinary frequency	70
"Spells"—dizziness	70
Appetite disturbances	70
Deceased libido	63
Cardiovascular disturbances	60
Sexual disturbances	60
Palpitations	59
Paresthesias	53
Nausea	48
Menstrual changes	41
Emotional complaints	
"Blue," low spirits, sadness	90
Crying	80
Feelings of guilt, hopelessness, unworthiness, unreality	65
Anxious or irritable	65
Anxiety	60
Fear of insanity, physical disease, death; rumination over the past, present, future	50
Psychic complaints	
"Morning worst time of day"	95
Poor concentration	91
No interest; no ambition	75
Indecisiveness	75
Poor memory	71
Suicidal thoughts; death wishes	35

tion rate by the Westergren method should be obtained to rule out temporal arteritis.

IMAGING STUDIES

Unless the headache history is clearly defined and the neurologic examination is essentially normal, imaging studies, including computed tomography (CT) scan of the head or magnetic resonance imaging (MRI) are advised.

CT Scan of the Head

CT scanning is the most reliable method of identifying intracranial lesions in the headache patient, and probably represents the greatest diagnostic advance for these patients in the past several decades. This noninvasive technique, using a computer coupled with a special radiographic device, produces detailed cross-sectional images of the brain. It can detect variations in tissue den-

sity that assist in detection of pathologic lesions. The CT scan can identify most space-occupying lesions, and aid in discriminating between neoplasms, abscesses, and hematomas. It is useful in detecting hydrocephalus, cerebral edema, infarction, hemorrhage, and occasionally arteriovenous malformations. CT scanning is not particularly effective in detecting aneurysms. However, aneurysms rarely produce headaches unless they leak or rupture, on which occasion the bleed will be demonstrated by the scan.

The CT scan provides information on the brain and its appendages that previously could not be obtained or that required invasive techniques such as cerebral angiography, pneumoencephalography, or ventriculography. In addition, its accuracy in detecting supratentorial lesions far exceeds that of radioisotope scanning. The availability of CT scanning as an outpatient procedure, with its noninvasive technique and low radiation exposure, makes it the most cost-effective of diagnostic tests in headache evaluation.

Following are indications for the use of CT scanning patients with recurrent headache:

1. Abnormal neurologic examination, especially if suspicious for intracranial mass lesion
2. Recent onset of persistent headache, exertional headache, personality change, seizures or loss of consciousness
3. Change in character of headache

The CT scan can also be of great value in the detection of acoustic neuromas. Evaluation for these tumors requires special computer cuts and contrast dye enhancement. Routine CT scanning of the headache to evaluate for supratentorial lesions, despite contrast enhancement, is inadequate to detect these tumors. If acoustic neuroma is suspected, CT scanning of the auditory canals should be obtained.

MRI

MRI is probably the most revolutionary method of disclosing occult organic lesions that cause headache. Lesions of the posterior fossa not visualized by other techniques, including CT scan, can occasionally be found by MRI.

MRI works by magnetic induction of nuclei of hydrogen atoms, within tissues from random distribution, into a uniform array. Radiowaves transmitted into the tissues being imaged set the nuclei into resonant oscillating motion. When the radiowaves are stopped, the hydrogen nuclei return to their original positions, emitting their own weak radiowaves that are picked up by antennas in the magnet. These waves are then transformed into electrical impulses and processed into images by computer, similar to the method used in CT scanning (5).

Table 19.5.
Classification of Headache*

Vascular Headache	Tension-Type Headaches	Traction and Inflammatory Headaches

Migraine
  With aura (classic)
  Without aura (common)
  Hemiplegic } Complicated
  Ophthalmoplegic } migraine
  Basilar artery
Cluster
Toxic vascular
Hypertensive
	Anxiety
	Depressive equivalents
	  and conversion reactions
	Cervical osteoarthritis
	Chronic myositis
		Mass lesions (tumors, edema, hematomas,
		  cerebral hemorrhage)
		Diseases of the eye, ear, nose, throat, teeth
		Arteritis, phlebitis, and cranial neuralgias
		Occlusive vascular disease
		Atypical facial pain
		TMJ disease

*Adapted from Diamond S, Dalessio DJ: *The Practicing Physician's Approach to Headache,* ed 5. Baltimore, Williams & Wilkins, 1992.

Imaging can be done in frontal, sagittal, or axial projections. Although the stages of MRI resemble those of CT scanning, there are important differences. The CT scan uses x rays to measure densities of various tissues, and MRI measures the physiologic function of atoms within tissues. This enables the MRI to differentiate normal structures for pathologic tissues. Also, MRI demonstrates soft tissues with greater resolution than CT scanning does, and may allow detection of tissue pathology at an earlier stage of disease.

MRI presents no known health hazards. Current FDA guidelines suggest that pregnant women in the first two trimesters of pregnancy should avoid MRI because the long-term effects of the magnetic field and radiowaves on the developing fetus are unknown. Additionally, patients with pacemakers or surgical steel clips from previous neurosurgery should not enter the MRI scanner.

Because of the lack of published studies specifically addressing the utility of MRI in headache patients, the clinical indications for MRI are uncertain. Brainstem and posterior fossa lesions, difficult to identify on CT scans because of bone artifacts, are well visualized on MRI scans. Soft tissue sensitivity is great enough to distinguish white and gray matter in the brain. Demyelinating lesions, such as those found in multiple sclerosis, can be detected. Brain tumors, infarcts, and hemorrhages are also easily delineated by MRI.

Recently, a group of 300 patients at the Diamond Headache Clinic were evaluated and treated for headache (6). As part of the diagnostic work-up, each patient underwent MRI of the brain. The investigation also included a control group of 300 randomly selected brain MRI studies. The goals of the study were as follows:

1. To determine any abnormal findings on MRI of the brain
2. To demonstrate any relationship between abnormal findings and length of headache history
3. To investigate any differences based on age or sex
4. To determine if excessive ergotamine use could lead to MRI changes

Scattered punctate and round areas of hyperintensity density (HID), distributed throughout the subcortical white matter, was demonstrated in 40 cases (13.2%). Only 2% had other abnormalities detected by MRI. Only 10 patients (3.3%) of the control group demonstrated punctate hyperintense lesions. An increased incidence of HID with advancing age was most obvious in age range distribution. "Normal" MRI was demonstrated in 58% of patients under age 40 years, but between the ages of 41 and 60 years, only 40% revealed normal MRI. HID was observed in 30% of patients under 40 years, and 57% of those patients between 41 and 60 years. The sex distribution of HID was not clinically significant. Eleven patients (27.5%) with a headache history of less than 6 years demonstrated HID. However, 29 patients (72.5%) with a headache history longer than 6 years revealed HID. In those patients overusing ergotamine, the difference in HID occurrences was insignificant. This finding excluded the vasoconstrictive effect of ergotamine as a causative mechanism.

CLASSIFICATION OF HEADACHE

Recently, the International Headache Society has developed a classification system for headache (7). A simpler categorization of headache types has been developed (Table 19.5), dividing these headaches into three groups—vascular, tension-type, and traction and inflammatory.

The category of vascular headache includes migraine, with or without aura, as well as cluster headache, toxic vascular headache, hypertensive headache, and more complicated forms of migraine, such as hemiplegic, ophthalmoplegic, and basilar artery migraine. The common pathway in these headaches is a tendency to vascular dilatation that provokes the headache phase. Toxic vascular headache refers to systemic vasodilation produced by fever, alcohol ingestion, poisons, carbon dioxide retention, and chemical vasodilators, such as the nitrates and nitrites. Hypertensive headache is associated with extreme elevations in systemic arterial pressure, such as hypertensive crisis of malignant hypertension. Cephalalgia in rarely seen with mild or moderate hypertenstion, and the diastolic pressure must be 110 mm Hg or greater to produce symptoms.

The typical description of tension-type (muscle contraction) headache is a dull, band-like, persistent pain. In the acute form, it is probably the most common form of headache, and is usually relieved by simple analgesics. These patients rarely seek professional help, except in the chronic form, when headache is frequently associated with depression or anxiety.

Traction and inflammatory headaches result from organic disease of the head, face, neck, brain, meninges, or vasculature. Mass lesions of the brain, including tumors, hematomas, abscesses, and cerebral edema, trigger traction headache. Traction and inflammatory headache can occur with subarachnoid hemorrhage, meningitis, arteritis, and disorders of the teeth, jaw, and neck. These disorders usually require specific therapy for the underlying disease.

Vascular Headache

Migraine Headache

Migraine has been defined by the International Headache Society Classification Committee as follows (7): "Idiopathic, recurring headache disorder manifesting in attacks lasting 4–72 hours. Typical characteristics of headache are unilateral location, pulsating quality, moderate and severe intensity, aggravation by routine physical activity, and association with nausea, photo-, and phono-phobia." Fifteen to twenty percent of migraine sufferers experience migraine with aura, in which the headache attack is preceded by "attacks of neurological symptoms unequivocally localizable to cerebral cortex or brain stem, usually gradually developed over 5–20 minutes and usually lasting less than 60 minutes. Headache, nausea, and/or photophobia usually follow neurological aura symptoms directly or after a free interval of less than an hour" (7).

The most frequent description of a migraine attack is a dull ache, progressively worsening into a throbbing pain. As it stabilizes, the headache may become constant and nonthrobbing. Migraine is unilateral about 70% of the time, usually affecting the frontal and temporal region. Some patients will note generalized headache, or pain localized to the occipital areas. The intensity of pain may vary between attacks and between patients. For most patients, the pain will require alteration of normal activities. Attacks can occur from every few days to less than once per year. The duration usually lasts from 4 hours to 2 days, with severe episodes lasting up to 6 days. Between attacks, the patients are headache-free.

Migraine is a common malady with a prevalence between 2% and 20% of the population, with women affected almost twice as often as men. In childhood, the incidence in males and females is equal.

The usual onset of migraine is before age 40, and migraine may begin during childhood. It tends to decrease with advancing age, and up to three-fourths of female migraineurs note relief after menopause. About 70% of migraine sufferers have a positive family history for migraine.

Hormonal factors play a role in migraine, with 70% of female migraineurs relating migraine attacks to menstruation. Many women note dramatic improvement in migraine during the last two trimesters of pregnancy. Both oral contraceptives and postmenopausal hormones can aggravate migraine.

The hallmark of migraine is the association of headache with gastrointestinal complaints. The more common gastrointestinal symptoms include anorexia, nausea, and vomiting, with occasional abdominal bloating and diarrhea. Photophobia and phonophobia are frequent associated symptoms of migraine, often forcing the migraine sufferer to seek refuge in a dark, quiet room. Alterations in fluid balance can occur, with peripheral edema and fluid retention noted. Prior to the onset of head pain, the migraine patient may note oliguria, often followed by polyuria as the attack resolves. Other signs less commonly observed are pallor, sweating, chills, and cold extremities. Migraine has been linked to a number of other medical conditions, including Raynaud's phenomenon, systemic lupus erythematosus, mitral valve prolapse, vasospastic (Prinzmetal's) angina, and stroke.

The pathogenesis of migraine remains obscure. The prevailing vascular theory, based on the pioneering work of Wolff (8) and his collaborative studies with Graham (9), is that migraine represents a disorder of cerebrovascular regulation. In the migraine with aura sequence, release of an as-yet-unidentified substance precipitates a cascade of events that includes platelet aggregation, release of platelet serotonin and thromboxane A_2, activation of prostaglandins and production of kinins, and the production of a localized sterile arteritis (10), causing symptomatic focal vasoconstriction. This is followed by reactive vasodilation, primarily in the extracranial cerebral circulation, stretching the pain-sensitive arterioles and producing the familiar throbbing headache of migraine.

In the past decade, studies by Lance et al. (11), Olesen et al. (12), and Kobari et al. (13) have promoted the neurogenic theory of migraine. This work emphasizes the significance of central nervous system neurotransmit-

Table 19.6.
Characteristics Useful in Distinguishing between Basilar Artery Migraine and Migraine with Aura

Characteristic	Basilar Artery Migraine	Migraine with Aura
Age of Onset	Childhood and early adolescence	Adolescence or early adult life
Frequency	Infrequent	Ranging through all degrees of frequency
Visual symptoms	Bilateral impairment or loss	Unilateral impairment or loss
Sensory symptoms	Bilateral, involving hands, feet, and mouth	Unilateral, involving hands, mouth, and tongue
Vertigo	Common	Rare
Ataxia (of gait)	Very common	Very rare
Speech disorder	Dysarthria	Dysphasia if on dominant side
Alteration of consciousness	Frequent	Very rare
Permanent sequelae	Very rare	Rare, but well recognized
Drop attacks	May occur	Do not occur
Origin	Posterior fossa lesions	Cerebral hemisphere lesions

ters (e.g., substance P) as the activators of intracerebral vasoconstriction and extracranial vasodilation.

Migraine without aura (nonclassic migraine) is seen in 85% of all migraine sufferers. In this type of migraine, no neurologic aura precedes the headache attack. It is not unusual, however, for patients to experience disturbances of mood or appetite in the 1–3 days preceding the attack.

In *migraine with aura (classic migraine),* distinct neurologic signs occur in the 15–30 min that precede the headache pain. Scotoma, or blind spots, are the most common aura symptom, but photopsia (flashes of light), teichopsia, or fortification spectra (bright borders resembling a wooden fort with a central blind spot) are also frequent. Other common visual aura symptoms include diplopia, micropsia, macropsia, and metamorphopsia. Nonvisual aura symptoms include paresthesias, olfactory hallucinations, and auditory hallucinations.

Complicated Migraine

Complicated migraine is defined by neurologic or visual symptoms that last beyond the head pain by more than 24 hours. The onset of the neurologic symptom may occur before the headache (aura) or during the pain phase. Complicated migraine can occur in any patient who suffers from migraine, just as migraine with aura and migraine without aura frequently occur in the same patient at different times. A small number of these patients suffer from residual neurologic deficit and stroke (14).

The physician should differentiate complicated migraine from *migraine accompagnee,* in which the neurologic symptoms begin during the pain phase and disappear before or shortly after the attack.

Basilar artery migraine, originally described by Bicker-

staff in 1961 (15), consists of bilateral, posterior, throbbing head pain preceded or accompanied by vertigo, tinnitus, hearing loss, ataxia, dysarthria, and occasionally bilateral sensory or motor symptoms (Table 19.6). Also, basilar artery migraine is occasionally associated with drop attacks, cranial nerve affections, loss of consciousness, and transient global amnesia. These symptoms are thought to represent vascular disturbances within the vertebrobasilar circulation. This syndrome is usually described in adolescent females with previous migraine attacks, but may also be present in younger males. In this age group, the constellation of symptoms may suggest drug intoxication or encephalitis. Basilar artery migraine in adults must be differentiated from thrombosis of cerebral veins and sinuses, subarachnoid hemorrhage, space-occupying lesions in the brainstem, and transient ischemic attacks of the vertebrobasilar system. The differentiation of basilar artery migraine from vertebrobasilar transient ischemic attacks is based on patient age, family history of migraine, risk factors for occlusive arterial disease, and previous migraine symptoms. Because cerebral infarction has been observed in patients with basilar artery migraine, invasive diagnostic work-up, including four-vessel arteriography, may be required.

Hemiplegic migraine consists of unilateral motor and/or sensory deficits beginning before or during the migraine attack, but frequently not resolving for days to weeks. A positive family history for this type of migraine is often elicited, although it can occur sporadically in migraine sufferers.

Paresis of the extraocular muscles characterizes *ophthalmoplegic migraine.* The most common symptom is diplopia developing during the course of a headache, and not a symptom of an aura. Usually, the third cranial nerve is involved, but the fourth and sixth may also be involved. The ocular paresis may survive the headache by days or weeks, but will rarely become permanent. To differentiate this condition from compression of the third nerve by a space-occupying lesion or aneurysm, CT scan and/or angiography must be used. These procedures are also indicated in the differential diagnosis of hemiplegia migraine.

Benign Orgasmic Cephalalgia

Benign orgasmic cephalalgia is a type of exertional headache triggered by sexual intercourse. It is usually of brief duration and recurs with each episode of orgasm. The pain is usually throbbing, although muscular pain is often reported. If the onset occurs during exertion, subarachnoid hemorrhage is suggested. Unlike subarachnoid hemorrhage, benign orgasmic cephalalgia has no accompanying hypertension or focal neurologic signs. Orgasmic cephalalgia is extremely responsive to therapy with indomethacin.

Cluster Headache

A variety of names are attributed to cluster headache, including histamine cephalalgia, Horton's cephalalgia, and migrainous neuralgia. Cluster is a form of headache that occurs in paroxysms of 2 weeks to 3 months, separated by long headache-free periods. Frequently, there is a seasonal incidence, with the cluster bouts occurring usually in spring and autumn. The individual attacks are severe, burning, and unilateral, usually localizing between or around the eye, and lasting from 10 min to 4 hours. During a paroxysm, attacks may occur from one to four times per day. Attacks frequently occur at night, awakening the patient from sleep. In contrast to migraine, there is no aura, and nausea and vomiting occur rarely.

Cluster headache is one of the most severe pains that has been observed. The pain may be so severe that the patient will contemplate suicide. It is usually described as constant and severe, and may be burning, tearing, or boring in quality. Cluster headache invariably occurs unilaterally, and usually affects the same side of the head in each bout. The pain may radiate ipsilaterally from the eye to the supraorbital region, temple, maxilla, and upper gum.

During an attack, patients may exhibit ptosis and miosis (partial Horner's syndrome), flushing or blanching of the face, injection of the conjunctiva, ipsilateral lacrimation, nasal congestion, and rhinorrhea. Focal neurologic signs, frequently seen in migraine, are rarely observed with cluster headache. Long-standing cluster sufferers are sometimes characterized by "leonine facies"—ruddy complexion, thick furrows across the forehead, telangiectasis, coarse cheek skin, and a square, thick chin.

Trigger factors for cluster are only implicated during the susceptible period. These include alcoholic beverages and other vasodilators, such as nitroglycerin. During the dormant periods, vasodilators are well tolerated.

In comparison with migraine (Table 19.7), cluster headache is uncommon, occurring in less than 2% of new patients in a headache clinic. Episodic cluster is predominantly a disease of young males, with a range of age at onset between 20 and 40 years, and an average of 25.5 years. Five to ten percent of cluster sufferers are females. Over 70% of cluster patients are cigarette smokers, and peptic ulcer disease is reported in 20% of cluster patients (16). Coronary artery disease may also be more common in these patients.

The etiology of cluster headaches remains uncertain. The sphenopalatine ganglion, when electrically stimulated, produces a syndrome similar to cluster headache; it is speculated that chronic irritation of the ganglion, possibly by cigarette smoke, may create unilateral hyperactivity. Nonspecific and repetitive stimuli of the ganglion may then induce attacks of cluster pain.

Vascular studies of cluster sufferers by Sakai and Meyer demonstrated that, during a cluster attack, there is increased cerebral blood flow, primarily contralateral to the headache (17). The asymmetry of blood flow suggests autonomic dysfunction. These authors also found that during the headache, the vasodilator response to carbon dioxide was impaired, although the vasoconstrictor response to oxygen was increased. This may explain the therapeutic role of oxygen in acute cluster headache.

Hormonal abnormalities have also been recognized and observed during cluster periods, as opposed to headache-free periods. Unexpectedly low levels of metenkephalin during the cluster attacks have also been observed, although the significance is unknown.

Chronic cluster headache is identical to episodic cluster headache with regard to the individual attacks and patient demographics. However, headache-free intervals of 2 weeks or longer are not seen. These headaches are also identical to episodic cluster headaches in location, duration, and accompanying symptoms, resulting in the misnomer "chronic cluster headache."

Two other syndromes are categorized as variants of cluster headache because of their unilaterality and the brief duration of individual attacks. *Chronic paroxysmal hemicrania* is a syndrome of strictly unilateral headache, never changing sides, without nausea or vomiting, with an attack frequency of 6–18/day. Attacks can be triggered by neck flexion or rotation. These patients have a dramatic response to indomethacin.

Cluster headache variant occurs almost exclusively in females (18). The average age at onset is 35 years. Unlike cluster patients, peptic ulcer disease is rare in this group. Similar to chronic paroxysmal hemicrania, it is also noted for its dramatic response to indomethacin. The pain can occur in three patterns: atypical cluster head-

Table 19.7.
Primary Distinguishing Features of Cluster and Migraine Headaches

Feature	Cluster	Migraine
Location of pain	Always unilateral, periorbital	Unilateral, occasionally bilateral
Age at onset	20–50 years	10–40 years
Sex incidence	90% male	65–70% female
Frequency of attacks	Daily for several weeks to several months*	Intermittent, 2–8 per month
Seasonal occurrence	More common in spring and fall	No variance
Number of attacks	1–6 per day	1–8 per month
Duration of pain	10 min to 3 hours	4–48 hours
Prodromes	Absent	25–30% of cases
Nausea and vomiting	2–5%	85%
Blurring of vision	Infrequent	Frequent
Lacrimation	Frequent	Infrequent
Nasal congestion	70%	Uncommon
Ptosis	30%	1–2%
Polyuria	2%	40%
Family history of vascular headaches	7%	90%
Miosis	50%	Absent
Chemical changes		
Decrease in plasma serotonin	None	80%
Rise in plasma histamine	90%	None
Rise in CSF acetylcholine	30%	None

*A small percentage of cluster headaches (2–3%) occur continuously and are refractory to all methods of treatment.

ache, multiple stabs and jabs throughout the day, and unilateral throbbing headache that is chronic, continuous, and aggravated by exertion.

TENSION-TYPE (MUSCLE CONTRACTION) HEADACHE

This group includes the syndromes of tension-type headaches, cervical arthritis, and mixed headache syndrome. Tension-type headache can be acute, as in a typical, episodic "tension headache," related to contraction of the head and neck muscles. It is usually relieved by over-the-counter analgesics and may be associated with fatigue and temporary stress situations. Chronic tension-type headache is part of a symptom complex due in part to psychological problems and is particularly present in those persons subject to depression. Because acute tension-type headaches respond well to simple analgesics, sufferers rarely consult a physician. Chronic tension-type headache usually manifests as a daily or almost daily headache, frequently lasting all day, and unresponsive to progressively larger amounts of analgesics.

Tension-type headache is described as a steady, non-throbbing ache occurring bitemporally at the occiput, or in a "hatband" distribution. The muscles of the head, neck, jaw, or upper back may be contracted and tender, and may contain localized tender nodules on palpation.

Predominantly seen in females, tension-type headache does occur in men. These headaches may occur in families, and are considered in some a learned pattern derived from the behavior of parents.

It is crucial to recognize that chronic tension-type headache may conceal a serious emotional disorder, such as depression. For many patients, the physical symptom of headache is more socially acceptable as compared to the symptoms of anxiety or depression.

Some modern headache researchers have theorized that chronic tension-type headache results from disturbances of the monoaminergic, serotonergic, and endorphin functions, involving the hypothalamus, brainstem, and spinal cord. These disturbances may be due to referred or a central pain phenomena from the intermingling of major circuits of the brain and spinal cord.

Because chronic tension-type headache is closely related to depression in a large percentage of patients, many associated symptoms of depression are observed. These include sleep disturbances, anorexia or excessive eating, decreased libido, and multiple somatic complaints. Biochemically, depression may be considered an illness involving depletion of biogenic amines and defects of neurotransmitters.

Cervical spine spondylosis may produce headache as a result of irritation of the structures of the spine, the adjacent musculature, and connective tissues. Pain is usually occipital, but may be anterior as a result of trigeminal nerve stimulation. Radiographs of the cervical spine will show osteoarthritic changes, with loss of the normal lordotic curve. Physical examination may reveal muscle spasm with increased tone and limited range of motion, and one or more tender areas on palpation of the posterior neck muscles.

The third major tension-type headache syndrome is the *mixed headache syndrome.* Patients with this type of headache pattern are the most frequently seen in a specialized headache clinic. This syndrome comprises the following symptoms: (1) daily, continuous headache, (2) a sick headache (migraine) occurring 1–10 times monthly, and (3) easy susceptibility to habituation to over-the-counter or prescribed analgesics and/or ergotamine tartrate (19). Depression is also a common finding in this group of patients.

Once the diagnosis of mixed headache has been established, the use of sedatives, tranquilizers, habituating analgesics, and narcotics should be avoided to prevent addiction that would perpetuate the problem. The use of ergotamine should be limited to relief of the sick headache, and must not be repeated less than every fourth day. Ergotamine should never be prescribed on a daily basis for the mixed headache syndrome in order to avoid ergotamine rebound headaches.

TRACTION AND INFLAMMATORY HEADACHES

Headache from intracranial sources is usually produced by inflammation, traction, displacement, or distention of pain-sensitive structures, including susceptible blood vessels. Headache is the initial symptom of brain tumor in 25–35% of patients, and occurs in up to 80% of patients with brain tumors. The headache seen with brain tumors is not characteristic, but is often associated with signs or symptoms of increased intracranial pressure, including seizures, sudden loss of consciousness, weakness, or changes in mental status.

The headache of *brain tumor* is often a deep, steady, dull, aching pain. It is intermittent in 90% of cases, does not interfere with sleep, may be worse in the early morning and is aggravated with coughing or straining. The pain is not as intense as with migraine or cluster, and is frequently relieved by minor analgesics. Nausea and vomiting are associated symptoms.

The headache of *brain abscess* is similar in quality to that of brain tumor. The presence of fever and leukocytosis with a brain abscess assists in the differential diagnosis.

Acute and chronic *subdural hematomas* frequently present with headache. Other common accompanying symptoms of subdural hematoma include altered consciousness, disorientation, drowsiness, and confusion. Although spontaneous subdural hematomas do occur, most cases are caused by head trauma, often minor injuries. The groups most susceptible to subdural hematomas are chronic alcoholics, the elderly, patients treated with anticoagulants, and patients with bleeding disorders. Diagnosis can be confirmed by a skull radiograph showing a midline shift of the calcified pineal gland, or by radionuclide brain scan, cerebral angiogram, or CT scan. CT scanning in chronic subdural hematomas may yield negative results during the second or third months, when the density of the hematoma is identical to that of surrounding brain tissue. During that period, radionuclide brain scan can be the most useful diagnostic test.

Postlumbar puncture headache occurs after one-fourth of spinal taps. It usually begins a few hours to several days after lumbar puncture and lasts for days to weeks. The pain is a dull, deep ache, usually bifrontal and suboccipital. It is exacerbated by head movement and erect posture. This headache has been related to a loss of CSF, secondary to leakage from a dural hole.

Elevated CSF pressure, either from acute hydrocephalus (ventricular obstruction or shunt malformation) or pseudotumor cerebri, may cause headache. Pseudotumor cerebri is a syndrome of increased intracranial pressure and papilledema, without focal neurologic signs, and with normal CSF composition and normal- or small-sized cerebral ventricles. This condition usually occurs in children or obese young women with a history of headache for several weeks. Etiologies of pseudotumor include obstruction of cerebral venous drainage, rarely by slowly evolving tumors; endocrine and more commonly metabolic dysfunction, such as obesity or pregnancy; exposure to exogenous agents; and systemic illness, such as sarcoidosis or monoclonal gammopathy (20). Because papilledema usually occurs with this disorder, more serious pathology must be ruled out before a diagnosis of pseudotumor can be made.

Temporal arteritis frequently presents with a severe, throbbing, persistent headache. Often the involved artery is distended and tender. Associated symptoms may include jaw claudication, ocular symptoms including partial or complete loss of vision, depression, and polymyalgia rheumatica. This condition is primarily a disease of patients older than 50 years. Erythrocyte sedimentation rate is frequently elevated in temporal arteritis, but definitive diagnosis is made by temporal artery biopsy.

Cranial neuritides (Table 19.8), particularly trigeminal neuralgia, will present with episodic, recurrent unilateral pain. Trigeminal neuralgia (*tic douloureux*) causes unilateral facial pain in the distribution of the second or third division of the trigeminal nerve. Involvement of the first division occurs less frequently. This syndrome is most common in older patients, although it may be observed in younger patients, usually with multiple sclerosis, vascular anomalies, or fifth-nerve tumors. The pain is usually described as a high-intensity jab lasting

Table 19.8.
Neuralgias: Signs and Symptoms

Trigeminal	Lancinating pain lasting second to minutes
	Maxillary-mandibular-opthalmic divisions, in that order
	Older ages
	Trigger area unilateral
Sphenopalatine ganglion	Sharp pain
	Lateral nose to frontotemporal area
	Older (40 years); females affected more often
	Often with lacrimation and rhinorrhea
	Unilateral
Glossopharyngeal	Deep, sharp pain
	Often ear–pharynx–roof of tongue
	Older patients (40 years)
	Unilateral
Geniculate ganglion	Sharp pain that is tic-like
	Tragus/external ear canal
	Unilateral
Gasserian ganglion	Post-herpetic
	Unilateral
	Aching pain
	Often ophthalmic division of trigeminal
	Weeks to years in duration
Dental	Short, throbbing pain
	Precipitated with thermal intraoral changes
Atypical pain	Pain does not follow anatomic distribution
	Constant with long duration, without trigger zones
	Younger patients

less than 30 sec, and is frequently triggered by trivial stimulation of the face around the nose and mouth. This stimulation may include touching the face, washing, chewing, shaving, or even talking. The avoidance of facial stimulation by the patient helps the clinician differentiate trigeminal neuralgia from other facial pain syndromes. Glossopharyngeal neuralgia is similar to trigeminal neuralgia except that the pain is usually located in the pharynx, tonsil, or ear, and is usually triggered by swallowing, yawning, or eating. Post-herpetic neuralgia frequently follow herpes zoster infection (shingles) in the elderly. The pain is described as an intense, aching, and burning pain with dysesthesia, and is unilateral. It is located in the trigeminal division that was previously infected with herpes zoster. *Atypical facial neuralgias* (or *atypical facial pain syndrome*) is the term used for facial pain syndromes that cannot otherwise be classified. The pain is usually a steady, diffuse, aching pain, lasting hours to days, without paroxysms or trigger zones. This condition is most commonly seen in 30- to 50-year-old women, and may be associated with depression. It may be differentiated from migraine without aura, which involves the face because of the lack of throbbing quality of the pain.

Post-traumatic headaches occur in one-third to one-half of patients incurring head injury. The pathogenesis of post-traumatic headache suggests an organic basis, probably acceleration injury of the brain. The headaches may mimic any type of chronic recurrent headache syndrome, but predominantly fit into three groups: (1) headaches that mimic migraine, (2) headaches that mimic tension-type headaches, and (3) headaches that mimic the mixed headache syndrome. In addition to the headache, symptoms may include lightheadedness, memory impairment, inability to concentrate, anxiety, and depression (Table 19.9). Work-up for this type of headache will usually include a CT scan to rule-out subdural hematoma, and a skull radiograph to evaluate for skull fracture.

Subarachnoid hemorrhage usually presents in a middle-aged individual, more frequently in females, with abrupt onset of an intense headache during exertion. The pain is generalized, and is associated with vomiting and often diarrhea, usually with alteration of consciousness. The patient appears critically ill, with meningeal signs on examination. Lumbar puncture and CT scan will confirm the diagnosis. If the patient survives, the headache will remain severe for a few days, then slowly diminish over a 1- to 2-week period. Massive subarachnoid hemorrhage is usually due to either rupture of an intracranial aneurysm, bleeding from a cerebral angioma, or the extension of an intracerebral hemorrhage in a hypertensive patient. Congenital aneurysms present most frequently on the internal carotid artery, the mid-

Table 19.9.
Symptoms Found in Post-Traumatic Syndrome

Lightheadedness or true vertigo
Hyperacusis
Tinnitus
Impaired memory
Reduced attention span
Heightened distractibility
Inattentiveness
Decreased ability to concentrate
Forgetfulness
Difficulty in turning from one subject to another
Deterioration of synthetic thinking
Inability to grasp new or abstract concepts
Insomnia
Lack of spontaneity accompanied by apathy and loss of
    initiative
Easy fatigability
Reduced motivation
Decreased libido
Alcohol intolerance
Increased sensitivity to weather or temperature change
Irritability
Anger outbursts
Emotional callousness
Blunting or lability of emotional response
Mood swings
Anxiety, depression, and frustration
Syncope

dle cerebral artery, and at the junction of the anterior communicating and anterior cerebral arteries. Subarachnoid hemorrhage due to a cerebral angioma is much less common than one from a ruptured aneurysm (21).

The onset of subarachnoid hemorrhage from an intracranial aneurysm usually occurs without previous warning. Aneurysms of the posterior communicating artery may present with headache in 20% of patients prior to hemorrhage, however. The pain is intermittent and boring in quality. As the aneurysm enlarges, an oculomotor palsy with a fixed, dilated pupil may result. Aneurysms of the internal carotid with the cavernous sinus may be associated with unilateral pain in or behind the eye. The pain may be increased by exertion and may be intermittent. Subarachnoid hemorrhage from a cerebral angioma is frequently preceded by symptoms of the cerebral lesion and focal neurologic signs.

The headache from subarachnoid hemorrhage is acute and persists for about a week. It is usually throbbing in character, is increased by head movement, and is frequently accompanied by meningeal signs, focal neurologic signs or altered consciousness, and arterial hypertension. Continuation or recurrence of the headache in the postbleeding period should raise the possibilities of recurrent bleeding usually occurring during the second week, cerebral edema, or acute hydrocephalus.

Ocular causes of headache are relatively rare, and include eyestrain (asthenopia), glaucoma, uveitis, and op-

tic neuritis. A thorough history can easily differentiate these causes from the recurrent headache disorders. Painful ophthalmoplegia syndromes, including Tolosa-Hunt syndrome and Raeder's paratrigeminal syndrome, may be confused with ophthalmoplegia migraine or cluster headache.

Tolosa-Hunt syndrome is characterized by a boring, intense, sharp, or aching ocular pain followed in several days by ophthalmoplegia and diplopia. It may be associated with granulomatous lesions or arteritis within the orbit. Raeder's paratrigeminal syndrome is manifested by unilateral, deep throbbing pain around the eye, forehead, and cheek that may awaken the patient. Horner's syndrome may also be present. This syndrome can easily be mistaken for cluster headache, except that the pain is usually constant. The pain is described as intense, sharp, and aching. Unequal pupil size and sensory loss may be noted. The causes of Raeder's paratrigeminal syndrome include tumors, injuries, and granulomatous lesions.

CONCLUSIONS

Headache is a common symptom that, although usually benign, may be the presenting complaint in life-threatening conditions. Headache may be classified as vascular, tension-type, or traction and inflammatory. A careful history and examination will usually lead to the establishment of proper diagnosis.

REFERENCES

1. Cypress BK: Patients' reasons for visiting physicians: National Ambulatory Medical Care Survey, United States, 1977–78. *Vital Health Stat* 13:1–128, 1981.
2. Diamond S, Dalessio DJ: Classification and mechanism(s) of headache. In Diamond S, Dalessio DJ (eds): *The Practicing Physician's Approach to Headache*, ed 5. Baltimore, Williams & Wilkins, 1992.
3. Goldstein J: Headache in AIDS. In Rose FC (ed): *Migraine, Clinical and Research Advances*, Basel, Karger, 1985, pp 138–143.
4. Grzelesskia-Rzymowski I, Bogucki A, Szmidt M, et al: Migraine in aspirin-sensitive asthmatics. *Allergoi Immunopathol* 13:13–16, 1985.
5. Diamond S, Dalessio DJ, Greenberg IM, Greenberg BM, Greenberg M: Additional studies are sometimes necessary in investigating headache. In Diamond S, Dalessio DJ (eds): *The Practicing Physician's Approach to Headache*, ed 5. Baltimore, Williams & Wilkins, 1992, pp 31–50.
6. Diamond S, Greenberg I, Freitag FG, Urban GJ: MRI changes in migraine. In Rose FC (ed): *New Advances in Headache Research*, ed 2. London, Smith-Gordon, 1991, pp 53–61.
7. Olesen JS: Classification and diagnostic criteria of headache disorders, cranial neuralgias and facial pain. *Cephalalgia* 8:1–96, 1988.

8. Wolff HG: *Headache and Other Head Pain,* ed 2. New York, Oxford University Press, 1963.

9. Graham JR, Wolff HG: Mechanism of migraine headache and action of ergotamine tartrate. *Arch Neurol Psychiatry* 39:737–740, 1938.

10. Sandler M: Monoamines and migraine: A path through the woods. In Diamond S, Dalessio DJ, Graham J et al (eds): *Vasoactive Substances Relevant to Migraine.* Springfield, IL, Charles C Thomas, 1975, pp 3–18.

11. Lance JW, Lambert GA, Goadsby PJ, et al: Brainstem influences in the cephalic circulation experimental data from cats and monkeys of relevance to the mechanism of migraine. *Headache* 23:258–265, 1983.

12. Olesen J, Lauritzen M, Tfelt-Hansen P, et al: Spreading cerebral oligemia in classical and normal cerebral blood flow in common migraine. *Headache* 22:242–248, 1982.

13. Kobari M, Meyer JS, Ichijo M, Imari A, Oravez WT: Hyperperfusion of cerebral cortex, thalamus, and basal ganglia during spontaneously occurring migraine headaches. *Headache* 29:282–289, 1988.

14. Spaccavento LJ, Solomon GD: Migraine as an etiology of stroke in young adults. *Headache* 24:19–22, 1984.

15. Bickerstaff E: Basilar artery migraine. *Lancet* 1:15–17, 1961.

16. Diamond S, Solomon GD, Freitag FG, et al: Demographics of cluster headache patients attending an outpatient headache clinic. *Headache* 26:314, 1986.

17. Sakai F, Meyer JS: Regional cerebral hemodynamics during migraine and cluster headache—Measured by the Xe inhalation method. *Headache* 18:122–133, 1978.

18. Medina JL, Diamond S: Cluster headache variant: Spectrum of a new headache syndrome. *Arch Neurol* 38:705–709, 1981.

19. Mathew NT, Stubits E, Nigam MP: Transformation of episodic migraine into daily headache: Analysis of factors. *Headache* 22:66–68, 1982.

20. Powers MJ, Schnur JA, Baldree ME: Pseudotumor cerebri due to partial obstruction of the sigmoid sinus by a cholesteatoma. *Arch Neurol* 43:519–521, 1986.

21. Bannister R: *Brain's Clinical Neurology,* ed 5. New York, Oxford University Press, 1978, pp 270–274.

CHAPTER **20**

MEDICAL MANAGEMENT OF HEADACHE PAIN
JOEL R. SAPER

IN THE previous chapter, the differential diagnosis of headache was reviewed with an emphasis upon the distinctive syndromes of migraine, muscle contraction headache, and cluster headache. This chapter provides the reader with an extensive survey of the medical management of headache as it pertains to the specific syndromes as well as to the transitional syndromes that are gaining increasing attention from headache specialists.

As our understanding of headaches changes, so too does our approach to treatment. In order to provide the proper perspective for the discussion that follows, it is important to provide this author's view of the changing attitudes toward headache pathogenesis as they influence the choices and development of treatment modalities.

In 1962, the Ad Hoc Committee on the Classification of Headache offered what was to become the standard classification for head pain disorders for the next 20 years (1). This report was based upon the premise of a clear distinction between migraine and tension headache, and focused on symptom-specific etiologies: vasculature in migraine and musculature in tension headache.

However, despite the many citations of the Ad Hoc Committee report and its traditional acceptance by researchers and clinicians alike, many authorities have been unable to reconcile the myriad of events and phenomena of migraine, tension headache, and cluster headache with the basic foundations of this classification (2). During the past several years, the emphasis on peripheral phenomena (blood vessels and muscles) and separateness between migraine and tension headache disorders has been challenged, and with this has come changing views on the treatment of this disorder.

Several authors (2–5) are now citing data that they believe support the view that migraine and tension headache are physiologically related entities, with a varied symptomatic expression reflecting a central disturbance of neuroreceptor function within the upper brainstem, limbic, and/or hypothalamic regions (2, 6).

The "central hypothesis" takes its support from the current understanding of brain mechanisms and the neurochemical and physiologic events that are purported to occur during headache (2, 5–8); the symptom overlap between migraine and tension headache (2–5, 8); the general acknowledgement that the clinical phenomena, including pain, cannot be satisfactorily or entirely explained by disturbances of the vascular or muscular structures alone (2–5, 8, 9); vascular flow studies that appear to challenge traditional views linking the preheadache and headache symptoms of migraine with specific changes in blood flow (10, 11); and therapeutic considerations that raise doubt as to the presumed mechanisms of well-known therapeutic agents (2, 12).

On this last point, drugs initially recognized to be useful for migraine or for muscle contraction headache may be of value in both disorders. Moreover, a large number of agents found useful in the treatment of tension headache, migraine, or both conditions do not demonstrate a consistent system (vascular or muscular) specificity sufficient to explain their effectiveness (2). In fact, the wide-ranging pharmacologic actions of drugs found useful in chronic headache disorders appear to share an influence on central brain mechanisms more than a specific vascular or muscular influence.

Thus, the perspectives on chronic headache are changing, and the villains of the past hundred years (the blood vessels and muscles) are now coming to be seen as possible victims, affected by chronic, intermittent, or continuous disturbances of central phenomena (2, 3, 6–8). Currently, the International Association for the Study of Headache is undertaking the first major attempt to reclassify headache since the Ad Hoc Committee report of 1963.

The following is an overview of the treatment of the primary headache conditions, including migraine, cluster headache, so-called tension headache, and chronic daily headache. Although the "separateness" concept still serves as the basis for treatment descriptions, the reader will soon note the substantial overlap of treatments between one headache entity and another, in part reflecting the transition period in understanding and terminology that currently exists.

GENERAL TREATMENT CONSIDERATIONS

In Chapter 21, the psychological therapies for headache are discussed. It is nonetheless critical to the success of any medical therapy for a proper physician/patient relationship to exist. Thus, the treatment of headache begins the moment the patient enters the office. Historically, patients claim that the medical profession reacts differently to the complaint of headache and chronic pain than to other similarly distressing illnesses. The merits of this claim aside, it is clear that helping such a patient is enhanced by conveying a sincere interest in their distress, understanding "the person" with the complaint, and establishing a worthwhile and frank communication forum.

A global recognition of the patient's life, emotional needs, and physiologic vulnerabilities is essential. Likewise, the physician's ability to enlist trust, allay anxiety and fear, and encourage cooperation are similarly important. In complex cases, the person, even more than the symptom, may require treatment, and the traditional focus of physicians on symptoms must make way for an emphasis on the individual first and the symptom second.

Although emotional factors are at times very important, in our need to explain that which is poorly understood, emotional phenomena may have been overemphasized as an etiologic basis for headache. Presumptions or premature emphasis on psychological elements early in the course of therapy is counterproductive and often clinically unfounded. Patients have come to feel defensive about these issues, because so many physicians are believed by patients to harbor preconceived notions as to the relevance of emotional considerations in the etiology of chronic headache.

The preventative as well as symptomatic treatment of chronic headache requires patience and innovativeness. Therapy in all cases must be modeled to meet individual differences in general health, psychological makeup, headache pattern, and patient compliance.

TREATMENT OF MIGRAINE

From its earliest recognition, migraine has defied a complete understanding of its pathophysiology, consistency of its diagnostic criteria, terminology, and reliability of treatment interventions. Although traditionally classified into *common* and *classic* forms, an expanded list of variants has evolved (3, 8, 9, 13). Also, differences of opinions exist as to whether classic migraine [forms with a preheadache (aura)] and *common* migraine (without a distinct, identifiable prodromal phase) are the same or different entities (14, 15).

Equally important is the growing recognition that many patients with migraine begin their headache years with acute intermittent "vascular"-type headache attacks, easily diagnosed as migraine by current criteria, but over the course of years evolve or "transform" into a chronic daily headache pattern that does not by current criteria fit the diagnosis of migraine (2, 8, 16, 17).

By traditional perspective, migraine is a common but periodic disorder, which undergoes natural remissions and spontaneous exacerbations. Prolonged uninterrupted use of preventative medications should be discouraged since remissions may not be appreciated when prolonged and successful therapy is continued indefinitely. Other nonpharmacologic treatments are of importance. Avoidance of migraine-provoking influences (3, 6, 8, 9), biofeedback, stress management, and adherence to life-style patterns that provide a regularity and sameness to the migraineur's daily activities may be important in many patients.

Symptomatic Treatment of Migraine

The pharmacologic symptomatic treatment of migraine should be considered when headaches occur infrequently and medications used for this approach are clinically acceptable (Table 20.1). The route of administration for symptomatic treatment may be as critical as the choice of medication. A delay of gastric absorption has been demonstrated in patients during both the acute phases of migraine and preheadache events, and can occur even in the absence of nausea and vomiting (6, 8). To abort a headache once begun, the use of one or more medications is usually required. The following are those noted to be of greatest value.

Ergotamine Tartrate and Other Alkaloids

Ergot alkaloids are estimated to be effective within the first 1–2 hr in up to 90% of cases when administered

**Table 20.1.
Criteria for Symptomatic Versus Preventive Treatment of Migraine**

Symptomatic Criteria
  Frequency less than 1–2 headaches/week
  General health does not contraindicate
    For ergot derivatives: coronary artery disease, severe hypertension, peripheral or cerebrovascular disease, etc.
    For analgesics containing aspirin: peptic ulcer disease, anticoagulant use, aspirin sensitive asthma, etc.
Preventive criteria
  Frequency greater than 1–2 headaches/week
Medical contraindications for symptomatic therapies. Failure of symptomatic therapies. When attacks occur with reliable, predictable regularity, at or around menstrual period, etc. Known substance abuse tendencies

---

parenterally; in 80% of patients given the rectal form; and in up to 50% of the patients given the oral form (8). Historically, the effects of ergotamine have been considered to be via an arterial vasoconstrictive influence. More recently, a central (brain) effect has been considered (12).

Ergotamine possesses a smooth muscle–stimulating effect capable of producing vasoconstriction, a mild central sympatholytic effect in the medulla, and a peripheral adrenergic effect (18). Ergotamine may also delay gastric emptying by its direct action on stomach musculature, and may at high levels produce endothelial damage.

Ergotamine alkaloids [ergotamine tartrate and dihydroergotamine (D.H.E. 45)] are available in intravenous, intramuscular, subcutaneous, oral, rectal, inhalant, and sublingual forms. The oral and sublingual forms are not as effective as parenteral or rectal routes. The sublingual forms (Ergomar, Wigrettes, and Ergostat) contain 2.0 mg of ergotamine tartrate. The oral and rectal routes contain ergotamine tartrate in combination with caffeine with or without belladonna and barbiturate.

The dose required to alleviate an evolving migraine is variable and depends in part upon the method of delivery. Parenteral treatment with dihydroergotamine (1–2 ml intramuscularly or 0.5–1.0 ml intravenously) is usually effective. (D.H.E. 45 is currently the only available parenteral form of ergot alkaloids.)

In rectal form, a suppository containing 2 mg of ergotamine tartrate (Cafergot or Wigraine) can be administered initially with a repeat dose in 1 hr, and a maximum dose daily of 4.0 mg. The starting dose of one-third to one-half of a suppository is advisable because of the likely adverse effects if excessive or too rapid absorption occurs.

In tablet form (Cafergot or Wigraine), a 1.0-mg tablet is administered as two tablets initially, followed by one tablet every 30 min until relief is obtained or until 5 mg have been taken. Sublingual tablets (Ergomar, Ergostat, Wigrettes) contain 2.0 mg of ergotamine tartrate. Although variability of the inhaled dose and concern over possible excessive pulmonary artery constriction has limited its usefulness, the inhalant form can be very effective.

Ergotamine and related alkaloids are contraindicated in patients with marked hypertension, peripheral vascular disease, ischemic heart disease, cardiac valvular abnormalities, collagen vascular disease, and thrombophlebitis, and in patients over the age of 60 (8). Caution must be exercised in patients with peptic ulcer disease, bradycardia, and renal and hepatic abnormalities. Concurrent infection or fever may also promote excessive vasoconstriction. Use of these compounds must be avoided in pregnancy.

Among the minor untoward reactions are nausea and vomiting, muscle achiness, diarrhea, and difficulty swallowing (usually benign). Abdominal cramps, chest pain, vertigo, and paresthesiae of hands and feet are estimated to occur in 5–50% of patients. Symptoms lasting several hours or less are not generally considered contraindications to use.

The more serious consequences to ergotamine usage occur when excessive dosages are employed or when the drug is used in the presence of a contraindication. Severe reactions have been reported at acceptable dosages in otherwise healthy patients (8, 9). Ergotamine tartrate may cause bradycardia and should be used with considerable caution in patients with preexisting bradycardia, or with combined usage with β-blocking drugs or others that may slow the heart rate.

Ergotism is a serious and well-known consequence of ergotamine overusage (8, 12). Susceptibility to ergotism is variable. Recently, dependency on ergotamine tartrate has been reported in patients taking ergotamine as infrequently as three times per week, with the development of "rebound" or "ergotamine headache" as a consequence. Ergotamine tartrate should be used no more than 2 days per week, since greater frequency of usage can lead to dependency and increasing headaches (12).

At this time, sumatriptan has been approved for use by the FDA. Sumatriptan (Imitrex) is a selective serotonin (5-HT$_1$) receptor agonist, studies of which appear to provide strong support for its efficacy in the symptomatic relief of migraine and cluster headache. It can be administered in parenteral and oral forms.

Isometheptene Mucate

Isometheptene mucate is a sympathomimetic agent in a combined form (Midrin) that exerts a beneficial effect on the acute attack of migraine (8). Midrin is a combination of 65 mg of isometheptene mucate, 325 mg of acetaminophen, and 100 mg of dichloralphenazone (a tranquilizer). It produces less gastrointestinal distress than ergotamine preparations, and in one controlled study (19) was noted to be superior to ergotamine tartrate and caffeine-preparations.

Midrin is an effective agent for the symptomatic treatment of mild to moderate migraine attacks, and is particularly useful in cases in which adverse effects to ergot medications exist. Although the general contraindications for the use of Midrin are the same as those for ergotamine, there exists a lesser likelihood of adverse responses. Mild sedation and gastrointestinal distress occur in some but not most patients. Generally the drug is well tolerated.

The dosage of Midrin is two capsules at the onset of an attack, followed by one or two capsules 30 min and 1 hr later, up to a maximum of five capsules per attack. Simultaneous administration of two aspirin at the onset of an attack or a nonsteroidal anti-inflammatory drug (NSAID) may enhance effectiveness.

The drug should not be used more than two or three times per week in order to avoid "rebound" effects.

Nonsteroidal Anti-Inflammatory Drugs

The NSAIDs have symptomatic as well as preventative value. A large numer of agents are available (20). Naproxen sodium (Anaprox) has been most widely evaluated (21–23). The dose of naproxen is 275 mg (one to two tablets), to be taken at onset of headache. Other agents include meclofenamate sodium (Meclomen) at 100–200 mg, indomethacin (Indocin) at 25–50 mg, or ibuprofen (Motrin) at 400–800 mg, all taken at onset of the attack.

Indocin is available in rectal suppository form, which has advantages for patients with nausea and vomiting.

Recently, ketorolac (Toradol) has been introduced and is available in oral and parenteral forms. Anecdotal experience suggests efficacy in the symptomatic treatment of migraine at dosages of 30–60 mg administered intramuscularly three times a day.

The NSAIDs have well known contraindications that generally include gastrointestinal or renal disease, or bleeding disturbances (20).

Analgesics

Although analgesics (narcotic and nonnarcotic) may benefit some patients during an acute migraine attack, the abuse potential for overuse is a sufficiently serious problem as to make the routine use of analgesics inappropriate for frequent headaches. This is particularly true of combination forms in which a narcotic or barbiturate ingredient is present. However, even the simple analgesics, when too frequently employed, can be troublesome.

Injectable narcotics are usually of greater value than oral medication, but the tendency for dependency must be emphasized. These drugs should not be employed as standard therapy for the acute migraine attack, unless other standard agents are of no value or are contraindicated, and the attacks are sufficiently infrequent as to justify this form of treatment. The physician must be alert to the somatic expression of the psychological despair and drug-seeking behavior as manifested through the complaint of headache. Discouraging the employment of injectable narcotics for the treatment of headache is worthwhile. In selected cases, however, narcotics may represent the most appropriate and safest treatment.

Phenothiazines, Other Antiemetics, and Related Medications

The phenothiazines may be effective as antiemetics and may also have some pain-relieving benefit. These and related substances can be administered in conjunction with symptomatic drugs and are most effective by parenteral or suppository route.

The dose of chlorpromazine (Thorazine) is 25–50 mg intramuscularly, rectally, or in tablet form. Promethazine (Phenergan) is administered in a dose of 25 mg intramuscularly or rectally, or 50 mg orally. This author generally avoids employing prochlorperazine (Compazine) because of the higher incidence of acute dystonic reactions associated with its use when compared to other agents, such as chlorpromazine.

(See later section on Special Therapeutic Considerations and Situations for recommendations on intravenous administration of phenothiazines for acute migraine.)

Reglan (metoclopramide hydrochloride) in dosages of 10 mg orally three times a day or in intravenous form can provide antiemetic effects and also may be of value in enhancing oral absorption. Hydroxyzine (Vistaril) in dosages of 50–100 mg orally or 75 mg intramuscularly may likewise be effective as an antiemetic and may enhance the benefit of other agents used to treat an attack. Hydroxyzine may also have primary analgesic effects (24).

The symptomatic usefulness of steroids should be noted (25). Prolonged refractory attacks may benefit from steroidal therapy. Prednisone in dosages of 40–60 mg administered orally for 3–5 days or 8–16 mg of dexamethasone by intramuscular administration may be used.

Patients should be administered steroids only when other less-troublesome agents are ineffective. When treated, patients should be informed of potential risks, including the possibility (though remote) of avascular necrosis of bone.

Intravenously administered dihydroergotamine has become the treatment of choice for severe, intractable headache (26). Further discussion can be found under "Special Therapeutic Considerations and Situations."

Finally, many of the drugs useful for migraine prevention, including β-blockers, tricyclic antidepressants, and calcium channel blockers, may have a value in symptomatic protocols.

PREVENTIVE PHARMACOLOGIC AGENTS IN THE TREATMENT OF MIGRAINE

The preventive medical management of migraine employs the daily use of one or a combination of medications that are presumed to block the biologic events leading up to migraine. Such a program should be considered when the frequency of migraine attacks exceeds the safety limitations for the use of symptomatic medications or concurrent medical conditions contraindicate the use of medications employed to abort headaches. Generally, more than four major attacks per month justifies a preventative program. Preventative treatment should be employed at intervals of 3–6 months followed by a gradual reduction of medication, since natural remissions of headache may not be recognized when preventative medication therapy is maintained.

β-Blockers

The most widely used and important group of drugs for the prevention of migraine are the β-blockers. Among the β-blocking agents that are useful in the prevention of migraine are propranolol (Inderal) and nadolol (Corgard), which are nonselective blocking agents, imposing a competitive blockade in both β_1- and β_2-adrenergic receptors (3, 8, 27). Selective β-blockers, including metoprolol (Lopressor) and timolol (Tenormin), which selectively block β_1-adrenergic receptors, may be of equal value (8, 28), although the nonselective blockers have historically been considered more effective.

Because of their β-adrenergic blocking action, these drugs were initially presumed to affect migraine via a blocking of the peripheral vasodilatory receptors, thereby interfering with the presumed dilatory phase of migraine. Many clinicians now believe that other influences are responsible for the antimigraine effects of these agents, and an effect on the central nervous system is considered likely by some (8).

Therapy with the β-blocking drugs requires individual dose determination, and one agent may be more effective for a particular patient than another similar medicine. Inderal comes in two forms, the short-acting original form and the new Inderal LA. In the short-acting form, treatment may begin at dosages between 20 and 40 mg given three to four times a day and increased up to a total dose of 400 mg/day, in three or four divided doses. Inderal LA is best employed in a twice-per-day regimen, beginning at 80 mg once or twice per day, and increasing to 160 mg twice a day as tolerated.

Corgard (40-mg tablet) is begun at a dose of 20 mg twice a day and increased to the point of tolerance, often up to 120–160 mg twice a day (240–320 mg total dose). Corgard appears particularly reliable and can be effective in some patients in a once-a-day dose regimen. It seems considerably less likely to produce the frequently encountered "central" effects often seen with propranolol, and appears at least as effective, and perhaps more so, than propranolol.

High-dose regimens may be of value in some cases, but if efficacy is not demonstrated at moderate dosages, higher dosage regimens are usually of little value (29). However, exceptions exist.

Most individuals taking β-blocking agents will experience an initial lowering of blood pressure and pulse rate, and some patients have an unexpected sensitivity, resulting in rather dramatic hypotension and bradycardia even at low dosages. Caution and patient monitoring are essential. Other common side effects, including depression and mental changes, are well known and can be found in standard sources. Slowly discontinuing the medication over several weeks after prolonged usage is advisable. Approximately 24–48 hr are required for complete dissipation of its effect after final discontinuance (8).

Methysergide and Other Ergot Agents

Methysergide (Sansert) is an effective preventative medication for migraine (6–8), with a beneficial response demonstrated in up to 50–65% of patients. At one time, methysergide was the standard bearer for the preventive control of migraine headaches. The exact mode by which methysergide exerts its effect remains unknown, but it may occupy serotonin reuptake sites on the blood vessel walls, thereby stabilizing both vasoconstriction and vasodilation. Like many of the migraine agents, including ergotamine tartrate, methysergide may have its greatest influence on central aminergic physiology (2).

The usual dose of methysergide is 2.0 mg once or twice per day up to a maximum of 8.0 mg/day in four divided doses. It should not be used in patients with peripheral vascular disease, coronary artery disease, hypertension, serious gastrointestinal distress, and pregnancy. Activation of peptic ulcer disease is possibly related to its enhancement of gastric acid secretion (8).

Methysergide should not be administered for more than 5–6 months without interruption of therapy for at least 1 to 2 months because of the potential development of fibrosis in the retroperitoneal region, lungs, and heart valves. These fibrotic reactions are estimated to occur in one of every 2000 cases. Although these changes tend to regress after discontinuance, they may not. A peripheral vascular occlusive reaction similar to Leriche's syndrome has been reported, and aggravation of preexisting angina pectoris is common. CT scan of the abdomen (with or without contrast enhancement), or MRI, chest x-ray, and cardiac exam are recommended after each 6 months of continuous therapy.

Adverse reactions of a mild to moderate degree occur frequently and thus limit methysergide's overall usefulness. The most common untoward reactions include transient muscle aching, abdominal distress, hallucinations, and a sense of swelling of face or throat. Frightening hallucinatory events after the first dose are not uncommon. Minor reactions are frequently transient, and continued use of the drug does not appear unsafe.

Two additional ergot derivatives are available and may in some instances be as effective as methysergide in migraine prophylaxis. Ergonovine maleate (Ergotrate) and methylergonovine (Methergine) can be used for short-term preventive treatment. Each is given in a dose of 0.2–0.4 mg t.i.d. Precautions and restrictions similar to those of methysergide are recommended.

The ergot alkaloids should be used in patients who do not respond to other preventive medications or when short-term prophylaxis is needed. Extended use should be determined by clinical necessity and with appropriate precautions and warnings. Care must be used to avoid these medications in patients with known risk of vascular disease.

Calcium Antagonists (Calcium Channel Blockers)

Increasing attention has focused on calcium antagonists in treatment of various headache conditions. The mechanism of effectiveness is unknown but may not be directly related to effects on blood vessels, since central effects are present (30–33).

The three available calcium antagonists are verapamil (Isoptin, Calan), diltiazem (Cardizem), and nifedipine (Procardia). Isoptin is usually administered beginning at 80 mg two or three times a day and increased to approximately 160 mg three to four times per day. The starting dose of diltiazem is 30 mg two or three times a day, increased to 90 mg three times per day if tolerated. Procardia may be begun at 10 mg three times per day and increased to 60–90 mg three times a day.

The calcium antagonists are of special benefit in patients who suffer from migraine and simultaneous vasoconstrictive tendencies such as Raynaud's phenomena/disease or asthma. β-Blocking agents aggravate these conditions.

Among the side effects of calcium antagonists are headache, (particularly with nifedipine), depression, vasomotor changes, tremor, gastrointestinal distress, dizziness, pedal edema, orthostatic hypotension, and bradycardia (particularly with verapamil and diltiazem). Numerous patients report an increase in headaches initially, with improvement occurring over several weeks. Periodic electrocardiographic evaluation is valuable, and special precautions in patients with bradycardia, hypotension, heart block, or vulnerability to heart failure are recommended.

The calcium channel blockers are generally considered safe and well tolerated. Their ultimate value in the prophylaxis of migraine remains to be determined.

Antidepressants

The tricyclic antidepressants (TCAs), particularly amitriptyline (Endep, Elavil), nortriptyline (Aventyl), doxepin (Sinequan, Adapin), and others, have been reported as effective in migraine prevention (3, 8), although their value in the treatment of daily chronic pain (tension headache) is better established (2, 34, 35). The usual dose of amitriptyline and doxepin ranges from 25 to 150 mg a day, often given in a single bedtime dose. Nortriptyline dosages range from 25 to 75 mg. Common side effects include sedation, dry mouth, urinary retention, constipation, blurred vision, intense dreaming with nightmares, weight gain, and hypotension. Contraindications include cardiac arrhythmias, narrow angle glaucoma, myocardial infarction, severe prostatism, and uncontrolled seizures.

Fluoxetine, well-accepted as an antidepressant, has gained substantial interest in the treatment of migraine.

Controlled studies are not yet available, though pending. Anecdotal use has suggested a value when fluoxetine is administered at a dose of 20–40 mg per day. Advantages include the absence of sedation and limited or absent weight-gain influence, in contrast to other antidepressants. Untoward reactions are many and include agitation, worsening of headache, GI distress, tremor, and adverse interactions with numerous other medications.

The monoamine oxidase–inhibiting antidepressants (MAOIs), particularly phenelzine (Nardil), can be quite effective in the prevention of migraine (3, 6, 8, 9). MAOIs influence the intracellular metabolism of biogenic amines, and disturbances of this system have been proposed in migraine (6). The usual dose of phenelzine is 15 mg three to four times per day, usually given in divided dosages beginning with 15 mg/day for several days, with a gradual increase in dose until benefit is achieved or safety limitations reached.

The most common side effects of the MAOIs include insomnia, orthostatic hypotension, anticholingergic effects, weight gain, and loss of sexual desire and/or orgasm (8). Insomnia can sometimes be avoided by administering all doses prior to noon.

Traditional concern over the use of MAOIs has waned during the past several years since it has been recognized that their use may be much safer and less restrictive than historically believed (36, 37). Moreover, combinations of MAOI and amitriptyline have been reported efficacious in both pain and depression disorders. MAOIs cannot be given with fluoxetine. Five weeks must transpire between the discontinuance of fluoxetine and the administration of MAOIs. Fluoxetine cannot be administered to patients who have previously taken MAOIs for at least 3 weeks following the discontinuation of MAOIs.

Simultaneous use of MAOIs with β-blockers and calcium channel blockers must be carried out with extreme caution, since severe orthostatic hypotension with syncope is frequently encountered.

Nonsteroidal Anti-Inflammatory Agents

The NSAIDs are useful in both the symptomatic and the preventative treatment of migraine (20–23). Naproxen sodium (Anaprox) has been most successfully established as an effective preventative agent. Indomethacin (Indocin) has shown its greatest value in the prevention of variants of cluster headache. The dose of naproxen sodium for migraine prevention is one or two 275-mg tablets twice a day. Gastrointestinal effects and long-term effects on renal function must be considered, and the drug should not be used in the presence of contraindications (20). The presumed mechanism is via an influence on prostaglandin and platelet metabolism.

The NSAIDs may be particularly valuable in the treatment of menstrual migraine (21).

Cyproheptadine

Although cyproheptadine (Periactin) has been used with minimal success alone in the prevention of migraine in adults, it is considered the treatment of choice for prevention of childhood migraine (8). Dosages range from 4 to 8 mg three to four times per day for adults and 4 mg two to three times per day in children. Weight gain is a common adverse effect when cyproheptadine is used prophylactically.

Clonidine

Clonidine hydrochloride (Catapres) is an antihypertensive agent possessing α-adrenergic stimulating properties. Clonidine has been studied in several trials (8) and has been found useful in some but not in others. The recommended dose is 0.2 mg given two to three times per day. This drug may be worthy of trial in patients with migraine who are withdrawing from narcotic analgesics or menopausal women experiencing headaches and vasomotor symptoms.

Bellergal/Anticonvulsants

Bellergal is a compound containing ergotamine tartrate, belladonna, and barbiturate. Bellergal-S is a sustained-release form of the same. The drug can be useful in some patients with migraine but should be used for only short-term intervention (such as around a menstrual period), since daily administration of ergotamine tartrate may result in dependency.

Patients with intermittent migraine or mixed syndromes may benefit from the anticonvulsants or antineuralgic agents, including valproate (Depakote), carbamazepine (Tegretol), phenytoin (Dilantin), and baclofen (Lioresal). Several reports have now suggested the efficacy of valproate in the prophylactic treatment of migraine, daily chronic headache, and cluster headache. Dosages range from 1000–2000 mg/day. Care must be given to avoid interaction with other drugs (increased sedation and cerebral suppression may occur in the presence of tricyclic antidepressants, neuroleptics, barbiturates, and benzodiazepines, among others).

Long-term effectiveness of preventative therapy has been established in a report by Raskin and Schwartz (38).

TREATMENT OF CLUSTER HEADACHE

Perhaps the most sinister of the well-recognized headache disorders, cluster headache is a severely painful affliction primarily affecting men (3, 6, 8, 9, 39, 40). In this sense, a cluster headache is distinct from the other primary headache disorders (migraine, tension headache, and combined headaches), which by most surveys affect women in a ratio of 3:1. Few headaches more challenge the clinician's knowledge, compassion, and pharmacotherapeutic skills than the cluster headache condition.

Cluster headaches can be divided into three major forms.

Episodic Cluster Headache This most well-known and common pattern is characterized by recurring bouts or clusters of headaches. During these cycles, typical headache attacks occur regularly and usually daily. Each cycle may last from weeks to months, and is then followed by a spontaneous remission, called the interim.

Chronic Cluster Headache Chronic cluster headache is divided into a *primary* form and a *secondary* form. In the absence of remission for 1 year or more, the term *chronic* is appropriate. Primary chronic cluster headache is characterized by recurring headache events for years without a remission. The *secondary* chronic cluster headache form is characterized by a pattern of typical recurring headache attacks that have become chronic but have evolved from an original episodic pattern.

Chronic Paroxysmal Hemicrania Chronic paroxysmal hemicrania is considered by many to be a true variant of cluster headache. It frequently affects children (8, 39). In 1974, Sjaastad and Dale (40) described this headache entity with striking similarity to cluster headaches. This disorder is quite similar to cluster headache despite some clinical differences. It primarily strikes young women, although not exclusively. Although often indistinguishable from cluster headache, headache events of chronic paroxysmal hemicrania may be shorter than those of a typical headache, generally occur with greater frequency (usually during the day), and rarely awaken patients from sleep.

During cluster headache cycles, one or more attacks occur daily with an average frequency of one to three attacks every 24 hr, each lasting from 20 min to 2 hr with residual distress for several hours after the termination of the most intense pain. The clinical features of attacks are well described in standard texts (3, 6, 8, 9, 39).

Although cycles of headaches occur randomly in the episodic form, they appear most common at times of season change. Seasonal sensitivity may in part relate to adaptational changes of hypothalamic function, which may be the pathophysiologic locus of cluster headache (8, 39). Periodic depression may occur in conjunction with cluster headaches.

The actual mechanism of cluster headache is unknown, but disturbances within the circuits of cranial nerve V, nervus intermedius, and sphenopalatine ganglion have been considered. Dysfunction of the hypothalamus, involving chronobiologic abnormalities, may be of importance in cluster headache.

General Treatment Considerations

The treatment of cluster headache requires above all persistence, diligence, innovation, and compassion along with a commitment to a variety of tools available to curb the pain and desperation associated with this condition. As in other headache disorders, the choice must take into account the age and health of the patient, frequency of the attacks, the expected duration of a cluster cycle, previous therapies, and a patient's daily activities and habits.

Patients with cluster headache must discontinue all alcohol products and avoid daytime napping. Normalization of sleep cycles can be accomplished naturally by medication therapy, including tricyclic antidepressants. Awakening at the same time each day is very important since prolonged sleeping appears to provoke attacks (8). This author asks all patients to discontinue smoking and in those in whom this goal is accomplished, increased control seems apparent although not yet formally established.

SYMPTOMATIC TREATMENT

Inhalation of 100% oxygen is an effective means of symptomatically relieving the pain in many patients (8, 39, 41, 42). Patients must be given a mask and employ 100% oxygen at 7 liters/min for a period of 15 min or more. Between 65 and 75% of episodic cluster patients, and 50% of chronic headache patients, will experience improvement.

In addition to oxygen, effective symptomatic management generally requires the use of an ergotamine alkaloid, which, if administered and absorbed promptly, can reverse most attacks within minutes. Standard oral tablets are impractical. Parenteral DHE and sumatriptan are likely to be useful, but impractical, for repetitive cluster headache attacks. DHE, when given in intravenous protocols (see later), may interrupt repetitive attacks for at least a time.

Although effective, ergot preparations must be used with great restraint because of the daily occurrence of attacks. Injectable narcotic analgesics are discouraged because of the obvious tendency for abuse with this headache pattern.

PREVENTIVE TREATMENT

The preventative therapy regimens are the most desirable treatment for cluster headache.

Prednisone

Prednisone is the most reliably effective drug for the immediate preventative control of cluster headache, and can dramatically prevent both chronic and episodic varieties within hours of first administration. Several regimens can be used. Kudrow (39) recommended a 3-week program starting with 40 mg for 5 days followed by a tapering course. This author employs a shorter regimen of 10 days beginning at 60 mg for four days and subsequently tapering (see Table 20.2) (8). Although some headache cycles can be terminated with such use, re-

Table 20.2.
Protocols for Prednisone Treatment of Cluster Headache

	10-Day Protocol[a]			
Day	8:00 AM	4:00 PM	Bedtime	
1	20 mg	20 mg	20 mg	= 60 mg/day
2	20 mg	20 mg	20 mg	= 60 mg/day
3	20 mg	20 mg	20 mg	= 60 mg/day
4	20 mg	20 mg	20 mg	= 60 mg/day
5	20 mg	15 mg	15 mg	= 50 mg/day
6	15 mg	15 mg	10 mg	= 40 mg/day
7	10 mg	10 mg	10 mg	= 30 mg/day
8	5 mg	5 mg	5 mg	= 15 mg/day
9	5 mg	0	5 mg	= 10 mg/day
10	5 mg	(finished)		= 5 mg/day

	7-Day Protocol[b]			
Day	8:00 AM	4:00 PM	Bedtime	
1	20 mg	20 mg	20 mg	= 60 mg/day
2	20 mg	20 mg	20 mg	= 60 mg/day
3	20 mg	15 mg	15 mg	= 50 mg/day
4	15 mg	15 mg	10 mg	= 40 mg/day
5	10 mg	10 mg	10 mg	= 30 mg/day
6	10 mg	5 mg	5 mg	= 20 mg/day
7	10 mg	(finished)		= 10 mg/day

[a]20 mg = 4 pills, 15 mg = 3 pills, 10 mg = 2 pills, 5 mg = 1 pill; total of 78 tablets needed.
[b]20 mg = 4 pills, 15 mg = 3 pills, 10 mg = 2 pills, 5 mg = 1 pill; total of 54 tablets needed.

emergence of headaches may occur as dosages fall to 15–20 mg/day. The risk from short-term usage in appropriate patients is small but the usual contraindications must be appreciated.

Steroid therapy is recommended in the following situations: to provide an immediate control, particularly in patients growing desperate from recurring attacks; to offer "insurance" treatment when patients are away from familiar medical care, such as when traveling; and during drug holidays from other medications.

Lithium Carbonate

Lithium carbonate (Eskalith, Lithobid, Lithane) can be effective in over 60% of cases (8, 39, 42–44). The usual starting dose is 300 mg administered two to four times per day. Therapeutic response does not necessarily correlate with blood levels, and serum levels exceeding 0.7 mEq/liter are rarely necessary for good results. Blood monitoring is appropriate to prevent toxicity. Lithium may have a direct effect on hypothalamic regulatory centers and may also influence enkephalinergic neuronal systems.

The adverse effects of lithium include nausea, vomiting, diarrhea, tremor, blurred vision, gait unsteadiness, and exacerbation of dermatologic conditions, including psoriasis. Hypothyroidism may occur with long-term use, particularly in women. Patients must avoid diuretics and salt-restrictive diets because of the increased risk of intoxication. Increased salt intake will reduce effectiveness.

During summer months, excessive salt loss through perspiration may result in lithium toxicity. Nephrotoxicity occurs in some patients even when lithium is maintained in the nontoxic range for short periods of time, although generally therapy is safe when given for short cycles. Other potentially nephrotoxic drugs such as NSAIDs should be used with caution during lithium treatment. Long-term, noninterrupted use in chronic headache patients should be discouraged. Frequent drug holidays and blood monitoring and alternate treatment programs are recommended.

Calcium Antagonists

Calcium antagonists, particularly verapamil, can be of great value in cluster headache (30, 31). This author has found verapamil (Isoptin, Calan) particularly valuable (42). Many patients do not benefit until the upper levels of treatment are reached, for example, at dosages of 120–160 mg of verapamil administered three or four times a day. Treatment effectiveness may require several weeks of administration.

Methysergide

Methysergide/Methylergonovine

Methysergide and methylergonovine can be effective in the prophylactic treatment of patients with cluster headache (see "Migraine Prophylaxis"). Use is appropriate in patients who do not respond to verapamil therapy and for those whose cluster cycles last less than 3–4 months, and in the absence of medical contraindications.

Valproate

Valproate may be of value in the prophylaxis of cluster headache as it is proposed to be in migraine. Dosages range between 1000 and 2000 mg per day in three or four divided doses.

Chlorpromazine

Chlorpromazine (Thorazine) in dosages ranging from 75 to several hundred milligrams per day has been reported useful in cluster headache (45). A sustained benefit for up to 6–8 months was demonstrated on maintenance levels of 75 mg per day. Not all authorities believe this drug to be similarly effective. It can be used as an adjunctive therapy in refractory patients and may be particularly useful for nocturnal attacks. Risks and long-term side effects are well known and must be considered.

Cyproheptadine

Cyproheptadine (Periactin) has not been proven useful for most cluster headache patients; however, occasional benefits are recognized. Because of its overall safety, its use as an adjunctive agent in difficult cases is recommended.

Nonsteroidal Anti-Inflammatory Agents

The NSAIDs may be effective for cluster headache (46), but appear to be most helpful for the variant called chronic paroxysmal hemicrania (CPH), which (by definition) is effectively treated with indomethacin (Indocin) at dosages of 25–50 mg three to four times per day. Whether other NSAIDs have similar benefits remains to be determined.

Other Therapies

Parenteral (intravenous) DHE administered for 3–5 days may significantly interrupt a cluster headache cycle, although return of the headaches may follow discontinuance of the treatment.

Histamine desensitization to alleviate cluster headache was first described in 1939 by Horton et al. (47). Although recent attention to this form of therapy exists (48), most clinicians informally surveyed by this author fail to recognize a major contribution from this therapy. In severely intractable cases, however, this intervention could be considered.

Sugery and other ablative procedures on the sphenopalatine ganglion, nervus intermedius, or the other branches or ganglia of cranial nerve V may be effective and appropriate in some patients (49, 50). At this time, however, surgical treatment cannot be generally recommended except in the most severe and intractable cases, when all other traditional treatments, including inpatient care, have been tried.

Cluster headache and its variants are distressing disorders and, when uncontrolled, pose a serious threat to the patient's will to endure. Inpatient-level care has been used in numerous intractable cases and is to be recommended for difficult cases.

Cluster headache inflicts the most ravaging type of painful distress, and this is often accompanied by intense emotional despair. A relationship to cyclical depression is possible (8). Patients will frequently experience a personality change along with other constitutional, emotional, and physiologic changes during these cycles. Aggressive intervention and a committed involvement of the physician until control is established are essential, and bring profound satisfaction to the patient and physician alike.

TENSION, CHRONIC DAILY, AND COMBINED HEADACHES

Tension-type headache is the new term for what has previously been called tension headache, muscle contraction headache, stress headache, and/or ordinary headache. The term "tension-type headache" as named in the New International Classification of Headache by the International Headache Society (IHS) recognizes the international controversy over the existence of the tension headache concept in general.

Although historically clinicians have used the term *tension headache* to characterize a daily or almost daily chronic headache disorder without vascular-type features and that is likely but not necessarily associated with provocation by stress or emotional factors, traditionally migraine and muscle contraction headaches have been considered distinct entities (9).

So imprecise have been the criteria for tension headache, and so casually has the diagnosis been rendered, that to many the diagnosis of tension headache or muscle contraction headache has become but a "wastebasket" diagnosis (2, 8). In many instances, the diagnosis has been applied to any headache disorder that ostensibly is not vascular (migraine, cluster) nor associated with identifiable structural disease, and that occurs when elements of stress, anxiety, or depression are evident.

A serious reappraisal of attitudes on this headache entity is underway, as was mentioned earlier (2, 16, 17). Research studies over the course of the past several years have raised serious challenges to traditional positions. Attention to the transformation from intermittent migraine to daily chronic headache and to central elements purported to be involved in this process is growing in importance and is considered as the basis for the clinical events and for treatment approaches.

With this in mind, and recognizing that a transition in our understanding and classification of this disorder is currently underway, treatment regimens are described. The reader will quickly note that considerable overlapping between treatments of this condition and migraine exists, and that treatment frequently involves combinations of drugs.

SYMPTOMATIC TREATMENT FOR "ACUTE" TENSION HEADACHE

Acute tension headache may in fact be a separate and distinct entity from that of the chronic form. Acute tension headache is perhaps of muscular origin and results in occasional, intermittent headache, whereas chronic "tension headache" is prolonged, sustained, and more likely to be daily rather than intermittent. Acute tension headache can be brought on by stress, posture, or injury. The symptoms are usually generalized, with occipitofrontal tightness or "band-like" pain, and rarely does the pain reach sufficient level to cause limitations of function (8).

The treatment for acute tension headache consists of mild analgesics (aspirin, acetaminophen) or NSAIDs. Simple muscle relaxants may also be of value.

TREATMENT FOR CHRONIC DAILY HEADACHE (TENSION-TYPE HEADACHE)

Symptomatic Treatment

From a therapeutic point of view, frequent, recurring headache patterns in which both muscular and vascular features coexist during a well-circumscribed attack are best treated with medications appropriate for the symptomatic alleviation of the predominant headache element. For acute muscular pain, simple analgesics, NSAIDs, or TCAs are useful. For acute migraine elements, ergotamine tartrate, Midrin, or other drugs mentioned in earlier sections are appropriate.

Preventive Treatment

Because most frequently chronic headaches forms result in daily or almost daily headache, preventative treatment is advisable.

The TCAs (see "Preventive Pharmacologic Agents in the Treatment of Migraine," above) are used on a daily basis (3, 8, 51). In addition to their value in daily pain states, these medications are particularly valuable in controlling accompanying depression as well as sleep disturbance, which are both frequently encountered in this population (2, 8). Dosages range from 25–150 mg at bedtime if tolerated. Treatment response may have little to do with existing depression or its elimination.

Tricyclic antidepressants can be readily combined with β-blocking agents (51), and in this regard propranolol and nadolol have been found useful. Periodic acute attacks of migraine that are encountered commonly on a background of daily chronic headache should be treated in the standard fashion as described earlier. The addition of NSAIDs, benzodiazepine therapy, and other drugs mentioned earlier in the treatment of migraine may also be necessary.

This population of patients is very complex. Analgesic overuse, psychological distress, and family and other complicating problems frequently render even the most appropriate pharmacotherapeutic intervention ineffective. In this author's experience, a comprehensive treatment program including inpatient-level care, psychotherapy, family involvement in treatment programs, dietary control, biofeedback, and several other interventions are frequently necessary to bring about satisfactory control of this difficult headache process.

HEADACHES IN CHILDREN

Children, like adults, get headaches. Migraine, mixed element headaches, cluster headache, and others seen in adulthood can be encountered in childhood (8). Of some interest is that the female/male ratio among children with headaches is 1:1, whereas a 3:1 ratio in favor of women is characteristic of most adult chronic headaches, except cluster headache, which is predominantly an illness of men (8).

The pharmacologic treatment of headache in children does not differ appreciably from that of adults. Cyproheptadine (Periactin) may be the treatment of first choice for the prevention of childhood migraine. Children appear to tolerate both preventive and symptomatic agents quite well. Tricyclic antidepressants, β-blockers, NSAIDs (particularly for chronic paroxysmal hemicrania), and symptomatic medications are all appropriate. Nonmedical interventions including biofeedback, dietary restriction, avoidance of excessive "junk food" intake, regular eating patterns, stress management, and family counseling may all represent important elements in the treatment of childhood headaches.

POST-TRAUMATIC CEPHALGIA

The incidence of headache following closed head injury varies from 33 to 80% and may take one of several clinical forms. Often the headache is a component of the *post-traumatic* or *postconcussion* syndrome, which represents a constellation of symptoms that can follow even mild head or flexion/extension injury (3, 8, 9). Among the nonheadache symptoms that are generally considered common in this condition are vertigo or nonspecific dizziness, personality change (most notably depression and anxiety), impairment of memory, reduced attention span, insomnia, and reduced motivation. Prolonged neuropsychological impairment can be documented in many patients who exhibit little in the way of objective dysfunction (52).

The headache may take the form of one of several patterns. Among these are: a generalized throbbing and/or nonthrobbing cephalgia; unilateral intermittent or continuous throbbing pain (similar to migraine); localized occipitocervical pain with neuralgic qualities; and unilateral intense intermittent cephalgia in the anterior triangle of the neck or in the orbital area, and resembling episodic cluster headache (8, 9). Frequently, an intermingling of two or more of these forms is present. Occipitocervical soreness and myofascial-type complaints often accompany the more specific headache patterns.

TREATMENT OF POST-TRAUMATIC HEADACHE

Important nonpharmacologic interventions such as counseling, biofeedback, physical therapy, transcutaneous electrical nerve stimulation treatment, and others are appropriate. A variety of pharmacologic interventions should be considered. For prophylaxis, a TCA, β-blocker, or calcium antagonist can be efficacious alone or in combination. Nonsteroidal anti-inflammatory agents, intermittently or prophylactically, may be useful. Intermittent acute headache events can be treated in the manner described earlier for symptomatic treatment of migraine. Focal tenderness often responds to local anesthesia with or without steroids. Neuralgic symptoms may be controlled with carbamazepine (Tegretol),

phenytoin (Dilantin), or baclofen (Lioresal). Local surgical procedures, including decompression or neurectomy, have been recommended in some patients.

Clinical experience, however, suggests that patients with post-traumatic headache require a comprehensive treatment program. Lingering symptoms that are often refractory to simple intervention are common.

SPECIAL THERAPEUTIC CONSIDERATIONS AND SITUATIONS

SPECIAL DRUG TECHNIQUES

The pharmacologic treatment of patients with chronic headache must be individually determined. Persistent and innovative attempts to develop appropriate treatment protocols is frequently necessary to bring about recognizable improvement.

Intravenous administration of dihydroergotamine at dosages ranging from 0.5–1.0 mg every 8 hours over a period of 3–5 days has now become the standard treatment of choice for intractable, persistent migraine, and related headaches. The treatment usually brings dramatic control over even the most refractory cases of migraine, including those aggravated by substance withdrawal. Though the value of treatment may not last beyond the administration of DHE, it provides an opportunity for time during which pain can be controlled and preventive interventions can be implemented.

Intravenous dihydroergotamine is best carried out in an inpatient setting and should be reserved for those patients in whom standard interventions are of little value.

Other intravenous protocols include the use of hydrocortisone and phenothiazine. Hydrocortisone can be given in a dose of 100 mg, administered in an IV "push" three times a day for 2–3 days. Chlorpromazine in a dose of 10–20 mg can be administered intravenously three times a day (consult *Handbook of Headache Management* for further details and prescribing information).

The MAIOs have proven useful in several of this author's most refractory cases. Although caution and special instructions to the patient are necessary, most patients can use these drugs without ill effects or undue risk.

In the symptomatic treatment of migraine, absorption from the gastrointestinal tract can prove to be the determining factor in establishing effectiveness. The use of metoclopramide (Reglan) 10 mg one to three times per day may be of value in enhancing the effectiveness of any of the oral tablets (8). Treatment with metoclopramide can precede the use of any of the oral agents by 10–15 min and can be helpful in avoiding some of the nausea that frequently occurs with the use of ergotamine tartrate or as part of the headache itself.

Inhalant forms of ergotamine tartrate or rectal forms are likewise useful in overcoming the gastrointestinal factors accompanying attacks.

Menstrual migraine represents a most difficult variation of migraine. Many women will experience their most severe headache at this time of the month and frequently it is superimposed upon other changes that occur as part of menses. Ergotamine tartrate is probably the most effective agent for the reversal of this headache, and preventive therapy that might include NSAIDs, Bellergal, β-blockers, and others may be necessary. Danazol (Danocrine) has been found useful anecdotally, but studies firmly establishing its efficacy are lacking.

Recently, the application of an estrogen patch several days prior to the onset of the menstrual headache has been found useful, through controlled studies are unavailable.

It is particularly important when using combinations of medications to exercise appropriate caution, periodic educational review, and diagnostic monitoring. Laboratory reviews to monitor biochemical parameters, electrocardiographic evaluation to assess QRS intervals and conduction disturbances, and blood level assessments are strongly recommended (53).

Despite the apparent reliability of an individual patient, noncompliance either intentionally or inadvertently is common (54). Periodic review of treatment regimens and appropriate counseling are likewise worthwhile and add measurably to the likelihood of treatment efficacy.

TREATMENT OF MEDICATION OVERUSE AND DEPENDENCY IN HEADACHE PATIENTS

Physicians and other health care professionals treating patients with headache and other chronic pain syndromes must confront a serious medication overuse problem in a large number of their patients. The extent of this problem is difficult to assess. In our center, it is estimated that at least one-half of the patients seeking help for headaches indulge in excessive use of medications to relieve their distress, and it is not unusual for first-time patients to report the consumption of 10–30 simple analgesic tablets per day, 6–8 mg of ergotamine tartrate daily, or the regular ingestion of large amounts of tranquilizing, hypnotic, or narcotic analgesics.

Aside from the important health consequences of the daily use of many of these agents, recent interest has focused on the "rebound" phenomenon in which daily or almost daily use of symptomatic agents enhances and worsens headache frequency (8, 12, 55). Personal experience suggests that this problem represents the most important single factor contributing to treatment refractoriness in long-standing headache patients, and several reports have documented the importance of this problem (56).

The headache patient who overuses medication presents a special challenge to the clinician, frequently forcing hospitalization to establish meaningful treatment intervention. Although cynicism toward the patient is common, it must be emphasized that patients with legitimate chronic headache syndromes experience years of torment as a result of their unsuccessfully treated disorders. Many awaken each morning and retire each night with pain, and many have sought various medical as well as nonmedical avenues of help, ranging from qualified health care to nonqualified sources promising quick and simple explanations and therapies. Many have turned to symptomatic drugs simply to "get through the day." Marital, employment, and other relationships suffer. The quality of life deteriorates, and, if present, preexisting psychological disturbances are intensified.

In many ways, patients with headache are trapped. If patients resort to excessive analgesics, they come under assault for their "abuse." If they simply "take to bed" or accept their disabling illness by withdrawing from functional status, families, and other activities, they are identified as psychologically impaired, unmotivated, and achieving "secondary gain."

The treatment of patients with medication overuse and headache is difficult and tenuous. Detoxification and removal of the offending agents from the treatment regimen are essential. Patients frequently fear that elimination of analgesics prior to the development of a preventive treatment program will result in their having little in the way of reliable control over headaches, and will thus resist the removal of analgesics prior to efficacious prevention. Ironically, effective prevention is generally not forthcoming until detoxification and removal of analgesics have occurred, thus providing for a classic "catch-22" dilemma. We have found that open communication and instruction on this point, the use of reasonable and flexible timetables, and the use of a comprehensive inpatient treatment setting are the key elements to successful transition from use of analgesics to more acceptable prophylaxis. Psychological as well as physiologic dependency must be confronted, as must the practical considerations regarding the patient's need to remain functional and maintain some limited control over their own painful events. Patients with headache will resist and are frequently frightened of treatment efforts that remove entirely their own ability to manage pain, and cooperative treatment regimens with careful monitoring and instruction appear most effective.

INPATIENT UNITS

In 1979, this author and associates established the first inpatient program directed to the treatment of headache. Over the course of the past few years, several other units have developed. The patient treatment program provides a comprehensive intervention that includes detoxification from overuse of symptomatic medications, aggressive pharmacotherapy, milieu treatment, dietary manipulation, identification and restriction from aggravating influences, psychological and family intervention, and educational programs. Chronic illnesses such as headache frequently require this degree of intervention for treatment success. Recently, this inpatient unit has been awarded national accreditation from the Commission on Accreditation of Rehabilitation Facilities (CARF). This marks the first inpatient pain unit directed at headache management to achieve accreditation status, and initiates the establishment of standards for units treating headache.

Recently, data from a prospective, long-term outcome study in refractory patients treated in this unit was presented. A statistically significant reduction in the major clinical variables, including headache frequency and intensity, excessive analgesic use, and disability, were noted (see Lake et al. 1990, under "Suggested Readings").

CONCLUSIONS

Headache, like other painful syndromes, is a difficult condition to treat. Nonetheless, it is currently estimated that with proper technique upward of 75% of chronic recurring headache patients can achieve successful control. No universally effective solution to this complicated health problem currently exists. It is clear that most of the pharmacologic agents described in this presentation provide an indirect influence on the mechanism of headache. No therapy, despite its support in treatment studies, can be relied upon to be universally effective or always satisfactory. Indeed, one of the more frustrating phenomena encountered in the treatment of patients with headache is that from patient to patient with this condition, effective treatment requires individual consideration and treatment planning.

Many patients will benefit from programs described above, including the comprehensive and multidisciplinary approaches now available in specialty centers and inpatient units. Headache is a disabling condition, and medical science has not, until recently, begun to address it in a fashion consistent with its widespread impact. However, despite the limitations in our current understanding as well as the historic prejudice directed toward patients with this condition, our current understanding as well as the treatment approaches described above can provide hope and relief for most patients who suffer from these disorders.

Unfortunately, not all patients can be satisfactorily helped. For some, it is because their condition exceeds current knowledge. For others the need to be sick or fear to be well can defeat even the most committed effort. Nevertheless, persistence, patience, and compassion will bring recognizable and satisfying relief for most who suffer from recurring headaches. Although the chronic headache patient is prone to isolation and despair, knowing that someone cares, understands, and is willing to help is mightily useful in chronic, poorly understood illnesses such as headache.

Finally, while the use of multiple medication regimens is to be discouraged under most circumstances, this, like all other aspects of treatment for difficult-to-treat illness, must be considered in perspective. Neurologists commonly employ multiple treatment regimens for the control of Parkinson's disease and epilepsy. Multiple treatment regimens are frequently necessary in the control of hypertension, ischemic heart disease, congestive heart failure, and multisystem disease. That such efforts are sometimes appropriate in the treatment of the most refractory headache patients seems similarly justifiable. Attitudes that infer that similar efforts are excessive or inappropriate for this disabling disorder may be more a reflection of bias than a fair appraisal of treatment need.

REFERENCES

1. Ad Hoc Committee on Classification of Headache: *Arch Neurol* 6:173–176, 1963.
2. Saper JR: Changing perspective on chronic headache. *Clin J Pain* 2:19–28, 1986.
3. Raskin NH, Appenzeller O: *Headache.* Philadelphia, WB Saunders 1980.
4. Featherstone HJ: Migraine and muscle contraction headaches: a continuum. *Headache* 25:194–198, 1984.
5. Cohen MJ: Psychophysiological studies of headache: is there a similarity between migraine and muscle contraction headache? *Headache* 18:189–196, 1978.
6. Lance JW: *Mechanism and Management of Headache,* ed 4. London, Butterworth Scientific, 1982.
7. Dalessio DJ, Camp WA, Goodell H, Wolff HG: Studies on headache. The mode of action of UML-491 and its relevance to the nature of vascular headache of the migraine type. *Arch Neurol* 4:235, 1961.
8. Saper JR: *Headache Disorders: Current Concepts and Treatment Strategies.* Littleton, MA, Wright, PSG, 1983.
9. Dalessio DJ: *Wolff's Headache and Other Head Pain,* ed 4. New York, Oxford University Press, 1980.
10. Olesen J, Lauritzen M, Tfelt-Hansen P, et al: Spreading cerebral oligemia in classical and normal cerebral blood flow in common migraine. *Headache* 22:242–248, 1982.
11. Olesen J, Tfelt-Hansen P, Henricksen L, et al: The common migraine attack may not be initiated by cerebral ischemia. *Lancet* 2:438–440, 1981.
12. Saper JR, Jones JM: Ergotamine tartrate dependency: features and possible mechanisms. *Clin Neuropharmacol* 9:244–256, 1986.
13. Blau JN: Migraine prodrome separated from aura: "complete migraine." *Br Med J* 281:658–660, 1980.
14. Wilkinson M, Blau JN: Are classical and common migraine different entities? *Headache* 25:211–221, 1985.
15. Olesen J: Are classical and common migraine different entities? *Headache* 25:213, 1985.
16. Mathew NT, Stubits E, Nigam M: Transformation of mi-

graine into daily headache: analysis of factors. *Headache* 22:66–68, 1982.

17. Saper JR, Johnson T, VanMeter M: "Mixed headache": a chronic headache complex. A study of 500 patients. *Headache* 23:143, 1983 (abstr).

18. Rall TW, Schliefer LS: Drugs affecting uterine motility. In Goodman LS, Gilman AG (eds): *Pharmacological Basis of Therapeutics*, ed 7. New York, Macmillan, 1985, pp 926–945.

19. Yuil GM, Swinburn WR, Liversedge LA: A double-blind crossover trial of isometheptane mucate compound and ergotamine in migraine. *Br J Clin Prac* 26:76–79, 1972.

20. Saper JR: Non-steroidal anti-inflammatory drugs. *Top Pain Manage* (newsletter) 1(3):9, 1985.

21. Saper JR: Naproxen sodium in the treatment of headache. *Top Pain Manage* (newsletter) 1(6):21–22, 1985.

22. Welch KMA, Ellis EJ, Keenan BA: Successful migraine prophylaxis with naproxen sodium. *Neurology* 35:1304–1310, 1985.

23. Pradalier A, Rancurl G, Dordain C, et al: Acute migraine attack therapy: comparison of naproxen sodium and ergotamine tartrate compound. *Cephalgia* 5:107–113, 1985.

24. Rumore MM, Schlichtine DA: Clinical efficacy of antihistaminics as analgesics. *Pain*, 25:7–22, 1986.

25. Gallagher RM: The emergency treatment of intractable migraine. *Headache* 26:74–75, 1986.

26. Raskin NH: Repetitive intravenous DHE as therapy for migraine. *Neurology* 36:995–997, 1986.

27. Sudilovsky A, Stern M, Mayer JH: Comparative efficacy of nadolol and propranolol in the prophylaxis of migraine. *J Headache* 26:311–312, 1986 (abstr).

28. Fanchamps A: Why do not all beta blockers prevent migraine? (Letter to the Editor). *Headache* 25:61–62, 1985.

29. Nadelmann JW, Phil M, Stevens J, Saper JR: Propranolol in prophylaxis of migraine. *Headache* 26:175–186, 1986.

30. Meyers JS, Hardenberg J: Clinical effectiveness of calcium entry blockers in the prophylactic treatment of migraine and cluster headache. *Headache* 26:266–277, 1983.

31. Meyer JS, Nancy M, Walker M, et al: Migraine and cluster headache treatment with calcium antagonists supports a vascular pathogenesis. *Headache* 25:358–367, 1985.

32. Solomon GD, Steel JG, Spaccavento LJ: Verapamil prophylaxis of migraine. A double blind placebo-controlled study. *JAMA* 250:2500–2502, 1983.

33. Saper JR: Calcium channel blockers. *Top Pain Manage* (newsletter) 1(2):7, 1985.

34. *AMA Drug Evaluations*, ed 6. New York, American Medical Association, 1986, pp 239–252.

35. Saper JR: Treatment of chronic headaches. In Conn HF (ed): *Conn's Current Therapy*. Philadelphia, WB Saunders, 1983, pp 724–732.

36. White K, Simpson G: Combined MAOI-tricyclic antidepressant treatment: a re-evaluation. *J Clin Psychopharmacol* 1:264–282, 1981.

37. Pare CMB, Halstrom C, Kline M, et al: Will amitriptyline prevent the "cheese" reaction of monoamine oxidase inhibitors? *Lancet* 2:183–186, 1982.

38. Raskin NH, Schwartz RK: Interval therapy of migraine: long term results. *Headache* 20:336–340, 1980.

39. Kudrow L: *Cluster Headache*. New York, Oxford University Press, 1980.

40. Sjaastad O, Dale I: A new ? clinical entity: "chronic paroxysmal hemicrania." *Headache* 14:105–108, 1974.

41. Fogan L: Treatment of cluster headache: a double blind comparison of oxygen vs. air inhalation. *Arch Neurol* 42:362–363, 1985.

42. Saper JR: Cluster headache: diagnosis and treatment. *Pain and Analgesia* (in press).

43. Ekbom K: Lithium in the treatment of chronic cluster headache (editorial). *Headache* 17:39–40, 1977.

44. Mathew NT: Clinical subtypes of cluster headache and responses to lithium therapy. *Headache* 18:26–30, 1978.

45. Caviness VS Jr, O'Brien P: Cluster headache: response to chlorpromazine. *Headache* 20:128–131, 1980.

46. Mathew NT: Indomethacin responsive headache syndromes. *Headache* 21:147–150, 1981.

47. Horton BT, McLean AR, Craig WM: The use of histamine in the treatment of specific types of headache. *Proc Staff Meetings Mayo Clin* 14:247, 1939.

48. Diamond S, Freitag FG, Prager J: Treatment of intractable cluster. *Headache* 26:42–46, 1986.

49. Watson CP, Morley TP, Richards JC, et al: The surgical treatment of chronic cluster headache. *Headache* 23:289–295, 1983.

50. Onofrio BM, Campbell JK: Surgical treatment of chronic cluster headache. *Mayo Clin Proc* 6:537–544, 1986.

51. Mathew NT: Prophylaxis of migraine and mixed headache: a randomized control study. *Headache* 21:105–109, 1981.

52. Stuss DT, Ely P, Heugenholtz H, et al: Subtle neuropsychological deficits in patients with good recovery after closed head injury. *Neurosurgery* 17:41–47, 1985.

53. Boehnert MT, Lovejoy FH: The value of the QRS duration vs. the serum drug level in predicting seizures and ventricular arrhythmias after an acute overdose of tricyclic antidepressants. *N Engl J Med* 313:474–479, 1985.

54. Packard RC, O'Connell P: Medication compliance among headache patients. *Headache* 26:30, 1986 (abstr).

55. Rapoport A: Analgesic rebound. *Top Pain Manage* (newsletter) 1(8):29–32, 1986.

56. Rapoport A, Weeks RE, Sheftell FD, et al: The "analgesic washout period": a critical variable in the evaluation of headache treatment of efficacy. *Neurology* 36(suppl):100–101, 1986.

Suggested Readings

Saper JR, Silberstein SD, Gordon CDG, Hamel RL: *Handbook of Headache Management*. Baltimore, Williams & Wilkins, 1992.

Silberstein SD (ed): Intractable headache: Inpatient and outpatient treatment strategies. *Neurology* (Suppl 2), 42:1–51.

Mathew NT (ed): Headache. *Neurol Clin* November, 1990.

Olesen J: Classification and diagnostic criteria for headache disorders, cranial neuralgias, and headache pain. *Cephalalgia* 8(Suppl 7):1–96, 1988.

The multinational oral sumatriptan and Cafergot comparative study group: A randomized, double-blind comparison of Cafergot and sumatriptan in the treatment of migraine. *Eur Neuro* 31:314–322, 1991.

Subcutaneous Sumatriptan International Study Group: Treatment of migraine attacks with sumatriptan. *N Engl J Med* 5:316–321, 1991.

The Oral Sumatriptan Dose-Defining Study Group: Sumatriptan—An oral dose-defining study. *Eur Neurol* 31:300–305, 1991.

The Oral Sumatriptan Multiple-Dose Study Group: Evaluation of a multiple-dose regimen of oral sumatriptan for the acute treatment of migraine. *Eur Neurol* 31:306–313, 1991.

Herring R, Kuritzky A: Sodium valproate in the prophylactic treatment of migraine: A double-blind study vs. placebo. *Cephalalgia* 12:81–84, 1992.

Silberstein SD, Shulman EA, Hopkins MM: Repetitive intra-venous DHE in the treatment of refractory headache. *Headache* 30:334–339, 1990.

Anonymous: Ketorolac tromethamine. *Med Lett* 32:79–81, 1990.

Lake AE, et al: Inpatient treatment for chronic daily headache: A prospective long-term outcome study. *Headache* 30:229, 1990.

Rapoport AM, Silberstein SD: Emergency treatment of headache. *Neurology* (Suppl 2), 42:1–51.

CHAPTER 21

PSYCHOLOGICAL MANAGEMENT OF HEADACHE PAIN

ANTHONY IEZZI
HENRY E. ADAMS
ROBERT N. PILON

ALTHOUGH HEADACHES are usually not a life-threatening health problem, they are a major health problem when considered from an epidemiologic point of view. An estimated 35 million Americans apparently suffer from headaches (1). In terms of the frequency for which individuals seek outpatient medical care, headache was found to be one of the top 14 health problems (2). The social and economic costs of headaches also attest to the debilitating nature of this health problem. According to a recent national survey, the *Nuprin Pain Report*, 7% of a cross-sectional sample reported experiencing headaches at least 100 days or more over a 1-year period (3).

Even though the prevalence and significance of headache pain is readily apparent and the literature is substantial on the etiology and treatment of headache (4–6), headache still remains an enigmatic health problem. The main emphasis of this chapter is on the psychological management of headache pain, although a brief review of the different headache types and their defining characteristics, the pathophysiology and etiology of the different headache types, and the assessment of headache also is presented. Initially, the successful management of chronic headache depends on a thorough assessment and accurate diagnosis of headache type and an understanding of the pathophysiology and etiology of headache type.

HEADACHE TYPES AND DEFINING CHARACTERISTICS

Useful information about etiology, mechanisms of pain, and treatment outcome requires an adequate headache classification system. The headache classification system provided by the Ad Hoc Committee of the National Institute of Neurological Disease and Blindness (NINDB) has been guiding the clinical and research activities in the headache field for the past 30 odd years (7). Fifteen headache types were identified and organized on the basis of pain mechanisms and on the presence or absence of prodromal symptoms. Unfortunately, the NINDB diagnostic criteria have been used extensively with little empirical evidence demonstrating their reliability and validity (8, 9).

In response to repeated criticism of the NINDB classification system, the International Headache Society (IHS) produced a new hierarchically organized classification system (10). Compared to the two-page document by the NINDB, the new classification system is comprehensively outlined in a 96-page document. It should be understood that the new classification system is based on the experience of experts rather than empirical data. Still, the IHS classification system is a heuristic research tool that attempts to increase the nosographic and epidemiologic foundation for the study of headache. A second edition is tentatively planned for release in 1993.

In addition to classifying headaches according to pain mechanism and the presence or absence of prodromal symptoms, the new headache classification system also classifies head pain according to frequency, location, and duration. Unlike the NINDB headache classification system, the IHS diagnostic criteria allow for multiple headache diagnoses in the same headache patient. For example, patients who have been diagnosed as having combined migraine and muscle contraction headache are now given a dual diagnosis of migraine headache and tension-type headache and coded in order of importance.

The initial reactions by clinicians and researchers to the IHS diagnostic criteria appear to be somewhat mixed. The criteria are complex and restrictive and clinicians may have some difficulty in applying the new criteria (11). Although the IHS criteria are thought to be exhaustive (12), the new IHS diagnostic criteria do not seem to radically change the diagnoses of the vast majority of headache patients that had originally been classified according to the NINDB criteria (13). In addition, there may be some difficulties in being able to distinguish between migraine and tension headache with the new classification system, more specifically, differentiating between migraine without aura and episodic tension-type headache (14). Only with further studies on the reliability and validity of the IHS diagnostic criteria will headache researchers and clinicians be able to evaluate its clinical utility.

Because of the fact that there are very little data on the new classification system, we will refer in this chapter primarily to the NINDB classification diagnostic terms. At the time this chapter was written, not one current psychological treatment study of headache had used the new IHS criteria. Readers are referred to Chapter 19 for more details on the IHS headache classification scheme. Only four headache types are discussed in this chapter: (1) migraine, (2) muscle contraction, (3) combined vascular and muscle contraction, and (4) headache of delusional, conversion, or hypochondriacal states. These four headache types are discussed because they are seen most frequently in the clinical context and because psychological factors have been implicated in their etiology, exacerbation, and maintenance.

Migraine

The following description of migraine headache is taken from the NINDB classification scheme (7):

> Recurrent attacks of headache, widely varied in intensity, frequency and duration. The attacks are commonly unilateral in onset; are usually associated with anorexia and, sometimes, with nausea and vomiting; in some are preceded by, or associated with, conspicuous sensory, motor, and mood disturbances; and are often familial.

A migraine headache episode may occur at any time of the day, but is common upon awakening. Frequency of migraine headache can vary from several times per week to several times per year. Duration of an episode is usually from 30 min to several hours, but migraine can occur for several days at a time. A fully developed migraine episode will usually interfere with a patient's regular daily activities.

Although the term *migraine* has often been used by the lay public as if it referred to a stereotypic pain phenomenon, migraine headache patients are a heterogeneous group. The migraine headache category can be further divided into five subtypes (7): (1) *classic migraine,* sharply defined headache with sensory and/or motor prodromes, (2) *common migraine,* similar to classic migraine except without a clear-cut prodrome or aura, (3) *cluster headache,* unexpected bouts of severe headaches, usually in clusters of two or three headache episodes lasting 20–90 min over several days, (4) *hemiplegic and opthalmoplegic migraine,* vascular headache with strong

sensory and motor phenomena that persist during and after the headache, and (5) *lower-half headache,* headache centered primarily in the lower face. Of patients who report migraine, approximately 85% tend to experience common migraine, and approximately 10% tend to experience classic migraine (15). According to the IHS classification system, classic migraine is referred to as migraine with aura; common migraine is referred to as migraine without aura (10).

The pathophysiology of migraine headache involves the cranial and cerebral vascular systems as well as the autonomic nervous system in some fashion (16, 17). The generally accepted pathophysiologic model of migraine, as suggested by Wolff (17), consists of a two-phase process. During the first phase, vasoconstriction of the cranial and cerebral arteries, with a subsequent reduction in blood supply to the brain, occurs. This initial phase is then followed by a vasodilation of cranial and cerebral arteries, including extracranial or scalp arteries. There then follows an inflammation of the arterial walls, vascular edema, and release of various local chemical and vasoactive substances. Actual head pain is believed to co-vary with the dilation of the extracranial arteries. More recent opinions implicate the serotonergic and adrenergic pain-modulating systems in the pathophysiologic model of migraine (17).

Although the pathophysiologic model of migraine headache has been fairly well established, the etiology remains somewhat equivocal. Exactly what initiates the two-phase pathophysiologic process is not known. Psychological distress or psychopathology (18, 19), stress (20), and neurovascular (17) and hormonal (21) factors have been implicated in the etiology of migraine. It is unlikely that any one of these factors is singularly responsible for migraines or can account for the heterogeneity of this disorder.

Muscle Contraction

Muscle contraction headache, also known as tension-type headache according to IHS criteria (10), results from sustained contraction of the muscles of the shoulders, neck, and scalp (7). A description of sensation of tightness or pressure in a "hat band" distribution is commonly reported with this type of headache. Duration of a muscle contraction headache episode ranges from a few hours to several weeks, with varying degrees of intensity but usually not interfering with routine activities. Muscle contraction head pain is usually located bilaterally and described as a dull ache (as opposed to the commonly reported sensation of throbbing in migraine headache). Patients will usually report a worsening of head pain as the day progresses. Clearly defined prodromes in patients with muscle contraction headache are not common. The prevalence of muscle contraction headache varies, but it has been reported that as many as 80% of individuals experiencing headaches suffer from muscle contraction headaches (22).

As mentioned earlier, the pathophysiology of muscle contraction headache involves sustained elevations of muscle activity in several muscle groups of the head, face and neck. These elevations in muscle activity are thought to occur in the absence of permanent structural change (7). Vascular changes have been also implicated in the pathophysiology of muscle contraction headache, but studies examining vascular changes have provided conflicting results (23). As is the case with migraine headache, exactly what initiates the pathophysiologic process of muscle contraction headache is unclear, but how an individual reacts to the stressors of daily living has been implicated in the etiology of muscle contraction headache. One fairly recent study found that although tension headache sufferers tended to experience a similar number of chronic stressors or daily hassles as compared to matched headache-free controls, headache sufferers tended to appraise stressful events and themselves more negatively (24). Personality style and emotional lability have been also considered in the etiology of muscle contraction headache (25); however, this contention has met with little empirical support.

Many authors are now challenging the view that muscle contraction headache and migraine headache are in fact separate diagnostic entities. It is not at all uncommon for a headache to begin as a muscle contraction headache and, as it becomes more severe, for migraine type features to occur. Migraine and muscle contraction headaches may be part of a continuum of benign recurring head pain that varies on a continuum of severity (26–28). Obviously, shared clinical features between muscle contraction and migraine headaches add to the diagnostic confusion.

Combined Vascular and Muscle Contraction

Combined vascular and muscle contraction headache (also referred to in the headache literature as mixed headache) is characterized by the expression of vascular and muscular symptoms (7). Adams et al. suggested that it may be more meaningful to think of patients with combined vascular and muscle contraction headache as individuals suffering from the two types of head pain independently (29), a viewpoint consistent with the new IHS classification scheme, which requires a dual diagnosis (10). As one might expect, the pathophysiology and etiology of combined vascular and muscle contraction headache involve a combination of vascular and muscle changes, as discussed earlier.

Headache of Delusional, Conversion, or Hypochondriacal States (Psychogenic headache)

The NINDB criteria for headache of delusional, conversion or hypochondriacal states are stated as follows (7):

Headaches of illnesses in which the prevailing clinical disorder is a delusional or a conversion reaction and a peripheral pain mechanism is nonexistent. Closely allied are the hypochondriacal reactions in which the peripheral disturbances relevant to headache are minimal. These also have been called "psychogenic" headaches.

The term *psychogenic headache* will be used in place of headache of delusional, conversion, or hypochondriacal states for reasons of convenience. In the IHS classification system, this type of headache would be diagnosed as tension-type headache associated with somatic, delusional or somatoform disorder (10).

A psychogenic headache tends to be relatively continuous in occurrence, with a waxing and waning quality; it is often described as a dull pain, and is located frontally and posteriorly, although on occasion some patients report that "it hurts all over my head, neck, and face." It is not unusual for patients to state that their pain travels—that is, that the pain moves from one area of the head to another, often in a fashion that is not consistent with an anatomic distribution. Associated symptoms commonly include anxiety and depression (30, 31). The prevalence of psychogenic headache is unknown, but is probably much greater than most clinicians have acknowledged. This lack of recognition may have contributed to the confusing nature of the muscle contraction headache literature.

Given the definition of psychogenic headache, there is no pathophysiologic process that can adequately explain psychogenic headache. Because there appears to be an absence of a pathophysiologic process, the etiology of headache very likely involves the role of social learning and psychological factors (32, 33). In other words, pain behavior is positively reinforced and "well" behavior is inadequately reinforced. Therefore, psychogenic headache can be viewed as a pain disorder reinforced by its consequences without the known peripheral pain mechanisms that are typical of migraine or muscle contraction headaches. The possible mechanism in the acquisition of psychogenic headache probably involves inappropriate positive reinforcement, modeling (e.g., family members who have headaches or other types of chronic pain), and/or avoidance conditioning (e.g., getting out of doing something aversive, such as school or work, by using pain as an excuse). Although these etiologic hypotheses appear reasonable, further empirical research is needed to determine their value and utility.

ASSESSMENT

A differential diagnosis of headache type involves the elimination of alternative medical (physical and physiologic) and psychological explanations of head pain. A comprehensive assessment requires collecting information from several sources (34): (1) an adequate medical examination, (2) a thorough interview with headache patient and significant other, (3) self-monitoring of head pain, and (4) performing a psychophysiologic assessment of the patient in headache and nonheadache states. A brief review of each assessment area is presented.

MEDICAL EXAMINATION

No treatment should ever begin on a headache patient who has not undergone a medical and neurologic work-up. Although organic causes of headaches are somewhat uncommon, psychological treatment of a headache patient with an organic disorder would be ineffective, and the consequences of choosing an inappropriate intervention can be very serious, to say the least. The medical diagnosis of headache type is made on the basis of behavioral symptoms and positive/negative findings on a series of medical tests. A physical examination involves an evaluation of blood pressure, eye function, cranial nerve function, and general sensory and motor function. Also included in a thorough medical examination, if indicated, is the use of laboratory studies (e.g., blood and urine analysis, skull radiographs, computed tomography scan, angiogram, and electroencephalogram). Even when psychological intervention of headache is initiated, a careful record of symptoms and results should be monitored; if any unusual or unexpected symptoms are observed and do not fit the case formulation, then consultation with the referring physician is strongly recommended.

INITIAL INTERVIEW

Interview information obtained from a headache patient allows the clinician to make a correct diagnosis, target psychological adjuncts to headache, establish rapport, and tailor a systematic treatment plan (34). Typically, a headache interview lasts anywhere from 1–1.5 hours and is usually conducted during the initial visit. The critical areas to be covered in the interview include a detailed history of head pain, family history of head pain and other chronic pain disorder, possible treatments (medical and psychological) received for head pain and their success, an evaluation of the patient's psychological adjustment in order to construct a functional analysis of head pain and other psychological difficulties that may be present, an examination of a patient's background history (e.g., history of sexual and physical abuse), and an evaluation of the reasons for seeking treatment.

An area often neglected in the interview process is in the report of observations provided by significant others. Significant others can often provide useful information about the patient's pain behavior (e.g., localizing a patient's environmental stress, providing a check on the patient's self-report of head pain). Interviewing significant others will help establish rapport with them, which will also increase the probability of getting them

to assist with the patient's treatment plan, and thereby increasing the possibility of positive therapeutic outcome.

A headache questionnaire can be administered to aid in the interview process. The critical areas assessed in a headache questionnaire are demographic information, headache history, current status and symptoms of headache, and location of head pain. In addition, circumstances surrounding the onset of headache, modeling influences, and the antecedents and consequences of headache are vital data. A headache questionnaire is useful in that it saves some of the clinician's therapy time, it is easy for the patient to complete, and it provides information that is more reliable than verbal report.

SELF-MONITORING

Self-monitoring or diary-keeping is a valuable component to the assessment and management of headache. On a daily basis, the patient is required to write the occurrence, intensity, degree of disability, duration, location, and associated symptoms of headache. Moreover, the type and amount of medications taken and other pain-relief strategies used are reported. Possible triggers, stressors, or mood states that may be associated with the patient's headaches are also noted. The patient is usually required to keep a diary for 1 month before treatment, throughout the whole treatment process, and during follow-up. It is our experience that patients comply well with self-monitoring; in fact, if the patient has problems with diary-keeping, then the patient is likely to neglect other aspects of treatment.

There are several advantages to using a headache diary. The data obtained from the patient are more objective and reliable than those obtained through global self-report. Diary-keeping facilitates the establishment of baseline levels of headache parameters and assesses treatment effectiveness. Finally, the functional relationship between antecedents and consequences of headache can be analyzed.

PSYCHOPHYSIOLOGY

The psychophysiologic evaluation is increasingly being used in the assessment and management of headache. This procedure essentially involves multichannel recording of multiple physiologic response systems. More specifically, physiologic activity (e.g., frontalis, trapezius, and splenius capitus electromyography, forehead and finger skin temperature, and cephalic blood-volume pulse) are assessed during baseline and in response to stress (e.g., "think of a typical day at work"). The most important aspect of the physiologic assessment is that the patient come in for an evaluation during both nonheadache and headache states (two 1-hour sessions). A psychophysiologic evaluation may be the only way to differentiate some headache types (e.g., the presence or absence of elevated electromyographic activity during a headache state to differentiate muscle contraction headache from psychogenic headache). The clinician can also observe the behavioral presentation of the patient in these two states. For example, a migraine headache patient in a headache state will often exhibit obvious tearing of eyes, temporal artery distention, and pallor, whereas a muscle contraction headache patient should exhibit stiffness of movement, muscle tightness, and squinting or frowning expression. Using video recordings, a recent study from our laboratory demonstrated that muscle contraction headache patients displayed specific muscle actions indicative of pain state (33). Among other facial actions, pursing of lips, facial grimacing, and slow eye blinks occurred more frequently during headache state.

PSYCHOLOGICAL MANAGEMENT OF HEADACHE PAIN

To date, there is no truly adequate treatment of chronic headache. Thus, "management" of headache is more accurate than "treatment" of headache, but as in the headache literature, in this chapter the two terms will be used interchangeably. Before discussing the different management strategies of headache, it should be noted that the clinician's choice of a particular intervention for a particular headache type needs to be made along several dimensions (35): (1) efficacy: does treatment achieve the desired results? (2) relative efficacy: is one treatment better than another? (3) generality: what proportion of a patient sample is able to derive benefit from treatment? (4) relative efficiency: which treatment works faster? (5) convenience: what treatment is easier to give and which is easier for the patient? and (5) cost. Because many different treatment strategies seem to be equally effective in the treatment of headache, then it becomes important to consider the cost-effectiveness of a particular intervention.

Psychological management of headache pain has included a divergent range of approaches, including insight-oriented therapy, modification of pain perception, self-relaxation, desensitization to or modification of stressful environment, assertiveness training, control of peripheral hand temperature, self-regulation of temporal artery, and reduction of tonic and phasic levels of muscle activity. For our purposes, headache intervention strategies can be classified into three major groups: relaxation training, biofeedback training, and cognitive techniques. Even though there is not enough literature to warrant the categorization of operant pain control techniques as a major treatment approach of headache, these techniques are also reviewed. The following sections discuss each treatment approach, giving a description of a procedure and its appropriateness for each headache type.

RELAXATION TRAINING

There are various forms of relaxation training, and the most commonly used technique is progressive muscular relaxation. This approach was originally developed by Jacobsen (36) and was popularized more recently by Bernstein and Borkovec (37). The rationale of this procedure involves the reduction of tonic states of muscular activity, learning to identify subtle differences in muscular tension, and a reduction of an overly active sympathetic nervous system. The ability to elicit the state of relaxation is ultimately implemented as an active skill to cope with situations that may trigger stress response.

Relaxation training requires the individual to alternately tense and relax a number of muscle groups throughout the whole body. The training sequence can involve as many as 10 1-hour sessions. An individual's training in relaxation progresses in turn from 16 muscle groups to 8 muscle groups to 4 muscle groups to 4 muscle groups through recall (no actual tensing, i.e., relaxation by remembering what it felt like when the muscle group had been previously relaxed), and cue-controlled relaxation (relaxation through recall and by counting backward from 10 to 1). Although the actual procedure becomes shorter as the training sequence progresses, by the end of the treatment regimen the individual should be able to elicit a state of physical and mental relaxation that is equivalent to that achieved by practicing relaxation with 16 muscle groups. Twice-daily practice at home is recommended to the individual and is assisted by having the individual listen to audiotaped versions of the training sessions. One investigation found that 10 sessions of progressive muscular relaxation with home practice tended to reduce headache activity in muscle contraction headache patients by about 35% more than another group receiving progressive muscular relaxation training without home practice (38).

Another variation of relaxation, which is similar to transcendental meditation, was proposed by Benson (39). He advocated a passive relaxation response wherein the individual is required to sit quietly and to repeat "one" as a form of mantra. No actual tensing of muscles even occurs with this approach. The elicitation of the passive relaxation response is believed to result in physiologic changes that are thought to reflect an integrated hypothalamic response. Finally, Schultz and Luthe (40) proposed a passive suggestive type of relaxation using visual and auditory aids (e.g., a beach scene) to induce mental, emotional, and somatic relaxation. This form of relaxation has come to be known as *autogenic training*.

Although relaxation training has been used to treat migraine, combined vascular and muscle contraction, and muscle contraction headaches, the most appropriate target population for this form of treatment appears to be muscle contraction headache. Discussion regarding the efficacy and cost-effectiveness of relaxation training is deferred to the next section on biofeedback because of the considerable treatment literature comparing relaxation training and biofeedback.

BIOFEEDBACK TRAINING

Biofeedback training is an approach that involves the individual in a continuous interchange with a physiologic monitoring device (e.g., polygraph). The goal of biofeedback is the self-regulation of a target physiologic state that often results in an improved psychological state. More specifically, during biofeedback training the individual is provided with information about physiologic activity via an auditory signal or visual display that is proportional to the change in physiologic activity. The individual's task is to modify the target response in the desired direction, usually in a trial-and-error manner. Success in modifying a target response is indicated by the feedback provided (e.g., a decrease in the loudness of a tone). Clinicians will also often use cognitive aids (e.g., various mental images and blanking the mind) to achieve the desired physiologic change. The ultimate goal of biofeedback is to teach the individual to achieve the desired physiologic response without the aid of a feedback apparatus (i.e., voluntary control).

Several biofeedback training techniques have been used with headache patients (41). Biofeedback training techniques can essentially be grouped into three different forms: (1) electromyographic (EMG) biofeedback, (2) thermal biofeedback, and (3) cephalic vasomotor feedback. Electromyographic biofeedback came about through the pioneering work of Budzinski and coworkers (42). Basically, they attached three surface electrodes, equidistant from each other on the midline of the forehead. In their original study, true feedback of frontalis muscle EMG in 15 subjects led to greater decreases in muscle activity than did pseudofeedback. This procedure was then applied to the treatment of muscle contraction headache subjects with substantial success (43). The rationale of EMG biofeedback is similar to that of relaxation training; EMG biofeedback is aimed at directly reducing elevated levels of muscle tension and indirectly reducing sympathetic nervous system activity.

Thermal biofeedback consists of attaching a temperature-sensitive thermistor to a finger and requiring an individual to increase his finger temperature. Although skin temperature is an indirect measure of peripheral blood volume, the rationale for this procedure is that an increased peripheral blood flow (i.e., peripheral hand vasodilation) is associated with decreased sympathetic tone and increased relaxation. In addition, it is assumed that by increasing blood flow to the periphery, blood flow to the extracranial vasculature will be decreased (this treatment approach was originally designed to treat migraine headache). Clinical research work with thermal biofeedback was made popular by the Menninger Foundation Clinic (44, 45). With thermal biofeedback, these authors also included autogenic training (i.e., during thermal biofeedback training the individual repeats phrases such as: "I feel quite relaxed," "I feel quiet," and "My arms and hands are heavy"). Of 62 patients, 74% of migraine headache sufferers were considered "improved" in the original study (44). Interestingly enough, unlike the enhanced treatment outcome of home practice of progressive muscular relaxation for muscle contraction headache subjects (38), home practice of thermal biofeedback does not appear to reduce headache activity in migraine headache subjects (46).

Cephalic vasomotor response feedback requires the placement of a photoelectric transducer on the extracranial artery (usually the zygomaticofacial branch). The aim of cephalic vasomotor response feedback is to teach the patient to reduce the tonic pain associated with excessively high blood volume via the reduction of pulse amplitude. In other words, the patient is taught to constrict his temporal artery so as to avoid vasodilation and the associated pain. Although the first investigation on the utility of cephalic vasomotor feedback was not focused on the treatment of headaches per se, Koppman et al. (47) conducted an investigation examining whether patients who suffered from migraine headache could learn to control the temporal artery pulse with the aid of biofeedback. Of nine patients who participated in 9–12 sessions (twice during each session), seven patients were able to reliably demonstrate "bidirectional" control of temporal artery blood flow, thus indicating that the subjects had learned to control their temporal artery pulse.

As with the development of any new therapy, initial enthusiastic claims from the biofeedback literature subsequently were tempered by more realistic and cautious expectations. Many of the enthusiastic claims were based on anecdotal case reports, uncontrolled group studies, and studies with major methodologic flaws (e.g., accurate definition of headache type omitted, biased representativeness of samples used, poor outcome measures). Despite the plethora of problems in the headache literature, some statements about the biofeedback treatment of headache can be made.

Much of what is known about the efficacy of headache treatment has been provided by the work of Blanchard and his associates (6, 48). They used "meta-analysis" to evaluate treatment effect across research studies (48). In meta-analysis, mean changes in headache measures across research studies form the unit of analysis. An average percentage of improvement in headache density (product of intensity and duration of headache pain) from baseline was calculated. Only treatment studies with five or more subjects per group were included in the meta-analysis. Although the authors pointed to the consistency of results across studies as evidence for the reproducibility of their general findings, the authors also acknowledged that the utility of meta-analysis is somewhat compromised by the different dependent measures, sample sizes, treatment protocols, and methodologic quality of underlying studies. Many of the evaluative statements of the headache treatment outcome literature presented are based on the work of Blanchard and his associates.

The muscle contraction headache literature indicates that relaxation training and frontal EMG biofeedback appear to be equally efficacious (6). The average percentage of improvement in muscle contraction headache patients treated with relaxation training (9 studies) and frontal EMG biofeedback (12 studies) was 59.2% and 60.9%, respectively. Interestingly, the combination of relaxation training and frontal EMG biofeedback resulted in an average percentage of improvement of 58.8% (6 studies); therefore, combining the two treatment approaches for muscle contraction headache did not lead to improved treatment outcome.

At this point it is worth repeating the criteria for choosing the best treatment for a particular headache type. If relaxation training and frontal EMG biofeedback appear to be equally efficacious (i.e., which treatment works best) and equally generalizable (i.e., what proportion of a patient sample achieves significant benefit from the treatment), headache therapy should be determined by the relative efficiency (i.e., which treatment works faster), convenience (i.e., which treatment is easier to administer and which is easier for the patient), and cost. Based on the literature and our own experience, the treatment of choice for muscle contraction headache is relaxation training. The results of a recent investigation suggested that muscle contraction headache patients should initially be treated with relaxation training; those who do not improve should proceed sequentially with frontal EMG biofeedback (49). This appears to be an appropriate recommendation; however, if the patient also fails to derive any benefit from frontal EMG biofeedback, then the clinician should reconsider the case formulation and reevaluation for psychogenic headache, which would require treatment with operant pain control techniques. In another study, Teders et al. (50) evaluated the comparative efficacy and cost-effectiveness of relaxation training for muscle contraction headache using a therapist-delivered relaxation treatment versus a procedure with minimal therapist-patient contact and based chiefly at home. Both procedures were highly effective and were equivalent in reducing headache complaints as assessed by measures of headache index, intensity, frequency, and medication consumption. Obviously, the minimal-contact, home-based treatment was found to be more cost-effective when relating total amount of therapist contact to headache improvement. The home-based relaxation package appears promising for the treatment of muscle contrac-

tion headache, and further research with this approach is needed.

The number of studies investigating the treatment of migraine headaches with relaxation training is relatively small (seven studies—see ref. 6). Depending on which study one considers, relaxation training appears to be either ineffective or beneficial, but overall, across seven studies, the average rate of improvement was 47.9%, which was not significantly different from combined thermal biofeedback and autogenic training (64.9%—see ref. 6). With regard to combined vascular and muscle contraction headache, one study obtained a 22% average improvement rate when using relaxation training alone (49). When relaxation training was combined with thermal biofeedback, however, the overall improvement rate rose to 54%. One other study worth mentioning examined the utility of group relaxation training (51). The authors of this investigation found that 70% of 98 patients improved using this treatment approach. Two major weaknesses in this study were noted: the lack of a control group and the lack of any follow-up data. Although the relatively high success rate of this study is impressive and appears promising, it is interesting that this study has apparently not been followed up with another investigation. It would appear at this time that relaxation training is cost-effective in the treatment of a substantial number of migraine headache patients (probably best for the common migraine headache); surely, for patients who derive no benefit from relaxation training, there are other interventions that can help.

Thermal biofeedback has been used rather extensively to manage migraine and combined vascular and muscle contraction headache. Thermal biofeedback *alone* does not appear to be helpful for either migraine or combined vascular and muscle contraction headache. The rate of improvement with thermal biofeedback (34.6%; seven studies) alone was significantly better than headache-monitoring alone (17.2%; six studies) and slightly but nonsignificantly better than psychological placebo (27.6%; five studies) (6). In another study by Blanchard and his colleagues, home-based treatment (thermal biofeedback and/or relaxation training) for migraine and combined migraine and muscle contraction headache patients was found to be four to six times more cost effective than a clinic-based treatment protocol (52). In addition, these significant reductions in headache activity held-up at a 2-year follow-up for 75% of vascular headache patients (53). In a meta-analysis comparing thermal biofeedback and/or relaxation training (35 studies) with propranolol (25 studies), similar rates of migraine headache improvement for both types of treatment were observed (54). Thus, thermal biofeedback combined with autogenic training and thermal biofeedback combined with relaxation training appear to be the treatments of choice for migraine and for combined vascular and muscle contraction headache.

The use of cephalic vasomotor biofeedback in the treatment of migraine and combined vascular and muscle contraction headache has been found to be effective. Friar and Beatty evaluated the therapeutic effects of eight sessions of cephalic vasomotor biofeedback training as compared to an attention control group (55). Post-training results indicated that the cephalic vasomotor biofeedback group demonstrated constriction of the extracranial arteries during a voluntary control assessment, whereas the attention-control group did not evidence vasoconstriction of the temporal artery. A significant reduction in the number of major headache attacks (headaches over 3 hours in duration) and total number of headaches per month in the treatment group was noted. Cephalic vasomotor biofeedback was also found to be superior to frontalis EMG feedback in reducing headache activity and medication intake in migraine headache patients (56). A number of experimental single-case studies evaluating cephalic vasomotor biofeedback have also been reported and indicate the clinical utility of this approach (57–59). Overall, the average rate of improvement in patients receiving cephalic vasomotor biofeedback was 42.3% (based on four studies), which was equal to relaxation training alone, thermal biofeedback alone, and psychological placebo, but significantly lower than thermal biofeedback combined with autogenic training (6). Which treatment of choice appears to be the best for migraine is uncertain. It would appear from a cost-effectiveness point of view that relaxation training should be the initial choice of treatment for migraine headache; any patient not improving should proceed to thermal biofeedback combined with autogenic training or cephalic vasomotor biofeedback. Although cephalic vasomotor biofeedback appears useful, one needs to consider that this kind of biofeedback training requires specialized equipment and a methodologic procedure that is still at the research state. In addition, for some migraine patients, voluntary control of the temporal artery may require an inordinate amount of training sessions (29).

COGNITIVE TECHNIQUES

The use of cognitive techniques in the treatment of headache is a fairly recent development. Much of the cognitive approach to treating headache borrows from the original work of Beck (60), Goldfried et al. (61), and Meichenbaum (62). Cognitive techniques have a much-expanded focus and are aimed at providing the patient with a general set of problem-solving or coping skills that will be used with a wide range of situations or stressors that can give rise to headaches. The rationale for this type of treatment emphasizes that disturbed emotional and behavioral responses are a direct function of specific maladaptive cognitions (e.g., the belief that one

should be a perfect manager or parent). A patient is encouraged to attribute the cause of his or her headaches to relatively specific cognitive aberrations rather than to external stimuli or complex inner dispositions. The therapist and patient focus on identifying cues that target tension and anxiety, how the patient responds when anxious, the patient's thoughts prior to becoming aware of tension, and how cognitions contribute to the patient's stress, tension, and emotional distress.

In reviewing the literature, it is difficult to evaluate studies using cognitive techniques because of the diversity in their approaches. Combinations of relaxation techniques, self-desensitization, thought stopping, rational thinking, experiential focusing and flooding, cognitive reappraisal, and others have been used. With this comment in mind, the first controlled evaluation of cognitive therapy for headaches was conducted by Holroyd et al. (63). Thirty-one muscle contraction headache subjects were randomly assigned to a waiting-list control group, frontal EMG biofeedback, or cognitive stress coping training. Holroyd et al.'s treatment consisted of teaching subjects to identify and subsequently modify maladaptive cognitive responses assumed to mediate headache. When subjects were able to reliably identify their antecedent and consequent cognitions, subjects were then taught to use cognitive reappraisal, attention deployment, and fantasy as a way of modifying their cognitions. Results indicated that subjects receiving cognitive therapy evidenced significantly greater reductions in headache activity (89% improvement rate), which were also maintained at a 2-year follow-up (64). Holroyd and his colleagues took their research a step further by examining a cognitive-behavioral, home-based treatment protocol versus amitriptyline in the management of muscle contraction headache. Both groups yielded significant improvements in recurrent muscle contraction headache; however, larger improvements in headache reduction, somatic complaints, and personal control were obtained with the psychological management package (65).

Knapp and Florin (66) assigned 20 long-term migraine patients to one of four training conditions: (1) 10 sessions of cephalic vasomotor biofeedback, (2) four sessions of cephalic vasomotor biofeedback and five sessions of cognitive stress coping training, (3) 10 sessions of cognitive stress coping training, and (4) five sessions of cognitive stress coping training and five sessions of cephalic vasomotor biofeedback. The study also included a waiting-list control group. The results indicated that all four treatment groups did equally well. In another study (67), migraine, muscle contraction, and combined vascular and muscle contraction headache groups received a cognitive-behavioral package (which was mostly based on Meichenbaum's work; see ref. 62). The results indicated that treatment gains were similar across all diagnostic groups. Finally, a more-recent investigation compared home-based relaxation training alone, home-based cognitive stress coping training plus relaxation, and office-based cognitive stress coping training and relaxation (68). All three groups were equally effective, and no significant differences in cost-effectiveness were noted. On the other hand, the addition of cognitive strategies to a home-based relaxation protocol for muscle contraction headache (69) and a home-based biofeedback protocol for migraine headache (70) did not add significantly to treatment outcome.

Although the results from several studies are mixed, the use of cognitive techniques appears promising in the treatment of all headache types except for psychogenic headache. Cognitive techniques seem to be equally efficacious in the treatment of headache when compared to other treatment modalities.

OPERANT PAIN-CONTROL TECHNIQUES

Although operant pain-control techniques have frequently been used to treat chronic pain disorders (e.g., low back pain), they have received little attention in the headache literature. Operant pain control techniques are based on suggestions by Fordyce (32). Essentially, pain is an experience that is influenced by physical and psychological factors. As remarked by Fordyce, the issue is not whether the pain is real or organic but what factors are influencing pain. Although pain is a physiologic process, it can be controlled and maintained by reinforcement. Therefore, if learning factors can influence the frequency, severity, and duration of pain, then it may be possible to extinguish learned components of pain, in this case, headache.

Following a functional analysis of headache and other pain behaviors, a clinician devises a pain control program and a behavioral contract (structured and formalized treatment goals and how to go about achieving them) is designed. The contract contains the following operant methods: *(1) extinction procedures*: the patient and significant other(s) will respond to pain behaviors with a neutral attitude; *(2) reinforcement of nonpain behaviors*: nonpain behaviors are to be reinforced with positive activities such as special meals, recreation, attention from significant other(s), and so on; *(3) reinforcement of competing responses during pain behavior*: patient will be encouraged to continue with ongoing activities even in the presence of pain; and *(4) therapist reinforcement*: therapist interaction is contingent on the decrease of pain behavior.

As of yet there are no control group outcome studies using operant pain-control techniques with headache. However, for illustration purposes, a case that was handled in our laboratory is presented (71). A 26-year-old female with a 13-year history of classic migraine headache was referred following hospitalization with severe head pain. Behavior assessment and analysis revealed that she received inordinant amounts of parental, social, and professional attention, as well as avoidance of school and work. The various treatments received by her included medication, acupuncture, chiropractic manipulation, psychotherapy, and even electroconvulsive shock. Following several trials of cephalic vasomotor feedback training, she was able to experience a decrease in headache, but treatment gains were lost following termination of each treatment program.

Self-monitoring data indicated that her headaches occurred five to seven times per week, lasted 8–12 hours per day, and were severely disabling. She avoided housework, meal preparation, working at her job as an L.P.N., socializing, and sexual activity. Domestic duties were completed by her parents and husband. Medications included, among others, as-needed injections of Demerol. Monitoring of the patient's pain behavior included verbal complaints, going to bed, cold compresses on her head, medication abuse, excuses from social obligations, and emergency room visits.

Her treatment consisted of having all the significant others completely ignore her pain behaviors, providing appropriate reinforcers by significant others for well behaviors, behavioral contracting that explicitly stated the above contingencies and expectations (with the cooperation of her physician and the patient's understanding that under no circumstances could she receive an injection of Demerol), muscle relaxation training as a procedure to handle daily stress or pain, and assertiveness training.

One month following treatment, the mean number of her daily pain behaviors went from 8 to below 1. Treatment results in the patient returning to work as an L.P.N. on a volunteer basis, maintaining an "A" average in a practical nursing program, walking 2 miles per day, and having been off all pain medication for slightly over a year. At 12-month follow-up, the client reported two headaches over the previous several months, and her husband had reported that their marital and sexual relationship had greatly improved. The results of this case study indicate the role of learning in migraine headache. This treatment approach has been also successfully used in the treatment of psychogenic headache in our laboratory. (For an excellent, detailed discussion on how to treat a psychogenic headache case, see ref. 72.) Obviously, it is too early to determine the efficacy of this treatment approach, but it does appear promising.

SUMMARY

To summarize the headache treatment literature, there is no treatment that is clearly more efficacious than another for any particular headache type. Relaxation training appears to be the most cost-effective treatment for headache. Home-based treatment also appears very promising. If relaxation training does not work, there are certainly a number of viable management options. Frontal EMG biofeedback can be used in the treatment of muscle contraction headache, and migraine and combined vascular and muscle contraction headache can be further treated with combined thermal biofeedback and autogenic training and cephalic vasomotor biofeedback. Cognitive techniques also appear useful in the treatment of muscle contraction headache. In addition, the use of operant pain-control techniques appears to be beneficial in the treatment of some migraine headache patients and surely is appropriate for psychogenic headache.

ISSUES IN THE PSYCHOLOGICAL MANAGEMENT OF HEADACHE PAIN

Despite the number of studies on the management of headache and the fact that a substantial number of headache patients improve following psychological treatment, several issues need to be addressed in the treatment literature. There is still little systematic research on predicting who responds to these treatments and who is more likely to relapse. Diamond and his coworkers conducted a 5-year retrospective study to examine the long-term effects of biofeedback (combined thermal and autogenic-training and frontal EMG biofeedback) on headache, and their results indicated that biofeedback training was significantly more effective in patients who were under age 18, female, and had no drug habituation problems (73). These characteristics are not a representative example of most headache patients seen in clinical practice.

Although biofeedback has received the most attention in the treatment literature, the clinical efficacy of biofeedback depends on the ability of the patient to demonstrate voluntary control (the ability to demonstrate bidirectional control of a physiologic response system without a feedback signal or on instruction). Clinicians usually include a voluntary control phase (e.g., patient is told to constrict his temporal artery) in their treatment, but very few studies ever evaluate or demonstrate true voluntary control. If no voluntary control can be demonstrated, then probably biofeedback at best has a nonspecific or placebo effect that has little to do with the hypothesized pain mechanisms of headache. Obviously, more research work investigating this issue of voluntary control is needed.

The treatment of headache will also become more successful as more is known about the mechanisms of headache pain and associated etiologic factors, which brings us back to the observation that the successful outcome of headache treatment is highly dependent on the thorough assessment and accurate diagnosis of headache. More attention needs to be paid to providing clear descriptions and definitions of headache. The criteria to be used must also undergo tests of validity and reliability. It is hoped that the new IHS classification scheme (10) will be instrumental in resolving many of the diagnostic quandaries currently faced by clinicians. The nature and

the parameters of the intervention strategies used with headache patients also need to be more clearly specified. The statement "more research of a controlled outcome nature is needed" is a cliche but very applicable to the headache treatment literature. Only with controlled outcome research will we be able to more clearly and effectively determine which are the treatments of choice for particular headache types.

REFERENCES

1. Bonica JJ: Pain research and therapy: Past and current status and future needs. In Ng L, Bonica JJ (eds): *Pain, Discomfort, and Humanitarian Care.* New York, Elsevier, 1980, p 1.
2. DeLozier JE, Gagnon RO: *National Ambulatory Medical Care Survey: 1973 Summary, United States,* May 1973–April 1974 (DHEW Publication No. HRA79–1772). Washington, D.C., U.S. Government Printing Office, 1975.
3. Taylor H, Curran NM: *The Nuprin Pain Report.* New York, Louis Harris, 1985, p 233.
4. Adams HE, Feuerstein M, Fowler JL: Migraine headache: Review of parameters, etiology, and intervention. *Psychol Bull* 87:217–237, 1980.
5. Blanchard EB: Long-term effects of behavioral treatment of chronic headache. *Behav Ther* 18:375–385, 1987.
6. Blanchard EB, Andrasik F: Psychological assessment and treatment of headache: Recent developments and emerging issues. *J Consult Clin Psychol* 50:859–879, 1982.
7. Ad Hoc Committee on the Classification of Headache of the National Institute of Neurological Diseases and Blindness. *Neurology* 12:127–128, 1962.
8. Turkat I, Brantley PJ, Orton K, Adams HE: Reliability of headache diagnosis. *J Behav Assess* 3:1–4, 1981.
9. Weeks RE, Rapoport AM: A critical look at reliability of headache diagnosis. *Ann Neurol* 22:148–149, 1987.
10. Headache Classification Committee of the International Headache Society: Classification and diagnostic criteria for headache disorders, cranial neuralgias, and facial pain. *Cephalagia* 8(Suppl 7):1–96, 1988.
11. Rapoport AM: The diagnosis of migraine and tension-type headache, then and now. *Neurology* 42(Suppl 2):11–15, 1992.
12. Rasmussen BK, Jensen R, Olesen J: A population-based analysis of the diagnostic criteria of the International Headache Society. *Cephalagia* 11:129–134, 1991.
13. Iversen HK, Langemark M, Andersson PG, Hansen PE, Olesen J: Clinical characteristics of migraine and episodic tension-type headache in relation to old and new diagnostic criteria. *Headache* 30:514–519, 1990.
14. Sheftell FD: Chronic daily headache. *Neurology* 42(Suppl 2):32–36, 1992.
15. Friedman AP: *Chronic Recurring Headache: A Multimedia Learning System.* Basel, Sandoz Pharmaceuticals, 1973.
16. Appel S, Kuritzky A, Zahavi I, Zigelman M, Akselrod S: Evidence for instability of the autonomic system in patients with migraine headache. *Headache* 32:10–17, 1992.
17. Silberstein SD: Advances in understanding the pathophysiology of headache. *Neurology* 42(Suppl 2):6–10, 1992.
18. Brandt J, Celentano D, Stewart W, Linet M, Folstein MF:

Personality and emotional disorder in a community sample of migraine headache sufferers. *Am J Psychiatry* 147:303–308, 1990.

19. Merikangas KR, Angst J, Isler H: Migraine and psychopathology. *Arch Gen Psychiatry* 147:849–853, 1990.
20. Kohler T, Haimerl C: Daily stress as a trigger of migraine attacks: Results of thirteen single-subject studies. *J Consult Clin Psychol* 58:870–872, 1990.
21. Silberstein SD: The role of sex hormones in headache. *Neurology* 42(Suppl 2):37–42, 1992.
22. Philips C: The modification of tension headache pain using EMG biofeedback. *Behav Res Ther* 15:119–129, 1977.
23. Haynes SN, Cuevas J, Gannon LR: The psychophysiological etiology of muscle contraction headache. *Headache* 22:122–132, 1982.
24. Holm JE, Holroyd KA, Hursey KG, Penzien DP: The role of stress in recurrent tension headache. *Headache* 26:160–167, 1986.
25. Martin MJ: Muscle-contraction (tension) headache. *Psychosomatics* 24:319–324, 1983.
26. Drummond PD: Predisposing, precipitating and relieving factors in different categories of headache. *Headache* 25:16–22, 1985.
27. Featherstone HJ: Migraine and muscle contraction headaches: A continuum. *Headache* 25:194–198, 1985.
28. Thompson JK, Haber JD, Figueroa JL, Adams HE: A replication and generalization of the psychobiological model of headache. *Headache* 20:199–203, 1980.
29. Adams HE, Brantley PJ, Thompson K: Biofeedback and headache: Methodological issues. In White L, Tursky B (eds): *Clinical Biofeedback: Efficacy and Mechanisms.* New York, Guilford Press, 1982, p 358.
30. Packard RC: Conversion headache. *Headache* 20:266–268, 1980.
31. Weatherhead AD: Psychogenic headache. *Headache* 20:47–54, 1980.
32. Fordyce W: *Behavioral Methods for Chronic Pain and Illness.* St. Louis, CV Mosby, 1976.
33. Iezzi A, Adams HE, Bugg F, Stokes GS: Facial expression of pain in muscle contraction headache patients. *J Psychopathol Behav Assess* 13:269–283, 1991.
34. Sturgis ET, Adams HE, Brantley PJ: The parameters, etiology and treatment of migraine headache. In Haynes SN, Gannon L (eds): *Psychosomatic Disorders: A Psychophysiological Approach to Etiology and Treatment.* New York, Praeger, 1981, p 485.
35. Blanchard EB, Ahles TA, Shaw ER: Behavioral treatment of headache. *Prog Behav Modif* 8:207–247, 1979.
36. Jacobsen, E: *Progressive Relaxation.* Chicago, University of Chicago Press, 1938.
37. Bernstein DA, Borkovec, TD: *Progressive Relaxation Training.* Champaign, IL, Research Press, 1973.
38. Blanchard EB, Nicholson NL, Taylor AE, Steffek BD, Radnitz CL, Appelbaum A: The role of regular home practice in the relaxation treatment of tension headache. *J Consult Clin Psychol* 59:467–470, 1991.
39. Benson H: *The Relaxation Response.* New York, William Morrow, 1975.
40. Schultz J, Luthe W: *Autogenic Therapy.* New York, Grune & Stratton, 1969.
41. Iezzi A, Adams HE, Sheck C: Biofeedback and psycholog-

ical management of migraine headache. In Tollison CD, Kunkel RS (eds): *Headache: Diagnosis and Interdisciplinary Treatment.* Baltimore, Urban & Schwarzenberg, in press.
42. Budzynski TH, Stoyva JM, Adler CS: Feedback-induced muscle relaxation: An application to tension headache. *J Behav Ther Exp Psychiatry* 1:205–211, 1970.
43. Budzynski TH, Stoyva JM, Adler CS, Mullaney DJ: EMG biofeedback and tension headache: A controlled outcome study. *Psychosom Med* 35:484–496, 1973.
44. Sargent JD, Green EE, Walters ED: The use of autogenic feedback training in a pilot study of migraine and tension headaches. *Headache* 12:120–124, 1972.
45. Sargent JD, Green EE, Walters ED: Preliminary report on the use of autogenic feedback training in the treatment of migraine and tension headaches. *Psychosom Med* 35:129–135, 1973.
46. Blanchard EB, Nicholson NL, Radnitz CL, Steffek BD, Appelbaum KA, Dentinger MP: The role of home practice in thermal biofeedback. *J Consult Clin Psychol* 59:507–512, 1991.
47. Koppman JW, McDonald RD, Kunzel MG: Voluntary regulation of temporal artery diameter by migraine patients. *Headache* 14:133–138, 1974.
48. Blanchard EB, Andrasik F, Ahles TA, O'Keeke D: Migraine and tension headaches: A meta-analytic review. *Behav Ther* 11:613–631, 1980.
49. Blanchard EB, Andrasik F, Neff DF, Teders SJ, Pallmeyer TP, Arena JG, et al: Sequential comparisons of relaxation training and biofeedback in the treatment of three kinds of chronic headache, or the machines may be necessary some of the time. *Behav Res Ther* 20:469–481, 1982.
50. Teders SJ, Blanchard EB, Andrasik F, Jurish SE, Neff DF, Arena JG: Relaxation and training for tension headache: Comparative efficacy and cost-effectiveness of a minimal therapist contact versus a therapist-delivered procedure. *Behav Ther* 11:613–631, 1984.
51. Hay KM, Madders J: Migraine treated by relaxation therapy. *J R Coll Gen Pract* 21:449–464, 1971.
52. Blanchard EB, Andrasik F, Appelbaum KA, Evans DD, Jurish SE, Teders SJ, et al: The efficacy and cost-effectiveness of minimal-therapist-contact, non-drug treatments of chronic migraine and tension headache. *Headache* 25:214–220, 1985.
53. Blanchard EB, Appelbaum KA, Guarnieri P, Neff DF, Andrasik F, Jaccard J, et al: Two studies of the long-term follow-up minimal therapist contact treatments of vascular and tension headache. *J Consult Clin Psychol* 56:427–432, 1988.
54. Holroyd KA, Penzien DB: Pharmacological versus non-pharmacological prophylaxis of recurrent migraine headache: A meta-analytic review of clinical trials. *Pain* 42:1–13, 1990.
55. Friar LR, Beatty J: Management of migraines by trained control of vasoconstriction. *J Consult Clin Psychol* 44:46–53, 1976.
56. Bild R, Adams HE: Modification of migraine headaches by cephalic blood volume pulse and EMG biofeedback. *J Consult Clin Psychol* 48:51–57, 1980.
57. Adams HE: Cephalic vasomotor feedback in the modification of migraine headaches. *Biofeedback Self Regul* 2:241–254, 1977.

58. Feuerstein M, Adams HE, Beiman I: Cephalic vasomotor and electromyographic feedback in the treatment of combined muscle contraction and migraine headaches in a geriatric case. *Headache* 16:232–237, 1976.
59. Sturgis ET, Tollison CD, Adams HE: Modification of combined migraine muscle-contraction headaches using BVP and EMG feedback. *J Appl Behav Anal* 11:215–233, 1978.
60. Beck AT: *Cognitive Therapy and the Emotional Disorders.* New York, International University Press, 1976.
61. Goldfried MR, Decentecco ET, Weinberg L: Systematic rational restructuring as a self-control technique. *Behav Ther* 5:247–254, 1974.
62. Meichenbaum D: *Cognitive Behavior Modification: An Integrative Approach.* New York, Plenum Press, 1977.
63. Holroyd KA, Andrasik F, Westbrook T: Cognitive control of tension headache. *Cogn Ther Res* 1:121–133, 1977.
64. Holroyd KA, Andrasik F: Do the effects of cognitive therapy endure? A two-year follow-up of tension headache sufferers treated with cognitive therapy or biofeedback. *Cogn Ther Res* 6:325–334, 1982.
65. Holroyd, KA, Nash JM, Pingel JD, Cordingly GE, Jerome A: A comparison of pharmcological (amitriptyline hcl) and nonpharmacological (cognitive-behavioral) therapies for chronic tension headaches. *J Consult Clin Psychol* 59:387–393, 1991.
66. Knapp TW, Florin I: The treatment of migraine headache by training in vasoconstriction of the temporal artery and a cognitive stress-coping training. *Behav Anal Modif* 4:267–274, 1981.
67. Bakal DA, Demjen S, Kaganov JA: Cognitive behavioral treatment of chronic headache. *Headache* 21:81–86, 1981.
68. Attanasio V, Andrasik F, Blanchard EB: Cognitive therapy and relaxation training in muscle-contraction headache: Efficacy and cost-effectiveness. *Headache* 27:254–260, 1987.
69. Appelbaum KA, Blanchard EB, Nicholson NL, Radnitz C, Kirsch C, Michultka D, et al: Controlled evaluation of the addition of cognitive strategies to a home-based relaxation protocol for tension headache. *Behav Ther* 21:293–303, 1990.
70. Blanchard EB, Appelbaum KA, Nicholson NL, Radnitz CL, Morrill B, Michultka D, et al: A controlled evaluation of the addition of cognitive therapy to a home-based biofeedback and relaxation treatment of vascular headache. *Headache* 30:371–376, 1990.
71. AuBuchon P, Haber JD, Adams HE: Can migraine headache be modified by operant pain techniques? *J Behav Ther Exp Psychiatry* 16:261–263, 1985.
72. Adams HE: Case formulations of chronic headaches. In Turkat ID (ed): *Behavioral Case Formulation.* New York, Plenum Press, 1985, p 89.
73. Diamond S, Medina J, Diamond-Falk J, DeVeno T: The value of biofeedback in the treatment of chronic headache: A five-year retrospective study. *Headache* 19:90–96, 1979.

CHAPTER 22

DIFFERENTIAL DIAGNOSIS AND MANAGEMENT OF OROFACIAL PAIN

KIM J. BURCHIEL
JEFFREY A. BURGESS

In this chapter we present a survey of the differential diagnosis of orofacial pain syndromes. No attempt has been made to produce an encyclopedic litany of exceptionally rare syndromes. Rather we discuss here the acute and chronic pain states that are seen with any frequency in a busy practice specializing in the treatment of orofacial pain problems. Where possible we have adhered to the Classification of Chronic Pain prepared by the International Association for the Study of Pain Subcommittee on Taxonomy (1). Emphasis is placed on diagnosis, although where appropriate, brief mention of relevant medical and surgical therapy is made. Specific discussions of therapy of orofacial pain can be found in Chapters 23 and 24. Primary headache syndromes and related disorders that produce craniofacial pain will not be addressed in this chapter; for this the reader is directed to Chapters 19–21.

NEURALGIAS OF THE HEAD AND FACE

TRIGEMINAL NEURALGIA (TIC DOULOUREUX)

Trigeminal neuralgia, or tic douloureux, can be divided into three subcategories: so-called "idiopathic" trigeminal neuralgia, atypical trigeminal neuralgia, and symptomatic trigeminal neuralgia (in patients with multiple sclerosis). This discussion will focus primarily on idiopathic, or essential, trigeminal neuralgia, because the other two varieties are simply minor exceptions to the general criteria for diagnosis.

Idiopathic Trigeminal Neuralgia

The term *idiopathic* implies that no known etiology can be ascribed to this variety of trigeminal neuralgia. Although not yet universally accepted, considerable evidence from the surgical treatment of trigeminal neuralgia indicates that the pathophysiology of this condition involves abnormal vascular cross-compression of the root entry zone of the trigeminal nerve (2). In the majority of patients, who by most criteria would be considered to have a diagnosis of idiopathic trigeminal neuralgia, distortion of the nerve by a blood vessel can be demonstrated at the time of surgical exposure. Typically an ectatic loop of the superior cerebellar artery or anterior inferior cerebellar artery impinges upon the nerve, and long-term pain-relief can be obtained by surgical repositioning of the vessel or by padding of the neurovascular point of contact with a small prosthetic implant. Although hypotheses have been advanced to relate this vascular compression to the pathophysiologic mechanism of the genesis of the pain of trigeminal neuralgia (3), these remain speculative. If we accept the principle that most trigeminal neuralgia results from vascular compression, then the majority of these patients would more appropriately be classified as having "secondary" trigeminal neuralgia (see below). Nevertheless, this group of patients forms the largest subset of those individuals with trigeminal neuralgia, and shares historical characteristics, physical signs, and neuroradiologic features that to some degree distinguish them from patients with trigeminal neuralgia secondary to clearly defined central nervous system (CNS) lesions. Thus, it seems prudent at this time, if only for semantic purposes, to discuss these patients under the rubric of "idiopathic."

The diagnosis of idiopathic trigeminal neuralgia can virtually always be made by a careful historical and physical examination of the patient. Trigeminal neuralgia is described as sudden, severe, agonizing, episodic but recurrent lancinating pains that are often "electric shock-like," in the distribution of one or more divisions of the fifth cranial nerve. Pain is felt superficially in the skin or buccal mucosa, and can often be triggered by light mechanical contact from a more or less restricted site, often in the perioral region. Duration of pain is usually brief, lasting only seconds, with repetition in bursts of several seconds to a minute or two, followed by a refractory period of 30 sec or so up to a few minutes. Episodes may occur at intervals of several or many times daily, or in rare instances, succeed one another almost continuously. Periodicity of the pain is characteristic, with episodes occurring as described for a few weeks to a month or two, followed by pain-free intervals of months or years with recurrence of another bout of pain in exactly the same region. Occasionally a mild flush may be noted during the paroxysms of pain. Patients also sometimes report that some relief is obtained by firm pressure with the hands around but not touching the trigger point. The pain is strictly limited to the distribution of the fifth nerve, usually involves one or two divisions, and is slightly more common on the right side. Pains are virtually always confined to one side of the face although occasionally treated patients or those in remission may experience contralateral typical neuralgic pain. Very rarely, bilateral trigeminal neuralgia can also be seen.

The prevalence of trigeminal neuralgia is relatively rare; the incidence per annum is for men 2.7/100,000, and for women 5.0/100,000. Age of onset is usually after the fourth decade, with peak onset during the fifth and sixth decades. Onset of pain before age 40 is uncommon and should at least suggest the possibility of multiple sclerosis.

In idiopathic trigeminal neuralgia, the neurologic examination is virtually always normal, although rarely some degree of trigeminal sensorimotor abnormality can be detected. Likewise, neuroradiologic studies such as computed tomography (CT) or magnetic resonance imaging (MRI) of the head are normal. Cerebral angiography is not necessary, even preoperatively, unless the neuroradiologic studies suggest a vascular abnormality, such as an aneurysm, arteriovenous malformation, or tumor.

Atypical Trigeminal Neuralgia

This clinical entity differs from typical trigeminal neuralgia in that in addition to the episodic lancinating pain, there exists a component of a more persistent aching or burning pain (4). In this setting, careful consideration should be given to the presence of structural pathology in the nerve, or to an extrinsic compressive lesion such as a tumor or vascular malformation (5, 6). This is particularly true if sensory loss is detected on the face. Patients with atypical features such as these should undergo CT or MRI scanning to rule out such pathology. If a cause for the pain can be determined, the patient would then be classified as having "secondary" neural-

gia (see below), although a distinct pathologic lesion will not be demonstrable in all cases. Cases that have atypical features but lack structural pathology would then fall into this group (i.e., atypical, or idiopathic, trigeminal neuralgia). The significance of this subgroup is that in comparison to more typical trigeminal neuralgia, affected patients present somewhat different historical features and are generally more refractory to therapy (5).

Symptomatic Trigeminal Neuralgia

Patients with multiple sclerosis (MS) can also develop trigeminal neuralgia. The description of the pain is similar to that with idiopathic trigeminal neuralgia, although atypical features of a constant pain component and sensory loss are more common. The pathology in these cases appears to be demyelination either in the nerve or in the brainstem within the descending tract of the trigeminal system (7). In patients less than 40 years of age with trigeminal neuralgia, not previously known to have MS, this diagnosis should at least be entertained, particularly if there is evidence of trigeminal sensorimotor dysfunction.

Nonsurgical Management

Approximately 70% of patients with trigeminal neuralgia will respond to pharmacologic therapy alone (8). Carbamazepine is the agent of choice and should be started at 100 mg (one half tablet) orally twice a day, increasing the dose by 100–200 mg every 3–4 days until pain relief is achieved, or toxicity develops, to a final maximum dose in the range of 1000–1200 mg/day. Because of its short serum half-life, carbamazepine administration should be spread out during the day in at least three or four doses. Rarely, carbamazepine may depress the peripheral leukocyte count, so a white blood cell count (WBC) should be obtained prior to initiation of therapy, and then every few weeks for the first few months of treatment. Perhaps a less serious but more insidious and pervasive toxicity of carbamazepine is the mental dulling and mild to moderate gait ataxia that are frequent accompaniments of drug treatment. In some patients, no degree of cognitive impairment or ataxia is acceptable, and this argues for discontinuance of carbamazepine and consideration of other therapeutic options.

It is important to point out that a response to carbamazepine is virtually pathognomonic for trigeminal neuralgia, and thus it represents, in effect, a "diagnostic" test with high reliability. Not infrequently, patients respond initially to carbamazepine therapy, only to become refractory even at toxic doses within the ensuing months or years. In these cases other medications can be substituted, but in our experience, at this point it is not likely the pain will come under control by pharmacologic means alone.

Other drugs that should be considered are diphenyl-hydantoin and baclofen. Diphenylhydantoin can be given once a day, and dosage ranges from 300–600 mg/day. Baclofen dose must be slowly increased from 5 mg (one half tablet) three times a day for 3 days, to 10 mg TID for 3 days, to 15 mg TID for 3 days, to 20 mg TID for 3 days, the usual dose being 40–80 mg/day. Both diphenylhydantoin and baclofen can cause mental slowing, ataxia, and in the case of baclofen, frank weakness. Both drugs can be given in combination or with carbamazepine, although this is not usually necessary. All three drugs must be slowly tapered when discontinued to avoid complications of CNS hyperexcitability (i.e., seizures).

Surgical Management

About 30% of patients with trigeminal neuralgia will not respond to pharmacologic therapy, will later become refractory to treatment, or will develop hypersensitivity reaction or other unacceptable toxic side effects of the drugs. These patients should then be considered for surgical treatment. Of the myriad surgical procedures available to patients with trigeminal neuralgia, perhaps three are currently the mainstays of surgical therapy: trigeminal gangliolysis, peripheral trigeminal neurectomy, and microvascular decompression of the trigeminal nerve.

Trigeminal Gangliolysis. Trigeminal gangliolysis can be performed by radiofrequency (RF) heating of a needle placed percutaneously through the foramen ovale into the ganglion, or either injection of glycerol into the cistern of Meckel's cave through a needle or 1- to 2-min inflation of a small Fogerty catheter balloon within Meckel's cave, both inserted by a transforaminal route. Both are minor procedures, performed with local or brief general anesthesia, have a very low incidence of morbidity or mortality, and in about 80–90% of patients, provide years of pain relief (9–15). All three procedures appear to depend, in part, on the production of some degree of trigeminal injury. These procedures appear to work as well for symptomatic trigeminal neuralgia as they do for the idiopathic type.

Neurectomy. Peripheral neurectomy of a branch of the trigeminal nerve, denervating the trigger area or the region in which pain is perceived, produces years of pain relief. Typically the supraorbital, infraorbital, or inferior alveolar (dental) nerves are avulsed for V1, V2, or V3 pain, respectively. This procedure is particularly useful in patients that may be too debilitated to undergo prolonged general anesthesia and microvascular decompression, and who are not sufficiently cooperative to tolerate a gangliolysis procedure (16).

Microvascular Decompression. Microvascular decompression (MVD) of the trigeminal nerve attacks what is considered by some to be the underlying cause of tri-geminal neuralgia alluded to above—that is, cross-compression of the nerve by an ectatic posterior fossa blood vessel. This is a major operation performed under general anesthesia, with a small risk of mortality. In approximately 70–80% of individuals this procedure produces long-lasting or even permanent pain-relief without sensory loss (2, 9).

There are many other surgical options for patients with trigeminal neuralgia, of which these simply reflect the most commonly performed at present. The reader is directed to more thorough discussions of the surgical approach to this disorder, which are beyond the scope of this chapter (17, 18).

Secondary Trigeminal Neuralgia

This entity, as noted above, constitutes a clinical syndrome of trigeminal neuralgia that is thought to be due to a definable structural pathologic lesion, such as tumor, aneurysm, or other vascular abnormality. These lesions are thought to produce a trigeminal neuropathy or neuritis by destruction, irritation, or demyelination of the nerve, and this in turn is responsible for the production of pain. It is much less common than idiopathic trigeminal neuralgia, representing only about 2% of cases of trigeminal neuralgia. The age of onset corresponds to the appearance of the tumor or vascular abnormality, and may be somewhat younger than with the idiopathic cases. Cases are equally distributed between males and females. The description of the pain is identical to that seen in primary trigeminal neuralgia, with the exception that nonparoxysmal pain of a dull or more constant type may occur. The timing and progression of the pains mimic primary trigeminal neuralgia, and the severity is equal.

Structural lesions that may produce this syndrome include tumors in Meckel's cave or in the cerebellopontine angle, which account for about 50% of cases. A partial list of associated conditions is given in Table 22.1. The likelihood of detecting one of these abnormalities is increased by documentation of hypesthesia in the trigeminal distribution, or depression of the corneal reflex (6). In these instances, a CT or MRI scan is mandatory.

Treatment in these cases is primarily directed at the offending structure or disorder, and pain-relief frequently requires surgical intervention. However, drug therapy, as described above for more typical pain, can be effective if a decision has been made to treat the neuralgia symptomatically and manage the patient conservatively.

Trigeminal Neuropathic Pain

Some 5–10% of patients will develop some degree of facial pain following facial fracture, or after reconstructive orthognathic surgery, and a further 1–5% of patients will do so after removal of impacted teeth. The quality

Table 22.1.
Partial List of Conditions Associated with Secondary Trigeminal Neuralgia

Tumors
  Meningioma
  Epidermoid tumor
  Acoustic neurinoma
  Nasopharyngeal carcinoma
  Metastatic tumors
  Brainstem glioma
Vascular lesions
  basilar artery or cavernous sinus aneurysm
  arteriovenous malformation
  tortuous basilar artery
Sarcoidosis
Connective tissue disease
  Scleroderma
Syringobulbia
Pseudotumor cerebri
Paget's disease or acromegaly
Amyloidosis
Toxins
Syphillis
Dejerine Sottas disease
Arnold Chiari malformation

of the pain is sharp, with episodic triggered paroxysms and dull throbbing or burning background pain. Signs of this condition include tender palpable nodules over peripheral nerves, or neurotropic effects. The course of the disorder is characterized by progression over a period of 6 months or so, then stabilization of the pain until treatment. The pathology is often vague, but may include neuromata, or trigeminal deafferentation (19, 20). This type of pain may also be termed *trigeminal neuropathic pain* to indicate that it is a pain probably related to peripheral nerve injury. Peripheral neuropathic pains are well known in noncranial neuropathies (e.g., diabetic or post-traumatic neuropathic pain), and these post-traumatic trigeminal neuralgias often are quite similar in description and resistance to treatment. A hypothesis has been put forward that proposes that the major difference between more typical trigeminal neuralgias and the trigeminal neuropathic pains is the *location* and *severity* of the nerve injury. That is, minimal injury of the trigeminal nerve at the root entry zone results in trigeminal neuralgia, whereas more distal injuries result in neuropathic pains (21). Atypical trigeminal neuralgia, an overlap syndrome, possibly results from more severe compression or injury of the trigeminal nerve that extends distal to the root entry zone.

"Atypical Facial Pain"

Unfortunately, the diagnosis of trigeminal neuropathic pain overlaps to some extent with the term "atypical facial pain," a catch-all diagnosis that is not useful from either a taxonomic, diagnostic, or therapeutic standpoint (see below, "Pain of Psychological Origin in the Head and Face"). The differential diagnosis of this type of pain is difficult because it lacks many of the characteristic attributes that signify primary or secondary (nontraumatic) trigeminal neuralgia. The differential diagnostic possibilities include idiopathic trigeminal neuralgia, secondary trigeminal neuralgia from intracranial lesions, post-herpetic neuralgia, odontalgia, and musculoskeletal pain.

In general, the more these pains resemble those of typical trigeminal neuralgia, the more likely patients will respond to the anticonvulsant medications such as carbamazepine and diphenylhydantoin. If the pain has a constant or burning character, a tricyclic antidepressant such as amitriptyline in doses of 100–150 mg at bedtime in combination with fluphenazine 1–2.5 mg PO BID represents a reasonable option. More recently, clonazepam 2–3 mg/day in divided doses has been shown to provide some relief.

If a discrete area of nerve injury ("neuroma") can be demonstrated, and the pain responds completely to local anesthetic block, surgical excision can be recommended. These problems are very complex, however. Detailed evaluation including psychological screening is essential, because the standard caveat in these cases is that further trigeminal deafferentation by neurectomy, gangliolysis, or rhizotomy is frequently unsuccessful in the management of this condition, and often worsens the pain state.

POST-HERPETIC NEURALGIA

Pain associated with an acute outbreak of herpetic lesions in the distribution of a branch or branches of the trigeminal nerve does not usually present a diagnostic dilemma. The etiologic agent is herpes zoster or varicella virus, and affects middle-aged to elderly individuals (males and females about equally). Pain is described as burning or tingling with occasionally lancinating components felt in the skin. The pain usually precedes the onset of herpetic eruption by 1 or 2 days, or may develop coincidentally with the eruption. The pain is severe and usually lasts 1 to several weeks (22).

Associated symptoms include malaise, low fever, and headaches. Clusters of small vesicles, almost invariably located in the distribution of the ophthalmic division of the trigeminal nerve, appear. Herpetic eruptions are often seen in patients undergoing treatment for systemic lymphoma, carcinomatous metastasis, or other conditions that predispose to or create immunosuppression. Elevated protein and pleocytosis of the spinal fluid are also observed. Corneal ulceration due to vesicles has been reported. The pathology of the lesions is small cell infiltrates in the affected skin and bullous cutaneous changes. Similar infiltrates in the trigeminal ganglion and root entry zone are also seen.

In the usual case spontaneous and permanent remission is the rule. In the older age group, however, progression to chronic (post-herpetic) neuralgia is more the rule.

Acute herpetic neuralgia can be managed symptomatically with oral or parenteral narcotic pain medication. Because of the limited duration of the syndrome, tricyclic and anticonvulsant medications are probably not appropriate. Some evidence indicates that repeated sympathetic blockade (i.e., stellate block) may reduce the acute pain as well as the incidence of post-herpetic neuralgia. Other agents that have been reported to be effective in the prevention of post-herpetic neuralgia, when given in the acute phase, include corticosteroids, amantadine, levodopa and benserazide, vidabarine, and interferon-alpha (22).

Chronic neuralgia that occurs in the distribution of one or more divisions of the fifth cranial nerve subsequent to an acute herpes zoster outbreak is described as post-herpetic neuralgia. Pain of this type is usually associated with chronic skin trophic changes or scarring and most commonly occurs in the first (ophthalmic) division. It is a relatively infrequent disorder, predominantly seen in patients in their fifties or older, and is more common in males. The quality of the pain is described as burning, tearing, crawling, or itching dysesthesia in the affected area, and is exacerbated by mechanical contact with the skin. The pain is moderate, but present constantly, and may last for years, although spontaneous remission can occur. Because of the chronic and unremitting nature of the pain, depression and irritability are common associated symptoms.

On examination the skin of the painful region may show scarring, loss of normal pigmentation, hypesthesia or hyperesthesia, hypalgesia, or hyperpathia (allodynia). In the early phase of the disorder, pathologically there are chronic inflammatory changes in the trigeminal ganglion and demyelination in the root entry zone. Later on, wallerian degeneration of the peripheral nerve fiber with fibrosis and a relative depletion of the large compared to than small myelinated and unmyelinated axons is seen (22).

Treatment of established post-herpetic neuralgia is difficult. Fortunately, there is a tendency for the pain to diminish with time. Medications that are effective for trigeminal neuralgia are of little benefit in this disorder, although carbamazepine or clonazepam may be useful in the treatment of any component of post-herpetic neuralgia described as being paroxysmal and lancinating. For the more typical constant burning dysesthetic pain, tricyclic antidepressant medications are probably the most effective choices for pharmacologic treatment. Amitriptyline 75 mg given at bedtime with fluphenazine 1 mg three times a day is a commonly used regimen (22, 23).

In light of the natural history of post-herpetic neural-gia, surgical therapy should be reserved for those patients with severe, unremitting pain that is refractory to medical management. Currently, stereotaxic trigeminal tractotomy and open radiofrequency tractotomy/nucleotomy are probably the only surgical procedures that have been shown, albeit in only a few cases, to be effective for the management of post-herpetic trigeminal neuralgia (23, 24).

GENICULATE NEURALGIA (VIITH CRANIAL NERVE)

The nervus intermedius is a component of the seventh (facial) cranial nerve that contains primary sensory afferent fibers whose somata are located in the geniculate ganglion. These fibers innervate part of the external canal and tympanic membrane, the skin of the angle between the ear and mastoid process, the tonsillar region, and some other deep structures of the head and neck. Severe lancinating pain felt within the territory of the nervous intermedius (i.e., deeply within the external auditory canal, auditory meatus, concha, or retroauricular region) constitutes geniculate neuralgia.

The clinical syndrome of geniculate neuralgia, or intermedius neuralgia, occurs in young or middle-aged adults, predominantly in women. The pain can be described as sharp, shock-like, lancinating, and located in the external auditory meatus with retroauricular radiation. Local tenderness in the pinna or external auditory canal may be present, and manifestations such as excessive salivation or nasal secretion, tinnitus, vertigo, or a bitter taste may accompany the pains.

This is an extremely rare entity, with only a few cases reported in the world's literature. Nevertheles, the syndrome is instructive because it demonstrates a pain syndrome due to involvement of the sensory component of the seventh cranial nerve, the nervus intermedius. Pain of this type must be differentiated from otic varieties of trigeminal and glossopharyngeal neuralgia (25, 26).

Geniculate neuralgia is not usually responsive to medical management; a surgical procedure is therefore required. The most efficacious technique has been surgical division of the nervus intermedius, glossopharyngeal, and upper two strands of the vagus nerve in the posterior fossa. Ideally, this procedure should be performed under local anesthesia such that electrical stimulation of cranial nerves VII, VIII, IX, and X can be achieved. If under these circumstances pain can be reproduced by stimulation only of VII, IX, and the upper fibers of X, then rhizotomy of these nerves should be carried out. Otherwise, a medullary tractotomy is the procedure of choice (25).

GLOSSOPHARYNGEAL NEURALGIA (IXTH CRANIAL NERVE)

Glossopharyngeal, or more appropriately *vago*glosso-pharyngeal, neuralgia is a rare syndrome that involves episodic bursts of pain in the sensory distribution of the ninth and tenth cranial nerves (27). The vagal and glossopharyngeal nerves are concerned with touch, pain, and temperature sensation in the posterior third of the tongue; tonsillar pillars and fossa; nasolaryngeal, orolaryngeal, and laryngeal pharynx, including the pyriform recess; larynx; eustachian tube; middle ear; external auditory canal; part of the pinna; and a small cutaneous area anterior and posterior to the pinna. Pains in these regions can be mild to severe, and may be described as sharp, stabbing, shock-like, hot, or burning. Other uncomfortable sensations, although not frankly painful, may occur in isolation or simply precede painful paroxysms. A dull aching or burning sensation may persist after an attack.

Swallowing, particularly of cold or acid fluids, often triggers the pain; less commonly chewing, eating, talking, or other movements that involve the oropharyngeal musculature also precipitate attacks. A discrete trigger point is commonly localizable on the fauces or tonsil, although this point may be absent. Individual pains may last from seconds to minutes, and may occur from a few per year to dozens per day. Episodes may last for weeks to months and subside spontaneously, although commonly there is recurrence of the pain.

Bradycardia, tachycardia, syncope, hypotension, or seizures may accompany the painful paroxysms. The cardiovascular effects are thought to be mediated by the carotid sinus nerve or its central connections via the glossopharyngeal or vagus nerves.

The pathophysiology of glossopharyngeal neuralgia is unknown. Vascular cross-compression by ectatic vessels in the region of the entry zones of the ninth and tenth cranial nerves, akin to what has been observed in the fifth nerve in trigeminal neuralgia, has been suggested as a possible etiology, however. A possible variant of this syndrome is neuralgia of the superior laryngeal nerve (vagus nerve neuralgia). In these cases paroxysms of unilateral lancinating pain radiate from the side of the thyroid cartilage or pyriform sinus to the angle of the jaw and occasionally to the ear. In all other aspects this syndrome is similar to glossopharyngeal neuralgia. The differential diagnosis for pains in this area includes carotidynia, Eagle's syndrome, or local lesions such as carcinoma.

Like trigeminal neuralgia, glossopharyngeal neuralgia typically does respond to anticonvulsant agents such as carbamazepine (28). If medical management fails to satisfactorily control the pain, the most promising approach has recently been to surgically explore the region of cranial nerve IX and X in the posterior fossa. Frequently, vascular loops impinging on the nerve can be identified and repositioned. This results in pain remission in the majority of cases (27). If no vascular cross-compression is identified, the ninth and upper one-half of the tenth nerve are divided. Again, this rhizotomy is effective in relieving pain in most cases. If the syndrome is attributed to the superior laryngeal nerve, then temporary relief may be obtained from analgesic nerve block, alcohol nerve block, or nerve section.

OCCIPITAL NEURALGIA

In contradistinction to other cranial neuralgias, occipital neuralgia is quite common. Paresthesias may occur in the occipital nerve distributions. Pain is usually deep, aching, or stabbing in the distribution of the second (greater occipital nerve) or third (lesser occipital nerve) cervical dorsal root—that is, unilaterally from the suboccipital area to the vertex (C2) or to the retromastoid and supra-auricular areas (C3). The temporal pattern of the pain is irregular, but usually worse later in the day, and may range from moderate to severe in intensity. A history of chronic recurring episodes is typical, although spontaneous cessation of the pain may also occur. Pains of this kind often occur after acceleration-deceleration injuries, and are more common in the third to fifth decades of life. Hyperesthesia of the scalp is a common complaint, and hypesthesia to pin prick in the C2–C3 region of the scalp or tenderness or Tinel's sign of the great occipital nerve may be found. Local anesthetic/corticosteroid block of the occipital nerve may produce effective temporary relief.

The pathophysiology of occipital neuralgia is unknown, although it may be secondary to trauma, including flexion-extension (whiplash) injuries. The mechanism may be related to increased muscle activity in the cervical region, or entrapment of the C2 root or dorsal root ganglion by paravertebral ligamentous structures (29, 30). The differential diagnosis of occipital neuralgia includes cluster headaches, posterior fossa, high cervical or foramen magnum tumors, herniated cervical intervertebral disk, uncomplicated flexion-extension injury, and metastatic neoplasm at the base of the skull.

Because occipital neuralgia is merely a symptom of radicular or peripheral nerve pathology, treatment varies with actual or supposed etiology. Treatment ranges from therapy directed at a specific lesion of the C1–C2 region such as Arnold-Chiari malformation, gout, or neoplasm to generalized disorders such as diabetes. Often a specific etiology can only be postulated, and in these cases a wide variety of treatments have been advocated such as rhizotomy, collar placement, massage, infrared heat, procaine and alcohol infiltrations, avulsion of the greater occipital nerve, traction, steroid injections, and excision or alcohol injection of all of the nerves in the back of the head (30). Another mechanism has been proposed, that being entrapment of the second or third cervical root and dorsal root ganglion either by ligamentous or fascial structures in their respective neural foramina, or by osteoarthritis and spondylosis in these areas (29, 30). Surgical exploration of the C2 or C3 foramen may demonstrate neural compression, which when relieved may result in pain remission without the need for a neurodestructive procedure.

OTHER FACIAL NEURALGIAS

These syndromes are unusual and are mentioned here only to complete the differential diagnostic possibilities in patient's with paroxysmal facial pain secondary to presumed neuralgia.

Sphenopalatine Neuralgia

Sphenopalatine neuralgia (Sluder's syndrome or lower-half headache) consists of paroxysmal pains that begin on the medial side of the nose or medial canthus of the eye and radiate to the roof of the mouth retroorbitally, or rarely to the ipsilateral neck, shoulder, and upper extremity (31). Attacks occur many times a day and are often precipitated by sneezing or preceded by a sensation of nasal congestion. Unilateral lacrimation and conjunctival injection may accompany the attacks. Cocaine injection into the sphenopalatine ganglion affords temporary relief. Vidian neuralgia, or Vail's syndrome, is a variant of sphenopalatine neuralgia. It is paroxysmal unilateral facial pain attributed to "irritation" of the vidian nerve, an afferent branch of the sphenopalatine ganglion. Pain may radiate backward into the ear, nape of the neck, and shoulder, and is occasionally associated with tinnitus and vertigo (31).

Raeder's Syndrome, or Paratrigeminal Neuralgia

Raeder's syndrome, or "paratrigeminal" neuralgia, is characterized by frontotemporal pain and oculosympathetic paresis (incomplete Horner's syndrome). The syndrome may be due to the proximity of the ophthalmic division of the fifth nerve to the ocular sympathetic fibers that travel with the carotid artery in the region of the cavernous sinus (32). Two types of pain result: a migrainous variant with episodic and recurrent pains lasting hours or days, and a "symptomatic," more persistent type, often secondary to an aneurysm or tumor in the region of the middle fossa or cavernous sinus.

CRANIOFACIAL PAIN OF MUSCULOSKELETAL ORIGIN

Craniofacial pain of musculoskeletal origin may arise from the muscles of mastication or the temporomandibular joint (TMJ), depending on the sites of pathology, or may be referred from the neck musculature (33). In this section we discuss chronic orofacial pain thought to originate specifically from the muscles of mastication or the TMJ. Information regarding head pain originating from the scalp muscles can be found in the appropriate sections in Chapters 19–21.

Chronic orofacial pain of musculoskeletal origin can be divided into four major subcategories: (1) temporomandibular pain and dysfunction syndromes (34) (also called myofacial pain and dysfunction syndromes) (35),

(2) specific myofacial disorders, (3) osteoarthritis of the temporomandibular joint, and (4) bone infections and tumors. Diagnosis in some cases may be confounded by the overlapping of conditions, pain referral from nonmasticatory muscles, lack of clear pathology, and psychosocial and behavioral factors contributing to symptom expression.

TEMPOROMANDIBULAR PAIN AND DYSFUNCTION SYNDROMES

Temporomandibular pain and dysfunction syndrome (TMPDS) has been equated by the IASP with myofascial pain and dysfunction syndrome (1). In contrast, some workers consider these conditions to be distinctly different entities, with TMPDS by definition associated with altered TMJ physiology, and myofascial pain and dysfunction syndrome (MPDS) primarily identified with sustained muscle activity (36). Practically, however, both conditions are characterized by the same triad of signs and symptoms: pain and tenderness of the masticatory muscles, joint sounds with jaw opening, and limited mandibular movement (37). Although the IASP has chosen to use the terms TMPDS and MPDS, the reader should be aware that the American Dental Association has recommended use of the term temporomandibular disorder (TMD) to define all conditions involving the temporomandibular joint and muscles of mastication. A number of recently proposed classification schemes present standardized terminology and diagnostic criteria for TMD (38, 39).

Diagnosis is based on the patient's history and clinical findings. In general, extensive radiographic evaluation is not necessary. Radiographic analysis with panography or tomography may be required to rule out degenerative joint disease or other forms of joint pathology, however (40), and in some complex cases, special procedures such as arthrography and CT scanning may be needed to define the nature of joint dysfunction or to rule-out other forms of muscular disease such as myofibrosis. Unless the history or clinical findings are suggestive of systemic muscle pathology, rheumatoid arthritis, or lupus erythematosus, laboratory blood studies are not generally useful. Additional laboratory tests such as surface or needle electromyography and thermography have been recommended to assess TMPDS, but the significance of the data gathered from such testing is not presently understood. Because psychosocial stressors may be easily assessed by detailed psychosocial interview, the use of more extensive psychometric testing is not generally necessary, unless to confirm or underscore a clinical impression.

Pain may be perceived on one or both sides of the face around the ear or in the cheek, jaw, or temple. Generally characterized as a dull, continuous, poorly localized ache of moderate intensity with a boring or gnawing quality, it may vary in degree of discomfort through the course of the day. Yawning, chewing, or moving the mandible will often result in stabs of severe pain and precipitate cramping or jaw-locking. Long-term pain may also include cyclical periods of remission.

In addition to pain, patients frequently report symptoms such as jaw muscle fatigue with chewing, episodic jaw-locking in either an open or closed position, and deviation with opening. Many patients note the presence of soft or hard clicking or popping joint sounds. If questioned, they may also relate grinding their teeth at night (bruxism) or keeping their teeth together during the day (clenching), or acknowledge other parafunctional habits (gum chewing or fingernail biting). There may be a history of trauma to the face or jaws (41), and onset may often be associated with recent psychosocial stress. Other signs and symptoms that have been irregularly associated with TMPDS include ear pain (42), headache (43), tinnitus and dizziness (44), malocclusion (45), and psychogenic pain.

TMPDS patients with chronic pain will display many of the psychological characteristics that have been observed for other chronic pain states including anxiety, stress, depression, anger, and frustration. They may also demonstrate assorted illness behaviors, including increased treatment seeking and medication use.

Examination will often reveal a limited mouth opening; although normal jaw opening is highly variable between individuals, an opening of less than 40 mm (or three finger widths) is generally considered restricted (46). Reduced jaw opening may be the result of muscle dysfunction, such as spasm or splinting (47), meniscal displacement, such as failure of the condylar head to capture the meniscus (reduce) during opening, or a combination of both conditions. Audible soft clicking or popping sounds resulting from meniscal reduction may occur at any point during jaw opening or closing and are not generally considered to be of significance. Hard clicking consistently occurring late in opening (greater than 25 mm) coupled with periodic closed locking may indicate pathologic change in the meniscus or joint, however. In these rare cases arthrography may be useful in defining the nature of meniscus function and potential pathology. Palpation of the jaw opening muscles, particularly the masseter, temporalis, and internal (lateral) pterygoid, will frequently elicit tenderness, but the pathophysiologic significance of such pain is presently unclear. Intraoral examination will sometimes demonstrate marked tooth attrition, cheek biting, or tongue indentations, findings associated with bruxism or clenching. In cases of dislocation of the meniscus there may be marked alteration in the occlusion.

The prevalence of TMPDS has been estimated to be between 10 and 15% of the population (48). It is a disease of the young (ages 15–45), with a three to five times greater incidence in females. Although TMPDS is generally acknowledged to be a psychophysiologic disease,

Table 22.2. Conditions to be Considered in Differential Diagnosis of TMPDS

Tumors
  Synovial chondromatosis
  Caronoid hyperplasia
  Sarcoma
Arthritis
  Infectious arthritis
  Traumatic arthritis
  Rheumatoid arthritis
  Osteoarthritis (degenerative joint disease)
  Psoriatic arthritis
  Juvenile rheumatoid arthritis
Connective tissue disease
  Systemic lupus erythematosus
  Dermatomyositis
Condylar agenesis
Myofascial disorders (myositis, fibrositis)
Myositis ossificans
Odontogenic or nonodontogenic infection
Otitis media
Parotitis
Reflex sympathetic dystrophy of the face
Elongated styloid process (Eagle's syndrome)
Pain of psychological origin in the face (psychogenic pain disorder)

its etiology remains unsettled. Fortunately, for approximately 80% of patients the condition is self-limiting. Conditions that must be considered in the differential diagnosis of TMPDS are presented in Table 22.2.

The American Dental Association has recommended that until differences concerning the etiology, pathophysiology, and diagnosis of TMPDS are resolved, treatment strategies should be conservative and noninvasive (49). Interventions that address the muscular component of the problem include psychophysiologic (habit control, hypnotherapy, relaxation therapy, and biofeedback), psychologic (counseling/stress management, communication/cognitive therapy, and behavioral modification), and pharmacologic (antidepressants, antianxiety agents, and muscle relaxants) modalities as well as message, physical exercises, physiotherapy, splints, transcutaneous electric neural stimulation (TENS), and myofunctional therapy. Relatively noninvasive strategies such as acupuncture and trigger-point injections may also be useful. Aggressive intervention with orthodontics or dental reconstruction is rarely necessary. In cases of severe TMJ dysfunction involving meniscus pathology, surgical therapy (e.g., disk repositioning and plication of the distal ligament, disk removal, or artificial meniscus implantation) may be indicated. The efficacy of the latter strategy, however, is increasingly being questioned because of premature breakdown and rejection. For greater detail about treatment methods the reader is referred to Chapters 23 and 24.

SPECIFIC OR DIFFUSE MYOFASCIAL PAIN SYNDROMES

The cardinal feature of what the IASP has described as "myofascial pain syndromes," on which diagnosis is based, is the presence of latent or active myofascial "trigger points" (1). These are discrete nodular areas of hyperirritable muscle or fascial tissue which, when compressed, predictably produce what has been termed a "jump sign" and a reproducible pain referral pattern (50). Satellite tender points may be found within the area of pain reference of the initial trigger point. The presence of multiple "trigger points" distinguishes this pain disorder from pain of other muscle conditions, such as TMPDS.

Pain, described as deep, aching, or pressure-like, may be induced by passive stretch, functional movements, strong voluntary contraction of shortened muscle, cold damp weather, trauma, hyperactivity or inactivity, fatigue, and emotional distress. Activation of an initial trigger point may excite satellite points within the zone of reference and trigger points within synergistic muscles (51). If myospasm becomes a feature of trigger point activation, associated orofacial symptoms may include limited opening or joint clicking. Evidence associating trigger points with specific or nonspecific pathologic features is limited (52), and there is virtually no experimental evidence supporting the presence of such discrete areas of pathophysiologic change within the muscles of mastication. Nonetheless, distinctive regions of tenderness described as trigger points have been reliably measured with a pressure algometer in the masseter and temporalis muscles (53). Laboratory procedures such as electromyography and thermography have not been thoroughly investigated in relation to masticatory trigger points and at present offer limited diagnostic utility. Blood studies yield no useful findings and are unnecessary unless there is suspicion that the condition is secondary to systemic disease. Radiography with soft tissue imaging has not demonstrated abnormalities and is not recommended.

Although myofascial pain associated with the masticatory musculature appears to be quite common, its epidemiologic characteristics are unknown. In a recent study of 296 patients with complaints of head and neck pain, 55.4% were found to have a primary diagnosis of myofascial pain syndrome based on the presence of multiple trigger points (54).

Myofascial pain syndromes may occur within an individual muscle ("specific" type) or involve several muscles ("diffuse" type). Synonyms for this condition include fibrositis (syndrome), myalgia, tenomyositis, muscular rheumatism, and nonarticular rheumatism. Conditions from which myofascial pain syndromes should be differentiated as listed in Table 22.3.

Specific myofascial pain syndromes involving the masticatory muscles respond well to stretch and spray techniques, trigger point compression, message, injec-

Table 22.3.
Conditions from which Myofascial Pain Syndromes Should be Differentiated

Temporomandibular pain and dysfunction syndrome
Myofascial pain and dysfunction syndrome
Connective tissue disease
   Systemic lupus erythematosis
   Dermatomyositis
Myositis ossificans
Odentogenic or nonodontogenic infection
The arthritides
Reflex sympathetic dystrophy of the face
Elongated styloid process
Pain of psychological origin in the face

tion, or acupuncture. Low-dose amitriptyline, 50–75 mg, may be helpful. The elimination of perpetuating postural or behavioral factors should be part of management strategy. Additional information concerning management of myofascial pain syndromes is found in Chapters 43 and 44.

OSTEOARTHRITIS AND THE TEMPOROMANDIBULAR JOINT

Pain is a frequent but not consistent finding in patients presenting with osteoarthritis of the TMJ. When present, it is often described as a deep ache within the ear or preauricular area of the face (with minimal radiation to surrounding regions) that increases in intensity from morning to evening and is exacerbated with use or cold weather. It may persist for months or years with cyclical periods of remission. Crepitus is the symptom most consistently related to osteoarthritis of the TMJ (55), but limitation of mandibular movement, presumably associated with muscle splinting, has also been reported (56). The sound of crepitus is distinctly different from clicking and has been described as a gristle, crackle, or soft-hard grating. It is assumed that damage to the soft tissue articulating components contributes to the noise, but the degree to which joint morphology, as opposed to degenerative change, contributes to the quality of sound is presently unknown. There is often a history of trauma. Patients with chronic osteoarthritis will appear to be less psychologically disturbed than those with myofascial conditions.

Diagnosis is based on history, the presence of crepitus revealed through stethoscopic evaluation, TMJ palpation pain (lateral and intrameatal), and radiographic interpretation. Change in the occlusion may aso be noted if joint degeneration has been rapid. Laboratory tests (e.g., blood or synovial fluid analysis) are not generally necessary, unless there is suspicion of infectious arthritis (bacterial, fungal, tubercular), connective tissue diseases (rheumatoid arthritis, systemic lupus erythematosus, dermatomyositis), or the rheumatoid varients (psoriatic arthritis, Reiter's syndrome, juvenile rheumatoid arthritis). Gross radiographic bone changes can be observed in panoramic and transcranial radiographs but tomograms are currently considered the most accurate means of assessing the full extent of pathology. Osseous changes include flattening of the condyle or eminence, osteophytes, marginal lipping of the anterior portion of the condyle, subarticular cystic changes or erosions in the lateral or superior portion of the condyle, sclerosis of marginal bone, and medullary distortions (57). Severe erosion of the TMJ is more indicative of connective tissue disease than osteoarthritis is. Joint-space narrowing has also been suggested as a sign of pathology, but this view remains controversial and unsupported. Other radiographic diagnostic techniques such as MRI and single photon emission computed tomography (SPECT) show promise for improving diagnostic capability.

Osteoarthritis of the TMJ is most likely to be observed in women after the age of 40 (58). It has, however, been reported in younger females (56). Epidemiologic studies suggest that between 4 and 14% of the population may have TMJ degenerative disease based on the presence of crepitus (59). Far fewer have pain or seek treatment. The histopathology of TMJ osteoarthritis is well documented, consisting of primary articular erosion and secondary joint-space dystrophic calcification in the absence of inflammation (60). Histopathologic studies suggest that degenerative change may be correlated with articular disk perforations or deformations (61).

The etiology of TMJ osteoarthritis is unknown. The literature identifies a plethora of causes that include age, various forms of trauma (62), and functional or dysfunctional loading. The effects of genetic predisposition, systemic disease, metabolic-endocrine processes, and inflammation have not been thoroughly investigated. Recent evidence suggests that osteoarthritis may be related to condylar dysfunction, particularly chronic anterior meniscus displacement (61). The hypothesis that osteoarthritis may result from intermittent joint clicking remains speculative, however. Conditions that should be considered in the differential diagnosis are listed in Table 22.4.

In general osteoarthritis of the temporomandibular joint follows a pattern similar to skeletal joints with symptoms lasting one to three years and including bone remodeling. The condition may be conservatively managed with therapeutic strategies outlined under "Temporomandibular Pain and Dysfunction Syndrome." In addition, anti-inflammatory medications and anesthetic injection into the joint may be helpful. Severe cases may require surgical management but recurrence is likely.

Bone Infections and Tumors

Orofacial pain resulting from infection and neoplasia is described as a constant, deep, aching sensation, some-

Table 22.4.
Conditions to be Considered in Differential Diagnosis of TMJ Osteoarthritis

Temporomandibular pain and dysfunction syndrome
Myofascial pain and dysfunction syndrome
    Infectious arthritis (bacterial, fungal, tubercular)
Connective tissue diseases
    Rheumatoid arthritis
    Systemic lupus erythematosus
    Dermatomyositis
Rheumatoid varients
    Psoriatic arthritis
    Reiter's syndrome
    Juvenile rheumatoid arthritis
Tramatic arthritis

times localized to the teeth but more often of a diffuse quality. Diagnosis is based on the patient's history and on laboratory, radiographic, and clinical findings. In cases of nonpurulent infection (osteitis), radiography may reveal demineralization or remineralization of the bone. Signs and symptoms associated with chronic osteomyelitis include paresthesia (if the condition involves the mandibular nerve canal), low-grade fever, elevated WBC and increased erythrocyte sedimentation rate (ESR) values, sinus tract formation, limitation of opening, and occasionally exposed bone. Bone death and necrosis results in a distinctive radiographic presentation, with islands of bone, termed *sequestra,* surrounded by demineralization. The condition may result from periapical tooth abcess, fracture, or surgical contamination. Osteoradionecrosis, one form of osteomyelitis, may result from radiation treatment to the jaws or from radiation treatment that is followed by trauma (e.g., tooth extraction).

When neoplastic activity in the mandible (osteogenic sarcoma) is the source of the pain, there may be concurrent altered skin sensation (e.g., hypesthesia, dyesthesia, or paresthesia over the chin or lower face). Chondrosarcoma, a relatively rare but exquisitely painful tumor, is most commonly found in the anterior maxilla. Diagnosis of neoplasm is straightforward and based on history and on clinical, laboratory, and radiographic findings.

LESIONS OF THE EAR, NOSE, AND ORAL CAVITY

Orofacial pain resulting from acute sinus infection can be mild to severe and is often described as an aching or throbbing or as a headache. Frontal or ethmoid sinus involvement generates bilateral forehead pain or pain felt between the eyes, whereas pain originating from the maxillary sinus is often experienced on one or both sides of the face in the upper cheek (zygoma) or the entire side of the face. Pain arising from chronic (as opposed to acute) maxillary sinusitis may be described as mild and continuous with a burning quality. Other associated symptoms may include a feeling of fullness in the face or, in cases of maxillary sinus involvement, tenderness of the maxillary premolar or molar teeth.

The diagnosis of chronic sinusitis is based on history and on clinical and radiographic findings. Forward bending or pressure applied over the affected sinus may intensify or exacerbate the pain in some cases. Examination may reveal hypertrophy or atrophy of the nasal mucosa and/or polyp formation. With maxillary involvement the upper teeth on the affected side will frequently be percussion-sensitive. Culture results of the nose or nasal discharge, however, are often negative (63). In these cases the examiner should be alert to the possibility of allergy or a reaction to irritating dusts or toxic chemicals. Standard radiography may demonstrate a fluid level but may not be helpful in assessing mucosal changes. CT may be necessary to rule-out neoplasm.

Acute sinusitis is prevalent in adults, with chronic sinusitis being less common. Males and females are equally affected. Inflammation of the sinus mucosal lining is considered to be the pathophysiologic mechanism responsible for facial pain genesis, and inflammation of elements of the superior alveolar nerve plexus the cause of tooth pain. Orofacial conditions that should be considered in the differential diagnosis include odontogenic infection and malignant disease.

Relief may be gained from antibiotics, decongestants, analgesics, moist heat, or lying down on the opposite side to promote drainage. Surgical lavage or drainage is necessary for intractable cases.

OROFACIAL PAIN OF ODONTOGENIC ORIGIN

Odontogenic pain or toothache, also termed *odontalgia*, is the commonest source of orofacial discomfort. Highly variable in presentation, odontogenic pain may be intermittent or continuous, spontaneous or induced, and will often simulate other pain syndromes. It is most often described as a mild to unbearable aching or sometimes throbbing sensation with a dull or depressing quality. The IASP has chosen to differentiate five varieties of odontalgia: pain due to dentinoenamel defects, pain arising from the pulp (e.g., pulpitis), pain arising from the periodontal structures (e.g., periapical periodontitis and abscess), pain not associated with lesions (e.g., atypical odontalgia), and cracked tooth syndrome. With the exception of pain due to dentinoenamel defects, all of these conditions can be chronic in nature. Because atypical odontalgia is not associated with a known pathophysiologic mechanism, we have elected to describe this condition under the classification "Pain of Psychogenic Origin in the Head and Face" (see below). A complete discussion of therapeutic considerations related to pain conditions of odontogenic origin is presented in Chapter 24.

Odontalgia: Toothache-Pulpitis

The term *pulpitis* implies that the etiology of this pain is due only to pulpal inflammation and not periapical infection. In these cases pain is very often poorly localized within the teeth, jaws, face, or head. It may occur spontaneously, or be activated (in severe cases exacerbated) by hot or cold stimuli. Pulpal pain is often perceived as a sharp or dull ache of moderate or severe intensity.

Diagnosis is based on clinical signs and radiologic findings. Examination and radiography will often reveal deep dental caries, sometimes with erosion into the pulp chamber or root canal. Application of stimulants such as cold, heat, or electricity and probing will induce pain. If inflammation progresses to infection and periodontal involvement, pain will be aggravated by percussion.

Differential diagnosis includes other forms of dental disease, trigeminal neuralgia, sinusitis, and migrainous headache syndromes.

Odontalgia: Toothache-Periapical Periodontitis and Abscess

Pain related to periodontal structures is similar in quality, occurrence, intensity, and duration to pain of pulpal origin. In contrast to pulpal pain, however, it is easily localized by the patient and diagnosis generally does not present difficulty. Pressure applied to the offending tooth will initiate or exacerbate tenderness. Associated symptoms may include localized redness, cellulitis, lymphadenitis, and drainage through the formation of a sinus tract. More severe complications can involve diffuse cellulitis and spread of the infection to parapharyngeal spaces with airway compromise, CNS with cerebral abscess, or endocardium (64). Radiographic data are useful for initial diagnosis and for defining extensive fascial plane involvement. In cases involving diffuse cellulitis, hematologic, histopathologic, and microbiologic laboratory tests may be necessary to augment diagnosis or to provide baseline information should the infection not respond to initial treatment. Differential diagnosis includes other dental disease, nonodontogenic infections, and neoplasia.

Cracked Tooth Syndrome

Pain originating from a tooth with a fine crack can be acute or chronic and is described as sharp or shock-like and of brief duration, often produced by biting or chewing. Upon examination, percussion directed laterally towards the affected tooth cusp will usually exacerbate the pain. A visible crack may sometimes be apparent or the cusp may move with manipulation. Radiography is not useful. The differential diagnosis includes other forms of toothache associated with the dentine or pulp.

OROFACIAL PAIN OF MUCOSAL ORIGIN

Mucosal diseases produce pain that is intermittent in nature, although the patient may experience chronic discomfort. There are, however, a number of conditions that may produce persistent facial pain of an aching quality, including chronic periodontitis, benign mucous membrane pemphigoid (BMMP), ulcerative lichen planus, major recurrent aphthous, Wegener's granulomatosis, and oral cancer with superimposed infection. Diagnosis in these cases is generally confirmed by history, examination, or laboratory findings (65).

One type of orofacial mucosal pain that may be encountered has been termed *burning mouth syndrome (glossodynia)*. The typical patient is a postmenopausal woman. The onset of the disorder is often associated with a prior dental procedure. In these cases, pain, described as a persistent, severe, burning sensation, may occur in the tongue or other mucosal tissues within the mouth, often in association with other altered sensations (e.g., taste or dryness) (66). It may fluctuate during the day. The etiology and pathophysiology of this disorder remain unknown. The condition has been associated with local irritation (ill-fitting dentures), xerostomia, systemic disease, and nutritional deficiencies (especially vitamin B_{12}, but also B_1, B_2, and B_6. Burning tongue has also been reported following the development of adenoid cystic carcinoma in the floor of the mouth. In addition, many workers consider burning mouth a psychogenic pain problem because symptoms are often associated with emotional upset in the absence of organic findings (see below).

PAIN OF PSYCHOLOGICAL ORIGIN IN THE HEAD AND FACE

The IASP has chosen to describe two general categories of pain of psychological origin in the head and face: "delusional or hallucinatory pain" and "hysterical or hypochondriacal" pain (1). Classification of a pain condition as such requires that there be no known physical cause or pathophysiologic mechanism and that there be proof of the presence of contributing psychological factors. As a result, these categories are roughly equivalent to what the American Psychiatric Association has described as "psychogenic pain disorder" (67).

Historically, *atypical facial pain,* or *prosopalgia,* has been the term most commonly used to describe diffuse, nonanatomic orofacial pain of unknown pathophysiology. In our opinion, the diagnosis of atypical facial pain should be made only on the following basis: (1) when other causes of facial pain have been considered and evaluated where appropriate, (2) when objective evidence for most of the facial pain syndromes is lacking, and (3) when specific antecedent psychologic or behavioral factors can be identified.

The predominant characteristic of psychologically induced pain is that it mimics pain of known pain syndromes. It is usually constant, often bilateral, and is not confined to the trigeminal distribution. The description

of the pain quality is often vague and variable, as is the location and precipitating factors. A constant aching or burning sensation is the dominant feature, paroxysmal pain being uncommon. Psychological features, such as delusions, hallucinations, multiple physical complaints with classic conversion or pseudoneurologic symptoms, exaggerated symptom reporting, excessive concern or fear of the symptoms, depression, illness behaviors, and excessive treatment seeking or medication use, are common. The patient often appears morose with evident suffering. Neurologic examination is usually normal except for some poorly localized tenderness and vague sensory loss in the painful region. Anticonvulsant medication is distinctly not helpful in these patients; psychiatric evaluation with psychotherapy and antidepressant medication are perhaps the only reasonable courses (26).

REFERENCES

1. Classification of chronic pain: Descriptions of chronic pain syndromes and definitions of chronic pain terms. *Pain (Suppl)* 3:1–225, 1986.
2. Jannetta PJ: Treatment of trigeminal neuralgia by suboccipital and transtentorial cranial operations. *Clin Neurosurg* 24:538–549, 1977.
3. Burchiel KJ: Abnormal impulse generation in focally demyelinated trigeminal roots. *J Neurosurg* 53:674–683, 1980.
4. Cusick JF: Atypical trigeminal neuralgia. *JAMA* 245:2328–2329, 1981.
5. Szapiro J Jr, Sindou M, Szapiro J: Prognostic factors in microvascular decompression for trigeminal neuralgia. *Neurosurgery* 17:920–929, 1985.
6. Bullitt E, Tew JM, Boyd J: Intracranial tumors in patients with facial pain. *J Neurosurg* 64:865–871, 1986.
7. Iragui VJ, Wiederholt WC, Romine JS: Evoked potentials in trigeminal neuralgia associated with multiple sclerosis. *Arch Neurol* 43:444–446, 1986.
8. Crill WE: Carbamazepine. *Ann Intern Med* 79:844–847, 1973.
9. Burchiel KJ, Steege TD, Howe JF, Loeser JD: Comparison of percutaneous radiofrequency gangliolysis and microvascular decompression of the trigeminal nerve for the surgical management of tic douloureux. *Neurosurgery* 9:111–119, 1981.
10. Sweet WH, Wepsic JG: Controlled thermocoagulation of trigeminal ganglion and rootlets for differential destruction of pain fibers: Part I. Trigeminal neuralgia. *J Neurosurg* 40:143–156, 1974.
11. Hakanson S: Tic douloureux treated by the injection of glycerol into the retrogasserian subarachnoid space: Long term results. *Acta Neurochir Suppl* 33:471–472, 1984.
12. Brown JA, Preul MC: Trigeminal depressor response during percutaneous microcompression of the trigeminal ganglion for trigeminal neuralgia. *Neurosurgery* 23:745–748, 1988.
13. Brown JA, Preul MC: Percutaneous trigeminal ganglion compression for trigeminal neuralgia. *J Neurosurg* 70:900–904, 1989.

14. Meglio M, Cioni B: Percutaneous procedures for trigeminal neuralgia: Microcompression versus radiofrequency thermocoagulation. Personal experience. *Pain* 38:9–16, 1989.

15. Lichtor T, Mullan JF: A 10-year follow-up review of percutaneous microcompression of the trigeminal ganglion. *J Neurosurg* 72:49–54, 1990.

16. Quinn JH: Repetitive peripheral neurectomies for neuralgia of second and third divisions of trigeminal neuralgia (tic douloureux). *Clin Neurosurg* 24:550–556, 1977.

17. Burchiel KJ: Surgical treatment of trigeminal neuralgia: Minor operative procedures. In Fromm GH (ed): *Trigeminal Neuralgia.* Mt. Kisko, New York; Futura, 1987, pp 71–99.

18. Burchiel KJ: Surgical treatment of trigeminal neuralgia: Major operative procedures. In Fromm GH (ed): *Trigeminal Neuralgia.* Mt. Kisko, New York; Futura, 1987, pp 101–119.

19. Goldstein NP, Gibilisco JA, Rushton JG: Trigeminal neuropathy and neuritis: A study of etiology with emphasis on dental causes. *JAMA* 184:458–462, 1963.

20. Thrus DC, Small M: How benign a symptom is face numbness? *Lancet* 2:851–853, 1970.

21. Burchiel KJ, Soldevilla FX, Loeser JD: Pathophysiology of atypical trigeminal neuralgia. Congress of Neurological Surgeons 1991 Annaul Meeting, program abstracts, p 258.

22. Loeser JD: Herpes zoster and postherpetic neuralgia. *Pain* 25:149–164, 1986.

23. Watson PN, Evans RJ: Postherpetic neuralgia: a review. *Arch Neurol* 43:836–840, 1986.

24. Nashold BS, Lopes H, Chodakiewitz J, Bronec P: Trigeminal DREZ for craniofacial pain. In Samii M (ed): *Surgery In and Around the Brain Stem and Third Ventricle.* Berlin, Springer-Verlag, 1986, pp 54–59.

25. White JC, Sweet WH: *Pain and the Neurosurgeon.* Springfield, IL, Charles C Thomas, 1969, pp 264–265.

26. Hart RG, Easton JD: Trigeminal neuralgia and other facial pains. Missouri Med 11:683–693, 1981.

27. Laha RK, Jannetta PJ: Glossopharyngeal neuralgia. *J Neurosurg* 47:316–320, 1977.

28. Ekbom KA, Westerberg CE: Carbomazepine in glossopharyngeal neuralgia. *Arch Neurol* 14:595–596, 1966.

29. Poletti CE: Proposed operation for occipital neuralgia: C-2 and C-3 root decompression. *Neurosurgery* 12:221–224, 1983.

30. Ehni G, Benner B: Occipital neuralgia and the C1-2 arthrosis syndrome. *J Neurosurg* 61:961–965, 1984.

31. Aubry M, Pialoux P: Sluder's syndrome. In Vinken PJ, Bruyn GW (eds): *Handbook of Clinical Neurology,* vol. 5. Amsterdam, Elsevier North Holland, 1968, pp 350–361.

32. Toussaint D: Raeder's syndrome. In Vinken PJ, Bruyn GW (eds): *Handbook of Clinical Neurology,* vol. 5. Amsterdam, Elsevier North Holland, 1968, pp 333–336.

33. Travell J: Temporomandibular joint pain referred from muscles of the head and neck. *J Prosthet Dent,* 10:745–763, 1960.

34. Schwartz L: *Disorders of the Temporomandibular Joint.* Philadelphia, W.B. Saunders, 1969.

35. Laskin D: Etiology of the pain-dysfunction syndrome. *J Am Dent Assoc* 70:147–153, 1969.

36. Moss RA, Garrett J: Temporomandibular joint dysfunction syndrome and myofascial pain dysfunction syndrome: A critical review. *J Oral Rehabil* 11:3–28, 1984.

37. Rugh JD, Solberg WK: Psychological implications in temporomandibular pain and dysfunction. *Oral Sci Rev* 7:3–30, 1976.

38. Truelove E, Sommers E, LeResche L, Dworkin S, Von Korff M: Clinical Diagnostic Criteria for TMD; New classification permits multiple diagnoses. *J Am Dent Assoc* 123:47–54, 1992.

39. American Academy of Craniomandibular Disorders, McNeill C (ed): *Craniomandibular Disorders: Guidelines for Evaluation, Diagnosis and Management.* Chicago, Quintessence Publishing, 1990.

40. Laskin D, Block S: Diagnosis and treatment of myofascial pain dysfunction (MPD) syndrome. *J Prosthet Dent* 56:75–84, 1986.

41. Burgess J: Symptom characteristics in TMD patients reporting blunt trauma and/or whiplash injury. *J Craniomandib Disorders Facial Oral Pain* 5:251–257, 1991.

42. Dolowitz DA, Ward JW, Fingerle CO, Smith C: The role of muscular incoordination in the pathogenesis of the temporomandibular joint syndrome. *Laryngoscope* 74:790–801, 1964.

43. Magnusson T, Carlsson GE: A two and one half year follow-up of changes in headache and mandibular dysfunction after stomatognathic treatment. *J Prosthet Dent* 49:398–402, 1983.

44. Sharov Y, Tzukert A, Refaeli, B, Isreal J: Muscle pain index in relation to pain dysfunction, and dizziness associated with the myofacial pain dysfunction syndrome. *Oral Surg* 46:742–747, 1978.

45. Agerberg G, Carlsson G: Symptoms of functional disturbances of the masticatory system. *Acta Odont Scand* 33:183–190, 1975.

46. Bell W: *Clinical Management of Temporomandibular Disorders.* Chicago, Year Book, 1982.

47. Griffin CT, Munro KK: Electromyography of the masseter and anterior temporalis muscles in patients with temporomandibular dysfunction. *Arch Oral Biol* 16:929–949, 1971.

48. Solberg W, Woo M, Houston J: Prevalence of mandibular dysfunction in young adults. *J Am Dent Assoc* 98:25–34, 1979.

49. Griffiths, RH: Report of the president's conference on the examination, diagnosis, and management of temporomandibular disorders. *J Am Dent Assoc* 106:75–77, 1983.

50. Travell J, Rinzler SH: The myofascial genesis of pain. *Postgrad Med* 11:425–434, 1952.

51. Travell JG, Simons DG: *Myofascial Pain and Dysfunction. The Trigger Point Manual.* Baltimore, Williams & Wilkins, 1983.

52. Awad EA: Interstitial myofibrositis: Hypothesis of the mechanism. *Arch Phys Med Rehabil* 54:449–453.

53. Reeves JL, Jaeger B, Graff-Radford SB: Reliability of the pressure algometer as a measure of myofascial trigger point sensitivity. *Pain* 24:313–321, 1986.

54. Fricton JR, Kroening R, Haley D, Siegert R: Myofascial pain syndrome of the head and neck: A review of clinical characteristics of 164 patients. *J Oral Surg Oral Pathol Oral Medicine* 60:615–623, 1985.

55. Shira RB: Temporomandibular degenerative joint disease. *Oral Surg* 40:1651–1682, 1975.

56. Ogus H: Degenerative disease of the temporomandibular joint in young persons. *Br J Oral Surg* 17:17–26, 1979–1980.

57. Wilkes DH: Structural and functional alterations of the temporomandibular joint. *Northwest Dent* 57:287–294, 1978.

58. Toller PA: Osteoarthrosis of the mandibular condyle. *Br Dent J* 134:223–231, 1973.

59. Gross A, Gale E: A prevalence study of the clinical signs associated with mandibular dysfunction. *J Am Dent Assoc* 107:932–936, 1983.

60. Moffett GC, Jonson LC, McCabe JB: Articular remodeling in the adult human temporomandibular joint. *Am J Anat* 115:119–142, 1964.

61. Wesstesson P-L, Rohlin M: Internal derangement of the temporomandibular joint: Morphologic description with correlation to joint function. *Oral Surg Oral Med Oral Pathol* 59:323–331, 1985.

62. Truelove E, Burgess J, Dworkin S, Lawton L, Sommers E, Shubert M: Incidence of trauma associated with temporomandibular disorders [Abstr]. *J Dent Res* 64:339, 1985.

63. Weinstein L: Diseases of the upper respiratory tract. In Wilson J (ed), *Harrison's Principles of Internal Medicine*. New York, McGraw-Hill, 1983, pp 1570–1571.

64. Hohl T, Whitacre R, Hooley J, Williams B (eds): *Diagnosis and Treatment of Odontogenic Infections*. Seattle, Stoma Press, 1983.

65. Wood NK, Goaz P (eds): *Differential Diagnosis of Oral Lesions*. St. Louis, C.V. Mosby, 1980.

66. Basker RM, Sturdee DW, Davenport JC: Patients with burning mouths—A clinical investigation of causative factors, including the climacteric and diabetes. *Br Dent J* 145:9–16, 1978.

67. American Psychiatric Association: *Quick Diagnostic and Statistical Manual (DSM-III)*. Washington, D.C., American Psychiatric Association, 1980.

CHAPTER 23

MEDICAL/NEUROSURGICAL MANAGEMENT OF OROFACIAL PAIN
RONALD BRISMAN

EFFECTIVE MEDICAL management of orofacial pain depends on appropriate diagnosis. Consultations from dental, otolaryngologic, and neurologic specialists are often necessary to find specific causes for the pain. Antibiotics, with or without drainage, may relieve infection of dental or periodontal structures. Malocclusion of the teeth that causes temporomandibular joint degeneration may need dental correction. Tumors of the trigeminal nerve are a rare cause of facial pain and often require neurosurgical intervention.

In many instances of orofacial pain, a specific cause and definitive cure cannot be achieved, and medical or surgical management focuses on the relief of pain and suffering.

Most orofacial pains of nondental origin are either neuralgic or atypical. The neuralgic pains are paroxysmal, episodic, unilateral, triggered by light touch about the mouth or face, and located in the distribution of the trigeminal or rarely the glossopharyngeal nerve. Atypical pains are continuous, burning, aching, or throbbing, often bilateral, and frequently distributed beyond the confines of one cranial nerve.

TRIGEMINAL NEURALGIA (TIC DOULOUREUX)

Episodic, triggered, severe, brief, lancinating paroxysms of pain, usually in the second and/or third divisions of the trigeminal nerve without loss of sensation, are characteristic of trigeminal neuralgia. A study showed that first-division pain occurred in 17.7% of patients, and was frequently accompanied by second division pain (1). At any one time, the condition is almost always unilateral, although 5–10% of patients will at some time in their lives have similar contralateral pain (2).

Multiple sclerosis occurs in 6% of patients with intractable trigeminal neuralgia (1). One should suspect the possibility of multiple sclerosis in patients with trigeminal neuralgia whose symptoms began before they were 45 years old and in those with bilateral symptoms (3, 4). Diagnostic tests for multiple sclerosis include cerebrospinal fluid examination for gamma-globulin and oligoclonal bands, visual-evoked responses, and magnetic resonance imaging (MRI). The physician should order these tests if multiple sclerosis is a possibility and he or she is considering microvascular decompression as treatment for the trigeminal neuralgia, because microvascular decompression is not appropriate for patients with multiple sclerosis.

Only a few patients with trigeminal neuralgia will have a brain tumor (1–5%) (1, 5), and many of these will have other neurologic abnormalities caused by the brain tumor (6). Rarely a patient with trigeminal neuralgia and no other signs or symptoms will have a brain tumor causing the trigeminal neuralgia (7). In those whose face pain is intractable enough to require a neurosurgical procedure, MRI can exclude the possibility of a brain tumor (8). A small tumor may cause trigeminal neuralgia, and MRI may not detect it unless gadolinium is given.

Carbamazepine (Tegretol) is so effective in treating trigeminal neuralgia (9, 10) that the diagnosis should be doubted if the patient does not show some response to this medication. Small doses of carbamazepine may help initially. Later, higher doses may no longer relieve the pain or may cause toxic side effects.

Carbamazepine is available in 200-mg tablets, 100-mg chewable tablets, and a suspension of 100 mg per 5 ml. The starting dose is usually 100 mg twice a day. The daily dose is increased by 100 mg or 200 mg until the patient gets relief. The usual maintenance dose is a total of 400–800 mg daily, which the patient takes in divided doses two to four times a day. It is rarely necessary to give more than 1200 mg daily. After the patient is free of pain for several weeks, the dose is reduced to the minimum necessary.

Patients should take carbamazepine right after a meal or with some milk to minimize the likelihood or severity of gastrointestinal disturbances such as nausea or vomiting.

Many unpleasant side effects can occur from carbamazepine. The most common are dizziness, drowsiness, unsteadiness, nausea, and vomiting, and are most likely to develop at the beginning of therapy or when the dose is too high. They usually subside when the dose is lowered. Central nervous system (CNS) toxicity is more likely to develop in the elderly (a group commonly afflicted with trigeminal neuralgia) and in those with multiple sclerosis. Physicians should not prescribe carbamazepine to those with a known sensitivity to tricyclic compounds. Carbamazepine may cause other toxic reactions. These include skin rashes, bone marrow suppression, and liver or renal impairment. A complete blood count and liver and renal chemistries before treatment, after 2 weeks, and at approximately 6-week intervals can help identify early toxicity. The medication should be stopped if there are significant alterations in these tests.

Aplastic anemia is a rare but sometimes fatal complication of carbamazepine therapy. In the medical literature, there are 20 cases (13 fatal) between 1964 and 1982 (11). Patients with abnormalities on the baseline blood and platelet counts and those taking other myelotoxic drugs are at increased risk for hematologic toxicity from carbamazepine (11). In these patients, the physician should avoid carbamazepine therapy or should monitor the blood counts more frequently (11). One should tell patients of signs and symptoms of early hematologic toxicity, such as fever, sore throat, ulcers in the mouth, pallor, easy bruising, and petechial or purpuric hemorrhage. Patients should report to the physician immediately if any of the above develop.

Carbamazepine has mildly anticholinergic effects and may worsen eye problems associated with elevated intraocular pressure. Patients with glaucoma who are also being treated with carbamazepine for trigeminal neuralgia should have their extraocular pressure carefully monitored.

Erythromycin, cimetidine, propoxyphene, isoniazid, or calcium-channel blockers may elevate carbamazepine blood levels, sometimes with toxicity.

It is easy to obtain blood levels for carbamazepine. Usual adult therapeutic levels are between 4 and 12 μg/ml.

If carbamazepine does not provide satisfactory pain relief, then baclofen (Lioresal) alone or in combination with carbamazepine may help (12). Gradually titrate the dose of baclofen for each individual. Start with an initial dose of 5 mg three times a day and increase every 3 days by a total daily dose of 15 mg until the patient is free of pain. The final daily dose is usually 40–80 mg. The most common adverse reactions are drowsiness, dizziness, and fatigue.

Although it is not effective in most patients (13), phenytoin (Dilantin) may help if treatment is not successful with carbamazepine and baclofen. The usual dose is 100 mg three times a day. Partial or even complete pain relief has occurred (14).

Clonazepam (Klonopin) is a benzodiazepine anticonvulsant that one study showed to be effective in 65% of cases of trigeminal neuralgia (15). The initial dose was 0.5 mg three times a day and was increased every 3 days by a total daily increment of 0.5–1 mg until pain was relieved. Severe and incapacitating somnolence or unsteadiness of gait developed in 9 of 25 patients.

Sodium valproate is an anticonvulsant that has decreased the symptoms of trigeminal neuralgia in 13 (65%) of 20 patients (16). The daily dose was 600–1200 mg per day. Four of the 13 responders also required other medications in addition to the sodium valproate. One patient was unable to tolerate sodium valproate because of persistent nausea.

Mephenesin carbamate and chlorphenesin carbamate (Maolate) are muscle relaxants that are now used infrequently but that have relieved pain in some patients with trigeminal neuralgia (17, 18).

A recent report indicates that pimozide, an antipsychotic drug that blocks dopaminergic receptors, may reduce symptoms of trigeminal neuralgia in patients who were refractory to other medical therapy (19). Oral doses were from 4–12 mg per day, and the trigeminal neuralgia score decreased by 78%. Adverse effects from pimozide occurred frequently. These were physical and mental retardation, hand tremors, memory impairment, involuntary movements during sleep (jerking), and slight Parkinson's disease manifestations.

Although physicians have used many medications in the treatment of trigeminal neuralgia, medical treatment is primarily treatment with carbamazepine because it is so effective. When carbamazepine does not suffice, either because it is no longer effective or because of adverse side effects, it is reasonable to offer baclofen. Most of the other medicines are either ineffective or associated with so many adverse effects that patients who continue to have severe and incapacitating pain in spite of carbamazepine and/or baclofen are best managed with neurosurgical procedures, especially the percutaneous ones.

Denervation of the sensory part of the trigeminal nerve can stop the pain of trigeminal neuralgia. Recurrent pain sometimes develops and is more likely if the denervation is peripheral to the gasserian ganglion or if it is partial. Denervation sometimes results in a new and unpleasant dysesthetic condition (anesthesia dolorosa), which occurs more frequently if the denervation is extensive. Fortunately, partial denervation also can relieve the pain of trigeminal neuralgia, and anesthesia dolorosa is much less likely to occur. Denervation of the cornea may result in keratitis, which if severe may cause impairment of vision. The surgeon can usually accomplish selective denervation, which spares the first division. This significantly lessens the risk of keratitis.

TREATMENT

Peripheral Denervation

Alcohol injection or neurectomy can produce peripheral denervation. The supraorbital, infraorbital, and mental nerves are readily accessible for such procedures. Pain usually recurs within 18 months; repeating the procedure is more difficult, less likely to work, and associated with an even shorter remission. Because of these drawbacks and the development of more effective percutaneous denervating procedures, peripheral denervations are rarely advisable. They may still be useful in those patients with first-division trigeminal neuralgia, because supraorbital denervation will not affect the cornea.

Radiofrequency Electrocoagulation

Controlled percutaneous radiofrequency electrocoagulation (RFE) is an important development in the neurosurgical treatment of trigeminal neuralgia because it allows for partial and selective denervation in a proximal (gasserian and retrogasserian) location (20–22). If there is recurrence, one can repeat the procedure without added risk or difficulty and with a similarly excellent chance of pain relief. Because of this, RFE is the procedure of choice for most patients with trigeminal neuralgia that is intractable in spite of appropriate medical treatment. This is especially the case for those with multiple sclerosis and for the elderly.

After prepping the face with alcohol and draping with a sterile towel, the surgeon marks Hartel coordinates on the face with a sterile marking pen. These are points just below the medial aspect of the pupil, on the zygoma 3 cm anterior to the tragus, and 2.5–3 cm lateral to the angle of the mouth. At the point lateral to the angle of the mouth, the surgeon inserts the cannula (Radionics) with 7 mm of uninsulated tip and directs it towards the foramen ovale.

Hartel coordinates and submentovertex and lateral skull radiographs are guides for cannula placement. Approximate target points are the midpoint of the foramen ovale as seen on the submentovertex radiograph and the clivus at its junction with the petrous bone as viewed on the lateral skull film. When position is proper, as verified by both radiographic projections, the surgeon (or anesthesiologist) induces slumber with intravenous medications and advances the cannula through the foramen ovale.

Final placement is between 5 mm anterior and 5 mm posterior to the clivus. First- or second-division lesions are easier to make if the cannula goes through the anteromedial half of the foramen ovale.

The patient's response to brief low-voltage stimulation confirms precise localization to a specific trigeminal division. By advancing the cannula deeper, the surgeon can often move it from third to second or first division.

In the original descriptions of the procedure, the surgeon made small incremental lesions until analgesia developed in the division of the triggered pain (21). Because this may cause too much analgesia and hypoesthesia, with an added risk of anesthesia dolorosa, it is better to make a more modest lesion. Heating for 65° C for 60 sec will often relieve pain and will rarely cause anesthesia dolorosa or unwanted corneal anesthesia, although recurrence is more likely following such a denervation (23).

When properly done, RFE is an extremely safe and effective treatment. Patients go home from the hospital a couple of hours after the procedure. Major complications with permanent morbidity are rare and have not occurred at all in a consecutive series of 723 procedures done by myself between 1976 and 1992.

RFE is not totally without risk of major complications (24). Infection may rarely occur, causing meningitis and/or brain abscess. Early suspicion and diagnosis of meningitis by cerebrospinal fluid (CSF) examination followed by vigorous treatment with appropriate antibiotics will minimize and usually prevent permanent sequelae. A few intracerebral hemorrhages associated with hypertension have also occurred during RFE (25). Careful monitoring of blood pressure and early treatment with intravenous medication can lessen the likelihood of this unusual development.

Glycerol

Glycerol injected into the retrogasserian subarachnoid space may provide relief of trigeminal neuralgia pain (26, 27). The initial technique for needle placement is similar to that used with RFE. For final localization, the surgeon may use water-soluble contrast material to define the size of the gasserian cistern (26) or the patient's response to electrical stimulation (28). Although small doses of glycerol (0.15–0.25 ml) rarely cause profound analgesia or anesthesia dolorosa, larger doses may produce both of these.

By being prepared to use either RFE or glycerol or perhaps both, the surgeon may maximize the effectiveness of either method and minimize the risk of complications (29, 30). If the response to electrical stimulation is in the desired division, one makes a modest RFE (65° C for 60 sec). If analgesia does not develop, there are three options: make another RF lesion (70–75° C for 30–45 sec), add a small dose of glycerol, or do nothing further. A free flow of CSF is a favorable situation for the use of glycerol. Patients who are fearful of postoperative dysesthesias or those who are difficult to examine for hypoalgesia are good candidates for no further lesioning. Sometimes the response to stimulation is not in the desired division. A deeper or more medial cannula position may facilitate a second- or first-division lesion. These maneuvers are not always successful. If CSF returns from the cannula, 0.25 ml of glycerol may give a good result; one may also add a light RFE (60–65° C for 30–45 sec).

Unwanted first division anesthesia may develop unexpectedly when the cannula is posterior to the clivus or stimulation produces a second- or first-division sensation. Smaller incremental lesions are needed, and the initial RFE should be at 55–60° C for 15 or 20 seconds. The surgeon should make further denervation at the same electrode position only after testing the awakened patient and noting the absence of first-division hypoalgesia.

In my experience with 520 patients with trigeminal neuralgia treated between 1976 and 1992 with percutaneous RFE with or without glycerol, I have found that 29% of the patients have required more that one procedure. Those who are younger at the time of the first procedure and those who live for a longer period are more likely to require another procedure. Of the first 157 patients (between 1976 and 1983), when I made a more denervating lesion, major dysesthesias occurred in 8% and keratitis in 2% (31). Between 1983 and 1992, patients received a milder denervation. Major dysesthesias occurred in only 2.5% of 366 patients, and none developed keratitis.

It is important to make the patient comfortable during the RFE/glycerol procedure. This will make patients more willing to undergo this procedure initially and subsequently if recurrence develops. It also provides better working conditions for the surgeon. Originally, I used intravenous fentanyl, droperidol, and methohexital to give the patient sedation and analgesia during the procedure. The early literature mentions these medications, and they became the anesthetic standard (21). More recently, I have found that patients are much more comfortable when they are premedicated with oral diazepam and given high doses of midazolam (average of 5.5 mg) as well as fentanyl and methohexital (32). A small dose of droperidol (1.25 mg) at the beginning of the procedure prevents nausea or vomiting.

During the percutaneous approach to the gasserian ganglion and retrogasserian rootlets, hemodynamic changes such as hypertension, tachycardia, and bradycardia often occur, especially when the cannula penetrates the foramen ovale or heats the nerve. Noninvasive monitoring of pulse, blood pressure, and electrocardiogram, and treatment of hypertension with small doses of hydralazine and bradycardia with atropine, can minimize the hemodynamic changes. Respiratory insufficiency may occur from medications given during the

procedure for analgesia and sedation. By using pulse oximetry to monitor oxygen saturation, encouraging the patient to breath deeply, administering nasal oxygen, and supporting the oral airway, the surgeon can prevent hypoxia (33).

Percutaneous Microcompression of the Trigeminal Ganglion

Percutaneous microcompression (PM) with a Fogarty balloon is a newer percutaneous method for denervating the trigeminal nerve and treating trigeminal neuralgia (34, 35). Although this procedure can relieve pain, complications are more common from PM than a moderate RFE/glycerol procedure (24). Percutaneous microcompression requires a larger needle than does RFE/glycerol, and facial hematomas are more likely to occur with PM. The percutaneous microcompression is less selective than RFE, and trigeminal motor loss, though it eventually resolves, occurs much more frequently with PM. The use of general anesthesia with PM also increases the complexity of the procedure and potential morbidity. Bradycardia is common during PM. One must monitor the EKG and have methods to counteract severe bradycardia.

Microvascular Decompression

Another important development in our understanding of trigeminal neuralgia is the recognition that a blood vessel may compress the trigeminal nerve close to its origin from the brainstem (36). This compression may cause trigeminal neuralgia, and decompression of the nerve away from the blood vessel may relieve pain (37).

There are several controversies associated with the above theory. There is dispute about the incidence of such compression. Although some detect it in 100% of patients with trigeminal neuralgia who do not have a tumor or multiple sclerosis (37), others find it in only 11% (38). The significance of the nerve/blood vessel relationship and the etiology of trigeminal neuralgia is also uncertain (39). Investigators have found contact between the trigeminal nerve and blood vessels in many people who do not have trigeminal neuralgia (40). During microvascular decompression, denervation occurs in some patients, and it is not clear how much pain relief is due to denervation, decompression, or spontaneous remission. This is an important consideration for evaluating any treatment for trigeminal neuralgia, no matter how intractable it initially appears to be.

The suboccipital craniectomy with direct exposure of the trigeminal nerve is a major neurosurgical procedure. It requires general anesthesia. I prefer the lateral or three-quarter prone position. The surgeon makes a vertical retromastoid incision and a circular craniectomy that is 4 cm in diameter. It is important that it extend superiorly to the transverse sinus and laterally to the sigmoid sinus. The surgeon waxes mastoid air cells thoroughly, then opens the dura with a cruciate incision.

If a three-quarter prone position is used initially, the table is now turned to place the head in a lateral position. This facilitates gentle retraction of the cerebellum, which is provided by a lightly applied self-retaining retractor. The initial exposure is at the superior lateral aspect of the cerebellum, which the surgeon retracts medially. The operating microscope with 275-mm objective is used.

The seventh and eighth nerves come first into view. The trigeminal nerve is more superior and deep. A narrow brain retractor provides proper exposure. The petrosal vein often has to be cauterized and divided. The arachnoid over the trigeminal nerve must be cut. Sometimes a blood vessel compresses the trigeminal nerve where it exits from the brainstem. This is usually a tortuous superior cerebellar artery. The surgeon decompresses the trigeminal nerve by placing a small prosthesis of either Ivalon foam sponge (Unipoint Industries, High Point, NC) or Teflon felt between the nerve and blood vessel. When there is no compression, one cuts the caudal third of the sensory part of the trigeminal nerve close to the pons.

Although the suboccipital microsurgical procedure provides pain relief for many patients, the chance of a serious operative complication is higher than from the percutaneous techniques (24). Under the best of circumstances, the risk of death or severely disabling stroke from the suboccipital procedure is approximately 1–2%. Facial palsy and ipsilateral hearing loss occur more frequently. Thirty percent of patients treated with Teflon felt developed aseptic meningitis (41). Because of this, one should reserve the suboccipital operation for those rare patients who have a posterior fossa tumor, or those few who persist with intractable trigeminal neuralgia in spite of appropriate management with medications and percutaneous procedures (radiofrequency and/or glycerol) (42).

The relative value of different procedures for treatment of trigeminal neuralgia is difficult to assess because of the lack of valid concurrent controls. A number of factors will influence the apparent effectiveness of a given treatment. Results will appear worse if recurrent pain is the measure of treatment failure rather than reoperation. Careful definitions of recurrent pain must specify duration and frequency of the pain and use of medication. The nature of the pain is also important, because patients with an atypical component to their trigeminal neuralgia may have a higher recurrence rate than those with pure trigeminal neuralgia (43). One must compare the degree of denervation (which is difficult to quantitate) in each treatment group, because patients with more denervation are less likely to develop recurrent pain. The duration and thoroughness of follow-up is most important, because the likelihood of

recurrence is directly proportional to the follow-up interval. One way to try to eliminate bias caused by losing patients from follow-up is to calculate Meier-Kaplan survival curves, which estimate probability of recurrence at specific intervals based on the actual numbers of patients available for follow-up at each interval (43–45).

ATYPICAL TRIGEMINAL NEURALGIA

Some patients with triggered paroxysmal pain in the trigeminal distribution have the atypical feature of constant pain that persists in between the paroxysms. Light touch may not always trigger the pain. Medications used for trigeminal neuralgia, especially carbamazepine, often help these patients. If medications do not relieve the pain, then radiofrequency and/or glycerol will often help, although the results are not so reliable as with pure trigeminal neuralgia.

TRIGEMINAL NEUROPATHY

Patients with trigeminal neuropathy show signs of trigeminal nerve dysfunction, such as hypoalgesia or hypoesthesia or impairment of muscles of mastication and deviation of the opened jaw to the side of the lesion. There may also be pain in the distribution of one or more divisions of the trigeminal nerve. This pain may be paroxysmal and triggered by light touch, but sometimes is continuous and not triggered. Dysfunction of other nearby cranial nerves may also occur and may cause impairment of extraocular movement, facial weakness, or eighth-nerve dysfunction. Tumors, infection, granuloma, vascular abnormalities, demyelinating disease, or viral infections are sometimes responsible.

Direct neurosurgical intervention is helpful for removal of intracranial tumors involving the fifth nerve, which are often benign (epidermoid, meningioma, or neurinoma) and may be in the middle or posterior cranial fossae. Peripheral tumors that involve the trigeminal nerve at the base of the skull are usually malignant and are more likely to cause atypical facial pains (6). An otolaryngologic approach usually provides adequate exposure for biopsy. These tumors often respond to radiotherapy.

VAGOGLOSSOPHARYNGEAL NEURALGIA

These patients have paroxysmal pain in the distribution of the glossopharyngeal and vagus nerves: the tonsillar pillars, base of the tongue, soft palate, and external auditory canal (46, 47). Swallowing, especially of cold drinks, or coughing triggers the pain. Triggered pain occurs less often with vagoglossopharyngeal neuralgia than with trigeminal neuralgia. Although patients with vagoglossopharyngeal neuralgia may have paroxysmal pain, they often have a more constant, dull, aching, burning or pressure sensation (48). Infrequently, syncope occurs with vagoglossopharyngeal neuralgia (48, 49).

The incidence of vagoglossopharyngeal neuralgia is approximately 0.04 per 100,000 people per year; that is one hundredth as often as trigeminal neuralgia. The average age of onset of vagoglossopharyngeal neuralgia is a little less than that of trigeminal neuralgia, although the age of onset has been anywhere from the third to the ninth decades (48). Eighty-three percent of patients with vagoglossopharyngeal neuralgia have left-sided pain (48). That is much more frequent than in trigeminal neuralgia, with which only 42% of the patients have pain on the left (50). Multiple sclerosis is extremely rare with vagoglossopharyngeal neuralgia and occurred in fewer than 0.3% of the cases. Brain tumor is much more common with vagoglossopharyngeal neuralgia and was present in 15–25% of patients (51). Approximately 11% of patients with vagoglossopharyngeal neuralgia will also have trigeminal neuralgia (48).

Local anesthetic throat sprays can sometimes provide temporary relief from vagoglossopharyngeal neuralgia. Carbamazepine often helps.

Surgical denervation can provide relief for intractable cases. One can do this denervation by a percutaneous RF technique (52). Denervation of the vagus nerve may produce difficulty in swallowing or vocal cord paralysis. Stimulation of the vagus nerve can cause bradycardia and hypotension. It is important to place the heating electrode in the anteromedial part of the foramen ovale, as confirmed by radiograph, and to monitor the electrocardiogram and blood pressure continuously during the procedure to prevent excessive damage to the vagus nerve (53). The surgeon should stop coagulation at any early sign of vagal impairment; otherwise severe hypotension and even cardiac arrest could develop (54).

If radiofrequency electrocoagulation is not successful, then the surgeon can section intracranially the glossopharyngeal nerve (51) and upper rootlets of the vagus nerve (55). This is particularly advisable in younger patients who do not have other major medical illness. Section of the ninth and upper 15–20% of the rootlets of the tenth cranial nerve provides excellent relief of pain with minimal morbidity (50, 51, 55).

Some have advocated microvascular decompression (56). Microvascular decompression is sometimes done alone or combined with partial nerve section (57). If there is no vascular compression, the surgeon may just cut the nerve (58). Sometimes it may not be possible to decompress the nerves without causing medullary compression. It is certainly preferable in this circumstance to cut the glossopharyngeal nerve and the upper part of the vagus nerve. In one of the early cases of microvascular decompression, the patient developed postoperative hypertension and intracranial hemorrhage and died (56).

GENICULATE NEURALGIA

This is pain in either the ear or the deeper structures of the face, orbit, or posterior nasal or palatal regions (59). Sometimes there is evidence of a herpetic rash in the auricle or external auditory canal, with possible facial palsy, hearing loss, vertigo, and tinnitus. Surgical section of the nervus intermedius may relieve this pain (60, 61).

Some are reluctant to operate on this condition because of the uncertainty of the diagnosis and the possible damage to the seventh and eighth nerves during the surgical procedure (62). Even with the operating microscope, surgeons could identify the nervus intermedius as a separate nerve bundle in only one out of five cases (63).

Perhaps the best possible surgical candidates are those with paroxysmal, intractable otalgia that physicians cannot satisfactorily manage with carbamazepine. One must differentiate geniculate neuralgia from glossopharyngeal neuralgia, which can also cause otalgia. Local anesthetics in the pharynx and tonsillar area may temporarily relieve the pain of glossopharyngeal neuralgia. Some recommend that surgeons perform posterior fossa surgery under local anesthesia so that they can stimulate the nervus intermedius. If this reproduces the otalgia, then section of the nervus intermedius may relieve the pain (60).

It is difficult to operate in the posterior fossa under local anesthesia and maintain the patient in an alertenough state to respond reliably to electrical stimulation. An alternative that one might consider when treating a patient with intractable paroxysmal otalgia is stimulation of the ninth nerve by a percutaneous approach. If this reproduces the otalgia, the nervus intermedius is not causing it. One could also temporarily block the ninth nerve at the same time with Xylocaine or Marcaine. If that relieves the pain, it would further suggest that the ninth nerve is responsible, and RF electrocoagulation of the ninth nerve can be carried out at the same time.

Section of the vestibular nerve (64), geniculate ganglion, and anterior 20% of the diameter of the motor portion of the facial nerve, where there are more sensory fibers, may help otalgia that does not respond to section of the nervus intermedius or of the glossopharyngeal nerve (65). A combined posterior cranial fossa and middle cranial fossa approach for exploration and/or section of the fifth, ninth, and tenth cranial nerves as well as the geniculate ganglion and nervus intermedius may relieve otalgia when glossopharyngeal neuralgia is not the working diagnosis (66).

ATYPICAL FACIAL PAIN

This pain is often continuous, not triggered, and not confined to the distribution of one cranial nerve. It is not usually paroxysmal and may be bilateral. Many symptoms of depression and anxiety are present in these patients (67–69). Atypical facial pain does not respond to carbamazepine but tricyclic or other kinds of antidepressants may be beneficial. Surgery is contraindicated because it does not help and often makes the patient worse (70).

VASCULAR DYSFUNCTION

There are some conditions associated with face pain that are probably a result of vascular dysfunction and that respond to medications for migraine. These include cluster headache, lower-half face pain, and carotidynia. Ergotamine may abort an acute attack, and methysergide, lithium carbonate, prednisone, or propranolol may help prevent further episodes; indomethacin and calcium-channel blockers may also be useful.

Cluster headache may involve the orbit and cheek as well as the head and affects men more often than women. During an attack, there are autonomic manifestations with conjunctival congestion, lacrimation, stuffiness in nasal passages, and occasionally ptosis or myosis associated with facial sweating and ipsilateral erythema. Patients often pace about during a cluster headache. Pain lasts for 20 min to 2 hours and recurs for a varying number of times every day for several weeks, then disappears and returns months or years later. Some have suggested that cluster headache is a form of geniculate neuralgia, and section of the nervus intermedius may relieve it (59, 63, 64). Others have not been able to confirm this. Retromastoid craniectomy with partial section of the main sensory root of the trigeminal nerve and sectioning of the nervus intermedius had limited value in the treatment of cluster headache (71).

Chronic cluster headache is a particularly severe and disabling form of the disease that occurs without remission and that may be intractable to standard medical treatment. Chronic cluster headache has responded well to both percutaneous RF trigeminal gangliorhizolysis (72) and trigeminal cisternal injection of glycerol (73).

Lower-half headache is more typical of migraine, except that the pain is in the face. This condition affects women more frequently than men. The face pain is throbbing and unilateral. Nausea, vomiting, and photophobia may be present. Menstruation and alcohol are frequent precipitating factors, and there is usually a family history of migraine.

Carotidynia is a syndrome of lateral neck pain that radiates to the side of the face. There is tenderness over the carotid artery in the neck (74, 75). The distribution of pain is not in the divisions of the trigeminal nerves, but rather along the branches of the external carotid artery. The pain is usually constant and dull with episodes of throbbing exacerbations. Palpation of the carotid artery aggravates the pain. Turning the neck or swallowing may also worsen the pain.

A painful condition of the internal carotid artery associated with oculosympathetic paralysis and anhidrosis of the forehead is a "pericarotid syndrome" (76). Pathogenetically associated conditions are migraine, cluster headache, infection, trauma, and dissecting internal carotid aneurysm. One of these is present in half of cases. Analgesics rather than vasoactive agents may provide symptomatic relief (76).

INFLAMMATORY VASCULAR DISEASES

Many patients with temporal arteritis will have pain and tenderness of the arteries of the scalp and face in addition to systemic disease, which may present with fever, malaise, anemia, or other protean manifestations (77). Vascular occlusion may cause blindness or infarction of the brain or facial structures. Temporal arteritis affects the elderly, and the sedimentation rate is almost always elevated. Superficial temporal artery biopsy establishes the diagnosis. The surgeon should obtain a large segment of the artery (4–6 cm) because pathologic abnormalities may be confined to short segments. An initial biopsy yielding negative results does not rule out the diagnosis, and contralateral biopsy is frequently positive. Corticosteroid therapy is beneficial.

Patients with Wegener's granulomatosis have systemic vasculitis. They may also have pain of the paranasal sinuses, orbit, or palate (78). Cranial neuropathy, mononeuritis multiplex, and infarction or hemorrhage of the brain may occur. Immunosuppressive therapy with cyclophosphamide is often effective.

REFLEX SYMPATHETIC DYSTROPHY (79)

Facial reflex sympathetic dystrophy may follow trauma to the face. Most of these patients have a constant, burning pain. Light touch makes it worse. Oral medication (phenoxybenzamine), repeated local anesthetic blocks of the stellate ganglion, or sympathectomy provide sympathetic denervation, which is the mainstay of treatment.

POST-HERPETIC NEURALGIA

As in other forms of trigeminal neuropathy, analgesia or hypoalgesia is usually present when patients have post-herpetic neuralgia of the trigeminal nerve. The appearance of vesicles establishes the diagnosis. Post-herpetic neuralgia of the face usually involves the first division of the trigeminal nerve. The pain is continuous and not triggered. Occasionally there is also a paroxysmal component.

Amitriptyline provides good to excellent pain relief in 67% of patients, as demonstrated by a double-blind crossover study (80). The analgesia may be independent of the antidepressant effect. The patient takes a single dose at bedtime, starting with 12.5–25 mg and increasing by half to one pill (25-mg size) every 2–5 days. Doses that are too high may sometimes result in increased pain, which is ameliorated after dose reduction. Patients over 65 years of age should take smaller doses, starting with 10 mg (81). Amitriptyline also helps patients sleep, and it is best to take it before going to bed at night.

Amitriptyline is an agent that elevates both noradrenaline and serotonin and is more effective in relieving the pain of post-herpetic neuralgia than is maprotiline, which elevates noradrenaline (81). Drugs like maprotiline and desipramine, a selective norepinephrine re-uptake inhibitor, may help some patients with postherpetic neuralgia (82), and may be tried when amitriptyline is not effective (81). Mood elevation is not the mechanism of desipramine-induced pain relief in postherpetic neuralgia (82).

Some physicians have given fluphenazine (Prolixin) 1 mg three times a day in addition to amitriptyline, but the possibility of tardive dyskinesia that may develop from the use of phenothiazines (such as fluphenazine) plus the uncertainty of their benefit should temper their use.

Several topical treatments may relieve pain in postherpetic neuralgia. These include capsaicin (83, 84), lidocaine cream (85), EMLA cream (a mixture of lidocaine and prilocaine in emulsion form) (86), aspirin and chloroform mixture (87), aspirin and Vaseline (88), aspirin and diethyl/ether mixture (89), and indomethacin stupe (90). The above treatments have certain limitations. Topical capsaicin often causes a burning discomfort. In a randomized double-blind study, topical capsaicin 0.025% was not superior to placebo in the treatment of post-herpetic neuralgia (91). Chloroform is not readily available and may have hepatic, renal, and cardiac toxicity (89). Application of aspirin and diethyl/ether in the ophthalmic area requires special care to avoid damage of the cornea by the evaporating diethyl ether (89). A study showed that mixtures of ether with indomethacin or diclofenac did not provide pain relief that was superior to placebo (89).

Transcutaneous nerve stimulation is a safe technique and has helped some of these patients (17). It is worth trying although it is frequently disappointing.

Although neurosurgical procedures do not usually provide relief, they may be beneficial if there is a paroxysmal, triggered component in a patient who is not analgesic. Nucleus caudalis dorsal root entry zone lesions achieved pain relief in 67% of nine patients with post-herpetic neuralgia (92). Favorable results following these dorsal root entry zone lesions in patients with face pain did not correlate with preoperative sensory loss. Positive results were more likely to occur in patients with sharp/electrical pain than in those with dull pain. Those with pain in the distribution of one trigeminal nerve were more likely to be helped than those with pain in all three divisions.

THALAMIC PAIN

Thalamic infarction can result in hemisensory dysfunction with agonizing, burning pain in the face as well as the rest of the body contralateral to the thalamic lesion. Tricyclic antidepressants and transcutaneous nerve stimulation (17) sometimes help. The pain may persist in spite of all treatment.

EAGLE'S SYNDROME (ELONGATED STYLOID PROCESS)

An elongated styloid process may be responsible for two clinical syndromes. The first "typical" form occurs after tonsillectomy and includes a sensation of a foreign body in the pharynx, pain in the ear, dysphagia, and a persistent sore throat (93). The second "atypical" syndrome is similar to that described for carotidynia (94). Palpation in the tonsillar fossa precipitates tenderness in the distribution of the symptomatic pain, and local anesthetics abolish the pain temporarily. Panoramic radiographs demonstrate the elongated styloid process. Some have recommended surgical reduction of the styloid process if symptoms are severe (93, 94).

In a more recent study (95), the radiologic finding of elongated styloid process and/or ossification of the stylomandibular or stylohyoid ligaments occurred in about 30% of edentulous patients. There was a statistically significant relationship between facial pain and pain on turning the neck, and radiologic evidence of anatomic aberrations in the styloid-stylohyoid complex. This relation existed only in women and was not present for the other Eagle's syndrome symptoms of pain on swallowing or tinnitus. The authors concluded that the finding of elongated styloid processes is of minor clinical importance.

SINUS DISEASE

Chronic sinus disease does not usually cause face pain, although an expanding mass can produce a dull, aching sensation. Sinus disease is much more likely to cause pain when it is acute. The pain of acute sinusitis is usually in the overlying face, which is often tender. In acute maxillary sinusitis, the patient may feel pain in the eye or teeth. Acute involvement of the frontal sinus causes pain in the forehead, and acute ethmoiditis causes pain in the bridge of the nose and between and behind the eyes. Infection requires treatment with appropriate antibiotics; surgical drainage is sometimes necessary.

TEMPOROMANDIBULAR JOINT DISEASE (96, 97)

Face pain and disturbance of mandibular movement are characteristic of myofascial pain-dysfunction (MPD) and temporomandibular joint (TMJ) dysfunction. The pain is a unilateral aching in the jaw with radiation to the face, ear, temple, and occasionally the lateral cervical or retro-orbital region. Tenderness may be in the muscles of mastication (MPD) or joint (TMJ). In only a few patients with pain, impaired mandibular movement, and tenderness are there organic abnormalities of the joint as demonstrated by imaging techniques. TMJ disease refers to this condition. Degenerative or rheumatoid arthritis, trauma, infection, or neoplasm may cause TMJ disease. Ankylosis or chronic dislocation may be present.

Treatment should usually be as conservative as possible. Massage, moist heat, muscle-relaxing exercises, biofeedback, or psychological counseling may relieve excessive muscle contraction. Dental maneuvers can correct obvious malocclusion. Non-narcotic analgesics, anti-inflammatory agents, antidepressants, muscle relaxants, and minor tranquilizers may be helpful. Some recommend local injections of trigger points in spastic muscles or intra-articular injections. Major surgical procedures on the joint may help those rare patients with very advanced disease.

CARCINOMA

Direct surgical excision and/or radiotherapy may relieve pain caused by malignant tumors of the face. Analgesics, including narcotics, are appropriate if non-narcotic analgesics are not effective and the patient has a limited life expectancy.

Neurosurgical procedures may help patients when medication cannot satisfactorily relieve their agonizing pain. Ablative maneuvers to denervate the trigeminal nerve are appropriate for pain in the distribution of the trigeminal nerve. Pain in the throat or pharynx may require denervation of the ninth and tenth cranial nerves. Interruption of the nervus intermedius may help pain in the auditory canal. Section of the appropriate cranial nerves and dorsal rhizotomies of C1, C2, C3, or C4 may alleviate neck pain. Trigeminal tractotomy and thalamotomy are alternative possibilities. Deep-brain stimulation (ventralis posteromedialis) combines the advantage of a small thalamotomy during passage of the stimulating electrode and the analgesic benefits of neuroaugmentation. Intraventricular infusion of small doses of morphine may be effective in some of these patients (98).

CONCLUSIONS

A careful, multidisciplinary diagnostic evaluation of the patient with face pain may help direct attention to a specific condition (such as infection, inflammation, malocclusion or, rarely, neoplasm) for which there is precise treatment. It is helpful to recognize the paroxysmal, triggered, episodic, and usually trigeminal neuralgic pain, which responds so well to carbamazepine and neurosurgical procedures. The percutaneous radiofrequency/glycerol partial denervation of the gasserian ganglion

and retrogasserian rootlets is an extraordinarily safe and effective procedure for trigeminal neuralgia. *Atypical* is the designation for pains that are constant, burning or aching, not triggered, and frequently beyond the confines of one cranial nerve. These patients are often depressed and may have myofascial or vascular dysfunction. If there is clinical depression, it should be treated. Some chronic orofacial pains, such as those caused by post-herpetic neuralgia, may respond favorably to tricyclic antidepressants even in patients who are not depressed.

REFERENCES

1. Brisman R: Cranial neuralgias and atypical facial pain. In Tollison CD, and Robert S Kunkel, editors (eds): *Headache: Diagnosis and Treatment*. Williams & Wilkins, Baltimore, MD, 1993.
2. Brisman R: Bilateral trigeminal neuralgia. *J Neurosurg* 67:44–48, 1987.
3. Brisman R: Trigeminal neuralgia and multiple sclerosis. *Arch Neurol* 44:379–381, 1987.
4. Rushton JG, Olafson RA: Trigeminal neuralgia associated with multiple sclerosis: Report of 35 cases. *Arch Neurol* 13:383–386, 1965.
5. Revilla AG: Tic douloureux and its relationship to tumors of the posterior fossa: Analysis of twenty-four cases. *J Neurosurg* 4:233–239, 1947.
6. Bullitt E, Tew JM, Boyd J: Intracranial tumors in patients with facial pain. *J Neurosurg* 64:865–871, 1986.
7. Brisman R: Trigeminal neuralgia and brain tumors. In Brisman R (ed): *Neurosurgical and Medical Management of Pain: Trigeminal Neuralgia, Chronic Pain, and Cancer Pain*. Boston, Kluwer, 1989, pp 65–70.
8. Tanaka A, Takaki T, Maruta Y: Neurinoma of the trigeminal root presenting as atypical trigeminal neuralgia: Diagnostic values of orbicularis oculi reflex and magnetic resonance imaging. A case report. *Neurosurgery* 21:733–736, 1987.
9. Blom S: Trigeminal neuralgia: Its treatment with a new anticonvulsant drug (G-32883). *Lancet* 1:839–840, 1962.
10. Rockliff BW, Davies EH: Controlled sequential trials of carbamazepine in trigeminal neuralgia. *Arch Neurol* 15:129–136, 1966.
11. Hart RG, Easton JD: Carbamazepine and hematological monitoring. *Ann Neurol* 11:309–312, 1982.
12. Fromm GH, Terrence CF, Chattha AS: Baclofen in the treatment of trigeminal neuralgia: Double-blind study and long-term follow-up. *Ann Neurol* 15:240–244, 1984.
13. White JC, Sweet WH: Trigeminal neuralgia, tic douloureux. In White JC, Sweet WH (eds): *Pain and the Neurosurgeon*. Springfield, Charles C Thomas, 1969, pp 123–178.
14. Braham J, Saiz A: Phenytoin in the treatment of trigeminal and other neuralgias. *Lancet* 2:892–893, 1960.
15. Court JE, Kase CS: Treatment of tic douloureux with a new anticonvulsant (clonazepam). *J Neurol Neurosurg Psychiatry* 39:297, 1976.
16. Peiris JB, Perera GLS, Devendra SV, Lionel NDW: Sodium valproate in trigeminal neuralgia. *Med J Aust* 2:278, 1980.

17. Dalessio DJ: The major neuralgias, postinfectious neuritis, intractable pain, and atypical facial pain. In Dalessio DJ (ed): *Wolff's Headache and Other Head Pain*, ed 4. Oxford University Press, New York, 1980, pp 233–255.

18. King RB: The value of mephenesin carbamate in the control of pain in patients with tic douloureux. *J Neurosurg* 25:153–158, 1966.

19. Lechin F, van der Difs B, Lechin ME, Amat J, Lechin AE, Cabrera A: Pimozide therapy for trigeminal neuralgia. *Arch Neurol* 46:960–963, 1989.

20. Nugent GR, Berry B: Trigeminal neuralgia treated by differential percutaneous radiofrequency coagulation of the Gasserian ganglion. *J Neurosurg* 40:517–523, 1974.

21. Sweet WH, Wepsic JG: Controlled thermocoagulation of trigeminal ganglion and rootlets for differential destruction of pain fibers: Part 1—Trigeminal neuralgia. *J Neurosurg* 39:143–156, 1974.

22. Tew JM, Tobler WD: Percutaneous rhizotomy in the treatment of intractable facial pain (trigeminal, glossopharyngeal, and vagal nerves). In Schmidek HH, Sweet WH (eds): *Operative Neurosurgical Techniques*, vol 2. New York, Grune & Stratton, 1982, pp 1083–1106.

23. Salar G, Mingrino S, Iob I: Alterations of facial sensitivity induced by percutaneous thermocoagulation for trigeminal neuralgia. *Surg Neurol* 19:126–130, 1983.

24. Brisman R: Complications of intracranial pain surgery. In Post KD, Friedman E, McCormick P (eds): *Postoperative Complications in Intracranial Neurosurgery*. New York, Thieme, 1993, pp 181–206.

25. Sweet WH, Poletti CE, Roberts JT: Dangerous rises in blood pressure upon heating of trigeminal rootlets: Increased bleeding times in patients with trigeminal neuralgia. *Neurosurgery* 17:843–844, 1985.

26. Häkanson S: Trigeminal neuralgia treated by the injection of glycerol into the trigeminal cistern. *Neurosurgery* 9:638–646, 1981.

27. Lunsford LD, Bennett MH: Percutaneous retrogasserian glycerol rhizotomy for tic douloureux: Part 1—Technique and results in 112 patients. *Neurosurgery* 14:424–430, 1984.

28. Sweet WH, Poletti CE, Macon JB: Treatment of trigeminal neuralgia and other facial pains by retrogasserian injection of glycerol. *Neurosurgery* 9:647–653, 1981.

29. Brisman R: Treatment of trigeminal neuralgia: Radiofrequency electrocoagulation with/without glycerol. *Contemp Neurosurg* 8:1–5, 1986.

30. Brisman R: Retrogasserian glycerol injection with or without radiofrequency electrocoagulation for trigeminal neuralgia. In Brisman R (ed): *Neurosurgical and Medical Management of Pain: Trigeminal Neuralgia, Chronic Pain, and Cancer Pain*. Boston, Kluwer, 1989, pp 51–56.

31. Brisman R: Treatment of trigeminal neuralgia by radiofrequency electrocoagulation. In Brisman R (ed): *Neurosurgical and Medical Management of Pain: Trigeminal Neuralgia, Chronic Pain, and Cancer Pain*. Boston, Kluwer, 1989, pp 41–49.

32. Brisman R: Analgesia and sedation during percutaneous radiofrequency electrocoagulation for trigeminal neuralgia. *Neurosurgery* 32:400–406, 1993.

33. Brisman R: Hemodynamic and respiratory monitoring during percutaneous radiofrequency electrocoagulation

34. Brown JA, Preul MC: Percutaneous trigeminal ganglion compression for trigeminal neuralgia. *J Neurosurg* 70:900–904, 1989.

35. Mullan S, Lichtor T: Percutaneous microcompresson of the trigeminal ganglion for trigeminal neuralgia. *J Neurosurg* 59:1007–1012, 1983.

36. Dandy WE: Concerning the cause of trigeminal neuralgia. *Am J Surg* 24:447–455, 1934.

37. Jannetta PJ: Microsurgical approach to the trigeminal nerve for tic douloureux. *Prog Neurol Surg* 7:180–200, 1976.

38. Adams CB, Kaye AH, Teddy PJ: The treatment of trigeminal neuralgia by posterior fossa microsurgery. *J Neurol Neurosurg Psychiatry* 45:1020–1026, 1982.

39. Adams CBT: Microvascular compression: An alternative view and hypothesis. *J Neurosurg* 57:1–12, 1989.

40. Hardy DG, Rhoton ALJ: Microsurgical relationships of the superior cerebellar artery and the trigeminal nerve. *J Neurosurg* 49:669–678, 1978.

41. Jannetta PJ: Trigeminal Neuralgia: Treatment by microvascular decompression. In Wilkins RH, Rengachary SS (eds): *Neurosurgery*, vol 3. New York, McGraw-Hill, 1985, pp 2357–2362.

42. Brisman R: Suboccipital craniectomy and treatment of trigeminal neuralgia. In Brisman R (ed): *Neurosurgical and Medical Management of Pain: Trigeminal Neuralgia, Chronic Pain, and Cancer Pain*. Boston, Kluwer, 1989, pp 57–63.

43. Latchaw JP, Hardy RW, Forsythe SB, Cook AF: Trigeminal neuralgia treated by radiofrequency coagulation. *J Neurosurg* 59:479–484, 1983.

44. Lee ET: Nonparametric methods of estimating survival functions. *Statistical Methods For Survival Data Analysis*. Belmont, CA, Lifetime Learning Publications, 1980, pp 75–156.

45. Piatt JHJ, Wilkins RH: Treatment of tic douloureux and hemifacial spasm by posterior fossa exploration: Therapeutic implications of various neurovascular relationships. *Neurosurgery* 14:462–471, 1984.

46. Harris W: Persistent pain in lesions of the peripheral and central nervous system. *Brain* 44:557–571, 1921.

47. Weisenburg TH: Cerebello-pontile tumor diagnosed for six years as tic douloureux. The symptoms of irritation of the ninth and twelfth cranial nerves. *JAMA* 54:1600–1604, 1910.

48. Rushton J, Stevens JC, Miller RH: Glossopharyngeal neuralgia (vagoglossopharyngeal). A study of 217 cases. *Arch Neurol* 38:201–205, 1981.

49. Bohm E, Strang RR: Glossopharyngeal neuralgia. *Brain* 85:371–388, 1962.

50. Brisman R: Neuralgia of the seventh, ninth, and tenth nerves. In Brisman R (ed): *Neurosurgical and Medical Management of Pain: Trigeminal Neuralgia, Chronic Pain, and Cancer Pain*. Boston, Kluwer, 1989, pp 83–90.

51. Dandy WE: Glossopharyngeal neuralgia (tic douloureux). Its diagnosis and treatment. *Arch Surg* 15:198–214, 1927.

52. Lazorthes Y, Verdie JC: Radiofrequency coagulation of the petrous ganglion in glossopharyngeal neuralgia. *Neurosurgery* 4:512–516, 1979.

53. Isamat F, Ferran E, Acebes JJ: Selective percutaneous ther-

for trigeminal neuralgia. Poster no. 1364. 59th Annual Meeting of AANS, New Orleans, 1991, p 550.

mocoagulation rhizotomy in essential glossopharyngeal neuralgia. *J Neurosurg* 23:575–580, 1981.

54. Ori C, Salar G, Giron G: Percutaneous glossopharyngeal thermocoagulation complicated by syncope and seizures. *Neurosurgery* 13:427–429, 1983.

55. Robson JT, Bonica J: The vagus nerve in surgical consideration of glossopharyngeal neuralgia. *J Neurosurg* 7:482–484, 1950.

56. Laha RK, Jannetta PJ: Glossopharyngeal neuralgia. *J Neurosurg* 47:316–320, 1977.

57. Fraioli B, Esposito V, Ferrante L, Trubiani L, Lunardi P: Microsurgical treatment of glossopharyngeal neuralgia: Case reports. *Neurosurgery* 25:630–632, 1989.

58. Sindou M, Henry JF, Blanchard P: Idiopathic (vago)-glossopharyngeal neuralgia: Analysis of 14 personal cases and literature review. *Neurochirurgie* 37:18–25, 1991.

59. Hunt JR: Geniculate neuralgia (neuralgia of the nervus facialis): A further contribution to the sensory system of the facial nerve and its neuralgic conditions. *AMA Arch Neurol Psychiatry* 37:253–285, 1937.

60. Furlow LT: Tic douloureux of the nervus intermedius (so-called idiopathic geniculate neuralgia). *JAMA* 119:255–259, 1942.

61. Wilson AA: Geniculate neuralgia: Report of a case relieved by intracranial section of the nerve of Wrisberg. *J Neurosurg* 7:473–481, 1950.

62. Stookey B, Ransohoff J: Geniculate ganglion neuralgia. In *Trigeminal Neuralgia: Its History and Treatment.* Springfield, IL, Charles C Thomas, 1959, pp 111–119.

63. Solomon S, Apfelbaum RI: Surgical decompression of the facial nerve in the treatment of chronic cluster headache. *Arch Neurol* 43:479–481, 1986.

64. Sachs EJ: The role of the nervus intermedius in facial neuralgia. Report of four cases with observations on the pathways for taste, lacrimation, and pain in the face. *J Neurosurg* 28:54–60, 1968.

65. Pulec JL: Geniculate neuralgia: Diagnosis and surgical management. *Laryngoscope* 86:955–964, 1976.

66. Rupa V, Saunders RL, Weider DJ: Geniculate neuralgia: The surgical management of primary otalgia. *J Neurosurg* 75:505–511, 1991.

67. Engle GL: "Psychogenic" pain and the pain prone patient. *Am J Med* 26:899–918, 1958.

68. Lesse SE: Atypical facial pain syndrome. *Arch Neurol* 3:122–123, 1960.

69. Weddington WW, Blazer D: Atypical facial pain and trigeminal neuralgia: A comparison study. *Psychosomatics* 20:348–349, 1979.

70. Brisman R: Trigeminal neuralgia and other facial pains: diagnosis, natural history, and nonsurgical treatment. In Brisman R (ed): *Neurosurgical and Medical Management of Pain: Trigeminal Neuralgia, Chronic Pain, and Cancer Pain.* Boston, Kluwer, 1989, pp 25–33.

71. Morgenlander JC, Wilkins RH: Surgical treatment of cluster headache. *J Neurosurg* 72:866–871, 1990.

72. Maxwell RE: Surgical control of chronic migrainous neuralgia by trigeminal ganglio-rhizolysis. *J Neurosurg* 57:459–466, 1982.

73. Hassenbusch SJ, Kunkel RS, Kosmorsky GS, Covington EC: Trigeminal cisternal injection of glycerol for treatment of chronic intractable cluster headaches. *Neurosurgery* 29:504–508, 1991.

74. Fay T: Atypical facial neuralgia, a syndrome of vascular pain. *Ann Otol Rhinol Laryngol* 41:1030–1062, 1932.

75. Orfei R, Meienberg O: Carotidynia: Report of eight cases and prospective evaluation of therapy. *J Neurol* 230:65–72, 1983.

76. Vijayan N, Watson C: Pericarotid syndrome. *Headache* 18:244–254, 1978.

77. Goodman BW: Temporal arteritis. *Am J Med* 67:839–852, 1979.

78. Wolff SM, Fauci AS, Horn RG, Dale DC: Wegener's granulomatosis. *Ann Intern Med* 81:513–525, 1974.

79. Jaeger B, Singer E, Kroening R: Reflex sympathetic dystrophy of the face. Report of two cases and a review of the literature. *Arch Neurol* 43:693–695, 1986.

80. Watson CP, Evans RJ, Reed K, Merskey H, Goldsmith L, Warsh J: Amitriptyline versus placebo in postherpetic neuralgia. *Neurology* 32:671–673, 1982.

81. Watson CPN, Chipman M, Reed K, Evans RJ, Birkett N: Amitriptyline versus maprotiline in postherpetic neuralgia: A randomized, double-blind, crossover trial. *Pain* 48:29–36, 1992.

82. Kishore-Kumar R, Max MB, Schafer SC, et al: Desipramine relieves postherpetic neuralgia. *Clin Pharmacol Ther* 47:305–312, 1990.

83. Bernstein JE, Bickers DR, Dahl MV, Roshal JY: Treatment of chronic postherpetic neuralgia with topical capsaicin. *Am Acad Dermatol* 17:93–96, 1987.

84. Watson CPN, Evans RJ, Watt VR: Post-herpetic neuralgia and topical capsaicin. *Pain* 33:333–340, 1988.

85. Rowbotham MC, Fields HL: Topical lidocaine reduces pain in post-herpetic neuralgia. *Pain* 39:297–301, 1989.

86. Stow PJ, Glynn CJ, Minor B: EMLA cream in the treatment of post-herpetic neuralgia. *Pain* 39:301–305, 1989.

87. King RB: Concerning the management of pain associated with herpes zoster and postherpetic neuralgia. *Pain* 33:73–78, 1988.

88. Kassirer MR: King and Robert, Concerning the management of pain associated with herpes zoster and of post-herpetic neuralgia, *Pain*, 33 (1988) 73–78. *Pain* 35:368–369, 1988.

89. De Benedittis G, Besana F, Lorenzetti A: A new topical treatment for acute herpetic neuralgia and post-herpetic neuralgia: The aspirin/diethyl ether mixture. An open-label study plus a double-blind controlled clinical trial. *Pain* 48:383–390, 1992.

90. Morimoto M, Inamori K, Hyodo M: The effect of indomethacin stupe for post-herpetic neuraliga—particularly in comparison with chloroform-aspirin solution. *Pain Suppl* 5:59, 1990.

91. Drake HF, Harries AJ, Gamester RE, Justins D: Randomized double-blind study of topical capsaicin for treatment of post-herpetic neuralgia. *Pain Suppl* 5:58, 1990.

92. Bernard EJJ, Nashold BSJ, Caputi F: Clinical review of nucleus caudalis dorsal root entry zone lesions for facial pain. *Appl Neurophysiol* 51:218–224, 1988.

93. Eagle WW: Elongated styloid process: Report of two cases. *Arch Otolaryngol* 25:584–587, 1937.

94. Eagle WW: Elongated styloid process: Further observations and a new syndrome. *Arch Otolaryngol* 47:630–640, 1948.

95. Keur JJ, Campbell JPS, McCarthy JF, Ralph WJ: The clinical significance of the elongated styloid process. *Oral Surg* 61:399–404, 1986.

96. Booth DF, Hagens GA, Altshuler JL: Facial pain. In Aronoff GM (ed): *Evaluation and Treatment of Chronic Pain.* Baltimore-Munich, Urban & Schwarzenberg, 1985, pp 131–147.

97. Guralnick W, Kaban LB, Merrill RG: Temporomandibular-joint afflictions. Medical progress. *N Engl J Med* 299:123–129, 1978.

98. Lenzi A, Galli G, Gandolfini M, Marini G: Intraventricular morphine in paraneoplastic painful syndrome of the cervicofacial region: Experience in thirty-eight cases. *Neurosurgery* 17:6–11, 1985.

CHAPTER 24

DENTAL MANAGEMENT OF OROFACIAL PAIN

JEROME D. BUXBAUM
NORBERT R. MYSLINSKI

TRADITIONALLY, DISCUSSIONS of nociception and pain as applied to the orofacial area have been fragmented and to a degree confusing. Part of the problem stems from the fact that some pathologic entities have, over the years, been given several different names. The more significant part of the problem is due to the inability of the professions to compartmentalize the vast array of pathologies that produce a similar orofacial symptom set. Included in this family of pathologies is temporomandibular dysfunction (TMD). As this is written, well over 100 pathologic and psychological entities have manifestations of orofacial discomfort (1). One of our aims is to attempt to organize this material in a logical and cogent manner so that the physician and dentist can easily use it to the betterment of their patients. To accomplish this purpose the chapter is divided into five sections: (1) physiologic background, (2) temporomandibular dysfunction (TMD), (3) other orofacial pathologies, (4) systemic pathologies, and (5) rare pathologies.

It may seem simplistic to state, but the single most important factor in the management of the orofacial pain patient is proper diagnosis. Yet our clinical experience has shown, and the literature supports the fact, that most orofacial patients have consulted multiple health specialists and have been treated without benefit of a reasonable work-up and diagnosis (2). It is not within the scope of this chapter to discuss diagnostic procedures in detail. It is appropriate to state that most orofacial chronic pain is multifactorial and requires the expertise of a team of health specialists to reach an accurate diagnosis and devise an appropriate treatment plan. This chapter focuses on the dentist's and physician's roles in the management of chronic orofacial pain. It emphasizes the importance of cooperation and interaction between the dentist and other medical specialists in the diagnosis and management of the chronic orofacial pain patient.

On the basis of the above statements, it is not surprising that a significant percentage of these patients have been subjected to nociceptive and/or pain sensations for extended periods. Patients with pain of approximately 6 months' or more duration become classified as "chronic pain" patients. The autonomic, psychologic, and therapeutic responses of these patients are markedly different from those of the acute pain patient. Even the nerve fiber pathway for acute nociception is different from the pathway for chronic pain. Indeed, chronic pain symptoms may persist long after the alleviation of the etiologic pathology (3). Hendler et al. have classified the characteristic differences between the acute and chronic pain patient, and Table 24.1 is a summary of these differences (3).

A discussion of chronic pain is a subject in itself. This statement notwithstanding, some aspects of chronic pain patients are germane to our discussion. Chronic pain patients can be grossly divided into three classes. Class I patients are those for whom a diagnostic work-up reveals objective reasons for their discomfort. An example of this class of patient would be one with an internal derangement of the temporomandibular joint that is confirmed by MRI studies. Class II chronic pain patients are those whose symptoms and history are highly indicative of a specific pathology. Regardless of this fact, the pathology can not be objectively demonstrated. An example of a class II chronic pain patient would be a subject with trigeminal neuralgia. In class III chronic pain patients the source or sources of the patient's symptoms cannot either be objectively demonstrated or logically inferred. Obviously, class III chronic pain patients present the greatest management problems. In addition, class III chronic pain patients have been divided into three subsets. These subsets are malingering, somatoform, and facetious disorders. In malingering disorders the symptoms are completely under the con-

Table 24.1.
Characteristics of Acute and Chronic Pain

Characteristic	Acute	Chronic
Onset	Current	Continuous or intermittent
Duration	Less than 6 months	6 months or more
Autonomic responses	Increased heart rate Increased stroke volume Increased blood pressure Pupillary dilation Increased muscle tension Decreased gut motility Decreased salivary flow Flight-or-fight response	Habituation of autonomic responses
Psychological aspects	Anxiety modified by cortical response; screening tests normal	Increased irritability Associated depression Somatic preoccupation Withdrawn from outside interests Decreased strength of relationships Occupational disability
Other changes	Screening tests normal	Decreased sleep Decreased libido Appetite changes Screening tests abnormal
Responsive to analgesic medication	Responsive	Not responsive

scious control of the patient. These actions are usually done for some tangible gain. In somatoform disorders the symptoms are not under conscious control. Factitious disorders are those wherein the symptoms are partially under conscious control, yet the only apparent purpose of the symptoms is for the subject to remain under treatment (4).

It is reasonable at this point for us to briefly state definitions of nociception and pain. Merskey defined pain as

> an unpleasant sensory and emotional experience associated with actual or potential tissue damage, or described in terms of such damage. Pain is always subjective. Each individual learns the application of the word through experiences related to injury in early life. It is unquestionably a sensation in a part of the body, but it is also always unpleasant and, therefore, also an emotional experience. (5)

There have been several theories proposed over the years in an effort to explain the many clinically observed aspects of "pain." One of these, the *specificity theory,* proposes that a pattern of specific pain receptors in the body tissues project to a brain center devoted to the sensation of pain. If we say that a specific sensory receptor responds to liminal noxious stimulation, it is a physiologic statement. To term this receptor a "pain" receptor is a psychological assumption. The former statement carries

the concept that there is a direct connection from the receptor to a cortical area where pain is received. It further implies that stimulation of the receptor must always elicit the sensation of pain and only pain. At present there is no substantive evidence to support the position that there is a special class of receptor-fiber units that are exclusively devoted to the detection and transmission of a pain modality. Burgess and Perl have discovered a small class of A-delta fibers that are specific for nociception (6). This small fiber group could not begin to account for the vast array of pain responses, however.

Even so, there are a broad spectrum of receptor-fiber units that are capable of responding to tissue injury. These receptors can physiologically be termed *nociceptors,* and their associated fibers *nociceptive fibers.* We therefore have nociceptive receptors but not pain receptors. If nociception is a response to tissue injury, what is pain? Pain is always a psychological event. The impulses in the nociceptive fibers are no more "pain" than the visual impulses from the retina are the perceptual impression of color and pattern that present to us when we have our eyes open. Pain is, in part, the psychological responses to nociceptive perception. Pain can exist without any demonstrable tissue injury, however (7, 8).

Epidemiologic studies of orofacial pain in a number of countries of the world have shown striking agreement. These studies indicate that approximately 50% of

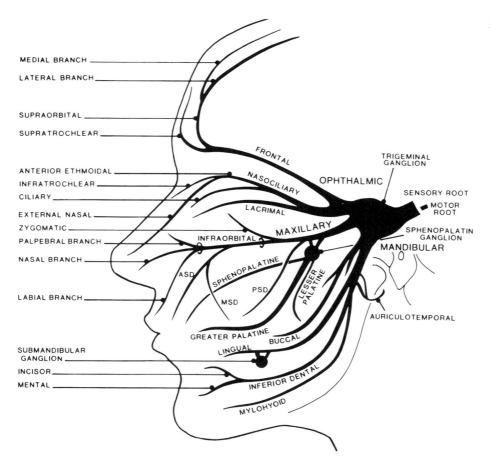

Figure 24.1. **Trigeminal innervation.**

the population displays one or more of the symptoms associated with orofacial pathology (9). More-recent studies have revealed that about 13% of the population have symptoms severe enough to warrant presentation for diagnosis and treatment (10). The problem of chronic orofacial pain is therefore significant in scope and presents major diagnostic and management problems.

PHYSIOLOGIC BACKGROUND

Orofacial Peripheral Nerves

The orofacial nociceptor fibers are found mainly in the trigeminal (fifth) nerve. Other cranial nerves contribute to the orofacial nociceptive spectrum, however. These include the facial (seventh) nerve, with receptors in the deep face; the glossopharyngeal (ninth) nerve, with receptors in the middle ear and pharynx; and the vagus (tenth) nerve, with receptors in the external auditory meatus.

The trigeminal nerve consists of three divisions—the ophthalmic, the maxillary, and the mandibular—each with many important branches (Fig. 24.1). The ophthalmic nerve is the smallest of the three divisions and has three main branches: the lacrimal, nasociliary, and frontal nerves. The branches of the maxillary nerve are the palatine, zygomatic, infraorbital, and superior den-

tal nerves. After giving off the nervus spinosus the mandibular nerve separates into anterior and posterior parts. The anterior part gives off the masseteric, deep temporal, lateral pterygoid, and buccal nerves. The posterior part gives off the auriculotemporal, lingual, inferior dental, incisor, and mental nerves.

Orofacial Central Pathways (Fig. 24.2)

First-Order Neurons

There are many similarities between the orofacial nociceptive system and the nociceptive system already described for the rest of the body. The primary afferents of the orofacial region have nonmyelinated (C-fiber range) and thinly myelinated (A-delta fiber range) peripheral processes that function as dendrites. C-nociceptor-fiber units are divided into two classes on the basis of their adaptive response to heat stimuli. A-nociceptor-fiber units have also been divided into two groups on the basis of their location and physiologic properties. For a more complete discussion of nociceptors the reader is directed to any of the recent texts on this subject (10).

The trigeminal nerve differs from the spinal nerves in a number of respects. It has a higher ratio of myelinated to unmyelinated fibers, a higher density of nociceptors

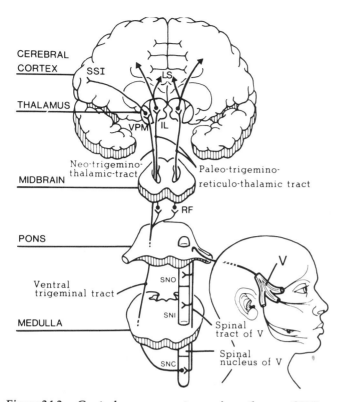

Figure 24.2. **Central nervous system pain pathways. SNC = subnucleus caudalis, SNI = subnucleus interpolaris, SNO = subnucleus oralis, RF = reticular formation, VPM = ventral posteromedial nucleus, IL = intralaminar nucleus, LS = limbic system, SSI = somatosensory cortex I.**

(especially around the mouth and nose), and shorter conduction distances. The last point leads to differences in the temporal dispersion of afferent activity reaching the central nervous system (CNS), which probably accounts for the absence of human reports of first and second pain sensations on the face (11).

The cell bodies of the first-order neurons are small and medium-sized pseudounipolar cells. They are located in the semilunar (trigeminal, gasserian) ganglion of the trigeminal nerve, which lies in a depression on the petrous portion of the temporal bone where it is situated lateral to the internal carotid artery and the posterior end of the cavernous venous sinus. Other afferent nerves associated with nociception in the orofacial area are the vagus, facial, glossopharyngeal, and first three cervical nerves.

The central or proximal processes of trigeminal neurons involved in the nociceptive process enter the brainstem and bend inferiorly to form a part of the spinal tract of the trigeminal nerve. This tract descends ipsilaterally through the pons and medulla to end in the third or fourth cervical segment. As it descends, its fibers pass to the spinal nucleus (or descending nucleus), which lies medial to it. Here they synapse in the substantia gela-

tinosa (laminae II and III) and the more superficial marginal layer (lamina I).

The spinal nucleus is divided into the subnucleus oralis (or rostralis), subnucleus interpolaris, and subnucleus caudalis (medullary dorsal horn). The subnucleus caudalis extends into the spinal cord and merges with the dorsal horn. Nociception is primarily relayed in the subnucleus caudalis, whereas tactile sensibility is primarily relayed in the more rostral subnucleus oralis and main sensory nuclei. Anatomic studies show that the superficial laminae of the subnucleus caudalis almost exclusively receive the small-diameter afferent fibers that can be stimulated by noxious orofacial stimuli. This anatomic arrangement is the basis for the trigeminal tractotomy operation, which is used for the relief of trigeminal neuralgia (12). The operation selectively interrupts the smaller fibers that extend caudal to the subnucleus caudalis but leaves intact the larger fibers that leave the spinal tract earlier to synapse in the more rostral sections of the trigeminal sensory complex. This produces an almost complete loss of orofacial pain sensibility but a less dramatic loss of touch. In the spinal tract the nerve fibers derived from the mandibular division of the trigeminal nerve run posteromedially, fibers from the ophthalmic division run laterally, and the maxillary division fibers run in between (13). This arrangement is constant, and allows for selective cutting during tractotomies.

Tooth pulp afferent fibers are different in that they project to all levels of the trigeminal spinal nucleus (14, 15). Whereas relay through the subnucleus caudalis is important for the transmission of nociception to higher centers, the importance of the relay through the subnucleus oralis and the main sensory nucleus is controversial and much less clear. Tooth pulp afferent fibers may be involved in the localization and discrimination of pulpal stimuli in referred pain mechanisms, or in reflex responses to pulpal stimuli. They may also be involved in non-nociceptive input, or "prepain," because it is now known that pain is not the only sensation experienced in stimulating human teeth, as was once thought. This is especially reasonable since Hu and Sessle found that the large tooth pulp fibers go to the main sensory nucleus and the subnucleus oralis (16).

Second-Order Neurons

There are two general types of nociceptive neurons in the subnucleus caudalis. One type consists of nociceptive-specific neurons that respond exclusively to noxious mechanical and thermal stimuli. The second type are the wide-dynamic range neurons that respond to non-noxious as well as noxious stimuli. Tooth pulp stimuli can activate not only both types of nociceptive neurons, but also the low-threshold mechanoreceptive neurons, which otherwise are only responsive to light touch, pressure, and facial hair movement.

These two types of nociceptive neurons are excellent candidates for the transmission cells described in the gate control theory of Melzack and Wall (17). They receive input from the nociceptive and non-nociceptive afferents, and mechanisms of convergence, central summation, inhibition, and descending control determine what sensory messages are relayed by these neurons.

These nociceptive neurons exist particularly in the superficial (layers II and III) and deep (layer V) parts of the subnucleus caudalis and in the adjacent reticular formation. From these locations some of the neurons connect with cranial motor nuclei or other subnuclei of the sensory complex. Other connections make up two major secondary pathways that cross ventromedial to the contralateral side and ascend to higher centers in the trigeminal lemniscus. These two trigeminothalamic pathways are analogous to the neo- and paleo-spinothalamic tracts that originate from the lower centers.

The neotrigeminothalamic pathway is epicritic in nature. It transmits information concerning sharp, pricking pain that is highly discriminative and localizable. It conveys this information in a point-to-point fashion to the medial part of the ventroposterior thalamic nucleus.

The paleotrigeminoreticulothalamic pathway is protopathic in nature. Its messages are consciously translated as poorly localized sensations usually described as aching or burning pain. It is this pathway that is most involved in chronic pain of the orofacial region. Some of this information goes directly to the intralaminar nuclei of the thalamus. The rest goes to two different zones of the reticular formation. The first zone is the lateral reticular formation lying immediately subjacent to the subnucleus caudalis. The second is the medial reticular formation, which receives convergent high-intensity input from all over the body and is responsible for the alerting response. This processed information is in turn transmitted to the intralaminar nuclei of the thalamus. The fact that input to this area is widely spread is of tremendous importance in the treatment of chronic pain. It means that impulses mediating pain can find a way around any localized destruction that the surgeon might produce.

Third-Order Neurons

The cell bodies of the thalamus and their ascending axons make up the third-order neurons. The axons from the ventroposterior thalamic nucleus pass through the internal limb of the internal capsule and corona radiata to terminate in the inferior portion (face area) of the postcentral gyrus of the parietal lobe (areas 3, 2, and 1). The orofacial region has a disproportionately large area of neuronal representation in the somatosensory cortex, thus producing a high level of sensory discrimination for this region. The intralaminar thalamic nuclei are at the origin of the diffuse thalamocortical projection system, which serves to activate (desynchronize) the cortex.

There are research data on nonhuman mammals to indicate a tooth pulp projection area within the face area of the primary somatosensory cortex. These neurons activated by pulp stimulation are located in deep cortex in the base of the central sulcus, and are of three types: those activated from one pulp alone, those activated from more than one pulp, and those activated from one pulp and its adjacent soft tissue (18, 19).

Electrical stimulation of the cortex in conscious humans does not often lead to a feeling of pain, however (20). Penfield and Boldrey found that out of more than 800 responses to direct electrical stimulation of the cortex only 11 were described as pain and none were of pain in the jaws or teeth (21). It is not yet possible to say at what anatomic level impulses from nociceptive stimuli reach consciousness and become pain. What happens in the cortex is complex and not well understood, but probably pain is localized and interpreted here, innervation densities; however, their numbers are not constant throughout life. A marked decrease in numbers of nerve fibers occurs during root resorption in deciduous teeth, and with age in permanent teeth. Pulp nerve degeneration is also associated with caries and poor dental restorations.

Although most tooth pain is acute, chronic pain can occur in both the pulp and dentin with such conditions as chronic pulpitis or cracked tooth syndrome.

TOOTH PULP

Nerve fibers enter the tooth via the apical foramen. They form a common pulpal nerve and proceed coronally through the radicular pulp, dividing several times. Some fibers terminate in the pulp proper, but many spread out toward the roof and walls of the coronal pulp and branch repeatedly on approaching the cell-free zone of Weil. Many fibers continue into the odontoblastic layer, and some may even proceed into the predentin and dentin layers.

Electrophysiologic recordings from the inferior dental nerve, the trigeminal ganglion, and the tooth itself have revealed that pulpal nerve fibers can be excited by a number of different stimuli, including thermal, osmotic, electric, and chemical (23). It is still not clear whether the response of single pulpal afferents is nonspecific or specific for one form of stimulation.

The response of pulpal nerve fibers to thermal stimulation and evaluated in terms of past experience.

Orofacial nociceptive information is also transmitted to the limbic system, mainly by way of the reticular formation. This system is largely responsible for the affective components of pain, including fear and aversion. Recent studies have used magnetic resonance imaging and positron emission tomography to objectively measure the CNS's response to injury and its associated pain response. These studies showed significantly increased activity in the cingulate gyrus, a component of the lim-

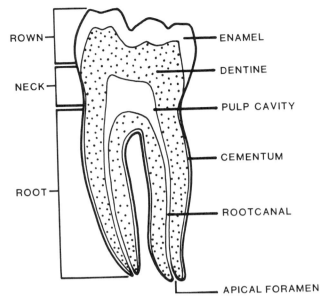

Figure 24.3. **Tooth anatomy.**

bic system. Unexpectedly, this increased activity was only ipsilateral (22).

TOOTH INNERVATION (FIG. 24.3)

The teeth are innervated primarily by the maxillary and mandibular branches of the trigeminal nerve. Muscle nerves such as the mylohyoid may be involved, and may be responsible for the incomplete anesthesia of the inferior dental and buccal nerves. Anatomic observations of the pulp have indicated unmyelinated as well as myelinated fibers. The myelinated fibers are mainly A-deltas, but A-betas have also been found. As for the unmyelinated fibers, there is still no physiologic evidence that they are nociceptive afferents. They may be autonomic efferent fibers that regulate the pulpal vasculature, or the unmyelinated pulpal component of the nerve fibers that are myelinated outside the pulp.

Both the deciduous and permanent teeth have similar innervation densities; however, their numbers are not constant throughout life. A marked decrease in numbers of nerve fibers occurs during root resorption in deciduous teeth, and with age in permanent teeth. Pulp nerve degeneration is also associated with caries and poor dental restorations.

Although most tooth pain is acute, chronic pain can occur in both the pulp and dentin with such conditions as chronic pulpitis or cracked tooth syndrome.

TOOTH PULP

Nerve fibers enter the tooth via the apical foramen. They form a common pulpal nerve and proceed coronally through the radicular pulp, dividing several times. Some fibers terminate in the pulp proper, but many spread out toward the roof and walls of the coronal pulp and branch repeatedly on approaching the cell-free zone of Weil. Many fibers continue into the odontoblastic layer, and some may even proceed into the predentin and dentin layers.

Electrophysiologic recordings from the inferior dental nerve, the trigeminal ganglion, and the tooth itself have revealed that pulpal nerve fibers can be excited by a number of different stimuli, including thermal, osmotic, electric, and chemical (23). It is still not clear whether the response of single pulpal afferents is nonspecific or specific for one form of stimulation.

The response of pulpal nerve fibers to thermal stimulation can be quite effective and is sometimes of a rhythmic nature, very similar to the throbbing seen with many types of toothaches. If a heat stimulus is repeated a number of times, prolonged afferent neural discharges can occur, which may suggest sensitization or damage to the pulp.

Like most other neural afferents in the body, the pulp afferents are sensitive to the chemical serotonin (5-hydroxytryptamine). Unlike the others, however, the pulp afferents are relatively insensitive to such endogenous chemicals as histamine, bradykinin, and substance P. Electrical stimulation is used clinically in pulp vitality testers. Unfortunately, many pulp testers do not deliver reproducible stimuli. The stimuli may also go beyond the pulpal tissue and produce pain by stimulating the periodontium. Nonvital teeth could also therefore respond falsely to the pulp tester. There also does not seem to be any correlation between electrical stimuli thresholds and the extent of pathology in the tooth. Bipolar, constant-current stimulators have been shown to produce less spread of excitation to extrapulpal tissues than the monopolar, constant-voltage stimulators do (24).

TOOTH DENTIN

In the past it has been very difficult to histologically preserve and identify neural elements of the tooth. Distinguishing them from connective tissue and odontoblastic processes has also been difficult. For these reasons there has been a prolonged controversy as to whether or not nerve fibers enter the dentin. Based on transection/degeneration experiments and retrograde transport of radioactive material, it is now accepted that they enter the inner layer of the dentin. There is still doubt, however, about how far they extend beyond that. Also, it is possible that some of these intradental nerve fibers are autonomic efferents that serve neurotrophic or metabolic support functions, and are not afferents at all. Gap junctions have been identified in the odontoblastic zone that may involve neural elements or odontoblasts or both. The existence of coupled nerve fibers is supported by the finding that sending a nerve impulse into the tooth antidromically may result in an orthodromic impulse in another nerve fiber (25).

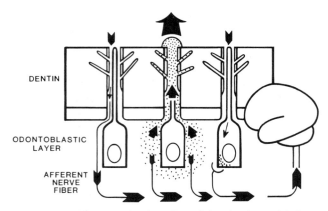

Figure 24.4. **Three main theories of dentinal sensitivity.**

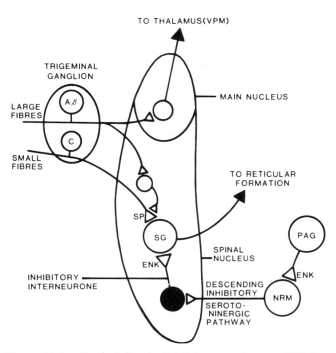

Figure 24.5. **Orofacial pain inhibitory pathways. VPM = ventral osteriomedial nucleus, SP = substance P, SG = substantia elatinosa, ENK = enkephalius, PAG = periaqueductal gray, RM = nucleus raphe magnus.**

Another controversy that has not yet been resolved concerns the basis for dentinal sensation. The neural theory, the odontoblastic transduction theory, and the hydrodynamic theory are all important attempts at explaining the mechanism of dentinal sensitivity (Fig. 24.4). The neural theory assumes that the intradentinal nerve fibers are in fact afferent fibers and that they are the morphologic substrate for dentinal sensitivity to enamel or dentinal stimuli. This is supported by electrophysiologic recordings of dentinal activity that disappears after transection of the inferior alveolar nerve (26). Contrary evidence includes the lack of intradental nerve fibers in deciduous teeth and the enamel-dentin junction, which are both nonetheless clinically sensitive. Also, a number of substances that normally either block or activate nociceptors have no effect when applied to the dentin. The odontoblast transduction theory attributes an active role to the odontoblast, which transmits its own excitation to adjacent nerve fibers. The neural crest origin of the odontoblast and its apparent tight gap relationship with nerve fibers are supporting evidence.

Probably the most accepted theory is the hydrodynamic theory (27). It is based on in-vitro findings regarding pressure changes produced in the pulp and on fluid flow through capillary tubes sealed in the pulps of recently extracted teeth. The theory states that stimuli to the enamel or dentin cause an outward or inward flow of dentinal tubular contents. This perturbation is transmitted to the pulp, causing a mechanical displacement that excites the pulpal nerve fibers. Most painful stimuli, whether drilling, air, temperature changes, osmotic changes, or the like, cause a change in flow. The amount of flow change is not always correlated with the pain, however, and certain substances that do not cause pain cause change in flow. Clearly the controversy is not resolved, and parts of all these theories could be true.

OROFACIAL ANALGESIC SYSTEMS (FIG. 24.5)

As with other parts of the body, the brain's own pain-suppressing systems, whether they be sensory interac-

tions or descending central control, are also effective on orofacial pain (28). Activation of large non-nociceptive fibers can suppress responses of trigeminal brainstem neurons to noxious stimuli. The trigeminal nociceptive neurons can also be suppressed by stimulation of certain brain sites, especially the periaqueductal gray matter in the midbrain and the nucleus raphe magnus in the medulla. The response of nociceptive neurons in the subnucleus caudalis can also be suppressed by local application of enkephalin, which is one of the neurotransmitters involved in descending pain suppression. Many important therapeutic procedures, such as narcotic analgesia, may exert their therapeutic effects by utilizing this natural pain-suppressing system. It is also suggested that dysfunction of this system may be a cause of chronic orofacial pain.

REFERRED PAIN, PROJECTED PAIN, AND NEUROMAS

Referred Pain

Pain that is perceived as occurring at a site distant from the source of tissue damage is known as referred pain. Well-known clinical examples include the left arm pain of angina pectoris and the left-sided chest pain and back pain of cholelithiasis. Referred pain also occurs in the orofacial region and is all the more significant because of the large number of anatomically discrete structures in this area (not the least of which are the 32 teeth).

Although the physiologic mechanism for referred pain

Table 24.2.
Some Common Areas of Referred Pain from the Masticatory Muscles

Muscle	Areas of Referred Pain
Anterior temporalis	Ipsilateral preauricular area and maxillary dentition
Sternocleidomastoid	Ipsilateral preauricular area, ear, side of the face from above the orbit to the angle of the mandible
Trapezius	Angle of the mandible and outer canthus of the eye
Masseter	Preauricular area, area above the orbit, maxillary and mandibular dentition ipsilaterally
Lateral pterygoid	Along the ala-tragus line from the preauricular area forward to the cuspid area ipsilaterally

is not completely understood, there is some anatomic and physiologic information relevant to this phenomenon. The most widely accepted concept is that there is central convergence of multiple afferent inputs with receptive fields covering a wide area of tissue. Evidence supporting this concept comes from a study in the cat that demonstrated that nociceptor-specific neurons of the trigeminal spinal nucleus receive multisynaptic input from high-threshold cervical afferents (29). The most likely explanation of referred pain therefore involves a central summation process. Impulses from the site of injury are transmitted into the spinal cord or subnucleus caudalis where they synapse with second-order neurons of the nociceptive pathway innervating the referred pain site. These referred impulses are then conducted to higher centers and the locale of the pain is perceived to be emanating from the referred area of the body. In most instances both the site of origin and the site of referred pain are found in the same dermatome or are developed from the same embryonic segment.

Regardless of the mechanism, pain referred to and from dental structures is a common clinical situation, and efforts have been made to identify the locations to which pain may commonly be referred in the orofacial region. Wolff electrically stimulated the teeth of volunteers in an effort to identify the sites to which pain from specific teeth may be referred (30). He found that stimulation of the lower posterior teeth produced a sensation of pain extending from the ipsilateral chin to the ipsilateral ear, including the posterior portion of the ipsilateral maxilla. Stimulation of the posterior maxillary teeth produced pain that was perceived in the ear, maxillary teeth and sinus, and temporal region. These results are in basic agreement with clinical experience, but there are situations in which pain may be referred to even more distant sites than those seen experimentally by Wolff. The most common clinical management problem caused by referred dental pain is in the localization of the offending tooth or other dental structure in the chronic facial pain patient. Standard endodontic tests such as percussion, palpation, thermal and electrical testing, and selective local anesthesia are extremely ef-

fective in identifying painful teeth. It is critical that teeth not be extracted without clearly identifying an irreversible pathologic condition. Although a patient may feel certain about the source of his pain he may be mistaken. Extraction of noninvolved teeth may exacerbate the problem by leading to a condition known as the *phantom tooth syndrome*. Occasionally, pain emanating from a pulpally involved tooth will produce a pain perceived by the patient as an "earache" or "headache" rather than a "toothache." It is therefore incumbent upon the practitioner who manages facial pain to either become familiar with the diagnosis of dental pain or call upon a dentist for assistance in facial pain of unclear origin. This may save the patient from unnecessary pain and medical procedures.

Just as pain may be referred from the teeth to other structures, pain from other sources may be perceived as a toothache. Clinical examples of this are sinusitis, cluster headaches, TMD, and periodontal disease. Countless healthy teeth have been extracted because of pain produced in those nearby structures.

Although the pain of angina pectoris may be referred to the left mandible and ear, there is generally associated chest pain. Thus very few patients mistake angina for toothache, yet this may occur (31). The above notwithstanding, referral of anginal pain to the angle of the mandible can be confused with TMD.

After the teeth, the most common source of referred maxillofacial pain is the temporomandibular joint with its associated structures. Although pain from the joint proper is generally perceived as being preauricular, many patients, either because of referred pain or through lack of knowledge of the existence or location of the temporomandibular joint (TMJ), believe they have an "earache" and initially seek medical attention (Table 24.2).

Projected Pain

Pain is most often initiated by noxious stimulation in which non-neural tissue damage is present or threatened. This non-neural tissue damage, through mechanisms yet undefined, causes stimulation of the free nerve endings of the nociceptor, thus initiating the neural signal that travels to various regions of the CNS by means of nociceptive pathways. The pain is perceived (with the exception of referred pain) as originating from the site of the noxious stimulation. A very different situation may occur when peripheral nerves are damaged, however.

When a nerve involved in a nociceptive pathway is injured in any way, including cutting, crushing, ischemia, or burns, one possible consequence is the development of pain that may become chronic. Although the neural damage may occur anywhere within the nociceptive pathway, the pain is perceived as originating in the dermatome supplied by the injured nerve. For example, injury to the cell body (in the trigeminal ganglion) of a neuron supplying the posterior mandibular teeth will produce a "toothache" in the patient's perception, regardless of the health or even presence of the tooth in question. This is known as *projected pain.*

An example of projected trigeminal pain occurs in tic douloureux, in which pathology in the region of the trigeminal ganglion may produce pain perceived as a toothache.

There are several possible mechanisms of projected pain, including neuroma formation, deafferentation, and development of epileptogenic foci.

Neuromas

When a nerve trunk is cut the proximal end begins regrowth in an attempt at reinnervation. To be successful the regenerating axons must find the proper neurilemma tubes and follow them to the original receptive field. If they do not, they may randomly overgrow into a disorganized bundle of intertwined intraneural and extraneural tissue and Schwann cells. These growths are called *neuromas.* The neurogenic pain that results is thought to be partly due to the ephaptic transfer of neural impulses generated by pressing or stretching the nerve tissue mass. This neurogenic pain in many cases is exacerbated by norepinephrine or sympathetic activity, in which case it is called *causalgia.*

Traumatic neuromas formed in scar tissue of the orofacial area usually produce no discomfort except when a certain mandibular movement stretches the affected scar tissue. The nociceptive response is greater in intensity than would be expected from the applied stimulus, and is quite faithful in incidence and duration. There are usually no accompanying sensory or motor symptoms indicative of a neural deficit. There is usually no visible or palpable mass. The pain can be temporarily arrested by a small injection of an anesthetic at the pain site. Sympathetic blockade is sometimes helpful in attenuating the pain, or if accessible, the traumatic neuroma can be surgically removed.

The placement of pressure on a neuroma produces pain projected to the dermatome supplied by the nerve in which it forms. Thus, neuroma formation in the infraorbital or alveolar nerves may produce pain perceived as a toothache. It is important to note that there may be spontaneous or evoked pain in a nerve regenerating properly. This pain generally may be expected to have a duration of up to 6 months.

Deafferentation

There is evidence that demonstrates that extracranial trigeminal nerve sectioning can produce retrograde degeneration of nervous tissue in the trigeminal ganglion and spinal nucleus (32–35). This degeneration includes cell necrosis and glial scarring. It is most prominent in the chief sensory nucleus and the rostral portions of the spinal nucleus and occurs 3–20 weeks after the injury.

Gregg has hypothesized that this central degeneration of neural elements produces an imbalance in the ratio of large sensory fibers to smaller (nociceptive) fibers (33). Therefore, according to the gate control theory, pain may be produced by an increase of the activity of small fibers in comparison to large fibers.

Development of Epileptogenic Foci

Another theory that can be applied to explain the occurrence of projected pain is based on the concept that long-lasting pain signals may be initiated spontaneously or by brief light touch. This has led to some authors to believe that reverberating circuits or epileptogenic foci are sometimes established following nerve injury. Although the exact mechanism by which this takes place is not known, it is believed that the efficacy of certain anticonvulsant drugs (i.e., phenytoin and carbamazepine) is based on their ability to reduce this neural reverberation. It has been shown that anticonvulsant medications reduce post-tetanic facilitation in the trigeminal ganglion, and this may account for their effectiveness in the control of tic douloureux and other trigeminal neuralgias (36).

A different theory that may be explain the phenomenon of pain evoked by light touch is that of neural crosstalk. It is postulated that following damage to a peripheral nerve one of two things may occur. One possibility is that the proximal end of a severed small fiber may regenerate and connect with the distal end of a large afferent nerve fiber, thus producing pain evoked by a light touch (35). Another possibility is that, following nerve damage, activity in the axon of a large afferent nerve fiber may induce activity in a small fiber axon as a result of the neural crosstalk phenomenon (35).

TEMPOROMANDIBULAR DYSFUNCTION AS A CAUSE OF OROFACIAL PAIN

DIFFERENTIAL DIAGNOSIS AND TREATMENT

The stomatognathic system is a closed system consisting of five parts: the TMJ, its associated neuromusculature, the dentition, the periodontium including its sen-

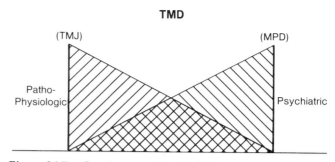

Figure 24.7.   Continuum of pathologies with typical TMD symptoms.

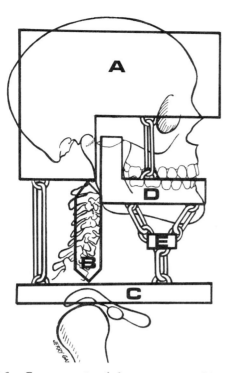

Figure 24.6.   Components of the stomatognathic system. A = skull, B = cervical section of the vertebral column, C = shoulder/sternum clavicular area, D = mandible, E = hyoid bone.

sorineural components, and the cervical-shoulder area (Fig. 24.6). It therefore, in varying degrees, involves all the structures from the skull superiorly to the sterno-cervical area inferiorly. Although the parts are not of equal importance, if present, they must all function within the physiologic tolerances of the patient in order to maintain orofacial health (37). Any change in one component of the system will have an immediate effect on one or more of the other components. These changes may or may not be of a magnitude to produce clinical symptoms.

Temporomandibular dysfunction syndrome is, at present, an ill-defined psychopathologic entity. Over 100 different pathologies may have the typical TMD symptoms of reduced mandibular range of motion, joint noises, myospasm, and pain. In order to organize this material in a cogent fashion it is logical to categorize these entities in a continuum (Fig. 24.7).

The pathologies to the left and right of the vertical lines in Figure 24.7 are discussed in other sections of this chapter. In this section we discuss those pathologies that effect the TMJ and its associated structures. The area at the left side of the continuum within the vertical lines represents pathologies of the articulating elements of the TMJ. Many authors use the term *temporomandibular joint disease* (TMJ disease) to describe these disabilities. Although most of these pathologies may be treated non-

surgically, some require surgical intervention. However, almost all of these joint disabilities will, over time, produce sequelae that result in disease on the right side of the continuum. The right side of the continuum represents neuromuscular-psychological pathologies. Moving from left to right, the pathophysiologic aspect decreases and the psychological aspect increases. In the literature, the term *myofacial pain dysfunction* (MPD) is used to categorize these items. Just as articulating structure pathologies can affect the neuromusculature, however, long-standing neuromuscular pathologies can produce disease in the articulating elements. We believe that the continuum represents a more logical way to visualize all of the interrelated disease entities, and the term *TMD* is a more comprehensive title for this syndrome.

The TMJ is a ginglymoarthrodial (rotating and translating) synovial joint. The articulating components are the condyle, the meniscus or articular disk, and the articular eminence of the temporal bone. The TMJ is a single joint with a bilateral articulation. Therefore, sensory input from receptors in the joint must be centrally integrated in a fashion similar to that of the vestibular sense. Unlike other synovial joints, the osseous parts of the TMJ (condyle and articular eminence) are both convex. This means that the biconcave disk is essential for normal joint function. The articulating bones are covered with fibrocartilage, which is usually found only in relatively immobile joints. Its purpose in the TMJ is to aid in preserving the condyle-disk-eminentia relationship (fibrocartilage is deformable).

Under normal function the condyle-disk relation is maintained by medial and lateral collateral ligaments that bind the two structures together. In addition, under loading, the osseous aspects of the joint deform the disk, producing a mechanical anulus that also contributes to preserving the integrity of the disk-bone relationship. For many years it was believed that the superior belly of the lateral pterygoid muscle was attached to the disk. Recent studies have shown that the superior belly of the lateral pterygoid is not attached to the disk. This muscle is inhibited during mandibular depression. It becomes active near the termination of mandibular elevation functioning to brace and stabilize the articular disk. The disk itself is divided into an anterior zone, thin intermediate zone, thicker posterior zone, and posterior attachment. The posterior attachment is contiguous with a number of otic structures. The disk is thicker posteriorly than anteriorly and medially more than laterally. The functional area is the thin intermediate zone. In function the anterior, then the anterior superior, then the posterior superior aspect of the condyle rotates against this thin intermediate zone as the mandible is depressed. The sequence is reversed in closure. This functional area of the disk is both avascular and aneural.

INTERNAL DERANGEMENTS

Internal derangements of the TMJ are a frequently encountered pathology. The term implies a lack of coordination between the disk, condyle, and the eminentia as described above. The disk tends to prolapse anteriorly or anteromedially. Internal derangements may be self-reducing or nonreducing. In the self-reducing derangement the disk is located anterior to the condyle in the closed mouth position. During opening an audible "click" represents the disk reducing into its normal position. There is almost always a reciprocal click on closure that corresponds to the disk relapsing into its anterior state. The closure click is usually less audible than the opening sound.

The signs and symptoms of patients with internal derangements are usually similar to those of TMD patients in general. These are a reduction in the range of mandibular motion, earache (more precisely pain and tenderness in the preauricular area), joint noises, myospasm, and headache. Some patients complain of a feeling of fullness in the ear. On opening, the mandible will usually deviate or deflect toward the affected side.

If the disk is anteriorly displaced, the condyle will, at least partially, function against the posterior attachment of the disk. This area has both a rich vascular and a rich neural supply. The posterior attachment is capable of fibrotic modification, however. This accounts for the fact that a percentage of patients with internal derangements will be asymptomatic.

Headache is a common symptom in TMD patients. According to Farrar and McCarty retro-orbital headache is also the most common of internal derangements (38). The above statement notwithstanding, headache is such a common symptom that it should not, without other joint signs and symptoms, be a major indicator of internal derangements.

Preauricular pain, often mistakenly reported by the patient as otic pain, is a frequent sign. In fact most TMD patients present initially to their physician believing they have otic involvement. It is essential that otic involvement be eliminated as a cause of the patient's symptom. The TMJ on the affected side is tender to palpation both directly and intermediately. In addition, there are usually multiple myospastic areas in the musculature associated with mandibular movement.

Because one of the cardinal symptoms of a reducing derangement is the reciprocal click, both sides of the TMJ should be auscultated to ascertain if clicks are present. Usually the earlier the click appears in the opening movement of the mandible the more amenable it is to nonsurgical management. If a click is demonstrated, the clinician should have the patient protrude the mandible and repeat the opening and closing movements. In most reducible derangements the click will disappear. This indicates that the derangement has reduced itself. In internal derangements the opening and closing clicks do not appear at the same point in the opening and closing cycle. If the click should appear at the same position in both opening and closing it is indicative of an anatomic abnormality rather than an internal derangement (39). It has been demonstrated both arthrographically and surgically that the opening click is the condyle slipping over the posterior attachment of the disk onto the thin intermediate zone. The fainter-sounding closing click is the condyle slipping posteriorly onto the posterior attachment of the disk.

Presumptive joint derangements can be verified by cine MRI studies or arthroscopic examination. If the only presenting symptom is noise in the joint, no treatment should be initiated. There is no evidence to indicate that clicks will progress into more acute TMD pathology.

The normal range of mandibular motion is approximately 50 mm vertically, 9 mm laterally, and at least 6 mm protrusively. The mandible should open without deviation. In the reducible internal derangement the degree of reduction in these parameters is variable. It usually depends on the extent of associated myospastic activity. The mandible may deviate toward the affected side until the disk prolapses into place and then complete the opening movement in a normal fashion.

In a percentage of patients who have reducing derangements and are not treated, the derangements will cease to reduce. The history would reveal the presence of a click that has now disappeared. There is almost always an increase in pain and a reduction in the mandibular range of motion. The mandible will deviate toward the affected side. This condition is known as a *closed lock*.

The treatment for a reducible internal derangement consists of the fabrication of an orthopedic repositioning appliance that maintains the mandible in a protruded position. Care must be exercised to be certain that there is no movement of the dentition during the period of joint therapy. A number of appliances are acceptable; the reader is referred to any of the texts on TMD management for the details of appliance construction. The myospastic areas are treated with trigger point injections of local anesthesia without vasoconstrictor and the external-use refrigerant sprays such as Fluori-Methane (Gebauer). Muscle relaxants and diazepam-type drugs are of little value. Nonsteroidal anti-inflammatory agents (NSAIDs) have proven helpful in providing symptomatic relief in association with the regimen outlined above. If reduction does occur, an effort should be made to evaluate the stomatognathic system to determine any correctable pathology that may have served as an etiologic base for the derangement.

If there is no symptomatic improvement within 3–4 months of nonsurgical therapy, the patient should undergo arthroscopic examination and treatment. Open-joint surgery should only be considered as a last resort. In the case of the closed-lock patient, arthroscopic studies should be obtained immediately. On the basis of the results of these tests either a surgical or nonsurgical treatment should be formulated. Cine MRI imaging offers an effective means of examining both the hard and soft tissues of the TM joint. It is noninvasive with excellent sensitivity and specificity capabilities. Cine MRI studies are the preferred diagnostic modality for confirming internal derangements of the TMJ. Arthroscopy allows direct visualization of the joint structures. It is an invasive procedure, however, and must be performed with extreme care. Perforations of the disk can only be revealed by arthrographic evaluation.

ARTHRITIDES

A traditional definition of arthritis is a disease entity that exists within the joint itself (40). A listing of arthritides that may affect the TMJ would include (1) osteoarthritis (arthrosis), (2) rheumatoid arthritis, (3) polyarthritis (e.g., gout, lupus erythematosus, Reiter's syndrome), (4) rheumatoid variants (e.g., psoriatic, juvenile), and (5) traumatic arthritis (41). Many authors equate the term *synovitis* with arthritis. This amalgamation of semantics fails when applied to the TMJ. One of the major signs of synovitis is swelling, and this symptom is not commonly associated with this joint (42). In the confirmed arthritic, the dentist's role is confined to restoring and maintaining the stomatognathic system in its optimal state of function.

Osteoarthritis

Osteoarthritis is also known as hypertrophic arthritis or degenerative joint disease (DJD). It is the most common form of joint disease affecting the TMJ (42). In clinical practice, osteoarthritic patients fall into one of two classes even though there may be only one pathohistologic profile of the disease.

In one group the patients are relatively asymptomatic, with the diagnosis of DJD being made rather serendipitously from routine radiographs. The condyle may show lipping or flattening, and Ely's cysts may be pres-

ent. On auscultation, crepitus is discernable. The disease is more often unilateral than bilateral. It is relatively common finding after the fifth decade of life.

The other group of osteoarthritic patients present with a variety of TMD symptoms. These include pain and tenderness over the TMJs, pain in the joint area on mastication, reduced range of mandibular opening, luxation and subluxation, bruxism, otic symptoms, dizziness, headache, deviation of the mandible toward the affected side, and pain and stiffness in the neck and shoulder areas.

The diagnostic work-up should include a complete examination by an otolaryngologist and appropriate blood studies. Cephalometrically corrected tomograms are especially revealing for this type of pathology. Whenever possible nonsurgical regimens should be tried as initial therapy. These regimens include eliminating any discrepancies between the mandibular closure position (dictated by the dentition) and the physiologic position (determined by the joint and its associated neuromusculature), orthopedic repositioning appliances to interdict any bruxing or clenching habits, and nonsteroidal anti-inflammatory medications. Surgical intervention should only be considered if these noinvasive procedures have proven to be ineffectual.

Rheumatoid Arthritis

The role of the dentist in rheumatoid arthritis is rather limited. The principal clinician obviously should be the rheumatologist. Rheumatoid arthritis patients may display limited range of mandibular movement and pain in the preauricular area. The clinician should be aware of patients who have developed an "open bite" in the anterior area. This sign can indicate the presence of rheumatoid arthritis in the TMJ. Open bites should not be corrected either surgically or by occlusal equilibration until rheumatoid arthritis has been completely eliminated as an etiologic possibility.

Traumatic Arthritis

Traumatic injury to the facial area may cause a chipping of the condyle without fracture. This condition produces chronic preauricular discomfort often accompanied with a reduction in the range of mandibular motion and some evidence of myospasm. Although a thorough history will usually reveal a moderate trauma to the joint, some patients cannot recall a precipitating event. The diagnosis is confirmed by means of transcranial and tomographic radiographs.

TUMORS

Although malignant tumors of the TMJ have been reported, most lesions of this joint are benign (44). Osteochondroma is the lesion most often encountered. The growth of the tumor produces an asymmetric condyle, and if the lesion is rapidly growing an ipsilateral posterior open bite may develop. These patients complain of preauricular pain on the affected side as well as a reduction in the range of mandibular motion and associated myospasms. When the preauricular area is palpated there is no rebound felt when a tumor is involved. This is opposite to the rebound that is associated with pain of myospastic origin. Diagnosis is confirmed radiographically. The patient should be referred immediately for a surgical consultation.

FRACTURES

Most fractures are of an acute nature and are therefore beyond the scope of this text. An undetected and untreated condylar fracture that heals in an abnormal position will place a strain on the remaining components of the stomatognathic system, however. Although the neuromusculature is capable of adaptation, this capability is not infinite. It will vary from individual to individual and in the same person during his or her lifetime. The reported symptoms are typical of TMD and include pain in the TMJ area, restricted mandibular movement, headache, and myospasm. Nonsurgical therapy to alleviate the strain on the system should always be attempted initially. Only when these nonsurgical measures have proven ineffective should surgical intervention be considered. The nonsurgical treatment plan should include physical therapy, mild stretching exercises, trigger point injections with a local anesthetic without any vasoconstrictor, refrigerant spray (e.g., Fluori-Methane), and the construction of an orthopedic repositioning appliance. It is important in these patients that any imbalance between the dentally dictated closure position and the neuromuscular closure position be eliminated.

NEUROMUSCULAR PATHOLOGIES

If the skeletal, traumatic, neoplastic, internal derangement, and infectious causes of orofacial pain are eliminated, there still remains 70–80% of the patients presenting with typical TMD symptoms (45). These are the patients with active myospastic areas, demonstrable trigger points, referred pain, occlusal disharmonies, parafunctional occlusal habits, emotion stress patterns, and a reduced range of mandibular movement.

The diagnosis and treatment of these TMD patients requires clinicians to use their full range of biologic and clinical knowledge and experience. It is essential to remember that, although a variety of therapeutic regimens may prove to be effective, there can only be one accurate diagnosis. The etiology of these patients' symptoms is usually multifactorial. We also believe that no definitive treatment should be initiated until the clinician has completed the diagnostic work-up and a presumptive diagnosis has been determined. The above statement notwithstanding, it is often necessary to initiate some emergency therapy to assist the acutely distressed pa-

tient. Even if the emergency measures alleviate the acute symptoms, they do not remove the responsibility of the clinician to discover the causes of the problem and to seek their remediation. It must always be remembered that many TMD patients are psychologically labile. It is often necessary to obtain counseling support (conducted by an appropriate specialist) coincident with the physical treatment of the stomatognathic system. The chronicity of "pain" in these patients is an important factor. Many of these patients' complaints originate as part of the "chronic pain pattern" and are not related to actual TMD pathology. These symptoms may continue to be manifested after all pathology in the stomatognathic system has been eliminated. We also emphatically believe that reversible treatments, when indicated, should be the initial treatment modes of choice. Irreversible procedures should be initiated usually only after all reversible techniques have been attempted without alleviating the patient's discomfort.

Etiologic Theories

The etiology of TMD of neuromuscular origin is unresolved at present. Several etiologic theories have evolved, however, and most TMD specialists will be devotees of one of these major schools of thought. Deboever has categorized these theories into five groups: mechanical displacement theory, muscle theory, neuromuscular theory, and the psychological and psychophysiologic theories (46).

Mechanical Displacement Theory (Costen's Theory)

The mechanical displacement theory is based on the observation that some TMD patients have overclosures of the mandible. This may be caused by the loss or improper eruption of the posterior dentition. The overclosure of the mandible is thought to place undue pressure on the auriculotemporal and chorda tympani nerves and the eustachian tube. Adherents of this theory place great emphasis on the visualization of equal anterior and posterior joint spaces on radiographic examination. The theory has been challenged on anatomic grounds.

Muscle Theory

The basis of the muscle theory is muscle hyperactivity. The hyperactivity serves as an initiator of myospasm, which then spreads to its primary and secondary referred pain sites. Although there is no basis for refutation of this theory, we believe this theory is narrow and restrictive. It does not take into account other viable causes of the TMD problem.

Neuromuscular Theory

The neuromuscular theory is based on a functional disharmony between the occlusal interface and a physiologic join-muscle position. The incompatibility leads to parafunctional habits such as grinding and clenching of the dentition (bruxism). The grinding and clenching may occur during the waking hours but are most often manifested during sleep. The bruxing habit leads to abnormal contractile states and hence myospastic activity. The theory covers many of the clinical TMD problems that are commonly seen and, indeed, may be the most popular theory. Its major weakness is that it does not explain why many patients with abnormalities in the occlusal interface do not have TMD problems.

Psychological and Psychophysiologic Theories

The basis of the psychological and psychophysiologic theories is that the patients under stress have increased tension and activity in the masticatory and associated musculature. Supporters of the psychological school believe that the syndrome is purely psychogenic and should be treated from a psychoanalytic point of view. Laskin has evolved a psychophysiologic approach to TMD problems (46). This theory states that myospastic activity is the primary cause of TMD symptoms. It is further believed that fatigue caused by tension-related oral habits is the major cause of the abnormal myospastic activity. The theory does take into account the necessity for physiologic harmony between the components of the stomatognathic system as well as the obvious influence that psychological factors have been in the TMD syndrome. At present there are too few data to unequivocally support this theory. We believe that its multifactorial base makes it far more rational than the other existing theories of TMD dysfunction, however.

It can be stated that the myofacial aspect of the syndrome is multifactorial, and there can be little doubt that the emotional status of the patient is one of the most important of these factors. For any lasting improvement in the patient's symptoms, however, all of the components of the stomatognathic system must also be functioning within the physiologic parameters of the patient. TMD has both a physical and an emotional aspect. Both must be accurately diagnosed and both must be treated.

Myospastic Cycle

Although there is a multiplicity of theories, the one common denominator in all of them is the presence of myospastic areas. The origin of muscle spasm is prolonged or abnormal muscle contraction. This abnormal muscle reaction is a response to one or more of three variables: alterations in skeletal muscle length, protective neuromuscular responses associated with occlusal relationships, and/or emotional stress. The two major effects of this abnormal muscle contraction are adenosine triphosphate (ATP) depletion and vasoconstriction. The cycle is diagramed in detail in Figure 24.8.

The cycle once started tends to perpetuate itself. In addition, once a muscle has been subjected to a myospastic episode it tends, for reasons not yet understood, to become more susceptible to future episodes. The nociceptive area may be in the muscle itself or it may be

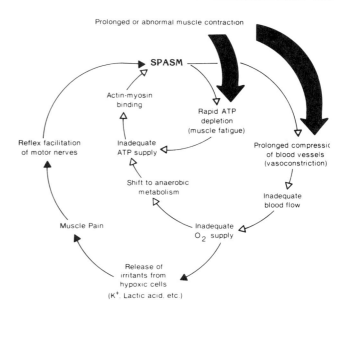

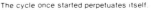

Figure 24.8. **The myospastic cycle.**

referred to orofacial areas. These referred pain sites have been meticulously mapped by Janet Travell, and the reader is referred to her text for exact referred site locations (47).

There are several techniques currently employed to break the cycle. These are refrigerant sprays (e.g., Fluori-Methane), trigger point injections using local anesthetics without any vasoconstrictor, mild stretching exercises, and ultrasonography. It is incumbent on the clinician to discover and treat the cause of the myospasm even if the above-noted measures temporarily break the cycle. Refrigerant sprays combined with mild stretching exercises are often effective in breaking the myospastic cycle. The technique employs sprays such as Fluori-Methane (Gebauer). The bottle is held about 6 inches from the affected area and the spray is applied in unidirectional parallel lines from insertion to origin. The skin should not be blanched. After spraying, the muscles are gently stretched by use of graduated rubber stoppers or tongue blades. The spray is repeated followed by stretching for about 10 additional min. The entire process is repeated four or five times per day.

Trigger point injection of anesthetic without vasoconstrictor is also an excellent technique for breaking myospasm. An aspirating syringe and 30-gauge needle is the usual delivery system. Care must be exercised to make certain not to deposit the solution into the vascular system.

TMD Work-Up

The diagnostic procedures involved in a TMD workup are both numerous and complex. They include a thorough systems review and history, an examination of the oral and perioral hard and soft tissues, a study of the occlusal relationships, measurement of the mandibular range of motion, patterns of mandibular movement, auscultation of the TMJ, palpation of the adnexal musculature of the joint, radiographs, MRI studies, deprogrammed occlusal analysis, electromyographic studies, and comprehensive hematologic tests. It is beyond the range of this work to discuss each of these entities in detail. For additional information the reader is referred to any one of a number of texts devoted to the diagnosis and treatment of temporomandibular pathologies. It is appropriate to elaborate on several basic diagnostic entities, however.

The mandibular range of motion can easily be measured by any clinician. Vertical movement is determined by first measuring the number of millimeters an upper central incisor overlaps its counterpart. The patient is then asked to open as far as possible and the interincisal dimension is recorded. The vertical range is the sum of these two parameters. Lateral excursions are the number of millimeters that the lower center incisors move either left or right from their central position. Protrusive excursion is the number of millimeters that the lower central incisors can move directly forward from their normal closure position. The normal values for these movements are as follows: the left and right lateral, 9.1 mm; protrusive, at least 6.1 mm; and vertical, 50.3 ± 6.9 mm (48).

Joint auscultation is performed by placement of a stethoscope over the preauricular areas and asking the patient to open, close, move left, move right, and protrude the mandible. Note should be made of the presence of any "clicks" or crepitus and where the sounds are detected in the opening and closing movements of the mandible. During opening and closing, the mandible should be observed to detect any deviation from the midline.

If TMD is suspected from the examination, the patient should be referred to an appropriate specialist. Muscle relaxants, tranquilizers, and narcotics are of little value in support of these patients. Symptoms can be temporarily best be handled medically by use of NSAIDs and tricyclic antidepressants.

OTHER OROFACIAL PATHOLOGIES (EXCLUDING THE TEMPOROMANDIBULAR JOINT AND ITS ADNEXAL STRUCTURES)

Although the single most common group of disorders that produce chronic facial pain are the musculoskeletal conditions collectively known as TMD, many other conditions are best treated by medical and surgical means and are not within the purview of the dentist or maxillofacial surgeon. On the other hand, there are some conditions that may best be managed by a combination of dental, medical, and psychological means.

Perhaps the best example of this multidisciplinary approach can be found in the neurogenic pain disorders (neuralgias). These include tic douloureux, post-traumatic trigeminal neuralgia, post-herpetic neuralgia, glossopharyngeal neuralgia, and multiple sclerosis neuralgia. Dental and maxillofacial surgical aspects of the treatment of these condition are described using post-traumatic neuralgia as an example. This condition responds best to these approaches. There are also atypical neuralgias.

POST-TRAUMATIC (POSTSURGICAL) NEURALGIAS

One common source of facial pain is produced by damage to the dental branches of the trigeminal nerve. Although this pain may be caused by infection, sports injuries, automobile accidents, or other accidental trauma, the majority of such injuries are brought about by dental extractions (49) and, to a lesser extent, other oral and maxillofacial surgical procedures (e.g., implants and orthognathic surgery) (50) and root canal therapy (51). The inferior and superior alveolar nerves travel precariously close to the surface in an area where infection, fractures, and traumatic injuries are common (52). These nerves are also subjected to the trauma of local anesthetic injections, which will, on rare occasion, produce a chronic pain condition. Furthermore, third-molar impactions often put pressure on the inferior alveolar nerve, causing some level of trauma. The psychological significance of the orofacial region and the symbolic importance of tooth extraction further complicate the management of post-traumatic neuralgias (53).

The pain of post-traumatic neuralgia may be severe at times. Generally, there is a persistent, nearly continuous low level of baseline pain with episodic bouts of severe pain brought about by the application of moderate to intense pressure to the site of the injury. The baseline pain is often described as deep, boring, and sometimes burning. Such daily activities as eating and wearing of dentures may be extremely difficult. This severe pain is usually described as being sharp. Complicating the pain of post-traumatic neuralgia are paresthesias and dysesthesias, which may also occur. In the event that the lingual nerve is damaged, usually from mandibular third-molar extraction, taste sensation may be impaired ipsilaterally.

Timing is a critical factor in the management of post-traumatic neuralgia, and the prognosis for this type of pain is highly dependent on the duration of the problem at the time of presentation. Acute post-traumatic neuralgias are quite common, and a certain degree of neurogenic pain probably accompanies most oral surgery and endodontic procedures without chronic sequelae. In contrast, chronic post-traumatic neuralgias may persist for decades, and the prognosis for satisfactory recovery from this condition deteriorates after 2 years' duration.

As described in the section on nerve regeneration following injury, several months may be required for complete recovery from peripheral nerve trauma under normal circumstances. Therefore, this kind of pain cannot be considered chronic until it extends beyond the expected healing period, generally held to be 6 months.

The first step in the management of postsurgical neuralgias actually occurs before the surgical procedure is performed. This involves making a definitive diagnosis before planning surgery and informing the patient that nerve damage involving pain may be a risk in the procedures. Those procedures that involve surgery near major nerve branches or extraction of deeply impacted teeth might be expected to produce more neuralgic pain than other procedures, but any oral and maxillofacial surgical procedure can cause this problem. By informing a patient of the possibility (although not a common one) that pain or paresthesia may last for several months following surgery, anxiety is reduced in the event nerve damage does occur.

It is well known that acute pain follows tooth extraction and other surgical procedures. In general, the treatment for this focuses on the use of analgesics, including the use of low doses of narcotics, such as codeine or other narcotic agents. Following the acute phase, however, pain may persist, especially if significant nerve damage took place. This pain is often combined with paresthesias that increase in severity as the nerve heals properly. At this time reassurance and non-narcotic analgesics are the best management techniques. If the pain and paresthesias do not improve or become more severe as the 6-month mark is reached, the pain may be considered chronic and appropriate management as described below should be initiated.

The introduction of the long-duration local anesthetic agent bupivacaine (Marcaine) has added a new dimension to the treatment of post-traumatic trigeminal neuralgias (54). Bupivacaine is an amide-type local anesthetic that is chemically similar to mepivacaine. The concentration best used in the management of chronic trigeminal pain is 0.5% with epinephrine 1:200,000. Bupivacaine is available in either cartridge or vial form. Generally one cartridge (1.8 ml) is sufficient to produce the desired anesthetic effect, but because of its low toxicity, up to 10 cartridges of bupivacaine may be safely administered at one time. Because of the possibility of intravascular injection, however, higher concentrations of vasoconstrictor should not be used.

In many cases, serial nerve blocks with bupivacaine are sufficient to satisfactorily manage post-traumatic trigeminal neuralgias (55). The following text describes the use of serial local anesthetic blocks of the branches of the trigeminal nerve.

During the initial block, anesthesia may be difficult to obtain and additional injections may be required. Along similar lines, the duration of anesthesia and analgesia may be relatively short.

The onset of anesthesia may also be somewhat delayed so that in emergency pain situations, lidocaine should be injected before bupivacaine. The duration of anesthetic action varies widely among individuals, but it generally lasts between 5 and 8 hours. The relief from neuralgic pain usually outlasts the anesthesia, however, with a duration of 12–24 hours being common. A diary should be kept by the patient to document the duration of pain relief and the general intensity of pain during the week following administration of the anesthetic.

At the next appointment (approximately 1 week later), the injection is repeated. This time the duration of neuralgia analgesia is somewhat greater. The injections are then continued in a series of increased intervals between blocks until the injections are required only once every several months.

In some cases, nerve blocks provide only partial relief for trigeminal neuralgias (this is especially true in cases of tic douloureux). Blocks then may serve as adjunctive therapy when combined with anticonvulsant medications (55). Because anticonvulsants may produce severe side effects, which are dose-dependent, the advantage of combined therapy is the reduction of anticonvulsant dosage required to achieve a therapeutic effect.

Furthermore, some patients do not benefit sufficiently from anesthetic blocks, anticonvulsants, or their combination. For these patients, a variety of surgical procedures is available. These procedures can be categorized as being either intracranial (i.e., at the level of the trigeminal ganglion or centrad) or extracranial (i.e., in the peripheral branches of the trigeminal nerve). The intracranial procedures are described in Chapter 23.

Gregg has pioneered the development of extracranial surgical procedures for trigeminal neuralgias (49, 52). There are two basic procedures available on a limited basis at this time: peripheral thermoneurolysis and neural decompression. The extracranial approach has several advantages over the intracranial one. Most importantly, there is no possibility of damaging intracranial contents, especially cranial nerves. There is also the advantage of easier access to the nerve and less discomfort during the procedure.

In this procedure a radiofrequency (RF) lesion is made in the mental nerve, inferior alveolar nerve, lingual nerves, or infraorbital nerve (52). These thermal lesions selectively destroy the nociceptive fibers while primarily sparing the larger fibers. The technique involves the localization of the damaged nerve by electrical stimulation of the needle probe. The probe is then heated to a controlled temperature (60–70° C) for 30 sec. This procedure may then be repeated. Radiofrequency lesions are highly effective in relieving pain without producing significant paresthesia. There is often recurrence of pain, however, and the procedures must be repeated every several years for continued relief in many cases.

Another type of oral surgery operation that may prove

Figure 24.9. Panorex radiograph at the time of presentation of a patient suffering from phantom tooth syndrome. The patient complained of pain in the left maxillary molar region that was not relieved by root canal therapy, apicoectomies, or extractions. In the past similiar conditions existed on the right side of the maxilla and mandible.

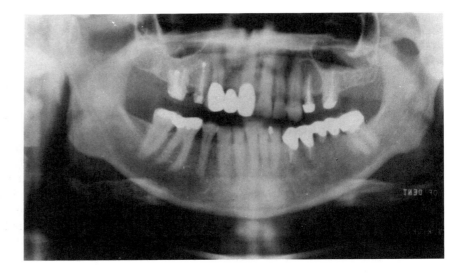

to be effective in those cases in which neuroma formation is a major problem is the neural decompression procedure (52). Such cases may be identified by the development of pain and paresthesia projected distally when pressure is placed over the site of the neuroma (Tinel's sign). In essence, the operation involves (1) exposure of the operative site, (2) removal of any tissue such as bony sequestra that may entrap the nerve, (3) removal of connective scar tissue, and (4) microsurgical repair of the nerve. As more cases are treated in this way, success rates, complication rates, and recurrence rates will be determined.

VASCULAR AND OTOLARYNGOLOGIC CAUSES

There are a number of painful vascular conditions of the face that either produce pain referred to the teeth or may on occasion affect oral vasculature, thus producing a perception of toothaches or TMD pain. These include facial migraine, cluster headache, angina pectoris, and temporal arteritis. These conditions must be recognized, and unnecessary tooth extraction must be prevented.

Likewise there are otolaryngologic diseases such as sinusitis, otitis, and tonsillitis that may be confused with tooth and jaw pain. Of special concern is the linkage, especially in the lay press, of TMD with auditory and vestibular dysfunction. Although treatment of TMD may relieve some ear symptoms, such as feelings of pain and fullness, others (such as tinnitus and hearing loss) are unlikely to improve.

PHANTOM TOOTH SYNDROME

Just as when a limb is amputated, the extraction of a tooth may produce the perception that the missing tooth is still present and perhaps painful (56, 57). The mechanism of phantom tooth pain is similar to that of other projected pains, involving neuroma formation, deafferentation, and epileptogenic foci. One aspect that may be unique to the pain associated with phantom body parts

(including teeth) is the psychological one. This is due to the sense of loss associated with a missing body part, as well as to perceived changes in body image.

In the phantom tooth syndrome there is either persistent pain in a tooth treated endodontically or toothache-like pain in the area of a previous extraction. Because there are potentially 32 teeth, all in close proximity, it is natural for a patient to think that the pain of a phantom tooth actually is caused by an adjacent tooth. The dentist must evaluate this possibility and at the same time recognize the fact that dental pain may be referred from dental and nondental structures. In some cases many teeth receive root canal therapy or extraction if the syndrome is not recognized (Fig. 24.9). There are several features of phantom tooth pain as defined by Marback et al. (58). First, the likelihood of phantom pain developing is greater if the tooth was painful before root canal treatment or extraction. This fact makes it essential to determine when the onset of any pain in the tooth in question occurred. Chronicity may be determined using this onset time as a guide. Second, the pain must persist after proper healing is expected (i.e., the pain must be chronic). Third, there must be pain on the palpation of the area. Fourth, there is often a lack of response to generally reliable therapy such as nerve blocks and analgesics. It is estimated that between 3 and 6% of the population undergoing endodontic or oral surgery procedures suffer from this problem.

Although it is correct to consider the phantom tooth syndrome a type of postsurgical neuralgia, its unique features warrant its designation as a discreet entity with management considerations of its own. One consideration of crucial importance is that a moratorium on further extractions or endodontic procedures should be placed on the patient until the nature of the problem can be addressed. The only exception is when teeth show a compelling need for such work based on radiographic or clinical information (not on the basis of subjective pain complaints alone). Because of the unusual nature of phantom tooth pain this condition may be considered an atypical facial neuralgia (57). Clinical experience suggests that psychological depression is often found in atypical facial pain patients (53). Thus, the management of this problem involves the skillful balance of nerve blocks, anticonvulsant medication, psychological counselling, and antidepressant medication (55). Surgery is not recommended until a thorough psychological evaluation has been undertaken.

Although the dentist is not a psychotherapist, he should be a sympathetic listener with whom a patient may develop a relationship based on trust. From a psychosocial history he should be able to broadly identify the nature and severity of a psychiatric problem and assist the therapist in management of the patient (53).

Phantom phenomena occur in orofacial regions other than the teeth. Phantom tongue has been described (59), and we have seen phantom pain following the removal of a salivary gland and a phantom mandible following hemimandibulectomy. The most commonly seen phantom situations occur following tooth extraction and root canal therapy, however.

One type of dental pain that may be particularly baffling is that due to a fracture of the tooth, and is known as the *cracked tooth syndrome* (60). The diagnosis is made primarily by symptoms amd may be supported by clinical detection of a fracture. Sometimes disclosing solutions may help to identify a crack. The tooth is painful when heavy pressure is placed on it as during mastication of hard foods (61, 62). In every other respect the tooth responds normally to all tests. The pain is of the sharp, shooting type (61, 62). The specific treatment depends on the extent of fracture. The goal of treatment is to prevent separation of the tooth segments by masticatory forces, however, and is often best accomplished by the fabrication of a cast metal crown (61, 62).

Pain from the Salivary Glands

Deep pain of the facial area may be caused by pathologic inflammation of the salivary glands, or *sialadenitis*. It most often originates in the excretory duct, and is caused by mechanical irritation of the duct followed by infection. Less frequently the inflammation results from the spread of infection from the oral cavity or the tonsils. The pain can be localized quite well by manual palpation and the presence of other signs of inflammation.

One of the most common causes of sialadenitis is the obstruction of the duct by calculi, or *sialothiasis*. Salivary stones occur most often with the submandibular duct and gland. When a salivary stone obstructs a duct, eating or other forms of salivary stimulation can increase pressure in the gland until salivary colic results. The pain may radiate to the ear and neck regions. Distention, compression, and mastication can accentuate the pain, and therefore may be mistaken for masticatory pain. If left untreated the stone may occasionally be shed. Some fibrosis may result together with a reduction in salivation. Surgical treatment may be required to remove the calculus.

Other possible causes of salivary gland pain include cystic degeneration, tumor formation, infectious mononucleosis, and neoplasia. With chronic inflammation the gland is permanently enlarged as a result of the exudate and proliferative changes in the stromal connective tissue. Compression interferes with the formation of saliva, and pressure from the fibrosing stroma produces atrophy of the acini.

Glossodynia (Burning Mouth and Burning Tongue)

Superficial, steady, and continuous are characteristics given to the somatic pain of the common oral complaint of glossodynia, or burning mouth and burning tongue. The immediate cause is the abrasive effect of the tissues rubbing against themselves, teeth, or ill-fitting dentures, bridges, or crowns. The location of the pain depends on which tissues are being rubbed anywhere, and this usually corresponds to the areas of greatest movement. The oral examination often reveals a clean hygienic mouth. Sometimes hyperemia, inflammation, and ulceration are seen. Infection of the irritated tissues may also complicate the condition.

Sometimes the complaint is cyclic in nature based on its inhibitory effect on movements. This inhibition permits some improvement of the tissue and decrease in pain. This in turn leads to an increase in rubbing and return of the pain.

Some causes are emotional tension, oral consciousness, dental appliances, and habits such as bruxism and tongue thrusting. One of the most common causes is xerostomia, which is an inadequate quantity or quality of saliva. Many modern medicines such as some diuretics, tranquilizers, muscle relaxants, antihypertensive agents, antihistamines, and other anticholinergic agents can alter and depress salivation. Radiation and the aging process can also depress salivation. Dietary influences and systemic conditions can also affect salivary functioning. An early sign of vitamin B_{12}, folic acid, or iron deficiency can be a pain and burning sensation in the tongue. The tip and margins of the tongue become smooth and red in these deficiencies.

All oral irritants can exacerbate the condition. Acidic juices, spices, hot liquids, strong coffee, and certain mouth washes can all increase the irritation.

This condition can be diagnosed by the application of a topical anesthetic, which should promptly and effectively arrest the pain. Deep or referred pains should not be affected.

Treatment includes the removal of any sharp cusps or sharp edges of the teeth that may cause irritation. It is only necessary to remove small amounts of tissue to restore comfort. Sources of irritation from bridges, crowns, partial dentures, and denture clasps should also be removed. Dentures may have to be adjusted, or new dentures may have to be made. Sliding pressures should be avoided and clasps placed carefully so as to avoid inviting the tongue to play with them. All oral irritants should be avoided.

Possible dietary causes should be considered, and any nutritional deficiencies rectified. Iron deficiency can be treated with 200 mg of ferrous sulfate twice daily, or folic acid deficiency with 5 mg of folic acid once a day. Artificial saliva, or *sialogogues*, can be used to reduce xerostomia. Psychological problems should be considered and stressful situations avoided or reduced. The patient should be reassured that the tongue symptoms do not indicate cancer. Despite all treatment, however, sometimes the pain persists. Fortunately, a relatively large percentage of these patients eventually exhibit spontaneous recovery.

Herpes Simplex

The herpes simplex viruses are usually divided into type 1 and type 2 viruses. The distinction between the infections caused by these two types of viruses, however, are not exact. There is overlap regarding the anatomic sites and clinical features.

Mucocutaneous lesions of the mouth and face are usually caused by herpes simplex type 1. The virus is virtually ubiquitous in the general population, and most individuals have prior exposure and some partial immunity. A primary infection called *acute herpetic stomatitis* may occur in life. There is malaise, raised temperature, and submandibular lymphadenitis. Vesicles occur and break down to form ulcers. The condition resolves itself in about 10 days. Primary infections can also be subclinical, but in both cases the individual continues to harbor the virus for life. Any patient debilitation can lead to outbreaks of herpes in the form of cold sores or fever blisters, usually on or near the lips. The first sign is a slight prodromal burning or tingling sensation followed by the formation of vesicles. These break down and become crusted over. Although the surface heals it can break down again because of the movement of the lips.

For the treatment of *primary* infections due to herpes simplex, acyclovir, an antiviral agent, appears to be significantly beneficial. Local therapy to ameliorate symptoms may include topical anesthetics such as viscous xylocaine or protective emollient mixtures such as Orabase (Hoyt). Bed rest, maintenance of adequate fluid intake, and a soft diet supplemented by proteins are recommended. Acetaminophen may also be used.

In the treatment of *secondary* or recurrent oral-labial herpetic lesions no existing antiviral agents are effective. There are nevertheless other forms of treatment that can be recommended. Symptomatically, bland emollient creams or ointments such as Herpecin-L (Campbell) or Blistex are recommended. The sooner and more often applied the better the results. During the prodrome, if the lesion has already developed, the emollient should be applied liberally as often as convenient or about every hour. Benzoin tincture or 70–90% topical alcohol can be also used. Where secondary infection is evident or likely, administration of antibiotic creams or ointments containing bacitracin, neomycin, or a combination of the two is recommended. Topical anesthetics applied to the oral lesions are helpful, especially prior to meals to alleviate pain while eating. Caustic or escharotic agents, such as phenol or silver nitrate, and topical corticosteroids are contraindicated in secondary herpes.

Type 1 herpes simplex infections are usually more severe in patients with impaired cellular immune functions. A simple blister of the lip may progress to an invasive oral-pharyngeal necrotizing lesion, esophagitis, pneumonia, or disseminated disease. Such patients should be referred for medical treatment.

OTHER SYSTEMIC PATHOLOGIES THAT MAY PRODUCE OROFACIAL NOCICEPTION

Although there are a number of systemic diseases that fall into this category, we have selected some of the more commonly encountered entities. These may be grossly classified into diseases of musculoskeletal origin and collagen disorders.

Musculoskeletal Disorders

Thoracic Outlet Syndrome

Thoracic outlet syndrome represents an abnormal compression of the brachial plexus produced by either a cervical rib or an abnormally tight anterior scalene muscle. At one time it was believed that the syndrome was fictitious, but it has now been validated and is seen in some post-traumatic patients. The symptoms include tingling in the fingers, diffuse pain, and myospasm in the shoulder and neck area that may be referred to the orofacial region. If thoracic outlet syndrome is suspected the patient should be checked for Adsen's sign. This is the absence of a pulse when the arm of the affected side is elevated above the head and the head rotated in the contralateral direction. If Adsen's sign is found the patient should be referred to an orthopedist or neurosurgeon for further evaluation.

Cervical Spondylosis

Spondylosis in its simplest form is defined as degenerative changes in the spine. These changes usually involve the cervical and lumbar regions (30). Although most individuals past the fifth decade of life will have demonstrable degenerative changes in the spinal cord, most of these subjects are asymptomatic. The predisposing factor for pain appears to be the size of the spinal

Table 24.3.
Dental Management of Orofacial Pain Patients

Treatment Modalities	Indications
Analgesic blocking—The use of local anesthetics to arrest pain input, interrupt cycling, resolve trigger point activity, or produce sympathetic blockade.	Pain of muscle origin Vascular pains Other visceral pains Neurogenic pains
Sensory stimulation—Stimulating non-nociceptive afferents to produce pain-inhibiting effects. This includes cutaneous (vibration, counter-irritation, hydrotherapy, vapocoolant therapy), and transcutaneous (TENS,[a] electro-acupuncture) stimulation.	Pains of dental origin Pains of muscle origin TMJ pains Other musculoskeletal pains Vascular pains Neurogenic pains
Physiotherapy—This includes cutaneous and deep massage, exercise, deep heat therapy, and trigger point therapy.	Pain of muscle origin TMJ pains Other musculoskeletal pains Other visceral pains
Medicinal therapy—This includes analgesics, anti-inflammatory agents analgesic balms, antibiotics, antiherpes agents, local anesthetics, anticonvulsants, neuroactive drugs, antianxiety drugs, muscle relaxants, antidepressant drugs, and vasoactive agents.	Cutaneous pains Mucogingival pains Pains of dental origin TMJ pains Other musculoskeletal pains Vascular pains Other visceral pains Neurogenic pains
Surgery—This includes TMJ surgeries such as eminectomies, condylectomies, condylotomies, disk repair and disk plication; and neurosurgeries such as peripheral thermoneurolysis and neural decompression.	TMJ pains Neurogenic pains

[a]TENS = transcutaneous electrical nerve stimulation.

canal. Narrower canals are predisposed to produce pain in the presence of spondylosis. The pain is produced on neck movement and may be referred to the orofacial area. Diagnosis is made by radiographic or magnetic resonance imaging, and the patient should be referred to an orthopedist or neurosurgeon.

Hyperextensive Trauma

As discussed in an earlier section of the chapter, the anterior aspect of the TMJ is its weakest section. Almost all hyperextensive-type injuries, such as whiplash, will produce symptom-producing injury to the joint or its adnexal structures. This injury is frequently overlooked by the physician because of the concentration on the coexistent pain in the neck, shoulder, and back area. It is suggested that all patients involved in whiplash-type traumas be evaluated for TMD as quickly as is practical.

Spastic Torticollis

Abnormal head posture associated with dyskinetic movements of the musculature of the neck are the distinguishing symptoms of this disorder. The etiology is unknown. It has been associated with psychiatric, kinesthetic, ocular, and neurologic disorders. The myospastic activity in the neck produces a profound response in the TMJ and its associated neuromusculature.

The patient requires simultaneous treatment by the dentist, psychiatrist, internist, and other appropriate medical specialties.

COLLAGEN DISORDERS

The proliferative collagen disorders lupus erythematosus and systemic sclerosis may produce facial pain and mandibular dysfunction or complicate the management of the facial pain patient. Temporomandibular joint inflammation similar to that found in rheumatoid arthritis may be a manifestation of the polyarthritis found in lupus and systemic sclerosis. A polymyositis involving the head and neck muscles may also be present. In addition, the skin tightness of systemic sclerosis can cause difficulties in all dental and oral surgical procedures.

Ehlers-Danlos syndrome is a disorder of collagen formation that produces joint hypermobility (among other problems). This syndrome may produce TMJ hypermobility with clicking and popping (61). Such patients are treated in basically the same way as others with TMJ disorders. The prognosis is not as favorable, however, and therapy must be continued beyond the time required by TMJ problems of other causes. Furthermore, excessive strain on the TMJ and other joints must be avoided. TMJ surgery is contraindicated because of excessive scar formation and poor healing.

RARE PATHOLOGIES

Damage to the auriculotemporal nerve produces the auriculotemporal, or Frey's syndrome. This involves a paradoxical gustatory reflex with unilateral burning pain in the temple or the temporomandibular joint area, associated with flushing and sweating when the patient eats. The skin may be hyperesthetic between attacks.

Eagle's syndrome induces a sensation of persistent raw throat, pain and difficulty in swallowing, pain referred to the auricular area, and limited neck movement. This syndrome is caused by an elongation of the styloid process or calcification of the stylohyoid ligament. Encroachment of the elongated styloid process on the carotid artery may produce carotid arteritis and carotodynia. Pain is sometimes referred through the face to the ophthalmic area. This encroachment on the carotid artery can also produce syncope when the head is turned from side to side. Diagnosis is confirmed by means of radiographic examination. Surgical intervention is the only accepted form of treatment.

Ernest's syndrome presents with a symptom set similar to Eagle's syndrome. The etiology of Ernest's syndrome is ossification of the stylomandibular ligament. Diagnosis is accomplished by administering local anesthesia into the area of insertion of the ligament. If Ernest's syndrome is the cause of the patient's discomfort, the symptoms will be eliminated by the local anesthetic. Treatment is identical with the diagnostic regimen, that is, a series of local anesthetic injections into the origin of the ligament. Surgical intervention is rarely required.

CONCLUSIONS

Although the subject of chronic orofacial pain is diverse and complex, we have attempted to present a rational, in-depth, organized discussion of the subject. In closing, Table 24.3 is presented to summarize much of the material in this chapter.

REFERENCES

1. McNeill C: Craniomandibular disorders: The state of the art. *J Prosthet Dent* 49:393–395, 1983.
2. Morgan DH, House LR, Hall WP, and Vamas SJ: *Diseases of the Temporomandibular Apparatus*, ed 2. St. Louis, CV Mosby, 1982, p 73.
3. Hendler NH, Long DM, Wise TM: *Diagnosis and Treatment of Chronic Pain*. Boston, John Wright PSG, 1982, pp 1–20.
4. Fishbein DA, et al: Munchausen syndrome presenting with chronic pain. *Pain* 35:91–94, 1988.
5. Merskey H: Pain terms: A list with definitions and notes on usage. Recommended by the IASP Subcommittee on Taxonomy. *Pain* 6:249–252, 1979.
6. Burgess PR, Perl ER: Myelinated afferent fibers responding specifically to noxious stimulation of the skin. *J Physical (London)* 190:541–562, 1967.
7. Weisenberg M (ed): *Pain, Clinical and Experimental Perspectives*. St. Louis, CV Mosby, 1975, p 132.
8. Buxbaum JD, Myslinski NR, Myers DE: *The Physiology, Pathophysiology, Diagnosis and Treatment of Temporomandibular Dysfunction and Related Pain*. Baltimore, University of Maryland, 2nd Edition, 1990.
9. Solberg WK, Clark GT: *Temporomandibular Joint Problems*. Chicago, Quintessence, 1980, p 17.
10. Duckro PW, Tait RC, Margolis RB, and Deshields TL: Prevalence of TMD symptoms in a large metropolitan area. *Cranio* 8:131–138, 1990.
11. Dubner R, Sessle BJ, Storey AT: *The Neural Basis of Oral and Facial Function*. New York, Plenum Press, 1978, pp 9–55.
12. Dubner R, Gobel S, Price DD: Peripheral and central trigeminal "pain" pathways. In Bonica JJ, Albe-Fessard D (eds): *Advances in Pain Research and Therapy*. New York, Raven, 1976, pp 137–148.
13. Kunc Z: Significance of fresh anatomic data on spinal trigeminal tract for possibility of selective tractotomies. In Knighton RS, Dumke PR (eds): *Pain*. London, Churchill Livingstone, 1966, pp 351–363.
14. Greenwood F: An electrophysiological study of the central connections of primary afferent nerve fibers from the dental pulp in the cat. *Arch Oral Biol* 18:771–785, 1973.
15. Vyklicky L, Keller O, Jastreboff P, et al: Spinal trigeminal tractotomy and nociceptive reactions evoked by tooth pulp stimulation in the cat. *J Physiol (Paris)* 73:379–386, 1977.
16. Hu JW, Sessle BJ: Trigeminal nociceptive and nonnociceptive neurons: Brain stem intranuclear projections and modulation by orofacial, periaqueductal gray and nucleus raphe magnus stimuli. *Brain Res* 170:547–552, 1979.
17. Melzack R, Wall PD: Pain mechanisms: A new theory. *Science* 150:971–979, 1965.
18. Anderson SA, Keller O, Roos A, et al: Cortical projection of tooth pulp afferents in the cat. In Anderson DJ, Matthews B (eds): *Pain in the Trigeminal Region*. Amsterdam, Elsevier/North Holland, 1977, pp 355–364.
19. Biedenbach MA, Van Hassel HJ, Brown AC: Tooth pulp-driven neurons in the somatosensory cortex of primates: Role in pain mechanisms including a review of the literature. *Pain* 7:31–50, 1979.
20. Albe-Fossard D: Central nervous mechanisms involved in pain and analgesia. In Lim RKS, Armstrong D, Pardo EG (eds): *Pharmacology of Pain*. Oxford, Pergamon Press, 1968, pp 131–168.
21. Penfield W, Boldrey R: Somatic motor and sensory representation in the cerebral cortex of man as studied by electrical stimulation. *Brain* 60:389–443, 1937.
22. Busbaum JA: *Imaging Pain. Frontiers of Pain Research in the Decade of the Brain*. National Academy of Sciences, Washington, DC, 1992, pp 50–60.
23. Matthews B: Responses of intradental nerves to electrical and thermal stimulation of teeth in dogs. *J Physiol (Lond)* 264:641–664, 1977.
24. Matthews B, Searle BN: Some observations on pulp testers. *Br Dent J* 137:307–312, 1974.
25. Matthews B, Holland GR: Couplings between nerves in teeth. *Brain Res* 98:354–358, 1975.

26. Scott D Jr: The arousal and suppression of pain in the tooth. *Int Dent J* 22:30–32, 1972.

27. Brannstrom M, Astrom A: The hydrodynamics of dentine: Its possible relationship to dentinal pain. *Int Dent J* 2:219–227, 1972.

28. Sessle BJ, Hu JW, Dubner R, Lucier GE: Functional properties of neurons trigeminal subnucleus caudalis of the cat. II. Modulation of responses to noxious and nonnoxious stimuli by perioaqueductal grey, nucleus raphe magnus, cerebral cortex and afferent influences, and effect of naloxone. *J Neurophysiol* 45:193–207, 1981.

29. Sessle BJ, Hu JW, Ahong G, Amano N: Responsiveness of trigeminal (V) brain stem neurons to cervical afferent stimulation. *J Dent Res* 64:284, 1985.

30. Dalessio D (ed): *Wolff's Headache and Other Head Pain.* New York, Oxford University Press, 1972, pp 463–476.

31. Tzukert A, Hasin Y, Sharar Y: Orofacial pain of cardiac origin. *Oral Surg* 51:484–486, 1981.

32. Tyndall DA, Gregg JM, Hawker JS: Evaluation of Peripheral nerve regeneration following crushing or transection injuries. *J Oral Maxillofac Surg* 42:314–318, 1984.

33. Gregg JM: Post-traumatic pain: Experimental trigeminal neuropathy. *J Oral Surg* 29:260–267, 1971.

34. Gobel S, Binck JM: Degenerative changes in primary trigeminal axons and in neurons in nucleus caudalis following tooth pulp extirpation in the cat. *Brain Res* 132:347–354, 1977.

35. Westrum LE, Canfield RC, Black RG: Transganglionic degeneration in the spinal trigeminal nucleus following removal of tooth pulp in adult cats. *Brain Res* 101:137–140, 1976.

36. Gardner WJ: Trigeminal neuralgia. In Hassler R, Walker AE (eds): *Trigeminal Neuralgia: Pathogenesis and Pathophysiology.* Philadelphia, WB Saunders, 1967, pp 153–174.

37. Buxbaum J, Myslinski N: *The Physiology, Pathophysiology, Diagnosis and Treatment of Temporomandibular Dysfunction and Related Facial Pain,* ed 2. Baltimore, University of Maryland, 1990.

38. Farrar WP, McCarty WL Jr: The TMJ dilemma. *J Alabama Dent Assoc* 63:19, 1979.

39. Helms CA, Katzberg RW, Dolwick MF: *Internal Derangements of the Temporomandibular Joint.* San Francisco, Radiology Research and Educational Foundation, Radiological Institute, 1983, p 34.

40. *Dorland's Illustrated Medical Dictionary,* ed 26. Philadelphia, WB Saunders, 1981.

41. Gibilisco JA: Temporomandibular joint dysfunction and treatment. *Dent Clin North Am* 27:459, 1983.

42. Gibilisco JA: Temporomandibular joint dysfunction and treatment. *Dent Clin North Am* 27:461, 1983.

43. Solberg WK, Clark GT: *Temporomandibular Joint Problems.* Chicago, Quintessence, 1980, p 123.

44. Solberg WK, Clark GT: *Temporomandibular Joint Problems.* Chicago, Quintessence, 1980, p 115.

45. Greene CS: The temporomandibular joint syndrome. *JAMA* 224:622, 1973.

46. Deboever J: Functional disturbances of the temporomandibular joint. *Oral Sci Rev* 2:140, 1973.

47. Travell JG, Simmons DG: *Myofascial Pain and Dysfunction: The Trigger Point Manual.* Baltimore, Williams & Wilkins, 1983.

48. Clark GT, Lynn P: Horizontal plane movements in controls and clinic patients with TMD. *J Prosthet Dent* 155:730–735, 1986.

49. Gregg JM: Post-traumatic trigeminal neuralgia: Response to physiologic, surgical and pharmacologic therapies. *Int Dent J* 23:43, 1978.

50. Rasmussen OC: Painful traumatic neuromas in theoral cavity. *Oral Surg* 49:191–195, 1980.

51. Siegel MA, Van Hassel H: Traumatic neuroma subsequent to endodontic therapy. *J Endodont* 11:179–180, 1985.

52. Gregg JM: Neurological disorders of the maxillofacial region. In Kruger GO (ed): *Textbook of Oral and Maxillofacial Surgery.* St. Louis, CV Mosby, 1979, pp 666–710.

53. Baile W, Myers DE: Psychological and behavioral dynamics in chronic atypical facial pain. *Anesthesia Prog* 33(5):252–257, 1986.

54. Moore PA: Bipivacaine: A long-lasting local anesthetic for dentistry. *Oral Surg* 58:369–374, 1984.

55. Myslinski NR, Myers DE: Drugs used in the treatment of facial pain. In: Holroyd SV, Wynn RL, Requa-Clark B (eds): *Clinical Pharmacology in Dental Practice,* ed 4. St. Louis, CV Mosby, 1988, 392–400.

56. Myers DE: Illustrative case of neurogenic toothache. *Headache.* 125:173–174, 1985.

57. Marback JJ: Phantom tooth pain. *J Endodont* 4:409–419, 1971.

58. Marback JJ, Hulbrock J, Hohn C, Segal AG: Incidence of phantom tooth pain: An atypical facial neuralgia. *Oral Surg* 53:190–193, 1982.

59. Hanowell ST, Kennedy SF: Phantom tongue pain and causalgia: Report of a case. *Anesth Analg* 58:436–438, 1979.

60. Cameron CE: Cracked tooth syndrome. *J Am Dent Assoc* 68:405, 1964.

61. Gibbs JW: Cuspal fracture odontalgia. *Dent Diagn* 60:156–160, 1954.

62. Silvestri AR: The undiagnosed split-root syndrome. *J Am Dent Assoc* 92:930–935, 1976.

63. Myers DE: Ehlers Danlos syndrome as a cause of TMJ disorders. *Anesthesia Prog* 33:23–24, 1985.

CHAPTER **25**

SPINAL SURGERY FOR PAIN MANAGEMENT

CLARK WATTS

SURGERY ON the spine for the management of pain is performed when pain arises from spinal or from extraspinal locations, and when pain is of neoplastic or of chronic non-neoplastic orgin. The surgery is of two types: *(1) Procedures designed to correct the cause of the pain.* An example would be a spinal fusion for pain secondary to chronic instability, or decompressive laminectomy for the pain of neurogenic claudication secondary to spinal stenosis. *(2) Surgery directed primarily to affect pain itself rather than the cause of the pain.* An example is the patient with a chronic "failed back" syndrome or widespread metastatic carcinoma who has an uncorrectable "lesion" requiring the surgeon to, in some way, modify the sensation of pain.

Techniques for pain modification are varied depending on the location of the pain and the neurologic status of the patient. The implantation of a dorsal column stimulator results in no change in the neurologic status of the patient, whereas a cordotomy or a lesion placed in the dorsal root entry zone may result in neurologic changes, both sensory and motor. All of these issues are dealt with in greater detail by other authors in other chapters. The purpose of this chapter is to give a thoughtful, some might even say *philosophical* analysis of the issues that should be considered by physician and patient alike in spinal surgery for pain management.

Surgeons who operate for pain management function constantly under the shadow cast by the dictum "if one operates for pain, pain is what one gets." This underscores the realization by these surgeons that patients who undergo surgery for the management of pain require a great deal of perioperative support, both medical and psychological. Often these patients are medical and psychological cripples by the time surgery is considered. More than one program of nonsurgical pain management has failed. These patients are often drug-dependent and have experienced more than one personal failure, whether it be the loss of family support or a negatively altered doctor-patient relationship.

The support that is required in the perioperative time is not unique to the perioperative state. In fact, if the support that is required at this time for successful management of the patient's pain had been available earlier in the patient's management, it is possible that the patient would not have suffered the failures bringing him to the surgeon in the first place. These concepts can be illustrated using as an example the experience of the patient with the chronic failed back syndrome.

This patient initially experiences an episode of back pain that does not respond to self-treatment consisting of a period of sedentary activity. The patient is then seen by a physician and complains of a nonspecific, but to the patient, disabling back pain, which is not very intellectually challenging to the busy physician. After a cursory examination that reveals little in the way of positive findings, the physician instructs the patient to return to sedentary activity with some medication; the physician makes no arrangements for a return appointment but does suggest that if the patient has not improved in a few days to call or return for another examination.

The patient at this time feels somewhat guilty for taking the physician's time but also feels some anger because at further cost to himself he has acquired little in the way of additional understanding of his problems. The interactions of these complex emotions along with lack of acceptance on the part of the patient's family, and possibly his employer, result in poor compliance. The patient does not improve.

After a few days the patient returns still complaining of the low backache that he now interprets as suffering. The physician at this point, finding nothing in the way of objective evidence of disease, must deal with his own emotional complexities. He is perturbed that his patient isn't better from what he considers a minor problem. There may be a sense of frustration that is transmitted to the patient in one way or another. The physician handles this problem, however, by proceeding to the next step, which is to obtain a battery of studies including blood tests (possibly an erythrocyte sedimentation rate), some radiographs, perhaps even a computerized tomographic (CT) scan or magnetic resonance imaging (MRI) despite finding nothing on the examination that would suggest that these studies will likely provide useful information.

If in fact this is what happens, the physician takes one of several avenues, all but one guaranteeing a continuation of the patient's relentless trip to the pain surgeon. The physician may tell the patient there is nothing wrong, even suggesting that the pain is simply "in the mind" of the patient, and dismiss him—whereupon the patient will seek some other health care provider, and the above scenario is repeated. Or the patient may be referred to a back surgeon, either a neurosurgeon or an orthopedic surgeon. More of this later.

Not often enough, the physician recognizes that he has more than a set of somatic complaints in this patient. He has a patient who needs education and direction. He will properly educate the patient about the biomechanics of the back and the interrelationships between those mechanics and the pain the patient is suffering. The physician will explain carefully, tactfully, and with a great deal of sensitivity the chronic effect that pain may have on the mind and on the patient's outlook on life. A careful analysis of the sociodynamics of the patient's life at home, at work, and at play will be conducted. The physician will develop a management protocol, skillfully incorporating into that protocol activities that the patient will understand and accept as useful to him and, just as importantly, as instructions from a knowing and caring physician. It is the resultant harmony in the doctor-patient relationship that will, as much as attention to the physical needs of the healing backache, guarantee success.

I noted above that one of the avenues available to the physician is to refer the patient to another physician for further evaluation, perhaps even a back surgeon. This is a critical step. In this referral it is important that the physician not suggest *rejection* of the patient but that he communicate an understandable desire to seek what is in the patient's best interest. The back surgeon, receiving the patient who has received unsuccessful medical management from a physician perceived as being insensitive or not knowledgeable, will face a number of pressures from both within and without the doctor-patient relationship, which too often results in the first of a number of surgical procedures not indicated, leading to the chronic failed back syndrome. The net result of these pressure is to bring into conflict noninterventional therapy, which I will call *inactive* and interventional therapy, which I will call *active*. The simplest way to analyze these pressures is to look at each one, and the contributors, individually.

The first contributor is the back surgeon himself. If he

recommends no surgery but rather continuation of the noninterventional or inactive management protocol that has already failed the patient, the surgeon has to admit the inability of his skills to be effective. This admission is hard for most physicians, especially surgeons, because of the general view that surgery is so definitive. The surgeon feels professionally impotent. This drives the surgeon to be less than objective about the "soft" signs that accompany the patient's story. The inconsequential findings on radiograph, CT scan, or myelography carry more weight in the deliberative process. Questionable additional studies such as epidural venography, discography, and the like are interpreted in the favor of intervention. The discrete lesion seen on the MRI scan may be considered dispositive, though there is little objective clinical correlation. Once the surgeon becomes committed, he proceeds aggressively, with his talents and skills, to apply the definitive management, intervention. It is the failure of ill-advised surgery that has driven the search for simpler, less-invasive techniques for the management of these patients, such as epidural and intradiscal steroids, chemonucleolysis, and the currently developing percutaneous nuclectomy. Although each of these techniques is effective in a narrowly defined group of patients, their simplicity and the pressures on the surgeon to intervene have resulted in their use in a wider group of patients, guaranteeing a higher degree of failure. It is this escalating failure coupled with, in some cases, serious complications that has resulted in rapid disenchantment with the procedures by both medical professionals and lay persons alike, and the acquisition by these procedures of poor reputations that may have been undeserved.

The conflict of inactive versus active therapy is contributed to by employers and third-party payers. They perceive the patient undergoing inactive treatment as receiving less than definitive management. They perceive the diagnosis to be uncertain. They are unable to accurately calculate, actuarially, their costs and to know with any acceptable (to them) degree of certainty when they will close the case file. On the other hand, they understand that if the patient has some form of intervention, they can calculate, based on past rates of success of the surgeon and the return-to-work rate of the patients, their costs and work-load scheduling responsibilities. They prefer the latter, apparently more-precise degree of certainty. It was, for example, the support of this group when told of the promises of chemonucleolysis that permitted the rather brief but astonishing degree of incorporation of this procedure into the standard surgical armamentarium of back surgeons. It is felt by some that the uncritical acceptance of chemonucleolysis on the part of employers and insurance companies, with its promise of more-rapid return to work even without promise of significant cost reduction, that as much as any other influence led to its rapid widespread use.

A third group that contributes to the conflict between active and inactive therapy for the patient with back pain is composed of the families and friends of the patient. The back surgeon who prescribes inactive treatment may be perceived by the family as uncaring and as senselessly prolonging the agony of the patient, whereas the surgeon who decides to intervene is perceived as just the opposite. In addition, the family may look on the patient who accepts additional inactive treatment by the back surgeon as being duped, or worse, as wishing to "punish" the family by requiring of them additional attention. Once again, the unknowing family, when presented with the option of active treatment, feels just the opposite about the patient.

And finally, what of the patient himself? The patient is suffering from pain. This is the reason he accepts the advice of the initially treating physician to see the back surgeon. If he learns nothing new about himself, if he receives no detailed treatment protocols by the surgeon, he feels additionally frustrated. He feels that health care professionals generally, and the surgeon specifically, really don't care. This attitude is readily transmitted to the surgeon. On the other hand, if the patient is offered surgery, he feels he is moving toward certain success. He is apprehensive about the additional risks of intervention, an increase in pain, and additional costs he will undertake, but the apprehension itself can lead to a curious reversal of priorities, enhancing the desire for more aggressive, more active treatment. This desire, along with the suggestion that chemonucleolysis is simpler and might get the patient back to work earlier with fewer risks, contributed to the acceptance by the public of this form of treatment.

Once the ill-advised intervention has occurred, failure is almost certain. This leads to additional interventions, and eventually intervention is not being undertaken to alleviate the cause of pain, but to alleviate the pain itself.

Do the ideas and concepts discussed above apply at this point? Yes, they do. Pain and suffering on the part of the patient will tend to push the patient and the physician to more active forms of therapy, to intervention for the pain itself. The same pressures, often with more intensity, come into play. The large number of pain management techniques and protocols underscore the disappointment felt by most who participate in these interventions, whether patient or physician. This disappointment drives the constant search for new means of management such as complex pain programs with biofeedback (nonsurgical) and chronically implanted central-nervous-system stimulating electrodes (surgical).

The thesis of this chapter is not that spinal surgery for pain management is not appropriate. Rather, it is that this surgery should be considered, in most cases, as intervention of a last resort. In some cases, it may be the most humane management technique. The patient with widespread cancer who has a few months left to live will certainly benefit the less she must use mind-dulling medication. On the other hand, large numbers of patients who fail surgery for chronic non–life-threatening pain speak to the need for extreme care and sensitivity on the part of the pain-management team in recommending such surgery, especially in view of risks of additional neurologic deficits brought on by surgery.

It is with this in mind that the reader should critically review techniques of spine surgery for pain presented in this book by extremely well-respected, experienced, and thoughtful surgeons.

CHAPTER 26

DIFFERENTIAL DIAGNOSIS AND MANAGEMENT OF CERVICAL SPINE PAIN

JOHN ARYANPUR
THOMAS B. DUCKER

"PAIN IN the neck" is such a common complaint and is so universally understood that the expression alone is used to described certain people, situations, and experiences. Within any given month approximately 10% of the population will experience pain in the neck, with or without radicular pain into the arms (1). More than one-third of the population can recall a significant episode of severe neck pain, often with radicular components (1). In epidemiologic studies, a history of significant stiff neck with or without arm pain has been found in one-half to three-quarters of all individuals (2–4). Often these people will see their physician with this complaint. The scope of this problem is therefore tremendous.

Fortunately, 70% of people with the complaint of new-onset neck pain who visit a doctor are well or improving within 1 month (2), and a majority of the remaining 30% obtain symptomatic relief with time and appropriate therapeutic interventions. Thus, only a small proportion of patients with acute neck pain go on to develop more chronic pain problems.

The human neck is evolutionarily an extremely complex structure with multiple bony, ligamentous, muscular, vascular, and neural components, all of which are capable of generating "neck pain." As such a structure, the neck can be affected by such processes as degenerative osteoarthritis, inflammatory diseases of muscle and ligament, vascular insufficiency, and neural compression syndromes, to mention only a few. Dermatomal, myotomal, and sclerotomal pain patterns may be distinguished.

More importantly, in a social sense the neck acts as a fulcrum from which our eyes, ears, nose, and mouth function to interact with our environment. Neck mobility is essential for the full appreciation of the world around us. More than we realize, the neck is active in common activities—nodding, turning, smiling, and shaking hands. Any disruption of its normal function may quickly be appreciated as uncomfortable, and even painful.

To complicate the situation, pathologic processes in other areas, such as the shoulder, the diaphragm, the heart, or the jaw, may cause pain that is referred to the neck—thus the complaint of "neck pain" in patients with acromioclavicular joint disease, diaphragmatic irritation, hypertension and myocardial infraction, or temporomandibular joint syndromes. Disease of the apical lung and pleura also may impinge upon the brachial plexus to give pain in a C8 or T1 distribution.

Finally, even the most minor discomfort in the neck may be colored by certain psychosocial and psychoneurotic factors, in which case the complaint of "pain in the neck" is in reality but a physical outlet for a variety of personal and psychological problems.

The differential diagnosis of cervical spine pain is therefore quite large, and it is often only with repeated office visits and multiple investigations and therapies that the proper diagnosis is made.

In the next few pages we review some basic aspects of cervical anatomy and biomechanics as well as bony and neurologic pathology and specific referred pain syndromes. Following that, diagnostic studies are outlined. From a synthesis of the above a list of differential diagnoses can in most cases be made, with the ultimate goals of focusing in upon the most appropriate diagnosis and treatment for each patient.

ANATOMY AND BIOMECHANICS

The neck is the most mobile region of the spine. Over 50% of all neck motion occurs at the atlanto-occipital and atlantoaxial joints; and the remaining 50% of neck motion is equally distributed through the C3-C7 segments. In quadriped animals the motion allowed at the atlanto-occipital and atlantoaxial joints is even greater than it is in humans.

Mechanically there are many places where the system may cause pain. In the seven cervical vertebrae there are 14 zygoapophyseal joints (usually referred to as facet joints) as well as five Luschka's joints (referred to as uncinate processes), and a muscular and ligamentous apparatus that is innervated not only by the eleventh cranial nerve but also by all of the eight cranial nerves on both sides. Muscle and ligamentous tears and sprains are by far the most common causes for neck pain, but other pathologies may exist as well. The facet joints and joints of Luschka are lined with synovial membrane, and are subject to the same inflammatory pain-producing pathologies as synovial joints elsewhere. The normal intervertebral disk absorbs axial loading pressures on the spine, serving as a "shock absorber." Disk rupture or degeneration or annulus tear can produce severe focal pain that may be difficult to diagnose and treat. Bony structures themselves may degenerate secondary to osteoporosis or metabolic or infiltrative processes, leading to pathologic fractures and pain. Finally, the neural tissues themselves may be a source of pain when compressed or irritated. These pathologic mechanisms are discussed in more detail below.

CERVICAL SPINE

The anatomy and relevant biomechanics of the cervical spine are most pertinent to clinical disorders if considered segmentally. Thus, the occiput-C1 region (comprising the occiput and C1 vertebrae, the joints between them, the muscles and ligaments affecting movement at these joints, and the spinal cord and nerve roots exiting at that level) may be considered an independent segment, and so on for the C1-C2, C2-C3, and remaining regions down C7-T1.

The seven small cervical vertebrae balance the 15-pound weight of the head and its contents. The center of weight of the skull is slightly anterior to the midaxis of the spine, and naturally causes the head to fall forward. For this reason there is constant tension on the posterior cervical musculature to hold the head in the upright position. Relaxation and contraction of this posterior musculature, aided by the upper one-third of the trapezius, allows cervical flexion and extension. The vast majority of this flexion and extension occurs at the atlanto-occipital joint, and this joint is commonly referred to as the "yes" joint. Conversion of the emotion of "yes" into the "yes" motion of the head is mediated by branches of the eleventh cranial nerve supplying the trapezius and sternocleidomastoid muscles, as well as by all eight cervical roots, including the C1 motor root, which exists at this level. There is no C1 sensory root.

Beneath this atlanto-occipital joint the neural anatomy is terribly complex. Within the spinal cord at that level there is the decussation of the long motor tracts as well as the descending spinal tract of the fifth cranial nerve, which is responsible for pain and temperature sensation over the face. The lower cranial nerve nuclei are also vulnerable at this location. Compression of the cord at this level can cause a variety of signs and symptoms (neck pain, limitation of flexion and extension, headaches, "onionskin" facial numbness, lower cranial nerve palsies, upper extremity weakness, and lower extremity spasticity) that may be diffuse enough to confuse even the best trained clinician. Suffice it to say that a patient presenting with complaints and physical findings as listed above should be suspected of having pathology at the occiput-C1 level.

Movement at the C1-C2 level is greatly influenced by the dens, which acts as a stable pin about which rotation may occur. The rotary movement of the atlantoaxial joint has led to its being referred to as the "no" joint. Again, motion through a cervical joint is controlled by one's emotions! Extremes of rotation, up to 80–100°, are possible at this joint.

The actual turning of the neck to produce a "no" movement is primarily a function of the sternocleidomastoid muscle. This muscle, with its attachments on the mastoid process at the base of the skull, clearly provides the major fulcrum for turning of the atlantoaxial joint. Posteriorly, the smaller capitis musculature, with attachments onto the spinous process of C2 extending up to the skull, acts primarily as a stabilizer and servo-mechanism balance system to maintain the head in proper alignment with the motions initiated by the stronger sternocleidomastoid muscle. Other posterior muscle groups, including the trapezius, complement this stabilizing action. Motor innervation for the sternocleidomastoid occurs primarily through the 11th cranial nerve, supplemented by small fibers from C2 and C3 to the lower half of the muscle. At the C1-C2 segment a sensory nerve component is present in the form of large C2 sensory nerve roots. These divide peripherally into several branches, the largest of which on each side is the greater occipital nerve. This nerve provides sensory innervation of the superior aspect of the neck and the entire posterior half of the hemicranium, including the occiput and superior parietal areas of the skull and scalp. The greater occipital nerve may be trapped peripherally as it passes through the thick fascial attachments of the posterior neck musculature over the occipital region. This can be a source of pain and tenderness on the posterior aspect of the head. Prolonged contraction of the posterior cervical musculature, due to stress or fatigue, can cause compression of both greater occipital nerves, contributing to the tension headache syndrome.

The C2-C3 segment is in a sense a transitional segment

between the hypermobile occiput-C2 area and the remaining cervical segments. The C2-C3 joint has multiple components: the intervertebral disk, the vertebral joints, and the zygoapophyseal joints. These limit the degrees of freedom at the segment, but also provide a degree of stability not present at higher levels. This joint will allow approximately 10° of motion in flexion and extension and 5–8° in rotation or lateral flexion. It is rarely involved in the degenerative arthritic changes that are so common at lower cervical levels.

The C3 vertebrae has the C3 nerve root above and the C4 nerve root below. The motor innervation of the diaphragm, and of the accessory muscles of respiration in the neck, basically comes from these two nerve roots. (Occasionally the C5 roots make several smaller contributions to this innervation.) These motor roots also contribute to the innervation of the intrinsic neck muscles, as do all motor roots in the cervical region. The sensory component of the C3 root supplies the superior half of the neck anteriorly, and can extend up to the angle of the jaw and ear. Below, the C4 dermatome covers the lower half of the neck, and will extend over the clavicles. C5 through C8 dermatomal patterns are carried primarily out through the brachial plexus into the upper extremities.

From the C3-C4 segment caudally the motion of each vertebra upon its adjacent vertebra is basically the same. All are associated with approximately 10° of rotation and/or lateral flexion. All have intervertebral disks and uncovertebral and zygoapophyseal joints. Although disease within any of these vertebrae, adjacent ligaments, or joint structures can cause focal pain, more commonly the pathologic process is associated with a prominent component of local nerve root irritation, and a strong radicular element is apparent. Pathology in the C4-T1 segments, therefore, commonly produces varying degrees of upper extremity pain and neurologic deficit. For this reason, the discussion of the caudal cervical segments simplifies to a neuroanatomic discussion of each of the individual cervical nerve roots that lead to the brachial plexus, although the specific organization of the brachial plexus complex's individual nerve root patterns are well recognized and easy to distinguish.

The C5 nerve root, which exits between the 4th and 5th cervical vertebrae, supplies the major innervation of the deltoid muscle. It also contributes to the biceps, the supra- and infra-spinatus, serratus anterior, and levator scapulae. All are muscles involved in stabilizing the shoulder and in abduction of the arm. The biceps reflex can be associated with the C5 nerve root, although in fact the C6 root may make a significant contribution. The sensory innervation of the C5 root is fairly specific, covering the shoulder and down the radial aspect of the arm to the mid-distal forearm.

The motor component of the C6 nerve root, which exits between the C5 and C6 vertebrae, is responsible for the innervation of the brachioradialis and biceps muscles, as well as the extensors of the wrist. Clinically, the brachioradialis reflex is linked with the C6 root—in truth the C5 root is also involved. The C6 dermatomal pattern is very specific and definitely involves the dorsal radial aspect of the dorsal surface of the index finger.

The C7 nerve root makes an important contribution to the posterior aspect of the brachial plexus, which leads directly into the radial nerve. For that reason C7 strongly influences the triceps musculature, as well as the extensors of the wrist and the intrinsic muscles of the hand. Its sensory dermatomal pattern always involves the middle finger, but can involve the index finger as well. The triceps reflex is subserved by this nerve root.

The C8 nerve root, which comes off beneath the 7th cervical vertebra just above the first thoracic vertebra and the 1st rib, contributes heavily to the inferior cord of the brachial plexus and the medial cord. Its primary myotome includes the flexors of the hand—it is responsible for grip. The sensory innervation of this root covers the ulnar aspects of the forearm and the dorsal and palmar ulnar aspects extending up over the fourth and fifth fingers. This differs from the sensory distribution of the ulnar nerve in that the latter covers only the ulnar half of the fourth finger and does not extend proximally beyond the palmar crease.

Although it exits outside the cervical spine at the T1-T2 region, the T1 nerve root obviously contributes to the brachial plexus and the intrinsic muscles of the hand. Its sensory contributions are into the axilla and down the medial aspect of the upper arm. There is no specific reflex associated with this nerve root.

SPINAL CORD

The relationship between the spinal cord and nerve roots at the C3-T1 levels is clinically important and is constant in the mid and lower cervical spine. The spinal cord lies within the vertebral canal, with nerve roots exiting via foramina at each level. The neural foramen at each level is bounded dorsolaterally by the facet joint capsule, anteromedially by the disk space and uncovertebral joints, and superiorly and inferiorly by the arches of the vertebra above and below. Each foramen can therefore be impinged upon in many ways. Degenerative changes leading to hypertrophy of the facet joint and/or the uncovertebral joints can often cause foraminal stenosis. The nucleus pulposis of the intervertebral disk is usually held in place by strong posterior longitudinal ligaments. Under certain extremes of pressure and stress, however, the disk material can herniate posteriorly or posterolaterally to impinge upon the spinal cord or nerve root. The neural foramina are slightly large at C2-C3 and become progressively smaller down to C6-C7. Generally speaking the foramina have an average vertical diameter of 10 mm and a transverse diameter of 5 mm. The nerve roots lie near the upper vertebral pedicle, and as they exit further they descend slightly toward the intervertebral joint space itself. Because the nerve roots themselves occupy only one-third of the cross-sectional area of the foraminal space, the actual shape of the foramen may be the most important consideration in determining its adequacy. A decrease in foraminal height is not as critical as a decrease in foraminal width. Consequently foraminal stenosis may be fairly advanced before the patient becomes symptomatic.

Cross-sectionally the normal spinal cord has a diameter in the lateral dimension of 12–13 mm throughout most of the cervical regions. In the anteroposterior (AP) dimension this diameter is generally less, from 8 to 9 mm. The spinal canal is largest in the high cervical region, and tapers progressively from there down. Assuming a normal AP diameter of 8–9 mm and allowing for the 1-mm thickness of cerebrospinal fluid and 1-mm thickness of dural coverings surrounding the cord anteriorly and posteriorly, a minimal spinal canal diameter of 12–13 mm is required to allow for a healthy, noncompressed spinal cord. Clinically, the AP diameter of the spinal canal is easily obtainable from plain films or computed tomography (CT), thus allowing quick estimates of the adequacy of the spinal canal. In practice, an AP diameter of 14 mm is considered normal, and anything less than that indicates a degree of central spinal stenosis with narrowing of the canal that could adversely effect the spinal cord.

Vascular Supply

The vertebral artery travels through the transverse foramina of the C8-C1 vertebrae, making a tight arch over the atlas as it pierces the dura between the atlas and occiput. The spinal cord and nerve roots derive their blood supply bilaterally from myeloradicular arteries that branch from each vertebral artery and accompany specific nerve roots toward the cord substance itself. In the neck there are often three or four of these arteries, the largest of which usually accompanies the C6 or C7 root and is usually larger on the left than the right. This is commonly termed the artery of the cervical enlargement. This supply feeds into bilateral contributions from the intracranial vertebral artery, which joins at the midline to form the anterior spinal artery. A system of parallel posterior spinal arteries also exists. Although anastomoses between anterior and posterior spinal arteries are numerous, in general the anterior spinal artery supplies blood to the anterior two-thirds of the cord (including the anterior and lateral funiculi and gray matter of the cord). The posterior spinal artery system supplies the posterior columns exclusively. In rare individuals the anterior spinal artery may be vestigial, and a single large myeloradicular artery may supply most of the cervical spinal cord. Embolic or thrombotic events, or occlusion of major spinal arteries or veins during surgical interventions or by trauma, can lead to spinal cord ischemia, and ultimately spinal infarction.

PATHOLOGY

Pathology within the cervical spine can involve the central nervous system and its adjacent nerve roots, the vertebral joints, or the bones themselves. When initially attempting to ascertain where the pathology lies, the first major division is between involvement of bony and soft tissue structures. In many cases both go hand in hand, and consequently may be difficult to tease apart. For discussion's sake we will begin centrally with problems of the spinal cord itself, and then proceed peripherally to quickly review pathology of the bones, joints, and muscles.

Clinically, the prototypical intrinsic spinal pathology is an expansile mass of the cord, and the simplest of central spinal masses is the syrinx. These can develop idiopathically or as a long-term sequela of spinal trauma, and may be initially associated with arm and facial pain and discomfort, especially at night. This latter is thought to be secondary to changes in differential pressure between syrinx and subarachnoid space that occur during recumbency. The pain then becomes less prominent as the neurologic deficit becomes more pronounced. There can be focal sensory loss on the face as well as over the trunk and limbs as a consequence of compression of the anterior white commissure and lateral spinothalamic tracts. Clumsy, wasted hands and a stiff gait reflect a combination of upper and lower motor neuron deficits in the upper extremities and pure upper motor neuron deficits in the lower extremities. Bowel and bladder problems may occur as well.

On occasion, a spinal cord cyst is associated with a tumor, such as an ependymoma. More frequently the tumor itself can develop cystic degeneration, as in astrocytomas of the cord.

Other degenerative processes besides intrinsic compressive cord lesions may lead to neurologic deficit and pain. Anterior motor horn cell loss, as in amyotrophic lateral sclerosis and polio, or ischemic processes of the cord may result in clinical syndromes that are difficult to distinguish from those of the more common spinal cord compressive syndromes.

Rather than being in the spinal cord itself, the mass may be centered along the meninges or adjacent nerve roots. These are locations at which meningiomas and neurofibromas are commonly found. Even though these tumors may initially develop on one root alone, they progress so slowly that the true pathology may not be fully appreciated. Again, the common initial symptom is often pain, but it is often only when spinal cord compression has reached the point of upper extremity weakness, myelopathy, or gait disturbance that the clinical syndrome is recognized.

Extradural processes as well may cause a syndrome identical to the one described above. By far the most common source of extradural compression is degenerative joint disease of the intervertebral joints. Normal degenerative joint changes lead, over time, to reactive pannus and bony spur formation that when severe can cause spinal cord or nerve root compression. These degenerative processes can be accelerated by coexistent disease, such as rheumatoid arthritis, which characteristically attacks predominantly the atlanto-occipital and atlantoaxial regions of the spine, leading to ligamentous laxity and spinal column instability as well as cord and nerve root compression. In contrast, ankylosing spondylitis causes calcification of joints and longitudinal spinal ligaments, leading to spinal fusion and abnormal bone formation that once again may compress neural tissues.

Other epidural masses such as metastatic tumors (usually from the breast or lung) and benign and malignant primary bone tumors may cause cord or root compression as above and can therefore be included in this category of extradural compressive masses.

Intervertebral disk herniation typically affects only a single nerve root. The herniation may be directly posterior into the canal to cause acute spinal cord compression and symptoms similar to those of other extradural lesions, however. In addition, joint and ligamentous pathology may cause pain independent of a compressive effect on neural tissue. Joints that are inflamed or unstable may produce focal, mechanical pain quite different from that of neural compression. Thus, a common clinical presentation is that of the patient with severe degenerative changes of the cervical spine who has both mechanical (joint and ligamentous) and radicular (neural compressive) pain components.

Intrinsic pathology of the bone, such as with osteoporotic fractures, bony tumors, or Pagets's disease of the spine, may produce focal pain. This pain may be exacerbated by neck movement, as is pain originating from the joints, but more commonly is not. Palpation of the involved vertebra, however, almost invariably reproduces the pain. The pain from bony lesions is characteristically described as dull or aching.

Finally, all the above pathologies may contribute to the development of cervical muscle spasm and irritation, making this a nearly universal accompaniment of all complaints of neck pain. Pain on movement and superficial palpation, and muscle tightness, are characteristic.

MEDICAL HISTORY

In evaluating a patient with cervical pain, as with any patient, the physician has the responsibility of directing the interview process. If this is skillfully done, in 70–80% of patients a reasonable initial diagnosis can be made even without a physical examination or further diagnostic studies. As always, open-ended questions yield the greatest information.

The interview begins as the patient enters the room, and his or her habitus, posture, and gait should be observed. Age, sex, and occupation are all readily ascertained. Next, a description of the pain is needed.

Pain always has at least three characteristics—onset, course, and severity. These need to be described in terms of location, exacerbating and relieving factors, quality, and severity. It is essential to have the patient begin by pointing to the painful area of the neck or arm. Once must literally have the patient stand up and show the examiner where he/she hurts. This will allow the examiner to sidestep any confusion the patient may have with anatomic description or terms.

Leading questions about particular activities (e.g., twisting the neck, running, doing sports, working, etc.) are useful. If the patient does not spontaneously provide descriptions of the type and severity of the pain then questions such as how sharp or dull, aching or burning, throbbing or cramping the pain is may be employed. Although it is important not to put words in the patient's mouth, certain general types of pain may indicate certain pathologies. For example, pain deep within the bone is usually described as dull and nagging, whereas fracture pain is sharp, severe, and immediately associated with muscle spasm. Pain that is worse at night can suggest a spinal cord tumor or mass. Pain that radiates sharply is usually radicular in origin.

Finally, patients may have initiated treatments on their own or sought advice elsewhere prior to being seen. Responses to over-the-counter drugs such as aspirin, Motrin, Tylenol, and the like are important. Some patient have seen physical therapists or chiropractors, and a knowledge of the response to such manipulations is always beneficial. As always, how the patient reacts to his/her disease psychologically is of paramount importance. If there is obvious secondary gain or malingering involved the examiner may do better to direct treatment toward these psychological factors.

It is also important to be cognizant of the many patterns of referred pain. As discussed earlier, numerous noncervical pathologies may cause various types of neck pain. Consequently, in difficult cases where no conspicuous cervical pathology can be held accountable for the patient's pain, consultation with colleagues in other specialties should be the rule rather than the exception.

CLINICAL EXAMINATION

In dealing with patients with neck pain, the physical examination must have two basic components. The first component must involve an examination of the anatomy and mechanics of the neck itself. The second component must include an accurate assessment of the patient's neurologic status.

ANATOMY AND MECHANICS OF THE NECK

In evaluating the mechanics of the neck it must be appreciated that, as described above, 50% of cervical motion occurs at the occipital C1 and C2 joints alone. Thus the "yes" and "no" motions may be intact in the face of many a severe cervical disorder. The first three cervical vertebrae are anatomically located behind the face and are covered by the jaw at the base of the skull. C4 through C7 are centrally placed, as are the vertebrae that make up the neck as we view it from the surface.

Grossly the neck should have a gentle lordotic curve, as in the lumbar region. Most patients should be able to easily extend their neck to look at the ceiling, and to flex their neck to look at the floor. A neck that is fixed and lacks motion has either mechanical or pain-evoked limitations to a full range of motion. The head compression, or Spurling's, test (5) is a valuable aid in localizing the level of the pathology (5). This maneuver causes compression of the vertebral bodies on one another and narrows the neural foramina. If this maneuver produces radicular pain a nerve root pathology is probable. If only local neck pain is elicited, however, joint or ligamentous disease is more likely. The reverse of compression (i.e., distraction) is often helpful as well. The radicular pain of a soft disk herniation or foraminal stenosis may be relieved by the opening of the foramina caused by cervical distraction. If pain is from joint disease, distraction will simply accentuate the pain as much as compression will..In cervical nerve root disorders due to either soft disk disease or osteophytes, extending the neck and turning the head to the side of the pain commonly reproduces the radicular pain symptoms. Patients will often volunteer that they will not turn or extend their neck because of this discomfort.

In addition to testing the range of motion of the neck the range of motion of the shoulder and upper extremity must be evaluated as well. In many cases, it is very difficult to distinguish between shoulder joint disorders and certain nerve root compression syndromes. Furthermore, with certain neck disorders weakness within the deltoid or biceps leads to shoulder stiffness and tightness, so the patient may in actuality have both problems. Nonetheless, if the patient has pain in the neck that radiates down the arm, it is useful for the patient and examiner to demonstrate that passive movement of the wrist, elbow, or shoulder will not reproduce the pain, thereby confirming that the upper extremity pain is not caused by pathology in the limb itself. If this is followed by measures that do reproduce the upper extremity pain (i.e., compression, extension, and rotation of the neck), ordering radiographs and other diagnostic studies of the neck will seem logical to the patient as well as reassuring to the physician.

NEUROLOGIC STATUS

The neurologic examination should be performed in a systematic way. The patient can be sitting on an examining table, although it may be found helpful to have the patient sitting in a chair. This way the examiner can walk around the patient to observe at many angles. A motor, sensory, and reflex examination can be done in a matter of a few minutes. The examiner begins by walking behind the patient and observing as he/she raises the arms above the head and lowers them back down. By looking at how the neck is held and at the mechanics of the neck and shoulders throughout this movement, one has already learned a good deal of information. Palpation of neck muscles and individual spinous processes may also yield valuable information regarding the origin of neck pain.

Next the patient is instructed to flex the arms at the elbows and to abduct at the shoulder, and to maintain this position. By exerting counterpressure the strength of the deltoid muscles may be tested simultaneously. This is essential because, although absolute strength is important, it is more crucial to detect an asymmetry in strength from side to side. The patient now lowers the arms to his/her side, keeping them flexed at the elbow. In this position biceps strength can be assessed. Again, one is looking above all for symmetry. Moving behind the patient, the patient's fist is then placed inside the examiner's hands with instructions to extend the arms, thus utilizing the triceps muscle. If the arm is only minimally flexed to begin with, the mechanical advantage will be with the examiner, and no patient will be able to overcome the examiner. A false impression of weakness might thus be given. It is therefore always crucial to examine individual muscles in positions that allow the patient maximal mechanical advantage. The triceps musculature has widespread innervation (C5-C8) so that asymmetry of the strength of this muscle is often a very sensitive indicator in patients with neurologic dysfunction. Finally the examiner faces the patient and has him/her extend the wrist, spread the fingers, and squeeze down tightly, all as a measure of the strength of the wrist extensors and intrinsic hand musculature. Although more-sophisticated motor examinations are possible, these simple maneuvers can be rapidly performed and will pick up the majority of upper extremity dysfunctions. The lower extremities can be tested in a similar fashion.

The sensory examination is best done with a safety pin. This will not cause bleeding, can be used to test the patient's ability to distinguish between sharp and dull, and can be discarded after each examination. Comparing dermatomal patterns from side to side is usually the best way to appreciate a subtle hypoalgesia. As discussed above, a simple way to remember dermatomal patterns is to think of C5 as covering the shoulder, C6 covering the thumb, C7 involving the index and middle fingers, and C8 the ring and little fingers. Often testing down onto the chest wall is helpful, and it is important to remember that the C4 dermatomal pattern on the anterior chest wall. Thus, a change in the sensation just below the clavicle may reflect a C4 sensory level deficit. Often, assessment of lower extremity proprioception is useful.

When cervical problems are suspected the reflex examination should include the upper and lower extremities as well as a comparison between the two. The biceps, triceps, and brachioradial reflexes are the significant deep tendon reflexes in the upper extremities. Inversion of the upper extremity reflexes or a positive Hoffman's sign are evidence of hyper-reflexia. Subsequent to this, lower extremity reflexes should be evaluated, especially at the knees. If the reflexes are perfectly normal in the upper extremities and at the knees, assessment of ankle and Babinski's reflexes are unlikely to yield much new information, and may be omitted in the interest of time. However, if any pathologic reflexes are noted then full lower extremity reflex assessment, including Babinski's reflex, is mandatory. The examination may be concluded by watching the patient walk from the examining room.

DIAGNOSTIC STUDIES

The investigation of any complaint of neck pain must first begin with plain films of the cervical spine. Any acute post-traumatic surgical pain, or persistent non-traumatic surgical pain, should be evaluated first using plain cervical spine x-rays. Often, plain films alone will show pathology such as bony erosion or degenerative osteoarthritis with osteophyte formation, which will guide further investigations and diagnostic decisions. If indicated, flexion and extension views of the cervical spine are indispensable in evaluating spinal stability radiographically. Oblique views allow visualization of the neural foramina. Other views such as the swimmer's view or the odontoid view may be tailored to the specific area being investigated.

With the plain film information in hand, further radiologic, electrophysiologic, or laboratory investigations may be ordered.

Any patient with a complaint or history suggestive of a radicular pattern who fails conservative therapy should be evaluated further. In the past this evaluation has consisted of myelography, with or without CT Scanning. Recently, magnetic resonance imaging (MRI) techniques have to a large degree supplanted this cervical myelogram. In general, following the plain x-ray evaluation of the patient with neck pain, the next radiologic study of choice should be an MRI scan. MRI studies, with the their ability to combine sagittal, axial, and coronal views of the cervical spine, allow for exquisite visualization of the spinal cord and nerve roots. Intra-

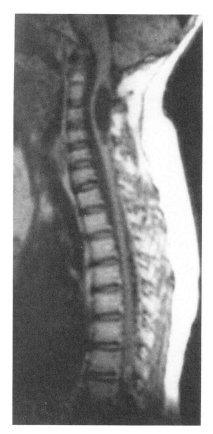

Figure 26.1.

spinal lesions such as herniated disks, osteophytes, and tumors are easily visualized using MRI techniques. Intrinsic diseases of the cervical spinal cord such as intramedullary tumors, syrinxes, or the Chiari malformations are in fact best visualized by MRI techniques (Fig. 26.1).

It should also be recognized, however, that if visualization of fine bony detail or bony destruction is desired, supplementation of MRI with CT scanning will be essential. Particularly in the area of osseus destructive lesions of the spinal column and bony osteophytes, MRI fails to provide enough bony detail to guide surgical intervention. In these circumstances, a high-resolution plain CT scan through the area of pathology is often an indispensable supplement to the MRI scan.

Although MRI has to a large degree supplanted myelography as an imaging modality, in certain patients the cervical myelogram is still indicated. Examples include patients with severe degenerative or postsurgical kyphosis in whom distortion of the normal anatomy prevents easy recognition of abnormalities using multiple plain or MRI formats. Another example is the patient who is suspected of having a cervical spinal arteriovenous malformation. In this case, MRI may miss the lesion altogether, and the diagnosis can only often times be made by detecting the classic serpiginous defect on the cervical myelogram.

Nuclear medicine studies, such as gallium- and leucocyte-tagged scans, are not capable of providing detailed anatomic information. They are useful, however, when infectious etiologies are suspected as a cause of neck pain. It is always necessary to remember that these are fairly nonspecific tests and that they may be positive for several months after surgery or other interventions.

Electrophysiologic testing utilizing electromyography (EMG) and nerve conduction velocity (NCV) testing techniques is indicated when evidence exists of damage to neural tissue. Decrease in motor potential and muscle groups and/or slowing of conduction velocities along nerves are among the many pathologic responses detected by these tests. In particular, EMG/NCV tests are useful in delineating the level and extent of neurologic injury. Nerve conduction velocities may be decreased relatively quickly after injury to the involved nerve, whereas electromyographic changes may take weeks to become apparent. For this reason, the nerve conduction velocity is a more sensitive test early in the disease course.

Laboratory investigations will supplement all the above tests. Determination of the complete blood count and differential, serum protein electrophoresis, the erythrocyte sedimentation rate, rheumatoid factor, or the serum calcium may be crucial to arriving at the final diagnosis.

Occasionally, a patient will be encountered in whom all investigations, including radiographic, electrophysiologic, and serologic, will be negative, despite the complaint of persistent neck pain. In such difficult patients, the use of diskography has gained some recent popularity. The percutaneous injection of the small amounts of radiographic contrast material into the cervical disk spaces may demonstrate annular tears or frank extrusion of contrast material, which could help localize the pathological level. Reproduction of the patient's pain with injection of a small amount of contrast material is also thought to be diagnostic of pathology at the injected level. It is possible to control for the effects of injection at one level by subsequently injecting a small amount of local anesthetic. Relief of the patient's typical neck pain following the intradiskal injection of local anesthetic is reported to be a highly specific test of diskogenic disease, and is reported to correlate well with relief of pain following subsequent surgery at that level. This technique has not yet been evaluated in a controlled fashion, and it remains to be seen whether such techniques find a wider applicability in the management of patients with intractable cervical pain.

Obviously, the individual tests described above will be ordered for each patient depending upon the details of the history, physical examination, and radiographic studies. As a rule, however, the sequence of diagnostic

Table 26.1.
Common Disorders of the Cervical Spinal Area Causing Neck and Upper Extremity Pain

Spinal cord compression due to tumor or syrinx

Intrinsic motor and sensory disorders of the cord (including torticollis, toxins, and viral, vascular, and metabolic diseases)

Extrinsic spinal cord neoplasms

Osteoarthritis

Nerve root irritations (soft and hard disk protrusions)

Traumatic injury to the cervical spine

Rheumatoid arthritis

Ankylosing spondylitis and diffuse idiopathic skeletal hyperostosis

Infections

evaluation should progress from plain spine films and simple serologic tests to more-extensive and -invasive evaluations only if the patient's neck pain persists. In over 90% of all patients with neck pain a simple plain spine series is sufficient to rule out serious pathology, and to reassure the patient that the episode of neck pain currently being experienced will most likely resolve with conservative therapy.

SPECIFIC CERVICAL PAIN SYNDROMES

Based upon With the history and physical examination, it should be possible to arrive at a tentative diagnosis. Diagnostic studies can bolster or refute these initial impressions. Certain disorders are common and should be familiar to every clinician. These are listed in Table 26.1, and are discussed individually. This table is in no way meant to be all-inclusive. Creating a huge differential diagnosis is not helpful in the day-to-day practice of treating cervical pain syndromes. Once again the key differential here is to determine whether the disease syndrome is primarily neurologic or bony in nature. Deciding this will allow a narrowing of the differential diagnosis list into manageable subclasses and will direct further studies that will allow the final diagnosis to be reached. Obviously there are other esoteric diseases that may cause pain in the neck and upper extremities. A full discussion of these disorders is beyond the scope of this chapter. For this the reader is referred to a more comprehensive text (6).

SPINAL CORD COMPRESSION

Compression of the spinal cord can occur from mass lesions either extrinsic or intrinsic to the cord itself. The most common intra-axial spinal mass lesions are syrinxes, and the most common primary spinal tumors are spinal ependymomas and spinal gliomas, respectively, accounting for 60% and 30% of all primary tumors (7).

The ependymoma literally starts from the central spinal canal, taking origin from vestigial ependymal cells lining this cavity. The tumor expands slowly to compress the spinal cord between it and the confines of the spinal canal.

Spinal gliomas arise from malignant transformation of astrocytes or other glial elements. These tumors are more infiltrative than ependymomas and are consequently much more difficult to deal with surgically.

The pain from such lesions is usually insidious in onset and is poorly localized. It is often worse at night or in the early morning, for reasons discussed above. It may occasionally be exacerbated by activity, leading to the speculation that increased blood supply to the tumor during exercise may aggravate any ongoing compression.

The key to arriving at the proper diagnosis is in recognizing that this pain is invariably associated with a defined but sometimes subtle neurologic deficit. There may be slight lower extremity hyper-reflexia, or subtle weakness of the upper extremities. Often, a cape-like distribution of sensory deficit over the shoulders and upper arms is the first appreciable evidence of neurologic problems. These deficits rapidly progress, however, to become more readily apparent. Soon there is loss of motor function and coordination in the hands. Invariably at some point in the progression of the syndrome lower extremity hyper-reflexia will develop, as will stiffness of gait and other signs of myelopathy.

There are often intradural tumors that may be associated, initially at least, predominantly with unilateral symptoms. These are tumors that usually lie within the dura but are extramedullary, the classic examples being neurofibromas and meningiomas. Here again, the history of night pain is common. These tumors may grow to totally envelop a single nerve root with no appreciable neurologic deficit on examination. Often, the patient presents with unilateral radicular pain and numbness only. Once again, as the mass grows and the spinal cord is compressed, signs and symptoms of myelopathy point the way to the correct diagnosis.

Once the tentative diagnosis of intrinsic spinal cord compression is reached, the diagnosis may be confirmed by radiologic studies. Intrathecally enhanced CT and MRI scans are most commonly available, and should be the radiologic studies of choice following the plain x-ray. Treatment of these lesions is surgical and, in the case of tumors, is often supplemental by local radiation.

INTRINSIC MOTOR AND SENSORY DISORDERS

Many primary neurologic disorders that can disrupt spinal cord function. When the disorder primarily involves the motor system it may disrupt spinal cord circuitry and cause a lack of balance between agonist and antagonist motor functions. This may cause constant paradoxical muscle spasms, or torticollis. This disorder can quickly be recognized by the patient's posturing. In severe torticollis there is almost constant head jerking to one side or the other, and the patient soon develops osteoarthritic changes in the facet and uncinate joints that may be a source of additional pain. Unfortunately, there is no good treatment for spontaneous idiopathic torticollis. Cutting the various motor roots that innervate the involved muscles can indeed reduce the constant and abnormal motor movement; however, this comes at the price of muscle denervation and associated atrophy. Such treatment is justified only in extreme cases. Other experimental procedures are being tested that may have more promise.

Toxins can affect the nervous system and cause severe burning pain as well as neurologic deficit. In our highly industrialized society the chance of significant exposure to potential neurotoxins is always present. The heavy metals lead and mercury, as well as more complex organic compounds, are in this group.

There are natural factors as well that have been implicated in neurologic disease. Recent reports of linkage between plants and amyotrophic lateral sclerosis (8) and the long-standing suspicions of a viral/infectious etiology for multiple sclerosis are prominent examples. Certain coral elements in the Caribbean, when eaten by fish and then by humans in the food cycle, may cause severe cervical pain. This is called *ciguatera*. Treatment of such conditions is directed toward ending exposure to the offending agent and providing supportive and curative care as needed.

On rare occasions, vascular insufficiency to the spinal cord can itself cause pain. This may occur as a result of surgery or trauma or pre-existent cardiovascular disease.

Characteristically the early stages of spinal cord ischemia will cause truncal pain that is poorly localized. Within a matter of hours, if not sooner, spinal infarction may occur, guaranteeing a devastating neurologic deficit and poor ultimate progress. Unfortunately we do not know a great deal about how these various metabolic, toxic, or infectious disorders bring about disease on a cellular level. Further advances will be required for rapid and more effective treatment and diagnosis of such disorders.

EXTRINSIC SPINAL CORD NEOPLASMS

Extra-axial neoplastic lesions of the cervical spine may cause mechanical symptoms and localized pain or may lead to neurologic deficit, depending on the site of origin of the process. Bony tumors may be divided into benign primary tumors of bone, malignant primary tumors of bone, and metastatic tumors to bone. Malignant tumor metastases to bone are far and away most common. A list of various tumor types is presented in Table 26.2.

Table 26.2.
Tumors of the Cervical Spine

Primary tumors
  Giant cell tumor
  Osteoblastoma
  Osteochondroma
  Eosinophilic granuloma
  Plasmacytoma
  Chondromyxoid fibroma
  Desmoid tumor
  Hemangioma
  Osteocartilaginous exostosis
  Rheumatoid pannus
Malignant tumors of the cervical spine
  Chordoma
  Chondrosarcoma
  Osteosarcoma
  Ewing's sarcoma
  Aggressive solitary plasmacytoma
  Hemangiopericytoma
Metastatic from solitary organs
  Breast
  Prostate
  Renal
  Gastrointestinal
  Thyroid
  Lung
  Nasopharyngeal
Hematogenous metastatic process
  Multiple myeloma
  Hodgkin's disease
  Lymphoma

Primary malignant bony tumors such as chordomas, osteosarcomas, and chondrosarcomas may occur in the cervical regions. Unfortunately the bones of the cervical spine can also be involved by metastatic tumor processes. Hematologic malignancies such as multiple myeloma or lymphoma very commonly involve the axial skeleton, causing bony destruction and neurologic deficit.

It is obvious that with such an extensive list of pathologic processes it would be impossible to formulate a "typical" clinical presentation. However, some typical clinical features exist that would allow the clinician a hint, however.

Pain deep within the bone itself is the most common clinical presentation of all of the above-listed processes. This complaint in any patient with previously diagnosed malignancy should trigger a full diagnostic work-up aimed at detection of possible bony metastases. The pain is initially mechanical in nature, and may be worse with motion. In addition there is often an element of night pain. The patient typically falls asleep only to be awakened in the middle of the night with a deep underlying gnawing pain, possibly due to tumor expansion. As the pain increases in severity a radicular component usually develops. If the tumor irritates adjacent nerve roots, a radiculopathy with definite motor and sensory loss becomes apparent. As the tumor expands into the spinal canal a cervical myelopathy will readily occur. Usually, however, the neurologic symptoms occur well after the onset of pain.

Fortunately the radiologic appearance of these diseases is fairly specific. Cervical spine films with oblique views followed by CT scanning will reveal osteolytic lesions, pathologic fractures, and abnormal soft tissue masses in the majority of cases. Definitive diagnosis requires tissue biopsy, either from the cervical lesion itself or, as is sometimes possible in metastatic lesions, from the primary tumor site itself. Multiple myeloma produces "punched out" osteolytic lesions of the spine as well as a severe generalized osteoporosis, and pathologic fractures may ensue. Appropriate hematologic evaluations will usually clinch the diagnosis in these cases.

In all cases in which the cervical spine is involved by tumor there are two important treatment considerations. Assuring the stability of the spine and maintaining neurologic functions are of paramount importance in planning treatment. Nonsurgical interventions such as radiation or chemotherapy and bracing are appropriate first-line treatments in many cases if a tissue diagnosis is already available. These may eliminate the need for surgical intervention. Close follow-up with radiologic studies and serial neurologic exams is necessary to detect progression of disease. If spinal stability or neurologic function is at risk, further consultation is required with specialists who are honestly interested in spinal surgical problems, be they neurologic or orthopedic surgeons. A variety of new techniques are now available to stabilize and decompress the spine, even in the most advanced of disease states. Patients with reasonable life expectancies (usually greater than 6 months) who are in medical condition to tolerate extensive operative procedures are candidates for these techniques. Unfortunately, for inpatients with a very limited prognosis as a result of extensive tumor spread or general poor health, simple bracing, supportive care, and radiation or chemotherapy are often all that is possible.

OSTEOARTHRITIS

In the vertebral column osteoarthritic changes are usually associated with intervertebral disk degeneration. Disk degeneration, resulting from trauma or advanced age, reduces the shock absorber effect of a well-hydrated intervertebral disk and causes abnormal stresses to be applied to the vertebral body, the adjacent uncinate process (joint of Luschka), and the posterior facet areas. Over time, reactive osteophyte formation occurs along the joint interfaces. The buildup of these bony spurs may extend directly posteriorly toward the spinal canal and cause cord compression and myelopathy. More commonly spur formation occurs at the uncinate process and facet joint, resulting thereby in neural foraminal stenosis. The most common sites of degenerative osteophytes are the C5-C6 and C6-C7 joint spaces.

Pure cervical osteoarthritis in itself (when not involving the nervous system) is not usually associated with a great number of symptoms. On occasion the patient may describe mechanical neck pain with radiation suggestive of but not corresponding to a radicular distribution. This may be associated with a variety of symptoms—headaches, shoulder pains, clicking sounds—that seem to be exacerbated by purely mechanical factors. For unclear reasons high cervical disk degeneration with joint collapse and osteoarthritic changes is commonly associated with a headache that at times is impossible to separate from a tension headache. Periodically the patient may suffer acute attacks with increased neck discomfort and severe muscle pains resembling acute torticollis. These episodes are often triggered by activity and physical exertion, and peak after 2–3 days, with total recovery within 7–10 days.

When the cervical osteoarthritis has progressed to cause nerve root compression, radicular pain and symptoms are common. Lesions of this type are often referred to as "hard" disks (to be discussed below). When the cervical osteoarthritis extends posteriorly and causes central canal stenosis, cord compression and cervical spondylotic myelopathy occur. The common term for this myelopathy is *cervical spondylosis*, and the classic references describing this disorder were written in 1967 and 1971 (9, 10). The combination of neck pain, increased lower extremity reflexes, stiff gait, and plain spine films showing osteophytic spurs is insufficient to make the presumptive diagnosis. The next diagnostic study of choice under these circumstances is the MRI scan. In some instances, bony anatomy may be insufficiently visualized, in which case a plain or intrathecally enhanced CT scan should be obtained. In all types of osteoarthritic disease, nonsteroidal anti-inflammatory medications often speed recovery from mechanical symptoms (such as local pain and muscle spasm) and are helpful in keeping the patient active. Once the osteoarthritic changes have progressed to cause problems related to compression of neural tissue, remission of the symptoms is rare. Anti-inflammatory medications and mechanical stabilization in bracing devices may prevent progression of symptoms for a long time; however, in the majority of cases well-planned operative decompressions will afford relief of symptoms and ensure that further neural tissue compression does not occur.

NERVE ROOT IRRITATIONS

The spinal cord is the conduit for carrying information to and from the brain. At the segmental level nerve roots gather information from the periphery and deliver motor messages to the trunk and limbs. Each of these nerve

roots exits through a foramen, and can be compressed by disk protrusion or osteophytes. Such compression will lead to pain in the distribution of the nerve root, and often locally as well. In explaining the problem to the patient it is often helpful to use the analogy of a telephone wire being rubbed on by a tree, which in turn produces static on the line.

Cervical radiculitis is a term applied when a nerve root is irritated and inflamed. The extension of this term, *cervical radiculopathy*, implies that damage to the root has produced a clinically appreciable motor or sensory neurologic deficit in the distribution of the root. Typically, patients with cervical root pain syndromes have neck pain made worse by extension and turning to the painful side. In addition, they will have pain that radiates either into the lower neck and shoulder (C4-C5 roots) or well down into the upper extremity (C8-T1 roots). C8 and C7 root irritation in particular cause significant arm pain. These patterns are described above in the anatomic section of this chapter. Unfortunately, differentiation between these patterns can sometimes be difficult in a clinical setting. For example, differentiation between C6 and C7 root involvement may be difficult at times. In both of these syndromes biceps and triceps strength is affected and the patterns of sensation loss are similar: C6 involvement causes sensation loss on the thumb and C7 on the middle finger. Either of these syndromes can cause sensation loss on the index finger, although the C7 syndrome does so more frequently.

The predominantly radicular nature of these patients' symptoms and complaints is the key element of the history and physical examination. Although the roots as they exit from the spinal canal can be compressed by numerous factors, by far the most common source of such irritation is either an acute disk herniation and/or a degenerative disk that in turn has caused focal osteoarthritic changes with foraminal stenosis. We commonly refer to these as "soft" and "hard" disk disease, respectively. The soft disk disorders tend to occur in patients under the age of 50. The hard disk/osteoarthritis spur formation tends to occur in the older population, although obviously there are no absolutes.

After obtaining a medical history and physical examination, diagnostic studies will often pinpoint which root is involved. Neurophysiologic studies such as EMG/NCV are helpful in pinpointing the level involved; however, diagnostic imaging is essential to making the correct diagnosis and in formulating treatment. In addition, in some patients (particularly those who have ill-defined neck and shoulder pain that is not clearly radicular in nature) plain shoulder films may be useful to rule out glenohumeral joint disease. The first and most basic diagnostic study, however, should be the plain cervical spine film with oblique views. In younger patients and in those who have normal-appearing plain x-rays, the next diagnostic study of choice is MRI, which will usually show the soft disks better than other diagnostic modalities will. In older patients and in those who have evidence of degenerative disk disease and spurs on plain films, the preferable next study is an intrathecally enhanced CT scan, which will allow better visualization of bony anatomy than MRI will.

Treatment of these lesions requires decompression of the affected root. In selected cases cervical bracing and traction or physical therapy may be of long-term benefit; however, in the vast majority this decompression is best accomplished surgically.

GOUT, MULTIPLE SCLEROSIS, AMYOTROPHIC LATERAL SCLEROSIS, SYRINGOMYELIA, KLIPPEL-FEIL SYNDROME

Gouty arthritis is associated with elevation of uric acid levels and deposits within various joints. Although the disease commonly affects such joints as the big toe, it definitely can influence the spinal axis, including the cervical spine. Patients with known gouty arthritis have an increased incidence of degenerative changes in the cervical spine. The radiographic appearance is identical to that of osteoarthritis. The symptoms cannot be differentiated from those of the cervical myeloradiculopathies, and the treatment is basically the same. In the acute episode of the presentation, confirmation of the uric acid levels and use of uricosuric agents is appropriate as well.

Multiple sclerosis can occur in conjunction with osteoarthritic changes in the cervical spine. It is true that the two diseases together can accentuate an existing myelopathy. Decompressive procedures are only half as successful in this condition as they are in the routine setting, and the chance of symptomatic relief after surgery is less than 50%. Consequently, in these settings, only 50% of patients truly benefit from any type of decompressive laminectomy, foraminotomy, anterior cervical diskectomy, or the like. It appears that when a fusion is done with an anterior diskectomy, the spine is slightly more stabilized and there are better results in the relief of not only the pain but the intrinsic neurologic problem. This probably is related to immobilization of the spinal cord, which is already diseased.

Amyotrophic lateral sclerosis can be present in patients with some pain caused by the associated arthritic changes that occur in the spine. The neurologic disease itself is painless. However, because of the imbalances along the spine caused by muscular weakness, however, arthritic changes can occur with some discomfort to the patients. Symptomatic treatment is all that is required. Rarely do any of these cases need operative surgery.

Syringomyelia was always thought to be a painless disease. In specific, patients experienced numbness in a cape-like distribution over the shoulders and arms, with muscle weakness primarily in the hands. Often they would have a myelopathy as well. However, as revealed by information obtained from MRI studies, however, syringomyelia usually presents initially as pain, often in a root fashion. This pain accompanies the initial development of the syrinx. As the syrinx enlarges, the pain fibers are destroyed and the patient has less pain. It is most beneficial to treat these patients early, with correction of the syrinx itself. This can be done by correcting the Arnold-Chiari malformation at the base of the skull if that exists and/or draining the syrinx into either the pleural or the peritoneal cavity. If the syrinx is adequately drained, patients will have less pain. Even with the most successful procedure, rarely is all the patient's discomfort obliterated.

When a patient has congenital blocked vertebrae, as in Klippel-Feil syndrome, there is an increased instance of osteoarthritic changes at an adjacent level, usually cephalad and rarely caudally. With an immobile joint in the cervical spine, the next superior joint often has accelerated degenerative changes with osteophyte formation. This can lead to a radiculitis and/or myelopathy. If the usual measures of physical therapy, proper exercises, and anti-inflammatory medications fail, then the patients often do require decompressive procedures on the nerve roots. If there is marked compression anteriorly, an anterior operation can be done. Rarely do patients require more-extensive fusions posteriorly.

CERVICAL TRAUMA

Cervical spine trauma is almost invariably diagnosed on the historic facts alone. In taking a history, details of the traumatic event should be recorded succinctly and accurately, because this may prove germane to further events in our current litigious society. The trauma itself may be divided into its neurologic, bony and ligamentous, and muscular components, and each may give rise to significant pain. The most frequent cervical spine traumatic event that causes pain is muscle sprain or strain, more commonly referred to as whiplash injury. Under normal conditions of wear and tear the cervical muscles modulate many of the forces being transmitted to the cervical spine via balanced contraction and relaxation. Rapid, large changes in motion or force, as occur in cervical spine injury, may exceed the capacity of the cervical musculature to compensate, leading to muscle strain and tears. Larger disruptive forces may cause bony and ligamentous damage in addition to the muscular injury. Classically the pain associated with muscle strain develops to a maximum after about 2–3 weeks. In the setting of trauma, local neck pain with spasm, and stiffness of cervical muscles, normal neurologic examination and normal diagnostic studies (if performed at all; usually plain films only) are the criteria that must be met before this diagnosis can be confidently made. If any one of these criteria is not met then other cervical spine injury beyond muscle spasm must be suspected, and further diagnostic work-up is appropriate and necessary. Similarly, traumatic neck pain that persists for more than 3 weeks after injury should raise a red flag, and should be considered suspicious of bony or ligamentous origin until proven otherwise.

Mild cases of cervical sprain are usually best treated with mild non-narcotic analgesics and application of heat packs. In more severe cases, decreasing cervical mobility with a bracing device such as a soft collar and the judicious use of antispasm medications such as cyclobenzaprine (Flexaril) or carisoprodol (Soma) may be required.

Trauma with bony or ligamentous disruption is caused by extreme abnormal movements or compressive forces in the neck. Although the head itself only weighs from 10 to 15 pounds, that weight alone is in extreme flexion and tension sufficient to damage bones. Furthermore, although protected from extremes of movement in flexion and extension by muscle and ligament, the cervical vertebrae are very vulnerable to axial compressive forces. These forces are commonly generated in diving and automobile accidents, thus accounting for the high percentage of cervical spine injury in such cases. The injury from such forces is variable, and may result in ligamentous tear, bony fracture, or dislocation and malalignment depending on the location and force vectors involved.

In general, bony and ligamentous cervical spine injuries can usually be classified into flexion, compression, or tension-type injuries. On rare occasions distraction injuries may occur, especially in the upper cervical and occipital areas. The pain associated with bony and ligamentous trauma is mechanical, sharp, and exacerbated by even the slightest cervical motion. In the absence of damage to neural structures, radicular or dysesthetic pain may not be present.

In the setting of trauma and neck pain, plain cervical spine films (particularly the lateral view) are essential. All seven cervical vertebrae must be visualized, as must be the occiput-C1 and C7-T1 junctions. Additional views such as oblique views are often helpful. Cooperative patients may have flexion and extension films (with careful monitoring of neurologic function at each position, of course) to further document the degree of instability. Generally the more abnormal the first lateral cervical spine radiograph, the lesser the need for further films. If the films initially appear normal and bony pathology is still suspected, then additional views such as oblique or flexion/extension should be attempted. If following adequate films any uncertainty remains regarding bony anatomy, CT scan becomes mandatory.

Trauma may leave the patient neurologically intact and with x-rays that are unimpressive. In these cases ligamentous and/or joint capsular tearing is usually the source of pain. In most cases the patients can localize the discomfort accurately to the level of the lesion. Local injection of damaged facets or ligaments with anesthetic agents is both diagnostic and therapeutic in this case.

In the neck with unstable bony disruption or significant malalignment secondary to trauma, skeletal tong traction must be initiated early to achieve stability. The only exceptions to this rule are disruption injuries causing distraction of the occiput from C1 or C2. In these cases the application of traction can worsen the distraction and literally "pull the head off." In all other instances, however, bony alignment with judicious use of traction, multiple sequential lateral cervical spine films, and close monitoring of neurologic status, is the appropriate course of action, and should be carried out as rapidly as feasible.

Finally, cervical spine trauma may result in injury to the nervous tissue itself. Although this most commonly occurs in the setting of cervical spine fractures, damage to neural structures may also occur independently of this, as in traumatic anterior spinal artery or central cord syndromes. Focal pain at the site of injury and the presence of neurologic deficit are presumptive evidence of traumatic cord/root injury. The classic picture is of flaccid plegia or paresis during the spinal shock phase that eventually gives way to spasticity and upper extremity lower motor neuron deficits. Proximal motor function may be preserved, but the fine motor control needed for adequate hand function is invariably lost. Numbness, clumsiness, and even complete paralysis of the hands is the rule rather than the exception in these situations, and hand dysfunction may even exceed lower extremity dysfunction. This is particularly true with central cord syndromes, where upper extremity lower motor neuron lesions figure prominently.

When there is neurologic deficit in the presence of spinal trauma, adequate visualization of the spinal cord/thecal sac is essential for planning further treatment. Bony fragments, herniated disks, and epidural hematomas may all cause persistent cord compression independent of that caused by the initial traumatic blow itself. Intrathecally enhanced CT or MRI scanning is therefore required.

Treatment centers around the dual needs to stabilize the spinal column and to alleviate ongoing neural compression. The institution of skeletal traction is a valuable first step toward stabilizing the spinal column, and may alleviate neural compression as well. Thus, judicious use of skeletal traction is the first treatment choice. Surgery, either to relieve ongoing neural compression or to internalize a stabilization construct, should be considered rapidly thereafter if the patient's clinical status will allow. This will be followed with 6 weeks to 3 months in a rigid cervical orthosis until the surgical fusion is stable.

RHEUMATOID ARTHRITIS

Rheumatoid arthritis is a chronic inflammatory disease of probable, although undefined, infectious etiology. Subsequent to the presumed infection, a broad immunologic response is generated that after prolonged periods of time leads to characteristic changes in many joints of the body. The prevalence of this disorder in the United States is roughly 1% of the population. Although juvenile forms exist, more frequently it is the elderly patient with rheumatoid arthritis who develops cervical spine pain and arthritic changes. The cervical spine is commonly involved, especially in the C1-C2 area. Inflammatory processes in this region cause exuberant pannus formation, bony destruction, and ligamentous laxity. Atlanto-occipital subluxation, basilar investigation, and atlantoaxial subluxation are frequent end results.

Mechanical neck pain is the initial presenting symptomatology. Occipital headache and muscle spasm can also occur. Extremes of bony and ligamentous instability may allow cord compression, resulting in lower cranial nerve palsies, myelopathy, and facial numbness. Trivial trauma in the presence of this instability may cause acute, devastating neurologic deficit. More commonly, the patient presents with simple neck pain and as followed over time develops a gait disturbance with myelopathy and associated changes.

The diagnosis of rheumatoid arthritis is often made on physical examination alone because the findings in patients with rheumatoid arthritis are multiple and characteristic. Confirmatory laboratory evidence is obtained by elevated erythrocyte sedimentation rate and rheumatoid factor screen. Radiologic evidence of rheumatoid arthritis is best obtained on plain spine films. Tomograms will also disclose the loss of bony tissue with further appreciation of atlantoaxial subluxation. More recently, with MRI, the actual pannus buildup in and around the dens can be seen. Treatment of the mechanical pain of cervical spine rheumatoid arthritis relies upon steroidal and nonsteroidal anti-inflammatory agents. The development of significant (usually greater than 1 cm) subluxation at C1-C2, spinal instability, or neurologic deficit warrants serious consideration of surgical decompressive/stabilization procedures. Such a procedure is a major operation for many of the senior patients involved, and the morbidity of the postsurgical bracing devices (i.e., the halo brace) is not insignificant in this population. Nonetheless, such treatment is warranted since the natural history of this disease in a patient with symptomatic neural compression is indeed most bleak.

Ankylosing Spondylitis

Ankylosing spondylitis is an inflammatory joint disorder with a striking predilection for the cartilaginous joints of the axial skeleton. The main pathologic features involve abnormal deposition of calcium and spontaneous fusion of the ligamentous and facet structures. Although ankylosing spondylitis is commonly associated with the lumbosacral spine, it may also advance to involve the neck. It is initially associated with gradual onset of pain and aching in the lower back and buttocks. Morning stiffness is often present; this tends to improve with exercise during the day. There may be an associated mild peripheral arthritis. Mechanical spine pain and restriction of mobility go hand in hand. Compression of neural structures is rare, and radicular and myelopathic pain patterns are therefore rarely present. The abnormally fused spine becomes brittle and is therefore fractured easily even with minor trauma. This may cause acute onset of neurologic complaints.

Diagnosis may be made on the basis of plain spine films. The high association of this disease with BLA-B27 antigen type warrants this type of testing as well.

Often confused with ankylosing spondylitis is a hyperostotic disorder that primarily affects the anterior longitudinal ligament of the spine. This is referred to as the *diffuse idiopathic skeletal hyperostosis (DISH)* syndrome. It has also been termed *Forrestier's disease* (11). Fortunately this unusual form of ankylosing hyperostosis does not require specific therapy outside of occasional nonsteroidal anti-inflammatory medications and continuous physical therapy modalities.

Infections

Although infections of the cervical spine are rare, the consequences of failure to make a proper diagnosis and initiate therapy in a timely fashion are so devastating that discussion is appropriate.

Whereas neoplastic processes usually begin in the bone and spare the disk space, infection is just the opposite; it usually begins in the disk space, with bony destruction occurring only later. The most common offending organisms are staphylococcal and streptococcal species, usually introduced into the area by iatrogenic means or by hematogenous spread from other foci. Other infectious organisms, such as tuberculosis, brucellosis, anaerobic bacteria, and fungi, are rare in this country except in specific host populations. Younger patients especially are susceptible to streptococcal infections, which may spread to the nasopharyngeal and tonsillar area and into the retropharyngeal space and on rare occasions become localized in a disk space. In the young adult the most common infection is usually staphylococcal. In the older person or in immunosuppressed individuals tuberculosis and other more indolent infections may be seen. Finally, select patients with severe immunosuppression may develop fungal infections of the spine.

When the infections occur within the spine there is relatively little systemic and/or immunologic response initially. Fever, sweats, and constitutional symptoms are common but not universal. Neck pain, with radiation to the shoulders and back of the head, is a predominant symptom of cervical spine infection. Invariably patients will have restricted range of motion of their neck and rather striking muscle spasms. These nonspecific complaints are often present for several weeks to months before the diagnosis is even entertained. If the infection tracks into the prevertebral space, dysphagia, dysphasia, and hoarseness may occur. Myelopathy is a late and ominous sign, indicative of epidural compression and possible epidural abscess.

Unfortunately, radiographic bony changes usually take 3–6 weeks to develop; thus the diagnosis of earlier, potentially more easily curable infection is difficult. Bone scanning with gallium or technetium or labeled white cells has become an important diagnostic adjuvant in these disorders. Elevated systemic white count as well as high erythrocyte sedimentation rate will point to possible infectious processes as well.

Making the proper microbiologic diagnosis may require aspiration or open biopsy and drainage. More recently more-aggressive care has been widely recommended. This protocol includes biopsy, drainage, curettage, and concomitant bony fusion occurring as the initial surgical procedure, and it has been very successful. The organism is identified, and appropriate antimicrobial coverage is continued for at least 6 weeks. After the cervical stabilization procedure, external immobilization with a rigid orthosis is commonly required.

CLINICAL CONCLUSIONS

The study of neck pain in cervical spine disorders is almost a specialty within itself, with rheumatologists, neurologists, orthopedic surgeons, and neurosurgeons all very interested in and committed to understanding these disorders. With a complaint so common as neck pain it is obvious that every patient cannot and should not see a specialist. Therefore some general guidelines should be outlined for the initiation of treatment of these patients.

Patients with pain in the neck with or without cord or root complaints will need to be seen on several occasions in order to make the proper diagnosis and assess treatment. The interval between these visits may vary, but in general should be proportionate to how ill the patient is. If the patient is suspected of harboring a serious neoplastic process or infection, or has suffered severe trauma with neurologic deficit, then hospitalization and more than two or three visits a day may be appropriate. The majority of patients with new-onset cervical pian will do well with an interval of 2–3 weeks between office visits. On the other hand, if the patient has a long-term complaint without impressive physical or radiographic findings, then the interval between visits can be 3–4 weeks, if not longer. The fundamental steps in managing the patient at each visit are basically the same, and are outlined below.

VISIT 1

Visit 1 includes the initial history and physical examination. Initial diagnostic testing, such as plain spine films, is often carried out at this time, although in most caes of simple neck pain from muscle sprain this is not indicated. It is wise at this time for the physician to give the patient an initial impression of what he/she believes the patient is suffering from. Treatment can be based upon diagnostic impression, and often times will be symptomatic only, such as with nonsteroidal anti-inflammatory medications. The neck may be immobilized with some type of collar or brace, with instructions to evaluate response to immobilization. The majority of patients will not require more than a single office visit.

VISIT 2

If the patient's neck pain has not improved after a sufficient period (usually 2–3 weeks) of initial treatment, several options exist. It is mandatory first, however, to re-examine the patient for evolution in signs and symptoms. If the patient is clinically stable at this point, medications could be changed to either another nonsteroidal anti-inflammatory medication or to stronger pain medications. Utilization of such modalities as exercise and physical therapy also may be appropriate at this time. At this second visit complete cervical spine films with flexion, extension, and oblique views should be obtained regardless of diagnostic impressions. This study remains the single most important diagnostic study available to us. While the cervical spine x-rays are being done, screening hematologic evaluation, including complete blood count, rheumatoid factor, or erythrocyte sedimentation rate, could also be obtained.

VISIT 3

If the patient has not responded to the second line of treatments after a reasonable time and all the studies obtained during the second office visit are normal, again repeat physical examination is warranted, and the differential diagnosis should be mentally reviewed. If the patient is clinically stable, medications should again be changed and additional studies ordered as below. In younger patients and those with normal cervical spine films, MRI is the next most important diagnostic study. This will point out soft tissue defects and herniated disks as well as visualize the neural elements. On the other hand, if there are significant arthritic changes, bony destruction, or malalignment on plain films, then the CT scan with or without intrathecal contrast is the study of choice.

VISIT 4

In some patients an acceptable diagnosis will still not have been reached even after repeat physical examination, plain films, CT scan, and/or MRI. At this time looking for clinical oddities is warranted. Patients who have had MRI studies should have CT studies next, and vice versa. Other testing, such as EMG/NCV and bone scans, may be appropriate in specific situations. Additional blood work is also done.

VISIT 5

If the patient is continuing to suffer from cervical spine pain at this point, now usually 2–3 months after initial presentation, then consultation and further diagnostic tests/procedures should be carried out. A more sophisticated mechanical examination of the neck by orthopedists or rheumatologists is warranted. A more detailed neurologic examination by neurologists or neurosurgeons is often appropriate as well. Further diagnostic studies also should be carried out, such as bone scanning, complete myelography, and lumbar puncture if indicated. Obviously, decisions need to be made on an individual basis. With each visit, if the patient is still failing to improve, medication changes should be considered. There are over a dozen nonsteroidal anti-inflammatory medications, and it is important to try many, for patients may very greatly in their response.

SUBSEQUENT PATIENT MANAGEMENT

Visits subsequent to the fifth one should be to either a competent rheumatologist or orthopedic surgeon or neurosurgeon, because the patient will probably not get well quickly, and further consultation and advice is needed. This is frequently the beginning of the chronic neck pain syndrome. It may be that nothing more can be done for the individual. It may also be that secondary gain or conversion disorders may be operative, especially in cases involving litigation and workers' compensation. In this case psychological evaluation should be seriously considered.

In any case, by following this guideline a logical and fairly complete evaluation of the patient with cervical spine pain will have been performed. In the vast majority of cases an appropriate diagnosis is obtained and appropriate treatments are started with excellent relief of symptoms.

REFERENCES

1. Lawrence J: Disc degeneration, its frequency and relationship to symptoms. *Ann Rheum Dis* 28:121, 1989.
2. British Association of Physical Medicine: Pain in the neck and arm. *Br Med J* 1:253, 1986.
3. Hult L: Cervical, dorsal and lumbar spinal syndromes. *Acta Orthop Scand (Suppl)* 17:1, 1954.
4. Hult L: The Munkford Investigation. *Acta Orthop Scand (Suppl)* 16:1, 1954.
5. Spurling RG, Scoville WB: Lateral rupture of the cervical intervertebral discs. *Surg Gynecol Obstet* 78:350, 1944.
6. Bland J: *Disorders of the Cervical Spine.* Philadelphia, WB Saunders, 1987, p 40.
7. Wilkins R, Regachary SP: *Neurosurgery.* New York, McGraw-Hill, 1985.
8. Spencer P, Nunn P, Hugan J, et al: Guam amyotrophic lateral sclerosis-parkinsonism-dementia linked to a plant excitant neurotoxin. *Science* 237:517–522, 1987.
9. Brain W: Cervical Spondylosis: Philadelphia, WB Saunders, 1967.
10. Wilkenson M: *Cervical Spondylosis: Its Early Diagnosis and Treatment.* Philadelphia, WB Saunders, 1971.
11. Rosnick D. Niawayama G: Radiographic and pathological features of spinal involvement in diffuse idiopathic skeletal hyperostosis (DISH). *Radiology* 119:558, 1978.

CHAPTER 27

DIFFERENTIAL DIAGNOSIS OF LOW BACK PAIN

JOHN A. McCULLOCH

THE FOLLOWING question is frequently asked by doctors at various stages of training and practice experience: "How can I assess and treat a patient with back pain when the diagnosis is so elusive?" It is hard on the ego to assess a patient and fail to arrive at a concrete diagnosis on which to base a treatment program. All too often, a treatment program for low back pain is based more on hope than on science. This should not be so. In today's medical world, our clinical skills and our investigative tools are such that we should be able to arrive at the correct diagnosis for most patients with "lumbago or sciatica." This chapter outlines the simple steps needed to assess a patient who presents with a complaint of low back pain.

ASSESSMENT METHOD

Do not initiate your assessment with a long list of time-consuming differential diagnoses on your menu. In family practice, this presents an overwhelming burden to the multitude of chief complaints heard during a day. Instead, adopt a simple, methodical approach. Your goal is to sort those patients who have mechanical or structural problems in the low back from those who have not. In a family practice setting, perhaps 20–25% of patients presenting with low back pain will have a source outside of the back as the cause of their symptoms. This fact presents many pitfalls for the unwary. For this reason, accurate evaluation requires a logical, step-by-step method. The foundation of this method is the clinical assessment, the good old-fashioned history and physical examination. Investigations such as magnetic resonance imaging (MRI), computed tomography (CT) scanning, and myelography should play a secondary role to clinical assessment. Today, our investigative tools are so sophisticated that one can find pathology in almost every patient whether or not the patient is sick (1, 2). Moreover, minor insignificant pathology can be-

come the red herring that causes you to miss the symptom-producing lesion.

CLINICAL APPROACH

In assessing a patient with a low back complaint, ask yourself five questions:

1. Is this a true physical disability or is there a setting and a pattern on history and physical examination to suggest a nonphysical or nonorganic problem?
2. Is this clinical presentation a diagnostic trap?
3. Is this a mechanical low back pain condition, and if so, what is the syndrome?
4. Are there clues to an anatomic level on history and physical examination?
5. After reviewing the results of investigation, what is the structural lesion and does it fit with the clinical syndrome?

Although these questions may not be answered sequentially during the history and physical examination, they ultimately must be answered sequentially before arriving at a diagnosis and prescribing a treatment program. That is to say, do not answer question 5 and plan a treatment program based on a radiographic diagnosis until you have satisfactory answers to each preceding question. Probably the biggest pitfall is to answer question 3 before you have satisfactorily answered questions 1 and 2. The answers to questions 1 and 2 should routinely be made outside the hospital, and before CT, myelography, MRI, and other sophisticated investigative modalities are used. The classic trap is to ignore questions 1 and 2 and admit a patient with a complaint of low back pain to the hospital, order sophisticated tests, and then prescribe a treatment plan based on false-positive radiographic findings.

Each of the five questions listed above will be dealt with in its own section.

QUESTION 1

Is this a true physical disability or is there a setting and a pattern on history and physical examination to suggest a nonphysical or nonorganic problem?

That medicine should concern itself with the whole person is often stated but frequently ignored. The hallmark of a good clinician is the ability not only to diagnose disease but also to assess the "whole patient." No test of the art of medicine is more demanding than the identification of the patient with a nonorganic or emotional component to a back disability.

To start, recognize the disability equation:

$$Disability = A + B + C$$

where

A = the physical component (disease)
B = the patient's emotional reaction
C = the situation the patient is in at the time of disability (e.g., compensation claim, motor vehicle accident)

Each patient presenting with a back disability may have some component of each of these entities entwined in their disability. For example, a patient presenting a collection of symptoms, with no physical disability evident on examination, should lead one to think of the other aspects of the equation and look for emotional disability or situational reactions.

A classification of nonorganic spinal pain is outlined in Table 27.1. The term *nonorganic* has been chosen over other terms such as nonphysical, functional, emotional, and psychogenic. The following definitions are used for the classification in Table 27.1.

1. Psychosomatic Spinal Pain. Psychosomatic spinal pain is defined as symptomatic physical change in tissues of the spine that has as its cause anxiety. The expression of anxiety is mediated as a prolonged and exaggerated state that eventually leads to structural change (spasm) in the muscles of the neck or low back.

2a. Psychogenic Spinal Pain. Psychogenic spinal pain is defined as the conversion or somatization of anxiety into pain located in the neck or back, unaccompanied by physical change in the tissues of these regions. The pain

Table 27.1.
Nonorganic Spinal Pain

1. Psychosomatic spinal pain
   a. Tension syndrome (fibrositis)
2. Psychogenic spinal pain
   a. Psychogenic spinal pain
   b. Psychogenic modification of organic spinal pain
3. Situational spinal pain
   a. Litigation reaction
   b. Exaggeration reaction

is variously known in the literature as conversion hysteria, psychogenic regional pain, traumatic or accident neurosis, and hypochondriasis.

The emotional upset brings pains to the back just as it may bring tears to the eyes. The reason for the conversion is found in complex psychodynamic mechanisms beyond the scope of this chapter. The reaction represents a sincere unconscious emotional illness that offers the patient the primary gain of solving inner conflicts, fears, and anxieties. Inherent in the conversion reaction is the concept of suggestion and hypnosis, the importance of which will become apparent later in this chapter.

2b. Psychogenic Modification of Organic Spinal Pain. Psychogenic modification of spinal pain is a sincere emotional reaction that modifies the appreciation of an organic pain. Usually, the organic pain by itself would not be disabling, but with the psychogenic modification a significant disability ensues. No associated physical change occurs as a result of anxiety, and a conversion reaction may or may not coexist (3).

An example is the patient burdened with life-situational pressures (mortgage payments, car payments) who, because of his physical illness, believes he cannot sustain the effort necessary to meet these demands. A resulting depression may occur, and the symptoms of fatigue, loss of appetite, insomnia, impotence, constipation, and the like so dominate the history that the underlying physical condition is missed. Other examples are patients with passive-dependent personality, drug or alcohol dependence, or psychosis who, in the face of a minor physical problem, use their illness to step out of the demands of the real world.

Some obsessive-compulsive patients cannot adjust to a minor physical problem, and this personality trait leads them to believe they have a significant disability.

3. Situational Spinal Pain. Situational spinal pain is a reaction whereby a patient, through a collection of symptoms, maintains a situation (with potential secondary gain) through overconcern (3a) or conscious effort (3b).

3a. Litigation Reaction. The litigation or compensation reaction is defined as overconcern by the patient for present and future health, arising out of a litigious or compensable event that initially affected health. The reaction manifests itself in patient's complaint of continuing neck or back pain coupled with a concern that, upon formal severance from his claim to compensation, deterioration in health may occur. The patient with this reaction is neither physically nor emotionally ill.

This reaction is not to be confused with the ambiguous terms *litigation neurosis* or *compensation neurosis.* Like "whiplash," these terms have no medical or legal value and should be dropped from our vocabulary. If a patient has a true neurosis arising out of a litigious or compensable event (accident), then those terms listed under *Psychogenic Spinal Pain (2a)* should be used for diagnostic purposes (e.g., traumatic neurosis or accident neurosis). If the patient's disability appears to be based more on his awareness of the commercial value of his symptoms, his reaction should not be legitimized by the use of the term neurosis in conjunction with the words "litigation" or "compensation" (thus *litigation reaction*).

3b. Exaggeration Reaction. Exaggeration reactions are attempts by the patient to appear ill or to magnify an existent illness. *Malingering* is a term frequently applied to the reaction, and is defined as "the conscious alteration of health for gain."

As is described below, it is possible for the physician to detect efforts to magnify pain, but it is not proper for him to assign motives (gain) to the patient. The lawyer involved is in a reversed role. He may raise doubts about the plaintiff's motives (gain), but he is in no position to clinically detect the effort to magnify or exaggerate. The choice of the word "malingering" implies proficiency in two professions, an uncommon occurrence. For this reason, the terms *malingering* and *conscious effort* are best not used by the physician when discussing nonorganic spinal pain.

Alteration of health in order to deceive, to evade responsibility, or to derive gain does occur. Those who would deny its occurrence deny the existence of human nature. The patient who tries to alter or reproduce symptoms or signs of a spinal problem may do so in a number of ways:

1. *Pretension:* No physical illness exists and the patient willfully fabricates symptoms and signs. Occurring infrequently in the military during wartime, it is a rare civilian event.
2. *Exaggeration:* Symptoms and signs of a spinal disability are magnified to represent more than they really do.
3. *Perseveration:* As a manifestation of back disability, perseveration is a continuing complaint by the patient after the physical cause of the disability has ceased to exist.
4. *Allegation:* Genuine disability is present, but the patient fraudulently ascribes these to some cause, associated with gain, knowing that, in fact, his condition is of different origin (e.g., a fall at home instead of at work).

Civilian nonorganic situational spinal pain is usually the exaggeration or perseveration type. Pretension and allegation are uncommon forms of gainful alteration of health in civilian practice. Like the patient with the litigation reaction, these patients are neither emotionally nor physically ill. They differ from patients with the litigation reaction, however, in that they are attempting to demonstrate physical illness through the effort of exaggeration or perseveration. The reason for this effort is usually, but not always, found in secondary financial gain.

CLINICAL DESCRIPTION

Before describing each of these entities, it is important to emphasize a few points. First, the above classification is a simplistic one that is useful only to the family practitioner or the spinal surgeon. It does not allow for the more-complex assessments done by psychologists, psychiatrists, and the like, but it does allow for a foundation on which to build clinical recognition of these entities so that the patient can be referred to others more skilled in the field. Second, one cannot rigidly define disability, because there are gray areas. There is a tendency for a nonorganic disability to fall largely into one category, however. Third, it is most important to determine if one of the following settings exist for nonorganic disabilities:

1. A patient who has had previous emotional problems is prone to have an emotional component to a disability. Symptoms such as fatigue, sleeplessness, agitation, gastrointestinal upset, and excessive sweating should signal that an emotional component is likely present.
2. A patient who is in a secondary gain situation such as a motor vehicle accident claim has the potential for these nonorganic reactions. It is important to establish the presence of such circumstances early in the patient encounter. If a patient states that low back pain started suddenly with an incident, it is important to document whether or not the incident is a claim type of accident and whether or not insurance and legal factors are involved. Conversely, if there is no secondary gain detected on history, it is unusual to arrive at a secondary gain diagnosis such as litigation reaction or exaggeration reaction.
3. A vague and confusing history, a baffling physical examination, and an elusive diagnosis signal a possible nonorganic diagnosis. Reflect on this before taking the expensive step of hospital admission and sophisticated testing.
4. A patient who quickly establishes an abnormal doctor-patient relationship has a potential nonorganic component to his disability. These abnormal doctor-patient relationships include a hostile or effusively complimentary patient, a patient who has had many other doctors involved in care prior to your assessment, a patient who fails to respond to standard conservative treatment measures, and a patient who is critical of other doctors.

Psychosomatic Spinal Pain

The psychosomatic phenomenon of muscle spasm arising out of tension states usually affects the neck, but may affect the low back. It should be known as the *orthopedic ulcer*, but more often is given the label of *fibrositis*. Patients with this problem are overtly strained and tense, as evidenced by facial expression. They are fidgety and restless and may sit on the edge of the chair while they wring their hands. Some of these patients will place their hands on their neck or back during the history and literally wring the area while describing the pain. They have a general feeling of restlessness and a specific feeling of a tightness in their neck with associated sensations of cracking and a constant feeling of the need to stretch out the neck and shoulder muscles. The pain is not specifically mechanical but does tend to accumulate with the day's activity, especially when that activity is carried out in the tension-producing environment (e.g., work).

The pain typically responds to chiropractic or physiotherapeutic intervention, but relief is usually temporary, a fact that makes the patient tend to seek prolonged care.

Physical examination reveals a good range of movement in the back, with a complaint of pain only if movement is done too quickly or carried to extremes. The significant physical finding is the presence of firm, tender muscles when the affected part is examined in a position of rest—the so-called "trigger-point." The patient may be able to demonstrate the "cracking" to the touch or auditory perception of the examiner.

No evidence of nerve root involvement exists in the lower extremities. Skin tenderness, the significance of which is explained below, is not a usual finding.

Psychogenic Spinal Pain

Patients with psychogenic spinal pain are emotionally ill. These patients often have a history of past illnesses replete with emotional problems. It follows that the history of the present illness contains a preponderance of emotional symptoms, and the description of the pain will not be typical of any organic condition. The patient is convinced that he is ill, and that conviction extends to the frequent demand for consultations with numerous doctors. Considerable financial hardship and aggravation will occur in some cases when these consultations take the patient great distances to and from major clinics or spas throughout the world. Throughout their constant demand for care, these patients notice times when their symptoms do improve. This is due to the institution of some new form of treatment that affects the patient through suggestion or hypnosis, a fact that makes placebo trial of little value in the evaluation of these problems.

It follows that because these patients are emotionally ill, no causative organic problem will be found on physical examination. The conversion reaction is associated with an upset body image appreciation such that a topographic unit (the back and leg), indifferent to matters of innervation or anatomic relationship, will contain physical findings of skin tenderness and dulled sensory appreciation (3). The somatization infrequently reaches the stage of weakness with wasting and depression of

all the reflexes in the contiguous part (e.g., an arm or leg).

The important observation on physical examination of this patient is the paucity of physical findings, which separates him from the magnifier and exaggerator, who by definition has many "physical" findings.

Psychogenic Modification of Organic Spinal Pain

Of all the nonorganic causes of spinal pain, the patient who psychogenically modifies organic pain presents the most difficult diagnostic and therapeutic challenge. Sometimes, but not always, the organic problem by itself would not be disabling. Thus, the historic and physical component of the disability related to the organicity is not significant. Those findings indicative of a physical illness will be appropriate and a quantitative guide to the extent of physical illness. The life-situational pressures or the personality of the patient modifies the disability to a significant point, however. Also, the psychogenic reaction interferes with response to treatment and leads to persistence of the disability. In a surgical practice, this failure to respond to conservative treatment is the classic indication for operative intervention. If the surgeon fails to recognize that the failure to respond to treatment is due in this instance to a psychogenic disability, he will gradually build a practice containing a number of spinal surgery failures. Psychogenic modifications are commonly seen in the patient with an inadequate personality. By definition, the patient's personality may limit advancement up the social, educational, and occupational ladder and confine him to the unskilled worker classification. Some of these patients can be found in the Workers' Compensation Board population and may be one of the reasons for poorer results of treatment sometimes obtained in the "Comp" patient.

These patients are seen with a minor physical problem (e.g., back strain), yet have a total disability. All attempts at treatment fail to return the patient to the work force. Frequent office visits reinforce the disability for the patient. If the doctor fails to recognize this maladaptive reaction and reinforcement, he may add a scar to or stick a needle into the back, which will not help the patient in any way.

Other psychogenic modifications come about through drug addiction and alcohol dependence. Occasionally, psychotic behavior will convert a minor physical problem into a prolonged disability. Physical examination will reveal the nature and extent of the physical impairment. Usually the physical impairment by itself would not be significantly disabling. The loss of movement in the back is minor, the limitation of straight leg raising is minimal, and the neurologic changes are of questionable significance. In the face of repeated assessments and a continuing statement of disability, the patient's minor physical problem may become magnified in the mind of the clinician who does not assess personality and life-situational factors.

Situational Spinal Pain—Litigation Reaction

The litigation reaction patient is neither physically nor emotionally ill. Thus, few emotional symptoms will be present on historic examination. The patient is in the process of litigation or under the care of the Worker's Compensation Board. These patients often state that they do not care about the litigious or compensation issue, yet they also state that they are afraid to settle or return to work for fear that further illness will develop. Their continuing complaints are rather vague and would not normally be incapacitating. If they are on treatment, they are not improving. Physically, there may be an increased awareness of the part as manifested by skin tenderness in the affected area, but no organic illness is detectable, and there is no attempt to exaggerate or magnify a disability.

Situational Spinal Pain—Exaggeration Reaction

Some or most of the following historic characteristics will be obtained from the exaggeration reaction patient. The most obvious historic point is the secondary gain situation, which usually involves the fault of someone else and/or payment of financial compensation. Other secondary gain situations can occur. The initiating event is usually a trivial or minor incident. There may be a latent period of hours or days between the incident and the onset of symptoms, during which time the patient speaks to friends and relatives and learns the commercial value of the injury.

The patient describes the pain with some degree of indifference as evidenced by a smile or a laugh when describing his severe disability. He is vague in describing and localizing the pain, giving the examiner the impression of someone struggling to remember a dream. Specificity and elaboration require memory for repetition, a quality not present to a significant degree in this type of patient. The individual wishes you to believe that this pain is unique and severe. This attempt to have you believe in the pain is often accompanied by a salesman-like attitude with many examples of the disability spontaneously listed. Inability to engage in sex is frequently mentioned.

In spite of the trivial initiating event, the disability may have been present for a long time. Three types of treatment patterns occur:

1. The patient follows a "straight line" course of treatment; he does not respond to the standard treatment, nor to the suggestion and hypnosis of treatment (i.e., he does not improve or he gets worse).
2. The patient is not on treatment because he is "allergic" to all medications prescribed, he "suffocates" in the neck or back braces, or he becomes ill in a physiotherapy setting.
3. The patient is not on treatment because he has not sought treatment.

Certain behavioral patterns become apparent after seeing a number of these patients. Some never appear for appointments in spite of weeks of notification. Others appear late for the appointment and do not apologize or state indifferently that the traffic was heavy. There may be an attempt to manipulate your feelings with a compliment about your reputation or your office. There may be an effort to play one doctor against another by making false statements about the other doctor. Finally, hostility may appear during the assessment. A patient truly ill will not be aware or afraid of exposure and will not be hostile unless provoked. A patient exaggerating a disability is suspicious. He may start out hostile, but the usual pattern is one of developing hostility as discrepancies in the history and physical examination are exposed. Examiners are advised, for obvious reasons, not to precipitate this final behavioral pattern.

The patient who is magnifying or exaggerating a disability can be exposed only through an adequate physical examination. Those physicians who do not physically examine patients will not recognize this reaction, which may explain the reluctance of the psychiatric community to accept this clinical entity.

The physical findings of exaggeration reaction are classified into those that demonstrate acting behavior, those that indicate anticipatory behavior, and those that fail to support the patient's claim to illness.

Acting Behavior

Exaggerating a disability requires acting by the patient. This acting may be general in nature, such as the Academy Award performances put on by some patients as they moan and groan through the examination, walk around the examining room with their eyes closed, and either reach for objects to support themselves or reach for their painful areas. The incongruity of this acting behavior may be evident when the patient mounts the examining table with considerable ease and/or dresses within minutes of the examination and smiles and waves goodbye as he leaves the office.

Specific examples of acting behavior are the rigid back, a condition that disappears on the examining table, the reduction of straight leg raising (SLR) in the supine position (Fig. 27.1A) that disappears in the sitting position (Fig. 27.1B), tender skin, and the paralyzed insensitive extremity. That these findings are a result of acting can be demonstrated through the use of distraction testing (Table 27.2). Using nonpainful, nonemotional, and nonsurprising examination techniques, it is possible not only to change the acting behavior but also to demonstrate normal physical function. It is my opinion that proper distraction testing that abolishes an acted physical finding and demonstrates normal physical function is a method of demonstrating exaggeration behavior. The best distraction test is simple observation of the pa-

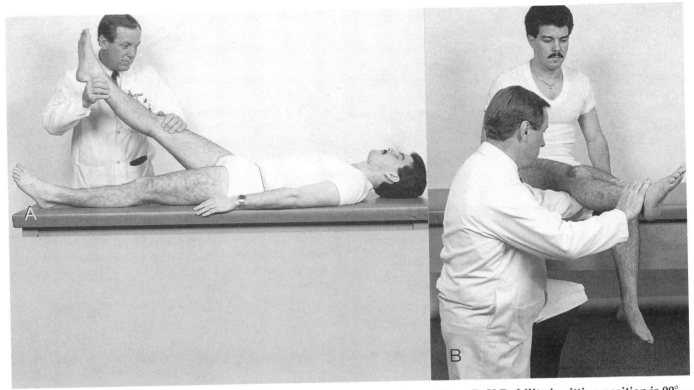

Figure 27.1. *A*, Patient demonstrating significant SLR reduction in supine position. *B*, SLR ability in sitting position is 90°—a difference from *A* that cannot be explained by root involvement, but rather represents magnification/exaggeration effort by the patient.

Table 27.2.
Demonstration of Acting Behavior

Condition	Response
Physical Finding (acting behavior)	Reduction in straight leg raising
Distraction Test (e.g., Flip test): nonpainful, nonemotional, nonsurprising	Normal straight leg raising (normal physical function)—sitting

tient as he gets undressed and moves about the examining room.

Varying degrees of acting behavior occur in different patients. In general, the more sophisticated the patient, the more sophisticated the acting behavior, and the more sophisticated the examiner must be.

Anticipatory Behavior

The second group of physical findings in this reaction represent anticipation on the part of the patient to the test situations. This anticipatory behavior leads to an appropriate response by the patient in an attempt to indicate illness. An example of this test is illustrated in Figure 27.2.

Contradictory Clinical Evidence

Statements by the patient to the effect that he is unable to work may not be supported by clinical observations. Some patients will say they are unable to drive, yet will have driven by themselves great distances to get to the examination. Some patients will say that they require frequent medication, yet will arrive from great distances without their medication. The patient who claims to be continuously wearing a collar or a brace should show signs of this wear on his body and the appliance. Patients with callouses on their hands and knees contradict their story of a prolonged inability to work. Other evidence of work may be in the form of paint stains or a particular distribution to their sunburn. Patients with nicotine stains on a grossly paralyzed limb should start to demonstrate similar stains on the opposite hand. Finally, those patients who demonstrate a prolonged and profound weakness in an extremity will not have associated wasting of that extremity.

It is important to stress that one swallow does not make a spring! The fact that a patient has one of these findings does not mean the patient should be classified as a exaggerator or litigant reactor. It is important to stress that a collection of symptoms and signs should be present with the appropriate clinical setting to make the diagnosis of exaggeration behavior. Waddell et al. (3) have documented the significant symptoms and signs

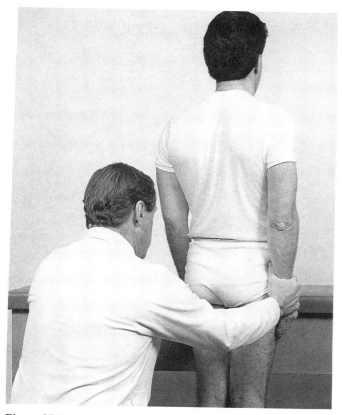

Figure 27.2. **Simulated movement testing. Holding the patient's arms fixed to the pelvis allows for rotation through the hip joints without moving the back. If the patient complains of back pain, this is considered anticipatory behavior, one of the many indications of nonorganic pain.**

Table 27.3.
Symptoms and Signs Suggesting a Nonorganic Component to Disability

Symptoms
1. Pain is multifocal in distribution and nonmechanical (present at rest)
2. Entire extremity is painful, numb, and/or weak
3. Extremity gives way (as a result the patient carries a cane)
4. Treatment response:
   a. No response
   b. "Allergic" to treatment
   c. Not on treatment
5. Multiple crises, multiple hospital admissions/investigations, multiple doctors

Signs
1. Tenderness is superficial (skin) or nonanatomic (e.g., over body of sacrum)
2. Simulated movement tests positive
3. Distraction tests positive
4. Whole leg weak or numb
5. "Academy Award" performance

that, when collected together, suggest that a nonorganic component to a disability is present. These symptoms and signs have been scientifically documented as valid and reproducible. As a screening mechanism they are an excellent substitute for pain drawings and psychological testing (Table 27.3).

CONCLUSIONS

Every human attends the school of survival. Sometimes the lessons lead patients to modify or magnify a physical disability at a conscious or unconscious level. One word of caution—the presence of one of these nonorganic reactions does not preclude an organic condition such as a herniated nucleus pulposus. The art of medicine is truly tested by a patient with a physical low back pain who modifies the disability with a nonorganic reaction of tension, hysteria, depression, or emotional factors.

QUESTION 2

Is this clinical presentation a diagnostic trap?
It is too easy, when trying to arrive at a mechanical diagnosis, to fall into the many traps in the differential

diagnosis of low back pain. An example is the young man in the early stages of ankylosing spondylitis who presents with vague sacroiliac joint pain and mild buttock and thigh discomfort who is thought to have a disk herniation. The patient with a retroperitoneal tumor invading the sacrum or sacral plexus may present with classic sciatica and also be misdiagnosed as having a disk herniation. It is not uncommon that patients with pathology within the peritoneal cavity will refer pain to the back.

To avoid missing these various diagnostic pitfalls, always ask yourself the second question: Is this clinical presentation a trap?

Two broad categories of disease are included in this question:

1. Back pain referred from outside the spine may come from within the peritoneal cavity (e.g., gastrointestinal tumors or ulcers) or from the retroperitoneal space (genitourinary conditions, abdominal aortic conditions, or primary or secondary tumors of the retroperitoneal space). These patients can be recognized clinically on the basis of two historic points. First, the pain is often nonmechanical in nature and troubles the patient just as much at rest as it does with activity. Second, the pain in the back often has the characteristics of the pain associated with the primary pathology.
2. Painful conditions arising from within the spinal column, including its neurologic content. This group is subdivided into the differential diagnosis of low back pain or lumbago (Table 27.4) and the differential diagnosis of radicular pain or sciatica (Table 27.5).

Table 27.4.
Differential Diagnosis of Nonmechanical Low Back Pain

1. Referred pain (e.g., from the abdomen or retroperitoneal space)
2. Infection—bone, disk, epidural space
3. Neoplasm
   a. Primary (e.g., multiple myeloma, osteoid osteroma)
   b. Secondary
4. Inflammation
5. Miscellaneous metabolic and vascular disorders such as osteopenias and Paget's disease

---

These patients have nonmechanical back pain or a pain more characteristic for the primary pathology. Radiating extremity pain is not common unless neurologic territory has been invaded by the disease process, which usually occurs late in the disease. Unfortunately, many of these conditions are not obvious on history and physical examination and are often missed on reviewing plain radiographs. The following diagnostic tests are useful as a screening mechanism:

1. Hemoglobin, hematocrit, white blood count, differential, and erythrocyte sedimentation rate
2. Serum chemistries, especially a fasting blood sugar, calcium, acid and alkaline phosphatase, and serum protein electrophoresis
3. Bone scan

These three screening tests can be completed outside of the hospital and almost routinely identify these conditions. MRI will start to play a bigger role in the diagnosis of these various nonmechanical conditions.

Although the most common cause of leg pain in a radicular distribution is a structural lesion in the lumbosacral region, there are many other causes of radiating leg discomfort that must be considered. Missing these conditions is probably the most common error made in a spine surgical practice. For example, the high sensitivity of today's investigative modalities is capable of showing a minor and insignificant herniated nucleus pulposus when in fact the patient has a conus tumor higher in the spinal canal. This situation is being abetted by the tendency to do a CT scan and skip myelography in an attempt to arrive at a structural diagnosis for mechanical low back pain. This may seem like a good idea to avoid the complications of myelography, but it will present problems unless you adhere to the following rule: An equivocal CT scan requires completion of myelography. Fortunately the issue is being resolved by the increasing use of MRI. Soon, all patients with low back pain who do not respond to usual conservative treatment measures will automatically have an outpatient

Table 27.5.
Differential Diagnosis of Sciatica

1. Intraspinal causes
   a. Proximal to disk—conus and cauda equina lesions (e.g., neurofibroma, ependymoma)
   b. Disk level
      Herniated nucleus pulposus
      Stenosis (canal or recess)
      Infection—osteomyelitis or diskitis (with nerve root pressure)
      Inflammation—arachnoiditis
      Neoplasm—benign or malignant with nerve root pressure
2. Extraspinal causes
   a. Pelvis
      Cardiovascular conditions (e.g., peripheral vascular disease)
      Gynecologic conditions
      Orthopedic conditions (e.g., osteoarthritis of hip)
      Sacroiliac joint disease
      Neoplasms
   b. Peripheral nerve lesions
      Neuropathy (diabetic, tumor, alcohol)
      Local sciatic nerve conditions (trauma, tumor)
      Inflammation (herpes zoster)

---

hematologic and serum screen, a bone scan, and MRI. (Is it far down the road that one day robots will deal with the structural lesion?)

ETIOLOGY OF RADIATING LEG PAIN

Space does not permit discussion of all the differential diagnoses of radiating leg pain, but three common conditions must be recognized: (1) cardiovascular conditions (peripheral vascular disease), (2) hip pathology, and (3) neuropathies.

Cardiovascular Conditions

Cardiovascular disorders in the form of peripheral vascular disease can cause leg discomfort that is easily confused with nerve root compression. Because these conditions tend to occur in the older patient population, they may coexist. Table 27.6 is an attempt to separate vascular claudication from neurogenic claudication.

Hip Pathology

Usually it is easy to diagnose conditions of the hip because they so commonly cause pain around the hip and specifically pain in the groin. In addition, walking causes a limp, and physical examination reveals a loss of internal rotation early in the disease. Occasionally, however, a patient with hip pathology will have no pain around the hip and will have only referred pain in the distal thigh. In these patients, it is easy to miss hip pathology unless one specifically examines the hip for loss of internal rotation. If there is any doubt, a radiograph of the pelvis must be taken.

Table 27.6.
Differential Diagnosis of Claudicant Leg Pain[a]

Findings	Vascular Claudication	Neurogenic Claudication
Pain		
Type	Sharp, cramping	Vague and variously described as radicular, heaviness, cramping
Location	Exercised muscles (usually excludes buttock)	Either typical radicular extremely diffuse (including buttock)
Radiation	Rare after onset	Common after onset, usually proximal to distal
Aggravation	Walking	Not only aggravated by walking, but also by standing
Relief	Stopping muscular activity even in the standing position	Walking in the forward flexed position more comfortably; once pain occurs, relief comes only with lying or sitting down
Time to relief	Quick (seconds to minutes)	Slow (many minutes)
Neurologic symptoms (paresthesia)	Not present	Commonly present
Straight leg raising tests	Negative	Mildly positive or negative
Neurologic examination	Negative	Mildly positive or negative
Vascular examination	Absent pulses	Pulses present

[a]Be wary of the patient when both conditions co-exist.

Neuropathies

The most easily missed diagnosis is diabetic mononeuropathy. Although it more commonly occurs in poorly controlled diabetes mellitus, it may occur in an undiagnosed late-onset diabetic. It is thought to be due to an ischemic episode affecting the peripheral nerve, and is characteristically manifested by acute onset with pain in a typical radicular distribution easily mimicking a disk herniation. If the peripheral neuropathy of diabetes is a mononeuropathy multiplex, a symmetrical polyneuropathy, or an autonomic neuropathy, the diagnosis is more readily apparent. The distinguishing features of diabetic mononeuropathy are as follows:

1. It occurs in the older patient with or without known diabetes.
2. There will be a history of the sudden onset of radicular pain with NO back pain.
3. The patient will describe nonmechanical leg pain; the patient is extremely uncomfortable at rest.
4. The pain is usually more severe than the pain associated with lateral recess stenosis or spinal stenosis, and of equal severity to the leg pain associated with a herniated nucleus pulposus.
5. The paresthetic discomfort often has a burning or uncomfortable characteristic to it.
6. Although the sensory symptoms predominate, it is my experience that mononeuropathy affecting the femoral or the lumbosacral nerve roots has a more significant motor and reflex component on examination. The diagnosis is supported with abnormal

blood sugar readings and electrical studies showing slower nerve conduction velocities and the presence of fibrillation potentials, positive waves at rest, and a decrease in the number of motor unit potentials on electromyography (EMG).

Conclusions

Although there are many other causes of extremity symptoms not listed in this table, it is important to recognize that the table includes most causes of lower-extremity pain. Extremity symptoms such as numbness and weakness, in the absence of pain, should suggest very strongly that a primary neurologic disorder is possible rather than a mechanical low back condition.

QUESTION 3

Is this a mechanical low back pain condition, and if so, what is the syndrome?

The two important words are "mechanical" and "syndrome." Mechanical pain is pain aggravated by activity such as bending and lifting, and relieved by rest. There may be specific complaints relative to household chores or specific work efforts. These mechanical pains, again, are usually relieved by rest. Although these statements seem straightforward, clinical assessment is not always easy. A poor historian may not be able to relate a history of mechanical aggravation or relief. In addition, if significant leg pain is present, implying a significant inflammatory response around the nerve root, then much rest will be needed before the patient describes a relief of leg pain. Significant mechanical back pain may sometimes be aggravated by simply rolling over in bed. To the unsophisticated historian, this may have the appearance of nonmechanical back pain. If one takes a careful history, however, and if a patient is a good historian, it is possible to determine that mechanical back pain is pain aggravated by activity and relieved by rest.

The second important word is "syndrome." It is much safer to make a syndrome diagnosis for mechanical low back pain and then, after investigation, try matching a structural lesion with the clinical syndrome. There are two reasons for taking this approach: (1) Today's investigative techniques are so sophisticated that it is possible to find MRI abnormalities whether a patient has symptoms or not, and (2) a patient may have an obvious structural lesion such as spondylolisthesis, yet may have an acute radicular syndrome due to a disk herniation at a level other than that of the spondylolisthesis. In fact, a patient with spondylolisthesis may have any one of the potential diagnoses discussed in this chapter. To focus on the structural lesion of spondylolisthesis shown on radiograph and ignore the history and physical examination will lead to errors in diagnosis and treatment.

There are basically two syndromes in mechanical low back pain (Table 27.7): (1) lumbago (mechanical instability) and (2) sciatica (radicular syndrome). Before enlarging on these syndromes, it is well to take a moment to reflect on the concept of "referred leg pain." Many state that leg pain that does not go below the knee and is associated with good SLR ability is likely referred leg pain. This idea is further entrenched if there is an absence of neurologic symptoms or signs. The gate control theory of pain is one of the theories used to explain referred pain. The phenomenon is thought to occur when painful stimuli are reflexively shifted around at the cord level. This shunting results in pain being felt in a myotomal or dermatomal distribution away from the back origin of the pain, such as in the leg. The concept is altogether too simplistic and needs to be reworked in light of new investigative techniques such as CT scanning and MRI. I predict that referred leg pain will be a lot less common than originally thought. It is more likely that patients labeled as having referred pain for their leg

radiations have various degrees of radicular pain due to nerve root encroachment by either bone or chronic disk herniations.

The diagnosis of referred leg pain should be reserved for the patient who has the following clinical presentation:

1. There is significant mechanical back pain present as the source of referral.
2. The leg pain affects both legs, is vague in its distribution, and has no radicular component.
3. The degree of referred leg discomfort varies directly with the back pain. When the back pain increases in severity, the referred leg pain occurs or increases in severity. Conversely, a decrease in back pain results in a decrease in the referral of pain. Referred pain is less likely to radiate below the knee.
4. There are no neurologic symptoms or signs in concert with the complaint of referred leg pain.

It is safer to assume that any patient with radiating leg pain, especially unilateral leg pain, has a radicular syndrome until proven otherwise.

LUMBAGO-MECHANICAL INSTABILITY

The lumbago-mechanical instability syndrome is easy to recognize. These patients present exclusively with lumbosacral backache aggravated by activities such as bending, lifting, and sitting. The pain may radiate toward either iliac crest, but does not radiate down into the buttock or legs. The pain is almost always relieved by various forms of rest, for example, reduced activity, weight reduction, corset support, or bedrest. Most patients have no trouble describing these relieving efforts.

Most importantly, there are no associated leg symptoms or signs.

UNILATERAL ACUTE RADICULAR SYNDROME

Before describing the unilateral acute radicular syndrome, it is important to note that the leg includes the buttock and sacroiliac joint areas proximally (Fig. 27.3). In fact, the younger patient may lateralize discomfort off the midline as high as the top of the sacroiliac joint or iliac crest region. Even this is considered leg pain in the young patient. Obviously, any pain below the buttock crease is to be considered leg pain. A radicular distribution to leg pain is just what it implies—not a diffuse, but a specific distribution to the pain that follows a radical distribution.

History

Approximately half the patients will attribute the onset of their acute radicular syndrome to some traumatic experience. This may be retrograde rationalization on the part of the patient. Experimental studies and careful statistical analysis of case histories do not support the concept that direct trauma or sudden weight-loading of the spine are routinely the causal agents of disk rupture,

Table 27.7.
Syndromes in Mechanical Low Back Pain

1. Lumbago–mechanical instability
2. Sciatica–radicular pain
   a. Unilateral acute radicular syndrome
   b. Bilateral acute radicular syndrome
   c. Unilateral chronic radicular syndrome
   d. Bilateral chronic radicular syndrome

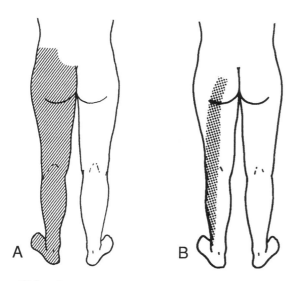

Figure 27.3. *A,* **When a spine surgeon talks of leg pain, he also includes any pain located in the buttock.** *B,* **The usual radicular distribution for L5 or S1 root lesion.**

although they may aggravate a pre-existing lesion. This aspect in the history becomes important when litigation or compensation is involved.

The younger the patient, the more likely sciatica is the only symptom. When asked specifically, many patients may state that they noted numbness in the calf or foot before the pain developed. This is a stage of root compression before the inflammatory radiculitis begins. The majority of patients, however, develop back pain that subsequently radiates to the buttock and then down the leg. Most patients report that as the sciatic pain increases, the back pain decreases in severity. The history of pain is spondylogenic in character—that is to say, the pain is aggravated by general and specific activities and is relieved by rest. Bending, stooping, lifting, coughing, sneezing, and straining at stool will intensify the pain. Infrequently, referral patterns of pain occur, such as perineal or testicular discomfort (pain or paresthesia) and lower abdominal discomfort. The former symptoms are likely due to irritation of lower sacral roots laterally or at the midline, and the latter may be due to muscular splinting of the pelvis.

Patients with acute radicular syndrome may complain of a dermatomal distribution to the paresthetic discomfort. It is interesting to note that although pain occurs in the buttock, thigh, and calf, the symptom in the foot is almost exclusively paresthesia.

Physical Examination

The Back

The posture is characteristic. The lumbar spine is flattened and slightly flexed. The patient often leans away from the side of his pain, and this sciatic scoliosis becomes more obvious on bending forward. The patient

is more comfortable standing with the affected hip and knee slightly flexed, a manner accentuated by asking the patient to flex forward (Fig. 27.4). He walks in obvious discomfort, sometimes holding his loin with his hands. The gait is slow and deliberate and is designed to avoid any unnecessary movement of the spine. With gross tension on the nerve root, the patient may not be able to put his heel on the ground, and walks slowly and painfully on tiptoe. Forward flexion may be permitted, so the hands reach the knees by virtue of flexion of the hip and knee joint. If the examiner keeps his fingertips on the spinous processes, it is observed that the lumbar spine is splinted and nonmobile. Limitation of flexion in such instances is therefore the result of root tension. The degree of flexion should be recorded by measuring the distance between the fingertips and the floor.

Extension is not significantly limited. A complaint of radiating leg pain on backward extension is usually indicative of a sequestered or extruded disk rupture.

Lateral flexion may be full and free, but in the presence of sciatic scoliosis, lateral flexion toward the concavity of the curve (side of sciatica) is limited.

The phenomenon of sciatic scoliosis and the relief of aggravation of pain on lateral flexion have been attributed to the position of the protrusion in relation to the nerve root (Fig. 27.5). This may be a simplistic explanation in view of the fact that the sciatic scoliosis dis-

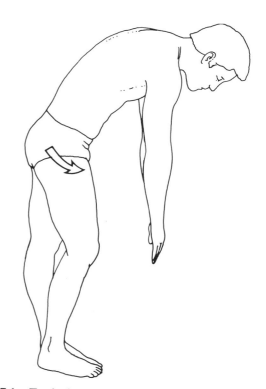

Figure 27.4. **Typical posture assumed by patient with herniated nucleus pulposus when forward flexion is attempted—flexion of knee on affected side and forward rotation of pelvis to affected side.**

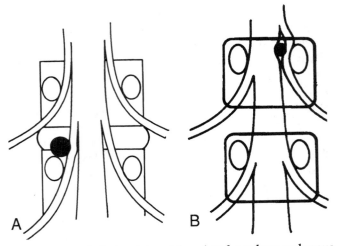

Figure 27.5.A, **Relationship of herniated nucleus pulposus (HNP) lateral to nerve root such that flexion to affected side increases pain.** *B,* **Not unusual location of HNP in axilla of nerve root such that flexion to opposite side increases pain.**

appears on recumbency, however. This observation, the loss of lateral curvature of the lumbar spine on recumbency, differentiates the sciatic list from structural scoliosis. On further assessment of the degree of root involvement present, it is imperative to test the extremities specifically for root tension, root irritation, and impairment of root conduction. These are the cardinal signs of lumbar root compromise.

Back Tenderness and Muscle Spasm. In the standing position, especially in the presence of scoliosis, muscle spasm can be observed. At rest, however, the spasm often subsides and there is little tenderness to be found in the back musculature. Selectively palpating and applying a lateral thrust to the spinous process may cause some back pain, and on rare occasions may produce leg pain. By and large, when the patient with acute radicular syndrome is at rest on the examining table, there is little to find in the back. The patient's major complaint is leg pain, and the majority of physical findings are in the extremity.

Extremities

Root Tension and Irritation. The term *root tension* denotes distortion of the emerging nerve root by an extradural lesion. The three most useful tests for the presence of root tension are limitation of SLR, crossover pain, and the bowstring sign, the latter also arising in part from root irritation.

When testing SLR, it is important not to hurt the patient. Never suddenly jerk the leg up in the air. The standard for SLR testing is a fully extended knee with the hip in slight internal rotation and adduction.

Figure 27.1A demonstrates a good way of doing the SLR test. An SLR test is considered "positive" when the test reproduces pain in the buttock or leg, which limits

SLR ability to something less than the normal of 90°. SLR in the acute radicular syndrome is significantly reduced (less than 50% of normal).

Two additional maneuvers are useful to support the finding of limitation of SLR:

1. Aggravation of pain by forced dorsiflexion of the ankle at the limit of SLR
2. Relief of pain by flexion of the knee and hip

Physiogenic sciatic pain due to nerve root compromise is always relieved by flexion of the knee and hip. Continuing to flex the patient's hip with the knee bent does not reproduce and aggravate sciatic pain. This phenomenon is seen only in the emotionally destroyed patient.

If SLR is permissible to 70° before leg pain is produced, the finding is equivocal for the acute radicular syndrome. Below this level the reproduction of leg pain on SLR, aggravated by dorsiflexion of the ankle and relieved by flexion of the knee, is strongly suggestive of tension on the L5 or S1 nerve roots. Reproduction of the sciatic pain in the affected extremity by raising the unaffected leg is irrefutable evidence of root tension in the acute radicular syndrome. This is known as *contralateral* or *crossed SLR pain.*

False-Positive SLR Test. Hamstring tightness may cloud the assessment of the SLR test. These patients generally have a tight body build (e.g., inability to fully extend the elbow). Their hamstring tightness–limiting SLR is bilateral, and the discomfort the patient feels is distal in the thigh in the region of the hamstring tendons. Hamstring tightness does not produce pain radiating below the knee. Finally, other physical findings of root tension, irritation, and compression are absent when hamstring tightness is the sole cause of decreased SLR ability.

False-Negative SLR Test. On occasion you will encounter a loose-jointed individual with sciatica due to an herniated nucleus pulposus. On SLR testing you may not be impressed with the minor degree of impaired SLR ability until you examine the unaffected leg and see the patient's ability to straight-leg-raise well beyond 90°.

Bowstring Sign. The bowstring sign is an important indication of root tension and irritation. To perform the test the examiner carries out SLR to the point at which the patient experiences some discomfort in the distribution of the sciatic nerve. At this level, the knee is allowed to flex and the patient's foot is allowed to rest on the examiner's shoulder (Fig. 27.6). The test demands sudden, firm pressure applied to the tibial nerve in the popliteal fossa. Do the test in the following stages: Apply firm pressure to the hamstrings—this will not hurt. Then, move your thumbs over to the tibial nerve. Apply sudden, firm pressure with your thumb over the nerve. A positive bowstring test is reproduction of radiating leg discomfort. Most commonly the radiating discomfort is pain felt proximally in the thigh and even into

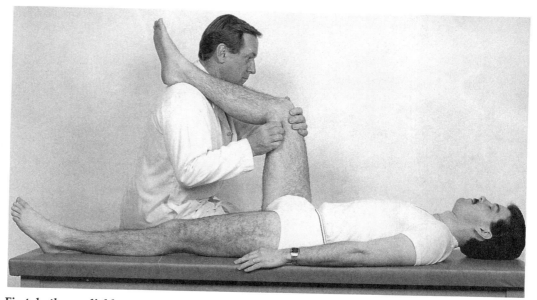

Figure 27.6. Bowstring test. First do the medial hamstrings (a), then the tibial nerve (b), then the lateral hamstrings (c), then the lateral popliteal nerve (d). A positive response at (b) and (d) equates with organic root irritation. A negative response at all four test sites is a negative test. A positive test at (a) and (c) is indicative of nonorganic reaction.

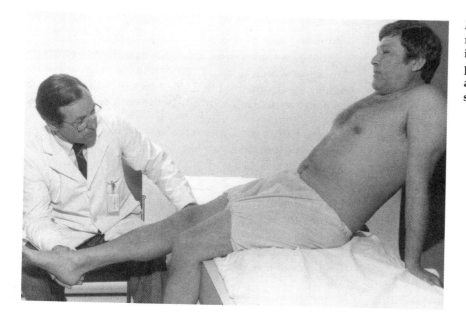

Figure 27.7. A positive flip test. Because of root tension, an attempt to straight leg raise in the sitting position causes buttock or leg pain and the patient flips back on the examining table to relieve the increased tension.

the back. Less commonly, radiating discomfort will travel distally, and this discomfort is more often paresthetic in nature than painful. It is important to emphasize that if the test only produces local pain in the popliteal fossa, it is of no significance. This demonstration of root irritation is probably the single most important sign in the diagnosis of tension and irritation of a nerve root by a ruptured intervertebral disk; unfortunately it is not always present in patients with herniated nucleus pulposus.

Tests to Verify SLR Reduction. When the patient sits with the legs dangling over the side of the bed, the hip and knee are both flexed to 90°. If the knee is now extended fully, the position assumed by the leg is equivalent to 90° of SLR. If the patient is suffering from root compromise, this will cause sudden, severe pain and the patient will lean backward to avoid tension on the nerve (Fig. 27.7). This is commonly referred to as the "positive flip test." With the psychogenic regional pain syndrome, the patient will permit the examiner to extend the knee of the painful leg without showing any response.

Sometimes crossover pain can be demonstrated only in the sitting position. If one crosses over pain from the

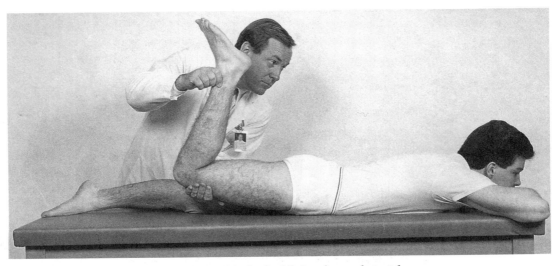

Figure 27.8. **Method of doing femoral stretch.**

Table 27.8.
Criteria for the Diagnosis of Acute Radicular Syndrome[a]

1. Leg pain (including buttock) is the dominant complaint when compared to back pain
2. Neurologic symptoms that are specific (e.g., paresthesia in a typical dermatomal distribution)
3. Significant SLR changes (any one or a combination of these)
   a. SLR less than 50% of normal
   b. Bowstring discomfort
   c. Crossover pain
4. Neurologic sign (see section on anatomic level)

[a]Three or four of these criteria must be present, the only exception being the young patients who are vary resistant to the effects of nerve root compression and thus may not have neurologic symptoms (criterion 2) or signs (criterion 4).

asymptomatic leg to the symptomatic leg in the sitting position, this is also considered a positive crossover sign and almost certainly indicative of an acute radicular syndrome.

Patients with acute radicular syndrome may also have tenderness over the sacroiliac joint and down the course of the sciatic nerve. This tenderness has led to the erroneous diagnosis of sacroiliac joint strain. It is very unusual in these patients to see any clinical or radiologic evidence of damage to the sacroiliac joint.

Femoral Nerve Stretch. With higher lumbar disk herniations and acute radicular syndromes, the SLR test may be negative, but the femoral stretch test will be positive. Figure 27.8 shows the femoral nerve stretch test. It is not nearly as satisfactory as an SLR test, but if this test re-produces radiating thigh pain, aggravated by knee flexion, then the test is considered positive.

Summary

Table 27.8 summarizes the historic and physical foundation on which to build the diagnosis of an acute radicular syndrome. Table 27.9 shows the differences in the acute radicular syndrome in the various age groups.

BILATERAL ACUTE RADICULAR SYNDROME
(CAUDA EQUINA SYNDROME)

Fortunately, the bilateral acute radicular syndrome is rare. It is usually due to a massive midline sequestered disk. The syndrome is manifested by the sudden onset of bilateral leg pain usually accompanied by bladder and bowel impairment. Perineal numbness is a predominant symptom. It is obviously an emergency and is a diagnosis that is rarely missed.

UNILATERAL CHRONIC RADICULAR SYNDROME

The difference between acuteness and chronicity in a radicular syndrome is often difficult to measure. The severity and the duration of the syndrome usually combine to distinguish acute from chronic radicular pain. Chronic unilateral radicular pain is usually a complaint for many months or more. It follows a typical radicular distribution, including pain below the knee, and is usually associated with much in the way of mechanical back pain. Both pains are usually aggravated by walking. Neurologic symptoms are less prevalent than in acute radicular syndrome, and are sometimes extremely diffuse and nonlocalizing. Straight leg raising ability is usually much better than 50% of normal, and bowstring discomfort and crossover pain are not seen in this syn-

Table 27.9.
Difference in Presentation of the Acute Radicular Syndrome in Various Age Groups

Presentation	Young (<30 years old)	Adult (35–55)	Older (60+)
Symptoms			
Leg Pain	Usually the only symptom	Some back pain (BP) but leg pain (LP) dominates	Usually BP but LP still dominates
Paresthesia	Often absent	Usually present	Almost always present
Signs			
SLR	Very positive (often 10–20%)	Less than 50% of normal	Occasionally good ability
Neurologic signs	Absent in at least 50% of patients	Sometimes absent	Rarely absent

drome. Neurologic findings are very few and usually not helpful in localizing the degree of nerve root involvement.

BILATERAL CHRONIC RADICULAR SYNDROME

To many, the bilateral chronic radicular syndrome is known as *neurogenic claudication*, which was summarized in Table 27.6. The structural lesion is almost always neurogenic claudication that causes spinal canal stenosis. This syndrome differs from the unilateral radicular syndrome in two ways:

1. Both legs are affected rather than one leg.
2. The pain of the bilateral radicular syndrome may not be a typical radicular-type pain. Some patients describe typical claudicant leg pain in a radicular distribution. Other patients describe a diffuse type of claudicant leg discomfort that cannot be localized to a radicular distribution.

Many other symptoms are present in this syndrome including weakness, "heaviness," and "rubberiness" in the legs. Numbness is also prevalent in this syndrome and is often of no value in localizing which nerve roots are compromised. There is a typical march phenomenon with the chronic bilateral radicular syndrome. Symptoms get much worse with prolonged walking, radiate further down the leg, and ultimately interfere with the ability of the patient to ambulate. Some patients may report noticing that if they attach themselves to a shopping cart and walk in the flexed position, they can get more distance before their leg symptoms appear. Characteristically, physical examination in chronic bilateral radicular syndrome reveals little. Straight leg raising is usually very good, and if the syndrome is due entirely to canal narrowing rather than lateral recess narrowing, there are limited neurologic findings except where the syndrome has significantly progressed. These patients will have significant weakness and are often wheelchair-bound.

QUESTION 4

Are there clues to an anatomic level on history and physical examination?

Is there an anatomic level clinically? There is an important intermediate question to consider between a syndrome diagnosis (question 3) and a structural diagnosis (question 5). If it is possible to determine an atomic level clinically, then any structural lesion has to be at the appropriate level or it cannot be considered a significant defect. A patient who has an anatomic level of S1 root involvement rarely should have a structural diagnosis localized to the L3-L4 interspace!

There are three ways to determine an anatomic level: distribution of leg pain, neurologic symptoms, and neurologic signs.

DISTRIBUTION OF LEG PAIN

Pain in the posterior thigh and posterior calf distribution incriminates the fifth lumbar root or the first sacral root. Whether this pain is posterior or posterolateral in the thigh and calf is of little use in separating fifth lumbar root lesions from first sacral root lesions. Pain down the anterior thigh, however, almost certainly incriminates the fourth lumbar nerve root or higher lumbar nerve roots, and excludes involvement of the fifth lumbar or first sacral roots.

NEUROLOGIC SYMPTOMS

A paresthetic discomfort with a dermatomal distribution is the most helpful historic feature in localizing an anatomic level. Paresthetic discomfort along the lateral edge of the foot incriminates the first sacral nerve root, paresthetic discomfort over the dorsum of the foot and the lateral calf incriminates the fifth lumbar nerve root, and paresthetic discomfort down the medial shin incriminates the fourth lumbar nerve root. In trying to use neurologic symptoms to determine an anatomic level, remember the following rule: the more distal the

Table 27.10.
Common Neurologic Changes in Acute Radicular Syndrome

	Root		
Change	L4	L5	S1
Motor weakness	Knee extension	Ankle dorsiflexion	Ankle plantar flexion
Sensory loss	Medial shin to knee	Dorsum of foot and lateral calf	Lateral border of foot and posterior calf
Reflex depression	Knee	Tibialis posterior	Ankle
Wasting	Thigh (no calf)	Calf (minimal thigh)	Calf (minimal thigh)

symptom, the more valuable it is as a determinant of an anatomic level.

NEUROLOGIC SIGNS

The diagnosis of acute radicular syndrome is in no way totally dependent on the demonstration of root impairment as reflected by signs of motor weakness or changes in sensory appreciation or reflex activity. The presence of such changes reinforces the diagnosis, however. The common neurologic changes are summarized in Table 27.10.

Changes in Reflex Activity

The ankle jerk may be diminished or absent with an S1 lesion. This is tested with the patient kneeling on a chair or sitting comfortably. (If a patient's sciatica is so severe that he cannot sit comfortably, then testing of the reflexes in the sitting position is invalid, because the guarding and posturing will depress the reflexes.) This explains the occasional depressed knee reflex seen in the presence of sciatica due to an L5-S1 disk protrusion. If the patient has suffered a previous attack of sciatic pain, with compression of the first sacral nerve sufficient enough to obliterate the ankle jerk, this may not return to normal. The absence of the ankle reflex therefore may be merely a remnant of a previous episode of disk rupture, and the present attack may be due to a disk rupture at another level.

With an L5 root compression, the tibialis posterior reflex (obtained by striking the tendon of the tibialis posterior near its point of insertion) may be absent. Diminution of the lateral hamstring jerk is also seen on occasion with an L5 root compromise, but multiple innervation of this muscle group makes this an unreliable reflex. With L4 and L3 lesions, the knee jerk may be diminished.

Wasting

Muscle wasting is rarely seen unless the symptoms have been present for more than 3 weeks. Very marked wasting is more suggestive of an extradural tumor or other neurologic diagnosis than of a disk rupture.

Always measure the girth of the thigh and the girth of the calf. This is a useful baseline from which to assess the progress of the lesion. Remember, if there is gross weakness of the gastrocnemii, the main venous pump of the affected extremity is no longer working, and these patients may even show some measure of ankle edema. The combination of calf tenderness due to S1 root irritation and the observation of a swollen ankle may give rise to the erroneous diagnosis of thrombophlebitis. For reasons unexplained this phenomenon is more common in far lateral disk herniations that must affect sympathetic postganglionic fibers.

Motor Loss

The weakness of the gastrocnemii is best demonstrated by getting the patient to rise on tiptoe five or six times. The patient is then asked if it requires more effort do this on the affected extremity. If the quadriceps is weak, the physician must be aware of this before ascribing the difficulty of tiptoe rising to weakness of the calf muscles; also, if sciatic pain is severe, the test cannot be performed by the patient.

The power of ankle dorsiflexion is best tested by applying full body weight to the dorsiflexed ankle. Testing the dorsiflexors by asking the patient to walk on his heels will only demonstrate marked weakness in this muscle group. Weakness of the flexor hallucis longus (S1) or weakness of the extensor hallucis longus (L5) is often the first evidence of motor involvement. The evertors of the foot may be weak with an L5 lesion. The gluteus maximus may become weak with lesions involving the first sacral nerve root and may be demonstrated by the sagging of one buttock crease when the patient stands. Weakness of the gluteus medius is seen with an L5 lesion and occasionally is marked enough to produce a Trendelenburg lurch, particularly noticeable when the patient is tired. When the gluteus medius is involved, there is frequently marked tenderness on pressure over the muscle near its point of insertion, and this may be confused with trochanteric bursitis or with gluteal tendonitis.

Quadriceps weakness is seen with an L4 lesion and can be assessed by the examiner placing his arm under

Table 27.11.
Structural Lesions in Mechanical Low Back Pain

1. Instability
   a. Intrinsic to disk–degenerative disk disease (DDD)
   b. Extrinsic to disk
      Facet joint disease (FJD)
      Spondylolisthesis
2. Soft tissue lesions–muscle spasm, ligamentous strain
3. Herniated nucleus pulposus (HNP)
4. Narrowing of spinal canal
   a. Spinal canal stenosis (SCS)
   b. Lateral recess stenosis (LRS)

Table 27.12.
Relationship of Syndromes and Structural Lesions

1. Lumbago	Degenerative Disk Disease (DDD)
	Facet joint dysfunction (FJD)
	Spondylolysis/spondylolisthesis
	Soft tissue
2. Unilateral acute radicular	Herniated nucleus pulposus (HNP)
	HNP + lateral recess stenosis (LRS)
3. Unilateral chronic radicular	LRS
	HNP
4. Bilateral acute radicular	Central HNP
5. Bilateral chronic radicular	Spinal canal spenosis (SCS)

the patient's knee and asking the patient to extend the knee against the resistance of the examiner's hand.

Sensory Impairment

The regions of sensory loss are reasonably constant. Within the sensory dermatomes, there appear to be areas more vulnerable to sensory loss than others. Loss of appreciation of pinprick is first noted in an S1 lesion below and behind the lateral malleolus and in an L5 lesion in the cleft between the first and second toes. Sensory appreciation is a subjective response and, as such, may sometimes be difficult to assess. Certain precautions must be followed. Sensory perception varies in different parts of the limb. Identical areas in each limb must be tested consecutively. The examination must be carried out as expeditiously as is compatible with accuracy, because the patient will soon tire of this form of examination and his answers may not be accurate. When the skin is pricked with a pin, the physiologic principle of recruitment is present. Thus, the overall sensory appreciation depends not only on the action of the pinprick, but also on the number of pinpricks experienced.

A sensory examination is only interpreted as positive when the sensory loss approximates one dermatomal distribution, and when the loss is not present in the adjacent dermatomes or the same contralateral dermatome.

QUESTION 5

After reviewing the results of investigation, what is the structural lesion and does it fit with the clinical syndrome?

The potential structural lesion diagnoses are listed in Table 27.11. This table covers only degenerative conditions of the spine; it omits postoperative scarring of arachnoid or nerve roots and fractures and dislocations. It is important to stress here that it is possible to have multiple syndromes related to a single structural lesion. For example, a degenerative spondylolisthesis can cause both mechanical instability (back pain) and bilateral claudicant leg pain as a result of encroachment on the

spinal canal. Table 27.12 links syndromes with structural lesions.

CONCLUSIONS

It is important to make a clear-cut syndrome diagnosis on the basis of a history and physical examination, and to match it to a clear-cut bona fide structural lesion on investigation. Failure to do this leads to wrong diagnoses and futile treatment interventions.

METHODS USED TO DOCUMENT THE STRUCTURAL LESION

Steps to document the presence of a structural lesion in mechanical low back pain should be taken only after a satisfactory answer has been obtained for questions 1, 2, and 3 above. Seeking a structural lesion in a patient with an unrecognized nonorganic problem is usually a waste of time and money, and is a danger to the patient.

False-positive investigative findings are easy to come by with today's sophisticated techniques. Before discussing each of these possible investigative procedures, it is assumed that a thorough history, physical examination, and other necessary investigations have satisfactorily answered questions 1 and 2.

PLAIN RADIOGRAPHS

It may not be necessary on the first assessment to do lumbar spine films, but if a patient does not quickly respond to treatment, anteroposterior, lateral, and oblique films should be obtained. Plain radiographs may demonstrate a narrowed disk space, facet joint disease, or spondylolisthesis, but one must not assume that one of these is the causative structural lesion.

In reading plain radiographs, look at the nonskeletal areas first. Review the retroperitoneal area in specific regard to the kidneys and ureters, and the abdominal aorta. Be sure that the psoas shadows are intact.

After reviewing the nonskeletal part of a lumbar spine

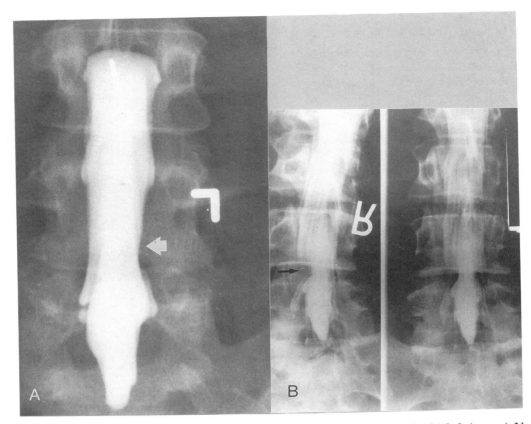

Figure 27.9. *A,* Oil-soluble contrast myelography showing defect in contrast column at L4-L5 left *(arrow).* Notice the lack of filling of nerve roots that made interpretation of apparent defect of L5-S1 left difficult (ultimately found to be not significant). *B,* Water-soluble contrast myelography showing large HNP central and left L4-L5. Notice how well nerve roots fill.

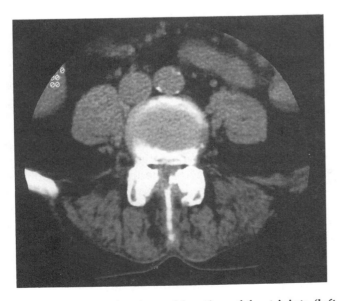

Figure 27.10. **CT showing subluxation of facet joints (left more than right) and canal stenosis.**

radiograph, consider the skeleton. Look at the sacroiliac joints, survey the pedicles and vertebral bodies for erosions, and finally consider the structural defects that are potential causes of the patient's syndrome. Such things as narrowing of the disk space and translation of vertebral bodies are important to note. Various measurements of plain radiographs are not helpful in assessment of canal or recess narrowing.

MYELOGRAPHY

This test is considered the gold standard by many. To me it is of historic importance only, having been replaced by MRI. Myelography should be considered only when adequate conservative treatment has failed, surgery is contemplated, and the clinician is unskilled in the interpretation of MRI.

Myelography has three purposes:

1. To rule out higher spine pathology
2. To localize the exact level of root involvement

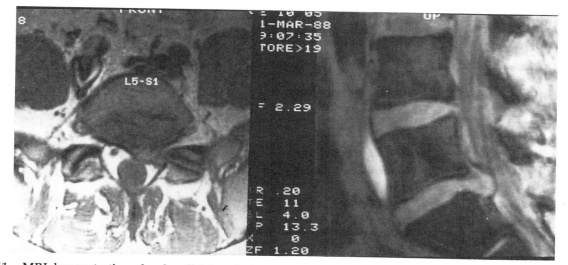

Figure 27.11. **MRI demonstrating a lumbar disk herniation. L5-S1 left axial view is T1-weighted, and sagittal view is gradient echo.**

3. To determine if any migration of disk material has occurred

It is not the purpose of this text to discuss in detail the radiologic changes that may be seen on myelography, but some general principles regarding interpretation of myelograms will now be described.

Myelography was introduced in 1921 by Sicard using iodized poppyseed oil injected into the epidural space (4). This is a logical place to put radiopaque material because the lesion is, indeed, an epidural lesion and should be demonstrated more easily by a radiopaque substance introduced into the epidural space. Difficulty in aspirating the radiopaque material at the conclusion of the epidural myelography, however, and the suggestion that this might give rise to root irritation at a later date persuaded surgeons to use the intrathecal injection of oil-soluble radiopaque compounds. Because these compounds are emulsified with the cerebrospinal fluid, it is not possible in the majority of instances to aspirate all of the dye injected.

Although many surgeons ordered oil myelograms, few themselves would undergo the procedure because of its difficulty and the postmyelographic complications. With the advent of water-soluble opaque materials and their refinement, however, myelography has become a much safer procedure.

The most popular water-soluble contrast material was metrizamide, but more recently this has been replaced by iohexol and iopamidol. These water-soluble compounds have several advantages over oil-soluble myelography in that the water-soluble contrast material is easier to inject and flows more readily through the nerve root sheaths. Obviously, it has a higher degree of sensitivity in documenting extradural lesions. Figure 27.9 is an example of oil- and water-soluble myelography.

Some neuroradiologists have popularized dynamic myelography. This entails flexion and extension of the patient on the fluoroscopic table with pictures being taken in these positions. Flexion supposedly opens up the spinal canal and reduces the degree of spinal stenosis encroachment on the contrast column. Conversely, extension decreases the dimensions of the spinal canal, and if a spinal stenotic lesion is present, more constriction of the contrast column will be evident on extension radiographs.

Myelography is still accompanied by some complications such as headache, nausea, and vomiting. More-severe complications such as convulsions and infections have also been reported after myelography.

COMPUTED TOMOGRAPHY

A few years ago, CT started to replace myelography. The tenure of CT was short-lived because of the advent of MRI, such that CT scanning is also mentioned as a historic footnote to the emergence of MRI as the test of first choice for investigation of degenerative conditions in the lumbar spine. Some might view this as a strong statement; it will soon be fact. Bell and others have published excellent articles on the overuse and pitfalls of routine CT scanning (1). Axial images are the most valuable and should be cut from L3 to the midportion of the sacrum. Therefore any lesion above or below these levels will not be documented by the CT scan. Many neuroradiologists believe that reconstructions are of value, but I am not convinced. Crude measurements from the CT scan can also give some impression as to the integrity of the spinal canal and the lateral recesses. Figure 27.10 demonstrates a narrowed spinal canal.

CT scanning is so simple, so readily available, and so nice to look at that many pitfalls await the unwary. Before embarking on treatment, especially surgery, be sure that the patient's clinical syndrome fits the structural lesion on CT scan. Remember you see nothing above L3 on routine scanning and you do not have sagittal sections of the spine. If there is any doubt, a myelogram must be combined with the CT scan to further document the structural lesion.

Magnetic Resonance Imaging

Magnetic resonance imaging is now the test of first choice for investigation of the patient with degenerative conditions of the spine. The procedure requires no x-ray radiation, and with the recent development of surface coils, the technique of MRI has improved to the point where it has become extremely sensitive in demonstrating soft tissue abnormalities in the lumbar spine. The major drawbacks to MRI are its cost, its time consumption, its propensity for false-positive results, and the claustrophobic effect it has on patients lying in the chamber for imaging purposes. These drawbacks have been overcome, however, and MRI is so useful in the investigation of a patient with mechanical low back conditions that it has replaced CT scanning and myelography. If only the insurance companies would recognize this! Figure 27.11 is an MRI scan demonstrating a lumbar disk herniation. MRI is limited in its outline of bony detail, a handicap not encountered with the CT scan. In the future a patient who has a mechanical low back pain syndrome, failing to respond to conservative treatment, will be investigated with an MRI scan, and if a clear-cut diagnosis is not evident the choice will be CT with myelography. Myelography by itself will be rarely ordered.

Nerve Root Infiltration

Nerve root infiltration is an investigative procedure that involves blocking the anterior primary ramus of a single nerve root. It is usually the fifth lumbar or first sacral nerve root that is blocked, but any root can be blocked. It is an investigative procedure that is useful only when one is sure that a radicular syndrome is present, but unsure of which nerve root is affected. It is of no value in trying to separate referred pain from radicular pain, or a herniated nucleus pulposus from lateral recess stenosis. Most often the procedure is used in chronic unilateral radicular syndrome (due to lateral recess stenosis) when structural recess stenosis lesions are noted at the level of the fifth lumbar and first sacral nerve roots and there are no clinical clues as to the anatomic level. The second indication for a nerve root infiltration is in the presence of scarring or arachnoiditis when trying to decide which root is most symptomatic.

The technique is accomplished in the prone position under image-intensifier control. A paraspinal approach is used to the fifth lumbar nerve root, catching it just as it exits under the pedicle of L5. The S1 nerve root is blocked through the posterior first sacral foramen. Under image-intensifier control, a long needle is slowly advanced toward the nerve root. When the nerve root is encountered, radiating discomfort down the leg will result. Usually this radiating discomfort is typical enough that the block can then be accomplished with 3 ml of 0.5% or 0.75% Marcaine, a long-acting anesthetic agent. On occasion, the radiating discomfort will not be striking, and water-soluble contrast material must be injected to be sure of needle placement.

Although radiography is used to assist in accomplishing a nerve root infiltration, the procedure is not a radiographic evaluation procedure. The first principle of nerve root infiltration is to obtain a good root block. That is to say, if a fifth lumbar nerve root is blocked, the patient should have a drop foot and numbness over the dorsum of the foot when the procedure is finished. Similarly, if the first sacral root is blocked, the patient should have numbness to pinprick sensation along the lateral border of the foot and weakness of plantar flexion. Once a good nerve root block is obtained, the patient is asked to participate in the activity that was most aggravating to him. Usually, the patient needs a cane for support because of the profound nature of the root block. Long-acting anesthetic agents last 4–6 hours, and at the end of that time the patient should record his impressions of relief or lack of relief of his symptoms with the root block. If you suspected the fifth lumbar nerve root as the culprit, and a good fifth lumbar nerve root block relieves the patient's pain, then the procedure has satisfactorily pinpointed the fifth lumbar nerve root as the source of symptoms. The appropriate surgical procedure can then be carried out with confidence.

Facet Joint Block

A facet joint block is a local anesthetic procedure to temporarily denervate the facet joint. This is accomplished by blocking the facet joint itself and the posterior primary ramus supply to the facet joint. Facet joint innervation from the posterior primary ramus is from multiple segments, and thus multiple blocks are required. It is routine to block the facet joint and posterior primary ramus at L3-L4, L4-L5, and L5-S1, and also to block the ascending posterior primary ramus branch coming out of the S1 foramen. Also, the procedure is done bilaterally.

Again, an image intensifier is used to guide needle placement. There is little in the way of radiating discomfort to help localize the block, and thus anatomic placement of the needle is important. Figure 27.12 shows such needle placement at the junction of the lateral edge of the superior facet and the superior edge of the transverse process. Here, the posterior primary ramus comes through a ligamentous tunnel to supply the facet joint at that level and send branches to adjacent levels. Next, a needle should be placed within the facet joint itself so that the joint can be blocked. Long-acting anesthetic

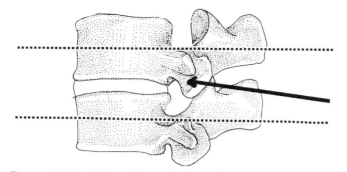

Figure 27.12. **Schematic rendering showing needle tip in correct location for block of facet joint nerve supply (see text).**

agents are also used for this procedure. After a satisfactory block is obtained, the patient is asked to participate in the activities that aggravated his pain and, at the end of 4–6 hours, to sit down and record his impressions of the effect of the procedure. If a patient has mechanical low back pain prior to the procedure that is abolished by the procedure, this suggests that the facet joints are the source of symptoms, and appropriate procedures can be prescribed.

Both nerve root infiltration and facet joint blocks are procedures that depend on patient response for evaluation. Obviously, if the patient is an abnormal responder (e.g., a patient with nonorganic pain), these two procedures are useless. Both will misguide you if you have missed the diagnosis of a nonorganic syndrome.

ELECTRODIAGNOSIS

There are three electrodiagnostic procedures that are used in the investigation of a patient with lumbar disk disease: electromyography (EMG), nerve conduction tests (NCTs), and sensory-evoked potentials.

Electromyography

EMG is a motor unit examination. Any disruption in the anterior horn, the nerve fiber, or the muscle fiber has the potential of producing an abnormal EMG. Thus, an abnormal EMG is indicative of lower motor dysfunction. Electromyographic examination for a lumbar spine abnormality includes needle electrode placements in the paraspinal muscles and specific extremity muscles. Electrical activity is recorded on insertion, at rest, and with voluntary contraction or stimulation. Normally, there is unsustained electrical discharge on insertion of the needle and no signal discharge (a silent EMG) at rest. With voluntary contraction, biphasic or triphasic forms of action potentials are seen. Theoretically, with lower motor nerve root dysfunction, insertional activity is abnormal in that more-positive sharp waves appear; at rest, there are fibrillation potentials and positive sharp waves; and with stimulation, the quantity of motor units recorded decreases and multiple polyphasic waves are

seen. Extending the theory further, in a herniated nucleus pulposus with single root involvement, the EMG findings will be localized to a single root. With spinal stenosis (multiple root involvement), there will be multiple root findings on EMG. In fact, EMG has a very low sensitivity and specificity in evaluating patients with lumbar disk disease. More blinded studies are required to determine the value of EMG in diagnosing lumbar disk disease. At present, there is over-reliance on EMGs when, instead, a good clinical history and physical examination can be more helpful.

Nerve Conduction Tests

Nerve conduction tests measure the speed at which nerve fibers conduct. They are useful in separating peripheral neuropathy from a radiculopathy (trying to answer question 2). In radiculopathy one should see normal NCT velocities, whereas in peripheral neuropathy NCT velocities are often slowed.

Sensory-Evoked Potentials

With the failure of EMG to play a significant role in the evaluation of lumbar disk disease, a search began for new electrodiagnostic fields. Probably the most interesting to date is somatosensory-evoked potentials, which focus on the sensory side of the nerve fiber. These highly sophisticated evaluations have been used for some time in scoliosis and major spine reconstructive surgery. The spinal-evoked potential is transmitted through the dorsal column and is detectible with receptors in the spine or on the skull. Theoretically, lesions of peripheral nerves will prolong the latency response of the sensory input, and root and cord lesions cause change in the wave form. Conflicting evaluations of this technique have appeared in the literature (5). At this stage, the technique is considered experimental, and is very sophisticated. Some authors see great promise in this approach to the evaluation of patients with lumbar disk disease, however.

OTHER TESTS OF LIMITED OR NO VALUE

There are three tests that I place in this classification: epidural venography, thermography, and ultrasonography.

Epidural Venography

In the early 1970s, epidural venography enjoyed a brief popularity. It represented an attempt at a more accurate diagnosis of disk lesions at the L5-S1 level, where an oil-based myelogram had at least a 25% false-negative rate. A secondary reason was the false-positive rate of oil-based myelography at the L4-L5 level. Epidural venography turned out to be a difficult technical exercise, however, and also stressful for the patient. Limitations resulting from previous surgery also detracted from its value. Eventually, epidural venography was displaced by the advent of water-soluble myelographic compound and CT scanning. It is largely un-heard-of as a test today.

Thermography

Many doctors have promoted and popularized thermography as a test of nerve root physiology. In theory, it states that pathology causing nerve root irritation will result in changes in skin temperature that can be detected with liquid cholesterol crystals or infrared photography. Although the principle is simple and attractive, there are limited blinded studies to support the claims of thermographers. In fact, a number of very good blinded studies have appeared that seriously question the clinical value of thermography (6, 7). Until thermography is submitted to more blinded studies on specificity and sensitivity, its use should be limited to experimental medicine only. Unfortunately, thermography has found its way into the courts and is being used extensively by judges and juries to determine financial awards. This is an unfortunate occurrence and one that should be halted until further blinded studies are completed.

Ultrasonography

In spite of excellent scientific efforts by Porter et al. in England (8), the use of ultrasonography for the evaluation of patients with mechanical low back pain has severe limitations. The technique is exacting and difficult because the bony cover of the spinal canal interferes with visualization of its soft tissue contents. It has become a useful tool during spine surgery for spine trauma in detecting residual fragments anterior to the dura. At this point, however, it is not a useful investigative tool for the ambulatory patient with mechanical low back pain.

CONCLUSIONS

The assessment of a patient with a low back disability does not need to be difficult. By keeping a simple system in mind, it is possible to arrive at a good clinical impression by asking yourself the five questions discussed at length in this chapter and committing yourself, eventually, to sequential answers.

Do not commit yourself to any major investigative step until questions 1 and 2 have been adequately answered. Then, if you are satisfied that you have a mechanical low back pain problem, dissect it into a syndrome first, an anatomic level second, and a structural lesion third. The structural lesion diagnosis should fully support the clinical syndrome and the anatomic level. If not, take one step back and repeat the history and physical examination. Listening to the patient's story, doing a thorough physical examination, and supporting your diagnosis with investigation is the best way to avoid erroneous diagnoses and ill-fated surgery.

REFERENCES

1. Bell GR, Rothman RH, Booth RE et al: A study of computer-assisted tomography. *Spine* 9:552–556, 1984.
2. Hitselberger W, Witten R: Abnormal myelograms in asymptomatic patients. *J Neurosurg* 28:204–206, 1968.
3. Waddell G, McCulloch JA, Kummel EC et al: Nonorganic physical signs in low back pain. *Spine* 5:117–125, 1980.
4. Sicard JL: Roentgenologic exploration of the central nervous system with iodized oil (Lipiodol). *Arch Neurol Psychiatry* 16:420–426, 1926.
5. Aminoff MJ et al: Dermatomal somatosensory evoked potentials in unilateral lumbosacral radiculopathy. *Ann Neurol* 17:171–176, 1985.
6. Mahoney L, McCulloch JA, Czima A: Thermography as a diagnostic aid in sciatica. *J Am Acad Thermol* 1:51–54,1985.
7. Mills GH, Davies GK, Getty CJM, Conay J: The evaluation of liquid crystal thermography in the investigation of nerve root compression due to lumbosacral lateral spinal stenosis. *Spine* 11:420–432, 1986.
8. Porter RW, Hubbert CS, Wicks M: The spinal canal in symptomatic lumbar disc lesions. *J Bone Joint Surg [Br]* 60:485–487, 1978.

CHAPTER 28

PAINFUL ARTHROPATHIES

J. LEONARD GOLDNER
JAMES NITKA
PATRICIA HOWSON
BRUCE TOBEY

SPINAL COLUMN AND SACROILIAC JOINTS

Pain arising from the spine may be related to the spinal joints, including the intervertebral disk complex; the facet joints, which have synovial coverings; the ligaments surrounding the vertebral bodies and the adjacent joints; the neural elements that are adjacent to the spine, protected by the posterior elements; and the pain receptors (nociceptors) that exist in the supporting ligaments. Many other extraneous factors that influence the severity and duration of pain are included in any discussion of painful joints, but the intent of this material is to describe the reasons for and the conditions that are known to produce pain.

DIAGNOSIS

A logical way to determine the cause of the complaints of the patient who describes back pain in any region of the spine is to gather data in a clear, concise, and knowledgeable way, perform a detailed and accurate physical examination, and order and interpret certain essential laboratory studies in order to assist in differentiating mechanical, inflammatory, neoplastic, metabolic, and vascular lesions from each other. In this way, a reasonable diagnosis is established and appropriate treatment initiated. This analysis includes a knowledge of the physiology of the pain and the alterations that occur when a pathologic lesion exists. Furthermore, the emotional, social, and administrative aspects of pain cannot be eliminated from the methods of management, but these aspects of the patients' complaints, along with their personality profile, are placed in proper perspective.

PATHOPHYSIOLOGY OF SPINAL JOINT PAIN

Pain related to vertebral disease is divided into two general categories: (*a*) pain associated with compression of or impingement on neural tissue that results in local or radicular sensations, and (*b*) pain related to stimulation of nociceptors of ligaments and muscle fascia causing referred pain in a myotome or sclerotome pattern.

Innervation of the Vertebral Ligament

The innervation of vertebral ligaments attached to the vertebral body is by a plexus of nerve fibers associated with the external and internal venous plexuses of the spine. Also, pain is conducted through the sinuvertebral nerve to innervate the posterior longitudinal ligament and the posterior aspect of the anulus fibrosis, and the ventral aspect of the dural sac. These nerve fibers travel with the vertebral veins into the vertebral bodies and innervate at least the posterior aspect of these structures. Each sinuvertebral nerve is composed of a somatic root from the ventral ramus and an autonomic root from the gray ramus communicans. This nerve supplies the adjacent vertebra and one or two levels above the origin of the nerve.

Innervation of the Annulus Fibrosis

The anterolateral aspect of the annulus fibrosus and the anterior longitudinal ligament are innervated by a series of nerve fibers from the ventral rami and from the sympathetic nerve chains. Also, free nerve endings have been described within the interspinous ligaments and the zygoapophyseal joints of the lumbar spine. These receptors are thought to represent type IV pain fibers. Very few of these have actually been found within the ligamentum flavum or the lumbodorsal fascia of the back. However, the muscles of the back contain abundant type IV nociceptor free nerve endings.

The assumption is that certain kinds of back pain originate with the nociceptor input, are conducted to the spinal cord, and are referred back to a dermatome distribution that coincides with a particular level of nociceptor nerve supply. Or, the fibers may conduct through the posterior sensory ganglion and be recognized as myotome or sclerotome sensations.

The origin of this stimulus is usually mechanical and is associated with abnormal activity or stress of the ligamentous and muscular structures around the disk complex that are attached to the vertebral elements opposite the intervetebral disk joint. Furthermore, pain arising from the fascia and ligaments in the thoracolumbar region may be referred to the lumbosacral region through the L4–5 or S1 nerve root distribution (1).

Referred Pain

Injection of hypertonic saline into the thoracolumbar fascia results in referred pain to the L4–S1 anatomic areas of the spine. Upper cervical sensory root irritation may result in headache, occipital numbness, and autonomic nervous system symptoms.

Radiculopathy is due to compression of a mixed nerve root by adjacent structures. The causes of nerve compression or disruption of soft tissue vary with each region of the spine and with each pathologic syndrome causing the root irritation. These lesions may cause a dermatome pattern as well as a sclerotome sensation. The latter is dull, deep, and aching, whereas the former is more likely hypesthesia, paresthesia, or hyperpathia.

CERVICAL SPINE ARTHROPATHY PAIN

Osteophytes

Cervical spine pain varies from chronic, intermittent, aching pain, as in cervical spondylosis, to sharp, lancinating pain with increased muscle tension and radicular distribution, noted in cervical osteoarthritis and degenerative intervertebral disk disease.

C1–C2 Instability (Congenital, Traumatic, or Rheumatoid Disease)

Atlantoaxial instability may initially present with occipital headache, upper neck pain (dull or sharp), and occasional cranial nerve involvement if the occipital compression is significant. Lower extremity paresthesias and dysesthesias as well as upper extremity paresthesias may also occur in an asymmetric manner. Paresthesias in all four extremities require careful review of the occipital cervical region. Electrical shocks may be associated with forceful flexion of the neck or percussion of the head with the neck in a neutral or a flexed position. This suggests instability of the atlas on the axis or possible stenosis. Pain receptors in the loose synovium, the inter-spinous ligaments, and the intervertebral disk complex cause unpleasant sensations, and cervical or occipital stenosis may cause spinal cord or cerebellar compression symptoms.

The position of the head and neck that causes pain depends on the location and severity of the pathologic lesion. Posterior compression is due to laminal arches, radicular canal stenosis, compression by the ligamen-

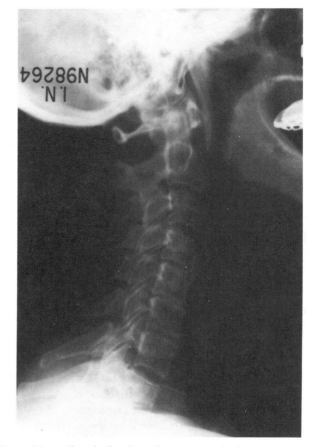

Figure 28.1. **Cervical spine of a 50-year-old female showing degenerative arthrosis of C4–C5. Nonoperative treatment did not relieve the neck symptoms or the radiculopathy. Anterior spine diskectomy and iliac bone arthrodesis resulted in reestablishment of the height of the nerve root foramina and fusion of the vertebral body interspaces.**

tum flavum, or combinations of these conditions causing compression. Extension of the head and neck may result in anterior compression by anterior osteophytes from the anulus or indentation from the posterior overgrowth of the zygoapophyseal joints and the anular ligaments (2).

With the head and neck in extension, posterior indentation occurs and anterior subluxation is diminished. With the head in flexion, anterior indentation occurs and posterior structures cause compression if the vertebral body displaces anteriorly.

Cervical Spine Stiffness and Neck Pain

Degenerative disease of the cervical interspaces results in narrowing, incongruity of the articulations, and irregularity of the articular facets and the synovial apophyseal joints (Fig. 28.1). The range of motion diminishes and pain may increase at the extremes of movement. The deep dull aching sensation is caused by abnormal stress on the nonelastic ligaments, by irritation of the synovial linings, and by instability and incongruity of the vertebral bodies and the facet joints. Very reactive hypertrophic osteophytes occur because of the narrowed intervertebral disk space and facet joints. The formation of osteophytes is associated with either instability or incongruity.

Mechanical Change. If encroachment on the spinal canal or the short radicular canals occurs, the classic findings of a degenerative cervical intervertebral disk syndrome result, with localized neck pain, decreased range of motion with or without radicular dermatome pain, and muscle weakness.

The severity of the neck and extremity pain is related to the patient's age and the rapidity of onset of the pathologic condition. The extent of the adaptation of the involved joints depends on the influence of other factors such as congenital synostosis of the cervical region, the hormonal and biochemical factors that influence the nerve receptors, and the coalition of the mucopolysaccarides and the proteoglycans that make up the nucleus and anulus of the cervical joints.

Biochemical Change. As the biochemical make up of the degenerating disk complex changes, the pain complaints become both mechanical and inflammatory. The mechanical and inflammatory irritation of the nociceptors in the anulus and the ligaments and the stimulation of the sinuvertebral nerves and the sensory roots cause varying degrees of pain that usually respond initially to anti-inflammatory medications and to intermittent periods of rest. Most patients with degenerative arthrosis of the cervical spine adapt to limited activity, use anti-inflammatories, and accommodate to the gradual onset of the condition. If the wear and degenerative changes occur relatively slowly, the healing and accommodation response is rapid enough to allow the patient to become relatively asymptomatic in a reasonable period of time.

Inflammatory Disease

Inflammatory disease of the cervical spine, such as rheumatoid arthritis, ankylosing spondylitis, or other collagen conditions, causes inflammatory reaction with pain that is eventually also associated with mechanical changes. The destructive lesions of rheumatoid disease may lead to encroachment on the spinal cord and the upper or lower cervical roots. Atlantoxial instability may require external support if the condition is mild or surgical stabilization if the condition is severe and progressive (3, 4).

Ankylosing spondylitis, on the other hand, results in spontaneous stabilization of the vertebral bodies and limited rotation of the head and neck. Once the spontaneous fusion occurs and the inflammatory condition subsides or goes into remission, the patient is comfortable but neck motion is limited. If the position of spontaneous fusion is in acute flexion, then corrective osteotomy and restabilization are necessary.

Benign or Malignant Lesions of the Cervical Spine

Benign or malignant cervical spine lesions are characterized by intermittent or continuous pain regardless of neck position or the time of day. The pain may be related to increased or constant pressure on nociceptors within the intervertebral disk bond or the osseous tissue; or radicular pain occurs as a result of encroachment on nerve roots or on the spinal cord.

Osteoid osteoma of the vertebral body or posterior spinal elements, for example, is usually associated with persistent or continuous or varying degrees of pain and may be partially or completely relieved by salicylates. A *giant cell tumor* of the cervical spine will be associated with intermittent pain, the range of motion will be diminished, and the pathologic lesion is progressive.

A *metastatic tumor* to the vertebral body and sparing the interspace may eventually involve the disk bond because of mechanical alterations. A *bacterial septicemia* may affect the interspace initially and the vertebral body secondarily and cause severe constant pain and limited motion.

Acute Neck Trauma

Traumatic cervical injuries may include acute herniation of the nucleus pulposus and be associated with intense paravertebral muscle tension, radicular dermatome changes with peripheral motor weakness, and dermatome deficiencies. If the spinal cord is involved by trauma or a central herniation of the disk, upper and lower extremity dysesthesias, paresthesias, and muscle weakness may be present.

Acute hyperextension of the cervical spine after a fall may cause hyperpathia along the C5–C8 dermatomes without evidence of fracture and without evidence of ruptured disk. This is particularly true in patients who have osteoarthrosis, small nerve root foramina, and limited elasticity of the neural tissue. This primary traumatic causalgia usually responds to limited activity and rest, but may require several months, and as much as a year, before the hypersensitivity reaches a point of equilibrium.

Management of Cervical Spine Arthropathies

Neck pain caused by mild degenerative arthrosis and facet joint involvement is managed by:

1. Regular active and relaxation exercises of the cervical spine.
2. Alteration of head and neck positions during work, recreational activities, and sleep. This may be done with contour pillow, feather pillow, and rearrangement of working habits. (5)

Before exercise is initiated, slow warm-up motion should be performed. Relaxation techniques should be acquired from a physical therapist so muscle tension associated with pain is relieved by massage and gentle activity and muscle tension associated with anxiety and stress is improved by behavioral modification.

Accessory methods are used to support the head and neck, maintain protection from intermittent cool and damp air, and provide protection of the neck during automobile riding. The soft molded neck collars are used to unload the neck, to provide moderate warmth, and to provide support and prevent sudden forceful flexion or extension when the patient is in an automobile.

Cervical spine traction for several hours at a time when the patient is in bed or intermittently with special arrangement of the apparatus using graduated weights, may be helpful. The bed traction apparatus should be arranged so that the pull is on the occiput, the strap under the chin is only supportive, the direction of pull is in slight flexion, and the head of the bed is elevated about 6 inches. A 6-pound weight is sufficient to provide the necessary traction and relaxation. Intermittment cervical traction is performed with greater weight, and the patient is usually in the sitting or standing position.

Intervertebral disk degeneration and pain and interbody pain may respond to methods already described and anti-inflammatory medications. However, if pain persists for several months, and if the condition is progressive and the range of motion is limited, then localized intervertebral disk excision and arthrodesis should be considered.

If neck pain and cervical radiculopathy are present, and if the condition does not respond to limited activity, traction, nonsteroidal anti-inflammatories, and observation for a reasonable period of time, then the necessary diagnostic studies are performed in order to determine if there is localized nerve root irritation. If the lesion is localized by imaging and electrical studies, and if the condition does not respond to traction, limited activities and pharmacologic agents, then anterior diskectomy and iliac bone graft to the interspace will eliminate the pain and provide a stable neck (6).

Referred Pain in the Cervical Region

Suboccipital headache may be associated with upper cervical disk degeneration or facet joint arthrosis. Primary shoulder disease may cause proximal tapezius pain that is confused with cervical lesion. Pulmonary and cardiac lesions may be referred to the supraclavicular or lateral neck area and suggest the occurrence of a cervical syndrome. A Parsonage-Turner neuronitis may be associated with severe neck and shoulder girdle pain and resemble a cervical arthropathy.

Thoracic Spine Arthropathy

Lesions affecting the intervertebral disks, the facet joints, or the soft tissue structures around the intervertebral spaces and the nerve root foramina of the thoracic spine may cause pain syndromes similar to those described for the cervical spine. However, the radicular pattern is less obvious because it remains confined to the chest wall, except in the case of a severe thoracic radiculopathy after herpes zoster, which may be readily defined and may remain painful for several months.

Degeneration of the intervertebral disks in the thoracic region may be associated with dermatome or sclerotome pain and with narrow interspaces on the radiograph.

The melted candle effect of ankylosing spondylitis may not be evident for several years after the origin of vague back pain.

Calcification of the intervertebral disks is noted in chondrocalcinosis and may be associated with acute pain followed by dull aching discomfort for many months.

The pain syndromes affecting the joints of the thoracic spine follow the same pattern in their pathologic changes as do those that have been described for the cervical spine.

Management of Thoracic Spine Arthropathy

The method of treatment depends upon the final diagnosis. Thoracic spine pain associated with osteopenia is managed by external corset support and an antiosteopenic medication program that includes Premarin, Provera, calcium, vitamin D, and limited exercise. The specific doses and the duration of treatment depend on the individual problem and the patient's complaints.

Thoracic pain associated with degenerative arthrosis may be improved by exercise, postural training, antiinflammatory medications, and external support. Weight reduction and support of large breasts are added considerations in order to manage this condition in certain individuals.

If ankylosis spondylitis is the cause of the thoracic pain, the appropriate anti-inflammatory medication may be helpful; the three-point brace may diminish pain moderately. This condition is usually self-limiting, although several years may pass before the pain is readily tolerated by the patient.

Lumbar and Lumbosacral Spine Arthropathy

The lesions affecting the intervertebral disks account for the greatest proportion of pain complaints referable to the low back. Intervertebral disks degeneration, facet joint arthrosis, radicular canal stenosis, and laminal arch and facet encroachment on the cauda equina are the major causes of progressive lumbar arthropathy.

The diagnosis of single or multiple intervertebral disk or facet joint disease in the lumbar or lumbosacral region follows the same pattern as already described for the cervical region. Careful history, a detailed physical and neurologic examination, specific laboratory tests, and the proper imaging studies will usually result in an accurate diagnosis. In the absence of any specific findings other than subjective complaints, the assumption is usually correct that the condition has to do with ligament attachment pain, early subtle intervertebral disk disease, or overuse syndromes that may be muscular-ligamentous in their origin (7).

Intervertebral disk disease varies according to the location of the pathologic lesion. An acute rupture of an intervertebral disk may cause nerve root irritation and not only back pain but also extremity pain. Neurologic changes indicate that the involved nerve root is being seriously compressed.

Management of Lumbar Spine Arthropathy

Options for treatment depend on the severity of the onset, the presence or absence of bowel or bladder involvement, and the degree of neurologic deficit.

If there is no bowel or bladder involvement, and if the neurologic deficit is not severe, then a program of non-operative management is usually adequate. Limited bedrest, anti-inflammatory medications, and avoidance of stress on the spine, including torque, flexion, and extension, will usually result in remission of the condition. However, if the neurologic findings progress, and if pain persists to the point where the patient is not able to function, then disk excision with or without spine fusion should be considered. The diskectomy alone is the usual method of management if there is no instability or incongruity of the interspace. However, if the disk bond is badly disrupted and damaged, then posterior and posterolateral spine fusion may be indicated (8).

If the first diskectomy fails and several months have elapsed since treatment, then an anterior diskectomy and fusion should be considered (9) (Fig. 28.2).

SACROILIAC JOINT ARTHROPATHY

Involvement of the sacroiliac joints by pathologic processes is relatively uncommon. Ankylosing spondylitis (Marie-Strumpell arthritis) is the most common specific condition affecting these joints. The onset of that syndrome is relatively slow and subtle, with vague complaints and a delayed diagnosis.

The history of early morning pain, limited chest expansion compared to the population average, radiograph showing sclerosis of the subchondral bone on either side of the sacroiliac joint, partial narrowing of the joints, and a positive HLA-B27 are the findings that will establish the diagnosis after the process has been present for several months or even years. Many patients who are affected by this condition have numerous diagnostic studies, particularly myelography, or currently computed tomography scan inspecting the nerve roots of the cauda equina, before a definite diagnosis is established.

The treatment is use of Indocin and other anti-inflammatories, a regular exercise program to attempt to maintain chest expansion, and occasionally a three-point brace to avoid the development of a kyphosis.

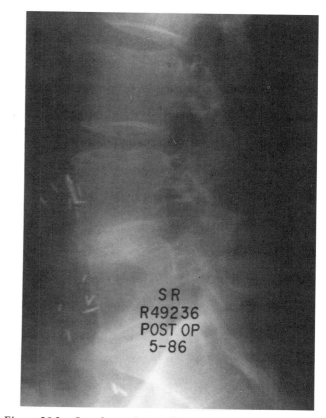

Figure 28.2. **Lumbar spine radiograph showing anterior intervertebral body arthrodesis for painful arthropathy at L4–L5 and L5–S1. This adult patient had two prior diskectomies at both interspaces. Extremity pain was improved but back pain persisted. Anterior diskectomy and iliac bone graft arthrodesis immobilizes the spine at this level, diminishes nerve root irritation, and eliminates interbody pain.**

HIP JOINT ARTHROPATHIES

The hip joints are a major cause of painful arthropathy.

PATHOLOGY

The most common cause of persistent hip pain is osteoarthrosis or degenerative arthrosis of the hip joint. The onset is usually subtle, but the symptoms gradually increase with time. The differential diagnosis early in the course of the disease includes trochanteric bursitis, syndovitis from trauma, pseudogout, iliopsoas bursitis, or pain at the insertion of the adductor tendons.

Other conditions, such as pain originating in the symphysis pubis, ischial tuberosity bursitis, or stress fracture associated with osteopenia, simulate the painful hip.

CLINICAL EXAMINATION

Limited rotation of the hip joint is the earliest clinical finding associated with osteoarthrosis or other pathology of the hip. A hip limp that consists of a shift of the

Figure 28.3. A, Preoperative degenerative arthrosis of both hips, probably associated with acetabular dysplasia, in a 55-year-old female. Pain was severe on the left, moderate on the right. The condition had been controlled with ibuprofen, but eventually the distorted gait and the fatigue associated with excessive energy expenditure in walking required a porous coated total hip replacement. B, Both hip joints have been replaced with porous coated total hip joints. The acetabulum is high-density polyethylene with metal-backed porous coated cobalt-chromium alloy. The femoral component is a cobalt-chromium-molybdenum alloy.

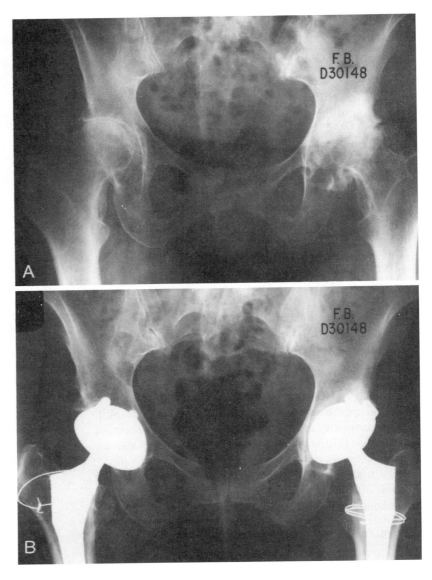

trunk to the involved side and pain on contraction of the gluteus medius are constant findings.

DIAGNOSTIC STUDIES

Radiographs demonstrate subchondral cyst formation either on the acetabular or the femoral side of the joint. Areas of increased density in the subchondral bone may occur, and osteophytes signifying narrowing of the articular cartilage are eventually obvious. Acetabular dysplasia, detected by a wide "teardrop" of the acetabulum, accounts for many changes in the hip joint that are not apparent in a younger individual. The pathologic changes may be superior or medial in relationship to the congruity of the femoral head and the acetabulum. Superior changes are more noticeable than medial alterations.

Additional diagnostic studies include aspiration of the hip joint for crystals, serologic studies with reference to possible rheumatoid disease, technetium-99 bone scan, tomography, magnetic resonance imaging (MRI), and computed tomography. These studies will usually allow a diagnosis and influence the ultimate treatment. *If asceptic necrosis is suspected, MRI is indicated.*

TREATMENT

If the condition is caused by a specific disease such as gout, psoriasis, ankylosing spondylitis, or rheumatoid disease, the primary disease should be treated.

The hip joint is unloaded by use of a cane in the opposite hand, and anti-inflammatories are helpful. Weight reduction, exercise activity to improve muscle tone, limited physical stress on the hip joint, and appropriate medication may protect the hip joint for many years.

More aggressive forms of therapy are:

1. Osteotomy of the femur and/or acetabulum.
2. Removal of osteochondral loose bodies if the condition is osteochondromatosis.

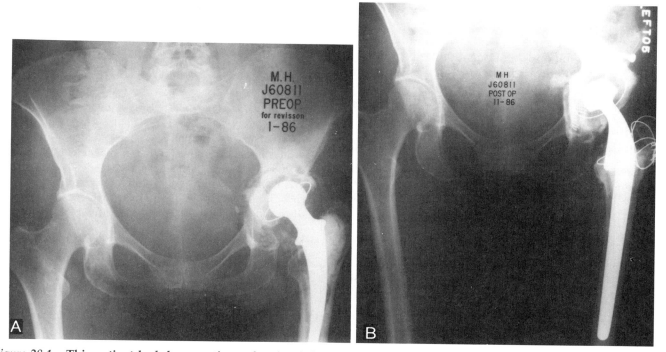

Figure 28.4. This patient had degenerative arthrosis of the left hip, that was severely incapacitating in 1970. A total hip replacement was performed at that time. A, Preoperative radiograph showing migration of the acetabulum superiorly and loosening of the femoral component in 1985. Bone absorption had resulted in both the acetabulum and the femur. B, A new prosthesis was inserted with iliac bone graft to the superior acetabulum. The bone graft is held by a screw. Additional bone was placed in the base of the acetabulum, and a large high-density polyethylene prosthesis was inserted over the reinforced bone graft with Gelfoam, vitallium mesh, and methacrylate. The femoral component replaced the absorbed neck and trochanteric region. The patient is pain-free, has a stable hip, and walks with minimal limp but is required to use a cane in the right hand to unload the left hip joint.

3. Excision of osteochondritis dessicans and drilling of the subchondral bone.
4. Prosthetic hip replacement.

Hip Arthroplasty

There are gradations of hip arthroplasty depending on the patient's age, the primary pathology involved in the hip joint, and the patient's general health.

Prosthetic Replacement of the Proximal End of the Femur

This procedure is performed by replacing the upper end of the femur with a stainless steel or alloy prosthesis. The A.T. Moore prosthesis has been used successfully for about 40 years. Its usual period of pain relief is about 15 years. The acetabular cartilage wears and additional surgical revision is necessary (see below).

Total Hip Replacement Without Methacrylate Using Porous Coated Acetabulum and Femoral Component

This prosthesis without methacrylate has been in use since about 1980. A large number of patients have had nonmethacrylate porous coated hip replacement from 1985 to the present time. The prosthesis without methacrylate has been inserted in a large number of patients, and currently the success rate is high. The patients may require as long as a year before thigh pain is diminished and stable ingrowth of tissue into the prosthesis has occurred. The longevity of the porous coated prosthesis is now known to last for at least 8 years with good ingrowth and good stability. In a small percentage of patients with porous coated prosthesis, however, stress shielding does occur at the upper end of the femoral shaft, and replacement and autologous and homologous bone grafting are necessary after 7–10 years.

Total Hip Replacement with Methacrylate

This procedure has been performed since 1968. The initial technique for inserting methacrylate allowed the prosthesis to survive for anywhere from 5 to 10 years. Replacement was frequently necessary within 10–15 years after the initial insertion of the prosthesis. Modern methacrylate cement insertion techniques have now assured the survival of the prosthesis to be longer than was thought originally, however. Although the procedure is not recommended for very young patients, it may be used for those over 60 years of age or for those who have systemic conditions such as renal disease or rheumatoid arthritis.

Figure 28.3*A* shows the preoperative condition of the

hip joints in a 55-year-old female with severe involvement on one side and a lesser amount on the other. Porous coat total joint hip replacements, including an acetabular cup and femoral component on both sides (Fig. 28.3*B*), have resulted in complete relief of pain, elimination of limp, and return of the patient to full activity, excluding axial loading such as running and jumping.

Total Hip Revision

The length of time that a high-density polyethylene-stainless steel-methacrylate fixed total hip joint will be painless and useful varies from patient to patient. Once the prosthesis shows evidence of loosening, settling, or methacrylate fracture, replacement is necessary.

Early replacement with a noncemented prosthesis or with a methacrylate-bonded prosthesis with supplementary bone graft and additional techniques for better bonding of the methacrylate will diminish the likelihood of rapid bone erosion in the future (Fig. 28.4).

References

1. Depalma A, Rothman R: *The Intervertebral Disc.* Philadelphia, WB Saunders, 1970.

2. Ferlic DC, Clayton ML, Leidholt JD, et al: Surgical treatment of the symptomatic unstable cervical spine in rheumatoid arthritis. *J Bone Joint Surg* 57A:349, 1975.

3. Bland JH, Davis BH, London MG, et al: Rheumatoid arthritis of the cervical spine. *Arch Intern Med* 112:130–136, 1963.

4. Fielding JW, Hensinger RN: The cervical spine. In Cruess RL, Rennier J (eds): *Adult Orthopaedics.* New York, Churchill Livingstone, 1984, pp. 747–765.

5. Gibson JW: Cervical syndromes: use of a comfortable cervical collar as an adjunct in their management. *South Med J* 67:205–208, 1974.

6. Robinson RA, Smith GW: The treatment of certain cervical-spine disorders by anterior removal of the intervertebral disc and interbody fusion. *J Bone Joint Surg* 40A:607, 1958.

7. Nachemson A, Bigos SJ: In Cruess RL, Rennier J (eds): *Adult Orthopaedics.* Churchill Livingstone, 1984, vol 2, pp 843–937.

8. Goldner JL: The role of spine fusion in management of low back pain. *Spine* 6:293–303, 1981, pp 293–303.

9. Goldner JL, Wood K, Urbaniak J: Anterior lumbar discectomy and interbody fusion: indications and technique. In Schmidek ED, Sweet (eds): *Operative Neurosurgical Technique.* New York, Grune & Stratton, 1982, vol II, p 1373–1379.

CHAPTER 29

Neuritis, Neuropathy, and Neuralgia

Benjamin L. Crue, Jr.

THOSE FAMILIAR with television advertising for presumably peripherally acting analgesics are accustomed to hearing the announcer extol their efficacy in "arthritis, neuritis, and neuralgia." Although this may be empirically correct (on occasion), it should remind us that much medical terminology may have a precise, specific meaning, but is often used in a much "looser" fashion that was originally intended, or that is medically correct.

The basic problem in communication lies usually in the definitions of terms used. Just what do we mean by the terms *neuropathy* and *chronic pain*? The problem of the taxonomy and classification of pain syndromes, and the difference between acute and chronic pain, has been tackled on numerous occasions by many authors, including myself, and reported almost ad nauseam (1–9). There remains considerable controversy over the "centralist" versus the "peripheralist" concept of chronic pain (2). I am a centralist and believe that to use the term *chronic pain* correctly is to imply a lack of clinical or experimental evidence of continued somatic or visceral peripheral nociceptive afferent input to the central nervous system. This is stated with the understanding that, in many chronic pain conditions, pain severity can be made worse (and the pains of neuralgia can be triggered) by several forms of "*non*nociceptive" peripheral afferent input, which have usually been considered central "perversions" of the normal patterns of sensory input. If this concept of chronic pain requiring a central underlying pain mechanism within the brain itself is accepted, then it can be logically stated that *all* "chronic pain" is *always* all basically psychosomatic (10). That is, the brain contains both the underlying central generator mechanism producing the chronic pain and the apparatus necessary for the chronic pain patient's conscious perception of the pain and the continued suffering that follows. It thus logically also follows that any therapeutic approach aimed at stopping any imaginary peripheral nociceptive input in patients with chronic pain can logically bring about a therapeutic improvement only through what we know as the "placebo" response. This is true of peripheral nerve blocks as well as such neurosurgical interventions as rhizotomy, chordotomy, and tractotomy.

The statement that all chronic pain is always all psychosomatic at first sounds fanatical. It must be understood, however, that it is merely a classification. That is, if it is not central pain, it should not be called *chronic* pain, no matter how long the pain has existed clinically. Our temporal classification of pain (outlined in Table 29.1) has been presented many times. Acute pain, subacute pain, recurrent pain (at times with underlying chronic ongoing pathology), and ongoing acute cancer pain are all believed to be related to nociceptive input, but the term *chronic pain* is reserved for those states that have no continued nociceptive input and hence are centrally generated and by definition psychosomatic.

The fact that I may well be in the minority in my view of chronic pain is well known, but the controversy continues, and I refer interested readers to a recent article by Brena, Crue, and Stieg that attempts to elucidate further this problem of definition of chronic pain (10).

For the purpose of a definition of neuropathy in the present chapter, we must discuss the meanings of the precise use of the words *neuritis, neuropathy,* and *neuralgia* (11). In 1958 Wartenberg offered a book entitled *Neuritis, Sensory Neuritis and Neuralgia* (12). Since then much has changed in our thinking about mechanisms underlying chronic pain (1, 13–19). I have been unable to find a more-recent work that deals specifically with this subject, however. Let us examine in terms of human pain the three suffixes attached to the stem *neuro*: *-itis, -opathy,* and *-algia.*

NEURITIS

Derived from the Greek, the suffix *-itis* denotes inflammation, not just infection. In a given case of peripheral neuritis, inflammation of a nerve can be due to bacterial

Table 29.1.
Temporal Classification of Pain Complaints

1. *Acute*: up to a few days in duration, mild or severe with cause known or unknown, presumed nociceptive input (the "fix-me" medical model)
2. *Subacute*: a few days to a few months in duration (although no longer an emergency, in most ways treat like acute pain)
3. *Recurrent acute*: recurrent or continued nociceptive input from underlying chronic pathologic process, i.e., arthritis (either rheumatoid or osteoarthritis)
4. *Ongoing acute*: due to uncontrolled malignant neoplastic disease, with *continued* nociceptive input
5. *Chronic*: benign, non-neoplastic, usually more than 6 months in duration; no longer any known nociceptive peripheral input, but pain often made more severe by any type of subsequent sensory input; basically a "central" pain, but with seemingly adequate coping by the patient
6. *Chronic intractable benign pain syndrome (CIBPS)*: chronic pain with poor patient coping; pain becomes central focus of the patient's existence (no known continued nociceptive peripheral input)

infection, but it appears that, when pain is involved, a disproportionate number of cases are due to other causes. For example, the herpes zoster virus in a person with shingles leads to pain in almost all cases. Inflammation can also accompany toxicity, and painful inflammation of the nerves, presumably the sensory portion, can be due to a whole host of toxins. It must be remembered that inflammation supposedly accompanies any type of injury or trauma, including compression such as that in the carpal tunnel syndrome with acute flare-up of pain in the median nerve at the wrist, or radiculoneuritis from nerve root compression from a herniated nucleus pulposus. This type of pain can be considered to have a neuritic basis. This neuritis or radiculoneuritis has been the object of many presently accepted therapeutic endeavors to decrease the inflammatory element of the painful syndrome. Specifically, the term *neuritis* means "peripheral neuritis." Nerve root inflammation is radiculoneuritis or radiculitis, inflammation within the spinal cord itself is myelitis, and inflammation within the cranial cavity is encephalitis or cerebritis. It is generally recognized that any sensory nerve can emit pain when it becomes inflamed, regardless of the cause. It becomes edematous and undergoes an infiltration of polynuclear leukocytes and, later, of lymphocytes and other monocytic cells.

There are two points to raise here. First, when we talk about an inflamed peripheral nerve, we are generally referring to an acute process. Although it may indeed be accompanied by a severe and, for a time, seemingly intractable pain, this classification of neuritis probably should be kept entirely for consideration of the etiologic agent and the mechanism underlying acute pain syndromes. There really is no evidence that neuritis plays any role in human chronic pain and suffering. Chronic pain due to continued nociceptive input probably does not exist, although it is a widely held myth within medicine. Second, in spite of our recent tremendous scientific advances in the use of neurophysiologic microelec-

trodes, electron microscopes, and special staining or isotope techniques, we still know very little as to how the inflammation in the nerve itself contributes to the increased barrage of nociceptive sensory input information that is apparently the underlying neurophysiologic mechanism leading to the acute pain. Even under the circumstances of neuritis, the awareness of pain when it is acute is still to be considered perception, and it must be remembered that even acute pain is not really limited to a primary sensory modality or sensation (14, 15).

Much work has been done to improve our understanding of some aspects of the neurochemical and neuropharmacologic activity resulting from acute trauma of peripheral tissues that give rise to severe acute clinical pain. In recent years studies of that old standby, aspirin, have been carried out in the periphery. Studies with histamine, then bradykinin, and more recently with the prostaglandins have led to an ever-increasing understanding of the whole arachidonic acid cascade and to the newer nonsteroidal anti-inflammatory analgesic agents that act in a number of ways to block the chain reaction in the periphery involving the prostaglandins and the leukotrienes. Yet much is still unknown concerning how neurochemistry and neuropharmacology relate to inflammation of neural tissue itself. This fuzzy area must include the finer peripheral elements, which are referred to as the chemoreceptor portion of the nociceptor apparatus. Just how they relate to the clinical syndromes of peripheral neuritis, which many clinicians almost automatically visualize as somehow having to do with larger sensory nerves, remains unidentified, even when we talk about this most common aspect of acute pain.

Over the last decade much new information has emerged about neural transmission as it relates to the endorphins, enkephalins, and other short peptide chains (20). The connection to the feedback loop descending to the region of the dorsal horn that modulates and apparently turns off subsequent nociceptive input has also received much attention (13). The endorphin system as yet plays no proven role in neuropathy and neuralgia (to be discussed below), however.

Activation of the acute pain-blocking feedback endorphin system to treat acute pain of great severity due to presumed afferent nociceptive input, regardless of the cause, is one of the possible and permissible uses of narcotics. Thus opiates and many of the newer synthetic narcotic-like compounds are certainly indicated in acute pain of clinical severity. Nevertheless, it has been well recognized that physicians often tend to undertreat the pain aspects and to be too conservative in the use of narcotics for patients in the recovery room after surgery, in the emergency room after injury, and in pain due to acute inflammation with neuritis, such as acute herpes zoster and the cutaneous lesions of shingles. Not only is there sound neuropharmacologic evidence that narcotics are effective with a central blocking mechanism, but also the accompanying sedation and euphoria can be helpful adjuncts in the treatments of severe acute clinical pain with presumed nociceptive input. Although it must always be stated that narcotic use should not be prolonged in nonterminal conditions, the fear of producing addiction generally has been stressed to a point that the frequent result is administration of the wrong narcotic in adequate doses over too long a time interval on a symptom-contingent rather than a time-contingent basis. Many physicians today unfortunately do not understand the optimal use of narcotics, even in acute pain associated with somatic or visceral tissue abnormalities with its neuritic component. This argument is being advanced as forcefully as possible, because I will later state that narcotics should have no role in either neuropathy or neuralgia.

Despite all the work that has been done on peripheral prostaglandins and central endorphins, the treatment of the inflamed nerve itself is still a confused issue. This is true for all of the therapeutic modalities that physical therapists can now provide, including diathermy, ultrasonography, and microwave. In general, for inflammation both of peripheral nerves (neuritis) and of joints (arthritis), it is still preferable to rest the afflicted part, and then to apply cold during the first few hours, and heat thereafter—or whatever sequence gives the most subjective relief on an empirical basis. For arthritis or synovitis, if the foregoing does not work after a reasonable length of time, injections of cortisone can be added. The inflamed nerves themselves in neuritis should *not* be the site of injection, however.

Pain of an ongoing nature seen with the invasion of malignant neoplasms into the perineurium of either peripheral nerves or frequently the brachial or the lumbosacral plexus should properly be included under neuritis rather than neuropathy. Although the mechanisms of pain from distended viscera, involvement of the peri-

osteum, bony metastases, or direct pressure on major nerve trunks have all been clearly demonstrated as causes of acute as well as continuing pain in terminal cancer, they probably always cause some type of inflammation in the nerve structures so affected. This is especially true when cancer of the lung or breast involves the brachial plexus and the perineurium is invaded, when carcinoma of the cervix involves the lumbosacral plexus, and when carcinoma of the rectum and sigmoid involves the presacral neural structures (21). Thus, such pain due to neoplasm should be classified as an acute pain problem, not only because of the hypothesized ongoing nociceptive input, but because the ongoing pain seen in cancer indicates some degree of neuritis in the involved sensory nerves.

It has always been interesting just how quickly even this fearsome pain can at times be turned off. For example, after hormonal manipulation through hypophysectomy in a hormone-sensitive metastatic tumor of the breast (22), the severe pain may be gone by the time the patient awakens from general anesthesia. The prompt cessation of pain after the injection into the pituitary gland under local anesthesia of larger amounts of alcohol than the sella turcica can be expected to hold gives rise to the hypothesis that at times this inflammation may be under the control of the hypothalamic structures rather than the pituitary gland itself. Be that as it may, "neuritis" comprises acute pain, subacute pain, recurrent acute pain, and the ongoing pain of malignancy (23).

NEUROPATHY

The suffix *-opathy* refers only to pathology, and neuropathy is usually used clinically in the sense of damaged nerve with no evidence of neuritis or inflammation. Neuropathy also has myriad causes, usually bringing to mind initially the concept of injury, such as post-traumatic neuropathy. However, the process may also be the end stage of neuritis, when the inflammation subsides; and if the sensory nerves or their coverings have sustained permanent damage, a form of neuropathy becomes a secondary stage that follows the neuritis. For instance, the end stage of herpes zoster or shingles after neuritis is usually a post-herpetic neuropathy. Because a number of patients with shingles proceed to a specific, painful syndrome known as *post-herpetic neuralgia*, we sometimes forget that most get over their acute neuritic pain and are left only with areas of temporary numbness and underlying neuropathy. Many patients suffering from difficult, chronic, post-herpetic neuralgic pain are very elderly and have severe underlying contributing emotional factors, concomitant diabetes, or a depressed immunosuppressive system from treatment of, for example, a pre-existing lymphoma. Nonetheless, most patients with herpes zoster neuritis end up with a neuropathy, and post-herpetic neuralgia does not develop to any great severity or for a long duration in the majority (24).

Some syndromes designated neuropathies are probably types of neuritis when they are painful. For example, diabetic neuropathy is well known and is usually painless, but when the sensory nerves are involved (usually in patients with juvenile diabetes, although persons with adult-onset diabetes can be so affected as well), it is often cited as the cause of the resultant pain. In all probability, these patients have neuritis. Some patients also may have a known diabetic neuropathy as well as a new episode of neuritis with pain; then, with clinically continued pain, they end up with chronic pain and *diabetic neuralgia*, a seldom-heard term.

Such a differentiation between neuritis, neuropathy, and neuralgia is necessary, in my opinion, because neuropathy is never painful. In fact, even in some neuritis patients a neuropathy develops without their ever having had pain associated with the original neuritis, provided that onset is slow enough or the virulence of the causal bacterial infection is low-grade. Three examples illustrate this possibility:

1. Many elderly people with cervical osteoarthritis may have never had any severe radicular pain from traumatic radiculoneuritis or radiculopathy and experience numbness of the hands from sensory nerve root involvement, as well as the atrophy from motor root involvement.

2. In Hansen's disease, especially before the advent of newer treatments with chemotherapeutic agents, the bacillus is of such low-grade virulence in its inflammatory response that profound numbness often develops and body parts are even lost as part of the slowly progressive neuritis leading to neuropathy without the patient's reporting any significant pain syndrome.

3. Most cases of tardy ulnar nerve palsy are of a nonpainful nature; repeated minor trauma at the elbow can often lead, without pain, to severe motor or sensory changes in the ulnar distribution in the hand. In fact, most experienced neurosurgeons will not perform an ulnar transplant at the elbow if there is much clinical pain, unless the motor or sensory deficits are also severe. The painful component frequently is not relieved for long, and the surgeon may be left postoperatively with a complaining patient in whom the central emotional factors potentiating the chronic pain syndrome have been recognized too late.

Some researchers believe that it is possible to have pain on the basis of a peripheral generator after nerves have undergone pathologic changes. This just does not make sense clinically, however, even after limb amputation. The phantom limb syndrome occurs almost universally, but only a small percentage of patients have a *painful* phantom limb. There is no good clinical evidence that, when phantom pain occurs, it is related to peripheral nociceptive input; in contrast, there is a tremendous amount of clinical evidence that it is related to central factors. Some neurophysiologists do not differentiate between the clinical entities of (1) phantom limb pain, (2) peripheral neuroma stump pain (especially when the patient attempts to wear a prosthesis), which may involve inflammation and nociceptive input generated by repeated trauma to the peripheral traumatic neuroma, and (3) chronic burning stump pain.

It must be admitted, however, that in some cases of neuropathy with damaged peripheral nerves, "crosstalk" may take place and may well contribute initially to the formation of a central "causalgia" syndrome (25).

If pathologic findings in a nerve per se are not a source of pain, we must revise our attitudes toward treatment of some of the clinical entities presently believed to be due to such changes. Our current state of medical knowledge sometimes leads to rather heroic therapeutic interventions, including surgery. For example, most cases of postlaminectomy or postmyelography "arachnoiditis" are, in fact, "arachnoidopathy." Although inflammation can occur initially, and although rare cases of progressive arachnoiditis from various etiologic agents may occur, most persons in whom arachnoiditis is diagnosed are the "failed back" patients who have undergone previous surgical intervention. After a while, the proper diagnosis almost certainly becomes arachnoidopathy with damage to the nerve roots within and without the canal, not arachnoiditis. These patients usually do not demonstrate nociceptive input from the condition. Many are being operated on inappropriately on the basis of modern scientific diagnostic techniques, such as computed tomography (CT) or magnetic resonance imaging (MRI) of the spine showing spinal or lateral recess "stenosis" that may or may not accompany the clumping of fibers on subsequent metrizamide myelography. Furthermore, positive thermographic results should not be taken as an indication for repeat laminectomy, especially in the absence of electromyographically demonstrated denervation fibrillations. The overwhelming evidence suggests that the majority of these patients have centrally generated chronic pain with underlying unresolved emotional conflicts. In any case of chronic pain, actively treating any neuropathy in the belief that one is treating the source of continuing nociceptive input is medically inappropriate.

There is no question but that the central mechanisms that we have been discussing in the establishment of central pain (to be discussed under neuralgia, rather than neuropathy) may relate to organic peripheral and/or organic central factors, and may not merely be due to centrally preprogrammed environmental factors. Thus, the pain seen in central syndromes in some cases clinically appears to be "much more organic" than in other syndromes. For example, trigeminal neuralgia,

Table 29.2.
Predisposing Central Factors to Chronic Pain

1. Organic lesion with CNS involvement:
   a. Pathologic (e.g., following stroke)
   b. Physiologic from abnormal peripheral input (e.g., major causalgia and reflex sympathetic dystrophy)
   c. Mixture of pathologic and physiologic (possible example: tic douloureux)
2. Possible "genetic" inherited defects, or at least individual differences in experiencing pain
3. "Functional" environmental factors from physiologically normal but psychologically often "abnormal" peripheral input from external milieu:
   a. Past input into memory storage including early nurturance ("psychosomatic")
   b. Reactive factors to acute pain (as often the etiologic trigger) ("somatopsychic")
   c. Mixture of the two (CIBPS syndrome)

and perhaps acute recurrent pain of some cases of migraine, may well be related to some form of sensoral epileptiform discharge and may respond to the anticonvulsants, and is certainly "organic." Although the chronic intractable benign pain syndrome with poor patient coping may be entirely central as well, it is usually considered "functional overlay" with no known continued peripheral pathophysiology or known continued nociceptive input, but in which both early nurturance and then later postinjury reactive factors might play a role from a psychogenic standpoint (Table 29.2). We are digressing from neuropathy, however, and getting into the next subject of central pain and neuralgia.

NEURALGIA

According to *Dorland's Illustrated Medical Dictionary*, *-algia* comes from the Greek *algos*, meaning "pain," and *ia*, meaning "condition": the word, therefore, suggests a painful condition. It goes on to define neuralgia as "paroxysmal pain which extends along the course of one or more nerves" and describes many varieties, distinguishing them by the anatomic part affected, the distribution of the nerve involved, and (even more unconvincingly) the etiology.

There are a number of things wrong with this definition. First, not all neuralgic pain is "paroxysmal"; in some cases it may be constant. Second, when one talks about the cause of any given case of neuralgia, it must be kept in mind that, although *etiology* and underlying neurophysiologic *mechanisms* are related sequentially, they are two different aspects of the problem and must never be confused. Third, defining neuralgia as pain of unknown origin in the distribution of a peripheral or cranial nerve implies that the cause of the pain may be within that cranial or peripheral sensory nerve and that, through biopsy, electron microscopy, or other yet-to-be invented techniques, one might find pathologic changes to explain the pain felt subjectively in the distribution of that sensory dermatome.

A quote from Wartenberg regarding neuralgia still il-

lustrates the present state of confusion regarding the use of the term (12):

> One is struck by the indiscriminate use of the term "neuralgia." It clearly illustrates the rampant confusion regarding this so extensively used term. This usage tacitly implies that any term which includes the word "neuralgia" or ends in "algia" signifies a definite morbid condition, and not merely pain in a certain area.
>
> The indiscriminate use of the term neuralgia to designate almost every undeterminable, and often not neurogenic [sic] painful affection is a menace to exact medical diagnosis. As a result, it is well nigh impossible to get a firm hold on the true meaning of the term. It covers so much that it has become almost useless for precise application.

I would like to suggest a different concept: *All neuralgia is centrally generated pain that is referred to the periphery*, at some part of the body image; thus neuralgia, of however short a duration, is central and is a form of chronic pain. Furthermore, as a centralist (who believes that the term *chronic pain* should *not* be used for a condition with continued nociceptive input), I would like to suggest conversely that all chronic pain is not only psychosomatic, but also basically a form of neuralgia.

This concept is not far from the schema proposed three decades ago by Ramzy and Wallerstein (26) (Fig. 29.1). In an attempt to give a hypothetic taxonomy to purely psychogenic (mental) and bodily pain, they subdivided the latter into somatic and neurotic categories. The somatic category included both peripheral (somatic) and internal (visceral) pain, which is equivalent to pain from continued nociceptive input and, per the temporal classification outlined in Table 29.1, comprises acute, subacute, recurrent acute, and ongoing cancer pain. Neuritis falls into this category for the purpose of this presentation. Ramzy and Wallerstein also delineated a second type, "neurotic bodily pain," involving memory. This can be considered "real" pain from a prior injury (or neuritis) that originally entailed nociceptive input, but for which no presently continuing underlying or-

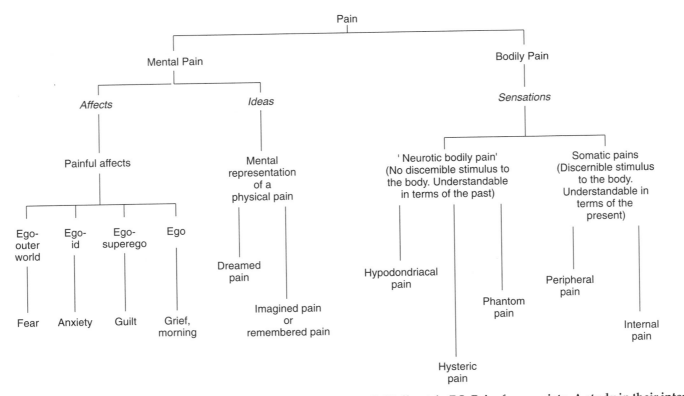

Figure 29.1. Psychoanalytic schematization of pain. (From Ramzy I, Wallerstein RS: Pain, fear, anxiety. A study in their inter-relationships. *Psychoanal Study Child* 13:147, 1958.)

ganic pathophysiologic process justifies the assumption that a "discernible stimulus to the body" provides continuing nociceptive input. This concept fits well with the definition by Pinsky of the chronic intractable benign pain syndrome, wherein it is suggested that there is no ongoing pathophysiology in the here and now—that is, no continued nociceptive input (27) (Table 29.3). Long ago, I suggested that this central mechanism of "neurotic bodily pain" could be relabeled *neuralgia* (28–30). This classification includes not only the few patients with hypochondriacal or hysterical features, or phantom limb pain, but also *all* patients with chronic pain.

In some forms of central neuralgia with a presently unknown etiology, such as idiopathic primary trigeminal neuralgia, the cause may be presumed to be peripheral. In secondary trigeminal neuralgia, acoustic tumors, entry zone multiple sclerosis, the carotid artery's beating under the trigeminal ganglion in the region of the foramen lacerum, and even pulsation of a smaller artery against the trigeminal root near the pons have all been listed as more-central but still peripheral etiologic agents. In all neuralgia, however, the mechanism is central. We have postulated that trigeminal neuralgia is a form of sensory epilepsy (repetitive, uncontrolled, epileptiform neuron firing) within the trigeminal nucleus in the brainstem (31–35). Hence, it is the drugs with anticonvulsant properties that have proved effective in treatment: first phenytoin (36), then mephanesin carba-

mate (37) (no longer available), then carbamazepine, and now recently baclofen. The anticonvulsants also seem to help in the paroxysmal jabs of pain after spinal cord injury, the lightning pains of tabes dorsalis, and post-herpetic neuralgia as well. They do not affect the constant pain of many chronic syndromes, however, especially the deafferentation hypersensitivity states, which often leads to the diagnoses of causalgia and reflex sympathetic dystrophy. For this type of constant "dysesthetic" chronic pain, often seen in post-herpetic neuralgia, the antidepressants amitriptyline and doxepin have given partial relief, presumably by a central analgesic action. Fortunately, the vast majority of neuralgic pain syndromes are of short duration and usually self-limiting (in spite of attempted therapy), and they do not become intractable. Consequently, therapeutic success has been attributed to virtually everything: nerve block, rhizotomy, transcutaneous electrical nerve stimulation, hypnosis, transcendental meditation, biofeedback, acupuncture, moxibustion, and even wearing a string of garlic. The last certainly is to be preferred to electroconvulsive therapy and depth electrode placement for stimulation, congulotomy, or even prefrontal lobotomy, which are still being done in this country without adequate trial of the pain team–oriented method of intensive treatment (38). Some patients and many physicians seem to be unable to accept that psychologically based treatment is indicated. The conflu-

Table 29.3.
Chronic Intractable Benign Pain Syndrome (CIBPS)

General characteristics of pain:
1. Cannot be shown to be causally related to the here and now with any active pathophysiologic or pathoanatomic process
2. Has an antecedent history of generally ineffective medical and surgical intervention in the pain problem
3. Has come to be accompanied by disturbed psychosocial function that includes the pain complaint and the epiphenomena that accompany it

Epiphenomena:
1. Substance use disorders of varying severity with their attendant CNS side effects
2. Multiple surgical procedures or pharmacologic treatments with their own morbid side effects (separate from those related above)
3. Escalated decrease in physical functioning related to accompanying pain and/or fear that this pain is a signal of increased bodily harm and damage
4. Escalated hopelessness and helplessness as persistent or increased dysphoria does not give way in the face of mounting numbers of "newer" or different treatment interventions
5. Emotional conflicts with medical care delivery personnel (doctors, nurses, therapists, technicians), which result in therapeutic goal interference
6. Interpersonal emotional conflicts with significant others
7. Lasting, unpleasant mood and affect changes
8. Decrease in feelings of self-esteem, self-worth, and self-confidence
9. Escalated withdrawal and loss of gratifications from psychosocial activity
10. Decreased ability to obtain pleasure from life, reflected in the presence of profound demoralization and, at times, significant depression

ence of attitudes agrees with the rationale "if there is something wrong in my head, fix it there," an approach that can lead to the use of essentially unproved chemical and surgical CNS treatments.

CONCLUSIONS

It is time that those in medicine live up to the dictum learned in medical school: "First do no harm!" When it comes to treating patients with chronic pain or the neuralgia syndromes of unknown etiology, we should always use the simpler, noninvasive, and nondestructive methods first (39), rather than try the newest therapeutic medication or operation available or even resort to them as a last desperate measure without adequately determining what we are trying to accomplish.

If the pain syndrome is chronic, then psychotherapy (40), however it may function as a therapeutic tool, is the best we presently have to offer (41). If physicians are not able to accept this concept, regardless of therapeutic outcome, patients who seek their advice will not have much chance of staying away from eventually harmful treatments. Group psychotherapy, usually by a trained pain team in the milieu of a multidisciplinary, interdisciplinary, comprehensive pain center, offers the best therapy presently available for these chronic pain syndromes.

It is obvious how complicated this can be, because we do not agree on definitions within the field of neurology and neurosurgery. It continues to lead to confusion. I

ask the interested reader to look through the recently published second edition of Dyck et al.'s two-volume set *Peripheral Neuropathy* (42). It is obvious at once that under the rubric of neuropathy are included many of the syndromes that I would refer to as neuritic or neuralgic. It must be admitted that there are esoteric causes of peripheral nerve damage that can on occasion be painful where it has not been proven that there is inflammation or a central mechanism. I contend, however, that the division of "neuropathy" into the concepts of neuritis, neuropathy, and neuralgia as presented above make a very useful clinical framework within which to consider treatment rationale in any given case of intractable pain (43). Perhaps one of the best examples of how confused we still are about this can be seen in a recent book, *Evaluation and Treatment of Chronic Pain*, edited by my good friend Gerald Aronoff (44). I wrote the foreword, in which I discussed the problem between the central and peripheral concepts of chronic pain; then neurologist Dave Agnew, in Chapter 4, carried this on, and appears to agree with me, when under the diagnosis of painful neurologic disorders he discusses the usual lack of pain in the truly neuropathic syndromes (45). Yet the editor himself joined with co-author Walter Panies in Chapter 5 of the same book when, under the title of "Painful Peripheral Neuropathies," he talked about pain in neuropathy, but included the "entrapment syndromes" and the "neuralgic syndromes" (46). No wonder students of human pain syndromes remain confused!

REFERENCES

1. Crue BL: A physiological view of the psychology of pain. *Bull LA Neurol Soc* 44:1, 1979.
2. Crue BL: The centralist concept of chronic pain. *Semin Neurol* 3:331–339, 1983.
3. Crue BL: Defining the chronic pain syndrome. In Long DM (ed): *Current Therapy in Neurosurgery*. Toronto, Ontario, BC Decker, 1985, pp 205–208.
4. Crue BL, Pinsky JJ: Chronic pain syndrome—Four aspects of the problem: New Hope Pain Center and Pain Research Foundation. In *New Approaches to Treatment of Chronic Pain*. Research #36. Monograph Series. Rockville, MD, National Institute on Drug Abuse, 1981, pp 137–168.
5. Crue BL: Multidisciplinary pain treatment programs—Current status. *J Clin Pain* 1:31–38, 1985.
6. Crue BL: Foreword. In Aronoff GM (ed): *Evaluation and Treatment of Chronic Pain*. Baltimore, Urban & Schwarzenberg, 1985, pp. *xv–xxi*.
7. Crue BL: Foreword. In Aronoff G (ed): *Pain Centers in the U.S.A.: A Revolution in Health Care*. (In press).
8. Crue BL: Historical perspectives. In Ghia JN (ed): *Organization of Pain Clinics and Function of Personnel*. Boston, Kluwer Academic, 1988.
9. Crue BL: Outpatient management of acute and chronic pain. In Wolcott MW (ed): *Ambulatory Surgery*. Philadelphia, JB Lippincott, 1988.
10. Brena S, Crue B, Stieg R: Comments on the classification of chronic pain: Its clinical significance. *Bull Clin Neurosci* 49:67–81, 1984.
11. Crue BL: Neuritis, neuropathy, and neuralgia. *Curr Concepts Pain* 1:3–10, 1983.
12. Wartenberg R: *Neuritis, Sensory Neuritis, Neuralgia*. New York, Oxford University Press, 1958.
13. Crue BL, Carregal EJA: Pain begins in the dorsal horn—With a proposed classification of the primary senses. In Crue BL (ed): *Pain Research and Treatment*. New York, Academic Press, 1975, pp 35–68.
14. Crue BL, Kenton B, Carregal EJA: Speculation concerning the possibility of a unitary peripheral cutaneous input system for pressure, hot-cold, and tissue damage: Discussion of relationship to pain. *Bull LA Neurol Soc* 41:13–42, 1976.
15. Crue BL, Kenton B, Carregal EJA: Review article—Neurophysiology of pain—Peripheral aspects. In Crue BL (ed): *Chronic Pain*. New York, Spectrum Publications, 1979, pp 59–96.
16. Crue BL, Kenton B, Carregal EJA, Pinsky JJ: The continuing crisis in pain research. In Crue BL (ed): *Chronic Pain*. New York, Spectrum Publications, 1979.
17. Crue BL, Saltzberg B: Dynamic pain. *Bull LA Neurol Soc* 44:127, 1979.
18. Crue BL: Neurophysiology and taxonomy of pain. In Brena S, Champman S (eds): *Management of Patients with Chronic Pain*. New York, Spectrum Publications, 1983, pp 21–36.
19. List CF: Cranial neuralgia—Introduction, definitions, anatomic and pathologic aspects. In Vinken PJ, Bruyn LW (eds): *Handbook of Neurology*, vol 5. Amsterdam, North Holland Publishing Co, 1968, pp 281–295.
20. Crue BL: Comments on recent neurochemical brain stem aspects of pain. In Crue BL (ed): *Chronic Pain*. New York, Spectrum Publications, 1979, pp 193–209.
21. Crue BL, Todd EM: A simplified technique of sacral rhizotomy for pelvic pain. *J Neurosurg* 21:835–837, 1964.
22. Freshwater DB, Crue BL, Shelden CH, Pudenz RH: Further experience with a technique of total extracapsular hypophysectomy. *Cancer* 10:105–110, 1957.
23. Crue BL: Treatment of patients with pain due to cancer. In Gross SC, Garb S (eds): *Cancer Treatment and Research in Humanistic Perspective*. New York, Springer-Verlag, 1985, pp 73–83.
24. Thomsen TC: *Shingles*. New York, Cross River Press, 1990.
25. Crue BL: Causalgia and the deafferentation syndromes. In Brena S, Chapman S (eds): *Management of Patients with Chronic Pain*. New York, Spectrum Publications, 1983, pp 73–83.
26. Ramzy I, Wallerstein RS: Pain, fear, anxiety. A study in their inter-relationships. *Psychoanal Study Child* 13:147, 1958.
27. Pinsky JJ, Crue BL: Intensive group psychotherapy. In Wall PD, Melzack R (eds): *Textbook of Pain*. New York, Churchill Livingstone, 1984, pp 823–831.
28. Crue BL, Carregal EA, Todd EM: Neuralgia: Consideration of central mechanisms. *Bull LA Neurol Soc* 29:107–132, 1964.
29. Crue BL, Todd EM, Carregal EJA: Cranial neuralgia—Neurophysiological considerations. In Vinken PJ, Bruyn GW (eds): *Handbook of Neurology*, vol 5. Amsterdam, North-Holland, 1968, pp 281–295.
30. Crue BL, Todd EM: Vagal neuralgia. In Vinken PJ, Bruyn GW (eds): *Handbook of Neurology*, vol 5. Amsterdam, North-Holland, 1968, pp 362–367.
31. Carregal E, Crue BL, Todd EM: Further observations of trigeminal antidromic potentials. *J Neurosurg* 20:277–288, 1963.
32. Crue BL, Shelden CH, Pudenz RH, Freshwater DB: Observations on the pain and trigger mechanism in trigeminal neuralgia. *Neurology* 6:196–207, 1956.
33. Crue BL, Sutin J: Delayed action potentials in the trigeminal system of cats. *J Neurosurg* 16:477—502, 1959.
34. Crue BL, Kilham OW, Carregal EJA, Todd EM: Peripheral trigeminal potentials. *Bull LA Neurol Soc* 32:17–29, 1967.
35. Crue BL, Carregal EJA: Postsynaptic repetitive neuron discharge in chronic neuralgia pain. *Adv Neurol* 4:643–649, 1974.
36. Crue BL, Todd EM, Carregal EJA: Observations on the present status of the compression procedure in trigeminal neuralgia. In Crue BL (ed): *Pain and Suffering—Selected Aspects*. Springfield, IL, Charles C Thomas, 1970, pp 47–63.
37. Crue BL, Todd EM, Lowe AG: Clinical use of mephensin carbamate (Tolseram) in trigeminal neuralgia. *Bull LA Neurol Soc* 30:212–215, 1965.
38. Pinsky JJ, Crue BL: Comments on psychosurgery for pain. In Crue BL (ed): *Chronic Pain*. New York, Spectrum Publications, 1979, pp 535–542.
40. Crue BL, Pinsky JJ: An approach to chronic pain of nonmalignant origin. *Postgrad Med J* 60:30–36, 1984.
41. Lee J: Lemons from a shady dealer. *Time* 23 May 1983, p 60.
42. Dyck PT, Thomas PK, Lambert EH, Bunge R: *Peripheral Neuropathy*, ed 2, Philadelphia, WB Saunders, 1984.
43. Crue BL: The Comprehensive Pain Program Approach. In

Tollison CD (ed): *Painful Cervical Trauma.* Baltimore, Williams & Wilkins, 1992, pp 230–257.

44. Aronoff GM (ed): *Evaluation and Treatment of Chronic Pain.* Baltimore, Urban & Schwarzenberg, 1985.

45. Agnew DC: Painful neurological disorders. In Aronoff GM (ed): *Evaluation and Treatment of Chronic Pain.* Baltimore, Urban & Schwarzenberg, 1985, pp 61–73.

46. Panis W, Aronoff GM: Painful peripheral neuropathies. In Aronoff GM (ed): *Evaluation and Treatment of Chronic Pain.* Baltimore, Urban & Schwarzenberg, 1985, pp 75–82.

CHAPTER **30**

LUMBAR SPINE AQUATIC REHABILITATION: A SPORTS MEDICINE APPROACH

ANDREW J. COLE
MARILOU MOSCHETTI
RICHARD E. EAGLESTON

ALTHOUGH MANY spine patients have been told by their physicians to swim for rehabilitation, exercise, and pain management, the role that the aquatic environment provides in spine rehabilitation has not been fully explored. The unique properties of water make it an ideal medium for rehabilitating spinal pain patients. A variety of methods may be used to integrate a water-based program into a comprehensive training regimen.

BACKGROUND

Aquatic activity is the most prevalent participation sport in the United States and is an extremely popular form of exercise for recreation, competition, and rehabilitation (1). Current estimates reveal over 28,000 people involved with U.S. Masters Swimming and over 2000 centers using aquatic techniques for rehabilitative purposes (2). The rising popularity of aquatic activities has resulted in ever-increasing numbers of spine and associated musculoskeletal injuries.

Land exercise, swimming, or an inappropriate aquatic rehabilitation program can cause a new spine injury or exacerbate a pre-existing spine disorder, but a properly designed aquatic program can help rehabilitate a patient with a spine injury. Aquatic stabilization techniques and swimming programs may be used in conjunction with an aggressive, comprehensive land-based spine stabilization program or as the sole rehabilitative tool (3, 4). Swimming skills alone will not determine the success or failure of an aquatic therapy candidate, because swim stroke proficiency is not a model for successful treatment (5).

Thorough comprehension of basic spine anatomy and biomechanics is necessary to understand the complex natural history of degenerative spine disease. A rehabilitation prescription can then be tailored to the patient's spine dysfunction and pain. Knowledge of the lumbar spine degenerative cascade ensures that potential problems are anticipated and addressed. An understanding of the cascade allows the astute clinician to more appropriately prescribe both land and aquatic rehabilitation programs.

LUMBAR SPINE ANATOMY, PATHOANATOMY, AND BIOMECHANICS OVERVIEW

A specific site in the spine is described by its general location: lumbar, thoracic, or cervical. Each of these regions contains a relatively constant number of motion segments. A motion segment consists of two vertebral bodies, an interposed disk, a pair of facet joints, and a variety of structures that bind them together. The central spinal canal, which transmits the spinal cord, and the segmental foramina, which form passages for the exiting nerve roots, are created by the structures that compose the motion segment (6–11).

The disk is made up of an outer anulus fibrosus and an inner nucleus pulposus. The anulus consists of 10–20 circumferential collagenous layers called *lamellae* that completely surround the nucleus pulposus (12). The fibers in each layer run parallel to one another. Although the direction of inclination alternates with each lamella, the fibers within each lamella are oriented 30° from the horizontal (13, 14). The outer half of the anulus, which

386

has great tensile strength, consists primarily of type I collagen. It has a vascular and a nervous supply. The inner half of the anulus is devoid of vascular or nervous input and consists primarily of type II collagen, which best accommodates pressure changes (15–17, 8, 18–21). The posterior and posterolateral portions of the anulus are thinnest (22–24) and are also the most common sites for "disk herniation" (8). The risk of herniation increases with activities that can cause repetitive microtrauma to the anulus and associated structures (25, 26). Repetitive or constant forward flexion loads the thinner posterior anulus, making a tear at this location more likely. Also, twisting motions are more likely to injure the anulus because resistance can be offered only by half of the available lamellae, those with their fibers oriented in the direction of the twist (8).

The annular fibers encapsulate the nucleus pulposus (12), a gelatinous structure which is primarily composed of proteoglycans, a substance which attracts and retains a significant amount of water (27, 28). The nucleus is devoid of a nervous or vascular supply. It relies on the diffusion of nutrients across the inner anulus or the vertebral cartilaginous endplate for its nutrition (29). The fluid nature of the nucleus helps to translate vertical pressure into circumferential tension in the anulus and attenuates the speed with which a particular force is transmitted to its neighboring motion segment (8). Therefore, any abnormal decrease in the water content of the nucleus or weakening of the annular fibers that contain it can change the biomechanics of the motion segment, resulting in spinal dysfunction and pain.

Each pair of facet joints that occupy the posterior portion of the motion segment consist of a superior and inferior cartilage lined articular process. The facet joint, a synovial joint that has a rich vascular and nervous supply, is surrounded by a tough collagenous capsule (9–11, 30–33). Normally the disk bears most if not all of the weight during standing, and the facets little or none. With abnormal loading situations or degeneration of the motion segment, however, the facets can help to support the load and become a source of pain (34–38).

Ligamentous and muscular structures reinforce and protect the motion segment from stressful loading situations. In particular, a series of muscles surrounding the spine help to control its motion. They work in concert with those positioning other associated structures such as the pelvis and lower extremities (39, 40). With proper training, the patient learns how to use these muscles and associated structures to better control lumbar motion, thus protecting the spine from stressful forces created by flexion, extension, and rotation—stresses potentially damaging to the motion segments. Finally, anterior shear forces created by the normal sacral inclination and lumbar lordosis are countered by the facet joints and iliolumbar ligaments, and are controlled by muscular forces (40–42).

The "degenerative cascade" concept that evolved from the work of Kirkaldy-Willis predicts anatomic, biomechanical, and clinical findings and tracks their evolution through time. The cascade is divided into three separate phases: (1) *dysfunction*, (2) *instability*, and (3) *stability*. During the dysfunction phase the disk develops annular laxity with disorganization of its annular lamellae. Small circumferential tears ensue, which then progress to radial tears. Nuclear peripheralization results because of annular and nuclear degeneration, which is enhanced by diminished diffusion of nutrients across the degenerating cartilage endplate. An alteration in normal motion segment biomechanics occurs. During the instability phase, the disk dehydrates further with progressive loss of disk height. There is increased movement within the affected motion segment. Osteophytosis results and helps minimize the impact that the altered biomechanics may have. During the stability phase, progressive fibrosis of the nucleus and continued osteophytosis occurs, resulting in progressive loss of disk space height, central stenosis, lateral recess stenosis, and foraminal stenosis (26, 43, 44).

Facet degeneration accompanies disk degeneration. Progressive motion of the facet joint results in facet synovitis and articular cartilage loss. During the instability phase, capsular laxity and subluxation occur. In response to the changes during instability, enlargement of the facets secondary to osteophytosis causes the fixed bony deformities seen during the stability phase. Enlargement of the superior articular facet narrows the lateral recess and foramen while enlargement of the inferior facet causes central stenosis (26, 43, 44).

CLINICAL DECISION-MAKING

The work-up and diagnosis of spine pain in athletes requires a thorough understanding of anatomy, physiology, and sport-specific functional biomechanics. After eliciting a careful history, with close attention to the specific mechanism of injury, a thorough yet directed musculoskeletal and neurologic examination of the injured structure and its contiguous supporting elements is performed. A functional evaluation is conducted in which the patient reproduces any painful motion. Finally, appropriate ancillary testing is ordered and the correct final diagnosis is confirmed.

When prescribing a rehabilitation plan, the sports spine physician must be aware that physiologic and psychological needs vary among different patient populations. For example, highly competitive athletes require alternative training regimes during their rehabilitation programs to maintain peak flexibility, strength, and aerobic conditioning. Recreational performers may be more flexible in this regard. The competitive athlete requires a specific training schedule and goals if he is to compete effectively during his particular athletic season.

On the other hand, a weekend athlete's needs are usually not as rigorous. Specific patient goals are met by tailoring the work-up and rehabilitation program to the level of athletic demand. Finally, changes in training routines and sports-specific mechanics require close cooperation among physician, patient, therapist, and coach (45).

REHABILITATION PROGRAMS: GENERAL THOUGHTS

The goal of the first phase of rehabilitation is to control inflammation and pain. Training must begin at the earliest possible moment so that the deleterious effects of inactivity do not hamper rapid recovery from a lumbar spine injury (46–53). Ice application (54), training in body mechanics to minimize pain associated with activities of daily living, and a trial of extension exercises (55) may be appropriate. Pain control can be further controlled by judicious use of medications such as nonsteroidal anti-inflammatory drugs (NSAIDs) (56). Selective epidural, nerve root, and facet injections that combine a local anesthetic and corticosteroid are powerful diagnostic and therapeutic tools. Using fluoroscopic guidance and radiographically visible contrast agents allows the medication to be placed precisely at the suspect tissue and thus confirm it as the source of pain (57). Therapeutic modalities including ultrasonography (58) and various forms of electrical stimulation (59) can help to treat pain and its causes. Additional therapeutic techniques such as mobilization and manipulation can help speed recovery by easing joint restrictions and improving soft tissue range of motion and neural function (60–64). Improved lumbar segmental mobility results.

Land-Based Lumbar Spine Dynamic Stabilization Exercise Programs

Once pain and inflammation are alleviated, exercise training, the second phase of the rehabilitation program, begins. Dynamic lumbar stabilization is a specific type of therapeutic exercise training that can help the patient gain dynamic control of lumbar spine forces, eliminate repetitive injury to the motion segments (i.e., disks, facets, and related structures), encourage healing of an injured segment, and possibly alter the degenerative process. The underlying premise is that the motion segment and its supporting soft tissues react to minimize applied stress and thereby reduce the risk of injury (65, 66).

Stabilization training begins from a neutral lumbar spine position, defined as a patient's least painful lumbar spine position—the one that minimizes segmental biomechanical stress. It is to be maintained during stressful spine situations such as repetitive motion or excessive single occurrence loads. A series of stabilization exercises is used to establish an engram (a cortically preprogrammed automatic multimuscular pattern of movement activated without conscious control) for muscle fusion (67). Muscle fusion results from the contraction of the muscles that maintain the neutral position of the lumbar spine and help protect it from various stresses. In addition to training the anterior muscles—rectus abdominis, internal oblique, external oblique, and transversus abdominis—particular attention is paid to the posterior muscle groups and their fascia—spinal extensors, gluteus maximus, trapezius, and dorsolumbar fascia. The lumbar longissimus and lumbar iliocostalis are particularly important because they generate a posterior shear force. This force counters anterior translation resulting from normal lumbar lordosis, sacral inclination, and flexion of the lumbar spine (41). Other relevant muscle groups include those that help control pelvic position—hamstrings, quadriceps, iliopsoas, rectus femoris, gastrocsoleus, and their associated groups—hip internal and external rotators and iliotibial band (25, 26, 66).

Soft tissue flexibility of the hamstring, quadriceps, iliopsoas, gastrocsoleus, and hip rotators and abductors allows optimal positioning of the pelvis to ensure that the most biomechanically sound neutral spine position is maintained. Stabilization training begins from this neutral spine position (25, 26, 66).

Once patients can find and maintain their neutral position in controlled static situations, training progresses to provide graded challenges in predictable and unpredictable situations during dynamic spine conditions. In addition, training of peripheral muscle groups occurs and a general aerobic conditioning program is added that incorporates neutral spine mechanics (25, 26, 66). In summary, the patient learns how to find neutral, incorporates biomechanically specific stabilization techniques, and develops adequate flexibility and strength to maintain neutral spine during dynamic functional activities. In so doing, the spine becomes a stable platform and force transmitter for peripheral joint action (5).

AQUATIC LUMBAR SPINE DYNAMIC STABILIZATION EXERCISE PROGRAMS

Spine stabilization principles used for land programs are also applicable in the water. Aquatic stabilization was first described by Richard Eagleston in 1987 (68). The goals of an aquatic stabilization program incorporate these same elements but take into account the properties of the aqueous medium. Thus, the risk of spine injury is minimized. Although the aquatic environment increases the potential number of training positions, certain exercises performed on land cannot be reproduced in water, and vice versa.

A number of factors should be considered when creating a detailed aquatic rehabilitation program designed for a specific patient's spine disorder. The diagnosis, arthrometry, positions that increase and decrease pain,

Table 30.1.
Contraindications for Aquatic Rehabilitation

1. Fever
2. Cardiac failure
3. Urinary infections
4. Bowel and/or bladder incontinence
5. Open wounds
6. Infectious diseases
7. Contagious skin conditions
8. Excessive fear of water
9. Severely weakened or deconditioned state
10. Uncontrolled seizures
11. Colostomy bag or catheter used by patient
12. Cognitive or functional impairment that would create a hazard to the patient in the pool
13. Poor endurance
14. Abnormal tone
15. Severe decreased range of motion that limits function

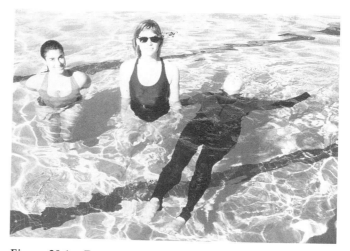

Figure 30.1. **Bouyancy provides depth-dependent, graded elimination of gravitational forces. In the vertical position, the more the patient's body is immersed, the greater the reduction in gravitational forces and axial load on the spine.**

initial level of conditioning, prior aquatic experience, response to land-based training, and level of athletic competition all need detailed evaluation. A transition from dry to wet exercise conditions eliminates dry risks, establishes a supportive training environment, provides a new therapeutic activity, decreases the risk of peripheral joint injury, and allows a return to a prior activity. Moving from dry to wet environments should also be considered if patients have an intolerance to axial or gravitational loads, or require increased support in the presence of a strength or proprioceptive deficit. Remaining in a water-supported environment is appropriate if the dry environment exacerbates symptoms or the patient has an exclusive preference for the water. Transition from a wet to a dry environment should occur if patients are doing well in the water and need to return to land to most efficiently meet functional training needs in order to attain their ultimate rehabilitative goals (5). See Table 30.1 for specific contraindications for aquatic rehabilitation.

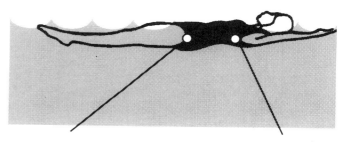

CENTER OF GRAVITY   CENTER OF BUOYANCY

Figure 30.2. **The center of bouyancy and the center of gravity are located in two separate positions.**

PROPERTIES OF WATER

Buoyancy was first described by Archimedes (ca. 287–212 BC), who noted that the force exerted on an immersed object is equal to the weight of the liquid it displaces (69, 70). This unique property of water allows for depth-dependent graded elimination of gravitational forces on the immersed patient (Fig. 30.1). When patients are vertically immersed up to their necks, a reduction of gravitational forces of approximately 90% occurs (71, 72). A center of buoyancy can be located in the region of the pleural cavity in supine patients. This center is distinct from the center of gravity, which is the

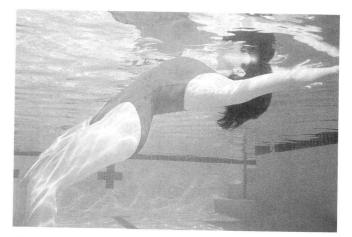

Figure 30.3. **A more-caudad center of gravity requires greater spine extension to keep the a patient afloat. This extended spinal position creates a potential pain problem for patient's with facet pain or foraminal stenosis.**

Figure 30.4. A more-cephalad center of gravity requires less spinal extension to deep the patient afloat but may increase intradiskal pressure and exacerbate diskogenic symptoms.

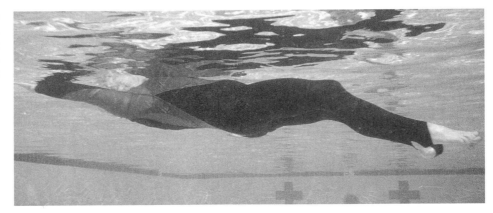

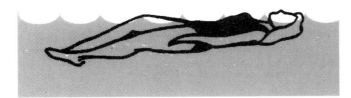

SPECIFIC GRAVITY IS LESS THAN 1.0 —
THUS THE HUMAN BODY WILL FLOAT

Figure 30.5. **The specific gravity of humans is less than that of water. Thus the human body floats in water.**

point through which the force of gravity acts, and which is located at the level of the second sacral segment or anterior superior iliac spine (Fig. 30.2). In water, the more caudad the center of gravity, the greater the amount of spine extension is required to keep the patient afloat (i.e., to place the center of buoyancy in an optimal position to balance downward forces at the center of gravity). This creates a potential pain problem for patients with facet pain or foraminal stenosis (Fig. 30.3). Conversely, a more cephalad center of gravity requires less spine extension to keep the patient afloat but may produce symptoms in patients suffering from diskogenic pain due to increased intradiskal pressures (3) (Fig. 30.4). Buoyancy increases with decreasing depth and will have a greater effect on body parts that are positioned to produce longer lever arms. Therefore, the direction of motion of the body part, up, down, or horizontal, dictates whether buoyant force is used to assist, resist, or support it, respectively (74–76). Patients performing stabilized hip motion with the knee extended while in the standing position will create a greater challenge to their neutral spine position during hip extension than when their knee is in flexion (Fig. 30.12B, C).

The *specific gravity* (i.e., the relative density) of an object is defined as its weight relative to the weight of an equal volume of water. The specific gravity of water is 1.0. Humans float because their specific gravity is less than that of water. In humans, specific gravity increases with greater bone density and muscle mass and reduced body fat. Specific gravity decreases with less bone density and muscle mass, and more body fat. Clearly, both buoyant forces and specific gravity play a critical role in patient positioning and energy consumption during aquatic therapeutic exercise programs (70, 74–77) (Fig. 30.5). The effect that gravity and buoyancy have on an immersed object is know as the *metacentric principle* (78). Gravity and buoyancy work in opposite directions: gravity downward and buoyancy upward. If these two forces are equal and opposite, no movement occurs. If, however, they are not equal, rotation of the object occurs until the forces once again balance. Therefore, careful assessment must be made of a patient's shape, specific gravity, and precise site of injury and pain to help avoid any undesirable movement through the injury site when positioning the patient for aquatic therapeutic exercise (78).

Hydrostatic Pressure is force per unit area and is measured in atmospheres. The greater the depth, the greater its effect on an immersed patient (Fig. 30.6). It may enhance proprioceptive feedback and improve patients' kinesthetic awareness. Hydrostatic pressure has many effects on the cardiovascular system, including increasing venous return and stroke volume. Hydrostatic pressure also has renal consequences such as changes in renal blood flow and ear, nose, and throat (ENT) effects, including changes in sinus pressure. Appropriate cardiac, renal, and ENT precautions must be observed (4, 70, 76, 77, 79–85, 100–102).

The frictional resistance of a fluid is called *viscosity*. Because water is more viscous than air, it offers a resistive force to movement that can assist in strengthening and conditioning patients as well as increasing their kinesthetic awareness. The faster the motion, the greater the resistance (70, 76).

Turbulence is a force differential created by movement and is a result of frontal resistance, laminar flow, and drag (eddies, tail suction). Frontal resistance impedes forward progress of any body part. Ideally, a layer of water flows smoothly down the body while it is in mo-

Hydrostatic Pressure in Water

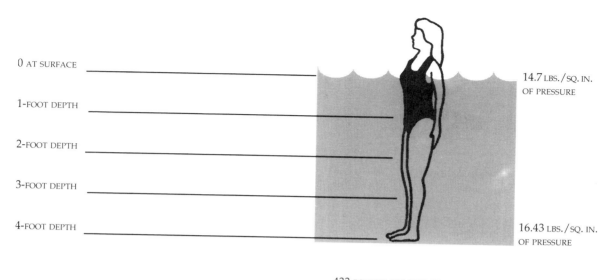

0 AT SURFACE

1-FOOT DEPTH

2-FOOT DEPTH

3-FOOT DEPTH

4-FOOT DEPTH

14.7 LBS./SQ. IN.
OF PRESSURE

16.43 LBS./SQ. IN.
OF PRESSURE

.433 POUNDS PER SQUARE INCH INCREASE IN HYDROSTATIC
PRESSURE FOR EVERY ONE FOOT OF INCREASE IN DEPTH

AT 33 FEET DEEP, PRESSURE IS TWICE AS MUCH AS IT IS AT THE SURFACE

Figure 30.6. **Hydrostatic pressure progressively increases at greater depths and thus produces depth-dependent physiologic consequences in the human body.**

FRONTAL RESISTANCE

LAMINAL FLOW

EDDIES

LAMINAL FLOW

EDDIES

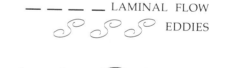

Figure 30.8. **Frontal resistance, laminar flow, and eddies created during prone swimming activities.**

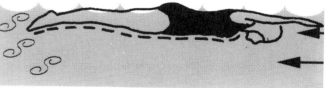

tion. This laminar flow produces small low-pressure areas called "eddies," "tail suctions," or "drag," which help dissipate frontal pressure caused when water is not able to "fill in" the streamlined parts of the body. Faster movement through water results in greater drag and resistance, which increase the muscular work required for movement. Motion-dependent drag and resistive forces provide the opportunity to create incremental challenges to various stabilized postures (76) (Figs. 30.7, 30.8).

Figure 30.7. **Frontal resistance, laminar flow, and eddies created during aquatic exercise programs in the vertical position.**

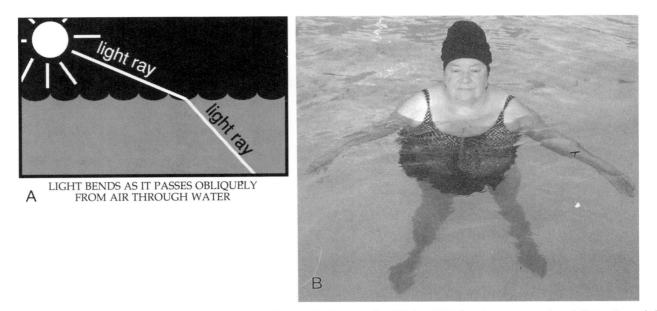

Figure 30.9. A, Refraction is a medium-dependent change in the speed of light. B, Refraction causes visual distortion of the submerged portion of the human body when viewed from above water.

Refraction is a medium-dependent change in the speed of light that causes visual distortion of submerged objects when viewed from above water. Refraction can make the acquisition of new skills, particularly those involving specific coordinated motions, more difficult. This effect is most profound in patients who have limited kinesthetic awareness (70) (Fig 30.9).

Water temperature can affect cognitive function as well as cardiac, respiratory, and muscular effort through a variety of mechanisms including various forms of heat transfer such as conduction, convection, and radiation. Oxygen consumption increases linearly with swimming speed, with the greatest consumption occurring in colder water, a phenomenon due almost entirely to the energy cost of shivering to maintain core temperature. Therefore, the optimal temperature range for swimming is 28–30° C (82–86° F). Within this range, the metabolic heat generated during exercise is easily transferred to the water without causing an even greater energy cost due to cold-water stress (4, 70, 76, 77, 79, 86, 87).

The advantages that aquatic programs offer are directly related to the properties of water. Graded elimination of gravitational forces through buoyancy allows the patient to train with decreased yet variable axial loads and shear forces. In essence, water increases the safety margin of patient postural error by decreasing the compressive and shear forces on the spine. The velocity of motion can be better controlled by water resistance, viscosity, buoyancy, and the training devices used. Buoyancy increases the available range of training positions. The psychological outlook of patients can be enhanced because rehabilitation occurs in a supportive environment. Many believe that a certain degree of pain

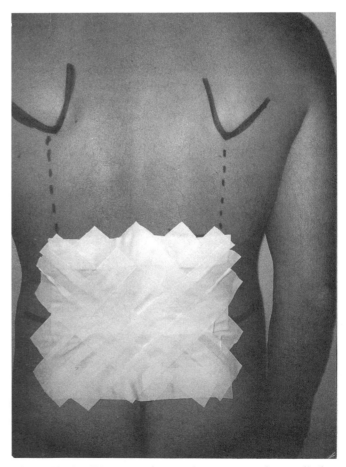

Figure 30.10. Waterproof strapping tape can be applied to the lumbar spine to reinforce lumbar proprioceptive awareness and help minimize lumbar rotation and lateral flexion.

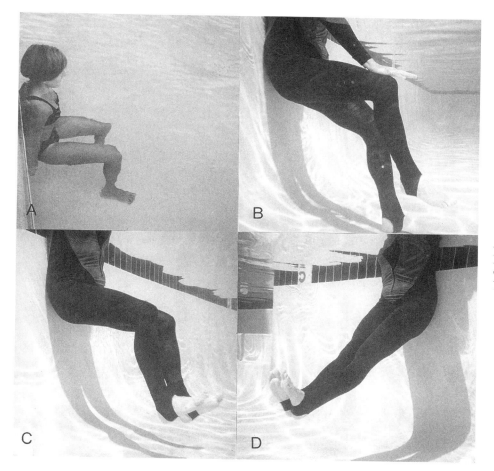

Figure 30.11. *A,* The wall sit develops isometric strength primarily in the quadriceps and hamstring groups. Abdominal muscles are trained to hold appropriate dynamic posture. *B,* Level 1 partial wall sit-ups train muscles activated in the wall sit and challenge contralateral gluteals, ipsilateral hip flexors, and rotational abdominals and paraspinals. *C,* Level 2 partial wall sit-ups train hip flexors and extensors bilaterally and isotonically. Higher-level isometric conditioning continues for abdominal and paraspinal muscle groups. *D,* Level 3 partial wall sit-ups provide an incrementally greater challenge to all groups described in Level 2 exercise.

attenuation takes place in the water because of the "sensory overload" generated by hydrostatic pressure, temperature, and turbulence (3–5, 75, 78, 88, 89).

Pool activity may provide the patient with full support by direct contact with a stationary device, semi-support by using a mobile floatation device or therapist assistance, or no support by eliminating any floatation assistance. The patient can be positioned in the vertical, supine, prone, or side-lying position. Activities performed in these positions with different levels of support include sitting, standing, floating (with no distance translation) and locomotion (with distance translation). The active body segment can be the upper body, lower body, both, or the trunk. The movement that occurs may be static (isometric), bilateral, reciprocal, or unilateral. An almost infinite variety of variables including speed, resistance, lever arm length, depth, time, equipment, and weight create an unlimited range of training options that progressively challenge neutral spine mechanics (90).

In general, patients are initially taught to maintain their unique neutral spine position by using floatation devices that reinforce proper positioning (3–5). Once sufficient kinesthetic awareness, flexibility, and strength are achieved, the devices are sequentially removed and

graded challenges are presented. In some cases a water-proof strapping tape is applied to the lumbar spine to reinforce lumbar proprioceptive awareness (91) (Fig. 30.10). Aquatic therapy program development includes closed-chain activity, performed in the shallow end of the pool with at least one foot on the pool bottom. It is here that the patient's six core-stabilization exercises are taught. These six core exercises have three levels of difficulty and have been designed to provide graded training of stabilization skills. They include the wall sit, partial wall sit-up, modified superman (hip extension in vertical position), walking backward, walking forward, and quadruped (prone position with graded arm and leg motion). Once mastered, a more-advanced program is provided. Eventually, patients can begin a swimming program that incorporates spine-stabilization techniques (3) (Figs. 30.11–30.14; Table 30.2).

AQUATIC DYNAMIC LUMBAR SPINE SWIMMING STABILIZATION PROGRAMS

Once stabilization skills have progressed, and a return to swimming is possible, a thorough analysis of stroke technique and its effect on spine motion is critical. The aquatic stabilization swimming program also incorpo-

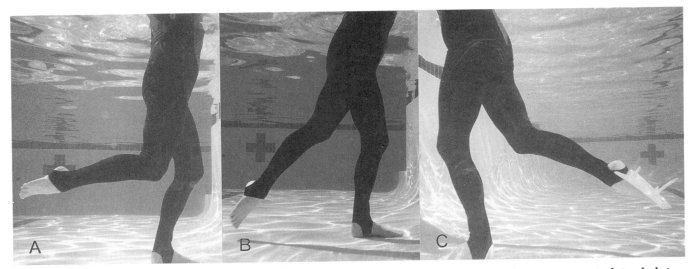

Figure 30.12. A, Level 1 modified superman develops strength in ipsolateral hip flexors and extensors, contralateral gluteus medius, as well as isometric strength in abdominal and paraspinal stabilizers. B, Level 2 modified superman provides an incrementally greater challenge to all groups described in Level 1. C, Level 3 modified superman again incrementally enhances resistive exercise and training duration of activity for muscle groups previously described for this component of the progression.

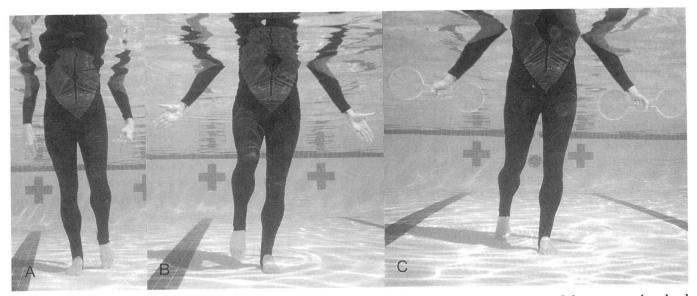

Figure 30.13. A, Level 1 walking forward isometrically strengthens the abdominal muscle groups and those groups involved in maintaining proper posture. Isotonic strengthening occurs in those muscles dynamically involved in gait. Walking backward provides a similar strengthening pattern with greater emphasis on isometric paraspinal muscle conditioning. B, Level 2 walking forward and backward provides incrementally greater challenge to all groups described in Level 1. C, Level 3 walking forward and backward incrementally enhances resistive exercise and training duration of activity for muscle groups previously described for this component of the progression.

rates land-based elements and takes into account the properties of the aqueous medium to minimize the risk of a spine injury. The goals of an aquatic stabilization swimming program are to minimize segmental trunk motion and shear forces; reinforce lumbar control; encourage hip, knee, and ankle propulsion; develop head and neck stability; and establish arm control and strength (3, 4).

PRONE SWIMMING

In prone swimming, the head should be midline. Breathing should occur by turning the head (i.e., rotat-

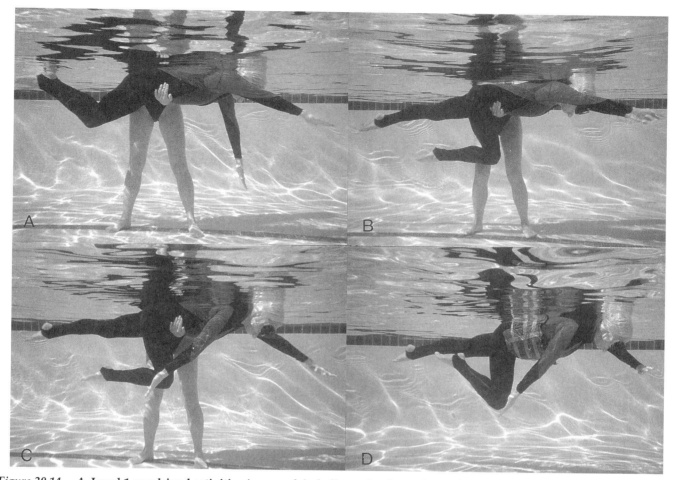

Figure 30.14. *A,* Level 1 quadriped activities (arms only) challenge lumbar spine stabilizer groups isometrically, and upper-extremity shoulder groups for flexion and extension isotonically. *B,* Level 1 quadriped activities (legs only) challenge lumbar spine stabilizer groups isometrically, and lower-extremity hip flexors and extensors isotonically. *C,* Level 2 quadriped activities incrementally isometrically challenge lumbar spine stabilizer groups and continue to isotonically train the upper- and lower-extremity groups previously described in Level 1. *D,* Level 3 quadriped exercise again increases the training intensity progression by requiring greater independence during performance of the exercise.

ing the head along the axial plane). There should be no craning (i.e., extending and rotating the cervical spine) (Fig. 30.15). Body roll also contributes to proper breathing mechanics and is essential in order to minimize dysfunctional cervical positioning and subsequent pain. The cervical spine should be kept in the neutral position along the sagittal plane because excessive extension causes the legs and torso to drop in the water, whereas excessive flexion can cause a struggle for air.

Upper-body arm position is evaluated by stroke phase (Table 30.3). Freestyle is broken into three phases. The *entry phase* includes both hand entry and hand submersion ("ride"). The *pull phase* incorporates insweep, outsweep, and finish components. The *recovery phase* includes exit and arm swing. There are several stroke defects that can cause poor lumbar mechanics. If the arm abducts beyond 180° during entry, lateral lumbar flexion is produced (Fig. 30.16). During the pull phase, de-

creased body rotation can cause lateral lumbar flexion and rotation, which stresses the lumbar spine. Inadequate triceps strength during the finish phase results in low arm recovery, which in turn generates secondary lateral lumbar flexion through the lumbar spine. During recovery, inadequate body roll causes the neck to crane, which results in a struggle for air and accompanying lateral flexion and rotation through the lumbar spine.

Trunk motion is closely monitored for any primary or secondary lumbar flexion, both sagittal and coronal, or for axial rotation. If not corrected by simple changes in stroke mechanics, additional proprioceptive cues can be provided by taping the lumbar spine region. The tape pulls on the skin each time the lumbar spine moves in a segmental manner—that is, when the patient generates excessive lumbar rotation or lateral lumbar flexion (91) (Fig. 30.10).

Flip turns are discouraged. Instead, stabilized turns

Table 30.2.
Aquatic Stabilization Exercises

Exercise	Level 1	Level 2	Level 3
Wall sit	Isometric 90° Hip 90° Knee 1-min Hold	Isometric 90°Hip 90° Knee 3-min Hold	Isometric 90° Hip 90° Knee 5-min Hold
Partial wall sit-up	Isometric Hip flexion Unilateral Alternating 90° hip 90° knee 5-sc hold 60 sec/side	Isotonic Hip flexion Bilateral Simultaneous 45° hip 90° knee Reps: 2 min	Isotonic Hip flexion Bilateral Simultaneous 45° hip 180° knee Reps: 3 min
Modified Superman	Face wall Hip Ext. to 20° Knee: 45° static Unilateral 60 sec/side	Face wall Hip ext. to 20° Knee: full ext. Unilateral 2 min/side	Face wall Hip ext. to 20° Knee: full ext. Unilateral 3 min/side 3 lbs/akle cuffs
Water walk backward	Palms at side 3 min Slow speed[2]	Palms forward Abduct arms 45° 5 min Moderate speed	Palms forward Abduct arms 45° Hand paddles 10 min Fast speed
Water walk forward	Palms at side 3 min Slow speed	Palms forward Abduct arms 45° 5 min Moderate speed	Palms forward Abduct arms 45° Hand paddles 10 min Fast speed
Quadruped	Therapist Assist Prone Mask/snorkle Alternating Arms only 1 min Alternating Legs only 1 min	Therapist Assist Prone Mask/snorkle Simultaneous/alternating Arm/leg 3 min	No assist Ski belt Prone Mask/snorkle Simultaneous/alternating Arm/leg 5 min

[a]Slow = 50% of potential maximum velocity; Moderate = 70% of potential maximum velocity; Fast = 85% of potential maximum velocity.

are employed in which the patient initially comes to a vertical position before turning. This vertical position allows the patient to stabilize the spine in preparation for changing direction. Eventually, a horizontal spin is incorporated into the turn and the vertical position is eliminated. Flip turns may then be resumed.

SUPINE SWIMMING

In the supine position, it is best to start with a simple kicking program with arms at the sides because adequate stabilization can thus be easily maintained. Often, the use of fins is suggested to improve propulsion. While a patient is supine, extension of the cervical spine will induce lumbar extension. On the other hand, cervical flexion will cause the patient to "sit" in the water with lowered leg position and decreased propulsion. Extremes of cervical extension (Fig. 30.17A) or flexion (Fig. 30.17B) are to be avoided in favor of a more-neutral stabilized cervical posture.

Problems with stroke technique can usually be solved with simple changes in stroke mechanics or by the addition of adaptive equipment. For example, a struggle for air can be resolved by the addition of a mask and snorkle. Trunk position can be improved by using the taping technique already mentioned. Poor propulsion can be remedied with an appropriate choice of fins. Hand paddles can provide better kinesthetic awareness of hand and arm position.

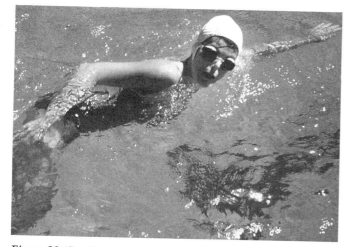

Figure 30.15. Crane breathing during the freestyle. The cervical spine extends and rotates during breathing.

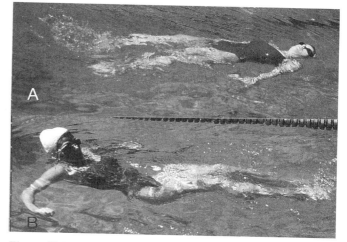

Figure 30.17. *A,* While the patient is supine, cervical spine extension induces lumbar extension. *B,* While the patient is supine, cervical spine flexion induces lumbar flexion and the patient "sits" in the water.

Table 30.3.
Swimming Stroke Phases (Freestyle)

I. *Entry phase*
   A. Hand entry
   B. Hand submersion ("ride")
II. *Pull phase*
   A. Insweep
   B. Outsweep
   C. Finish
III. *Recovery phase*
   A. Exit
   B. Arm swing

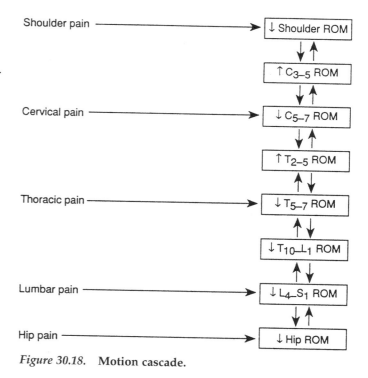

Figure 30.18. Motion cascade.

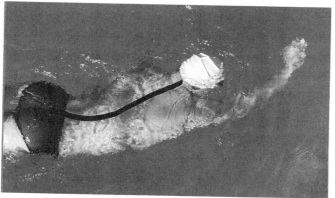

Figure 30.16. The swimmer's arm abducts beyond 180° during the entry phase of freestyle. This stroke defect creates lateral lumbar flexion and lumbar segmental rotation.

ADVANCED AQUATIC ACTIVITIES

Once basic stroke mechanics can be performed in a spine-safe manner, more complicated and challenging strokes and training regimes may be initiated. Patients might begin rigorous sculling programs for enhanced aerobic benefit. Or, aquatic running programs might be added (98, 99). The spine can be challenged with varied and graded axial loads by varying the depth at which patients train. A variety of other exercise options exist. The critical factor common to all aquatic therapeutic exercise programs is that they be performed with the lumbar spine well stabilized and in neutral position (67, 94–97).

THE MOTION CASCADE AND THE RELATIONSHIP BETWEEN THE SPINE AND PERIPHERAL JOINTS

Peripheral joint dysfunction can set off a cascading series of motion changes throughout the spinal axis. In particular, the cervicothoracic and thoracolumbar transition zones are most commonly affected because they are the junctions between the more-mobile and less-mobile sections of the spine (92). Figure 30.18 presents this "motion cascade." For example, a shoulder injury such as rotator cuff tendonitis results in guarding and decreased shoulder range of motion (93). The swimmer's arm cannot abduct and extend as it normally would during recovery, resulting in decreased body roll, increased lumbar segmental motion, and an abnormally low head position from which to breathe. Compensatory adaptive changes, which include cervical extension and rotation (Fig. 30.15) facilitated by increased range of motion from C3–C5, then occur. The C5–T1 segments ultimately become hypomobile to compensate, and mid and low cervical pain results. Compensatory hypermobility from T2–T5 and hypomobility from T5–T7 and T10–L1 begin. Primary cervical, thoracic, and lumbar injuries and pain influence the spinal axis in a similar fashion. Hip, pelvis, and lumbar spine pain result in hypomobility of L4–S1 and ultimately at the T10–L1 transition zone. Adaptive changes then proceed up the axis and may even set the stage for a compensatory change in shoulder mechanics and ultimately cause a shoulder injury. Identification of the initial injury is important so that treatment can eliminate that problem as well as the secondary compensatory sites of dysfunction.

CONCLUSIONS

Repetitive microtrauma from aquatic rehabilitation and the land-based flexibility and strength programs that are performed without attention to proper spine mechanics can either cause or contribute to spine injury and pain. Because the spinal axis is essentially a force transmitter for peripheral joint motion, both direct spinal injury and altered biomechanics at sites distant from the spine can change spinal mechanics and cause dysfunction and pain. A series of aquatic stabilization exercises has been designed that incorporates the intrinsic properties of water and enhances rehabilitative efforts. Once these exercises are mastered, injured patients can soon be advanced to spine-safe swimming or other high-level aquatic training activities. Swimming programs, in particular, require that close attention be paid to proper swim-stroke biomechanics and to the effect that abnormal mechanics may have on the spine. This attention ensures the most-rapid rehabilitation of painful spinal disorders.

REFERENCES

1. Canadian Olympic Association Report, Autumn, 1982.
2. United States Master's Swimming and YMCA of America (Unpublished data).
3. Cole AJ, Moschetti ML, Eagleston RE: Getting backs in the swim. *Rehab Mgmt* (August/September):62–71, 1992
4. Eagleston RE: Health South Physical Therapy of Portola Valley, Inc. (Unpublished data) 1991.
5. Moschetti ML, AquaTechnics Consulting Group, (Unpublished data) 1992
6. Yong-Hing K, Kirkaldy-Willis WH: The three-joint complex. In Weinstein JN, Wiesel SW (eds): *The Lumbar Spine.* Philadelphia, WB Saunders, 1990, pp 80–87.
7. Bogduk N, Twomey LT: The lumbar vertebrae. In *Clinical Anatomy of the Lumbar Spine,* ed 2. Melbourne, Churchill Livingstone, 1991, pp 1–10.
8. Bogduk N, Twomey LT: The inter-body joints and the intervertebral discs. In *Clinical Anatomy of the Lumbar Spine,* ed 2. Melbourne, Churchill Livingstone, 1991, pp 11–25.
9. Rauschning W: Anatomy and pathology of the lumbar spine. In Frymoyer JW (ed): *The Adult Spine: Principles and Practice.* New York, Raven Press, 1991, pp 1465–1486.
10. Pope MH, Wilder DG, Krag MH: Biomechanics of the lumbar spine: A. Basic principles. In Frymoyer JW (ed): *The Adult Spine: Principles and Practice.* New York, Raven Press, 1991, pp 1487–1501.
11. Goel VK, Weinstein JN, Okuma T: Biomechanics of the lumbar spine: B. Surgical principles. In Frymoyer JW (ed): *The Adult Spine: Principles and Practice.* New York, Raven Press, 1991, pp 1503–1521.
12. Taylor JR: The development and adult structure of lumbar intervertebral discs. *J Man Med* 5:43–47, 1990.
13. Hickey DS, Hunkins SWL: X-ray diffraction studies of the arrangement of collagen fibres in human fetal intervertebral disc. *J Anat* 131:81–90, 1980.
14. Hickey DS, Hunkins DWL: Relation between the structure of the annulus fibrosus and the function and failure of the intervertebral disc. *Spine* 5:100–116, 1980.
15. Crock HV, Goldwasser M, Yoshizawa H: Vascular anatomy related to the intervertebral disc. In Ghosh P (ed): *The Biology of the Intervertebral Disc.* Boca Raton, CRC Press, 1988, pp 109–133.
16. Bogduk N: The innervation of the intervertebral disc. The Biology of the Intervertebral Disc. In Ghosh P (ed): *The Biology of the Intervertebral Disc.* Boca Raton, CRC Press, 1988, pp 135–149.
17. Eyre DR: Collagens of the disc. In Ghosh P (ed): *The Biology of the Intervertebral Disc.* Boca Raton, CRC Press, 1988, pp 171–188.
18. Bailey AJ, Herbert CM, Jayson MIV: Collagen of the intervertebral disc. In Jayson MIV (ed): *The Lumbar Spine and Backache.* New York, Grune & Stratton, 1976, pp 327–340.
19. Comper WD, Laurent TC: Physiological function of connective tissue polysaccharides. *Phys Rev* 58:255–315, 1978.

20. Eyre D, Muir H: Type I and Type II collagen in intervertebral disk. Interchanging radial distribution in annulus fibrosus. *J Biochem* 157:267–270, 1976.
21. Maroudas A, Nachemson A, Stockwell R, Urban J: Some factors involved in the nutrition of the intervertebral disc. *J Anat* 120:113–130, 1975.
22. Armstrong JR: *Lumbar Disc Lesions,* ed 3. Edinburgh, Livingstone, 1965, p 13.
23. Jayson MIV, Barks JS: Structural changes in the intervertebral disc. *Ann Rheum Dis* 32:10–15, 1973.
24. Peacock A: Observations on the pre-natal development of the intervertebral disc in man. *J Anat* 85:260–274, 1951.
25. Saal JA, Saal JS: Later stage management of lumber spine problems. In Herring SA (ed): *Low Back Pain.* Philadelphia, WB Saunders, 1991, pp 205–221.
26. Saal JS: Pathoanatomy, the Degenerative Cascade. Presented at the annual meeting of The Injured Worker Dilemma: Definitive Solutions, San Francisco, 1989.
27. Beard HK, Stevens RL: Biochemical changes in the intervertebral disc. In Jayson MIV (ed): *The Lumbar Spine and Backache,* ed 2. London, Pitman, 1980, pp 407–436.
28. Gower WE, Pedrini V: Age related variation in protein polysaccharides from human nucleus pulposus, annulus fibrosus and costal cartilage. *J Bone Joint Surg [Am]* 51:1154–1162, 1969.
29. Bogduk N, Twomey LT: Blood supply of the lumbar spine. In *Clinical Anatomy of the Lumbar Spine,* ed 2. Melbourne, Churchill Livingstone, 1991, pp 121–128.
30. Bogduk N, Twomey LT: The zygapophysial joints. In *Clinical Anatomy of the Lumbar Spine,* ed 2. Melbourne, Churchill Livingstone, 1991, pp 27–34.
31. Taylor JR, Twomey LT: Age changes in lumbar zygapophyseal joints. *Spine* 11:739–745, 1986.
32. Twomey LT, Taylor JR: Age changes in the lumbar articular triad. *Aust J Physiol* 31:106–112, 1985.
33. Giles LGF: Innervation of the zygapophyseal joints and associated structures (from L3 to S1). In Satterfield TS (ed): *Anatomical Basis of Low Back Pain.* Baltimore, Williams & Wilkins, 1989, pp 58–66.
34. Nachemson A: The influence of spinal movements on the lumbar intradiscal pressure and on the tensile stresses in the annulus fibrosus. *Acta Orthrop Scand* 33:183–207, 1963.
35. Adams MA, Hutton WC: The effect of posture on the role of the apophyseal joints in resisting intervertebral compression force. *J Bone Joint Surg [Br]* 62:358–362, 1980.
36. Adams MA, Hutton WC: The mechanical function of the lumbar apophyseal joints. *Spine* 8:327–330, 1983.
37. Yang KH, King AI: Mechanism of facet load transmission as a hypothesis for low-back pain. *Spine* 9:557–565, 1984.
38. Bogduk N, Twomey LT: Movements of the lumbar spine. In *Clinical Anatomy of the Lumbar Spine,* ed 2. Melbourne, Churchill Livingstone, 1991, pp 65–81.
39. Bogduk N, Twomey LT: The ligaments of the lumbar spine. In *Clinical Anatomy of the Lumbar Spine,* ed 2. Melbourne, Churchill Livingstone, 1991, pp 35–44.
40. Bogduk N, Twomey LT: The lumbar muscles and their fascia. In *Clinical Anatomy of the Lumbar Spine,* ed 2. Melbourne, Churchill Livingstone, 1991, pp 83–105.
41. Bogduk N, Twomey LT: The lumbar lordosis and the vertebral canal. In *Clinical Anatomy of the Lumbar Spine,* ed 2. Melbourne, Churchill Livingstone, 1991, pp 45–52.
42. Bogduk N, Twomey LT: Pathology of mechanical lumbar back pain. In *Clinical Anatomy of the Lumbar Spine,* ed 2. Melbourne, Churchill Livingstone, 1991, pp 161–173.
43. Yong-Hing D, Kirkaldy-Willis W: The pathophysiology of degenerative disease of the lumbar spine. *Orthop Clin Am* 14:491–503, 1983.
44. Kirkaldy-Willis WH: The three phases of the spectrum of degenerative disease. In Kirkaldy-Willis WH (ed): *Managing Low Back Pain,* ed 2. New York, Churchill Livingstone, 1988, pp 117–131.
45. Saal J: Rehabilitation of the injured athlete. In DeLisa J (ed): *Rehabilitation Medicine: Principles and Practice.* Philadelphia, JB Lippincott, 1988, pp 840–864.
46. Deyo RA, Diehl AK, Rosenthal M: How many days of bed rest for acute low back pain? A randomized critical trial. *N Engl J Med* 315:1064–1070, 1986.
47. Akeson V, Woo S, Amiel D: The connective tissue response to immobility: Biomechanical changes in periarticular connective tissue of the immobilized rabbit knee. *Clin Orthop* 93:356, 1973.
48. Finsterbush A, Friedman B: Reversibility of joint changes produces by immobilization in rabbits. *Clin Orthop* 111:290, 1975.
49. Hettingger T, Mueller EA: Muskelleistung und muskeltraining. *Arbeitsphysiologie* 15:111, 1953.
50. Paulos LE, Payne FC, Rosenberg TD: Rehabilitation after anterior cruciate ligament surgery. In Jackson D, Drew D (eds): *The Anterior Cruciate Deficient Knee.* St. Louis, CV Mosby, 1987, pp 291–314.
51. Zarins B: Soft tissue injury and repair-biochemical aspects. *Int J Sports Med* 3(Suppl 1):9, 1982.
52. Frank G, Woo S, Amiel D, Harwood F, Gomez M, Akeson W: Medial collateral ligament healing. A multidisciplinary assessment in rabbits. *Am J Sports Med* 11:379, 1983.
53. Leach R: The prevention and rehabilitation of soft tissue injuries. *Int J Sports Med* 3(Suppl 1):18, 1982.
54. Eldred E, Lindsky DF, Buchwald JS: The effect of cooling on mammalian muscle spindles. *Exp Neurol* 2:144–157, 1960.
55. McKenzie R: *Mechanical Disorders and Treatment of Lumbar Spine Disorders.* New Zealand, Spinal Publications, 1981.
56. Robinson JP, Brown PB: Medications in low back pain. In Herring SW (ed): *Low Back Pain.* Philadelphia, WB Saunders, 1991, pp 97–126.
57. Gamburd RS: The use of selective injections in the lumbar spine. In Herring SW (ed): *Low Back Pain.* Philadelphia, WB Saunders, 1991, pp 79–96.
58. Cole AJ, Eagleston RE: Ultrasound and diathermy in sportsmedicine. *Phys Sportsmed* (Accepted for publication).
59. Windsor RE, Lester JP, Herring SA: Electrical stimulation in clinical practice. *Phys Sportsmed* 21:85–96, 1993.
60. Paris S: Mobilization of the spine. *Phys Ther* 59:988–995, 1979.
61. Korr IM: Neurochemical and neurotrophic consequences of nerve deformation. In Glasgow EF et al (eds): *Aspects of Manipulative Therapy.* Melbourne, Churchill Livingstone, 1985, pp 64–71.
62. Wyke B, Polacek P: Articular neurology: The present position. *J Bone Joint Surg [Br]* 57:401, 1975.

63. Ward R: Headache: An osteopathic perspective. *J Am Osteopath Assoc* 81:458–466, 1982.

64. Frank C, Akeson W, Woo S et al: Physiology and therapeutic value of passive joint motion. *Clin Orthop Rel Res* 185:113–125, 1984.

65. Saal JA, Saal JS: Later stage management of lumbar spine problems. In Herring SW (ed): *Low Back Pain*. Philadelphia, WB Saunders, 1991, pp 205–221.

66. Saal JA: Dynamic muscular stabilization in the nonoperative treatment of lumbar pain syndromes. *Orthop Rev* 19:691–700, 1990.

67. Kottke FJ, Stillwell GK, Lehmann JF: Therapeutic exercise to develop neuromuscular coordination. In Kottke FJ, Stillwell GK, Lehmann JF (eds): *Krusen's Handbook of Physical Medicine and Rehabilitation*, ed 3. Philadelphia, WB Saunders, 1982, pp 403–426.

68. Eagleston R: Aquatic stabilization programs. Presented at The Challenge of the Lumbar Spine, San Francisco, March, 1987.

69. Martin R: Swimming: Forces on aquatic animals and humans. In Vaughan CL (ed): *Biomechanics of Sport*. Boca Raton, CRC Press, 1989, pp 35–51.

70. Miller F: Fluids. In Miller F (ed): *College Physics*, ed 4. New York, Harcourt Brace Jovanovich, 1977, pp 271–298.

71. Department of Health and Human Services: *Aqua Dynamics—Water Exercises are the New Way To Stay in Shape*. Washington, DC, Department of Health and Human Services, 1986.

72. Harrison R, Bulstrode S: Percentage weight bearing during partial immersion in the hydrotherapy pool. *Physiol Pract* 3:60–63, 1987.

73. Skinner AT, Thompson AM: *Duffield's Exercise in Water*. London, Bailliere Tindall, 1983.

74. Genuario S, Negso J: The use of a swimming pool in the rehabilitation and reconditioning of athletic injuries. *Contemp Orthop* 20:381–387, 1990.

75. Haralson K: Therapeutic pool programs, clinical management. *Phys Ther* 5:10–13, 1985.

76. Krieghbaum E, Barthels K: *A Qualitative Approach for Studying Human Movement*, ed 2. Minneapolis, Burgess Publishing, 1985, pp 421–467.

77. McArdle W, Katch F, Katch V: Energy expenditure during walking, jogging, running, and swimming. In McArdle W, Katch F, Katch V (eds): *Exercise Physiology: Energy, Nutrition, and Human Performance*. Philadelphia, Lea & Febiger, 1986, pp 158–185.

78. Campion M: Introduction to hydrotherapy. In Campion M (ed): *Adult Hydrotherapy: A Practical Approach*. London, Heinemann Medical Books, 1990, pp 3–20.

79. Martin W, Montgomery J, Snell P et al: Cardiovascular adaptations to intensive swim training in sedentary middle-aged men and women. *Circulation* 75:323–330, 1987.

80. Arborelius M Jr, Balldin U, Lilja B et al: Hemodynamic changes in man during immersion with head above water. *Aero Med* 43:592–598, 1972.

81. Holmer I: Physiology of swimming man. *Acta Pysiol Scand Suppl* 407:1–55, 1974.

82. Bove A: Cardiovascular disorders and diving. In Bove A (ed): *Diving Medicine*. Philadelphia, WB Saunders, 1990, pp 239–248.

83. Bove A, Davis J: Pulmonary barotrauma. In Bove A (ed): *Diving Medicine*. Philadelphia, WB Saunders, 1990, pp 188–191.

84. Farmer J Jr: Ear and sinus problems in diving. In Bove A (ed): *Diving Medicine*. Philadelphia, WB Saunders, 1990, pp 200–222.

85. Neuman T: Pulmonary disorders in diving. In Bove A (ed): *Diving Medicine*. Philadelphia, WB Saunders, 1990, pp 233–238.

86. Nodel E et al: Energy exchanges of swimming man. *J Appl Phys* 36:465, 1974.

87. Astrand P, Rodahl K: Applied sports psychology. In Astrand P, Rodahl K (eds): *Textbook of Work Physiology: Physiological Bases of Exercise*, ed 3. New York, McGraw-Hill, 1986, pp 654–657.

88. Kolb M: Principles of underwater exercise. *Phys Ther Rev* 37:361–365, 1957.

89. Walsh MT: Hydrotherapy: The use of water as a therapeutic agent. In Michlovitz S (ed): *Thermal Agents in Rehabilitation*, ed 2. Philadelphia, FA Davis, 1990, pp 109–133.

90. Cole AJ, Eagleston RE, Moschetti ML: The Portola Valley Scale: A classification system for aquatic exercise. (In press).

91. Cole AJ, Eagleston RE, Moschetti ML: Lumbar torque: A new proprioceptive approach. Presented as a Poster Session at the Annual Meeting of the North American Spine Society, August 1–3, 1991. Presented at the annual meeting of the North American Spine Society, Keystone, CO, 1991.

92. Paris S: The spine and swimming. In Hockschuler S (ed): *Spine: State of the Art Reviews*. Philadelphia, Hanley & Belfus, 1990, pp 351–358.

93. Scovazzo M, Browne A, Pink M, et al: The painful shoulder during freestyle swimming: An electromyographic cinematographic analysis of twelve muscles. *Am J Sports Med* 19:577–582, 1991.

94. Councilman J: *The Science of Swimming*. Englewood Cliffs, NJ, Prentice Hall, 1968, p 457.

95. Farfan HF: Effects of torsion on the intervertebral joints. *Can J Surg* 12:336–341, 1969.

96. Farfan HF, Cossette JW, Robertson GH et al: The effects of torsion on the lumbar intervertebral joints: The role of torsion in the production of disc degeneration. *J Bone Joint Surg [Am]* 52:468–497, 1970.

97. Maglischo E: *Swimming Faster*, ed 1. Bakersfield, Mayfield Publishing, 1982, p 472.

98. Wilder R, Brennan D, Schotte D: Standard measure for exercise prescription for aqua running. *Am J Sports Med* 21:45–48, 1993.

99. Brennan D, Wilder R: *Deep Water Running: An Instructor's Manual*. Houston, Houston International Running Center, 1991.

100. Epstein M: Cardiovascular and renal effects of head-out water immersion in man. *Circ Res* 39:5, 619–628, 1976.

101. Risch, Koubenec, Beckmann, Lange, Gauer: The effect of graded immersion on heart volume, central venous pressure, pulmonary blood distribution and heart rate in man. *Pflugers Arc* 375:115–118, 1978.

102. Becker B: The physiologic consequences of aquatic exercise. The American Academy of Physical Medicine and Rehabilitation, San Francisco, November 16, 1992.

CHAPTER 31

GYNECOLOGIC PAIN

J. GREG JOHNSON

Pᴇʟᴠɪᴄ ᴘᴀɪɴ in the female patient is a common symptom that often leads her to seek gynecologic consultation. Symptoms of pelvic pain along with vaginal bleeding are the two most common reasons for a woman to seek gynecologic consultation. Pelvic pain can be a disabling problem, accounting for many lost work days and having severe impact on the psychosocial inter-relationships of the female patient. I attempt here to describe and delineate a practical approach to the recognition and management of gynecologic or pelvic pain.

Because the pelvis contains all of the female genital organs and also includes portions of the urinary tract and gastrointestinal tract, it is sometimes quite difficult to differentiate in a clinical setting the origin of pelvic pain. Possible etiologies of nongynecologic pelvic pain include diseases of the gastrointestinal tract (including appendicitis, diverticulitis, ulcerative colitis, and other inflammatory bowel diseases) and functional disturbances, or the so-called spastic colon. One must also differentiate pain that originates from the urinary tract. This may include ureteral stones, urinary tract infections, and trigonitis. The urinary tract infection is easily diagnosed by urinalysis and culture, whereas the other disorders may need further radiographic and cystoscopic evaluation. This discussion does not include the work-up and management of urologic conditions.

Pain arising in the female genital tract may be of multiple origins. It may vary from an early intrauterine pregnancy to an ectopic pregnancy to infectious or inflammatory disease of the uterus, tubes, and ovaries, to neoplasia or various endocrinologic abnormalities. Included also in this discussion is pelvic pain for which one cannot find a readily identifiable cause. Pelvic pain without obvious pathology is a significant problem requiring a multidisciplinary solution.

Women presenting with pelvic pain can usually be categorized as those with acute, severe onset of pain or as those whose pain is of a more chronic, nagging nature. Those with acute, severe pain usually have had the onset of the pain within the last few hours or days, and it has become so severe that it is incapacitating. In these patients, one must consider the possibility of an ectopic pregnancy, an ovarian cyst with torsion or rupture, and acute pelvic inflammatory disease. The patient with chronic pelvic pain is more likely to have endometriosis, a neoplasm, or chronic pelvic inflammatory disease, or to fall into the category of pelvic pain without obvious pathology.

DIAGNOSTIC TOOLS IN GYNECOLOGY

Two of the more useful tools available in gynecology are ultrasonography and laparoscopy. With the development and progression of these two tools, visualizing the pelvis, both noninvasively and invasively, has become an easier task.

Ultrasound is defined as mechanical radiant energy with a frequency rate above the audible range. The use of ultrasonography as a diagnostic tool is a major advancement in the investigation of pelvic abnormalities and disease. With the development of real-time ultrasonography, the image has become very much like watching a TV in black and white. Ultrasonography has the ability to visualize tissue interfaces, which radiography is incapable of doing. This provides us with an anatomic picture of an object with the body cavity. Ultrasonography has greatly enhanced our diagnostic capabilities in gynecology and in general is superior to standard radiographic procedures, including computed tomography (CT) scan, in imaging the pelvic organs.

Laparoscopy, although an invasive procedure, is relatively safe and, in experienced hands, simple. With the use of fiberoptics, one is allowed to directly visualize the pelvis to delineate and diagnose conditions that may present a similar clinical picture. With the progression of technique in laparoscopy, it is even possible to do more and more operative procedures through the laparoscope, thus sparing the patient the major trauma of laparotomy. In diagnosis, the development of laparoscopy has greatly enhanced our early diagnosis of such conditions as pelvic inflammatory disease, ectopic pregnancy, and pelvic endometriosis. One may also delineate between functional and pathologic ovarian growths or cysts. The laparoscope is also useful in the management of malignant neoplasms of the pelvis.

These two procedures are referred to frequently in the following discussion because they are both very helpful in diagnosing the causes of pelvic pain.

ECTOPIC PREGNANCY

Implantation of the fertilized ovum outside of the uterine cavity is known as *ectopic pregnancy*. Although the vast majority of these will occur in the fallopian tube, ectopic pregnancies can also occur in the ovary, pelvis, and other parts of the abdominal cavity. Ectopic pregnancy is definitely on the rise, with the overall incidence exceeding 1%. The increase that is seen in pelvic infections and pelvic inflammatory disease, the use of intrauterine devices, and the increasing rate of tubal surgery have all led to the increased incidence of ectopic pregnancy.

The patient with an ectopic pregnancy may have a variety of symptoms that can be confused with an early intrauterine pregnancy, spontaneous abortion, or pelvic inflammatory disease. It is imperative to recognize the possibility of an ectopic pregnancy early, because if one can diagnose it in the unruptured state, the fallopian tube can be preserved for future fertility. Commonly, the patient will present with a history of missed period, vaginal bleeding, and abdominal pain. The pain may be variable. If it is early in the pregnancy, the pain may be of a mild, nagging nature. If it is later and impending rupture is occurring, however, the pain will be severe. On examination in the unruptured state, the patient will have adnexal tenderness, usually on the side of the ectopic pregnancy, but this tenderness may be bilateral. There is frequently tenderness upon motion of the cervix also. If the ectopic pregnancy has ruptured, this may be accompanied by hypotension and shock with signs of intra-abdominal hemorrhage. These signs include weakness, dizziness, abdominal distention, hypotension, and tachycardia. If the bleeding has been profuse, there may be shoulder pain, which is an ominous sign.

Newer diagnostic techniques, including ultrasonography, quantitative human chorionic gonadotropin (HCG) assays, and laparoscopy, are very helpful in the early diagnosis of an ectopic pregnancy. If one is presented with a woman who has a history of a missed period, a positive pregnancy test, and abdominal pain, it is useful to obtain ultrasound examination. With the advent of vaginal ultrasonography, one should see the gestational sac and early development of an embryo within 4 weeks of the last menstrual period. By 6 weeks following the last menstrual period, one should see definite fetal cardiac activity if there is an intrauterine pregnancy. If the gestational sac and embryo are not seen at ultrasonography at the appropriate times, it is helpful to obtain a quantitative HCG assay. An HCG titer of greater than 2000 MIU/ml with absence of an intrauterine pregnancy on vaginal ultrasonography should lead one to the diagnosis of ectopic pregnancy (1). With these diagnostic tools, when one suspects an ectopic pregnancy, it is usually beneficial to proceed with laparoscopy prior to laparotomy to definitely establish the diagnosis. With the laparoscope, one can directly visualize the uterus, tubes, and ovaries to determine, without major surgery, the correctness of the diagnosis. If an ectopic pregnancy is found, it is then necessary to proceed with definitive surgery to remove it. In the unruptured state, this may be done by a linear salpingostomy with removal of only the ectopic pregnancy from the fallopian tube. If the fallopian tube has ruptured, however, it is usually necessary to remove at least that portion of the fallopian tube that is involved with the ectopic pregnancy. With modern reconstructive surgery, it is preferable to be conservative and save as much of the fallopian tube as possible, because it may lend itself to repair at a future date. Recently, several investigators have treated ectopic pregnancies medically using different regimens of methotrexate (1).

Ovarian and abdominal pregnancies are rare, but may present as a surgical emergency with an acute abdomen and massive internal hemorrhage. Diagnosis preoperatively may be difficult, and it is necessary to proceed with laparotomy based on the patient's signs and symptoms.

UTERINE CAUSES OF GYNECOLOGIC PAIN

Dysmenorrhea is that pain that occurs with the menstrual period. This usually includes lower abdominal pain and low back pain associated with menstruation. In the past, this has been divided into primary and secondary dysmenorrhea, with primary dysmenorrhea being that for which no etiology could be found, and secondary dysmenorrhea the painful menstruation associated with a variety of pathologic conditions. In a patient with primary dysmenorrhea, the pain begins near or at the onset of menstrual flow and will usually become increasingly worse during the first or second day of the menstrual period, gradually diminishing as the menstrual flow diminishes. Women with dysmenorrhea have been documented to have increased levels of prostaglandins in their endometrium and menstrual discharge (2). This information is important because of the development of prostaglandin synthetase inhibitors that can block the production of prostaglandins. These substances not only reduce the level of prostaglandin but also have some analgesic effect of their own in most cases. In the office experience, it is useful to give a trial of the various prostaglandin synthetase inhibitors to find one to which the individual will respond. It is unusual with primary dysmenorrhea to find a patient who does not respond to one of the variety of available prostaglandin synthetase inhibitors. Use of oral contraceptives in the patient with dysmenorrhea may additionally benefit her with pain relief by reducing the amount of menstrual discharge and relieving intrauterine pressure. Benign tumors of the uterus may produce secondary dysmenorrhea that initially will present with pain similar to that of primary dysmenorrhea. Usually on pelvic examination, these tumors are palpable, but in the early stages they may not be readily apparent. The most common of these tumors are leiomyoma and adenomyosis. Other less common tumors will produce a similar picture. Adenomyosis, also known as *internal endometriosis,* is a condition in which the glands grow into the myometrium or muscle layer of the uterus, producing swelling and inflammation within the wall of the uterus. Because this is endometrial tissue, it is under the control of the hormonal cycle and will initially cause pain at the time of menses. As the condition progresses, the pain may occur at other times during the menstrual cycle. There is also usually associated increased flow at the time of menstruation.

On pelvic exam, one may find an enlarged, boggy, tender uterus that is symmetrical and globular in shape. Adenomyosis usually occurs in the patient at the upper end of her reproductive years, in the later thirties and early forties. The definitive treatment for this condition, and the only definite way to make the diagnosis, is hysterectomy and pathologic examination.

Leiomyoma of the uterus may occur at any time during the reproductive years, but is more common as women age. This is probably the most common benign disease in women. Twenty percent of women at age 40 will have developed uterine leiomyomas. The vast majority of these cases are asymptomatic and require no therapy; if the woman reaches menopause, these tumors will decrease in size after removal of the influence of estrogen. The most common sign of a problem with leiomyomas is that of increasing and irregular menstrual flow. At times this flow can be very heavy, producing an associated anemia. If the leiomyomas increase in size rapidly, they can produce sudden, sharp pain, particularly if there is degeneration within the center of an enlarging fibroid. More commonly, the patient will complain of a painful pressure sensation in the pelvis that is of a nagging nature.

As the fibroids become larger, they are more easily palpable on pelvic examination. Surgical management is indicated when the leiomyomas are producing significant pain or significant abnormal uterine bleeding, or when they become so large that they are greater than the size of a 12-week pregnancy. At this time, ureteral compression can occur. It is also difficult to differentiate between a tumor originating in the ovary and a tumor originating in the uterus when these tumors become this large. In the young woman who desires further child-bearing, a myomectomy can be performed. Gonadotro-

pin-releasing hormone (GNRH) agonists can reduce the size of leiomyomas by suppressing pituitary production of follicle-stimulating hormone (FSH) and luteinizing hormone (LH). This is useful prior to pregnancy or surgery.

Malignant tumors of the uterus usually do not present with pain as a significant symptom. Cancer of the endometrium will initially present with abnormal uterine bleeding, and only late in its course will pain be a significant symptom. Other malignant tumors of the uterus are rare, and it can also be stated that only late in their course would pelvic pain be a significant problem.

OVARIAN CAUSES OF GYNECOLOGIC PAIN

This section considers those conditions that are unique to the ovary, not including inflammatory or infectious causes of ovarian pain. One may have a non-neoplastic ovarian cyst, such as the follicular cyst, corpus luteum cyst, and theca-lutein cyst. Usually these are of no clinical significance, but must be included in the differential diagnosis in ruling out neoplastic ovarian tumors. A neoplasm may be either benign or malignant. Most benign ovarian tumors occur in women in their reproductive years, but they may occur at any age. Malignancy is most common in the postmenopausal women, but can be seen in young women in their teens and twenties, and must be included in the differential diagnosis of ovarian tumors.

Follicular cysts occur when the ovarian follicle does not rupture at the time of ovulation and there is a subsequent accumulation of fluid within the follicle. Follicular cysts are usually small, rarely becoming larger than 5 cm. They are confined to one ovary and will usually not cause any symptoms. The patient, however, may complain of fullness and occasionally a sharp pain in the area of the involved ovary. If these cysts are found at the time of pelvic examination, there may be tenderness present that is of a mild to moderate nature. Following this cyst through one to two menstrual cycles will usually result in spontaneous resolution of the cyst. Occasionally, spontaneous rupture will occur, producing a sharp pain that may last several hours. Typically, these patients present with a history of a sharp, stabbing pain that is now somewhat better, and on pelvic examination, the findings are essentially normal. One rare occasions, the cyst may be involved in torsion of the adnexa, leading to a picture similar to that of an acute abdomen. It may be accompanied by fever, chills, severe abdominal pain, an elevated white blood cell count, and an extremely tender unilateral pelvic mass. When this occurs, emergency surgical treatment is necessary, with removal of the involved adnexa because of the thrombosis that occurs in the ovarian vessels.

A patient may also develop a corpus luteum cyst after ovulation. After release of the egg, the corpus luteum remains and, for reasons unknown, may produce an excessive amount of fluid within the corpus luteum. This may lead to cyst formation, usually in the range of 5 cm or less, with symptoms similar to those of the follicular cyst. Rarely, rupture of a corpus luteum cyst may produce severe intra-abdominal hemorrhage that requires immediate surgical attention. A patient may also have a persistent corpus luteum cyst, known as *Halban's syndrome*, that is characterized by amenorrhea followed by irregular uterine bleeding, pelvic pain, and a tender adnexal mass. In this case, a pregnancy test is negative. The corpus luteum may occur within the menstrual cycle or early in pregnancy, and it is at this time that it can be confused with an ectopic pregnancy. Following the cyst through one to two menstrual cycles or through early pregnancy will result in resolution.

A theca-lutein cyst develops in the absence of ovulation and is more commonly bilateral. These cysts occur as a result of elevations of the gonadotropin level. As with follicular cysts, the theca-lutein cyst will usually regress spontaneously.

Ovarian neoplasms, as previously stated, may occur in any age group, with benign tumors occurring more frequently in women in their reproductive years. Fortunately, the vast majority of ovarian tumors are benign. Unfortunately, there are no specific symptoms related to ovarian malignancy.

The patient with an ovarian neoplasm will usually present with a dull, chronic discomfort that produces fullness and pressure in the pelvis without severe pain. In the younger woman, the findings of adnexal mass do not clearly establish the diagnosis of ovarian neoplasia, as can be seen from the previous discussion. In postmenopausal woman, however, the finding of a mass in the pelvis warrants immediate surgical attention for diagnosis of possible pathology. If one sees a young woman in her reproductive years with an adnexal mass that is producing a mild to moderate degree of discomfort, one may choose to follow her through one or two menstrual cycles to see if it will regress spontaneously. A mass of greater than 6 cm, however, is usually an ovarian neoplasm and may be handled by laparoscopic examination and further surgical intervention as necessary.

Ovarian malignancies, unfortunately, produce few specific symptoms in their early stages. This makes early detection and thus improved outcome very difficult. A woman with an ovarian malignancy may present complaining only of a vague pelvic discomfort and gastrointestinal distress with nausea, dyspepsia, and vague lower abdominal discomfort. It is not until later in the progression of ovarian cancer that the patient will have increasingly severe abdominal and pelvic pain, which, by that time, is usually accompanied by ascites and abdominal distention. Severe pain in the early stages of ovarian cancer usually is related to a complication of torsion or rupture of the cystic structure. A thorough discussion of the types of ovarian neoplasia is left for a gynecology textbook.

Associated with the ovary are paraovarian cysts. These result from incomplete resolution of embryologic structures related to the mesonephros and metanephros. These cysts are usually asymptomatic and small but may distend, producing a large, painful mass in the adnexa. Ultrasound examination may be helpful in differentiating the simple-type cyst, that is, the follicular or corpus luteum cyst, from the more complex ovarian neoplasm, which may have a more echogenic appearance. One may also be able to distinguish areas of calcification within the ovary that indicate an ovarian neoplasm is present. Ultrasonography cannot, however, distinguish a benign from a malignant mass. Radiographic examination may be very helpful in distinguishing the nature of an ovarian or pelvic mass. Computerized tomography, in my experience, has not been helpful in delineating the type of pelvic tumor present, but may demonstrate metastatic disease.

Occasionally at laparoscopy done for pelvic pain, one will see an ovary that has a thickened capsule and is filled with multiple small cysts. This patient's pain may be due to the distention of the ovarian capsule by functional cysts. These patients may have a variation of the polycystic ovarian syndrome, which results from tonic elevations of luteinizing hormone. These patients respond well to oral contraceptives by suppression of ovarian function or diminished gonadotropin output secondary to the oral contraceptive.

ENDOMETRIOSIS

Endometriosis is one of the more intriguing causes of pelvic pain. It occurs when the endometrium locates in areas outside the uterine cavity. Endometriosis is a common finding during gynecologic surgery. The incidence is difficult to establish because women with endometriosis may be asymptomatic. This may occur anywhere within the body, but is most frequent in the pelvic organs. The most common pelvic location of endometriosis is the ovary, but it may be found on any of the peritoneal surfaces covering the bladder and the cul-de-sac, particularly along the uterosacral ligaments, the fallopian tubes, the round ligaments, and the broad ligaments. Commonly, one finds endometriotic lesions in the appendix, cecum, and small intestine. The umbilicus, bladder, and ureter, previous laparotomy scars, and the vagina, vulva, and cervix may also be included. Interestingly, endometriosis has been described in the lung, pleura, kidney, spleen, gallbladder, and brains.

Typically, these lesions appear as powder burn areas

with dark brown or black pigmentation that may have a hemosiderin-laden fluid within the lesion and are surrounded by fibrosis. Lesions may vary from a few millimeters to much larger lesions in the centimeter range, and may turn into endometriomas within the ovary, producing large cystic structures with old blood that has been broken down into a chocolate-like material.

The most common symptom of endometriosis is pelvic pain and dysmenorrhea. Also common is dyspareunia. Most women have some degree of pelvic pain; however, it is interesting that one woman with extensive disease may have few or no symptoms and another with minimal disease may have severe pelvic pain. Also associated with this condition is a history of infertility and abnormal uterine bleeding. Frequently one will see a patient whose pain initially began with her menstrual period, but instead of having the onset and diminution synchronously with the menstrual period, the dysmenorrhea will become progressively worse as the menstrual period continues and may take several days beyond the menstrual period to diminish. As the endometriosis spreads and progresses within the pelvis, the pelvic pain will increase and become dissociated with the menstrual period. As previously stated, the nature and severity of the pain associated with endometriosis is quite variable. Pain with intercourse may occur as the disease involves the cul-de-sac and uterosacral ligaments and produces pelvic adhesions and scarring within the pelvis. In approximately one-third of women, abnormal uterine bleeding will occur, primarily characterized by premenstrual spotting. Infertility is common and may occur in as many as 40% of these patients (3).

On physical examination, one may find tenderness in the uterus, cul-de-sac, or adnexa. There may be some thickening and nodularity along the uterosacral ligaments posterior to the uterus. If there is scarring and adhesion formation, there may be fixation of the uterus and adnexa. If endometriomas are present, these will present as tender cystic masses. In other cases, however, physical findings will be those of a normal pelvis. There can be significant pain without significant physical findings.

The only definitive way to diagnose endometriosis is by direct visualization either by laparoscopy or by laparotomy. Ultrasonography and laboratory evaluation are of no value in diagnosing endometriosis with absence of physical findings.

The management of endometriosis depends on several factors, including the woman's age and desire for childbearing and the extent or severity of the endometriosis. In the young, infertile woman with mild endometriosis, an expectant therapy approach is appropriate. One must correct other causes of infertility during this time and then, if no pregnancy occurs, medical or surgical alternatives may be instituted.

Medical therapy initially included androgens and estrogens and then progestins and eventually progressed to estrogen-progestin combination therapy (pseudopregnancy). The symptoms improved in over half the cases and pregnancy rates were 40–50% with this therapy. With the addition of danazol to the medical therapeutic regimen of endometriosis, use of the pseudopregnancy therapy has decreased. In young women who are not desirous of childbearing, low-dose contraceptive therapy will usually relieve the pain.

GNRH analogs and danazol are both used to treat endometriosis. These drugs produce their effect by reducing the production of gonadotropins from the pituitary, which then produces atrophy in the normal endometrium and endometriotic implants. In addition danazol has some androgenic effects, which can be bothersome. The average duration of therapy is 6 months, with symptomatic improvement in women with mild to moderate disease in the range of 72–100% and improvement of disease by laparoscopy in the range of 85–95%. Pregnancy rates following danazol therapy vary from 28 to 60% (4). A small study of nafarelin (a GNRH analog) in patients with endometriosis and infertility found the nafarelin group to have a higher pregnancy rate than the danazol group (29% vs. 13%) (5). In a patient who is having significant pain but does not desire pregnancy in the near future, a 6-month course of danazol or a GNRH agonist followed by a low-dose oral contraceptive may be very effective.

Conservative surgical therapy of severe endometriosis is indicated when an adnexal mass is present or symptoms that are not responding to medical therapy in a patient who desires pregnancy. At surgery, one should attempt to resect endometriomas and remove as much endometriosis, either by excision or cauterization, as can be done safely without injury to bowel, bladder, or ureters. Any disease in the cul-de-sac should be carefully removed.

In the patient who has completed her reproductive function, definitive surgical therapy is warranted. Abdominal hysterectomy with bilateral salpingo-oophorectomy can be done in women for whom childbearing is not a consideration. Also, in those women without children who have progressive severe disease that has been refractory to medical or conservative surgical therapy, definitive surgery should be considered.

Some gynecologists consider central pelvic pain to be a clear indication for presacral neurectomy. This procedure has decreased in use in recent years, but may still be of value at the time of conservative surgery for endometriosis. In addition, laser ablation of the uterosacral ligaments at laparoscopy will relieve central pelvic pain for up to 2 years. Along the same lines, a number of surgeons believe that uterine suspension is desirable in the patient who has had surgery for pelvic endometriosis.

INFECTIOUS CAUSES FOR GYNECOLOGIC PAIN

Thanks to the sexual revolution, we are in the midst of an epidemic of sexually transmitted diseases. Although there are several such diseases that can cause clinical problems, most of these are localized problems within the lower genital tract and do not produce significant pain other than the local irritation and inflammation within the vagina or vulva. Included in these, but not exclusively limited to these, are trichomoniasis and herpetic infections. These can be recognized either by microscopic examination of a vaginal discharge or by visualization of vulvar or vaginal lesions characteristic of herpes simplex II. The two most common agents producing pelvic inflammatory disease are gonorrhea and chlamydia. The term *pelvic inflammatory disease* refers to an infection in the endometrium, ovary, or fallopian tube. Previously gonorrhea was the most common organism producing pelvic inflammatory disease; however, in the past decade chlamydial infections have become more common than gonococcal infections. It is currently estimated by the Centers for Disease Control that there are 4 million chlamydial infections annually in the United States. Either of these organisms may produce the classic signs and symptoms of pelvic inflammatory disease, which may than lead to chronic pelvic pain.

The patient with gonococcal or chlamydial infection varies from being asymptomatic to developing severe pelvic inflammatory disease and pelvic abscess formation. To prevent the sequelae of pelvic inflammatory disease with destruction of the fallopian tube, it is imperative to diagnose this entity early in its course.

Unfortunately, it may be easy to confuse acute salpingitis with acute appendicitis, ectopic pregnancy, or pelvic endometriosis. Typically, the patient with acute salpingitis will have bilateral lower abdominal tenderness that usually begins shortly after a menstrual period. The pain becomes progressively worse over several days to the point where the patient is having severe pelvic pain at the time of presentation. Although patients with pelvic inflammatory disease at any stage may be asymptomatic and afebrile and have a normal white blood cell count, in the acute phase typically the patient will have an elevated temperature that may be quite high, in the range of 102–104°. At this point, the white blood cell count is usually elevated. As the infection progresses further, the patient may develop an ileus with nausea and vomiting and may develop the Fitz-Hugh–Curtis syndrome with right upper quadrant pain from perihepatitis. On examination, the patient will usually have bilateral lower abdominal tenderness with guarding and rebound present, depending on the degree of pelvic peritonitis. On pelvic exam, there will be a profuse yellow discharge and a great deal of tenderness with motion of the cervix. The adnexa may feel thickened and will be very tender on both sides, but it may be difficult to delineate a mass because of the patient's guarding and tenderness.

In contrast, in the patient with acute appendicitis, the abdominal pain is usually migratory and will localize in the right lower quadrant. The classic pain of pelvic inflammatory disease is bilateral. Bowel symptoms occur late in the course of the disease of acute salpingitis only after severe peritonitis has developed. Tenderness upon motion of the cervix may be present in acute appendicitis, particularly if the appendix is low in the abdomen or in the pelvis, or in ectopic pregnancy.

In women with pelvic inflammatory disease, laboratory studies may not be particularly helpful, as has been previously mentioned. A significant number of patients with acute salpingitis will have normal white blood cell counts. Cultures of the endocervix are useful, but take several days to report; in particular, the chlamydial culture requires very careful handling for it to be valid. Laparoscopy is very useful in the patient with a confusing picture, in that one may visualize the fallopian tubes and see erythema and a purulent discharge from the fimbria and rule-out an ectopic pregnancy or endometriosis. One may also visualize the appendix and rule-out appendicitis at the same time.

Appropriate medical therapy should be instituted as soon as one makes the diagnosis of pelvic inflammatory disease. Antibiotic therapy for gonococcal and chlamydial infection may be found by referring to the latest recommendations of the Centers for Disease Control.

The patient with chronic pelvic inflammatory disease will usually have exacerbation of her symptoms after each menstrual period, which then gradually abate into her cycle. These patients should initially be tried on a course of antibiotics with each menstrual period, but if they fail to respond after two to three cycles, it may be necessary to surgically correct their problem. This may be done by laparoscopy or laparotomy, depending on the severity of the pelvic adhesions. In more-extreme cases with the formation of pelvic abscess, appropriate surgical intervention is necessary in a timely fashion. This may necessitate the drainage of the abscess or, in more-severe cases, definitive surgery with total abdominal hysterectomy and bilateral salpingo-oophorectomy.

UNEXPLAINED CAUSES OF PELVIC PAIN

After careful and thorough evaluation to eliminate the possibility of organic causes of pelvic pain, one will still be left with a group of patients in whom the etiology of the pain is not readily apparent. These patients will have been carefully screened with appropriate radiographic, ultrasonographic, and laparoscopic procedures, but no organic cause for the pain can be found. This leads one to conclude that there is an underlying psychological cause for this pain. This is not necessarily the case, however. As our knowledge of physiology progresses, the syndrome of primary dysmenorrhea, for example, which was once thought to be a psychosomatic problem, has been found to be related to the excessive secretion of prostaglandins.

Numerous authors have attempted to attribute chronic pelvic pain without obvious pathology to a vascular or autonomic nervous system disorder (6, 7). Renaer, in a comprehensive review article in 1980, concluded that although a good percentage of patients with chronic pelvic pain without obvious pathology present radiographic signs of passive pelvic congestion, there are a certain percentage who do not present these signs. He also concluded that many persons who do not complain of pain may also have radiographic signs of passive pelvic congestion (8).

Typically, patients in this category are in their twenties and thirties, married (or in this day and age probably divorced) with children, and have a number of psychosomatic complaints along with their pelvic pain. Generally they will also complain of nervous tension, fatigue, constipation, diarrhea, and bowel irritability. Dyspareunia is also a common complaint. In my experience, although tenderness may be elicited upon initial examination of the uterus and adnexa, if one is able to distract the patient with conversation, this tenderness may diminish or dissipate.

The psychological aspects of chronic pelvic pain certainly cannot be underplayed. Studies have shown significant prevalence of major depression, substance abuse, adult sexual dysfunction, and somatization in patients with chronic pelvic pain. In women who have undergone laparoscopy and in whom no pathology has been demonstrated, there is a definite difference in response to psychological questionnaires. Women who have chronic pelvic pain and are laparoscopically "negative" are significantly less positive about themselves and their male partners; they feel less sexually attractive and less physically attractive, and are more anxious. They tend to have fewer orgasms than women in a control group do. These women also have a poorer relationship with their families (9). I find that these women are generally under a great deal of stress either because of an unhappy marriage, divorce, stressful job situations, or overwhelming demands of motherhood. Numerous studies have found a significant relationship between childhood physical and sexual abuse and chronic pelvic pain. Nineteen to sixty-four percent of patients with chronic pelvic pain studied had experienced some form of childhood sexual abuse (10–13).

With these factors in mind, it is important for the physician to maintain an open attitude toward these patients. One must be prepared to take the symptoms seriously but not alarm the patient, thereby producing a "cancer mentality." A thorough evaluation must be done, but when one cannot find an organic cause for the pain syndrome, one must be prepared to take a multi-

disciplinary approach to helping these patients. Even in this modern era, psychiatric evaluation is considered to be taboo by some. The gynecologist should gently probe the patient's lifestyle and sexual history looking for situational problems that might be producing the chronic pain syndrome. It is helpful to have a psychologist or psychiatrist with whom the patient will feel comfortable in exploring these possibilities. As part of this, it may be necessary to look for personality disorders through the standard testing mechanisms. Frequently one will find associated depression and anxiety. Availability of a chronic pain center is of great benefit in helping these patients to deal with their pain, and to accept therapeutic modalities that improve their response to stressful situations and enable them to better live their lives with this entity of chronic pelvic pain without obvious pathology. A clinical trial of integrated therapies including equal attention to somatic, psychological, dietary, and environmental factors can significantly improve pelvic pain symptoms (13).

CONCLUSIONS

The majority of women entering the gynecologist's office with a complaint of pelvic pain will have an organic reason for this pain. One must thoroughly evaluate cases of pelvic pain. Medical trials with oral contraceptives, prostaglandin synthetase inhibitors, and antibiotics are appropriate. If these fail to improve the pain, however, a thorough evaluation including laparoscopic examination is warranted. Any organic findings should then be corrected in the appropriate manner. In patients with chronic pelvic pain without obvious pathology, one should look very carefully for environmental causes.

REFERENCES

1. Stovall TG, Ling LW: Some new approaches to ectopic pregnancy. *Contemp Obstet Gynecol* 37:35, 1992.
2. Pickels BR, Hall WJ, Best FA et al: Prostaglandins in endometrium and menstrual flow from normal and dysmenorrheic subjects. *J Obstet Gynecol [Br]* 72:185, 1965.
3. Kitchen JD: Endometriosis. In Sciarra JJ, Droegenueller W (eds): *Gynecology and Obstetrics*, vol 1. Philadelphia, Harper & Rowe, 1985, p 10.
4. Butler L, Wilson E, Belisle S et al: Collaborative study of pregnancy rates following danazol therapy of stage I endometriosis. *Fertil Steril* 41:373, 1984.
5. Barlow DH: Nafarelin in the treatment of infertility caused by endometriosis. *Am J Obstet Gynecol* 162:576–579, 1990.
6. Taylor HC: The problem of pelvic pain. In Meigs JV (ed): *Problems in Gynecology*, vol 3. New York, Grune & Stratton, 1957, pp 191–207.
7. Hobbs JT: The pelvic congestion syndrome. *Practitioner.* 216:529–540, 1976.
8. Renaer M: Chronic pelvic pain without obvious pathology

in women—Personal observations and review of the problem. *J Obstet Gynecol Reproduct Biol* 10:415–463, 1980.

9. Beard RW, Belsey EN, Lieberman BA et al: Pelvic pain in women. *Am J Obstet Gynecol* 128:556, 1977.

10. Walker E, Katon W, Harrop-Griffiths J et al: Relationship of chronic pelvic pain to psychiatric diagnoses and childhood sexual abuse. *Am J Psychiatry* 145:1, 1988.

11. Harrop-Griffiths J, Katon W, Walker E et al: The associa-tion of chronic pelvic pain, psychiatric diagnoses and childhood sexual abuse. *Obstet Gynecol* 71:589, 1988.

12. Rapkin AJ, Kames LD, Dark LL et al: History of physical and sexual abuse in women with chronic pelvic pain. *Obstet Gynecol* 76:92, 1990.

13. Peters AAW, vanDorst E, Jellis B et al: A randomized clinical trial to compare two different approaches in women with chronic pelvic pain. *Obstet Gynecol* 77:740, 1991.

CHAPTER 32
PAIN IN THE MALE GENITALIA

TERRENCE R. MALLOY
CHARLES WITTEN
JERALD B. GILBERT

IN ASSESSING pain in the male genitalia, the physician has to be aware of the many areas from which pain can be referred to the male genitalia. Because of the anatomy and nerve supply, pain is often felt in the genitalia that originates at some distance. It is not uncommon, for example, for men to complain of pain in the glans penis. This pain is rarely caused by a lesion in the glans but is referred from such diffuse organs as the ureter, bladder, trigone, or prostate.

In assessing the management of pain in the male, the physician has to utilize all the classic investigative modalities to identify the causal agent. It is imperative that a complete history and thorough physical examination be done along with appropriate laboratory and radiologic studies in order to delineate the exact etiology of the patient's discomfort. In assessing this problem, the anatomy of the male genitalia must be carefully considered.

ANATOMY

The kidney, renal pelvis, and ureter are retroperitoneal organs lying beneath the diaphragm, traversing caudally to the area of the bladder and prostate. The renal pelvis tapers to become the ureter, which crosses the pelvic inlet anterior to the bifurcation of the common iliac artery (1). The ureter descends to the level of the ischial spine where it proceeds anteriorly and medially to enter the bladder at its lateral border. Proximal to where the ureter enters the bladder it is crossed by the vas deferens. The ureter traverses the bladder muscle to open in the region of the bladder neck at the trigone.

The urinary bladder is a pelvic organ that is posterior to the pubic bones and anterior to the sacrum (2). Its lateral attachments are the arteries coming from the internal iliac artery. Distally the bladder neck joins into the prostate to become the prostatic urethra. The urethra

is anchored at this area by the urogenital diaphragm. The puboprostatic ligaments secure the prostate to the symphysis pubis. The bladder and prostate are separated from the rectum posteriorly by Denonvilliers' fascia. In this area lies the vas deferens and the seminal vesicles. Anteriorly, the dome of the bladder is covered with parietal peritoneum, which is in direct contact with small and large bowel.

The efferent nerve supply to the bladder originates from the vesicle plexus, which arises from the inferior hypogastric plexus. Multiple branches accompany the vesicle artery to the bladder, delivering further branches to the seminal vesicles. Sympathetic fibers that arise from the lower two thoracic and the upper two lumbar segments of the cord synapse in the bladder wall to provide motor fibers to the same muscles of the sphincters at the bladder neck and inhibition fibers to the detrussor muscles of the bladder. Parasympathetic efferent fibers arise from the second through the fourth sacral segments. They produce the pelvic splanchnic nerves, which provide excitory synapses to the detrussor muscle and inhibit the smooth muscle sphincter. The majority of efferent sensory fibers from the bladder and proximal urethra pass via the pelvic splanchnic nerves. Some efferent nerves travel with the sympathetic supply via the hypogastric plexus, however, and enter the first and second lumbar segments of the spinal cord. Bladder pain fibers can be stimulated by distension or spasm of the bladder wall, ureteral obstruction, inflammation, or malignant growth. Because of the dual afferent supply, simple division of the appropriate sympathetic nerves or division of the superior hypogastric plexus does not materially alter bladder pain. Additionally, although bilateral anterior cordotomy may transect pain fibers in the anterior columns, these efferents that sense filling of the bladder travel in the posterior fasciculus gracilis and allow the patient to be aware of filling and the need to micturate.

The prostate gland is a pear-shaped organ in the adult male that can vary in size from 10 to 100 g (2). It is a fibromuscular and glandular structure that surrounds the prostatic urethra and is bounded superiorly by the bladder neck and inferiorly by the urogenital diaphragm. The prostate is surrounded by a fibrous capsule as well as an outer fibrous sheath. Anteriorly, the prostate is attached to the pubic symphysis by the puboprostatic ligaments. Posteriorly, the prostate is separated from the rectal ampulla by the rectovesicle septum called Denonvilliers' fascia. Laterally, the prostate is suspended by the anterior fibers of the levator ani muscles. The prostate is divided into a central zone and a much larger peripheral zone that constitutes 95% of the glandular structure. The remaining 5% forms the transition zone, which lies superior to the verumontanum and is the site of the origin of benign prostatic hyperplasia.

The arterial blood supply to the prostate is from the branches of the inferior vesical and middle rectal arteries. Veins from the prostatic venous complex situated between the capsule and the fibrous sheath traverse with the arteries. The venous complex receives the deep dorsal vein of the penis and numerous vesicle veins that eventually drain to the internal iliac vein or the vertebral veins called Batson's plexus.

The efferent nerve supply to the prostate forms a prostatic plexus that arises from the inferior hypogastric plexus. Large nerves enter the base and side of the prostate with branches distributed to the prostate, seminal vesicles, prostatic urethra, ejaculatory ducts, corpora cavernosa, corpus spongiosum, and membranous and penile urethra. Sympathetic fibers provide the glandular elements with secretory function. They also innervate the prostatic capsule. Parasympathetic nerves arise via the pelvic splanchnics and supply most of the muscular stroma of the prostate.

The male urethra, unlike the female, serves a dual capacity as a urinary conduit and a participant in sexual function. It extends from the bladder outlet to the meatus within the glans penis. It is divided into three main components: prostatic urethra, membranous urethra, and penile urethra (3).

The prostatic urethra is a wide distensible organ averaging 3 cm in length. A median longitudinal ridge arises posteriorly at the bladder neck. The verumontanum is found at the distal portion of the prostatic urethra. The utricle has a slit-like orifice through which ejaculatory ducts open into the prostatic urethra. Prostatic sinuses are found on either side of the crista urethralis with additional prostatic ducts on the floor of the prostatic urethra.

The membranous urethra passes through the genitourinary diaphragm. It is enveloped in skeletal and smooth muscle components, the skeletal muscle components forming the external or voluntary urinary sphincter. This area is approximately 2 cm in length extending from the apex of the prostate to the bulbous portion of the urethra.

The longest portion of the urethra, the penile urethra, is contained within the corpus spongiosum and averages 15 cm in length. Proximally a fusiform segment is called the *bulbous urethra*. Terminally the urethra traverses the glans penis where it is termed the *fossa navicularis* and then tapers to the external urinary meatus.

Muscular elements of the prostatomembranous urethra receive innervation from autonomic and somatic nervous systems. Parasympathetic and sympathetic fibers are found throughout the entire length of the urethra. Somatic fibers derive branches mainly from the pudendal nerve supply and its branches, including muscular branches from the perineal nerve. The afferent supply to the urethra is similar to that of the bladder.

The penis arises embryologically from paired genital tubercles that form the paired corpora cavernosa and their crura. The root of the penis is situated in the superficial perineal pouch and provides fixation stability to the penis. The body of the penis is composed of two corpora cavernosa and a corpora spongiosum urethra. The glans penis is the distal extension of the corpus spongiosum. The corpora cavernosa traverse the penis on the dorsal side, with the corpus spongiosum urethra being on the ventral surface of the penis. These structures are surrounded by dense connective tissue labeled *Buck's fascia*. The corpora cavernosa diverge proximally to form the crura, which attach to the pubic arch at each ischial tuberosity. In this area they are surrounded by fibers of the ischiocavernosus muscle.

The skin of the penis is easily distensible and is based on loose fascial connections to the glans penis and to the Buck's fascia. At the distal end, the skin folds on itself to be the foreskin, which overlaps the glans penis.

Arterial supply to the penis is derived from the internal pudendal arteries branching from the right and left internal iliac arteries. Three main branches constitute the deep penile arteries, the urethral artery, and the bulbar artery. There is also a branch of the deep dorsal artery of the penis that runs on the dorsal surface of the corpora cavernosa with the dorsal veins and nerve supply. This structure is called the *neurovascular bundle*. Venous drainage from the penis is via the cavernosa veins, the deep dorsal veins, and the superficial dorsal vein. The deep dorsal vein empties into the prostatic plexus whereas the superficial veins enter the external pudendal vein.

The nerve supply of the penis is derived from the pelvic plexus made up of sacral parasympathetics and sympathetic fibers from the hypogastric plexuses via the pudendal nerve. These fibers form the perineal nerve, which supplies muscular branches to the perineum and sensory nerves to the posterior scrotum. The pudendal nerve also has a dorsal component that innervates the penis. The ilioinguinal nerve also contributes sensory innervation to the skin of the proximal penis and scrotum.

The spermatic cord structures consist of the artery and vein to the testicle, vas deferens, and artery and vein to the vas. These structures arise from the testicle, traversing the scrotum to enter the external inguinal ring. The ilioinguinal nerve traverses the inguinal canal along the floor separated from the structures by loose areolar tissue. The inguinal canal extends from the internal to the external inguinal ring. The transversalis fascia forms the internal spermatic fascia, the internal oblique fibers create a continuum with the cremasteric muscle fibers that surround the cord structures, and the aponeurosis of the external oblique is continued into the cord structures as the external spermatic fascia that arises at the external ring.

Deep to these layers, the lining of parietal peritoneum that descended with the testicles through the inguinal canal forms the tunica vaginalis. The arterial supply to the spermatic cord structures are the testicular, the cremasteric, and the vasal arteries. Testicular veins form the pampiniform plexus. Lymphatic vessels ascend to the lumbar lymphatics. Nerves include the genital branch of the genitofemoral nerve and the testicular plexus, which is composed of fibers from the renal and aorta plexus as well as the superior and inferior hypogastric plexuses.

The scrotum is partitioned into two compartments by a medial septum with each half containing a testicle, epididymis, and lower portions of the spermatic cord structures. Beneath the skin of the scrotum is the dartos muscle, which replaces the superficial fat and Colle's fascia. The external spermatic fascia, cremasteric muscle fibers, and internal spermatic fascia are the next layers encountered in dissecting the scrotum. The tunica vaginalis is deep to all these structures surrounding the testicle. This is normally sealed from the peritoneum shortly after the testicles descend in utero. The scrotal blood supply is derived from branches of the external pudendal artery that perfuse the anterior scrotum. The posterior scrotum is perfused by branches of the internal pudendal artery. Additional vascular supply comes from the cremasteric and testicular branches that traverse the spermatic cord. Lymphatic drainage from the scrotum is the superficial inguinal nodes. The nerve supply to the scrotum is provided by the ilioinguinal and genital branches of the genitofemoral nerve. The perineal division of the pudendal nerve supplies the cutaneous branches to the posterior scrotal wall. Additionally, the posterior femoral cutaneous nerve has fibers to the posterior scrotal skin.

The testicle is an egg-like structure approximately 5 cm by 3 cm by 3 cm in size (2). The tunica vaginalis

covers the testes. The tunica albuginea forms a capsule around the testicle and supplies numerous septa that divide the testicle into approximately 400 lobules. These converge toward the upper pole. Each lobule is associated with two or more seminiferous tubules that produce spermatozoa. These tubules form the rete testis, which connects by straight tubular recti into the epididymis via efferent ductules. The blood supply to the testis is supplied from the internal spermatic arteries, which arise bilaterally from the aorta just below the origin of the renal arteries. These spermatic vessels traverse the inguinal canal where they anastomose with the cremasteric and vasal arteries that arise from the hypogastric arteries. The venous return is via a network of small veins called the *pampiniform plexus* that forms spermatic veins within or proximal to the inguinal canal. The right spermatic vein drains directly to the vena cava, whereas the left spermatic vein ascends to join the left renal vein. Lymphatic drainage is via retroperitoneal nodes. The testicular nerve plexus travels within the spermatic arteries and veins to the testicles and branches are distributed to the epididymis and vas deferens. Afferent pain fibers from the testicle travel in corresponding plexuses with their origins in the dorsal roots of the tenth and eleventh thoracic nerves. This afferent innervation plays an essential role in referred pain mechanisms from renal and arterial pain syndromes.

The epididymis has three segments: head, body, and tail. The head is found in the upper pole of the testicle. The body is located posterior to the testicle. The tail is attached to the inferior pole of the testicle. The head of the epididymis consists of convoluted efferent ductules that form lobules. These lobules empty into one duct forming the body of the epididymis. The vas deferens is a thick muscular duct 2–3 mm in diameter and approximately 18 inches long that is connected to the epididymis. The vas deferens travels through the spermatic cord into the inguinal canal ascending to pass extraperitoneally around the lateral margins of the inferior epigastric artery and eventually to the lateral wall of the pelvis. It crosses the ureter at the level of the ischial spine and then proceeds medially and inferiorly onto the posterior surface of the bladder where it terminates as the ampulla of the vas deferens. The inferior end of the ampulla narrows and joins the duct of the seminal vesicle forming the ejaculatory duct, which traverses the prostate to open into the prostatic urethra at the crista urethralis. The vas deferens derives its own blood supply from the hypogastric artery.

The seminal vesicles are convoluted glandular sacs approximately 4 cm in length and 1 cm in width located lateral to the vas deferens on the posterior bladder wall. They form an accessory sexual gland storing fluid critical for sperm survival that includes high levels of fructose. The seminal vesicles are supplied by nerves from the vesicle plexus, the prostatic plexus, and the lower portion of the inferior hypogastric plexus. Efferent fibers pass to the ejaculatory ducts in the vas deferens. Contraction of the seminal vesicles and seminal ejaculation are caused by sympathetic innervation, which also constricts the internal urethral sphincter and relaxes the detrusor to prevent retrograde ejaculation.

The bulbourethral glands, located on each side of the membranous urethra between the fascial layers of the urogenital diaphragm, have ducts that run distally into the corpus spongiosum before entering into the bulbous urethra. These glands provide a mucoid secretion to seminal fluid.

The male perineum is divided into the anal and urogenital triangles. The borders include the pubic symphysis anteriorly, ischial tuberosities laterally, and coccyx posteriorly. The perineal body is located centrally between the bulbous urethra and anus. A median ridge, the perineal raphe, passes from the anus anteriorly to become the median raphe of the scrotum and the ventral raphe of the penis. The urogenital triangle is marked posteriorly along a border to which Colle's fascia attaches. Below Colle's fascia, the bulbospongiosus muscle is located in the midline surrounding the bulb of the penis. On either side are the ischiocavernosus muscles, which cover the crura of the penis as they attach to the ischial and pubic arches. The superficial transversus perinea muscles run from the perineal body to the inferior pubic rami. The perineal membrane is located deep to the superficial space. The sphincter urethrae surrounds this membranous urethra and forms the external voluntary sphincter. Arterial supply to the region is derived from the internal pudendal artery, which travels through Alcock's canal with the pudendal nerve to supply muscles of the perineum, scrotum, penis, and urethra.

Specific mention must be made of the autonomic innervation to the pelvis. The pelvic portion of the sympathetic trunk is continuous with the abdominal portion descending anteriorly to the sacrum and posteriorly to the rectum. Four to five segments communicate to the sacral and coccygeal spinal nerves as well as branches to the efferent somatic plexus, particularly the pelvic plexus. The pelvic splanchnic nerves constitute the sacral part of the parasympathetic system and are preganglionic fibers from the sacral roots S2–S4. Branches pass to the pelvic plexus and then to the pelvic viscera. There are additional parasympathetic fibers that ascend to the hypogastric plexus and the inferior mesenteric plexus. Somatic nerves from the thoracolumbar cord derive branches to the ilioinguinal and genitofemoral nerves. From the sacral cords arise fibers that lead to the pudendal nerve and the posterior femoral cutaneous nerve.

Referred pain is an especially important component in dealing with disorders of the male genitalia. Viscera, which are insensitive to cutting or burning but do respond to tension or contraction, will be perceived as pain in the region of skin or tissue distal to the organ effected. The afferent fibers from the referred pain site enter the spinal cord at the same segment as those pain fibers from the viscus itself. In the case of renal and ureteral pain, referred discomfort is a common presenting symptom. The distribution of afferent fibers with autonomic nerves is such that renal pain is felt either at the costovertebral angle, flank, or lower quadrant of the abdomen or even in the inguinal and scrotal areas. Somatic sensory fibers from the groin, bladder, proximal urethra, and genitalia may enter the cord at the same level as the autonomic fibers from the kidney and portions of the ureter: namely, the tenth thoracic through the second lumbar segments. With ureteral colic, pain is conducted through the visceral afferent fibers in a fashion similar to that of the kidney. Colic in the ureter as a result of distension or inflammation is referred to contiguous areas innervated by segments T11–L2. This cutaneous referral produces pain that often commences in the back or flank and progresses anteriorly and inferiorly into the area of the groin and genitalia. Ureteral pain may also be perceived in the anterior aspects of the upper thigh along the femoral branches of the genitofemoral nerve (L1, L2). The testicles may be retracted by activation of the cremasteric reflex via the genital branch of the genitofemoral nerve.

RENAL AND URETERAL PAIN

Pain derived from the kidney and ureter is often perceived as genital pain. It is essential to obtain a good history as to the onset and duration of the pain in addition to the exact description of the origin, length, duration, and movement of the pain. The history provides clues as to what diagnostic studies to perform. These include intravenous urography and ultrasound studies of the kidney and ureter to determine if there is obstruction (4). The most common cause of renal and ureteral pain is colic associated with stone passage. It also may be found with severe hematuria or inflammation, however (5).

Treatment is initiated to relieve pain and determine the exact cause of the obstruction. Pain relief is mandatory. Narcotics administered intravenously, intramuscularly, or orally may be effective. Once pain is relieved the patient can usually effectively increase fluid intake. If nausea is present, intravenous fluids are required to allow for hydration. The pain from renal or ureteral pathology will usually be perceived as pain or discomfort in the ipsilateral flank, lower quadrant, inguinal region, or scrotum. At times pain may also be felt on the anterior thigh of the affected side (6). Antispasmodics are sometimes helpful along with narcotics for relief. Anticholinergics may produce relaxation of ureteral spasms or bladder spasms. Heat may produce relief (warm tub baths). Urinary output should be monitored carefully so that the patient does not become dehydrated.

Nerve blocks are not especially effective in the treatment of renal or ureteral pain. The major source of relief of pain is the removal of the offending agent (i.e., stone or infection) with establishment of adequate urinary drainage past the obstruction. This can be achieved in many ways. Removal of a stone, if present, can be accomplished with the cystoscope and ureteroscopy in a retrograde fashion. The stone can be managed by basket extraction, ultrasound disintegration of the stone, electrohydraulic destruction of the stone, or laser lithotripsey (7). The stone may be pushed back to the kidney where it can be treated with extracorporeal shock-wave lithotripsey or percutaneous endoscopy and antegrade stone removal. Throughout all these procedures, it is essential to have adequate urinary drainage, which will prevent further pain.

If the cause of ureteral obstruction is not immediately evident or complete ureteral obstruction is present, cystoscopy, retrograde pyelography, and retrograde catheterization with a double "J" ureteral stent may provide the diagnosis and the urinary drainage required for relief of the pain (8, 9). If retrograde catheterization is not possible, percutaneous drainage of the affected collecting system should be accomplished via percutaneous nephrostomy placement. This will effectively divert the urine, relieving pain as well as allowing diagnostic and therapeutic interventions (10).

In many instances, renal or ureteral pain will subside with the passage of a stone or the correction of urinary infection. It is important that after the pain has subsided, follow-up studies are obtained to make sure that the anatomic integrity of the upper urinary tract has returned to normal.

BLADDER PAIN

Pain from conditions in the male bladder is usually perceived as suprapubic fullness, pain, urinary frequency, hematuria, or urinary incontinence. The pain, however, may be referred to the penis and felt as discomfort in the perineum, scrotum, or glans penis. These are aspects of referred pain induced by the nerve supply from the scrotum passing adjacent to the bladder.

The primary management of pain caused by the bladder is urinary drainage. In the male, obstruction may occur with failure to empty completely. Drainage by catheter will usually give instantaneous relief. In those patients not suffering from urinary retention, frequency and spasms are the next most disabling symptoms. Anticholinergics and various antispasmodics or analgesics may be used. The primary cause of pain should be ascertained whether it be infection, bleeding, or obstruction. In conditions associated with infections such as

cystitis, prompt intervention with appropriate antibiotics will usually produce relief of pain within 6–12 hours. Urine cultures should be obtained where possible so definitive antibiotic therapy can be established. Once the pain has subsided, diagnostic tests should be undertaken to determine the etiology and source of the infection. Intravenous pyelography, cystography, and/or ultrasonography of the bladder should be accomplished. Cystoscopy should be performed to ascertain if there are anatomic obstructions or conditions within the bladder that have caused the discomfort such as stones, malignancies, or anatomic obstructions of the ureteral orifices. When there are obstructive elements at the bladder outlet such as prostate enlargement or urethral obstruction, surgery is required to prevent further pain in the bladder. With inflammatory conditions, subsequent urinary cultures are required to establish the fact that infection has been eliminated. If a prompt response to inflammatory conditions is not achieved, cystoscopy with bladder biopsy is essential because carcinoma in situ may mimic inflammatory conditions.

PROSTATE PAIN

Pain from the prostate is perceived in the external genitalia at the head of the penis or in the scrotum, the perineum, and possibly the anterior thigh (12). Patients will complain of suprapubic tenderness or aching. Additional symptoms may be noticed with pain on ejaculation or shortly after sexual activity. Urinary frequency, urgency, or double voiding may also be perceived (13).

A meticulous history and physical examination will usually reveal the prostate as the source of pain. Urinalysis is essential with urine culture because it is often difficult to isolate offending organisms in prostatitis.

On a physical examination, the abdomen may be slightly distended, and there may be tenderness over the bladder. Examination of the external genitalia and scrotum will be essentially normal. Rectal examination, however, will often reveal a swollen or tender prostate. Prostatic massage may be helpful in the diagnosis with the expression of prostatic fluid. This then can be examined microscopically and cultures can be obtained. Transrectal ultrasound examinations may also be made, which can reveal prostatic abscesses or other abnormalities of the prostatic anatomy.

Prostatitis may affect men of any age and is not confined to the elderly. The treatment and relief of pain consists of proper introduction of appropriate antibiotics and the use of urinary analgesics and antispasmodics. The patient should be told to soak in warm water and to urinate while sitting in the tub. This often relieves the severe urgency and dysuria associated with prostatitis.

In pain caused by obstruction from the prostate, the symptom complex will usually be that of bladder outlet obstruction. The patient will notice nocturia, frequency, severe urgency, and at times double voiding. Double voiding is a symptom complex in which the patient voids and within 5 min has to void again with a considerable amount of urine being passed on the second occasion. With an obstructed prostate, use of antispasmodics may cause urinary retention. The primary relief of pain is delivered by urinary diversion with a catheter or a suprapubic cystotomy. Surgery should be undertaken to relieve the prostatic obstruction. The prostatic obstruction may be caused by benign or malignant causes. Follow-up studies should be done with malignant specimens to properly treat carcinoma of the prostate.

The principles of pain management remain, however, to obtain temporary urinary diversion from the bladder and then proceed with elimination of a prostatic obstruction.

Care should be taken, however, to assure that the pain is caused by prostatic obstruction and not from prostatic irritation, which is seen in conditions such as prostatitis, prostatosis, and prostatodynia. In these conditions, spasms of the prostate will often mimic prostatic obstruction. Surgery in these patients may remove tissue but the symptoms complex will still be there. This is especially true of males below the age of 50, unfortunately in whom transurethral resection of the prostate is performed but the pain complex continues.

Urodynamics and intravenous urography are advised in all patients under 50 years of age who are suffering with symptoms of prostatic pain. If the intravenous pyelogram (IVP) shows normal upper tracts with no evidence of ureteral obstruction and complete emptying of the bladder, care should be exercised in considering surgery. Urodynamics should also be obtained, which will demonstrate whether the bladder is emptying properly. Urine flowmetry can be employed to assess the patient's ability to empty his bladder in a timely fashion. In prostatic obstruction the flow rates will be below 10 ml per second, whereas in prostatitis flow will often be faster but interrupted by nerve spasms.

In many individuals, after an acute infection has been eliminated from the prostate, they will continue with long-term pain and discomfort in the perineum, genitals, or suprapubic area (15). This symptom complex is often referred to as *prostatodynia*. Treatment for this condition should be symptomatic to include analgesics and positive reinforcement. Sometimes the symptom complex becomes severe, and the patients will suffer severe depressive episodes. Referral to pain centers is often required to train the individual to live with chronic pain. Far too often physicians feel surgery will correct this symptom complex, and procedures are done to no avail. If there are not signs of obvious bladder outlet obstruction from the prostate or severe active infection, surgery will rarely be curative. Reinforcement to the patient of the benign nature of the condition is essential. Often patients feel they have an undiscovered malignancy. Prostatic biopsies to rule-out carcinoma of the prostate should be undertaken on these patients who do not respond to conventional therapy.

URETHRAL PAIN

Pain emanating from conditions originating in the urethra are usually perceived as dysuria, frequency, or pain in the scrotum or perineum. The urethra is usually affected by inflammatory conditions, most often sexually transmitted diseases (STDs) (16, 17).

Important in the treatment of STDs is the proper history and good physical examination including a proper urinalysis and a smear of urethral secretions (18). When STDs are present, prompt treatment with appropriate antibiotics will usually produce immediate relief of pain. Urinary analgesics may be used to relieve the dysuria and frequency. Hot sitz baths are often helpful for the discomfort. In acute conditions with severe symptoms, urinary obstruction may result. A temporary catheterization or suprapubic cystotomy may be required. Urethroscopy may be necessary if the condition does not promptly resolve.

The urethra may also be involved in chronic conditions derived from repeated infections or trauma (19). Most notably these conditions may lead to urethral strictures, which are ring-like constrictions of the urethral diameter. The patient will complain of a narrowed stream, increased frequency, and a decreased force of urinary evacuation. The physician may make the diagnosis by observing the patient void. A thin dribbling or erratic stream will often be indicative of a urethral stricture.

Treatment of urethral strictures consists of proximal urinary diversion by enlarging the urethral caliber and inserting a foley catheter or by a suprapubic cystotomy. The initial form of therapy for urethral strictures is urethroscopy with either internal urethrotomy using a surgical knife or with laser urethrotomy using the KTP 532 laser (20). This will open the stricture so that it may be dilated. Laser urethrotomy vaporizes the entire circumference of the stricture back to the original urethral muscle. Internal urethrotomy has been effective in approximately 50% of patients with chronic intermittent catheterization and may improve long-term results (21). KTP laser urethrotomy has been successful in approximately 65% of patients when followed for 1 year. Urethral strictures often recur or reform even with the appropriate therapy. Repeat urethrotomies or laser urethrotomy may be required; in resistant cases surgical urethroplasty may be required to obtain a proper urethral diameter (22, 23).

Generally, painful conditions of the urethra can be managed conservatively until definitive diagnostic tests reveal the etiology of the problem.

TESTICLE AND EPIDIDYMIS PAIN

Pathologic conditions of the testicle and epididymis will usually be perceived as pain within the scrotum or pain in the inguinal area. The patient may also note difficulty voiding because of referred pain or dysuria. The patient may exhibit raised temperatures and a sense of malaise.

The diagnosis is made by careful history and physical examination. Urinalysis will often reveal inflammatory conditions associated with early epididymitis or orchitis (24). In young men, careful examination has to be made to distinguish between acute epididymo-orchitis and orchitis of testicular torsion. Testicular torsion may be intermittent, and when it does occur is a surgical emergency. Classically in distinguishing torsion from epididymitis, the patient's testicle is found to be elevated in the scrotum close to the external inguinal ring. The testicle may be de-torsed in a counterclockwise fashion. In epididymitis, there is tenderness along the epididymis or testicle. The testicle will usually hang in a dependent portion of the scrotum.

Certain diagnostic tests can distinguish the pain of torsion of the testicle from epididymo-orchitis. In torsion, the urinalysis will usually be normal. With torsion, there is usually no temperature elevation. Radioactive testicular scans will be diagnostic showing decreased blood supply to the affected testicle when torsion is present. Doppler ultrasonography of the testicle will also show decreased vascular supply to the testicle (25). It should be emphasized that in a young male, when the diagnosis is questionable, scrotal exploration must be accomplished without delay to rule-out torsion. If epididymaorchitis is found, there are no serious sequelae. If a patient is treated conservatively for epididymo-orchitis when in fact he has torsion of the testicle, however, he will lose function in that testicle. For medicolegal reasons, the physician must be careful that he is not dealing with a torsion of the testicle. If surgery is undertaken for torsion, the patient should undergo orchiopexy of both the affected testicle and the contralateral organ. Testicular torsion may occur on the contralateral side at a later date if surgery is not performed.

Cancer of the testicle is a common problem in males ranging in age from 20 to 40 years (26). In most cases, the early cancer may be asymptomatic. It may be associated with acute infection and/or hemorrhage into the testicle or epididymis, however. In any suspicious mass in the testicle that is associated with epididymitis, the patient should be treated appropriately with antibiotics. It is mandatory to do proper follow-up studies once the inflammatory condition has subsided to rule-out carcinoma of the testicle. Ultrasonography of any testicular mass should be performed in doubtful cases to rule-out carcinoma. In any doubtful cases, the testicle should undergo inguinal exploration with temporary occlusion of the spermatic artery and vein so that the testicle may

be delivered into the surgical field. The mass in the testicle then can be viewed; if there is a tumor present, orchiectomy will be performed. When one is in doubt, the testicle may be isolated on sterile towels and a biopsy may be obtained for frozen section.

It has to be emphasized that all testicular masses that persist after treatment must be investigated until an exact etiology is determined.

Trauma to the testicle may occur from athletic events, accidents, or injuries. In most instances the testicle can be treated by elevation and ice to the scrotum. Immobilization will usually stop bleeding and allow for resolution of the problem. Testicular scans and ultrasonography may be done to verify that there is a good blood supply to the affected organ. If a portion of the testicle has been fractured, scrotal exploration with excision of the necrotic portion of the testicle and anastomosis of the tunica albuginea will preserve testicular function. As with other testicular conditions, a high index of suspicion is required to prevent long-term complications of the gonad (28).

Testicular pain may also be experienced when the testicle appears to be normal with no signs of testicular torsion. This may occur with torsion of the appendis testis. These are small structures that will cause temporary pain when torsed, but the testicle will be in a normal position and the testicular scan will show normal blood supply.

In dealing with patients with testicular or epididymal pain, careful physical examination is imperative. If the physical examination is normal and there is no tenderness over the testicle or epididymis, referred pain must be considered. The prostate gland should be carefully examined because prostatitis will often be perceived as pain in the scrotum or testicle. Renal or ureteral colic at times will only be perceived as testicular pain. Appropriate radiologic studies will often reveal the cause of the ureteral or renal pathology.

If no pathology is found, a chronic pain syndrome may be considered. Chronic orchialgia is a syndrome characterized by chronic testicular or scrotal pain lasting 6 months or longer. There is no clear etiology. These patients have minimal or no voiding complaints and minimal objective evidence of pathology on physical examination. The work-up should include urinalysis and urine culture followed by scrotal ultrasonography. If these studies are negative, a chronic pain syndrome may be hypothesized, and referral to a pain clinic is in order. Successful treatment may require a multidisciplinary approach and may include biofeedback, regional nerve blocks, or other forms of therapy (29).

SCROTUM PAIN

Pain within the scrotum that is not directly related to the testicle or epididymis may be caused by referred pain from other structures in the genitourinary tract.

A hydrocele is a benign enlargement of the scrotum that consists of fluid within the tunica vaginalis (30). The fluid can enlarge to cause chronic pain or a heavy dragging sensation within the scrotum. In patients presenting with hydrocele, physical examination of the testicle may not be possible because of the size of the scrotum. Ultrasonography should be done to rule-out testicular neoplasm. If the hydrocele is large and causing symptoms, hydrocelectomy may be performed. This operation may be done through a scrotal or an inguinal approach. The hydrocele sac is excised and sutured so that it will not reform.

In an acute situation, relief from pain in the scrotum due to a hydrocele may be obtained by placing ice on the scrotum. Drainage of a hydrocele by needle aspiration may be accomplished but is not recommended. This will cause an initial decrease in the size of the hydrocele but the fluid will usually reform. The hydrocele may become infected, which could lead to orchitis and epididymo-orchitis.

Varicoceles may produce pain and discomfort within the scrotum (31). A varicocele is a dilated collection of veins usually found on the left side of the scrotum. The left side is seen most often because the left spermatic vein travels upward to drain into the left renal vein. If the valves become incompetent, the patient will notice a sensation of fullness or heaviness, and a mass in the left side of the scrotum, especially on being erect. Varicoceles may be bilateral. The diagnosis can be made by having the patient stand and proform a Valsalva maneuver. This may produce a sac of "worm-like" veins in the scrotum, which produce the varicocele. Unilateral right-sided varicoceles and acute varicoceles that do not reduce with recumbency should raise the issue of a potential malignancy. This also may indicate inferior vena caval obstruction by malignancy or thrombosis. Appropriate radiologic studies should be undertaken to establish the etiology of the obstruction that is causing the varicocele.

When a varicocele produces pain, the treatment should consist of ice and reduction of exertion. Long-term relief is produced by having the varicocele repaired surgically or by embolizing the testicular vein. These procedures are advised for pain relief and when the patient is suffering from infertility. In younger patients, long-term reduction in the size of the testicle has been noted when varicoceles are present. When varicoceles are found, especially in young men, surgery should be recommended to prevent testicular atrophy and to protect fertility.

PENIS PAIN

Pain within the penis is commonly associated with inflammatory conditions or obstructive conditions in other areas of the genitourinary tract. A meticulous history should be obtained to determine the etiology and duration of the pain perceived in the penis. Physical examination may reveal the etiology of the discomfort. Referred pain may be felt in the penis from the kidney, ureter, bladder, or prostate.

Primary conditions that cause pain in the penis are varied. In the uncircumcised male, the foreskin may cause irritation or constriction of the glans penis. When the foreskin cannot be retracted, the condition is called *phimosis*. The treatment in the short term is ice and mild analgesics. Obviously, circumcision is the preferred means of therapy.

When the foreskin is retracted and then cannot be placed back over the glans penis, the condition is called *paraphimosis*. The treatment of this condition consists of ice and manual retraction to bring the foreskin over the glans. If this is impossible, local anesthesia can be used on the dorsum of the penis, and a dorsal slit can be made with a scalpel or scissors on the constricting band, which will relieve the stenosis and allow the foreskin to be replaced over the glans penis. The long-term therapy is a properly performed circumcision.

Other conditions are seen in the uncircumcised male. Chronic irritation of the glans penis can produce balanitis or malignancies of the penis (34). Meatal stenosis may produce narrowing of the urinary stream. Condyloma acuminata may form beneath the foreskin. Recent studies have shown that STDs are much more prevalent in the uncircumcised male. When any of these conditions are noted, circumcision should be performed to allow for primary treatment of the pathology and to prevent recurrence. Carcinoma of the penis has not been noted in males circumcised at birth. In any patient suffering with conditions of inflammation, pain, or pain of the glans penis, circumcision should be considered if the foreskin is present.

Peyronie's disease is a condition of the penis in which fibrous plaques form on the tunica albuginea of the corpora cavernosa (35). This condition can be mild and may only be noticed as a fibrous band on the penis when it becomes erect. With progression, however, it may lead to severe pain within the penis and/or penile angulation with erection and eventual impotence. If the Peyronie's plaque becomes large, the penis may angulate 90° with an erection. The diagnosis of Peyronie's disease is made by a careful physical examination. In the early stages of the disease, conservative treatment with vitamin E, steroid injections, or Tomoxifen is warranted. Ultrasonic treatment may be attempted. When the condition becomes more severe, surgical removal of the plaque with grafting to the excised area, or surgical excision of the tunica albuginea to provide straightening, may be undertaken. The grafts may be done with dermal patch grafts or various artificial vascular grafts. In severe cases, especially those accompanied by impotence, the patient may only improve with a penile prosthesis (37).

The patient should be reassured that Peyronie's disease is not a malignant condition and does not progress to carcinoma of the penis.

Priapism is an emergency condition in which the penis sustains a prolonged painful erection that will not detumesce. This may be seen in patients suffering with chronic diseases such as leukemia or with various congenital diseases such as sickle cell trait or sickle cell disease (38). The etiology may be unknown in patients who engage in repeated strenuous sexual activity, patients using narcotics or sexual stimulants, and those patients on intracavernosal pharmacologic treatment for erectile impotence. In the initial stages of priapism, the management of pain should consist of sedation and pain relief. Intracavernosal injections of diluted alpha-adrenergic agonists such as epinephrine or phenylephrine will produce prompt detumescence. If these are unsuccessful, more-invasive treatments may be necessary such as grafts between the corpora spongiosum and corpora cavernosa to relieve the vascular obstruction. Prior to surgical intervention, spinal or caudal anesthesia may be undertaken to attempt to relieve the priapism (39–42). In either case, priapism can be a surgical emergency and the patient should be treated with narcotic pain relief, sedation, and prompt efforts to obtain detumescence of the penis.

Prompt efforts at reduction of priapism are important, because if priapism is not relieved the penis will scar and the patient may suffer erectile impotence. Prompt surgical treatment with detumescence is essential if erectile ability is to be maintained.

At times the penis will be involved with pain caused from neuralgias involving the ilioinguinal, iliohypogastric, or genitofemoral nerves. These nerves may have been traumatized from injuries or previous surgery. The pain may be referred to the penile shaft. The diagnosis should consist of careful inspection to rule-out primary etiologies within the penis causing the pain.

Inflammatory conditions of the penis and STDs to the penis are becoming more prevalent. Condyloma acuminata is rapidly becoming the number one STD of the 1990s. Condylomata are caused by human papilloma viruses, which are easily disseminated to sexual partners. Most of the condylomata are caused by benign HPV viruses 6 and 11. However, HPVs 16, 18, and 31 are associated with condylomata, which may produce precancerous lesions in the female cervix (43). Males exhibiting condylomata of the penis must have careful treatment of both themselves and their sexual partners to guarantee total treatment. Condylomata have been treated in multiple fashions including surgical excision, local caustic agents such as podophylin, and cryosurgery. For the past 10 years, laser therapy with either the CO_2, KTP 532, or neodymium YAG laser have proven to be the most efficacious means of removing the condylomata and destroying the virus surrounding them in what appears to be normal skin (44, 45). The patient must be examined with magnification after a dilute acetic acid solution has been placed over the penis and scrotum. Acetic acid (3–5%) is applied and then allowed to dry. Using magnification the skin is carefully inspected. Suspicious lesions are biopsied for pathology and HPV virus typing. In any areas that are positive, the lesion should be treated. Discomfort from condylomata is usually associated with itching or bleeding. Condylomata may be present in the urethra. When they are present, urethroscopy should be performed to ascertain that the condylomata have not progressed into the bulbous or prostatic urethra or bladder neck. The neodymium YAG laser is effective in eliminating condylomata within the urethra and bladder. In any patients with dysuria, frequency, or a bloody discharge, urethral condyloma should be suspected.

CONCLUSIONS

The management of pain in the male genitalia is essentially concerned with proper diagnosis of the pain. Local treatments may not be effective because of the fact that the etiologic agent may be in a distal organ. Once the diagnosis is established, proper treatment can be obtained to relieve the discomfort.

REFERENCES

1. Bo WJ, Krueger WA: Gross anatomy of the kidney: Cross and coronal-section anatomy. In *Surgical Anatomy of the Kidney*. Mt. Kisco, NY, Futura Press, 1982, p 1.
2. Tanagho EA: Anatomy of the lower tract. In Harrison JH, Giddes RF, Perlmutter AD, Stamey TA, Walsh PC (eds): *Campbell's Urology*. Philadelphia, WB Saunders, 1986, p 46.
3. Warwick R, Williams DL: The male urethra. In *Gray's Anatomy*. Philadelphia, WB Saunders, 1973, p 1334.
4. Cameran DO, Azimi F: The value of excretory urography in the diagnosis of acute pyelonephritis. *J Urol* 112:546, 1974.
5. Smith DR, Raney FL: Radiculitis distress as a mimic of renal pain. *J Urol* 116:269, 1976.
6. Dowd JB: Flank pain in non-urologic disease. *Med Clin North Am* 47:437, 1963.
7. Dretler SP: An evaluation of ureteral laser lithotripsey: 225 consecutive patients. *J Urol* 143:267, 1990.
8. Andriola GL, Bettmann MA, Garnick MD, Richie JP: Indwelling double J ureteral stents for temporary and permanent urinary drainage: Experience with 87 patients. *J Urol* 131:239, 1984.
9. Mardis HK, Kroeger RM, Hepperlen TW, Mazer MJ, Kammandel H: Polyethylene double-pigtail ureteral stents. *Urol Clin North Am* 9:95, 1982.
10. Stable DB: Percutaneous nephrostomy techniques, indications, and results. *Urol Clin North Am* 9:15, 1982.
11. Stamey TA: *Pathogenesis and Treatment of Urinary Tract Infections*. Philadelphia, Williams & Wilkins, 1980.
12. Meares EM: Prostatitis syndromes: New perspective about old woes. *J Urol* 123:141, 1980.

13. Drach GW, Fair WR, Meares EM, Stamey TA: Classifications of benign diseases associated with prostatic pain: Prostatitis or prostatodynia [Letter]. *J. Urol* 120:266, 1978.

14. Schaeffer AJ, Wendel EF, Dunn JK, Grayhack JT: Prevalence and significance of prostatic inflammation. *J. Urol* 125:215, 1981.

15. Meares EM, Stamey TA: Bacteriologic localization patterns in bacterial prostatitis and urethritis. *Invest Urol* 5:492, 1968.

16. Bowie WR: Non-gonococcal urethritis. *Urol Clin North Am* 22:55, 1984.

17. Harrison WG: Gonococcal urethritis. *Urol Clin North Am* 11:45, 1984.

18. Centers for Disease Control: Sexually transmitted disease treatment guidelines. Morb Mort Wk Rep Fep 31:335, 1982.

19. Mitchell TP: Injuries to the urethra. *Br J Urol* 40:649, 1968.

20. Turek PJ, Malloy TR, Cendron M, Carpiniello VL, Wein AJ: KTP-532 laser ablation of urethral strictures. *Urology* 40:330–334, 1992.

21. Robertson GS, Everitt N, Lamprecht JR, Brett M, Flynn JT: Treatment of recurrent urethral strictures using clean intermittent catheterization. *Br J Urol* 68:89–92, 1991.

22. Badenoch AW: A pull-through operation for impassable traumatic strictures of the urethra. *Br J Urol* 22:404, 1950.

23. Waterhouse K, Abrahams J, Gruber H et al: The transpubic approach to the lower urinary tract. *J Urol* 109:486, 1976.

24. Berger RE: Nongonococcal urethritis and related syndromes. *Monogr Urol* 3:99, 1982.

25. Zoeller, Gerhard, Ringert, Rolf-Hermann: Color-coded duplex sonography for diagnosis of testicular torsion. *J Urol* 146:1288, 1991.

26. Donahue JP (ed): *Testis Tumor*. Baltimore, Williams & Wilkins, 1983.

27. LaNasa JA, Lange EI: Disorders of the scrotum and its contents. In Resnick Mi, Older Ra (eds): *Diagnosis of Genitourinary Disease*. New York, Thieme-Stratton, 1982, p 433.

28. McDougal WS, Persky L: *Traumatic Injuries of the Genitourinary System*. Baltimore, Williams & Wilkins, 1981.

29. Costabile A, Hahn M, Hahn M, David G: Chronic orchialgia in the pain prone patient: The clinical perspective. *J Urol* 146:1571, 1991.

30. Marshall FF: *The Management of Hydroceles*. Houston, AUA

31. Cockett ATK, Koshiba K: The scrotum and its contents. In Cockett ATK, Koshiba K (eds): *Manual of Urologic Surgery*. New York, Springer-Verlag, 1979, p 221.

32. Williams RD: Renal perirenal and ureteral neoplasms. In *Adult and Pediatric Urology*. New York, Mosby Year Book, 1991, p 579.

33. Takihara H, Sakatoku J, Fujii M, Nasu T, Cosentino MJ, Cockett ATK: Significance of testicular size measurements in andrology. I. A new orchidometer and its clinical application. *Fertil Steril* 39:836, 1983.

34. Baker BH, Spratt JS, Perez-Mesa C et al: Carcinoma of the penis. *J Urol* 116:548, 1976.

35. Metz P, Ebbehoj J, Uhrenholdt A, Wagner G: Peyronie's erectile failure. *J Urol* 130:1103, 1983.

36. Herwig K: Retroperitoneal Fibrosis with Tomoxifen. *J Surg* April 1991.

37. Malloy TR, Carpiniello VL, Wein AJ: Advanced Peyronie's disease treated with the inflatable penile prosthesis. *J Urol* 125:327, 1981.

38. Baran M, Leiter E: The management of priapism in sickle cell anemia. *J Urol* 119:610, 1978.

39. Ercole CJ, Pontes JE, Pierce JM: Changing surgical concepts in the treatment of priapism. *J Urol* 125:210, 1981.

40. Winter CC: Cure of idiopathic priapism. New procedure for creating fistula in glans and corpora cavernosa. *Urology* 8:389, 1976.

41. Sayer J, Parsons CL: Successful treatment of priapism with intracorporeal epinephrine. *J Urol* 140:827, 1988.

42. Dittrich A, Albrecht K, Bar-Moshe O, Vandendris M: Treatment of pharmacological priapism with phenylephrine. *J Urol* 146:323, 1991.

43. Gupta JW, Saito K, Saito A, Fu YS, Keerti SV: Human papillomaviruses and the pathogenesis of cervical neoplasia. *Cancer* 64:2104, 1989.

44. Grussendorf-Conen EJ, de Villiers E, Gissman L: Human papilloma virus genomes in penile smears of health men. *Lancet* 76:1092, 1986.

45. Fuselier HA Jr, McBurney EI, Brannan W, Randrup ER: Treatment of condyloma acuminata with carbon dioxide laser. *Urology* 15:265, 1980.

46. Malloy TR, Wein AJ: Laser treatment of bladder carcinoma and genital condylomata. *Urol Clin North Am* 13:121, 1987.

Update Series Vol. 1, Lesson 9, American Urological Association, 1982.

CHAPTER **33**

PHYSICAL MANAGEMENT OF MALIGNANT PAIN
THERESA FERRER-BRECHNER

THE PHYSICAL management of malignant pain involves the expert orchestration of currently available modalities so that they will provide pain relief commensurate with the natural progression of disease and the now-prolonged life expectancy of patients with cancer. Serious commitment to providing pain relief should last throughout the patient's life expectancy if pain persists or recurs. This review plans to give the clinician who deals with patients suffering from malignant pain the ability to maximize their use of currently available pain-relieving modalities as well as keep them abreast with recently innovated modalities.

Although this chapter is primarily aimed toward the physical management of malignant pain, it by no means ignores the fact that simultaneous psychological evaluation and management is of equal importance. The management of cancer-related pain is best dealt with by an interdisciplinary/multidisciplinary approach between physicians, psychologists, and other health care professionals. This milieu of pain specialists can create a program that has increased chances of maximizing efficacy of physical modalities specific for malignant pain. In dealing with malignant pain, we need to remember that cancer is not a static disease, but progressive at variable rates. Therefore, physical modalities should be planned according to the known natural progression of the disease.

The physical modalities currently available for the treatment of cancer pain are numerous. The choice of modality is influenced largely by the specialty of the physician who happens to be taking care of the patient at the time of pain complaint. The oncologist, who traditionally manages the patient's pain problem initially, needs to master the pharmacologic approach, as well as understand other available options if pharmacologic approaches no longer provide adequate pain relief. To maximize the use of an interdisciplinary approach for malignant pain treatment, the primary physician should fully understand the role of various available modalities, identifying specialists who can lend expertise in performing procedures that are outside his/her scope of practice. Since there are only four or five cancer pain clinics in the entire United States, the responsibility of managing cancer pain primarily falls on internists and oncologists medically managing these patients.

This chapter deals with the physical evaluation and management of patients with malignant pain. Current and recent modes of therapy are presented with the concept of a graduated somatic approach, that is, utilizing less invasive, less risky approaches before more invasive, high-risk modalities are utilized.

PHYSICAL EVALUATION

A competent physical evaluation of the cancer patient with pain includes a thorough neurologic examination; appropriate radiologic workup, including repeat computed tomography (CT) scan and magnetic resonance imaging (MRI); assessment of functional capacity; understanding of pain language; assessment of previous analgesics and adjunctive drugs used; and, if necessary, utilization of prognostic and diagnostic nerve blocks. Although oncologic modalities are no longer utilized, further workup to clearly define the pathophysiology of pain is of paramount importance.

NEUROLOGIC EVALUATION

Neurologic evaluation is necessary to understand the underlying cause of pain. The various causes of pain have been identified by Foley (1), and include the two main causes of pain in the patient with malignancy (Table 33.1): pain secondary to direct tumor invasion, and pain secondary to cancer-directed therapy. It is of paramount importance to determine the predominant cause of the patient's pain, since it will dictate the mode of therapy. For example group I patients primarily suffer from nociceptive pain, and group II from deafferentation pain. The management of these two types of

Table 33.1.
Pain Syndromes Associated with Cancer

I. Due to direct tumor invasion
   A. Bone metastasis
      1. Base of the skull
      2. Sphenoid
      3. Vertebral body
         a. C2
         b. C7–T1
         c. L1
      4. Sacral syndrome
   B. Nerve encroachment
      1. Peripheral nerves: neuropathy
      2. Plexus: branchial, lumbar, sacral
      3. Root: leptomeningeal
      4. Spinal cord: compression
II. Due to therapy
   A. Postsurgical
      1. Radical neck dissection
      2. Thoracotomy
      3. Mastectomy
      4. Phantom limb
   B. Chemotherapy
      1. Neuropathies
      2. Aseptic necrosis of femoral head
      3. Herpes zoster and postherpetic neuralgia
   C. Radiation therapy
      1. Myelopathy
      2. Necrosis
      3. Fibrosis
      4. Secondary tumors

pain are entirely different, the first group responding well to narcotic analgesics, and the second group to drugs such as tricyclic antidepressants and anticonvulsants, but not to narcotic analgesics. Deafferentation pain is characterized by decreased response to pinprick sensation, hyperesthesias, and dysesthesias in the painful area as a result of destruction of large somatic fibers from viral diseases, surgical trauma, chemotherapy, or neural compression. This destruction results in the functional loss of the somatic fibers that normally inhibit small nociceptive C fibers in the periphery of the involved area. Neurologic exam is also necessary to document the extent of neural compression from tumor invasion, and is helpful in planning the extent of neuroablation, as well as documenting the extent of any altered sensory function prior to a neuroablative procedure. In addition, repeated neurologic exam will document any impending neurologic catastrophe, such as spinal cord compression, during the course of treating the pain.

Assessment of Pain Experience

Assessment of somatic pain in patients with malignancy is difficult because it is often mixed with "suffering" or the affective/emotional aspect of the pain experience. The patient with malignancy and pain need not be subjected to lengthy methods of assessing pain experience used more commonly in chronic nonmalignant pain. However, semi-quantitative methods of assessing pain severity and pain experience must be attempted to appropriately assess the impact on treatment outcome. Some suggestions for easily applicable pain assessment tools for cancer patients are the Pain Visual Analog Scale (2), which measures pain severity, and the McGill Pain Questionnaire (3), which measures the sensory and affective dimension of pain experience. Both of these tests can be easily filled out repeatedly by patients with malignancy and pain.

To successfully physically manage malignant pain, one has to decrease not only the somatic or sensory aspect, but also the affective aspect of pain experience. We have shown that somatic treatments such as pharmacologic treatment and neurolytic blocks only decrease the sensory dimension, and not the affective dimension, of the pain experience (4). Therefore, repeated evaluation of the pain experience during the course of treatment is important in directing changes of therapy.

Another useful method of assessing pain in cancer patients is to use a daily diary, which yields information on medication compliance, sleep patterns, diurnal variation of pain, and types of activities that increase or decrease pain. Assessment of previous analgesics lays important groundwork for planning subsequent pharmacologic tailoring. Types of previous medications used, duration of analgesia, and side effects encountered with each medication should be elicited from the patient.

Diagnostic Nerve Blocks

Prognostic and diagnostic nerve blocks can also be an important aspect of the total evaluation of the patient's pain. The pathophysiology of pain and the extent of dermatomes involved can be determined by the use of carefully administered neural blocking procedures with varying concentrations of local anesthetics. Sympathetic mediated pain secondary to reactive causalgia, lymphatic distention, and deafferentation pain can be blocked by sympathetic ganglion blocks. The ganglia can be blocked with low concentrations of local anesthetic (e.g., 0.5% lidocaine or 0.25% bupivicaine), at various locations: for head and neck pain, upper and middle cervical ganglion block; for upper extremities, stellate ganglion block; for lower extremities, paravertebral sympathetic ganglion block. Somatic nerve-mediated pain can be blocked by administration of a higher concentration of local anesthetic (e.g., 1% lidocaine, 0.5% bupivicaine), into somatic nerves or epidural space. This is particularly helpful in determining whether neurolytic somatic nerve blocks can be helpful in patients with pain secondary to multiple rib metastases, chest wall or

Table 33.2.
Currently Available Physical Treatments for Malignant Pain

I. Pharmacologic tailoring
   A. Nonnarcotic and narcotic analgesics
     1. Oral
     2. Intravenous/intramuscular
     3. Epidural/intrathecal
   B. Adjuvant drugs
     1. Antidepressants
     2. Anxiolytics
     3. Anticonvulsants
     4. Steroids
     5. Antihistamines
     6. Dextroamphetamine
     7. Phenothiazines
     8. Caffeine
II. Modulation of pain pathway
   A. Central stimulation: periventricular or thalamic capsule stimulation
   B. Dorsal column stimulation
   C. Peripheral stimulation: transcutaneous electrical nerve stimulation, acupuncture
III. Neuroablation
   A. Chemical: injection of neurolytic solutions
     1. Spinal block
     2. Epidural block
     3. Somatic nerve block
     4. Sympathetic ganglion block
     5. Peripheral nerve block
   B. Surgical
     1. Percutaneous or open chordotomy
     2. Surgical rhizotomy
     3. Dorsal root entry zone lesions
     4. Median myelotomy
     5. Hypophysectomy

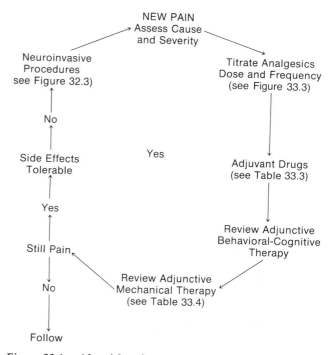

Figure 33.1. **Algorithm for managing malignant pain.**

PHYSICAL TREATMENTS

Table 33.2 lists the general types of current physical treatments for the alleviation of malignant pain. Description of some of these modalities has been dealt with in previous chapters. Since malignancy is not a stable disease, but is typically progressive, the use of a single modality frequently fails to give a lasting or "permanent" solution to the pain problem. Often, a combination of the various modalities is necessary over the course of the disease. Understanding the life history of the specific cancer inducing the pain will provide better information in orchestrating the various types of physical modalities available for pain control. Recently, a consensus group for cancer pain management suggested a decision tree for managing malignancy pain, taking into consideration various causes of cancer pain, factors that can influence the pain experience, and currently available modalities (5). A synopsis of this algorithm is presented in Figure 33.1.

INDIVIDUALIZED PHARMACOLOGIC TAILORING

In this section, both standard and current novel approaches in drug therapy are discussed as they apply to malignant pain therapy. Although drug therapy has been the mainstay of treatment for malignant pain, it remains the mode most fraught with controversy. Unfortunately, most physicians have been taught primarily to use narcotic analgesics for the relief of acute pain (i.e., postoperative pain, post-trauma pain, pain from procedures). Therefore, physicians expect to use narcotic analgesics only for a limited period of time, becoming

abdominal wall metastases, or somatic nerve compression due to vertebral metastases.

When determining the prognosis of neurolytic blocks with local anesthetics, appropriate semiquantitative pain scales and careful sensory examination should be documented before and after injection of the local anesthetic. At least 50% reduction in pain and absence of intolerable side effects should be present before chemical neurolysis is entertained. If a patient is a candidate for a neurolytic block, a diagnostic block with local anesthetic should be done 24–48 hr before to determine the volume of neurolytic agent necessary. Prior to any diagnostic block, platelet count, prothrombin time, bleeding time, and thromboplastin time should be determined. This is particularly important in patients receiving epidural blocks, where the danger of epidural hematoma with coagulopathy can lead to severe neurologic deficits if not treated immediately with surgical intervention. In addition, if impending spinal cord compression is suspected, a CT scan or MRI should be done before an epidural or spinal injection is attempted.

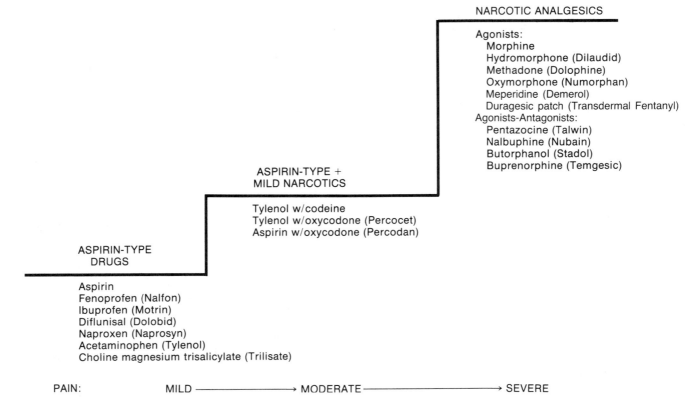

Figure 33.2. **Ladder of commonly used drugs for malignant pain.**

increasingly uncomfortable in extending their use for long periods of time in patients with malignant pain. There is difficulty in understanding the individualized development of tolerance with prolonged use. Often patients are labeled "addicted" when the requirements for analgesia naturally increases. Risk of substance abuse with chronic opioid use in patients with chronic non-cancer pain or cancer patients has not been substantiated. In reviewing the use of narcotics in a cancer pain clinic, the major factor for increased drug intake is substantiated progression of metastatic disease (6). In addition, monitoring the incidence of narcotic addiction in 39,946 hospitalized medical patients revealed that of 11,882 who received at least one narcotic preparation, there were only 4 cases of reasonably well-documented addiction in patients without prior addiction history (7). For physicians to effectively begin using narcotic analgesia in cancer patients, the fear of inducing addiction in cancer patients should be eradicated.

To effectively use narcotic analgesics for malignant pain, several factors need to be examined: choice of drug; method of administration; route of drug administration; and development of tolerance with prolonged use. In this review, only analgesic studies done in cancer pain are addressed since the review of pharmacology of analgesics for other pain models has been given elsewhere.

Figure 33.2 illustrates the ladder of analgesic drugs for oral use utilized for malignant pain. (*a*) aspirin-type drugs, including the nonsteroidal anti-inflammatory drugs (NSAIDs); (*b*) aspirin-type drugs combined with mild narcotics; and (*c*) narcotic analgesics.

Aspirin-Type Drugs

Nonnarcotic analgesics are used primarily for mild malignancy pain as the first line of analgesic (8, 9). This class includes aspirin, acetaminophen, and NSAIDs. Their use in malignancy pain is limited because aspirin beyond 1300 mg has a "ceiling" effect; therefore further increase in dosage will not increase peak analgesia, but may increase duration (10). In addition, malignancy pain rarely stays at a mild level, but more commonly proceeds to moderate or severe pain. Increasing the dose to more than 4 g/day of aspirin produces gastrointestinal side effects or salicylate intoxication in a majority of patients. Unfortunately, the majority of studies on mild analgesics have been done in postoperative, dental, or other acute pain models, and have rarely been done on patients with malignancy pain.

Acetaminophen has been found to be equieffective and equipotent to aspirin in malignancy pain, and their time-effect curves virtually overlap (11). As with aspirin, a ceiling effect is also obtained past a 1000-mg dose. Acetaminophen has fewer side effects than aspirin, but with overdosage can induce hepatotoxicity. A daily dose over 4–6 g is not recommended because of this dangerous side effect, especially in cancer patients with liver involvement.

Aspirin-Type Drugs with Mild Narcotics

The second step in the analgesic ladder is the use of mild narcotics in combination with aspirin or acetaminophen. A majority of analgesic studies done with this group again have been in postoperative, postpartum, or dental pain models, and not on chronic malignant pain. Moertel et al. probably performed the only study comparing a number of oral analgesics in outpatients with malignant pain (12). Codeine (65 mg) and pentazocine (50 mg) were not significantly different than aspirin (600 mg) and propoxyphene hydrochloride (65 mg) was found to be slightly less effective than aspirin (650 mg).

Combinations of opiate and antipyretics are known to produce analgesia by two mechanisms: opioids bind to opiate receptors in the central nervous system, and the antipyretics act peripherally. Therefore, an additive analgesic effect is produced with this combination, usually substantially greater than when either drug is administered by itself. This combination also results in reduction of side effects. Specifically, in malignant pain, factorial studies indicate that the combination of 600 mg of aspirin and 32 mg codeine clearly produces more significant analgesia than either one alone (13). For those with chronic pain, repetitive dosing of codeine with acetaminophen over a period of 8 days produced a greater analgesic effect than is seen with a single-dose study (14). Although the subjects did not have malignant pain, it demonstrates that differences in efficacy can be secondary to repetitive dosing, common in patients with malignant pain, and that results seen with single-dose acute pain models do not necessarily apply to chronic cancer pain models.

In 100 outpatients with cancer pain who self-administered medications in a drug crossover study, Moertel et al. found that codeine (65 mg), oxycodone (9.76 mg), and pentazocine (25 mg) produced statistically significant increases in the analgesia when added to aspirin, but propoxyphene napsylate added to aspirin failed to increase analgesia (12).

Nonsteroidal anti-inflammatory drugs are known to be more efficacious than aspirin and acetaminophen and are known to enhance narcotic analgesia more than aspirin and acetaminophen. Specifically, in a double-blind study in patients with malignant pain, addition of ibuprofen (600 mg) to methadone (2–5 and 5 mg) was clearly superior to methadone given alone in the same doses (15). Although newer NSAIDs have mushroomed, studies on their use for chronic malignancy pain is lacking, despite the fact that research for better analgesics in this area is of priority.

Narcotic Analgesics

Narcotics are the basic mainstay of therapy for managing moderate to severe acute and chronic malignant pain. For a complete review of the principles of various narcotics used in cancer pain, the reader is referred to a recently published guide on the topic (16). This guide promotes nine principles for the individualization of narcotic analgesics:

1. Individualize dose by choosing the route of administration to fit the patient's needs, titrating the dose to analgesia, and respecting the wide variation in optimal analgesic for the cancer patient.
2. Administer the analgesic on a time-contingent, not pain-contingent, basis.
3. Become familiar with the dose and time course of potent narcotics.
4. Be aware of the potential hazards of pentazocine (Talwin) and meperidine (Demerol). Pentazocine is an agonist-antagonist drug in oral form and, therefore, will precipitate withdrawal in patients taking pure agonist opioids. Meperidine (Demerol) is short acting and has poor oral to intramuscular potency. Its metabolic by-product, normeperidine, can induce central nervous system stimulation, possibly leading to convulsions (17), especially in patients with compromised kidney function.
5. Recognize and treat side effects appropriately.
6. Use drug combinations that enhance analgesia without increasing side effects.
7. Do not use placebos to assess the nature of the pain.
8. Watch for the development of tolerance and treat appropriately.
9. Be aware of the development of physical dependence and prevent withdrawal.

To remove the myths that hamper most physicians in appropriately prescribing adequate narcotic analgesics in malignant pain, the definitions of tolerance, physical dependence, and psychological dependence (*"addiction"*) should be clearly understood. It is inhuman to label cancer patients "addicts," especially if this is the main reason for their undertreatment with analgesics.

Adjuvant Drugs

There are some atypical types of malignant pain that may not respond even to high doses of narcotics. In these situations, the use of adjuvant drugs or procedures becomes of paramount importance (Table 33.3). Merely increasing narcotic dose with this atypical narcotic-resistant pain syndrome will just increase narcotic toxicity without increasing analgesia.

Patients with progressive bone metastasis may require adjuvant use of NSAIDs for their antiprostaglandin E_2 effect, or epidural steroids for painful nerve root or plexus compression resulting in neural edema. Patients with smooth muscle spasm (rectal, pancreatic, parotid, and salivary glands) may also not respond well to narcotics and may require adjuvant anticholinergic drugs such as atropine (0.2–0.4 mg). Deafferentation resulting in neuropathic pain (postherpetic neuralgia, postmastectomy and post-thoracotomy pain), is best treated

Table 33.3.
Adjuvant Drugs for Malignant Pain

Problem	Adjuvant Drug
Nociceptive pain	
Bone pain	NSAIDs
	L-dopa
Visceral pain	ASA
	Acetaminophen
Deafferentation pain	
Burning pain	Tricyclic antidepressants
Shooting pain	Anticonvulsants
Nausea and vomiting	Hydroxyzine
Sedation	Dextroamphetamine
Painful neural compression	Steroids
Increased intracranial pressure	Steroids

with the use of tricyclic antidepressants with or without phenothiazine (18, 19). The analgesic effect of amitriptyline is better seen at lower doses (25–150 mg) than their antidepressant effects in patients with chronic pain.

Another group of patients whose pain may not respond well to narcotics are patients with headaches secondary to increased intrathecal pressure. Narcotic administration can cause CO_2 accumulation, which further increases intracranial pressure. This condition is best treated with systemic or oral steroids. Skeletal muscle spasm due to malignant infiltration of the posterior fossa or paraspinal muscles can be best treated with drugs such as Flexeril.

Other adjuvant drugs that can be useful for cancer pain are:

1. Anticonvulsants (phenytoin, carbamazepine, sodium valproate, clonazepam) for brief shooting or lancinating pain secondary to chronic neuralgias such as postherpetic neuralgia, intercostal neuralgia, traumatic neuralgias (20).
2. Dextroamphetamine, which has been shown to increase analgesia when given with narcotics (21) as well as reduce the sedative effects of narcotics in patients with malignant pain.
3. Antihistamines such as hydroxyzine (Vistaril) in a 25–50-mg dose, which has analgesic, antiemetic, and sedative actions and, therefore, is ideal for patients who have pain, anxiety, and nausea.

Drugs that should be avoided in the management of cancer pain are sedative-hypnotic drugs, benzodiazepines, cannabinoids, and cocaine, because of nonexistent or poor analgesic effect in the face of intolerable side effects.

New Techniques in Narcotic Administration

Newer methods of drug delivery have recently been innovated in an attempt to improve the management of cancer pain. These include: (*a*) sublingual; (*b*) continuous subcutaneous infusion; (*c*) transdermal; (*d*) continuous spinal or epidural opioid infusion; and (*e*) intraventricular injection. In addition, the use of patient-controlled analgesia (PCA) has innovated the use of intravenous morphine administration, giving the patients better control of their pain. Not all of these methods have undergone adequate clinical trials in patients with malignancy pain.

The sublingual area is rich in blood and lymphatic vessels, making it ideal for rapid absorption (22). The ideal drugs for sublingual administration are methadone, fentanyl, or buprenorphine, because of their high partition coefficient, a measure of lipid solubility. To maximize the proportion of unionized opioids in the sublingual cavity, the pH of the dosing solution can be raised to enhance absorption. The absorption of levorphanol or methadone was significantly increased when the pH of the solution was increased from 6.5 to 8.5 (23).

Continuous subcutaneous infusion (CSCI) can be a relatively simple, safe, and effective method of pain control in children and adults. A portable infusion pump is attached to a 27-gauge butterfly needle and inserted in the subcutaneous tissue, usually in the chest area (24). Most opioids can be used for CSCI except meperidine and pentazocine, which can be irritating to tissues. The ideal volume of infusion seems to be <1 ml/hr to prevent local irritation.

Transdermal delivery, the newest method of opioid delivery, can offer several advantages for patients with chronic malignancy pain. However, absorption of drugs applied to the skin surface is a challenging problem. The opioid must have high lipid solubility to penetrate the skin to the capillaries, adequate water solubility to allow highly concentrated solutions (>1.0 mg/ml) to be incorporated in the reservoir, and a high relative analgesic potency since it reduces the bulk of the reservoir. The ideal drug presently being studied is fentanyl, which is found to appear in the plasma 2–3 hr after application of the patch and reaches steady state plasma level after 12 hr (25).

Continuous spinal or epidural opioid infusion was introduced in the 1970s for the management of acute pain due to postoperative, obstetric, and chronic benign and malignant pain (26). The advantages of centrally administered opioids include a prolonged analgesia with lower doses when compared to systemic opioid administration. In contrast to the use of local anesthetics in the epidural or intrathecal space, opioid analgesia is free of sympathetic motor and proprioceptive adverse effects. Administration of opioids centrally does produce adverse effects of nausea and vomiting, pruritus, and delayed respiratory depression in narcotic-naive patients. The analgesic effects of centrally administered opioids are dose dependent, naloxone reversible, and subject to tolerance development (27). Several factors determine

Table 33.4.
Adjunctive Mechanical Treatments

Physical and occupational therapy
    Orthotic/prosthetic devices
    Improve functionality
Peripheral stimulation–produced analgesia
    Transcutaneous electrical nerve stimulation
    Acupuncture

the clinical response to spinal opioids: relative analgesic potency, receptor selectivity pharmacokinetics in cerebrospinal fluid (CSF) and spinal cord, and tolerance to opioids. Although morphine is the most common opioid injected into the epidural or intrathecal space, no controlled studies have compared graded doses of spinal opioid to obtain relative potency estimates. Receptor selectivity for mu, kappa, and delta receptor types in the spinal cord has been studied in animal models. Selection of opioids for specific receptors in the spinal cord can be used to obviate tolerance by switching the patient to another narcotic of different receptor specificity (27). Morphine, the narcotic commonly used for epidural and intrathecal administration, binds primarily to mu receptors. After tolerance to intrathecal morphine developed in rats and primates, administration of DADL, a β-receptor ligand, induced significant analgesia (28). Respiratory depression in a morphine-tolerant cancer patient with an intrathecal bolus of DADL, reversed by naloxone, was recently reported (29).

Pharmacokinetics of intrathecally or epidurally administered opioids is affected by lipid solubility and ionization of the opioid in CSF. In comparing cisternal concentration of morphine and methadone after lumbar subarachnoid injections, morphine reached the cisternal CSF 180 min after injection, whereas methadone did not (30). The lipid solubility of methadone results from its rapid uptake into the spinal cord, leaving little in the CSF to move supraspinally. This results in more rapid, but shorter duration, analgesia with methadone in comparison to morphine.

Opioids can be administered intrathecally or epidurally in single doses, repetitive doses, or continuous infusion. Single-dose injection of morphine and β-endorphin in the intrathecal space at the second and third lumbar space induced peak analgesia in 30 min that lasted for periods averaging 20 hr (31, 32). Cancer patients who were not narcotic naive did not suffer from respiratory depression, hypotension, hypothermia, or catatonia. Chronic intraspinal or epidural opioid infusions can be accomplished by repetitive or continuous infusion into an open or closed system. A catheter can be implanted into the epidural or intrathecal space and connected into an Omaya reservoir or a custom device

(33). A high-precision pump with a 50-ml reservoir can be implanted subcutaneously (34). Chronic administration of epidural narcotics leads to tolerance. The average increase of intrathecal morphine dose over a 12-week period was 2–6.6 mg/day (35).

Acute complications include nausea, pruritus, respiratory depression, and urinary retention. Complications with chronic implantation include mechanical problems such as catheter displacement and development of CSF hygromas with fluid collection under the pump and along the catheter tract (34, 36). The use of chronic intrathecal or epidural opioid infusion seems to be ideal if the life expectancy is 2–3 months (37).

Patient-controlled analgesia is a new method for intravenous opioid delivery, where the patient is able to demand an opioid dose directly from a drug-dispensing system that will administer a preset dose of the opioid. By administering small doses by triggering a push-button device at frequent intervals, the patient can theoretically titrate analgesia against pain (38). Thus, PCA is innovative by providing individualized pharmacologic tailoring and patient autonomy. There are several PCA devices commercially available at present. Some ideal characteristics are ease of programmability, availability of a printout, and a sounding device that responds to both active or inactive trigger. Various narcotics have been administered to post-operative patients by this technique (39, 40). The use of PCA has also been compared between intravenous and epidural routes of narcotic administration (41).

MODULATION OF PAIN PATHWAY

Modulation of pain pathway in human beings is performed by stimulation of three sites: the periventricular/periaqueductal gray matter in the brain, the dorsal column in the spinal cord, and the periphery, by percutaneous stimulation (acupuncture) and transcutaneous electrical nerve stimulation (TENS). TENS and acupuncture are considered adjunctive mechanical treatments for malignant pain (see Table 33.4).

Deep brain stimulation has been mainly applied to therapy of chronic noncancer pain (42), and was thought to have minimal application to therapy of pain due to malignancy (43), since a majority of these patients have become tolerant to exogenous opiates. This impression is challenged by a recent study. Seventeen patients with intractable pain secondary to progressive malignancy and tolerant to high doses of systemic or epidural narcotics were treated with electrical stimulation of the brain (44). Thirteen of the 17 patients achieved virtually complete pain relief, and 13 patients withdrew themselves totally from the exogenous narcotics within 2 weeks of deep brain stimulation. This successful analgesia with deep brain stimulation in narcotic-tolerant patients may be secondary to a nonopioid mechanism and not due to the accepted opioid mechanism. There-

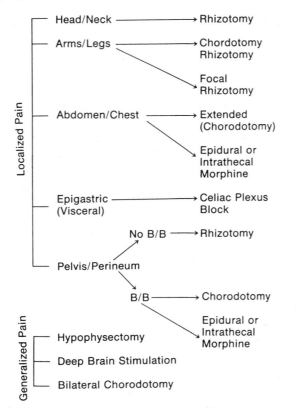

Figure 33.3. **Neuroinvasive procedures. Rhizotomy may be surgical or chemical. B/B = bladder and bowel function.**

fore, deep brain stimulation may be an excellent alternative for the relief of intractable pain due to malignancy, even in those unresponsive or tolerant to the analgesic effect of opiates.

Dorsal column stimulation has been used in patients with malignant pain, but is reported to have only 50% efficacy (45). Phantom pain appears to respond better to this treatment than pain due to peripheral nerve lesions and acute pain (46).

Peripheral stimulation-induced analgesia by TENS or acupuncture has not been adequately studied in patients with malignant pain. In a noncontrolled study, TENS was found effective in 96% of patients with malignant pain during the first 10 days, decreasing to 11% by the end of 1 month (47).

NEUROABLATIVE PROCEDURES

Neuroablation can be performed by chemical or neurosurgical techniques (see Fig. 33.3). Neurosurgical techniques for pain control have been covered in Chapter 17 and are not dealt with in this review, with two exceptions.

Neurosurgical Procedures

Two neurosurgical techniques warrant special attention since these procedures have been widely used for the management of malignant pain: percutaneous chordotomy and hypophysectomy.

Percutaneous chordotomy, the interruption of the ascending spinothalamic tract, is usually done with stereotaxic technique at the cervical or thoracic level. After needle position confirmation, a lesion can be made by radiofrequency. In patients with malignant pain, 80% efficacy is reported immediately after the procedure, but this deteriorates to 60% in just a few weeks (48). Chordotomy is ideal in patients with unilateral pain in a dermatomal level below T10–T12, but who still have intact bowel and bladder function, intact motor function, and a life expectancy of 6 months to 1 year. One must use caution in patients with restricted pulmonary function on the ipsilateral side of the pain, since the spinothalamic tract decussates contralaterally, whereas motor fibers do not. If motor fibers to the intercostal nerves on the opposite side are affected by the chordotomy, the remaining normal lung function can deteriorate.

Hypophysectomy has been recommended for the management of pain due to hormone-dependent prostate or breast cancer. This can be accomplished by a trans-sphenoidal approach with injection of various destructive substances such as alcohol, water, or yttrium (49–51). Success is quoted in between 74 and 94% of patients with malignant pain, but long-term studies to demise have not been carried out.

Chemical Neurolysis

The use of neurolytic blocks by injection of various concentrations of neurolytic agents into the epidural, intrathecal, ganglia, and peripheral nerves has been used for more than 50 years (52). The most common agents used are phenol or alcohol, the concentration and volume being dependent on the site of injection. The type of neurolytic block performed is dependent on the site of injection and the pathophysiology of pain (Table 33.5). Distinguishing between nociceptive and deafferentation pain must be accomplished by neurologic examination and differential nerve blocking procedure prior to chemical neurolysis.

Further deafferentation with neuroablation must be avoided if the cause of pain is due to previous deafferentation, since the pain may get worse 3–6 months later. Neurolysis can be used only if the classic pharmacologic treatment of deafferentation does not produce adequate pain relief, and if life expectancy is less than 3–6 months.

To understand fully the indications and limitations of neurolytic block, discussion of available neurolytic agents and the success and limitations of commonly used neurolytic blocks is necessary.

Alcohol is perhaps the longest used neurolytic agent, initially used by Daglioti in 1936. It is used in concentration of 50–100%, depending on the site of injection (Table 33.6). Phenol, on the other hand, is available in concentrations of 4–10%, dissolved in 10–100% glycerol (Table 33.6). The differences between these two agents are best shown when they are injected intrathecally. One

Table 33.5.
Choices for Neurolytic Block Sites

	Nociceptive pain	Deafferentiation pain
Head and neck	Somatic nerve block of peripheral nerves	Upper and middle cervical ganglion block
Upper extremities	Cervical epidural or intrathecal block	Stellate ganglion block
Chest wall and thoracic viscera	Intercostal nerve block	Thoracic epidural or intrathecal block
	Thoracic epidural/ intrathecal block	
Abdomen		
Viscera	Celiac plexus block	Celiac plexus block
Wall	Thoracic epidural/ intrathecal block	
	Intercostal nerve block	
Lower extremities	Intrathecal phenol	Lumbar sympathetic block
	Epidural/intrathecal morphine	
Perineal	Intrathecal block	Caudal block
	Intrathecal/epidural morphine	
	Caudal block	

Table 33.6.
Concentrations of Neurolytic Agents

	Alcohol	Phenol
Intrathecal	100%	4–15% in glycerol
Epidural	30%	10% in 10% glycerol
	100%	7% in water
Celiac plexus	50%	—
Sympathetic ganglion	50%	10% in 10% glycerol
Pituitary	100%	7% in water

hundred per cent alcohol is hypobaric and 4–5% phenol in absolute glycerin is hyperbaric in relationship to the CSF specific gravity. Therefore, when alcohol is used, the patient is positioned so that the dorsal roots to be blocked are in the most superior position (53). With phenol, the patient is positioned so that the dorsal roots to be blocked are in the most dependent position (54). Alcohol, on injection, produces burning pain, sometimes making it difficult for the patient to maintain their critical position. Phenol, on the other hand, is not painful on injection, and is better tolerated by the patient. Success rates for intrathecal phenol and alcohol do not differ significantly, ranging from 46 to 63% despite decades of use.

Complications of intrathecal neurolysis are primarily those of bladder, bowel, and motor paresis (55). If intact bladder and/or bladder function exists, epidural or intrathecal morphine or percutaneous chordotomy may be a more appropriate alternative.

Epidural neurolysis with phenol or alcohol has been introduced as an alternative to intrathecal block, especially indicated for wide segmental block (56). The ideal application of this technique is in patients with chest or abdominal trunk pain. Concentrations for alcohol used for epidural neurolysis range from 30 to 100%, and for phenol, 6–10%. Meaningful successful outcome of epidural neurolysis has not been adequately studied, but isolated reports indicate wide variations ranging from 33 to 90% success (54, 55, 57).

Another important neurolytic block for malignant pain that warrants special attention is celiac plexus block (58). Celiac plexus block is ideal for relief of malignant pain secondary to pancreatic carcinoma, retroperitoneal metastasis, peritoneal carcinomatoses, colon carcinoma, gastric carcinoma, and liver and spleen capsular distention. The needle is placed anterior to vertebral bodies T12–L1 under fluroroscopic guidance or CT scan and 40–50 ml of 50% alcohol are injected. The reported success rate ranges from 57 to 94% (58, 59).

Unfortunately, a majority of oncologists and surgeons are not aware of this procedure, and continue to manage their patients with narcotics, often aggravating impending colon obstruction with narcotic-induced ileus. Celiac plexus block can also be easily performed under direct vision during an exploratory laparotomy. This is particularly indicated if pancreatic carcinoma is diagnosed during exploration, since no oncologic therapy in the past 30 years has succeeded in prolonging the life expectancy of this group of patients.

ORCHESTRATION OF PHYSICAL TREATMENTS

To orchestrate the physical treatments available for malignant pain, one has to take into consideration several factors: life expectancy, natural history of the patient's malignancy, stage of the disease, rapidity of progression, and acceptability of procedures to the patient and family. Sensitivity to the patient's and family's goals and degree of acceptance of the progressive disease are of paramount importance in planning treatment. Since malignant pain can be stable, progressive, persistent, or recurrent at various stages, the physician placed in charge of controlling the pain should have a commitment to the patient until demise. Modalities should be made available to the patient for the persistent quest for pain relief.

Several principles useful for successful orchestration of modalities are:

1. Be sensitive to the changing needs of the patient as the disease progresses. Increased narcotic intake is associated with sudden progression of the disease, and not due to "addiction" potential in patients with malignant pain.
2. Start with a noninvasive, low-risk approach before proceeding to a more invasive, high-risk approach (see Fig. 33.1).
3. Relief of pain in one area may result in the awareness of pain in other areas.
4. The risk versus benefit ratio in every step should be explained to the patient and family, and the ultimate choice of alternatives be given to the patient.
5. Respect the patient's decision, even if it is not similar to yours. The ultimate goal of treatment is to provide comfort without sacrificing functions important to the patient and his/her family.

The orchestration of physical modalities is best illustrated by an actual case presentation. A 32-year-old female with cervical carcinoma metastatic to the sacral plexus and pelvic area was referred to the pain clinic because of persistent lower pelvic and perineal pain. The patient had undergone a total radical abdominal hysterectomy 4 months prior to admission, received radiation postoperatively, and was presently receiving chemotherapy. The patient still had intact bowel function, but had intermittent urinary incontinence. Computed tomography scan revealed a recurrent tumor anterior to the sacrum, beginning to erode into the sacral bone. The patient was receiving Tylenol with codeine, two tablets every 4 hr, whenever pain became severe. She was averaging 10–15 tablets/day; her pain decreased 30–40% for 2–3 hr after ingestion of the drug. She had become totally inactive, staying in bed most of the day. She took Valium (10 mg) at night for sleep, which only gave her 3–4 hr of sleep until she was awakened by the pain.

The first step in the treatment was analgesic tailoring. The patient was changed to the next step in the analgesic ladder (see Fig 33.2) and given Percocet, two tablets given on a time-contingent, around-the-clock approach. Valium was discontinued and substituted with amitriptyline, (25 mg before sleep). This maneuver immediately decreased her pain level to 25% as measured by the Visual Analog Scale, a level acceptable to her. She was able to increase her activity during the day, spending more time with her children.

Two months later, she developed acute herpes zoster in her neck and arm after receiving a chemotherapeutic regimen. She was treated with intravenous acyclovir and steroids, but the lesions and pain persisted. On the third week, stellate ganglion block was performed at 3-day intervals, with 0.5% lidocaine and 80 mg Depo-Medrol (60, 61). After three blocks, her lesions resolved and pain subsided dramatically.

The patient did well until 1 month later when her perineal and pelvic pain escalated, with Percocet no longer providing pain relief. Urinary incontinence became complete and an indwelling catheter was inserted. Computed tomography scan showed further erosion of the tumor into the anterior scaral table. The patient still maintained anal spincter control.

Percocet was discontinued and methadone (5 mg, q4h) was started. This provided 50% relief. An epidural catheter was inserted at the L4–L5 level and directed downward. Morphine (5 mg) was injected, producing pain relief for 17 hr. A neurosurgeon was consulted for implantation of an indwelling epidural catheter with a portacath. The patient and family were instructed on how to continue morphine injections into the portacath at home. The patient obtained satisfactory pain relief until 2 months later.

At that time, the dose of epidural morphine was escalated to 20 mg every 6 hr, and failed to produce adequate pain relief. Repeat CT scan revealed further progression of metastasis. Bowel spincter control was lost at this point. Intrathecal phenol injection was presented to the patient as an alternative and was accepted. Phenol (2 ml of 5% in absolute glycerol) was injected intrathecally with the patient in a sitting position, relieving 75% of her pain. She was taught how to use patient-controlled analgesia, and went home with a portable device. She died at home 1 month later, pain free.

REFERENCES

1. Foley KM: Pain syndromes in patients with cancer. In Bonica JJ, Ventafridda V (eds): *Advances in Pain Research and Therapy*. New York, Raven Press, 1979, vol 2, pp 59–75.
2. Wallenstein SL, Heidrich G, Kaiko R, et al: Clinical evaluation of mild analgesics: the measurement of clinical pain. *Br J Clin Pharmacol* 10(suppl):3195–3275, 1980.
3. Graham C, Bond SS, Gerkovich MM, et al: Use of the McGill Pain Questionnaire in the assessment of cancer pain: replicability and consistency. *Pain* 8:377–387, 1980.
4. Cohen R, Brechner T: The role and timing of neural blockade in the multidisciplinary management of cancer pain. In Gamez Q, Egay L (eds): *Proceedings of the 8th World Congress of Anesthesiology*. New York, Elsevier, 1984, pp 381–386.
5. Cleeland CS, Ratondi A, Brechner T, et al: A model for the treatment of cancer pain. 1:209–215, 1986.
6. Kanner RM, Foley KM: Patterns of narcotic drug use in cancer pain clinics. *Ann NY Acad Sci* 362:162–165, 1981.
7. Porter J, Jeck H: Addiction rate in patients treated with narcotics. *N Engl J Med* 302:123, 1980.
8. Foley KM: The treatment of cancer pain. *N Engl J Med* 313:84–95, 1985.
9. Moertel CC, Ahmann DL, Taylor WF, Schwartaul N: A comparative evaluation of marketed analgesic drugs. *N Engl J Med* 287:815–815, 1972.
10. Wallenstein SL: Analgesic studies of aspirin in cancer patients. In: *Proceedings of the Aspirin Symposium*. London, Aspirin Foundation, 1975, pp 5–10.
11. Houde RW, Wallenstein SL, Beaver WT: Clinical measure-

ment of pain. In deStevens G (ed): *Anglesics*. New York, Academic Press, 1965, pp 75–122.

12. Moertel CG, Ahmann DL, Taylor WF, et al: Relief of pain by oral medications: a controlled evaluation of analgesic combinations. *JAMA* 229:55–59, 1974.

13. Matts SGF: A clinical comparison of panadeine Co, a soluble codeine Co and soluble aspirin in the relief of pain. *Br J Clin Pract* 20:515–517, 1966.

14. Kaiko RF, Foley KM, Gabrinski PY, et al: Central nervous system excitatory effects of meperidine in cancer patients. *Ann Neurol* 13:180–185, 1983.

15. Ferrer-Brechner T, Ganz P: Ibuprofen (Motrin, ®) as an analgesic potentiator of methadone (Dolophene, ®) in cancer patients. *Am J Med* 77(1A):78–83, 1984.

16. Payne R, Max M, Inturrisi C, et al: *Principles of Analgesic Use in the Treatment of Acute Pain and Chronic Cancer Pain: A Concise Guide to Medical Practice*. Washington, DC, The American Pain Society, 1987.

17. Reidenberg MM: Central nervous system excitatory effects of meperidine in cancer patients. *Ann Neurol* 13:180–185, 1983.

18. Watson CT, Evans RV, Reed K, et al: Amitriptyline versus placebo in postherpetic neuralgia. *Neurology* 32:671–673, 1982.

19. Max MB, Culnane M, Schafer SC, et al: Amitriptyline relieves diabetic neuropathy pain in patients with normal or depressed mood. *Neurology* 37:589–596, 1987.

20. Swerdlow M: Anticonvulsant drugs and chronic pain. *Clin Neuropharmacol* 7:51–82, 1984.

21. Forrest WH, Brown BW, Brown CR, et al: Dextroamphetamine with morphine for the treatment of postoperative pain. *N Engl J Med* 296:712–715, 1977.

22. Slattery PJ, Boas RA: Newer methods of delivery of opiates for the relief of pain. *Drugs* 30:539–551, 1985.

23. Inturrisi C: Newer methods of opioid drug delivery. International Association for the Study of Pain, Refresher Courses, August 2, 1987, 27–39.

24. Coyle N, Mauskop A, Maggard J, et al: Continuous subcutaneous infusions of opiates in cancer patients with pain. *Oncol Nurs Forum* 13:53–57, 1986.

25. Gourlay GK, Plummer JL, Kowalski DA, et al: An evaluation of the pharmacokinetics and efficacy of transdermal fentanyl in the treatment of postoperative pain. *Pain Suppl* 4:S229, 1987.

26. Cousins MJ, Mather LE: Intrathecal and epidural administration of opioids. *Anesthesiology* 61:276–310, 1984.

27. Yaksh TL, Atchison SR, Durant PAC: Characteristics of action and pharmacology of intrathecally administered D-Ala²-D-Leu⁵-enkephalin. In Foley KM, Inturrisi CE (eds): *Advances in Pain Research and Therapy*. New York, Raven Press, 1986, vol 8, pp 303–314.

28. Lord JAH, Waterford AA, Hughes J, et al: Endogenous opioid peptides: multiple agonists and receptors. *Nature* 267:495–499, 1977.

29. Onofrio BM, Yaksh TL: Intrathecal delta-receptor ligand products analgesia in man. *Lancet* 1:1386–1387, 1983.

30. Payne R, Inturrisi CE: CSF distribution of morphine, methadone and sucrose after intrathecal injection. *Life Sci* 37:1134–1137, 1985.

31. Omaya T, Jen T, Yamaga R: Profound analgesic effects of endorphin in man. *Lancet* 1:122–124, 1980.

32. Wang JK, Nauss LA, Thomas JE: Pain relief by intrathecally applied morphine in man. *Anesthesiology* 50:149–151, 1979.

33. Poletti CE, Cohen AM, Todd DP, et al: Cancer pain relieved by long term epidural morphine with permanent indwelling systems for self administration. *J Neurosurg* 55:581–584, 1981.

34. Coombs, PW, Saunders RL, Pageau MG: Continuous intrapsinal opioid analgesia: technical aspects of an implantable infusion system. *Reg Anaesth* 7:110–113, 1982.

35. Coombs, DW, Saunders RL, Gaylor MS, et al: Relief of continuous chronic pain by intraspinal opioid infusion via an implanted reservoir. *JAMA* 250:2336–2339, 1983.

36. Greenberg HS, Layton PB, Schroeder, et al: Continuous intrathecal morphine for intractable cancer pain. *Neurology* 33(S2):226, 1983.

37. Greenberg H, Enssinger W, Taren J, et al: Benefit from and tolerance to continuous intrathecal infusion of morphine for intractable cancer pain. *J Neurosurg* 57:360–364, 1982.

38. Keeri-Szanto M, Heaman S: Postoperative demand analgesia. *Surg Gynecol Obstet* 134:647–651, 1972.

39. Harmer M, Slattery PS, Rosen M, et al: Intramuscular on demand analgesia: double blind controlled trial of pethedene, buprenorphine, morphine and meptazinal. *Br Med J* 286:680–682, 1983.

40. Kay B: Postoperative pain relief: use of an on-demand analgesia computer (ODAC) and a comparison of the rate of fentanyl and alfentanyl. *Anesthesia* 36:949–951, 1981.

41. Tamsen A, Sjoestroem S, Hartvig P: The Uppsala experience of patient controlled analgesia. In Foley KM, Inturrissi CE (eds): *Advances in Pain Research and Therapy*. Raven Press, New York, 1986, vol 8, pp 325–331.

42. Young RF, Feldman RA, Kroening R, et al: Electrical stimulation of the brain in the treatment of chronic pain in man. In Kruger L, Liebeskind JC (eds): *Advances in Pain Research and Therapy*. New York, Raven Press, 1984, vol 6, pp 289–303.

43. Mayerson BA, Boethius J, Carlsson AM: Alleviation of malignant pain by electrical stimulation in the periventricular-periaqueductal region: pain relief as related to stimulation sites. In Bonica JS, Liebeskind JC, Albe-Fessard D (eds): *Advances in Pain Research and Therapy*. New York, Raven Press, 1979, vol 3, pp 523–533.

44. Young RF, Brechner T: Electrical stimulation of the brain for relief of intractable pain due to cancer. *Cancer* 57:1266–1272, 1986.

45. Long DM, Erickson DE: Stimulation of the posterior columns of the spinal cord for relief of intractable pain. *Surg Neurol* 4(1):134–141, 1975.

46. Krainick JR, Thoden U: Experience with dorsal column stimulation (DSC) in the operative treatment of chronic intractable pain. *J Neurosurg Sci* 18(3):187–189, 1974.

47. Ventafridda V, Sganzeria EP, Fochi C, et al: Transcutaneous stimulation in cancer pain. In Bonica JJ, Ventafridda V (eds): *Advances in Pain Research and Therapy*. New York, Raven Press, 1979, vol 2, pp 509–515.

48. Rosumoff HF, Carrall F, Brown J, et al: Percutaneous radiofrequency cervical chordotomy technique. *J Neurosurg* 23:639, 1965.

49. Katz J, Levin AB: Treatment of diffuse metastatic cancer

pain by instillation of alcohol into the sella turcica. *Anesthesiology* 46(2):115–121, 1977.
50. Lipton S, Miles J, Williams N, et al: Pituitary injection of alcohol for widespread cancer pain. *Pain* 5(1):73–82, 1978.
51. Fitzpatrick JM, Gardiner RA, William JP, et al: Pituitary ablation in the relief of pain in advanced prostatic carcinoma. *Br Med J (Clin Res)* 284:75–76, 1981.
52. Swerdlow J: Subarachnoid and extradural neurolytic block. In Bonica JJ, Ventafridda V (eds): *Advances in Pain Research and Therapy.* New York, Raven Press, 1979, vol 2, pp 325–337.
53. Swerdlow M: Current views on intrathecal neurolysis. *Anesthesia* 33:733, 1978.
54. Ferrer-Brechner T: Epidural and intrathecal phenol neurolyses for cancer pain: review of rationale and techniques. *Reg Anaesth* 8(8):14–20, 1981.
55. Wood K: The use of phenol as a neurolytic agent: a review. *Pain* 5:205, 1978.
56. Colpitts MR, Levy BA, Lawrence M: Treatment of cancer-related pain with phenol epidural block (abstr). In *Proceedings of the World Congress on Pain,* Montreal, 1978. *Pain* Suppl 4, 1987.
57. Korevaar WC, Kline MT, Donnelly CC: Thoracic epidural neurolyses using alcohol. *Pain* Suppl 4:5133, 1987.
58. Thompson GE, Moore DC, Bridenbaugh LD, et al: Abdominal pain and alcohol celiac plexus nerve block. *Anesth Analg* 56(1):1–5, 1977.
59. Hankemeier U: Neurolytic celiac plexus block for cancer-related upper abdominal pain using the unilateral puncture technique and lateral position. *Pain* Suppl 4:135, 1987.
60. Tenicela R, Lovasek D, Eaglstein W: Treatment of herpes zoster with sympathetic blocks. *Clin J Pain* 1:63–67, 1985.
61. Perkins HM, Hanalon PR: Epidural injection of local anesthetic for the relief of pain secondary to herpes zoster. *Arch Surg* 113:253–254, 1978.

CHAPTER **34**

PSYCHOLOGICAL MANAGEMENT OF MALIGNANT PAIN

BLAKE H. TEARNAN
CLAY H. WARD

PAIN RELATED to cancer and its treatment is a national health problem (1). It has been estimated that hundreds of thousands nationally and millions worldwide are affected. Over 15% of patients with nonmetastatic cancer report significant pain. Depending on the type of cancer, as many as one-third of patients with metastatic disease and greater than two-thirds of terminally ill patients report pain severe enough to interfere with their social and physical activity and overall enjoyment of life (2). Cancer pain can also produce disturbances in sleep and appetite, causing adverse effects on the health status of patients.

The severity of the problem is reflected in the public's view of cancer as a very painful disease, equal to the pain caused by a myocardial infarction. Survey data suggest that a significant minority of patients would delay or avoid treatment because of expected pain (3). Most persons questioned indicated cancer pain would be a sufficient reason to end one's life. A recent survey of first-year medical students showed that 95% indicated that the vast majority of cancer patients experience pain, and nearly 40% of the students felt cancer pain was untreatable (4).

The psychological treatment of cancer pain requires a basic understanding of cancer and the physical basis of cancer pain. It is also important for the behavioral clinician to recognize the difference between assessment and treatment of chronic benign pain and pain of malignant origin. Cancer is a generic term that is used to describe a variety of different diseases that share in common the distortion of cell development leading to invasion of surrounding tissues and metastases. The primary site of cancer (e.g., lung, breast, prostate) determines many of its features, including rate of development, response to medical therapies, spread of disease, and the course, severity, and quality of pain. Foley found that 85% of patients with primary bone tumors,

52% of patients with breast cancer, 80% with cancer of the oral cavity, 75% of men and 70% of women with cancer of the genitourinary system, and 45% with cancer of the lung had pain, in contrast to 20% with lymphomas and only 5% with leukemias (6). Taken as a whole, nearly one-third of all hospitalized cancer patients have pain requiring the use of analgesics, and close to two-thirds of terminally ill patients report significant pain (7).

Cancer pain can result from diverse causes because of its multiple and primary metastatic sites. Foley reported that 78% of hospitalized cancer pain patients had pain due to direct tumor involvement, with 50% caused by bone involvement, 25% caused by nerve compression, and 3% due to invasion of hollow viscus (7). She discovered that only 19% of patients had iatrogenically produced pain (e.g., radiation, chemotherapy, and surgery). Similar results were found in patients with advanced cancer (8). Most patients had multiple mechanisms for their pain.

Cancer pain caused by nerve damage or compression is similar in many ways to nerve-related pain of benign origin (8). Treatment-related pain can resemble the neuropathic pain associated with diabetes. Tumor invasion of bone produces pain this is different from most noncancerous pain syndromes. Patients often describe this pain as severe and throbbing. Unfortunately, it appears to be the most difficult type of cancer pain to manage, even with multimodal therapies.

Cancer pain is usually better managed early in the course of the disease when pain is not present. As the disease progresses, pain problems increase. Daut and Cleeland found that only 6% of cancer patients with nonmetastatic disease reported pain, whereas 33% of patients with metastases had pain (2). The severity of the pain reported by patients with advanced disease is also generally higher than that of patients at initial diagnosis. Significant pain problems can occur early in the course of cancer, however. Greenwald, Bergner, and Renica reported on the prevalence and pain characteristics of four cancers (9). A very high proportion of their subjects were interviewed within 6 months of their initial diagnosis. They found that nearly 65% of patients reported their worst pain in the preceding week to be slight, moderate, or very bad and that about 45% reported pain they would characterize as moderate to bad at its worst. Approximately 35% of the respondents reported that their typical pain was moderate or very bad.

Interestingly, the authors found only a weak association between stage (progression) and pain prevalence. They suggested that most physicians alter their pain therapies to provide greater relief to patients with later-stage illness, and patients with postoperative pain in the early course of their disease may be experiencing pain more typical of untreated patients in advanced stages. They speculated that patients with early-stage disease might benefit from early, more-aggressive pain therapies.

Pain ratings of severity for the majority of cancer patients are moderate. Patients surveyed rated their pain at its worse close to the midpoint or lower on conventional pain scales. This contrasts with the widely held belief by health care providers and the general public that cancer is extremely painful (3). Comparing the severity of pain across different diseases, patients with metastatic cancer rated their worst pain at about the same level as patients with rheumatoid arthritis (2). Both the cancer and arthritic patients rated their worst pain at a significantly lower level than patients with chronic benign pain. Dalton and Feuerstein also found that patients with chronic noncancer pain reported lower pain intensity scores than cancer patients even though nearly 85% of the cancer patients had metastatic disease (10). The relationship between pain and life adjustment problems for patients with chronic benign pain is well known. Many of these patients report difficulties in their marriage, work, and recreational activities. They also admit to significant levels of depression and other mood disturbances (11). Surprisingly, cancer pain does not appear to be strongly related to psychosocial problems, negative mood in particular. In one study, patients with advanced disease and moderate to severe pain at initial contact were interviewed and completed ratings of pain severity, mood, and activity (12). Patients completed the same scales for 5 consecutive months. The relationships among pain ratings and mood measures were examined. A significant but small correlation between pain severity and measures of negative mood was found. More compellingly, patients with end-stage disease and poorly controlled pain reported very little mood disturbance at any assessment period, although these data suggest modest association between psychological variables and cancer pain. The absence of significant psychosocial problems speaks little to the role psychological variables may have had in mediating both a positive and a negative response to the pain patients experienced. There is ample evidence implicating the role of expectancy, affective distress, symptom interpretation, and perceived controllability in the perception and report of cancer pain (13). Few empirical studies have been conducted to demonstrate a consistent relationship, however (10).

Aside from the impact cancer pain may have on overall adjustment, there is significant evidence to show that cancer patients are at risk for developing problems including depression, marital stress, fatigue, body image concerns, and anxiety: in many patients these problems are enduring (14). The comprehensive assessment and treatment of the cancer pain patient should be directed at pain reduction and amelioration of significant psychosocial problems.

Most psychologically based therapies for cancer pain are based on a chronic benign pain model wherein the absence of progressive disease is assumed. The fundamental principles and goals of treatment are helpful to many patients with active disease. Cancer pain is unique in many ways, however, which suggests that many therapies currently being used to treat chronic benign pain do not apply or have to be qualified. For example, when pain is persistent but benign, complaints of pain can result in social alienation or may be reinforced by family members. Treatment efforts need to be aimed at discouraging the patient from reporting pain and teaching family members to ignore the patient's pain complaints. Continual reporting of pain that is benign and stable contributes little information that is diagnostically or therapeutically useful. Patients with cancer pain need to report pain, however, and medical staff and family members should listen to their complaints. New pain complaints can signal a change in disease status, and reporting of pain is a prerequisite for proper titration of analgesics.

This is not to imply that clinicians should throw the baby out with the bath water by ignoring the role that social reinforcement and other positive consequences play in exacerbating and maintaining cancer pain behavior. Instead of attempting to eliminate the reinforcement of all pain behaviors, however, distinguishing pain behaviors that are clearly inappropriate or excessive would be an alternative therapeutic goal.

Cancer pain therapies also differ in the use of increased physical activity, which is a mainstay in the rehabilitation of chronic benign pain. Encouraging cancer patients to increase their physical activity can be counterproductive. Some patients experience pain only when active. Patients in pain due to vertebral metastases may endanger themselves if physically active.

The meaning of pain for the cancer patient also differs. More than a reminder of chronic debilitation and discomfort, it represents the presence of a life-threatening disease. The anxiety and uncertainty this may generate can influence the total pain experience and make it more difficult for the patient to cope.

Perhaps the most significant difference is the role analgesic and palliative medications play in the relief of pain. Elimination of analgesic medications has been advocated as an appropriate treatment goal for chronic benign pain patients. This goal is motivated by concern about psychological addiction, physical dependence, and the depressant and mental-blurring effects of narcotics. Although it is beyond the scope of this chapter to examine the use of analgesics in chronic pain, it must be emphasized that reduction of the analgesics is rarely a goal for the patient with progressive malignant disease. Quite the contrary, patients need to be taught to recognize the role that analgesics play in pain control and how and when to take them. They also need to be taught how to request needed analgesics so that they are most likely to receive them.

Many cancer patients are undermedicated for pain (15, 16). Physicians are often reluctant to prescribe analgesics in effective doses because of concerns about addiction and the rapid development of narcotic tolerance and respiratory depression. Much of the problem of undermedication, however, has its basis in patient's beliefs and attitudes. For instance, patients may refuse to follow a medication schedule carefully designed to maintain effective blood levels of analgesics: instead, they take the medications only when pain is unbearable because they do not want to think of themselves as addicts. They may not wish to report that the medications they are taking are not effective because to do so would "bother the doctor." Some patients may want to avoid taking narcotics because of the belief that narcotic dependence is acknowledging that their disease is beyond hope (17).

The psychological management of cancer pain should never be used as a substitute for analgesics. Its use to ease staff's concern about narcotic addiction is rarely in the patient's best interest. If patients volunteer that they want to reduce their analgesics after some success with psychological management, this can be attempted on a trial basis following medical consultation.

Identifying patients appropriate for psychological intervention of cancer pain is a difficult task. There are no empirical guidelines to assist the clinician. Some clinicians have suggested that patients whose pain is adequately controlled by analgesics with few side effects are poor candidates for behavioral treatment. Few of them are motivated to expend the time and effort to learn behavioral methods. At the other extreme are patients with severe pain that limits their capacity to learn new skills. The best candidates appear to be patients with

moderate pain that is not adequately controlled by analgesics. Further research should help to clarify this issue as well as establish psychological variables as integral to the successful management of cancer pain.

ASSESSMENT OF THE PAIN PROBLEM

The aim of assessment is twofold. First, the clinician must pinpoint and define the entire domain of pain behaviors across cognitive, overt behavioral, and physiologic response dimensions. Second, stimuli associated with the occurrence and recurrence or exacerbation of the pain behavior need to be identified. This requires knowledge of frequently occurring controlling variables unique to cancer pain and attention to the multitude of factors that can affect the assessment process and influence a patient's report of pain.

Inherent in this approach to assessment is the recognition that cancer pain is not directly linked to nociceptive input. Factors other than underlying pathology are important contributors to the pain experience and need to be understood within a multidimensional context.

RESPONSE DIMENSIONS

Cognitive Responses

The assessment of cancer pain requires an understanding of the patient's cognitions, including an analysis of cognitive errors and self-statements. Cognitive errors refer to maladaptive patterns of thinking that are unrealistic and distorted. They are assumed to be causally related to the maintenance and exacerbation of the pain complaint and can interfere with treatment. Cancer pain patients can present several different types of cognitive errors. Frequently observed are thoughts that they can do nothing to reduce their pain, that they should have better control over their pain, that pain is inevitable and should be tolerated. Self-statements are thoughts patients may have regarding their pain, such as "the pain is frightening," or "it hurts so bad." Self-statements are internal dialogues patients have that reflect the cognitive appraisal of their pain state. Self-statements differ from cognitive errors in that they have not been analyzed to represent some underlying belief system or faulty logic such as "I will never be able to overcome this problem." Both cognitive errors and self-statements can be assessed during the interview by direct questioning, but often the most reliable method is to have patients self-monitor their pain and thoughts. The patient is instructed to use pain diaries to record any thoughts or feelings that accompany the pain when it is at its worst (18). The thought that pain signals an increase in spread of cancer may not be a cognitive error per se, but still can be challenged on the grounds that many factors influence pain perception.

Overt Behavioral Responses

The pain behavior of cancer patients can include the verbal and nonverbal responses patients use to communicate the experience of pain, such as facial grimacing, limping, bracing, and groaning. Estimates of physical activity are also useful. Measures of time spent in bed, physical exercise, amount of housework, and the like have all been employed with chronic pain patients (19). Because cancer patients may be physically disabled as a result of their disease or the effects of treatment, the use of activity measures should be limited to the range of behaviors in which patients are physically capable of engaging but that are restricted because of pain.

The amount and type of pain medication use is another overt behavioral measure of pain this is frequently reported. The milligram dosage per day and the specific type of palliative drug prescribed or taken should be recorded. Analgesic orders vary with practice setting, and patients may not accurately report levels of pain to their physicians. Patients do not always take the medications as prescribed; consequently the reliability of medication use as a measure of the pain experience is questionable.

Overt pain behavior can be collected through direct observation by others such as nursing personnel, other therapists, and the patient's significant others. Simple rating sheets can be constructed for use on a time-sampling basis, or the behaviors can be recorded at the end of a specific period. Unfortunately, systematic ratings can be costly in terms of observation time, interference with other procedures, and training observers to an acceptable reliability criterion. Although recording sheets used once daily are more convenient and practical, there is some loss of reliability due to memory interference.

The self-report of overt pain behaviors can also be gathered. This includes the self-monitoring of pain behaviors or information obtained from pain behavior inventories or by interview. The problem of reliability with any self-report instrument is well known; these measures are easily obtainable, economical, and sometimes the only instruments used, however, especially with cancer patients. One very useful self-report measure of overt pain behavior is the rating of how much pain interferes with activity levels. It has been shown to be significantly correlated with mood, pain intensity, and physical disability in cancer patients (5).

It deserves mention that any self-report instrument used with cancer patients should be simple and brief. Many patients are quite ill and obtunded because of their disease or high narcotic doses and will not be able to follow complicated instructions, or will be too fatigued to complete lengthy measures. An additional reason for simplicity is patient compliance. Patients do not always share the clinician's enthusiasm for comprehensive data bases.

Sensory-Physiologic Responses

The final response system is physiologic. Measures of heart rate, muscular activity, respiration, and other responses have been used to estimate autonomic arousal and pain severity. Unfortunately, the usefulness of these measures, with the possible exception of muscular activity, is of questionable value, especially in chronic pain. Most reports have not shown a clear relationship between physiologic measures and degree of pain (20).

Instead, clinicians have relied on patients' descriptions of the sensory-physiologic aspects of their pain, including intensity, temporal aspects, location, and quality (21). Intensity measures are usually simple numeric rating scales of subjective pain intensity. They normally require the patient to rate his or her average, worst, least, and present pain on a 10-point scale or an equivalent visual analogue scale without numeric anchors during a specific period such as the last week or month. The temporal aspects of the patient's pain are usually assessed for frequency and duration. Most cancer patients will complain of constant, daily pain. Fluctuations in the pain most likely occur and should be documented, however. Location parameters of the pain are collected by having patients shade the location of their pain on the front and back of human figures, or simply by describing where the affected area is located. The patient can be asked to indicate if the pain is deep or shallow. Finally, the measure of pain quality is obtained by asking patients to describe their pain using words such as "burning," "stabbing," and "cramping."

Pain quality ratings have been shown to be a useful alternative to assessing pain intensity with cancer patients. Tearnan and Cleeland found that cancer patients who reported high levels of pain intensity tended to use certain sensory words such as "sharp," "gnawing," and "pressing" more frequently than patients who rated their pain intensity lower (22). In addition, it was found that without the aid of word lists as prompts, patients' word usage overall was limited to a few sensory descriptions. Very few evaluative words and virtually no affective descriptors were used.

Physiologic data can be obtained with the use of sophisticated instrumentation such as electromyographic recordings. Usually, however, patients are simply asked to describe their pain and its location or they are instructed in self-monitoring. Again, the use of some procedures is limited with cancer patients. A great deal depends on the physical status of the patient, as well as what is permissible and appropriate in the setting in which the cancer patient is being treated. Early interventions are important in terms of establishing baselines and learning skills that will be useful when pain levels are more severe. One method of collecting ongoing pain intensity ratings as well as other measures of pain by nursing and additional health care staff for use with inpatients is to place a recording sheet directly in the patient's chart with clear instructions (23).

PAIN PRECIPITATORS

One of the most important aspects of assessment is examining the relationships among the exacerbation of pain and various cognitive, behavioral, physiologic, emotional, and environmental stimuli that aggravate or trigger the pain state. Clinicians using numerous examples of verbal and imaginal prompts to systematically explore potential cognitive antecedents will yield more than those who ask the simple question, "Are there any thoughts or images that seem to make your pain worse?" Examples of cognitive antecedents cancer patients have identified include images of fire, a red-hot poker, or a sharp knife, and thoughts that the pain is all-consuming and out of control and nothing can be done to control it, as well as "I must be weak-minded because I cannot tolerate the pain." Many cognitive antecedents will also be useful in defining the cognitive response of pain. Whether they should be included as antecedent stimuli is based on the presumption that they may also exacerbate or trigger the pain state.

By far the largest category of antecedent stimuli are behaviors cancer patients engage in that contribute to the onset or worsening of pain. These behaviors can include certain bodily movements such as bending, twisting, coughing, and reaching as well as activities such as walking, getting out of bed, eating, standing, and sitting. Cancer patients with vertebral metastases will experience pain with many movements and may have to confine themselves to bed because of the dangers of fracture, whereas patients with prostatic disease may experience pain whenever they engage in weight-bearing activities. Each cancer patient will differ, and only a thorough assessment will uncover the particular behaviors that contribute to the experience of pain.

Physiologic pain precipitants include the disease, but also disease- and treatment-related adverse effects that make patients more vulnerable or intolerant to pain sensation. For example, fatigue, nausea, weakness, and dry mouth are commonly observed. In addition, the ingestion of stimulants or other substances can substantially alter biochemistry and modify the pain response.

Emotional upset can also be related to the patient's pain complaint. It is well understood that anxiety and depression can alter the experience of pain. The cancer patient who has just been informed that his or her disease has progressed and metastasized to another location will undoubtedly be anxious and report higher levels of pain, especially because the pain can serve as a constant reminder of the disease process. Questions that elicit information about changes in intensity and suffering in relation to emotional arousal need to be a standard part of the assessment protocol. It is interesting

that a recent study by Dalton and Feuerstein showed little relationship between levels of trait anxiety and pain intensity ratings for cancer patients (24). A significant correlation between trait anxiety and composite pain score was observed in a group of chronic noncancer patients, however. Obviously, this finding needs to be replicated because it is at odds with a wealth of data demonstrating the connection between pain and heightened emotional activity.

Environmental factors can often precipitate pain, and many are unique to the hospital setting. For example, patients may complain that their pain seems to worsen when they are alone or when the doctors are making their rounds. Frequently, patients state that their pain is hardest to cope with when they are not comfortable because their bed is cold or too hard or there is too much noise in the hallways for them to rest properly (23). Staff or family behaviors can also be correlated with pain and should be assessed.

Antecedent events must be operationally defined and reliability must be understood between clinician and patient and/or staff. Simplicity and specificity are the rules of a good behavioral description. Too often patients and staff are asked to monitor pain and not the presence or absence of antecedent events without being sure what to look for.

COPING STRATEGIES

It is also important to identify the behaviors that patients engage in to cope with pain. This is important because coping strategies may provide clues to the maintenance of the pain problem and frequently occurring complications of cancer pain such as depression. Tearnan and Lewandowski found that chronic benign pain patients who relied on passive coping modalities, such as hoping or praying the pain will go away and using pain medication, tended to complain of significantly higher levels of anxiety, depression, activity avoidance, maladaptic beliefs, and overall impairment than patients who used more active methods of managing their pain (e.g., stretching) (25). Other researchers have also found that passive methods of coping with pain are related to impairment. There is also a strong association between the tendency to catastrophize and avoidance of activities because of pain, depression, and maladaptive beliefs about pain (25). Although the coping strategies of cancer patients have not been examined closely, similar findings most likely exist.

Coping strategies should be assessed across similar categories used to systematically explore pain antecedents. That is, the cognitive, behavioral, and physiologic strategies for managing pain should be examined. These can include self-statements, ignoring the pain, praying, and distraction. Behavioral coping strategies can include bed rest, physical or social activities as distractors, use of heating pads, ice, and warm baths. Medication and alcohol are common physiologic methods used to diminish pain. The type and amount of mediation must always be assessed.

Self-monitoring is an effective method of gathering information concerning pain coping strategies. Questionnaires and direct interviewing can produce useful information, however.

CONSEQUENCES

The immediate consequences of the patients' pain behavior need to be assessed to determine if medical staff or significant others are reinforcing behaviors that are clearly inappropriate or excessive. Spouses who are solicitous and pay more attention to pain behaviors will obviously impact the pain experience differently than spouses who punish or ignore their spouses reports of pain. It will be recalled that most pain behaviors emitted by cancer patients should be attended to because pain can signal new or recurrent disease, and communication of pain is necessary for the titration of analgesics. Pain behaviors that foster unneeded dependency and helplessness or seem unreasonable may be targets for later intervention, however. The differentiation of maladaptive pain behaviors and appropriate pain responses is very important in cancer pain patients.

The patient might also engage in certain behaviors that could reinforce or punish wellness behaviors. For example, cancer pain patients who overextend themselves physically, causing their pain to increase sharply, may avoid engaging in the activity in the future.

ONSET, HISTORY, AND DEVELOPMENT

A thorough assessment strategy should examine the onset, history, and development of the pain complaint. This information is important because it helps the clinician put the problem in perspective and may lead to the discovery of antecedent stimuli that were overlooked. The knowledge of previous therapy attempts is also important to know because steps need be taken to correct the inadequacies of past failures and build on previous successes. Analyzing the development of the patient's pain problem will provide clues regarding past coping attempts and over what time frame changes in the pain occurred.

OTHER COMPLICATIONS

Cancer pain can produce adverse changes in mood, work, family, physical activity, and interpersonal relationships (5). These are areas that need to be routinely evaluated to determine the overall impact of the pain problem on the patient's life. These changes, if pronounced, can compromise the patient's response to medical treatment and interfere significantly with the quality of life. They can also amplify the pain experience. Ratings of pain interference in mood, pleasant activities, and overall enjoyment of life can be used in ad-

dition to more-traditional assessment tools. Interviews with significant others can also provide worthwhile information regarding the impact pain has had on the family and marriage. The patient's psychosocial history of coping with other problems is an important factor to consider in terms of understanding how they will respond to pain, health care professionals, and family members. It is usually more beneficial to build on the patient's strengths because cancer patients are rarely motivated to change major aspects of their personality.

FORMULATION

Formulating a treatment plan and making predictions regarding the patient's response to intervention is the final step in the assessment process. This is accomplished by generating several hypotheses about the onset, development, and maintenance of the patient's pain complaint and proposing a treatment intervention based on these conclusions that would most likely result in the desired change. For instance, cancer patients who report that anxiety exacerbates their pain, and report diminished pain after receiving diazepam, might be good candidates for relaxation/biofeedback therapy.

INSTRUMENTS

Numerous instruments can assist the clinician in the assessment process. Some have been designed specially for pain assessment, and others are used primarily for determining the patient's level of mood and personality disturbance. Most are self-report measures. Cancer patients are often unable to complete a comprehensive test battery or lengthy test, such as the Minnesota Multiphasic Personality Inventory 2 (MMPI-2), because of their medical status. The best assessment tool for this population is one that can be easily understood with minimal instructions and is relatively short. It should require little administrative supervision by staff. The health care staff should find the instrument useful and easily interpretable. Finally, it should include items that sample pain behaviors as well as mood disturbance.

The Pain Research Group at the University of Wisconsin Medical School developed the Wisconsin Brief Pain Inventory (BPI) for the specific purpose of administration to cancer pain patients (26). The BPI is a short questionnaire that usually requires only 10 min for the patient to complete. It includes several types of items such as whether or not the patient has had any surgery in the last month; front and back human figures with instructions for the patient in pain to shade the painful area; numeric ratings of worst, average, least, and present pain intensity; requests for the patient to describe any pain diminishers or antecedents that have been associated with pain relief or exacerbation; current pain treatments; and questions regarding response to treatment. In addition, the patient is also instructed to rate several pain adjectives, such as "throbbing" and "burning," on a scale of 0 to 10. Another section of the questionnaire includes several items that ask patients how much they feel their pain has interfered with their mood, general activity, walking ability, normal work, relations with other people, sleep, and enjoyment of life. Finally, the questionnaire contains a shortened version of the Profile of Mood States (POMS) that has been shown to be statistically equivalent to the complete scale (27). The POMS was included to screen for mood disturbance. The BPI has demonstrated respectable validity and reliability and has been shown to be a useful pre- and post-treatment measure (26).

GENERAL ISSUES

Several other issues need to be considered and addressed when assessing the cancer pain patient. These matters can significantly affect an evaluation, and unless the clinician is cognizant of their presence they can lead to spurious conclusions and/or disrupt the assessment process.

Setting

Most cancer patients in pain are inpatients or outpatients at medical centers. They are receiving ongoing cancer therapy or palliative care, or are being evaluated periodically for recurrence of their disease. In most cases when conventional therapy fails to relieve pain, a member of a liaison service specializing in pain is requested to consult. The role of a consultant in a medical setting is that of an expert who is expected to render an opinion quickly without consuming too much of the patient's time. Under these circumstances, lengthy procedures are unsuitable because the consultant often has to present recommendations after only one session. This necessitates a streamlined version of an ideal assessment. If the consultant is expected to treat the patient, he or she can afford more elaborate procedures but is still limited by the brief residence of inpatients and by the physical and mental incapacitation of many cancer patients.

The clinician should be sensitive to the patient's primary care providers, who may not share their enthusiasm for psychological control of pain and may see the intervention as an interference. Unfortunately, these negative opinions can sometimes be communicated to the patient and compliance can be reduced. Frequent physician updates on the patient's progress and rationale for particular assessment and treatment protocols can help eliminate many obstacles.

Overcoming a Reluctance to Participate

Cancer pain patients are medical patients. Often the patient's beliefs about the role of a psychologist or other behavioral clinician run counter to their expectations for being treated for medical problems. As a result, some patients are reluctant to participate in assessment or treatment. DeGood discussed practical ways in which

to overcome this barrier and increase compliance with chronic pain patients (28). His suggestions can be applied to cancer patients in pain. In brief, he first explains to patients that he is a psychologist and reassures them that often pain produces changes in one's life that can affect work, mood, and so forth. According to DeGood, this usually helps to de-escalate the implicit message that "the referral was because the doctor thinks the pain is all in my head." Although the credibility of cancer patients is rarely questioned regarding the organic basis of their pain, they may have a history of diagnostic procedures in which nothing was discovered, and may believe that the severity of the pain and their inability to tolerate it is related to psychological weakness. DeGood mentions that this initial explanation also helps challenge the belief that because psychological variables may be correlated with the exacerbation of pain this makes the physical problem less legitimate.

DeGood recommends that the interview initially focus on physical symptoms. This helps reduce the defensiveness of the patient and establish the credibility of the behavioral clinician. He advised that when assessing other aspects of the pain complaint, such as depression, these topics be introduced with a statement to the effect that "pain often makes us feel. . . ." Patients are often reluctant to admit to emotional problems because doing so confirms the belief that something is wrong mentally. Finally, we have found that cancer patients need to be assured that their participation in no way indicates that their medical therapy, including the use of analgesic medications, will be jeopardized.

Factors Affecting the Report of Pain

Numerous factors can influence a patient's report of pain. The clinician should be familiar with the more frequently occurring factors because they can significantly affect how cancer patients communicate their pain. For instance, the patient's history can influence how pain is reported. Patients who have received support in the past from health care professionals for their pain problem and for requesting medication will be more inclined to admit to pain.

Often cancer patients are reluctant to report pain because of beliefs that discourage disclosure (5). One study found that many cancer patients do not complain of pain because they believe there is a social stigma attached to people who do (29). Other patients admit that they do not want to bother their doctor or distract him or her from medical treatment. Our society also reinforces the notion that a good patient does not complain when in pain, and a complainer is one who has lost self-control. Unfortunately, health care professions sometimes directly reinforce these beliefs (23).

The nature of the pain itself can also influence a patient's report. A patient who has severe pain may be more motivated to admit to pain and request medications than patients experiencing mild or moderate pain. Yet, certain pain locations, such as rectal or genital areas, can discourage reports of pain because of personal embarrassment (30). Patients will generally acknowledge pain more readily if it is constant as opposed to episodic. The expectation of pain-free periods can increase the patient's tolerance level (23). Finally, patients experiencing significant interferences in mood and physical activity because of their pain may be more likely to communicate their experience.

The stage of disease may also affect the report of pain. Abrams wrote an intriguing paper in which she observed that cancer patients are less likely to communicate to others as their disease progresses (31). She found that newly diagnosed patients are optimistic and hopeful concerning treatment and anxiety is lessened by direct answers to questions. As the disease advances, there is a change in what patients desire to know and to whom they direct their questions. Patients sometimes develop a fear of abandonment by their physician that is manifested in becoming compliant and uncomplaining. In the terminal stages, communication becomes minimal and support from others is more important. Although Abrams did not address the issue of pain communication specifically, the points she raised certainly have many implications for pain assessment.

Other variables influencing the pain report of cancer and chronic pain patients that have been mentioned in the literature include neuroticism (32), level of awareness and education (33), depression and chronicity (34), use of certain medications (35), desire to manipulate treatment (36), and staff support of pain complaints (35). Each of these factors should be considered in the assessment process.

PSYCHOLOGICAL TREATMENT APPROACHES

Psychological interventions have received increasing attention in the management of cancer pain (37–40). These approaches are similar to psychological treatments used in the management of chronic, nonmalignant pain. The application of therapies shown to be effective in the management of chronic, nonmalignant pain to the management of cancer pain is a logical extension of theory and clinical practice. There appears to be fewer distinctions than once thought for psychological interventions between benign and malignant pain (13); however, it should be reemphasized that cancer pain is distinct in many ways. Consequently, treatments shown to be effective in treating chronic, nonmalignant pain cannot be assumed to be equally efficacious in treating cancer pain. The purpose of this section is to discuss treatment-related issues and briefly outline psychological approaches that appear to have promise in the management of cancer pain. There is still a paucity of empirical literature to support the efficacy of any particular psychological intervention in the management of cancer pain. We believe that enhancement of existing medical pain control techniques will be the most important impact of psychological pain control techniques for cancer patients.

Psychological cancer pain control techniques can be implemented by individuals with a wide variety of professional backgrounds who have appropriate training and a core of interpersonal skills typically associated with successful behavioral change (41). Our experience indicates that oncology nurses can be readily trained to effectively teach and implement the majority of psychological pain control techniques. Hypnosis might be the exception that is reserved for induction by professional psychological or other specially trained staff, but even this restriction is based more on caution than common sense or empirical evidence.

Training of staff members in psychological pain management should include an educational component covering psychological assessment, conceptualization, and treatment of cancer pain; a skills acquisition and rehearsal component with behavioral modeling, rehearsal, feedback, and reinforcement of practice; and training in general factors of behavior change and psychotherapy. Once treatment is implemented, follow-up consultations are important so that treatment effectiveness can be measured and, if necessary, adjustments in the treatment plan can be recommended. Ongoing assessment and evaluation of treatment effectiveness is especially important given the complex nature and changing clinical presentation of cancer pain.

Ongoing assessment and evaluation also is important from another perspective. An assessment that fails to consider ongoing changes in disease, person, or situation variables is often responsible for treatment failure. The spectrum and variety of cancer pain patients necessitates the understanding of the temporal setting and origin of the pain in order to determine the most effective therapeutic approach (6). It is the selection and combination of psychological pain control techniques tailored to the specific characteristics of the individual cancer pain patient that determines successful intervention.

Cancer pain patients experience both acute and chronic pain that may be due to the disease itself and/or its treatment. At least four different types of cancer pain patients can be identified, each with different treatment requirements (6, 38). One group consists of *patients with no active disease but chronic, persistent post-treatment pain*. These patients are free of active disease, but may have pain due to postsurgical scarring, neuropathy induced by chemotherapy, or postradiation myelopathy or fibrosis. Because the disease has been arrested, these patients are not good candidates for continued narcotic medications. Instead, the treatment approach should be similar to interventions used for patients with chronic, nonmalignant pain.

Patients with acute treatment-related pain or those preparing for cancer therapy that will produce pain represent a second group of pain patients. Pain in these patients is often adequately controlled by properly prescribed analgesics (6). Some will experience pain that is refractory to traditional medical management, however, or the patient might have problems with the medication side effects. Psychological approaches to pain control might be of benefit to this subgroup of patients. In addition, psychological approaches might also be useful for reducing anticipatory anxiety with patients undergoing painful and frightening treatment procedures.

A third group of cancer patients are *those with chronic pain due to active disease with a prognosis of at least several months.* Patients with an indefinite prognosis are often good candidates for psychological pain-control techniques. Most individuals in this group are receiving narcotic and other analgesic drugs. They may want to continue working or managing their households, continue with avocational activities, and/or have an active family life. To stay active, they may want to reduce their use of analgesic medications to minimize side effects, primarily mental blurring. Many will elect to learn psychological control techniques to increase their sense of control over some aspect of their disease. Some patients might also want to manage other areas of disease-related discomforts such as nausea, sleep disturbances, and procedurally related anxiety. Unlike the patient with arrested disease, but like the patient preparing for painful treatment procedures, the appropriate use of narcotic medication is important. Issues of addiction, tolerance, dependence, scheduling, and sufficient plasma levels needs to be reviewed on an individual basis.

A fourth group of patients are *those in the terminal stages of illness.* With this group of patients, it is very important to review all available medical management techniques for potential benefit to the individual. Psychological pain-control techniques may still be useful, but it is important to recognize factors that might limit the applicability of some techniques. The patient's memory and concentration is often impaired by brain metastases, medications, emotional distress, and fatigue. There will often not be sufficient time to teach psychological pain management techniques unless the process was begun at an earlier stage of disease.

Which psychological pain control techniques are most effective for each group of cancer pain patients is uncertain. With the exception of patients in the terminal stages of illness, most psychological approaches to pain management seem applicable.

PSYCHOTHERAPY

Psychotherapy as an approach to pain control is based on the assumption that the perception of pain occurs within a personal and interpersonal context. The general premise is that dealing with critical intra- and inter-personal issues will reduce the impact of pain. It has been argued that psychotherapy aimed at relieving the emotional distress, anxiety, or depression associated with either the diagnosis of cancer or cancer pain can often have a favorable influence on the patient's experience of pain (37, 40, 42). The management of psychiatric aspects of cancer pain has received increasing attention in the medical literature (43, 44). The advantage of psychological interventions is that there are usually no negative side effects.

Suggested psychotherapy techniques include education and reality orientation, support, reassurance, encouragement, group and family therapy, and activities designed to facilitate enrichment of remaining time such as activities planning and participation, goal setting, and positive expectations. Unfortunately, there is no direct empirical evidence for the benefits of psychotherapy in reducing cancer pain. Psychotherapy and psychosocial interventions have been shown to be effective in ameliorating emotional distress and improving the quality of life (45–48); however, the direct effect of such interventions on cancer pain has not been demonstrated.

HYPNOSIS

Hypnosis is probably the oldest and most widely used psychological approach to pain management for cancer patients. Numerous clinical reports have appeared in the literature over the last three decades to support its efficacy in treating cancer pain (49–56). Hypnosis has also been reported to be effective in treating emotional distress, anxiety, or treatment-related discomfort in cancer patients (57). Although the literature reports that 20–50% of cancer patients benefit from hypnosis (40), this evidence is largely anecdotal and based on uncontrolled studies.

Hypnotic pain-reduction techniques overlap somewhat with relaxation and cognitive-behavioral techniques. The five major techniques that have been used for analgesia and the treatment of cancer pain are anesthesia, direct diminution, sensory substitution, displacement, and dissociation (58, 59). The technique of anesthesia refers to hypnotic suggestions that render a body area numb and insensitive to pain.

Direct diminution and sensory substitution are techniques that change the meaning of pain so that it is less important and painful. Direct diminution employs suggestions that focus on the lessening of the intensity of the pain. These suggestions often use metaphors, such as "turning down the volume" or "dimming the brightness." Sensory substitution also tries to modify painful stimuli, but the suggestions focus more on creating a sensory substitution or reinterpretation of the sensation. For example, the painful sensation might be reinterpreted as a sensation such as coldness, tingling, or itching. Barber indicated that both of these techniques are effective and easier to use than anesthesia because they allow the patient to still know the pain is present, and the sensations are not necessarily pleasant (59). Consequently, the suggestion seems more plausible to the patient. Barber also argues that these techniques are most effective when the suggestions incorporate the qualities of the patient's subjective experience of pain. We have found this technique to be beneficial when the location of the pain has secondary psychological meaning, such as breast cancer pain.

Displacement suggestions are used to displace the pain from one body area to another. The applicability of this technique is limited primarily to pain that is well localized and painful by virtue of its localization. A change in the quality or intensity is sometimes achieved by changing the location. This technique can be very useful for patients in terminal stages.

Dissociation refers to hypnotic suggestions to create a sense of dissociation from the pain. Often this technique is used with individuals confined to a bed. The suggestions are used to dissociate the body of pain from the patient's awareness. Patients are still able to perceive and describe the pain, but there is less affective involvement and it is less distressing.

Post-hypnotic suggestions and self-hypnosis are additional techniques that are used to extend the pain relief. These techniques appear useful in rehabilitation where the goal is to maintain activity levels. Post-hypnotic suggestions attempt to establish a cue that initiates the pain-relief experience. For example, one suggestion might instruct the patient that whenever they think about a particular activity they "will discover at the same time how comfortable and relaxed they really feel." Other post-hypnotic suggestions are based on functional cues, such as the perception of pain. Self-hypnosis is thought to be especially effective in creating long-term pain relief (59).

Despite numerous shortcomings, including the absence of comparison groups, a few studies examining the use of hypnosis in the treatment of cancer pain deserve mention. An early uncontrolled study by Butler showed that 5 out of 12 patients benefitted from hypnosis, and that depth of trance was the critical factor in determining the effectiveness of hypnosis in relieving pain (60). Depth of trance and a high degree of hypnotic susceptibility have been cited by others as important in hypnotic pain relief (61, 62). Finer, however, suggested that depth of trace is not important, but that susceptibility is the major determinant of effectiveness (63). Susceptibility is often uncertain and difficult to predict without actually hypnotizing the patient (63). Clearly, research is needed to resolve the role of depth of trance and individual differences in susceptibility in the use of hypnosis to treat cancer pain.

Kellerman et al. used a hypnotic induction with suggestions of muscle relaxation, rhythmic breathing, and pleasant imagery (64). When their subjects appeared to be deeply relaxed, they gave post-hypnotic suggestions of reduced discomfort, greater mastery during painful medial procedures, and an increased sense of well-being. Based on self-report, the hypnosis was effective in reducing anxiety and discomfort in 16 adolescents undergoing painful medical procedures. Unfortunately, there were no objective behavioral observations of anxiety or discomfort during the procedures and no control groups.

Zelter and LeBaron presented data from a controlled study on the use of hypnosis in pediatric cancer patients undergoing bone marrow aspirations and lumbar puncture (65). Their study included both subjective self-report and objective ratings of anxiety and pain. They compared hypnosis consisting of imagery and fantasy to a nonhypnotic technique of deep breathing, distraction, and practice sessions. Both treatment procedures were effective in reducing pain and anxiety, but hypnosis was significantly more effective.

A study by Spiegal and Bloom evaluated the effectiveness of hypnosis in treating disease-related breast cancer pain (66). Patients were randomly assigned to a control group, a weekly support group, or a support group with self-hypnosis exercises. The difference between support groups was a weekly training session in self-hypnosis lasting 10–15 min that used sensory substitution by having the patients imagine competing sensations in the affected areas. Self-report measures of pain at 4- and 13-month follow-ups revealed that the self-hypnosis group had the lowest pain ratings. Conclusions regarding the superiority of self-hypnosis are tempered by the facts that both treatment groups showed smaller increases in pain over time compared to the control group and that direct statistical analyses of group means was not reported, however. Thus, the results suggest that psychological interventions, including self-hypnosis, are effective, but little can be concluded about the comparative benefits of hypnosis.

As stated earlier, controlled studies on the effectiveness of hypnosis in treating cancer pain are lacking. Furthermore, available studies are deficient in ways that limit conclusions regarding the effectiveness of hypnosis in treating cancer-related pain. In addition to the problems common to most research on psychological approaches to cancer pain, such as the absence of control groups and failure to use multimodal and objective pain measures, there are several difficulties specific to hypnosis. A major problem is the lack of standardized and clearly defined hypnotic induction and therapeutic techniques. Hilgard and Hilgard have suggested that research on hypnosis should measure hypnotic susceptibility prior to treatment, clearly define and delineate hypnotic inductions and therapeutic techniques, and use more objective, multimodal measures (53). A measure of depth of trace would also be useful.

RELAXATION TRAINING

There are several techniques for inducing a state of physiologic and mental relaxation, ranging from passive techniques such as yoga and meditation to the more active relaxation technique of progressive muscle relaxation (67). The two most commonly used relaxation procedures are progressive muscle and autogenic relaxation. *Progressive muscle relaxation* consists of systematically tensing and relaxing 14–16 muscle groups (68–70). The introduction, exact order, and number of muscle groups involved varies, but common to all protocols is approximately 10 sec of tensing followed by 10–15 sec of relaxation. Although therapeutic implementation is relatively easy, a certain degree of training and experience in the techniques is important to ensure effectiveness (68–70).

Autogenic relaxation is a more passive relaxation technique (71, 72). In autogenic relaxation, the patient is instructed to use self-statements and visual images to achieve relaxation. Typically, autogenic relaxation exercises begin with suggestions of heaviness, warmth, and relaxation of specific muscle groups until the whole body is involved. Often additional phrases are added to quiet emotions and mental states such as "I feel at ease" and "My mind is quiet and calm."

Most relaxation techniques adhere to a format of 6–10 weekly sessions in which the techniques are modeled and rehearsed, coupled with daily home practice for 15–30 min. Patients are often given an audiotape to facilitate home practice; however, it is very important to ensure that the individual has mastered the technique. In this respect, audiotapes are best viewed as adjuncts rather than substitutes for supervised instruction when there is a chance to monitor progress, provide feedback, and solve problems that arise. Often relaxation procedures, especially autogenic and meditation techniques, produce a feeling of depersonalization that may be distressing to some individuals. Adequate patient preparation can help prevent any distress associated with feelings of deep relaxation. The relaxation techniques are relatively easy to master provided the therapist has an adequate understanding of learning theory principles.

BIOFEEDBACK

Biofeedback is a technique that uses instrumentation to provide feedback of physiologic responses. The feedback is useful in learning self-regulation of the physiologic response. The most common types of biofeedback are electromyographic (EMG), skin temperature, skin conductance, and electroencephalographic (EEG). Like relaxation techniques, biofeedback is thought to reduce sympathetically mediated responses and/or affective responses, such as anger or anxiety, that induce, facilitate, or maintain the pain.

Relaxation techniques and biofeedback appear to be equally efficacious (73) and are often used in conjunction with each other. Several studies have shown relaxation and biofeedback techniques to be beneficial in the management of side effects from chemotherapy (74, 75) and in treating insomnia secondary to cancer (76). Unfortunately, direct empirical evidence of effectiveness in treating cancer pain is limited to two uncontrolled studies (77, 78). In the first study, the combined use of EMG and EEG biofeedback was evaluated in seven cancer patients (77). Their results showed significant reductions in pain during biofeedback sessions, but generalization of pain reduction to the home environment was only demonstrated in two patients. In a follow-up study using EMG and skin conductance biofeedback on five patients who completed the study, three patients were able to reduce their analgesic medication intake and two patients were able to achieve pain reduction in their daily activities (78). Although these studies were uncontrolled, it is noteworthy that these patients were seriously ill and most were considered to be nonresponders to other pain management approaches.

COGNITIVE APPROACHES

Turk and Rennert have proposed a cognitive–social learning approach to the management of cancer pain (79). One of the major assumptions of cognitive approaches to pain management is that the experience of pain is based partly on its appraisal and psychological significance to the individual. The individual's evaluation of the pain is influenced by cognitive coping resources, beliefs, and attitudes, as well as other cognitive factors. As noted earlier, negative expectations and anticipatory fears such as unavoidable pain, loss of control, disfigurements, and subjective perceptions of rejection are common among cancer patients. These cognitions will likely have a negative impact on the cancer pain problem and contribute to increased distress. The goal of cognitive approaches to pain management is to modify thoughts, beliefs, and behaviors that may be contributing to the pain problem and to teach specific cognitive coping skills to deal with pain (37). Cognitive techniques have been effective in treating chronic, benign pain problems (18).

Obviously, there is a cognitive component to most forms of psychological pain management. Guided or self-directed imagery, controlled attentional focus, fantasy, and self-statements are commonly used in relaxation training and hypnosis. Cognitive techniques also consist of several additional types of procedures, however, such as cognitive distraction, attention diversion techniques, cognitive coping strategies, and restructuring strategies. Distraction and attention diversion techniques can be divided into the broad categories of environmental stimulation techniques, such as social activities, and cognitive strategies, such as focusing attention on nonpainful sensations, positive thoughts, pleasant images, or aspects of the environment (18, 37).

Cognitive restructuring and coping strategies generally involve reconceptualization of the pain. The patient's thoughts and feelings associated with the pain experience are evaluated. Thoughts and feelings that have a negative effect on the experience of pain are targeted for change (80). Such cognitive restructuring requires a certain degree of skill in eliciting cognitions contributing to the pain problem, as well as an active collaboration between clinician and patient. Other cognitive techniques include covert self-reinforcement for mastery of acute pain episodes, imagery rehearsal of coping skills, and use of imagery for covert desensitization or exposure to procedures and activities that are painful but necessary for treatment or daily living skills.

BEHAVIORAL APPROACHES

Although operant approaches in treating chronic pain are well established (81) and are a mainstay of psychological approaches to treating chronic pain, little attention has been focused on the role of environmental reinforcement on cancer-related pain and pain behavior. Ahles et al. provided some evidence for the operant reinforcement of pain behaviors in cancer patients by significant others (82). Yet, as noted above, the report of pain is important in the assessment of the disease process and, in most cases, should not be ignored. This is the fundamental difference between cancer pain and chronic, benign pain in which pain complaints are of little therapeutic value. This difference will limit the use of operant approaches for cancer pain patients.

Medication scheduling is one area wherein operant control of cancer pain may be significant. Contingent reinforcement for pain behavior and the experience of pain is often maintained by pain-contingent analgesic administration (81). Often pain-contingent administration of analgesics occurs because of physician and patient concerns about tolerance or dependence. The use of contingent scheduling of medication eliminates reinforcement for the experience or demonstration of pain.

Contingent reinforcers for the experience of pain and/or pain behaviors may often be overlooked in cancer pain treatment. Ahles has noted that operant variables are often of little importance for patients in the terminal stages of illness, yet may be an important factor for patients who experience pain for extended periods (37). Operant factors are likely to be especially important in patients who experience chronic pain but do not have active disease. This area has largely been ignored and needs greater clinical and research attention.

Other behavioral approaches might also be useful in the management of cancer pain either by themselves or in conjunction with other treatment approaches. Incentive programs might be useful to increase compliance with treatment, such as taking medication, home practice of relaxation techniques, and so on. Audiovisual presentations of modeling might be useful in acute treatment-related pain. Contracting to maintain activity level and participation in social events might be beneficial for increasing adaptive functioning despite pain. Exposure, modeling, and other behavioral approaches might be useful in treating pain, as well as anxiety- or depression-associated and cancer disease and treatment. These techniques could be effective in reducing pain and suffering in cancer patients.

STAFF EDUCATION AND SKILLS TRAINING

In some cases, the focus of treatment is not on the patient but on the staff. As already mentioned, pain-contingent administration of narcotics by staff might be an important factor in maintaining the intensity of cancer pain. Physician concerns about addiction, respiratory depression, and tolerance can contribute to inadequate control of cancer pain with analgesics. Also, patients might not request pain medication because of negative reactions by staff to prior requests. The important point is that attitudes and misconceptions by physicians and other health care professionals can interfere with the administration of analgesic medication and how patients cope with their pain (15, 83–85).

Educational skills training programs focusing on information regarding the administration of narcotics and other analgesic drugs, information on the pathophysiology of cancer pain, and concerns about narcotic addiction, tolerance, and respiratory distress could have a positive impact on the treatment of cancer pain. Hauck found that participation in an educational program on cancer pain management resulted in an increase in knowledge about the pharmacology of analgesics and more-positive attitudes toward cancer pain patients (86). Unfortunately, no direct assessment was conducted of pain management, actual behavior toward patients, or the patients' perception of staffs' attitude toward them. In addition to health care professionals, such a program could be extended to patients and their families because they often have similar attitudes, misconceptions, or behaviors that interfere with pain management.

COMPREHENSIVE TREATMENT PACKAGES

Comprehensive treatment programs are likely to be the most effective method for managing cancer pain. One approach has been suggested by Turk and Rennert (79). They outlined a treatment package based on cognitive-social learning principles. They described four components to their treatment package. The first phase is a *pretreatment preparation* that provides an overview of the program with an introduction to the notion that pain can be influenced by a variety of cognitive, affective, social, and behavioral factors. Patients are also provided with the expectation that specific skills can be learned to minimize the negative impact of these factors on their pain. A secondary purpose of the pretreatment preparation is to reassure patients that such a referral does not indicate that they are crazy or that their pain is "in their heads." In a sense, this initial phase is designed to enhance the patient's motivational level and assess for potential factors that might interfere with their cooperation in the treatment program.

Turk and Rennert described the second phase of treatment as a *conceptualization-translation* component. The primary goal of this phase is to educate the patient on the multidimensional nature of pain and the rationale behind various treatment procedures. This phase is designed to provide a framework for understanding the interaction between the experience of pain and sensory-physiologic, affective, and cognitive responses. Patients are also taught problem-solving skills and how to break large, overwhelming problems into smaller component parts. This phase of treatment focuses on reconceptualization of nonspecific, vague, and seemingly overwhelming pain-related and non–pain-related problems into specific and concrete problems that can be solved.

The third phase of treatment involves actual *training in cognitive and behavioral strategies to reduce pain and minimize stress*. Patients are taught relaxation and attention diversion techniques. In addition to focusing on pain reduction, an emphasis of this phase in treatment is to enhance the individual's sense of control and personal mastery. The fourth phase is essentially a *continuation of rehearsal and practice to consolidate the pain-control techniques and reinforce a sense of personal control*. Turk and Rennert suggest that a stress inoculation procedure is useful at this point in treatment. This involves having the individual imagine himself experiencing pain and then using the previously learned coping techniques. Another useful technique is to have the patient take the role of an instructor and teach the coping techniques to the clinician, who takes the role of a new patient.

A final element of the treatment package is *homework tasks of gradually increasing difficulty*. For example, the patient might be instructed to practice pain-control techniques only when pain is low at first, then to gradually shift the use of pain-control techniques when pain is more severe. The point is to ensure that the patient is experiencing success in order to increase his or her sense of competence and confidence in the techniques. Turk and Rennert reported that this approach to cancer pain management is effective; unfortunately they present no data to support this conclusion (79). Although the program appears to have face validity for being an effective treatment for cancer pain, conclusions regarding efficacy must await empirical verification.

Jay et al. (87) and Varni et al. (88) have used cognitive behavioral interventions to develop a comprehensive treatment approach to treat pain and distress in children undergoing painful medical procedures. Their intervention, labeled the Cognitive Behavior Therapy Package (CBTP), incorporates five behavioral treatment components: filmed modeling, breathing exercises, positive reinforcement, imagery/distraction, and behavior rehearsal (39, 88). In a controlled treatment outcome study, pediatric cancer patients receiving the CBTP showed significantly lower levels of behavioral distress (e.g., crying, screaming), self-reported pain, and physiologic reactivity during bone marrow procedures than either a control or Valium-treatment group (88). This research is praiseworthy, not only because it supports the efficacy of psychological approaches to cancer pain, but also because it represents one of the few controlled treatment outcome studies in this area.

TREATMENT ISSUES

In summary, there are a variety of psychological interventions available for use in the management of cancer pain. The problem is not the lack of approaches but rather the dearth of empirical evidence to confirm efficacy or to establish the applicability and generalizability of psychological approaches to cancer pain. Research on treatment-related acute pain in adult cancer patients has almost been entirely ignored, although some research has focused on treatment-related acute pain in pediatric cancer patients (39). The studies on disease-related chronic pain are limited by a lack of rigorous scientific methodology, especially appropriate control groups, quantitative and multimodal pain measures, and evaluation of process variables or mechanisms of change.

Some of the limitations in current research on the psychological management of cancer pain are undoubtedly related to inherent difficulties in conducting research on cancer patients (89) and the incomplete conceptual understanding of important psychological aspects of cancer pain. Although there is ultimately no substitute for controlled treatment outcome studies, one approach to advancing knowledge in this area is through the use of time-series methodology (64). Barlow et al. have detailed the application of single-case designs and time-series methodology to document change in clinical practice (90). Because clinicians are currently employing psychological interventions, considerable knowledge could be gained from more-systematic evaluation of treatment responses in individuals. Specific interventions could be compared, as well as the efficacy of combined treatments for different types of cancer pain problems and patient variables. Such information would be extremely valuable in planning and justifying the commitment of time and resources for controlled treatment outcome studies.

CONCLUSIONS

The diverse expressions of pain associated with cancer necessitate that behavioral assessment and the resulting psychological treatment plan be based not only on a thorough understanding of the pain complaint, but also on an adequate knowledge of the disease itself and its stage of progression. In all cases, comprehensive psychological and medical therapies must be evaluated for potential benefit to the patient. The specific needs of cancer patients will require some reorientation by clinicians with experience in treating chronic pain.

Psychological pain management techniques have a place in the comprehensive management of cancer pain; however, psychological techniques should always be considered as alternative and adjunct pain-management therapies rather than substitutes for medical pain management. We suggest that relatively simple behavioral skills training can be surprisingly effective in pain reduction, that a package of different psychological techniques appropriately selected for the individual has distinct advantages over any skill presented in isolation, and that cancer patients, as a group, are well motivated to learn and practice these skills. Psychological approaches have some advantages over other methods of treating cancer pain, because pain control can be achieved without unpleasant or destructive side effects. In fact, psychological pain control techniques may also facilitate life-enhancing immune system functioning, psychological adjustment, and health-promoting cognitions and behavior (91). There is definitely a need for empirical research in this area. The research thus far seems to indicate that psychological interventions can provide a wide range of beneficial services to cancer patients and their families, including pain management.

REFERENCES

1. National Institute of Health: Report of the Panel on Pain to the National Advisory NINDS Council (NIH 79-1912). Washington, D.C., Government Printing Office, 1979.
2. Daut RL, Cleeland CS: The prevalence and severity of pain in cancer. *Cancer* 50:1903–1918, 1982.
3. Levin CN, Cleeland CS, Dar R: Public attitudes towards cancer pain. *Cancer* 56:2337–2339, 1985.
4. Weissman DE, Dahl JL: Attitudes about cancer pain: A survey of Wisconsin's first-year medical students, *J Pain Symptom Manag* 5:345–349, 1990.
5. Cleeland CS: The impact of pain on the patient with cancer. *Cancer* 54:2635–2641, 1984.
6. Foley KM: Assessment of pain. *Clin Oncol* 3:17–31, 1984.
7. Foley KM: Pain syndromes in patients with cancer. In Bonica JJ, Ventafredda V (eds): *Advances in Pain Research and Therapy*. New York, Raven Press, 1979, vol 2, p 59.
8. Schwettmann RS, Shacham S, Cleeland CS: Relating cancer pain to its physical basis. Presented at the annual meeting of the American Pain Society, Chicago, IL, 1983.
9. Greenwald HP, Bonica JJ, Bergner M: The prevalence of pain four cancers. *Cancer* 60:2563–2569, 1987.
10. Dalton JA, Feuerstein M: Biobehavioral factors in cancer pain. *Pain* 33:137–147, 1988.
11. Turk D, Holzman AD: Chronic pain: Interfaces among physical, psychological, and social parameters. In Holzman AD, Turk DC (eds): *Pain Management: A Handbook of Psychological Treatment Approaches*. New York, Pergamon Press, 1986, pp 1–9.
12. Shacham S, Reinhardt LC, Raubertas RF, Cleeland CS: Emotional state and pain: Intraindividual and interindividual measure of association. *J Behav Med* 6:405–419, 1983.
13. Turk DC, Fernandez E: On the putative uniqueness of cancer pain: Do psychological principles apply? *Behav Res Ther* 28:1–13, 1990.
14. Telch CF, Telch MJ: Group coping skills instruction and supportive group therapy for cancer patients: A comparison of strategies. *J Consult Clin Psychol* 54:802–808, 1986.
15. Bonica JJ: Cancer pain: A major national health problem. *Cancer Nurs* 1:313–316, 1978.
16. Marks RM, Sacher EJ: Undertreatment of medical inpatients with narcotic analgesics. *Ann Intern Med* 78:173–181, 1973.
17. Twycross RG, Lacks SA: *Symptom Control in Advanced Cancer: Pain Relief*. London, Pitman, 1985.
18. Turk D, Meichenbaum D, Genest M: *Pain and Behavioral Medicine*. New York, Guilford Press, 1983.
19. Keefe FJ, Brown C, Scott DS, Ziesat H: The behavioral assessment of chronic pain. In Keefe FJ, Blumenthal JA (eds): *Assessment Strategies in Behavioral Medicine*. New York, Grune & Stratton, 1982.
20. Hilgard ER: Pain as a puzzle for psychology and physiology. *Am J Psychol* 24:103–113, 1969.
21. Melzack R (ed): *Pain Measurement and Assessment*. New York, Raven Press, 1983.
22. Tearnan BH, Cleeland CS: The unaided use of pain descriptors by patients with cancer pain. *J Pain Symptom Manag* 5 (4), 1990.
23. McCaffery M: *Nursing Management of the Patient with Pain*, ed 2. Philadelphia, JB Lippincott, 1979.
24. Dalton JA, Feuerstein M: Fear, alexithymia and cancer pain. *Pain* 38:159–170, 1989.
25. Tearnan BH, Lewandowski MJ: The Behavioral Assessment of Pain Questionnaire (BAP): The development and validation of a self-report instrument for assessing pain. *Am J Pain Manag Assess* 2:181–191, 1992.
26. Daut RL, Cleeland CS, Flanery RC: Development of the Wisconsin Brief Pain Questionnaire to assess pain in cancer and other diseases. *Pain* 17:197–210, 1983.
27. Shacham S: A shortened version of the Profile of Mood States. *J Pers Assess* 47:305–306, 1983.
28. DeGood DE: Reducing medical patients' reluctance to participate in psychological therapies: The initial session. *Professional Psychol Res Pract* 14:570–579, 1983.
29. Jacox A, Stewart M: *Psychosocial Contingencies of the Pain Experience*. Iowa City, The University of Iowa Press, 1973.
30. Hardy JD: The nature of pain. *J Chronic Dis* 7:22–51, 1956.
31. Abrams RD: The patient with cancer—his changing pattern of communication. *N Engl J Med* 274:317–322, 1966.
32. Bond MR: Pain and personality in cancer patients. In Bonica JJ, Albe Fossard D (eds): *Advances in Pain Research and Therapy*. New York, Raven Press, 1976, vol 1, pp 311–316.
33. Moses R, Cividoli N: Differential levels of awareness of illness: Their relation to some salient features in cancer patients. *Ann N Y Acad Sci* 125:884, 1966.
34. Kremer EF, Block A, Gaylor M: Behavioral approaches to

treatment of chronic pain: The inaccuracy of patient self-report measures. *Arch Phys Med Rehabil* 62:188–191, 1981.

35. Kremer EF, Block A, Atkinson JH: Assessment of pain behavior: Factors that distort self-report. In Melzack R (ed): *Pain Measurement and Assessment*. New York, Raven Press, 1983.

36. Ignelzi RJ, Kremer EF, Atkinson JH: Patient pain intensity report to different health professionals. Presented at the annual meeting of the Association for Advancement of Behavior Therapy, New York, November 1980.

37. Ahles TA: Psychological approaches to the management of cancer-related pain. *Semin Oncol Nurs* 1:141–146, 1985. Bonica JJ: Cancer pain. In Bonica JJ (ed): *Pain*. New York, Raven Press, 1980, pp 335–362.

38. Cleeland CS, Tearnan BH: Behavioral control of pain. In Holzman AD, Turk DC (eds): *Pain Management: A Handbook of Psychological Treatment Approaches*. New York, Pergamon Press, 1986, pp 193–212.

39. Jay SM, Elliot C, Varni JW: Acute and chronic pain in adults and children with cancer. *J Consult Clin Psychol* 54:601–607, 1986.

40. Noyles R Jr: Treatment of cancer pain. *Psychosom Med* 43:57–70, 1981.

41. Kendall PC, Norton-Ford JD: *Clinical Psychology: Scientific and Professional Dimensions*. New York, John Wiley & Sons, 1982.

42. Bond MR: Psychologic and psychiatric techniques for the relief of advanced cancer pain. In Bonica JJ, Ventatridda V (eds): *Advances in Pain Research and Therapy*. New York, Raven Press, 1979, vol 2, pp. 215–222.

43. Breitsart, W: Psychiatric management of cancer pain. *Cancer* 63:2336–2342, 1989.

44. Massie MJ, Holland JC: The cancer patient with pain. Psychiatric complications and their management. *J Pain Symptom Manag* 7:99–109, 1992.

45. Feinstein AD: Psychological interventions in the treatment of cancer. *Clin Psychol Rev* 3:1–14, 1983.

46. Jay, SM, Elliot, C., Varni, JW: Acute and chronic pain in adults and children with cancer. *Journal of Consulting and Clinical Psychology* 54, 601–607, 1986.

47. Gordon WA, Freidenbergs I, Diller L, et al: Efficacy of psychosocial intervention with cancer patients. *J Consult Clin Psychol* 48:743–759, 1980.

48. Shapiro A: Psychotherapy as adjunct treatment for cancer patients. *Am J Clin Hypn* 25:150–155, 1983.

49. Ament P: Concepts in the use of hypnosis for pain relief in cancer. *J Med* 13:233–240, 1982.

50. Barber J, Gitelson J: Cancer pain: psychological management using hypnosis. *Cancer* 30:130–135, 1980.

51. Butler B: The use of hypnosis in the care of cancer patient, part I. *Br J Med Hypn* 6:2–12, 1954.

52. Cangello VM: Hypnosis for the patient with cancer. *Am J Clin Hypn* 4:215–226, 1962.

53. Hilgard ER, Hilgard JR: *Hypnosis in the Relief of Pain*. Los Altos, CA, William Kaufmann, 1975.

54. Koerner ME: Using hypnosis to relieve pain of terminal cancer. *Hypn Q* 20:39–46, 1977.

55. LaBaw W, Holton C, Tewell K, Eccles D: The use of self-hypnosis by children with cancer. *Am J Clin Hypn* 7:308–319, 1975.

56. Levitan, AA: The use of hypnosis with cancer patients. *10*, 119–131, 1992.

57. Hilgard JR, LeBaron S: Relief of anxiety and pain in children and adolescents with cancer: quantitative measures and clinical observations. *Int J Clin Exp Hypn* 30:417–442, 1982.

58. Araoz DL: Use of hypnotic techniques with oncology patients. *J Psychosoc Oncol* 1:47–54, 1983.

59. Barber J: Hypnotic analgesia. In Holzman AD, Turk DC (eds): *Pain Management: A Handbook of Psychological Treatment Approaches*. New York, Pergamon Press, 1986, pp 151–167.

60. Butler B: The use of hypnosis in the care of cancer patient, part II. *Br J Med Hypn* 6:2–12, 1955.

61. Hilgard ER, Morgan AH: Heart rate and blood pressure in the study of laboratory pain in man under normal conditions and as influenced by hypnosis. *Acta Neurol Exp* 35:741–759, 1975.

62. Reeves JL, Redd WH, Storm FK, Minagawa RY: Hypnosis in the control of pain during hyperthermia treatment of cancer. In Bonica JJ (ed): *Advances in Pain Research and Therapy*. New York, Raven Press, 1983, vol 5, pp 857–861.

63. Finer B: Hypnotherapy in pain of advanced cancer. In Bonica JJ, Ventafridda V (eds): *Advances in Pain Research and Therapy*. New York, Raven Press, 1979, vol 2, pp 223–229.

64. Kellerman J, Zeltzer L, Ellenberg L, Dash J: Adolescents with cancer: hypnosis for the reduction of the acute pain and anxiety associated with medical procedures. *J Adoles Health Care* 4:85–90, 1983.

65. Zelter L, LeBaron S: Hypnosis and nonhypnotic techniques for reduction of pain and anxiety during painful procedures in children and adolescents with cancer. *J Pediatr* 101:1032–1035, 1982.

66. Spiegel D, Bloom JR: Group therapy and hypnosis reduce metastatic breast carcinoma pain. *Psychosom Med* 45:333–339, 1983.

67. Woolfolk RL, Lehrer PM (eds): *Principles and Practice of Stress Management*, New York, Guilford Press, 1984.

68. Bernstein DA, Borkovec TD: *Progressive Relocation Training: A Manual For the Helping Professions*. Champaign, IL, Research Press, 1973.

69. Jacobson E: *Progressive Relaxation*. New York, Avon, 1938.

70. Rimm DC, Masters JC: *Behavioral Therapy: Techniques and Empirical Findings*, ed 2. New York, Academic Press, 1979.

71. Norris PA, Fahrion SL: Autogenic biofeedback in psychophysiological therapy and stress management. In Woolfolk RL, Lehrer PM (eds): *Principles and Practice of Stress Management*. New York, Guilford Press, 1984, pp 220–254.

72. Schultz JH, Luthe W: *Autogenic Therapy, Vol 1: Autogenic Methods*, New York, Grune & Stratton, 1969.

73. Silver BV, Blanchard EB: Biofeedback and relaxation training in the treatment of psychophysiological disorders: or, are the machines really necessary? *J Behav Med* 1:217–239, 1978.

74. Lyles JN, Burish TG, Krozely MG, Oldham RK: Efficacy of relaxation training and guided imagery in reducing the aversiveness of cancer chemotherapy. *J Consult Clin Psychol* 50:509–524, 1982.

75. Redd WH, Andrykowski MA: Behavioral intervention in

cancer treatment: controlling aversion to chemotherapy. *J Consult Clin Psychol* 50:1018–1029, 1982.

76. Cannici J, Malcolm R, Peck LA: Treatment of insomnia in cancer patients using muscle relaxation training. *J Behav Ther Exp Psychiatry* 14:251–256, 1983.

77. Fotopoulos SS, Graham C, Cook MR: Psychophysiologic control of cancer pain. In Bonica JJ, Ventafridda V (eds): *Advances in Pain Research and Therapy*. New York, Raven Press, 1979, vol 2 pp 231–243.

78. Fotopoulos SS, Cook MR, Graham C, et al: Cancer pain: evaluation of electromyographic and electrodermal feedback. *Prog Clin Biol Res* 132D:33–53, 1983.

79. Turk DC, Rennert D: Pain and the terminally ill cancer patient: a cognitive social learning perspective. In Sobel HJ (ed): *Behavior Therapy in Terminal Care*. Cambridge, MA, Ballinger, 1981, pp 95–123.

80. Holzman AD, Turk DC, Kerns RD Jr.: The cognitive-behavioral approach to the management of chronic pain. In Holzman AD, Turk DC (eds): *Pain Management: A Handbook of Psychological Treatment Approaches*. New York, Pergamon Press, 1986, pp 31–50.

81. Fordyce W: *Behavioral Methods for Chronic Pain and Illness*. St. Louis, CV Mosby, 1976.

82. Ahles TA, Blanchard EB, Ruckdeschel JC: The multidimensional nature of cancer-related pain. *Pain* 17:277–288, 1983.

83. Bagley C, Falinski E, Garnizo N, Hooker L: Pain management: a pilot project. *Cancer Nurs* 5:191–199, 1982.

84. Jacox AK, Rogers AG: The nursing management of pain. In Marino LB (ed): *Cancer Nursing*. St. Louis, CV Mosby, 1981, pp 381–404.

85. Cleeland CS, Cleeland LM, Dar R, Rienhardt LC: Factors influencing physicians' management of cancer pain. *Cancer* 58:796–800, 1986.

86. Hauck SL: Pain problem for the person with cancer. *Cancer Nurs* 9:66–76, 1986.

87. Jay SM, Elliot CM, Ozolins M, Olson R, Pruitt S: Behavioral management of children's distress during painful medical procedures. *Behav Res Ther* 23:513–520, 1985.

88. Varni JW, Jay SM, Masek BJ, Thompson KL: Cognitive-behavioral assessment and management of pediatric pain. In Holzman AD, Turk DC (eds): *Pain Management: A Handbook of Psychological Treatment Approaches*. New York, Pergamon Press, 1986, pp 168–192.

89. Ahles TA, Cohen RE, Blanchard EB: Difficulties inherent in conducting behavioral research with cancer patients. *Behav Ther* 1:69–70, 1984.

90. Barlow DH, Hayes SC, Nelson RD: *The Scientist Practitioner: Research and Accountability in Clinical and Educational Settings*. New York, Pergamon Press, 1985.

91. Gruber, BL, Hall, NR, Hersh, SP & Dubois, P: Immune system and psychological changes in metastatic cancer patients using relaxation and guided imagery. A pilot study. *Scandinavian Journal of Behavior Therapy*, 17, 25–46, 1988.

CHAPTER 35
NEUROSURGICAL TREATMENT OF PAIN RELATED TO CANCER
STEPHEN R. FREIDBERG

PAIN, A common symptom of disease, is valuable because it may initiate or direct a search for underlying disease. The ideal way to eliminate pain is to treat the underlying disease. However, sometimes the primary underlying disease is not or cannot be treated adequately, and pain persists, becomes chronic, and is the focal point of a wretched existence that requires attention.

Pain caused by benign disease must be differentiated from pain caused by malignant disease. Chronic pain of benign origin presents a specific constellation of symptoms. Frequently, secondary gain occurs either consciously or subconsciously. Does the pain permit a long-desired change in occupation or marital relationship? Is the basic problem severe underlying depression? Surgical attempts at relief of pain of benign origin invariably fail, and the problem is managed best by a behavior modification program in a pain clinic (1).

Chronic pain caused by malignant disease requires a different therapeutic approach. Although the patient is frequently ill and depressed, the evaluation and treatment of pain as an isolated entity are usually fairly straightforward (2). In the last decade, improvements have been made in the treatment of cancer by surgery, chemotherapy, and radiotherapy. These modalities together with a clearer understanding of the mechanism of action and more effective delivery of pain-controlling medication have substantially reduced the need for neurosurgical methods to relieve pain. In some instances, however, a carefully chosen neurosurgical operation provides excellent palliation of pain with low risk and low morbidity (3, 4). Neurosurgical treatment of pain may be *ablative*, with destruction of neural tissue, or *augmentative*, with stimulation of neural tissue or more effective delivery of medication.

To experience pain, a patient must have a peripheral lesion exciting pain receptors. This sensation is transmitted through the central nervous system to the brain, where the stimulus is recorded as pain. Therefore, it is theoretically possible to divide the neural connection between the peripheral nerve and the brain and alleviate the pain. Although ablative surgery is effective in selected patients, unfortunately it is not the solution for all patients. Psychodynamic factors can embellish the sensation of pain, creating a clinical situation that demands treatment (5). Alternatively, some patients may tolerate the pain.

A clinically proved approach to the problem of pain associated with cancer is presented in this chapter. Procedures being investigated, which are currently not appropriate in a general neurosurgical practice, are discussed.

ABLATIVE NEUROSURGERY

Virtually every neural structure has at one time or another been sectioned in an attempt to relieve pain.

PERIPHERAL NEURECTOMY

Peripheral neurectomy (Fig. 35.1*J*) is rarely effective. A lesion is not commonly found in the dermatomic area of a single nerve because of the overlap of innervation from adjacent nerves. Sectioning many nerves, as is possible with intercostal nerves, leaves the denervated area with a numb sensation and almost certainly with persistent pain. Nerves with important functional innervation in the extremities cannot be sectioned safely.

NERVE ROOT SECTION (RHIZOTOMY)

Nerve root section (Fig. 35.1*I*) usually does not help relieve pain. No important motor nerves are present at the thoracic level, and the operation is associated with low morbidity. In two series of patients with cancer who underwent thoracic rhizotomy (6, 7), results were disappointing in terms of relief of pain.

Arbit et al. have used an extradural approach to the nerve roots, anterior and sympathetic as well as posterior, with excellent and good results in 93% of patients

Figure 35.1. *A–K.* Diagrammatic representation of neurosurgical operations for relief of pain. References to each specific section are detailed in the text. (Copyright © 1986, the Lahey Clinic Medical Center, Burlington, MA.)

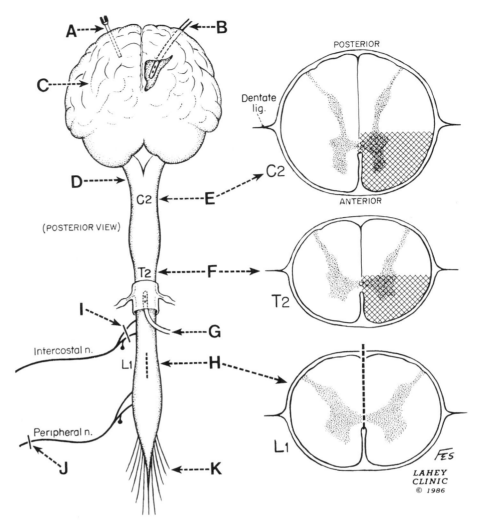

(8). They stress that small, thinly myelinated fibers related to pain conduction run with the motor roots, and sympathetic nerves play a role in the transmission of visceral pain. Computed tomography (CT) or magnetic resonance imaging (MRI) is used to accurately localize the involved nerve roots. This is a less stressful operation than an intradural rhizotomy. Care must be taken to avoid injuring radicular arteries in the T1–4 and T11–L1 watershed areas.

Rhizotomy, however, does provide excellent relief of pain in specific limited clinical situations. Infiltration of the brachial plexus in patients with carcinoma of the breast is an extremely painful condition. Section of the dorsal root, if it involves C5, C6, C7, and C8, renders the arm sensory deprived and useless. We have used rhizotomy to treat two patients with invasion of the brachial plexus from carcinoma of the breast, one with an amputation at the shoulder and one who had total loss of function of the brachial plexus as a result of her disease. Dorsal rhizotomy was performed with a long hemilaminectomy on the involved side from C3 to C8, with excellent relief of pain and no change in the clinical status. These results would not have been possible had the patient had a neurologically functioning limb.

Patients with nerve root involvement with epidural cancer may benefit from root section carried out at the time of laminectomy.

A sacral rhizotomy (Fig. 35.1K) performed with alcohol is effective for perianal, perineal, and genital pain associated with carcinoma of the rectum, bladder, or genitalia (4). Sacral rhizotomy is easily carried out in the radiology department with a needle inserted into the L5–S1 interspace under fluoroscopic control. Because alcohol is hypobaric compared with cerebrospinal fluid, the patient is positioned with the head down. Absolute (95%) ethanol is injected in aliquots of 0.25 ml until a maximum of 2 ml is injected or until the sensory level, which begins in the perianal and genital areas (S4 and S5), rises to S2 on the posterior calf. The level will descend to S3 on the posterior thigh several hours after the procedure. The level must not rise to S1 because weakness of plantar flexion of the ankle and sensory loss on the sole of the foot will be produced. A contraindication to this procedure is a short dural sac ending at L5 rather than in the sacrum. In this situation, the S1 roots will be bathed in alcohol. A myelogram using 1 ml of contrast material is always performed before injecting alcohol, and the procedure is stopped if the sac ends at L5. A sacral rhizotomy can be carried out without motor loss, but loss of sphincter control is invariable. Many of these patients already have a colostomy. Bladder function in patients who have had extensive pelvic surgery is frequently compromised, and a permanent Foley catheter may be necessary after rhizotomy. The ideal patient for this procedure is one with both fecal and urinary diversion. Some physicians (9) prefer to perform this operation using hyperbaric phenol mixed with iophendylate (Pantopaque) or glycerin. In selected patients, this procedure provides long-lasting, excellent relief of pain with minimal acceptable morbidity.

Commissural Myelotomy

Commissural myelotomy (Fig. 35.1*H*) is used in some medical centers for treatment of pain in the pelvic area. An incision is made in the lumbar spinal cord over several segments. The incision sections the commissural fibers in the ventral white matter before they enter the spinothalamic tract. The surgeon must be certain the incision is at the correct level. Although Sourek (10) described the correlation between vertebral and spinal cord levels, a discrepancy may exist, and the cord level selected may not be completely accurate. Even with use of the operating microscope, paraparesis or dorsal column dysfunction is possible. We rarely perform this operation.

Gildenberg and Hirshberg (11) described limited myelotomy at either the level of C1 or the thoracolumbar junction. Schvarcz (12) described an extralemniscal tract in the center of the spinal cord at the cervicomedullary junction. Destroying this tract provided relief of pain. I have no personal experience with the limited myelotomy.

Anterolateral Cordotomy

Anterolateral cordotomy remains the mainstay of treatment to relieve pain associated with cancer (4). The spinothalamic tract is sectioned after the fibers have crossed in the anterior commissure of the spinal cord. The lesion is, therefore, made on the side opposite the pain. Unlike commissural myelotomy, anterolateral cordotomy does not require selecting an exact level, but the level must be sufficiently craniad to the site of the pain to produce a satisfactorily high sensory level to pain and temperature. As always, careful selection of patients is the key to a safe, effective operation, the result of which usually lasts for several years. The sensory loss is well tolerated by the patient.

The ideal patient for cordotomy is one with pain that is clearly unilateral in the lower part of the body. An open T2 cordotomy (Fig. 35.1*F*) contralateral to the pain

produces a midthoracic sensory level to pinprick and temperature with analgesia. Weakness of the leg on the side of the cordotomy is a possibility. Disturbance in sphincter control is usually transient.

One of the problems related to cordotomy is that pain near the midline, even if dominant on only one side, frequently becomes clinically serious on the opposite side after relief of pain from cordotomy (13). Minor contralateral pain becomes magnified, and the patient requires relief of pain on the other side. Bilateral pain or pain developing on the second side requires bilateral cordotomy, usually carried out at T3 with at least a week between operations. Physiologically, bilateral cordotomy is a more serious operation than unilateral cordotomy. The patient is likely to experience severe autonomic dysfunction with sphincter dysfunction and orthostatic hypotension, which may require elastic stockings and fludrocortisone (Florinef) to maintain blood pressure.

Pain in the upper extremity or in the chest wall produces a more difficult clinical problem than pain in the lower extremity. For pain at the higher level, cordotomy must be performed at C2 (Fig. 35.1*E*). Because the ventral gray matter of the anterior horn of the spinal cord is sectioned along with the spinothalamic tract, unacceptable motor deficit in the arm is produced if the incision is made at a level where the anterior horn is clinically important. Therefore, the lesion cannot be made between C4 and T1. For pain in the chest wall, a satisfactorily high sensory level can usually be obtained with C2 cordotomy. A problem may arise in the presence of a pneumonectomy on the painful side or damage to the residual lung by tumor or radiation or both. The lung on the nonpainful side may be compromised as a result of chronic lung disease. A C2 cordotomy may interfere with function of the ipsilateral phrenic nerve, which will reduce pulmonary function severely on the nonpainful side (14). Unilateral cordotomy not only interferes with the motor component of respiration but also decreases the central response to inspired CO_2 (15). Krieger and Rosomoff (16) demonstrated the danger of performing bilateral cordotomy at a high cervical level. The dangers of severe pulmonary insufficiency, impairment of automatic control of respiration (Ondine's curse), and autonomic dysfunction make this operation unjustified.

Although cordotomy may be performed at either C2 or T2, a standard open operation by a hemilaminectomy at T2 is preferred (17). The physiologic morbidity associated with cordotomy at T2 is considerably less than at C2. The surgical technique at C2 is the same if the level of pain demands this approach.

Some neurosurgeons (18, 19) prefer to carry out cordotomy with a percutaneous technique using a radiofrequency current to produce a lesion. It can be performed with the patient under local anesthesia, a benefit in an ill patient. The main advantage is the ability to manipulate the lesion while testing the patient, an especially important point if the pain is in the upper extremity or brachial plexus (20). It is extremely difficult to obtain a level this high with open cordotomy. With no operative complications, patients have been satisfied, but when the procedure is unsuccessful, patients become uncomfortable. The incidence of hemiparesis and respiratory difficulty is also higher with percutaneous than with open cordotomy. The high cervical percutaneous procedure is currently reserved for patients with pain high in the upper extremity and in the brachial plexus. Gildenberg and associates (21) described a high thoracic percutaneous technique, and Hardy and co-workers (22) described a microsurgical approach to the anterior cervical area using a variation of Cloward's technique. I have no personal experience with these last two procedures.

Kanpolat et al. have used CT-guided techniques to improve localization for percutaneous cordotomy (23). They had good results in 20 of 21 patients. In addition to the cordotomy they used the CT-guided technique to perform extralemniscal myelotomy and trigeminal tractotomy-nucleotomy with encouraging results.

Medullary Tractotomy (Fig. 35.1D)

Pain related to cancer of the head and neck is difficult to treat. Fortunately, improved methods of treatment of the underlying disease make this an infrequent clinical problem. Percutaneous trigeminal rhizotomy or posterior fossa trigeminal root section may relieve the pain. However, because of the complex sensory innervation of the face, destruction of the fifth cranial nerve may not be adequate. In this situation, a lesion made in the descending tract of the trigeminal root in the medulla produces satisfactory relief of pain. The open operation was designed by Sjöqvist in 1938 (24). Stereotaxic procedures have been performed since 1972 in interested centers (25).

Rostral Mesencephalotomy

Bosch reported a series of 33 patients with cancer and 7 with deafferentation pain (26). Stereotactic radiofrequency lesions were produced in the rostral portion of the mesencephalon involving the medial lemniscus, the spinothalamic tract, and the quintothalamic tract. The indications are unilateral pain. The major benefit of this procedure is that pain in the head and neck and cervical area is treatable. The lesions were unilateral in 31 patients and bilateral in 2. The author used ventriculography landmarks. He felt, at the time, that CT and MRI was not sufficiently accurate. The results in the cancer group were good in 87.9% of patients. There was one death in a patient who had bilateral lesions made in one sitting. The morbidity was otherwise not serious.

DREZ

The Duke University neurosurgical group extended their work with DREZ lesions for deafferentation facial pain secondary to cancer (27). They produced the lesion by coagulating the entire ipsilateral nucleus caudalis including the afferent fibers of the descending tract and the secondary neurons at the level of the obex to the dorsal rootlets of C2. All of the five patients had immediate good to excellent pain relief. One excellent result held at 2 months. A good result held for 40 months. One early excellent and two good results had fallen to fair at 8–12 months. No patient had poor results, and none had serious morbidity from the operation. The authors concluded that patients with less preoperative objective sensory loss will have better results. Pain of burning quality appears to respond better than aching pain.

Hypophysectomy

Hypophysectomy (removal of the pituitary gland) effectively relieves bone pain in patients with carcinoma of the breast and prostate. Objective shrinkage of tumor is seen in 50% of patients with breast cancer and in 30% of patients with prostate cancer. Relief of pain, however, is obtained in 70% of patients in each group (28). The mechanism of pain relief is not completely understood but may be related to a hypothalamic mechanism triggered by removal of the pituitary gland. After the pituitary gland has been removed, changes are noted in the pituitary stalk and hypothalamus. Total hypophysectomy is not necessary for pain relief (29). Permanent postoperative diabetes insipidus correlates well with good pain relief (30). Since pain relief is not reversed with injection of naloxone (Narcan), it is probably not mediated through changes in the endorphin system. Moricca (31) carried out hypophysectomy by injection of alcohol into the pituitary gland in patients with a wide variety of malignant processes with uniformly good results. Zervas and Gordy (32) performed the operation with a radiofrequency probe technique. I have carried out hypophysectomy through a transsphenoidal approach.

Lesions of the Brain (Fig. 35.1C)

Cingulotomy

A patient's perception of pain may be altered by creating a lesion in the bilateral frontal lobe or cingulum. These lesions do not produce relief of pain but rather apathy, thereby relieving the terror and anxiety brought on by the cancer and the pain. Hurt and Ballantine (33) achieved satisfactory short-term relief of pain after cingulotomy in 18 of 32 patients with cancer, and satisfactory long-term relief of pain was achieved in two of nine. The lesions can be produced by an open or percutaneous technique. Because of the social pressure against leukotomy in the United States, this operation is performed infrequently.

Thalamotomy

Hitchcock and Teixeira (34) reported their experience with lesions produced stereotaxically in the centromedian and basal nuclei of the thalamus and reviewed the literature on thalamotomy for control of chronic pain. They believed the centromedian lesion was associated with the best rate of success for both immediate and long-term results. In all of their eight patients with malignant disease, centromedian thalamotomy yielded complete relief compared with only four of six patients who had basal thalamotomy. If adequate relief of pain was not obtained with unilateral thalamotomy, a contralateral lesion was created with little morbidity. The results of thalamotomy in patients with cancer were better than in those with benign disease.

ALCOHOL BLOCK OF THE CELIAC PLEXUS

Local metastases are common in patients with cancer of the upper abdominal viscera, that is, pancreas, gallbladder, liver, stomach, and colon, and produce pain in the region of the upper abdomen or back or both. This sensation of pain is conducted by the splanchnic nerves, which contain autonomic and pain fibers. The sensation through these fibers can be interrupted by block of the celiac plexus.

Gorbitz and Leavens (35) described the technique of celiac plexus block. It is valuable in patients in whom tumor is confined to the viscera. The injection of alcohol is painful and involves the risk of vascular or visceral perforation. They stressed that the needle should be placed under radiographic control with intravenous neuroleptanesthesia (35). Should a somatic component to the pain be present, further ablative treatment may be necessary after relief of visceral pain by the celiac block.

AUGMENTATIVE NEUROSURGERY (NONABLATIVE PROCEDURES)

The last decade has produced a clearer understanding of the endogenous endorphin system (36). Endorphins are opiates produced in the body that bind to specific receptors in the central nervous system. These are the receptors for opiates administered exogenously and are thought to represent the mechanism by which narcotics relieve pain. Exogenous opiates administered locally to the central nervous system bind with receptors and produce analgesia in doses far lower than with systemic administration and without the severe side effects associated with systemic narcotics. This observation forms the basis of spinal and intraventricular administration of narcotics.

SPINAL MORPHINE

Endorphin receptors are present in the substantia gelatinosa of the dorsal gray matter of the spinal cord (37, 38). Preservative-free morphine sulfate (2–5 mg in 2–5 ml of saline solution) is administered every 8–12 hr in the epidural or subarachnoid space through an indwelling catheter (39) (Fig. 35.1G). When the procedure is effective, the patient experiences relief of pain with little systemic effect. The catheter can be placed percutaneously through a Tuohy needle (Becton-Dickinson, Rutherford, NJ 07070) or by limited laminectomy. The reservoir attached to the proximal portion of the catheter, which is tunneled beneath the skin, varies from a simple externalized Broviac type, to an implanted Ommaya system (American Heyer-Schults, Division of American Hospital Supply Corporation, Goleta, CA 93117), which requires intermittent and transcutaneous injections, to a totally implantable Infusaid pump (Infusaid, Norwood, MA) (40).

Disagreement exists regarding the optimal method of administering the narcotic. Shetter and colleagues (40) reported less tolerance, and ultimately a lower necessary dose of narcotic, with continuous rather than intermittent infusion. Intermittent instillation using an externalized catheter or an implanted reservoir has the benefits of simplicity and low initial cost. When installed, the device can be serviced by the patient, family member, or visiting nurse. The necessary medication, syringes, and needles are readily available from local pharmacies. The implanted pump is considerably more expensive initially and demands periodic refilling by a physician (41). It does, however, free the patient from having injections several times a day.

Most investigators have used preservative-free morphine. Coombs and associates (42) used hydromorphone (Dilaudid) in a patient sensitive to morphine and changed to clonidine (Catapres) when tolerance to the hydromorphone developed. They hypothesized that different subgroups of drugs may have different profiles of receptor affinity (42). The ability to lower the equivalent dose of medication may prolong the effectiveness of this system and reduce the side effects.

INTRAVENTRICULAR NARCOTICS

In an admittedly preliminary study, Lobato and coworkers (43) produced satisfactory analgesia with intraventricular injection of morphine (Fig. 35.1B). An Ommaya reservoir, which can be inserted with the patient under local anesthesia, is used. The patient's family can be instructed in the method of administering the drug for home use. A dose of 0.5–1.0 mg every 12–24 hr has sufficed in most instances with a low complication rate, few serious side effects, and minimal intolerance. The effect is not reversed by naloxone. The authors therefore postulate that a nonopiate analgesic system is being activated (43). This is currently an experimental approach to relief of pain, but it does hold promise.

ELECTRICAL STIMULATION OF THE SPINAL CORD

In 1965, Melzack and Wall (44) proposed the gate control theory of transmission of pain. They postulated the presence of an inhibitory synapse in the substantia gelatinosa of the dorsal gray matter of the spinal cord, which is activated by stimulation of large myelinated peripheral afferent fibers. The inhibitory synapse acts on the synapse of the small unmyelinated fibers carrying impulses of pain from the periphery to the second-order neuron crossing in the ventral white commissure and forming the ventral spinothalamic tract. This would "close the gate" on the transmission and sensation of pain. With reasoning analogous to that of cordotomy, namely, that the incision need only be cephalad to the level of the pain, a high thoracic or cervical level of implantation was usually chosen. Based on this theory, the medical electronic industry produced an array of sophisticated electronic devices that could stimulate the dorsal spinal cord either epidurally or from the subarachnoid space (45). The totally implanted spinal cord stimulators are powered by the transcutaneous activation of an induction coil. Eventually it was possible to install the electrodes percutaneously with a needle and embed the entire system using local anesthesia (46). Unfortunately, this technique never produced adequate results for the severe pain related to cancer. Some physicians (47, 48) still advocate this as treatment for pain of benign origin.

Transcutaneous nerve stimulation is a simple and harmless widely used modality that stimulates peripheral nerves through the intact skin. The mechanism is probably similar to that of acupuncture. Unfortunately, the technique is not effective for cancer pain (49).

ELECTRICAL STIMULATION OF THE BRAIN (FIG. 35.1A)

Richardson (50) investigated the relief of pain after stereotaxically implanting electrodes into deep brain structures. Stimulation of the periventricular gray and periaqueductal gray matter (PVG-PAG) increases levels of β-endorphins and enkephalins in the ventricular fluid. This effect is reversed by naloxone. He postulated that the β-endorphin is activated by the stimulation, subsequently inhibiting input in the dorsal horn of the spinal cord (50). Activating this system is beneficial for pain produced outside of the central nervous system, that is, pain that enters the central nervous system through the dorsal horn of the spinal cord. Richardson recommended ablative procedures initially for cancer and brain stimulation when ablation is not appropriate, such as pain in the upper extremity, midline area, and head and neck. For pain caused by neural deafferentation, stimulation in the internal capsule produces better results.

Young and Brechner (51) substantiated these findings by stimulating the PVG-PAG in 17 patients with cancer and obtained good results in 13. They noted that relief of pain produced by stimulation of the PVG-PAG lasted several hours longer than the stimulation procedure, implicating a humeral mechanism. Stimulation of thalamic nuclei is helpful for deafferentation pain, does not increase levels of endorphins, and does not result in relief of pain that exceeds the time of stimulation. Stimulation techniques hold promise but at present are being performed in only a few academic centers.

CONCLUSIONS

Pain can be a devastating accompaniment of disseminated cancer. The initial treatment of disease is aimed at the treatment of the tumor either systemically or locally. Analgesics are the first response to the pain. When treatment of the disease and medical treatment of the pain are not effective, neurosurgical procedures judiciously applied can produce gratifying comfort and palliation associated with a low incidence of morbidity and few side effects.

REFERENCES

1. Friedberg SR: The neurosurgeon's approach to pain. In Aronoff GM (ed): *Evaluation and Treatment of Chronic Pain.* Baltimore, Urban & Schwarzenberg. 1985, pp 319–331.
2. Black P: Neurosurgical management of cancer pain. *Semin Oncol* 12:438–444, 1985.
3. Foley KM: The treatment of cancer pain. *N Engl J Med* 313:84–95, 1985.
4. Freidberg SR: Neurosurgical treatment of pain caused by cancer. *Med Clin North Am* 59:481–485, 1975.
5. Cleeland CS: The impact of pain on the patient with cancer. *Cancer* 54(11 suppl):2635–2641, 1984.
6. Loeser JD: Dorsal rhizotomy for the relief of chronic pain. *J Neurosurg* 36:745–750, 1972.
7. Onofrio BM, Campa HK: Evaluation of rhizotomy: review of 12 years' experience. *J Neurosurg* 36:751–755, 1972.
8. Arbit E, Galicich JH, Burt M, Mallya K: Modified open thoracic rhizotomy for treatment of intractable chest wall pain of malignant etiology. *Ann Thorac Surg* 48:820–823, 1989.
9. Nathan PW, Scott TG: Intrathecal phenol for intractable pain: safety and dangers of the method. *Lancet* 1:76–80, 1958.
10. Sourek K: Commissural myelotomy. *J Neurosurg* 31:524–527, 1969.
11. Gildenberg PL, Hirshberg RM: Limited myelotomy for the treatment of intractable cancer pain. *J Neurol Neurosurg Psychiatry* 47:94–96, 1984.
12. Schvarcz JR: Sterotactic extralemniscal myelotomy. *J Neurol Neurosurg Psychiatry* 39:53–57, 1976.
13. Nathan PW: Results of antero-lateral cordotomy for pain in cancer. *J Neurol Neurosurg Psychiatry* 26:353–362, 1963.
14. Mullan S, Hosobuchi Y: Respiratory hazards of high cer-

vical percutaneous cordotomy. *J Neurosurg* 28:291–297, 1968.

15. Parker JF, Freidberg SR, Andrews JL Jr: Pulmonary dysfunction after unilateral percutaneous cervical cordotomy. *Lahey Clin Found Bull* 26:105–114, 1977.

16. Krieger AJ, Rosomoff HL: Sleep-induced apnea. Part 1: A respiratory and autonomic dysfunction syndrome following bilateral percutaneous cervical cordotomy. *J Neurosurg* 40:168–180, 1974.

17. Spiller WG, Martin E: Treatment of persistent pain of organic origin in the lower part of the body by division of the anterolateral column of the spinal cord. *JAMA* 58:1489–1490, 1912.

18. Mullan S: Percutaneous cordotomy: *J Neurosurg* 35:360–366, 1971.

19. Siegfried J, Kühner A, Sturm V: Neurosurgical treatment of cancer pain. *Recent Results Cancer Res* 89:148–156, 1984.

20. Takaoka Y, Freidberg SR: Electrode carrier for percutaneous cordotomy. *J Neurosurg* 40:786, 1974.

21. Gildenberg PL, Lin PM, Polakoff PP II, Flitter MA: Anterior percutaneous cervical cordotomy: determination of target point and calculation of angle of insertion. Technical note. *J Neurosurg* 28:173–177, 1968.

22. Hardy J, LeClercq TA, Mercky F: Microsurgical cordotomy by the anterior approach: technical note. *J Neurosurg* 41:640–643, 1974.

23. Kanpolat Y, Deda H, Akyar S, Caglar S: C.T.–guided pain procedures. *Neurochirurgie* 36:394–398, 1990.

24. Sjöqvist O: Cited by White JC, Sweet WH: *Pain—Its Mechanisms and Neurosurgical Control.* Springfield, IL, Charles C Thomas, 1955, p 450.

25. Hitchcock ER, Schvarcz JR: Stereotaxic trigeminal tractotomy for post-herpetic facial pain. *J Neurosurg* 37:412–417, 1972.

26. Bosch DA: Stereotactic rostral mesencephalotomy in cancer pain and deafferentation pain. *J Neurosurg* 75:747–751, 1991.

27. Rossitch E, Zeidman SM, Nashold BS: Nucleus caudalis DREZ for facial pain due to cancer. *Br J Neurosurg* 3:45–50, 1989.

28. Ramirez LF, Levin AB: Pain relief after hypophysectomy. *Neurosurgery* 14:499–504, 1984.

29. LaRossa JT, Strong MS, Melby JC: Endocrinologically incomplete transethmoidal, trans-sphenoidal hypophysectomy with relief of bone pain in breast cancer. *N Engl J Med* 298:1332–1335, 1978.

30. Levin AB, Katz J, Benson RC, Jones AG: Treatment of pain of diffuse metastatic cancer by stereotactic chemical hypophysectomy: long term results and observations on mechanism of action. *Neurosurgery* 6:258–262, 1980.

31. Moricca G: Chemical hypophysectomy for cancer pain. In Bonica JJ (ed): *Advances in Neurology: International Symposium on Pain.* New York, Raven Press, 1974, vol 4, pp 707–714.

32. Zervas NT, Gordy PD: Radiofrequency hypophysectomy for metastatic breast and prostatic carcinoma. *Surg Clin North Am* 47:1279–1285, 1967.

33. Hurt RW, Ballantine HT Jr: Stereotactic anterior cingulate lesions for persistent pain: a report on 68 cases. *Clin Neurosurg* 21:334–351, 1973.

34. Hitchcock ER, Teixeira MJ: A comparison of results from center-median and basal thalamotomies for pain. *Surg Neurol* 15:341–351, 1981.

35. Gorbitz C, Leavens ME: Alcohol block of the celiac plexus for control of upper abdominal pain caused by cancer and pancreatitis: technical note. *J Neurosurg* 34:575–579, 1971.

36. Snyder SH: Opiate receptors in the brain. *N Engl J Med* 296:266–271, 1977.

37. Yaksh TL: Spinal pharmacology of pain and its modulation. *Clin Neurosurg* 31:291–303, 1983.

38. Behar M, Magora F, Olshwang D, Davidson JT: Epidural morphine in treatment of pain. *Lancet* 1:527–529, 1979.

39. Poletti CE, Cohen AM, Todd DP, Ojemann RG, Sweet WH, Zervas NT: Cancer pain relieved by long-term epidural morphine with permanent indwelling systems for self-administration. *J Neurosurg* 55:581–584, 1981.

40. Shetter AG, Hadley MN, Wilkinson E: Administration of intraspinal morphine sulfate for the treatment of intractable cancer pain. *Neurosurgery* 18:740–747, 1986.

41. Krames ES, Gershow J, Glassberg A, Kenefick T, Lyons A, Taylor P, Wilkie D: Continuous infusion of spinally administered narcotics for the relief of pain due to malignant disorders. *Cancer* 56:696–702, 1985.

42. Coombs DW, Saunders RL, Fratkin JD, Jensen LE, Murphy CA: Continuous intrathecal hydromorphone and clonidine for intractable cancer pain. *J Neurosurg* 64:890–894, 1986.

43. Lobato RD, Madrid JL, Fatela LV, Rivas JJ, Reig E, Lamas E: Intraventricular morphine for control of pain in terminal cancer patients. *J Neurosurg* 59:627–633, 1983.

44. Melzack R, Wall PD: Pain mechanisms: a new therapy. *Science* 150:971–979, 1965.

45. Sweet WH, Wepsic JG: Stimulation of the posterior columns of the spinal cord for pain control: indications, technique, and results. *Clin Neurosurg* 21:278–310, 1973.

46. Zumpano BJ, Saunders RL: Percutaneous epidural dorsal column stimulation: technical note. *J Neurosurg* 45:459–460, 1976.

47. Young RF: Evaluation of dorsal column stimulation in the treatment of chronic pain. *Neurosurgery* 3:373–379, 1978.

48. Urban BJ, Nashold BS Jr: Percutaneous epidural stimulation of the spinal cord for relief of pain: long-term results. *J Neurosurg* 48:323–328, 1978.

49. Long DM: Stimulation of the peripheral nervous system for pain control. *Clin Neurosurg* 31:323–343, 1983.

50. Richardson DE: Intracranial stimulation for the control of chronic pain. *Clin Neurosurg* 31:316–322, 1983.

51. Young RF, Brechner T: Electrical stimulation of the brain for relief of intractable pain due to cancer. *Cancer* 57:1266–1272, 1986.

CHAPTER **36**

PALLIATION OF PAIN SECONDARY TO MALIGNANCY BY RADIATION THERAPY

RICHARD H. FITZGERALD, JR.

RECENT DISCUSSIONS of chronic pain have become eclectic and inclusive of the contributions of diverse disciplines in understanding and addressing the mechanisms of pain (1). Among those involved in chronic pain clinics, among non-oncologic physicians (2), and among psychologists and other care givers, however, there is little understanding of the contributions of irradiation in caring for patients with pain (3, 4). Approximately one million persons in the United States will be diagnosed with malignancy every year for the foreseeable future (5). Fifty to sixty percent of those patients will have some reason for radiation treatments during their lifetime (6). Many will be treated for cure, many more will be treated for palliation. In 1990 more than 12 million persons underwent treatment for malignancy in the United States (7). It is a paradox that the use of radiation therapy has had such little consideration among those who make the treatment of nonmalignant pain their life's endeavor. By not understanding that radiation therapy palliates and often completely relieves cancer-related pain and discomforting symptoms, appropriate referral may be delayed or omitted. Some treatises on cancer pain address radiation therapy only to accentuate the very uncommon, and even rare neurologic complications of radiation therapy (8). This is regrettable because radiation palliation is often very long-lasting and contributes to the comfort of hundreds of thousands of patients each year (9). There is no nonpharmacologic technique, technology, or agent that benefits the pain management of as many patients with malignancy as does radiation therapy.

Chronic pain treatment by any method is an attempt to restore function and mobility while lessening the appreciation of painful stimuli, or the stimulus itself. Palliation, from the Latin *pallium*, means that clinical signs or symptoms are lessened or abated without the complete cure of the disease process. This is what separates acute medicine from the chronic care of disease states. Most infectious diseases and trauma are acute processes that may be painful but that are often associated with complete restoration of function. The chronic care of degenerative or autoimmune illnesses and geriatric organ decline requires a completely different temperament and approach for empathic and effective caregiving. It is hoped that this discussion will introduce to some, and clarify for others, the discipline known as Radiation Oncology and the tool of radiation therapy in the treatment of chronic cancer pain.

The technical and therapeutic aspects of the use of radiation distinguish the specific purview of the radiation oncologist, a physician who, after completing a prescribed residency, may be certified by the American Board of Radiology in Radiation Oncology. This is a specialty distinct from diagnostic radiology, though using some of the same tools. It is separate from surgical and medical oncology though often employing some limited surgery for radioisotope application. Very often systemic chemotherapy is given concurrent with irradiation in the curative approach to some malignancies. The radiation oncologist should be conversant with the pathophysiology of malignancy and the capabilities, strengths and weaknesses of other disciplines in managing cancer-related pain. An appreciation of the pharmacology of analgesics and the usefulness and prudent use of diagnostic tests to elucidate sites or processes causative in pain are paramount. The radiation oncologist needs the complementing capabilities of modern therapy equipment, physicists, and technologists.

Irradiation for pain control is a major part of the practice of radiation oncology (10). In 1896, 1 year following the description of Roentgen's x-ray, Grubbe in Chicago described the use of x-ray for palliation (11). The evolution of radiation as a therapeutic tool has been empiric, and the long iteration has resulted in the supporting sciences of radiation biology and radiation physics (11). Detailed descriptions of cell kinetics and the radiation biology and physics of high-energy ionizing radiation are beyond the realm of this discussion (12). Briefly, the energy deposited when an x-ray photon interacts with tissue results in a complex chain of molecular events that produce free radical formation, ionization of atomic structure, molecular alteration, and disruption of DNA. The resultant biochemical changes result in cell death.

Radiation can be provided in several forms, including external x-rays of varying energy, Cobalt gamma rays, particulate energy (most often in the form of electrons, which also are commonly available in several energies), and less often the internal application of radioactive substances. The subtleties and distinctions of these beams are not germane to this discussion. The particular form of radiation is chosen by the radiation oncologist to irradiate the abnormal tissue volume while attempting to minimize treatment of normal, healthy structures.

Many cancers, including the larynx and other upper aerodigestive mucosal malignancies (13), cervix (14), prostate (15), and Hodgkin's disease (16), are curable by radiation therapy alone, especially in earlier stages. Most early breast carcinomas can be removed with a quite limited volume of adjacent normal breast, and—with modern radiation therapy to the residual same breast—obviate the need for total breast removal (17–19). Pain may be a component of the initial manifestation of malignancy while still curable by irradiation. Then, through a process of a protracted course of curative irradiation, the accompanying pain is most often completely ameliorated. When cure is no longer possible, irradiation is considered palliative. This discussion will address the palliative role of radiation.

The art of using radiation therapy for palliation is not easily taught or learned. It is often more difficult to deliver palliative than curative doses of radiation (20). The reasons for this are many, not the least of which is the different mindset needed to plan for and implement palliation. Palliation cannot be done in an emotional vacuum (2) and requires more than technical excellence (20).

For most patients with cancer-related pain, anti-inflammatory, opiate, and neuroleptic medications are necessary and remain so in varying amounts. Radiation therapy is a local modality of treatment, and when there is a dominant area of concern, radiation should be used to address pain in the form of somatic or sensory discomfort, functional deficit, or the psychological burden of reckoning with a mass or symptom. Judicious use of all the tools in the palliative armamentarium requires a particular knowledge base that allows one to decide not to employ a particular modality when it is not likely to be of benefit.

The goal in management of cancer-related pain is to extend comfort and prolong life, not to extend death (21, 22). Prolongation of the life of a suffering patient with incurable cancer is not palliation. Relief of suffering remains distinct and often exclusive from the prolongation of life (20).

All patients possess a premorbid history of personality traits; social, environmental, and familial mechanisms of conflict resolution; and perceptions of secondary gain. Incurable cancer will often remove the mask or patina of secondary gain, but not always. The symptoms are usually real and quite literally life-threatening. Survival with malignancy is often not predictable, and when treatment is predicated only on the expected duration of survival, patients can suffer literally and figuratively. Survival in a pain-free state after irradiation for isolated bone metastases may be experienced for many months and even many years (9, 23, 24). Radiation therapy is appropriate when a major disability is likely to be alleviated by irradiation. One must recognize that, as with the use of analgesic drugs (8), the fundamental dictum of the use of palliative irradiation is individualization without rigidity. The side effects of irradiation are directly dependent on the region of the body and volume of tissue treated and dose administered in each treatment session. There is a less predictable toxicity depending on the general state of health or debility of the patient, nutritional status, other medical illnesses, concurrent medications, and prior surgical or radiation procedures. Acute toxicity is manifested primarily as mucosal reaction limited to the area treated (e.g., nausea with abdominal and diarrhea with pelvic treatments).

Table 36.1 lists a comprehensive schema of the potential side effects of radiation (39). Please note that this is a broad compendium and is presented for the elucidation of the reader. Just as medication has potential adverse effects and surgery has attendant morbidity, irradiation sometimes can be associated with acute and chronic sequelae. It is the judicious use of any therapy that identifies the expert. Recognizing that all forms of therapeutic endeavor have some attendant cost and potential detriment, the goal in palliating cancer pain is to minimize cost and treatment-related morbidity while maximizing the degree and duration of improvement.

In Table 36.1, acute toxicity is considered. Morbidity scores 4 and 5 are exceptionally unusual. In clinical practice, one structures a treatment regimen with all attempts to minimize acute and late adverse effects. Toxicity scores of 0–2 are most often the extent of adverse acute effects, whereas a zero morbidity for chronic effects is the ideal (Table 36.2) (39).

The side effects and toxicity noted are much less likely to be observed or experienced with the doses most often employed in palliative circumstances. The radiation on-

Table 36.1.
Acute Radiation Morbidity Scoring Criteria (RTOG)[a]

Organ/Tissue	0	Score			
		Grade 1	Grade 2	Grade 3	Grade 4
Skin	No change over baseline	Follicular, faint or dull erythema, epilation, dry desquamation, decreased sweating	Tender or bright erythema, patchy moist desquamation, moderate edema	Confluent, moist desquamation other than skin folds, pitting edema	Ulceration, hemorrhage, necrosis
Mucous membrane	No change over baseline	Injection, may experience mild pain not requiring analgesic	Pathy mucositis that may produce an inflammatory serosanguinous discharge, may experience moderate pain requiring analgesic	Confluent fibrinous mucositis; may include severe pain requiring narcotic	Ulceration, hemorrhage, or necrosis
Eye	No change	Mild conjunctivitis with or without scleral injection, increased tearing	Moderate conjunctivitis with or without keratitis requiring steroids or antibiotics, dry eye requiring artificial tears, iritis with photophobia	Severe keratitis with corneal ulceration, objective decrease in visual acuity or in visual fields, acute glaucoma, panophthalmitis	Loss of vision (unilateral or bilateral)
Ear	No change over baseline	Mild external otitis with erythema, pruritis, secondary to dry desquamation not requiring medication. Audiogram unchanged from baseline	Moderate external otitis requiring topical medication, serous otitis medius, hypoacusis on testing only	Severe external otitis with discharge or moist desquamation, symptomatic hypoacusis, tinnitus, not drug-related	Deafness
Salivary gland	No change over baseline	Mild mouth dryness; slightly thickened saliva; may have slightly altered taste such as metallic; these changes not reflected in alteration in baseline feeding behavior, such as increased use of liquids with meals	Moderate to complete dryness; thick, sticky saliva, markedly altered taste	—	Acute salivary gland necrosis
Pharynx and esophagus	No change over baseline	Mild dysphagia or odynophagia; may require topical anesthetic or nonnarcotic analgesics; may require soft diet	Moderate dysphagia or odynophagia; may require narcotic analgesics; may require purée or liquid diet	Severe dysphagia or odynophagia with dehydration or weight loss (>15% from pretreatment baseline) requiring NG feeding tube, IV fluids, or hyperalimentation	Complete obstruction, ulceration, perforation, fistula
Larynx	No change over baseline	Mild or intermittent hoarseness; cough not requiring antitussive; erythema of mucosa	Persistent hoarseness but able to vocalize; referred ear pain, sore throat, patchy fibrinous exudate or mild arythenoid edema not requiring narcotic; cough requiring antitussive	Whispered speech, throat pain or referred ear pain requiring narcotic; confluent fibrinous exudate, marked arytenoid edema	Marked dyspnea; stridor or hemoptysis with tracheostomy or intubation necessary
Upper GI	No change	Anorexia with ≤5% weight loss from pretreatment baseline; nausea not requiring antiemetics; abdominal discomfort not requiring parasympatholytic drugs or analgesics	Anorexia with ≤15% weight loss from pretreatment baseline; nausea or vomiting requiring antiemetics; abdominal pain requiring analgesics	Anorexia with >15% weight loss from pretreatment baseline or requiring NG tube or parenteral support; nausea or vomiting requiring NG tube or parenteral support; abdominal pain, severe despite medication; hematemesis or melena; abdominal distention (flat plate radiograph demonstrated distended bowel loops)	Ileus, subacute or acute obstruction, perforation, GI bleeding requiring transfusion; abdominal pain requiring tube decompression or bowel diversion
Lower GI including pelvis	No change	Increased frequency or change in quality of bowel habits not requiring medication; rectal discomfort not requiring analgesics	Diarrhea requiring parasympatholytic drugs (e.g., diphenoxylate); mucous discharge not necessitating sanitary pads; rectal or abdominal pain requiring analgesics	Diarrhea requiring parenteral support; severe mucous or blood discharge necessitating sanitary pads; abdominal distention (flat plate radiograph demonstrates distended bowel loops)	Acute or subacute obstruction, fistula or perforation, GI bleeding requiring transfusion, abdominal pain or tenesmus requiring tube decompression or bowel diversion

Table 36.1.
(Continued)

Organ/Tissue	0	Score			
		Grade 1	Grade 2	Grade 3	Grade 4
Lung	No change	Mild symptoms of dry cough or dyspnea on exertion	Persistent cough requiring narcotic, antitussive agents; dyspnea with minimal effort but not at rest	Severe cough unresponsive to narcotic antitussive agent or dyspnea at rest; clinical or radiologic evidence of acute pneumonitis; intermittent O_2 or steroids may be required	Severe respiratory insufficiency; continuous oxygen or assisted ventilation
Genitourinary	No change	Frequency of urination or nocturia twice pretreatment habit; dysuria, urgency not requiring medication	Frequency of urination or nocturia less frequent than every hour; dysuria, urgency, bladder spasm requiring local anesthetic (e.g., phenazopyridine)	Frequency with urgency and nocturia hourly or more frequently; dysuria, pelvic pain, or bladder spasm requiring regular, frequent narcotic; gross hematuria with or without clot passage	Hematuria requiring transfusion; acute bladder obstruction not secondary to clot passage, ulceration, or necrosis
Heart	No change over baseline	Asymptomatic but objective evidence of EKG changes or pericardial abnormalities without evidence of other heart disease	Symptomatic with EKG changes and radiologic findings of congestive heart failure or pericardial disease; no specific treatment required	Congestive heart failure, angina pectoris, pericardial disease responding to therapy	Congestive heart failure, angina pectoris, pericardial disease, arrhythmias not responsive to nonsurgical measures
CNS	No change	Fully functional status (able to work) with minor neurologic findings; no medication needed	Neurologic findings sufficient to require home care; nursing assistance may be required; medication including steroids; antiseizure agents may be required	Neurologic findings requiring hospitalization for initial management	Serious neurologic impairment that includes paralysis coma, or seizures >3 per wk despite medication; hospitalization required
Hematologic WBC ($\times$ 1000)	$\geq$4.0	3.0–<4.0	2.0–<3.0	1.0–<2.0	<1.0
Platelets ($\times$ 1000)	>100	75–<100	50–<75	25–<50	<25 or spontaneous bleeding
Neutrophils ($\times$ 1000)	$\geq$1.9	1.5–<1.9	1.0–<1.5	0.5–<1.0	<0.5 or sepsis
Hemoglobin (GM %)	>11	11–9.5	<9.5–7.5	<7.5–5.0	—
Hematocrit (%)	$\geq$32	20–<32	20	Packed cell transfusion required	—

Guidelines:
The acute morbidity criteria are used to score/grade toxicity from radiation therapy. The criteria are relevant from day 1, the commencement of therapy, through day 90. Thereafter, the EORTC/RTOG Criteria for Late Effects are to be utilized.
The evaluator must attempt to discriminate between disease and treatment-related signs and symptoms.
An accurate baseline evaluation prior to commencement of therapy is necessary.
All toxicities of Grade 3, 4, or 5 must be verified by the principal investigator (Any toxicity that caused death is graded 5).
[a]*From Perez CA, Brady LW: Overview. In Perez CA, Brady LW (eds): Principles and Practice of Radiation Oncology. Philadelphia, JB Lippincott, 1992, pp 1–63.*

cologist chooses his treatment mindful of the goals of the particular problem to be addressed in the individual patient.

Radiation dose fractionation schedules vary among radiation oncologists and radiation centers. Dose schedules are arrived at by complex formulae, factoring in the area to be treated, prior and current therapies, concurrent illnesses, and the judgement of the treating physician (25–28). Radiation therapy is most often used to palliate bone pain, neuropathic pain, headache, visceral pain, and soft tissue pain (Table 36.3). In addition, but not within the scope of this chapter, it can be used to treat bleeding (e.g., from lung carcinoma or malignancy involving the rectum, bladder, or cervix). Radiation can be used to treat skin or nodal disease, which are the source of much psychological pain for patients, family, and caregivers. The nursing care required to attend to fungating skin lesions can be markedly assisted by decreasing bleeding, drainage, and discharge. Often, large masses are associated with fever and debility and contribute to cachexia. Treatment of such large masses may provide substantial comfort and palliation (20). Paresis due to brain metastases is most often treated with radiation. Other common concerns of radiation palliation

Table 36.2.
Late Radiation Morbidity Scoring Scheme (RTOG, EORTC)

Organ/Tissue	0	Grade 1	Grade 2	Grade 3	Grade 4	Grade 5
Skin	None	Slight atrophy, pigmentation change, some hair loss	Patchy atrophy, moderate telangiectasia, total hair loss	Marked atrophy, gross telangiectasia	Ulceration	Death directly related to radiation late effect
Subcutaneous tissue	None	Slight induration (fibrosis) and loss of subcutaneous fat	Moderate fibrosis but asymptomatic, slight field contracture; <10% linear reduction	Severe induration and loss of subcutaneous tissue; field contracture >10% linear measurement	Necrosis	
Mucous membrane	None	Slight atrophy and dryness	Moderate atrophy and telangiectasia, little mucus	Marked atrophy with complete dryness, severe telangiectasia	Ulceration	
Salivary glands	None	Slight dryness of mouth, good response on stimulation	Moderate dryness of mouth, poor response on stimulation	Complete dryness of mouth, no response on stimulation	Fibrosis	
Spinal cord	None	Mild L'hermitte's sign	Severe L'hermitte's sign	Objective neurologic findings at or below cord level treated	Mono-, paraquadriplegia	
Brain	None	Mild headache, slight lethargy	Moderate headache, great lethargy	Severe headache, severe CNS dysfunction (partial loss of power or dyskinesia)	Seizures or paralysis, coma	
Eye	None	Asymptomatic cataract, minor corneal ulceration or keratitis	Symptomatic cataract, moderate corneal ulceration, minor retinopathy or glaucoma	Severe keratitis, severe retinopathy or detachment, severe glaucoma	Panophthalmitis, blindness	
Larynx	None	Hoarseness, slight arytenoid edema	Moderate arytenoid edema, chondritis	Severe edema, severe chondritis	Necrosis	
Lung	None	Asymptomatic or mild symptoms (dry cough), slight radiographic appearances	Moderate symptomatic fibrosis or pneumonitis (severe cough); low-grade fever, patchy radiographic appearances	Severe symptomatic fibrosis or pneumonitis, dense radiographic changes	Severe respiratory insufficiency, continuous O_2, assisted ventilation	
Heart	None	Asymptomatic or mild symptoms, transient T-wave inversion and ST changes, sinus tachycardia >110 (at rest)	Moderate angina on effort, mild pericarditis, normal heart size, persistent abnormality T wave and ST changes, low ORS	Severe angina, pericardial effusion, constrictive pericarditis, moderate heart failure, cardiac enlargement, EKG abnormalities	Tamponade, severe heart failure, severe constrictive pericarditis	
Esophagus	None	Mild fibrosis, slight difficulty in swallowing solids, no pain on swallowing	Unable to take solid food normally, swallowing semisolid food, dilatation may be indicated	Severe fibrosis, able to swallow only liquids, may have pain on swallowing; dilatation required	Necrosis, perforation, fistula	
Small/large intestine	None	Mild diarrhea, mild cramping, bowel movement 5 times daily, slight rectal discharge or bleeding	Moderate diarrhea and colic, bowel movement >5 times daily, excessive rectal mucus or intermittent bleeding	Obstruction or bleeding requiring surgery	Necrosis, perforation, fistula	
Liver	None	Mild lassitude, nausea, dyspepsia, slightly abnormal liver function	Moderate symptoms, some abnormal liver function tests, secrum albumin normal	Disabling hepatitic insufficiency, liver function tests grossly abnormal, low albumin, edema or ascites	Necrosis, hepatic coma or encephalopathy	
Kidney	None	Transient albuminuria, no hypertension, mild impairment renal function, urea 25–35 mg%, creatinine 1.5–2.0 mg%, creatinine clearance >75%	Persistent moderate albuminuria (2+); mild hypertension, no related anemia, moderate impairment renal function; urea >36–60 mg%, creatinine clearance (50–74%)	Severe albuminuria, severe hypertension, persistent anemia (<100%), severe renal failure, urea >60 mg%, creatinine >4.0 mg%, creatinine clearance <50%	Malignant hypertension, uremic coma; urea >100%	

Table 36.2.
(Continued)

Organ/Tissue	0	Grade 1	Grade 2	Grade 3	Grade 4	Grade 5
Bladder	None	Slight epithelial atrophy, mild telangiectasia (microscopic hematuria)	Moderate frequency, generalized telangiectasia, intermittent macroscopic hematuria	Severe frequency and dysuria, severe generalized telangiectasia (often with petechiae), frequent hematuria, reduction in bladder capacity (<150 ml)	Necrosis, contracted bladder (capacity <100 ml), severe hemorrhagic cystitis	
Bone	None	Asymptomatic, no growth retardation, reduced bone density	Moderate pain or tenderness, growth retardation, irregular bone sclerosis	Severe pain or tenderness, complete arrest of bone growth, dense bone sclerosis	Necrosis, spontaneous fracture	
Joint	None	Mild joint stiffness, slight limitation of movement	Moderate stiffness, intermittent or moderate joint pain, moderate limitation of movement	Severe joint stiffness, pain with severe limitation of movement	Necrosis, complete fixation	

ªFrom Perez CA, Brady LW: Overview. In Perez CA, Brady LW (eds): *Principles and Practice of Radiation Oncology*. Philadelphia, JB Lippincott, 1992, pp 1–63.

Table 36.3.
Radiation Therapy Palliation

Pain
  Bone
  Pathologic fracture prophylaxis
  Spinal cord compression
  Neuropathic pain
  Headache
  Viscera
  Soft tissue masses
Symptoms and Signs
  Bleeding
  Visceral obstruction
  Cough
  Swallowing
  Vessel compression
  Nerve entrapment
  Paresis
  Retinal (choroid) deposit
  Skin masses

are relief of cough, prevention of fistula, and easing of swallowing. Cranial nerves may be compressed as they exit through the base of the skull because of osseous metastases. Treatment of the base of the skull can release the compression and stabilize or improve the deficit (29). Retinal metastases and resultant loss of a portion of the visual field may be treated, with possible restoration of vision (30).

BONE PAIN

Mature bone is associated with nociceptor fibers in the endosteum and periosteum, supporting vascular structures, and ligamentous and muscular attachments. Bone metastases are seen in up to 84% of patients with incurable disease depending on the site of the primary malignancy and the intensity of analysis (10). Pain is usually aching and often worsened with movement (31). Pain may be the result of chemical mediators produced by the malignancy. A prostaglandin or other kinin is thought to be associated and may explain the rather rapid onset of pain relief in some patients following the initiation of irradiation (8, 32). The observation of a brisk response allows the conclusion that a chemical mediator is being produced in a lesser quantity by disruption of the metabolism of the irradiated tumor cell. Just as often, however, pain relief is delayed for 1–4 weeks and may be due to an actual reduction in the bulk of tumor deposits and release of pressure on entrapped or compressed nerves or surrounding sensitive structures (32). Repeatedly, it has been demonstrated that 80% of patients treated with radiation for cancer-related bone pain will achieve relief (25). Furthermore, up to 70% of those patients will remain pain-free in the area irradiated for the remainder of their life (10, 29). Some patients with metastatic bone disease may live for many years (9, 23). For example, Bagshaw found that among his patients with metastatic prostate carcinoma there was a 2-year median survival and a maximum survival of 8 years (23).

Some diseases have a propensity for bone metastases and often demonstrate substantial and prolonged relief after irradiation. Among these are prostate carcinoma, breast carcinoma, multiple myeloma, and lymphoma. Patients with a solitary bone metastasis and little or no other evidence of metastasis should be offered aggressive treatment in contradistinction to patients with advanced multiorgan metastases.

The benefits of decreasing pain include less obtundation and constipation from narcotics, improved mobility, and less attendant depression and anxiety.

PATHOLOGIC FRACTURE

Most bone metastases occur in the area of active blood-producing red marrow with its associated rich vascular supply. The proximal-most weight-bearing areas of the femur and acetabulum, which make up the functioning ball and socket joint of the hip, are very often involved. Radiographic demonstration of lytic defects in those bones is a harbinger of possible fracture. Approximately 10% of people with metastases in this area develop pathologic fractures (25). Those at higher risk are patients with cortical defects greater than 2.5 cm and those who have lost more than 50% of the bony cortex (25). By recognizing that full function and stability may never be returned to those bones, and by counseling the patient to modify activity in spite of pain improvement, it is possible to avoid completely pathologic fracture in many patients (25). Obviously, the economic drain of being bedfast and the loss of productivity and increased cost of surgical repair of a pathologic fracture of the proximal femur are much better anticipated and prevented.

Pathologic fractures of the central axial skeleton, especially of vertebrae, are associated with severe debility and are a special concern of spinal cord compression.

SPINAL CORD COMPRESSION

The spinal cord is encased in a rigid bony structure with little room for extraneous tissue. The spinal cord is quite sensitive to the loss of blood supply. Ischemia results in death of the spinal cord distal to the site of obstruction.

Anatomically, there are two common patterns of compression recognized. The usual form is due to direct extension posteriorly of a malignant mass from the involved vertebral bone. A second, less common means of spinal cord compression is by direct extension of soft tissue disease through an intervertebral foramen. Direct metastases to the epidural space or spinal cord is rare (33). A limited vascular supply and rigid envelope of bone contribute to the sensitivity of the cord to ischemia (34, 35). Early recognition and intervention is critical to restore and maintain function. Treatment can be surgical or by means of radiation therapy, depending on the availability of technology, the rapidity of change, and the site of the primary malignancy (36). Findlay reviewed 1816 patients with spinal cord compression and reported that only 25% were referred for treatment when still able to walk. Of those patients treated with surgery, 48% remained ambulatory following surgical decompression. Of those patients who received surgery followed by irradiation, 67% remained ambulatory. Of those patients treated with radiation therapy only, 79%

remained able to walk (25). Posterior decompression of the spinal laminae will decompress the spinal cord in the area of resection. It will not address the bulk and distortion coming from the vertebra in the anterior aspect of the spinal canal ventral to the spinal cord. Anterior approaches to the spinal canal through the neck or thorax are becoming commonplace. Such a procedure is more demanding on the patient and the surgeon, and often requires stabilization by means of a prostheses to strut the surgical or neoplastic defect. After any surgical decompression, irradiation is appropriate to further safeguard the spinal cord by treating the encroaching malignancy.

All tissues have an innate individual tolerance to irradiation that depends on whether treatment consists of one or a few large fractions or of multiple smaller doses delivered over a longer period. The tolerance of the spinal cord exceeds the dose needed most often to relieve bone pain. Retreatment courses pose a complex problem in that additional doses may cumulatively approach or exceed spinal cord tolerance. Spinal cord injury and death by malignancy is orders of magnitude more problematic and common than irradiation-induced damage.

Injury to any tissue during a therapeutic endeavor is to be avoided whenever possible. An occasional patient will be seen who has severe vertebral pain or impending spinal cord compression in an area already irradiated. The therapeutic dilemma then arises of whether to further treat with the goal of improving mobility and pain by reducing the tumor volume, or to address the pain only with greater doses of analgesics while watching paresis worsen. These circumstances call for philosophic, practical, and prudent analyses of the individual patient's prognosis and desires. This is the crux of why palliative treatment is demanding on the care giver.

NEUROPATHIC INVOLVEMENT

The origin and course of the brachial and lumbar sacral plexuses are intimately associated with bone and soft tissue. Direct invasion or compression of these structures results in severe and complex pain patterns. The violation of nerve trunks by malignancy causes a pain more akin to causalgia. When nerves are actually invaded or infiltrated and disrupted, irradiation-associated palliation is usually less than complete and may be minimal. At times, however, treatment can be quite gratifying and irradiation should not be withheld because of the anatomic location of the disease only. Some malignancies (e.g., the lymphomas and small cell carcinoma of the lung) are more quickly responsive to irradiation.

HEADACHE

The brain is within the rigid bony calvarium, which does not allow the brain to expand after insult or injury.

Metastases to the cerebral cortex can produce mass effect and an increase in intracranial pressure. By decreasing the bulk of the metastases by irradiation, and by decreasing any attendant edema by corticosteroids, headache pain can often be alleviated. Headache can be an accompaniment of the superior vena caval syndrome. Venous drainage from the upper extremities and head is afforded by a large vein just proximal to the heart, the superior vena cava. Central mediastinal masses that compress the superior vena cava result in a syndrome of edema of the arms, neck and face, and a throbbing headache presumably due to edema of the brain and meninges. Irradiation of the mediastinum with resultant decrease of the obstruction can quickly relieve headache and improve the comfort of patients with superior vena cava syndrome (20). Less commonly are other thin-walled, low-pressure venous structures compressed (e.g., the axillary vein or inferior vena cava). Minimal change in the radius of the lumen of a vessel can result in substantial improvement in blood flow and comfort.

VISCERAL PAIN

Pleural infiltration and pleuritic pain may be improved by irradiation of the area of concern. Often it is difficult to distinguish between pleural or associated rib pain. The capsule of the liver (Glisson's capsule) may be infiltrated or stretched by neoplastic enlargement of the liver. Although not commonly done because of the gravity of the physical state of the patient population with advanced liver metastases, treatment of the liver and Glisson's capsule can result in greater patient comfort with a corresponding decrease in the need for narcotics and improvement in sensorium and function (37, 38).

The spleen may be enlarged because of infiltration by lymphoma or leukemia. Splenomegaly can be uncomfortable and associated with shortness of breath and distension of the abdomen which is, in itself, uncomfortable. Irradiation of the spleen in this circumstance is indicated to effect improvement in patient comfort.

Occasionally, the bowel or mesentery will be involved with lymphoma; irradiation of that section of bowel or the entire abdominal or pelvic cavity may result in improvement in comfort. Ovarian and colonic carcinoma can widely involve omentum, but these conditions are much less subject to manipulation by irradiation of the abdomen.

Organs high in the abdomen, especially the pancreas, can directly invade and infiltrate the prevertebral soft tissue and splanchnic nerve plexus. This results in a severe, deep, boring pain that is quite debilitating and often the dominant site of concern. Irradiation may improve the comfort of these patients. If the pain is not severe, it may be more indicative of mass effect than of nerve infiltration, and treatment may obviate the occurrence of severe pain throughout the course of the patient's life (20).

SOFT TISSUE MASSES

Direct, contiguous extension of disease into soft tissue, or metastases to tight compartments or areas associated with muscular activity, are painful and debilitating. Low pelvic and perineal occurrence of malignancy, such as prostate or rectum cancer, may make it impossible to sit. Metastases to groin nodes or the axillary soft tissue compartment allows for easy maceration of the overlying skin. This becomes tight and thin and can be associated with compression of vascular and neural structures with attendant morbidity. Irradiation of these masses will result in a decrease in the mass and release of the associated pressures on other structures.

CONCLUSIONS

Until mechanisms that will prevent the development of malignancy are established, major lifestyle changes regarding cigarettes and diet are implemented, and mechanisms for earlier diagnosis are developed, palliation of patients with advanced malignancy will remain a problem of great magnitude. Radiation therapy is one tool in the armamentarium of caregivers who have chosen to relieve the chronic pain and suffering of patients with malignancy.

REFERENCES

1. Tollison CD (ed): *Handbook of Chronic Pain Management.* Baltimore, Williams & Wilkins, 1989.
2. Torpie RJ: Paliation of the patient with cancer: Treatment of Mind and Body. In Perez CA, Brady L (eds): *Principles and Practice of Radiation Oncology*. Philadelphia, JB Lippincott, 1987, pp 1283–1286.
3. Payne R, Foley K (eds): Cancer Pain, Medical Clinics of North America, March 1987, Saunders.
4. Arter OE, Racz GR: Pain management of the oncologic patient. *Semin Surg Oncol* 6:162–172, 1990.
5. Boring CC, Squires TS, Tong T: Cancer statistics, 1992. *CA-A Cancer J Civil* 42:19–38, 1992.
6. Intersociety Council for Radiation Oncology: Radiation Oncology in Integrated Cancer Management, 1991. This is a monograph, fifth edition, December 1991, Philadelphia, PA, published by the Intersociety Council.
7. *Curing Cancer with Radiation Therapy*. American Society for Therapeutic Radiation and Oncology, 1990.
8. Foley KM: Diagnosis and treatment of cancer pain. In Holleb A, Fink D, Murphy G (eds): *American Cancer Society Textbook of Clinical Oncology*, 1991. (textbook) Atlanta, GA. published by American Cancer Society.
9. Schocker JD, Brady LW: Radiation therapy for bone metastasis. *Clin Orthop Rel Res* 169:38–43, 1982.

10. Tong D, Gillik L, Hendrickson F: The palliation of osseus metastases: Final study by the Radiation Therapy Oncology Group. *Cancer* 50:893–899, 1982.

11. Kaplan HS: Radiobiology's contribution to radiotherapy: Promise or mirage? Failla Memorial Lecture. *Radiat Res* 43:460–476, 1970.

12. Fletcher GH: Keynote address: The scientific basis of the present and future practice of clinical radiotherapy. *Int J Radiat Oncol Biol Phys* 9:1073–1082, 1983.

13. Million RR, Cassisi N (eds): *Management of Head and Neck Cancer—A multidisciplinary Approach.* Philadelphia, JB Lippincott, 1984.

14. Perez CA, Kuske RR, Camel HM et al: Analysis of pelvic tumor control and impact on survival in carcinoma of the uterine cervix treated with radiation therapy alone. *Int J Radiat Oncol Biol Phys* 14:613–621, 1988.

15. Hanks GE, Leibel S et al: Patterns of care studies: Dose-response of observations to local control of adenocarcinoma of the prostate. *Int J Radiat Oncol Biol Phys* 11:153, 1985.

16. Hoppe RT: Radiation therapy in the management of Hodgkin's disease. *Semin Oncol* 17:704, 1990.

17. Harris JR, Hellman S: Primary radiation for early breast cancer. *Cancer* 51(Suppl 12):2547–2552, 1983.

18. Montague ED: Conservation surgery and radiation therapy in the treatment of operable breast cancer. *Cancer* 53:700–704, 1984.

19. Fisher B, Redmond C, Poisson R et al: Eight year results of a randomized clinical trial comparing total mastectomy and lumpectomy with our without irradiation in the treatment of breast cancer. *N Engl J Med* 320:822–828, 1989.

20. Buschke F, Parker RG: Palliative radiation therapy of the patient with incurable cancer. In Buschke F, Parker RG: *Radiation Therapy in Cancer Management.* New York, Grune & Stratton, 1972, pp 363–373.

21. Kübler-Ross E: *On Death and Dying.* New York, Macmillan, 1969.

22. Kagan, AR: Radiation therapy in palliative cancer management. In Perez CA, Brady LW (eds): *Principles and Practice of Radiation Oncology.* Philadelphia, JB Lippincott, 1992, pp 1495–1507.

23. Wazer DE, Willett BL: Clinical considerations in palliative treatment of metastatic prostate carcinoma. *Int J Radiat Oncol Biol Phys* 13:145–146, 1987.

24. Dunphy JE: Annual discourse on caring for the patient with cancer. *N Engl J Med* 295:313–319, 1976.

25. Bates T: A review of local radiotherapy in the treatment of bone metastases and cord compression. *Int J Radiat Oncol Biol Phys* 23:217–221, 1992.

26. Maher EJ, Coia L et al: Treatment strategies in advanced and metastatic cancer: Differences in attitude between the USA, Canada and Europe. *Int J Radiat Oncol Biol Phys* 23:239–244, 1992.

27. Priestman TJ, Bullimore JA, Godden TP et al: The Royal College of Radiologists fractionation survey. *Clin Oncol* 1:39–46, 1989.

28. Scher HI, Yagoda A: Bone metastases: Pathogenesis, treatment and rationale for using resorption inhibitors. *Am J Med* 82:6–28, 1987.

29. Vikram B, Chu F: Radiation therapy for metastases to the base of the skull. *Radiology* 130:465–468, 1979.

30. Brady LW, Shields JA et al: Malignant intraocular tumors. *Cancer* 49:578, 1982.

31. Kanner R: Pain treatment. In Dutcher JP, Wiervik PH (eds): *Handbook of Hematologic and Oncologic Emergencies.* New York, Plenum, 1987.

32. Nielsen OS, Munro AJ, Tannock IF: Bone metastases: Pathophysiology and management policy. *J Clin Oncol* 9:509–524, 1991.

33. Cairncross JG, Posner JB: Neurologic complications of systemic cancer. In Yarbro JW, Bornstein RS (eds): *Oncologic Emergencies.* New York, Grune & Stratton, 1988, pp 75–96.

34. Gilbert H, Apuzzo M et al: Neoplastic epidural spinal cord compression. *JAMA* 240:2771–2773, 1978.

35. Delaney TF, Olfield EH: Spinal cord compression. In DeVita V, Hellman S, Rosenberg S (eds). *Cancer Principles and Practice of Oncology.* Philadelphia, JB Lippincott, 1989, pp 1978–1986.

36. Bruchman JE, Bloomer WE: Management of spinal cord compression. *Semin Oncol* 5:135, 1978.

37. Borgelt BB, Gelber R et al: The palliation of lupatic metastases. Results of ROTG pilot study. *Int J Radiat Oncol Biol Phys* 7:587–591, 1981.

38. Sherman DM et al: Palliation of hepatic metastases. *Cancer* 41:2013–2017, 1978.

39. Perez CA, Brady LW: Overview. In Perez CA, Brady LW (eds): *Principles and Practice of Radiation Oncology.* Philadelphia, JB Lippincott, 1992, pp 1–63.

CHAPTER 37

PERIPHERAL NEUROPATHY

DAVID R. CORNBLATH
JONATHAN D. GLASS

THIS CHAPTER considers the diagnosis and management of peripheral neuropathies in which pain is a dominant feature. Although pain is a sensory phenomenon, these neuropathies usually affect both sensory and motor fibers; in some, autonomic neuropathy may be prominent. Pathologically, the majority of these disorders are distal symmetric axonal degenerations (1), but a few are systemic vascular disorders with involvement of the peripheral nervous system. Pain is rare in demyelinating neuropathies. Entrapment neuropathies and mononeuropathies are discussed in other chapters in this volume.

Three main points are relevant to the evaluation and treatment of painful peripheral neuropathy. First, because these disorders have in common dysfunction of small myelinated and unmyelinated fibers, patients present with a stereotypical account of their pain. Second, the differential diagnoses of patients with painful peripheral neuropathy are few. The section below addressing the individual disorders concentrates on aids to diagnosis, because specific information about these disorders can be found elsewhere (2). Third, treatment is initially directed at the underlying cause of the neuropathy, if known. If the underlying etiology is not known, therapy for the pain is undertaken but is only symptomatic.

SYMPTOMS AND SIGNS

The symptoms of pain in patients with peripheral neuropathy are stereotypical and, classically, are either positive or negative (3); individual patients may experience both. *Positive symptoms* may include *paresthesias* (abnormal spontaneous sensations) such as tingling, the feeling as though "novocaine is wearing off," or the feeling that the limb is "asleep." More annoying are *dysesthesias*, in which the presentation of ordinary stimuli results in disagreeable sensation. Dysesthesias are the most distressing symptom, because the limbs are normally in continuous contact with stimuli. This is particularly troublesome at night when the feet are elevated and the

bed sheets touch the feet. Dysesthetic pain is distinctive: burning, raw, and searing. It has also been described as an unfamiliar sensation on the surface of the skin. Many patients find that activity exacerbates dysesthesia.

Patients may also have *negative symptoms*: numbness, a "wooden" feeling, or a feeling that the limb is wrapped in cotton or encased in cement. Some patients feel as if they are walking on stilts. Negative symptoms rarely trouble patients because pain is absent. When sensory loss is particularly severe, however, patients may discover that they are unable to locate their feet unless they look at them, or patients may develop painless injuries.

Physical examination of patients with painful peripheral neuropathy almost always uncovers distal sensory abnormalities, particularly among those modalities that reflect small myelinated and unmyelinated fiber function (i.e., pain and temperature). Many of these patients have relatively intact large-fiber function (i.e., position and vibration sense, strength, and reflexes). Touch is variably affected and may induce dysesthesias. When examining these patients, several questions should be asked. First, are the patient's symptoms positive or negative? Second, is the threshold for perception of a stimulus normal or raised at a specific location? Third, is dysesthesia or hyperpathia (exaggerated responses to a painful stimuli) present?

Two mechanisms are hypothesized necessary for the generation of peripheral nerve pain (4). First, there must be increased impulse generation in nerve fibers, most likely in small myelinated or unmyelinated fibers. Second, unmyelinated fibers must be abnormal. This may happen either "externally," as with a compressive lesion, or "internally," as with a peripheral neuropathy.

What is the evidence for these hypotheses? Microneurographic recordings of human nerve impulses reveal that perception of pain is associated with nerve impulses that are conducted at velocities consistent with those of C-fibers (5). Dyck and colleagues found that pain in the foot was related to the presence of acute fiber break-

463

down in myelinated fibers and that the ratio of remaining large and small fibers is not correlated to pain (6). Brown and colleagues found that in patients with painful diabetic neuropathy the number of myelinated fibers was reduced by two-thirds, especially the small myelinated fibers (7). Nevertheless, the total number of unmyelinated fibers was normal in these patients but, based on morphologic criteria, these were assumed to represent regenerating sprouts, which implied previous fiber breakdown. Said and co-workers found that diabetic patients who do not have spontaneous pain but who do experience painless injuries have almost no unmyelinated fibers and a moderate reduction in the small myelinated fiber population (8), suggesting that the primary problem in peripheral nerve pain is the small myelinated and unmyelinated fibers. These data, however, do not allow a clear understanding of the role of large myelinated fibers in the generation of peripheral nerve pain. The gate theory implies that loss of large myelinated fibers alone may leave small myelinated and unmyelinated fibers free to generate painful impulses (9). This is not the case in most diseases in which large fibers are preferentially lost, however, because they are not associated with spontaneous pain (10). Large myelinated fibers are likely to play a role in pain modulation, but are not necessary for pain generation.

Over the last several years, the possible role of the sympathetic nervous system in painful peripheral neuropathy has gained increasing attention. Although a role for the sympathetic nervous system in sympathetically mediated pain syndromes (causalgia) is not debated, the contribution of the sympathetic nervous system to distal axonal degenerations causing pain is less well-defined. Clinical and experimental observations do suggest that the sympathetic nervous system is involved in painful neuropathy syndromes (11), but the precise translation of this into therapeutics is still undefined.

Because pain in peripheral neuropathies depends on abnormalities of unmyelinated and small myelinated fibers, autonomic function, which is subserved by a similar nerve-fiber class, can also be affected. Thus, symptoms such as orthostatic hypotension, gastrointestinal dysautonomia, impotence, changes in sweat pattern, gustatory sweating, and bladder dysfunction should be sought and directed therapies should be applied, especially for orthostatic hypotension (12). Equally important is that the presence of dysautonomia provides clues to diagnosis.

DIFFERENTIAL DIAGNOSIS

As stated above, the differential diagnosis of predominantly painful peripheral neuropathy is limited (Table 37.1), and in many patients the correct diagnosis may be obtained from the history and physical examination alone. Further evaluation, including blood and urine

Table 37.1.
Causes of Painful Peripheral Neuropathy

AIDS	Guillain-Barré syndrome
Alcohol	Insulinoma
Amyloidois	Ischemia
Cancer	Malnutrition
Diabetes	Porphyria
Drugs	Sjögren's syndrome
Dysproteinemias	Toxins
Fabry's disease	Uremia

studies and electrodiagnostic testing, may be required to confirm the diagnosis. Nerve biopsy is necessary in only a small proportion of patients.

Diabetes is the most common cause of painful peripheral neuropathy. In diabetics who develop painful peripheral neuropathy, the history of diabetes is usually well established. In most of these patients, the neuropathy begins after many years of suboptimally controlled diabetes. Other "end-organ" diseases, such as retinopathy and nephropathy, are frequently present. A more-difficult clinical situation occurs when diabetes has not been previously diagnosed but is suspected in a patient with a painful peripheral neuropathy. Some of these patients have metabolic abnormalities consistent with diabetes and meet criteria outlined by the American Diabetes Association. In others, an abnormal glucose tolerance test suggests diabetes. In these patients, the probability that the painful neuropathy is caused by glucose intolerance is further strengthened by the presence of other neurologic complications suggestive of sustained hyperglycemia, such as impotence and carpal tunnel or lateral femoral cutaneous nerve entrapments. In these circumstances, the neuropathy is presumptively related to glucose intolerance, and treatment can be instituted.

The best therapy now available for painful diabetic peripheral neuropathy is improved glucose control (13). In diabetics already taking insulin, improved control may require more-frequent administration of insulin or frequent dose adjustments based on glucometer readings. In diabetics previously treated with oral agents or diet, insulin therapy may have to be initiated.

Antiglycemic therapy alone may be sufficient to alleviate the pain due to diabetic neuropathy (14, 15). Moreover, in some patients with diabetic neuropathy, pain may spontaneously resolve (16). Two hypotheses have been proposed to explain spontaneous improvement. First, nerves may regenerate through improved glucose control. Second, fibers may continue to degenerate, and so impulses can no longer be spontaneously generated. Because spontaneous pain may remit spontaneously, only short-acting symptomatic drugs should be used.

Patients whose pain is continuous and aggravating are managed in other ways. Several new therapies for diabetic neuropathy are now under investigation, including aldose reductase inhibitors, gangliosides, and neurotrophic growth factors.

Malnutrition from alcoholism, gastrointestinal disease or surgery, improper diet, or other causes can produce painful neuropathy (17). The disorder begins with dysesthesia and progresses to weakness and sensory loss. Pain on the soles of the feet is particularly distressing, and the term *burning feet* has been used in various disorders associated with malnutrition. Deficiencies of the B vitamins, especially thiamine, pyridoxine, pantothenic acid, and cyanocobalamin, are most commonly associated with neuropathy. Lack of other dietary constituents such as niacin is also associated with painful neuropathy. In many of these patients, it is difficult to ascribe the neuropathy to the lack of a single vitamin. Most individuals are multiply vitamin-deficient, and the symptoms and signs of individual vitamin deficiencies may overlap; also, laboratory measurements of the vitamins may not truly reflect tissue stores or utilization. Thus, treatment will involve multivitamin replacement and a balanced, high-calorie diet.

Two points deserve further consideration. The precise role of *alcohol* in the production of peripheral neuropathy is still debated. The evidence has been summarized and suggests that alcohol alone is not toxic to peripheral nerves (17). Because most alcoholics are also malnourished, it is difficult to ascribe cause and effect. In addition to that mentioned above, treatment includes abstinence from alcohol. In B_{12} *deficiency*, the peripheral nerve abnormalities are minor and are far overshadowed by the spinal cord disease. Thus, routine treatment of patients with painful peripheral neuropathy with B_{12} injections is unwarranted.

Amyloidosis is another cause of painful peripheral neuropathy. About 30% of those patients with amyloidosis have peripheral neuropathy that is usually painful (18). These patients may present with neurologic dysfunction, especially distal dysesthesia, but after a detailed history is taken, it emerges that a systemic disorder is present, manifested by weight loss and fatigue. Many also show evidence of other neurologic abnormalities such as autonomic insufficiency, impotence, and carpal tunnel syndrome. A monoclonal protein in serum or urine suggests the diagnosis, which is confirmed by biopsy. Of the currently available diagnostic techniques, immunofixation electrophoresis is the most sensitive. There is no proven therapy for amyloidosis; patients have a progressive neurologic decline but usually die from general medical problems.

Several pathogenetic types of neuropathy can be encountered in patients infected with *human immunodeficiency virus (HIV) infection*, including demyelinating, vasculitic, infectious, and distal symmetric degeneration (19). Neuropathy can also occur as a consequence of treatment with certain anti-retroviral medications. Pain is a prominent feature in cytomegalovirus-associated polyradiculoneuritis, and can be present in mononeuropathy multiplex caused by vasculitis. In these cases, treatment of the underlying disorder with antiviral agents or immunosuppression may alleviate the pain. Far more common than these disorders is the painful, predominantly sensory neuropathy seen in patients with late or end-stage acquired immunodeficiency syndrome (AIDS) (20). These patients complain of dysesthetic and spontaneous pain in the toes and over the dorsal surfaces of the feet. Examination shows elevated sensory thresholds distally and often the patient experiences severe discomfort when a cool surface or vibrating tuning fork is placed on the foot. Deep tendon reflexes are likely to be absent at the ankles but accentuated at the knees because of the myelopathy that is frequently present. The pathogenesis is unknown. Pathologic studies do not suggest that the syndrome is caused by infection of lumbosacral dorsal root ganglia with cytomegalovirus, and HIV cannot be isolated from the peripheral nerve in the majority of cases. Quantitative morphometric analysis of distal peripheral nerves has shown a disproportionate loss of unmyelinated fibers (21). The painful neuropathy of AIDS may respond symptomatically to the same regimens used in other painful neuropathies (see below). We have had little success with topical therapies such as capsaicin or lidocaine cream. Fortunately, many patients experience a spontaneous resolution of their pain as nerve fiber loss progresses.

Several *toxins and drugs* can cause a painful neuropathy. Patients with arsenic intoxication present with an acute gastrointestinal disturbance that is followed by a painful neuropathy (22). There may be remissions, particularly while the patient is in the hospital, and relapses, suggesting repeated exposure. The neuropathy is a distal axonal degeneration; however, there are reports of patients with arsenic intoxication who present with a disorder resembling acute inflammatory demyelinating polyneuropathy (Guillain-Barré syndrome). The diagnosis of arsenic intoxication is confirmed by measurement of arsenic in urine, hair, and nails. Unfortunately, the neuropathy may progress after exposure is discontinued. Thallium intoxication also produces a painful peripheral neuropathy (22). These patients also develop an acute gastrointestinal disturbance, followed by painful neuropathy. Hair loss, which occurs several weeks after initial exposure, is a diagnostic finding. Urine collection for measurement of thallium establishes the diagnosis. For both of these toxic neuropathies, removal of the toxin is the only proven therapy.

Metronidazole (23, 24), misonidazole (25), nitrofurantoin (26), 2′,3′-dideoxyinosine (27, 28), and 2′,3′-dideoxycytidine (29, 30) have all been associated with peripheral neuropathy, particularly when given over a long time. These drug-induced neuropathies reverse when the treatment is stopped, if nerve damage is not severe. Nitrofurantoin neuropathy is especially common in patients with uremia (31) and may mimic uremic neuropathy.

Uremic neuropathy can occasionally be painful, especially at its onset (32). These patients will have been uremic for at least several months, and many improve with either more-vigorous dialysis or transplantation (33).

Abnormalities of serum proteins have been associated with peripheral neuropathies, and a proportion of these are painful at onset (34). The neuropathy may precede the signs of a systemic illness so that careful testing of serum and urine for the presence of abnormal proteins is warranted in any patient with painful peripheral neuropathy. The neuropathy associated with multiple myeloma typically presents as a distal symmetric axonal degeneration with pain as a major component. Cryoglobulinemia can also cause a painful peripheral neuropathy. Clues helpful in diagnosis are Raynaud's phenomenon, bleeding diatheses, and digital ulcers. If cryoglobulinemia is suspected, special care must be taken when examining serum for the presence of cryoglobulins. Treatment is directed at the underlying cause of the cryoglobulinemia. Macroglobulinemia primarily affects elderly patients and presents with fatigue, weight loss, anemia, lymphadenopathy, organomegaly, and an elevated erythrocyte sedimentation rate. The polyneuropathy of macroglobulinemia usually develops after the illness is well-established. Immunosuppressants and plasmapheresis are the treatments of choice.

Patients with dorsal root ganglionopathy develop progressive sensory loss, areflexia, and ataxia, and some experience pain as a major symptom. The sensory disturbance is usually asymmetric and frequently affects the face. Electrodiagnostic studies are distinctive, with absence of sensory action potentials but normal motor conduction studies and electromyography. The differential diagnosis of dorsal root ganglionopathy is limited. The most frequently encountered disorders causing this syndrome are *Sjögren's syndrome* (35), *pyridoxine intoxication* (36), and *carcinoma* (37). Pain associated with progressive asymmetric sensory loss raises the likelihood that carcinoma is the cause, particularly that of the lung, breast, or ovary.

Sjögren's syndrome has also been associated with a painful sensory neuropathy (38, 39). Close questioning may be necessary to elicit from these patients the symptoms of dry eyes (keroconjunctivitis sicca) and dry mouth (xerostomia) that have gone unrecognized for years. Laboratory evidence suggesting Sjögren's syndrome (Ro antibody, positive ANA, a positive Rose Bengal test, or an inflammatory lip biopsy) is helpful in the differential diagnosis. Treatment with immunosuppressants has provided mixed results.

Porphyritic neuropathy may begin with pain (40). Painful paresthesias may be felt anywhere on the body, rapidly followed by weakness that frequently affects proximal upper extremities. These patients' presentations may mimic those of Guillain-Barré syndrome. A positive family history, associated episodes of abdominal pain, or psychiatric disturbance suggests the diagnosis of porphyria. The Watson-Schwartz test is diagnostic during acute episodes. Further testing is needed to define the specific metabolic abnormality. Treatment of the primary disorder consists of glucose infusion and hematin, with propranolol used to control the dysautonomia. In treating the pain, it is essential to be aware of the drugs contraindicated in these patients (41). Chlorpromazine, meperidine, and morphine may be safely used when pain is severe. The former has the advantage of also helping the psychiatric disturbance that accompanies the illness.

Fabry's disease (ceramide trihexosidase deficiency) is an X-linked genetic disorder in which young men and boys commonly complain of spontaneous pain in the feet and legs (42). A typical patient has spontaneous episodes of distal extremity pain that are brought on by emotional stimuli associated with vasomotor instability of the legs. Examination may show no evidence of neuropathy, however. A characteristic rash, renal disease, and evidence of accelerated vascular disease—hypertension, stroke, and myocardial infarction—all suggest the diagnosis, which is confirmed by enzyme assay in leukocytes or cultured skin fibroblasts. Clinical trials of enzyme replacement are underway.

Patients with *insulinoma* may develop a severe peripheral neuropathy that is frequently painful (43). Although motor signs predominate, painful paresthesia is common. The neuropathy usually develops after a prolonged period of hypoglycemia in which cerebral symptoms overshadow the neuropathy. Diagnosis is suggested by low random blood sugars and hypoglycemia during a prolonged fast.

Multiple *mononeuropathies* may present with pain in the distribution of named nerves. There are a large number of causes of this syndrome, the most common being vascular compromise (2). Treatment of the underlying disease is usually all that is required.

Patients with acute inflammatory demyelinating polyneuropathy *(Guillain-Barré syndrome)* may have pain as one of their presenting complaints (44). Usually pain is a deep-seated back pain that is resistent to non-narcotic analgesics. No satisfactory explanation exists for this pain, which usually subsides within a week or two.

TREATMENT

The treatment of pain secondary to a peripheral neuropathy is multifaceted. The first and most successful treatment is that of the underlying etiology of the neuropathy. In many cases, this alone will relieve the pain. For example, in diabetes, improved glucose control, either by more-frequent insulin injections or by the use of the subcutaneous insulin pump (15), has been reported to alleviate pain completely. In alcoholic/nutritional neuropathy, abstinence from alcohol and vitamin replacement will usually be sufficient to relieve the pain.

In several of the disorders listed above, such as drug-induced or toxic neuropathies, pain is a transitory phenomenon if the toxin is removed. In these and in other disorders wherein primary treatment of the neuropathy can be expected eventually to alleviate the pain, the use of analgesics alone is frequently sufficient. Aspirin, acetaminophen, nonsteroidal anti-inflammatory drugs (NSAIDS), and narcotic analgesics are used. Although many physicians are reluctant to use narcotics in these cases, if it is known that the disorder will be short-lived, then hesitancy about the use of these agents is unnecessary.

Nonpharmacologic therapies may also be tried. These include transcutaneous electrical nerve stimulation (TENS), immersion of dysesthetic skin in cold water, and the wearing of tight stockings to alleviate dysesthesias that develop in the evening when the feet are elevated. Although the efficacy of these modalities has not been proven in controlled trials, individuals may find any or all of them beneficial, and so they are worth trying.

Last, and the most difficult problem, is to treat chronic neuropathic pain due to peripheral neuropathy. The literature contains small well-controlled studies as well as numerous anecdotal reports, both of which taken together provide guidelines for therapy. The general principle is to give a single medication until the maximum dose is reached, as determined by either evidence of drug toxicity or failure to relieve symptoms. If unsuccessful, that agent is discontinued and a second agent is given in accord with the same principle. If no single agent is effective, then combinations of medications are tried.

In published studies, the most effective agent for treating the chronic pain associated with peripheral neuropathy is amitriptyline (45). Although low doses are used at first, the effective dose in most studies has ranged from 75 to 150 mg/day. Side effects are a potential problem and need to be monitored. Two other tricyclic antidepressants, desipramine and imipramine, have also been tried but are usually less effective than amitriptyline, when compared in the same patient. Anti-convulsant medications, such as carbamazapine (46), phenytoin, and clonazepam, have also been used with varying degrees of success. Most physicians have abandoned use of phenothiozines as an additive agent (47).

Three recently reported therapies deserve special mention. Local anesthetic drugs have now been used in several studies. Initially, Kastrup and colleagues (48, 49) reported improvement in chronic painful diabetic neuropathy following intravenous infusion of lidocaine. The effectiveness of intravenous lidocaine for pain treatment has been replicated in a study of post-herpetic neuralgia (50). In diabetic neuropathy, pain relief may last from 1 to 30 days. Because of the inconvenience and potential side effects of intravenous lidocaine, oral mexiletine has also been tried, with early promising results (51, 52). Further well-designed studies of this agent are eagerly awaited.

Topical capsaicin cream has been studied extensively, but the results are conflicting, with some studies providing encouraging results (53) and other studies suggesting negative results (54, 55). Anecdotal experience, however, suggests that topical capsaicin is not a useful agent.

A number of case reports have described the use of agents that improve blood flow to alleviate the pain of diabetic neuropathy (56–59). These individual case reports do not provide enough information to allow conclusions as to the effectiveness of this form of therapy. Further investigations are clearly needed.

As described above, the pain from peripheral neuropathies may spontaneously resolve. This information is important for two reasons. First, because these patients are frequently depressed at the thought that their pain will last forever, this knowledge can be transmitted to them to reassure them that with time it is likely that they will improve. Second, it is worth attempting a trial of medication withdrawal every few months in the hope that the pain will have spontaneously resolved.

REFERENCES

1. Griffin JW, Cornblath DR: Diseases of the peripheral nervous system. In Rosenberg RN (ed): *Comprehensive Neurology.* New York, Raven Press, 1991, p 421.
2. Dyck PJ, Thomas PK, Griffin JW, Low PA, Poduslo J (eds): *Peripheral Neuropathy*, ed 3. Philadelphia, WB Saunders, 1993.
3. Matthews B: *Holmes's Introduction to Clinical Neurology*, ed 3. Baltimore, Williams & Wilkins, 1968.
4. Asbury AK, Fields HL: Pain due to peripheral nerve damage: An hypothesis. *Neurology* 34:1587–1590, 1984.
5. Torebjork HE, Hallin RG: Identification of afferent C units in intact human skin nerves. *Brain Res* 67:387–403, 1974.
6. Dyck PJ, Lambert EH, O'Brien PC: Pain in peripheral neuropathy related to rate and kind of fiber degeneration. *Neurology* 26:466–477, 1976.
7. Brown MJ, Martin JR, Asbury AK: Painful diabetic neuropathy: A morphometric study. *Arch Neurol* 33:164–171, 1976.
8. Said G, Slama G, Selva J: Progressive centripetal degeneration of axons in small fibre diabetic polyneuropathy. *Brain* 106:791–807, 1983.
9. Melzack RA, Wall PD: Pain mechanisms: A new theory. *Science* 150:971–979, 1965.

10. Dyck PJ, Lambert EH, Nichols PC: Quantitative measurement of sensation related to compound action potential and number and sizes of myelinated and unmyelinated fibers of sural nerve in health, Friedrich's ataxia, hereditary sensory neuropathy, and tabes dorsalis. In Cobb WA (ed): *Handbook of Electroencephalography and Clinical Neurophysiology*, vol 9. Amsterdam, Elsevier, 1971, p 83.

11. Bennett GJ: The role of the sympathetic nervous system in painful peripheral neuropathy. *Pain* 45:221–223, 1991.

12. Low PA (ed): *Clinical Anatomic Disorders*. Boston, Little Brown, 1993.

13. Committee on Health Care Issues American Neurological Association: Does improved control of glycemia prevent or ameliorate diabetic polyneuropathy? *Ann Neurol* 19:288–290, 1986.

14. Archer AG, Watkins PJ, Thomas PK, Sharma AK, Payan J: The natural history of acute painful diabetic neuropathy. *J Neurol Neurosurg Psychiatry* 46:491–499, 1983.

15. Boulton AJM, Drury J, Clark B, Ward JD: Continuous subcutaneous insulin infusion in the management of painful diabetic neuropathy. *Diabetes Care* 5:386–390, 1986.

16. Mayne M: The short term prognosis of diabetic neuropathy. *Diabetes* 17:270–273, 1968.

17. Victor M: Polyneuropathy due to nutritional deficiency and alcoholism. In Dyck PJ, Thomas PK, Lambert EH, Bunge R (eds): *Peripheral Neuropathies*, vol 2, ed 2. Philadelphia, WB Saunders, 1984.

18. Kelly JJ, Kyle RA, O'Brien PC, Dyck PJ: The natural history of peripheral neuropathy in primary systemic amyloidosis. *Ann Neurol* 6:1–7, 1979.

19. Cornblath DR, McArthur JC, Parry G, Griffin JW: Peripheral neuropathies in human immunodeficiency virus infection. In Dyck PJ, Thomas PK, Griffin JW, Low PA, Poduslo J (eds): *Peripheral Neuropathy*, ed 3. Philadelphia, WB Saunders, 1992, pp 1343–1353.

20. Cornblath DR, McArthur JC: Predominantly sensory neuropathy in patients with AIDS and AIDS-related complex. *Neurology* 38:794–796, 1988.

21. Griffin JW, Crawford TO, Glass JD, Tyor WR, Price DL, Cornblath DR, McArthur JC: Neuropathology of painful sensory neuropathy in AIDS. *Brain*, in press.

22. Windebank AJ, McCall JT, Dyck PJ: Metal neuropathy. In Dyck PJ, Thomas PK, Lambert EH, Bunge R (eds): *Peripheral Neuropathy*, ed 2. Philadelphia, WB Saunders, 1984, p 2133.

23. Bradley WG, Karlsson IJ, Rassol CG: Metronidazole neuropathy. *Br Med J* 2:610–611, 1977.

24. Coxon A, Pallis CA: Metronidazole neuropathy. *J Neurol Neurosurg Psychiatry* 39:403–405, 1976.

25. Dische S, Saunders MI, Lee ME, Adams GR, Flockhart IR: Clinical testing of the radiosensitizer Ro 07-0582: Experience with multiple doses. *Br J Cancer* 35:567–579, 1977.

26. Olivarius BdeF: Polyneuropathy due to nitrofurantoin therapy. *Ugeskr Laegerl* 118:753–755, 1956.

27. Lambert JS, Seidlin M, Reichman RC, Plank CS, Laverty M, Morse GD, Knupp C, McLaren C, Pettinelli C, Valentine FT, Dolin R: 2′,3′-dideoxyinosine (ddI) in patients with the acquired immunodeficiency syndrome or AIDS-related complex. A phase I trial. *N Engl J Med* 322:1333–1340, 1990.

28. Cooley TP, Kunches LM, Saunders CA, Ritter JK, Perkins CJ, McLaren C, McCaffrey RP, Liebman HA: Once-daily administration of 2′,3′-dideoxyinosine (ddI) in patients with the acquired immunodeficiency syndrome or AIDS-related complex. *N Engl J Med* 322:1340–1345, 1990.

29. Dubinsky RM, Yarchoan R, Dalakas M, Broder S: Reversible axonal neuropathy from the treatment of AIDS and related disorders with 2′,3′-dideoxycytidine (ddC). *Muscle Nerve* 12:856–860, 1989.

30. Merigan TC, Skowron G, Bozzette SA, Richman d, Uttamchandani R, Fischl M, Schooley R, Hirsch M, Soo W, Pettinelli C, Schaumburg H, the DDC Study Group of the AIDS Clinical Trials Group: Circulating p24 antigen levels and responses to dideoxycytidine in human immunodeficiency virus (HIV) infections: A phase I and II study. *Ann Intern Med* 110:189–195, 1989.

31. Tyler HR: Neurologic disorders in renal failure. *Am J Med* 44:734–748, 1968.

32. Nielsen VK: The peripheral nerve function in chronic renal failure. VII. Longitudinal course during terminal renal failure and regular hemodialysis. *Acta Med Scand* 195:155–162, 1974.

33. Asbury AK: Uremic neuropathy. In Dyck PJ, Thomas PK, Lambert EH, Bunge R (eds): *Peripheral Neuropathies*, vol 2, ed 2. Philadelphia, WB Saunders, 1984, p 1811.

34. McLeod JG, Walsh JC, Pollard JD: Neuropathies associated with paraproteinemias and dysproteinemias. In Dyck PJ, Thomas PK, Lambert EH, Bunge R (eds): *Peripheral Neuropathy*, ed 2. Philadelphia, WB Saunders, 1984, p 1847.

35. Griffin JW, Cornblath DR, Alexander E, Campbell J, Low PA, Bird S, Feldman EL: Ataxic sensory neuropathy and dorsal root ganglionitis associated with Sjögren's syndrome. *Ann Neurol* 27:304–315, 1990.

36. Schaumburg H, Kaplan J, Windebank A, Vick N, Rasmus S, Pleasure D, Brown MJ: Sensory neuropathy from pyridoxine abuse: A new megavitamin syndrome. *N Engl J Med* 309:445–448, 1983.

37. Horwich MS, Cho L, Porro RS, Posner JB: Subacute sensory neuropathy: a remote effect of carcinoma. *Ann Neurol* 2:7–19, 1977.

38. Kaltrieder HB, Talal N: The neuropathy of Sjogren's syndrome: trigeminal nerve involvement. *Ann Intern Med* 70:751–762, 1969.

39. Windebank AJ, Blexrud MD, Dyck PJ, Daube JR, Karnes JL: The syndrome of acute sensory neuropathy: clinical features and electrophysiologic and pathologic changes. *Neurology* 40:584–591, 1990.

40. Ridley A: Porphyric neuropathy. In Dyck PJ, Thomas PK, Lambert EH, Bunge R (eds): *Peripheral Neuropathy*, ed 2, Philadelphia, WB Saunders, 1984, p 1704.

41. Eales L, Dowdle EB: Porphyria and dangerous life-threatening drugs. *S Afr Med J* 56:914–917, 1979.

42. Brady RO: Fabry disease. In Dyck PJ, Thomas PK, Lambert EH, Bunge R (eds): *Peripheral Neuropathy*, ed 2. Philadelphia, WB Saunders, 1984, p 1717.

43. Jaspan JB, Wollman RL, Bernstein L, Rubinstein AH: Hypoglycemic peripheral neuropathy in association with insulinonia: Implication of glucopenia rather than hyperinsulinism. *Medicine* 61:33–44, 1982.

44. Ropper AH, Shahani BT: Pain in Guillain-Barré syndrome. *Arch Neurol* 41:511–514, 1984.

45. Max MB, Lynch SA, Muir J, Shoaf SE, Smoller B, Dubner R: Effects of desipramine, amitriptyline, and fluoxetine on pain in diabetic neuropathy. *N Engl J Med* 326:1250–1256, 1992.

46. Rull JA, Quibrera R, Gonzalez-Millan H, Castaneda DL: Symptomatic treatment of peripheral diabetic neuropathy with carbamazepine (Tegretol): Double blind crossover trial. *Diabetologia* 5:215–218, 1969.

47. Davis JL, Lewis SB, Gerich JE: Peripheral diabetic neuropathy treated with amitriptyline and fluphenazine. *JAMA* 238:2291–2292, 1977.

48. Kastrup J, Petersen P, Dejgard A, Hilsted J, Angelo HR: Treatment of chronic painful diabetic neuropathy with intravenous lidocaine infusion. *Br Med J* 292:173, 1986.

49. Kastrup J, Petersen P, Dejgard A, Angelo HR, Histed J: Intravenous lidocaine infusion—A new treatment of chronic painful diabetic neuropathy? *Pain* 28:69–75, 1987.

50. Rowbotham MC, Reisner-Keller LA, Fields HL: Both intravenous lidocaine and morphine reduce the pain of postherpetic neuralgia. *Neurology* 41:1024–1028, 1991.

51. Fross RD: Mexiletine, an oral local anesthetic, for treatment of neuropathic pain [Abstr]. *Neurology* 42(Suppl 3):162, 1992.

52. Dejgard A, Petersen P, Kastrup J: Mexiletine for treatment of chronic painful diabetic neuropathy. *Lancet* 1:9–10, 1988.

53. Tandan R, Lewis GA, Krusinski PB, Badger GB, Fries TJ: Topical capsaicin in painful diabetic neuropathy. Controlled study with long-term follow-up. *Diabetes Care* 15:8–14, 1992.

54. Chad DA, Aronin N, Lundstrom R, McKeon P, et al: Does capsaicin relieve the pain of diabetic neuropathy? *Pain* 42:387–388, 1990.

55. Low PA, Opfer-Gehrking TL, Dyck PJ, Litchy WJ, O'Brien PC: Double-blind, placebo-controlled study of the application of Axsain cream in chronic distal painful neuropathy [Abstr]. *Neurology* 42(Suppl 3):410, 1992.

56. Sindrup SH, Grodum E, BEck-Nielsen H: Concentration-response relationship in peroxetine treatment of diabetic neuropathy symptoms: A patient-blinded dose-escalation study. *Ther Drug Monit* 13:408–414, 1991.

57. Cohen SM, Mathews T: Pentoxifylline in treatment of distal diabetic neuropathy. *Angiology* 42:741–746, 1991.

58. Shindo H, Tawata M, Aida K, Onaya T: Clinical efficacy of a stable prostacyclin analog, iloprost, in diabetic neuropathy. *Prostaglandins* 41:85–96, 1991.

59. Theesen KA, Marsh WR: Relief of diabetic neuropathy with fluoxetine. *DICP* 23:572–574, 1989.

CHAPTER 38

ENTRAPMENT AND COMPRESSION NEUROPATHIES

STEPHEN R. CONWAY
H. ROYDEN JONES, JR.

THE TERMS *entrapment neuropathy* and *compression neuropathy* are often used interchangeably, although they are really separate entities. The term *entrapment* is appropriate to use when mechanical distortion of a nerve occurs within a fibro-osseous tunnel or as a consequence of a constricting fibrous band. With entrapment, nerve damage may result from angulation and stretch as well as compression. The term also implies that the distortion occurs at a particular site that is potentially correctable by surgery (1). In contradistinction, *compression* neuropathies result from pressure applied to a nerve through the skin, as in Saturday night palsy, during operation from retractors, or from soft tissue sources, such as hematomas.

In either entity, nerve damage can result from high-grade pressure exerted over a short period of time or low-grade pressure exerted chronically. For example, ulnar compression neuropathy can occur acutely after coma, administration of anesthesia, or repeated low-grade trauma, such as habitually leaning on the elbows. Similarly, entrapment neuropathies can develop acutely or gradually. Generalized polyneuropathies may predispose to compression (hereditary liability to pressure palsies) or entrapment (as in diabetics). Other systemic conditions such as rheumatoid arthritis, can result in entrapment syndromes by causing deformities in joints and ligaments.

Two types of pain are characteristic of compression and entrapment syndromes. When sensory fibers from the skin are disrupted, dysesthesias usually occur appropriate to all or part of the cutaneous distribution of the nerve. In addition, poorly localized pain frequently occurs as a result of disruption of sensory afferent nerves from structures, such as joint capsules, that do not have dermatomal representation. For example, deep pain is often a prominent symptom of entrapment of the anterior interosseous nerve (a pure motor nerve) and

not infrequently accompanies carpal tunnel syndrome (in addition to the typical sensory dysesthesias).

The diagnosis of entrapment and compression neuropathies is greatly aided by electromyography (EMG), which consists of nerve conduction studies and needle examination of muscle. Nerve conduction studies help to determine the site of nerve compression or entrapment and the presence or absence of conduction block, and the needle examination is useful to estimate the degree of acute and chronic axonal loss if any. With this information an accurate prognosis can be determined. The recovery from pure demyelinative lesions, for example, is likely to be quicker and more complete than the recovery from lesions associated with axonal loss.

MEDIAN NERVE

CARPAL TUNNEL SYNDROME

Carpal tunnel syndrome refers to the constellation of symptoms and signs resulting from compression of the median nerve within the carpal tunnel. It is by far the most common entrapment neuropathy seen in clinical practice and serves as a model for entrapment neuropathies.

Anatomy

The boundaries of the carpal tunnel are formed by the carpal bones and the superficial border of the thick ligamentous flexor retinaculum, which is attached medially to the hamate and pisiform bones and laterally to the trapezium and scaphoid bones. The contents of the canal include the median nerve, blood vessels, and the flexor tendons of the hands and their sheaths. The median nerve gives off its palmar cutaneous branch before entering the tunnel. This branch courses superficial to the flexor retinaculum, and thus its injury during operation can result in persistent pain that can be mistaken for inadequate decompression of the median nerve itself

(2). The flexor tendons are surrounded by synovial tissue that permits smooth gliding. The synovial tissue, however, is susceptible to hypertrophy and degeneration, which can narrow the effective space within the canal.

Venous and arterial vessels within the carpal tunnel compose part of a complex interrelated pressure system (3). Any increase in pressure can reduce venous outflow, raise intrafunicular pressure within the nerve, and consequently endanger the flow in the nutrient arteries to the median nerve. When hypoxia reaches a critical level, pain fibers become hyperexcitable and discharge spontaneously. Within the carpal tunnel the median nerve is composed of small funiculi that are well separated by epineural tissue packing (3). These funiculi can be compressed selectively, resulting in symptoms in only a segment of the distribution of the nerve.

Clinical Features

Carpal tunnel syndrome occurs most often in middle-aged women. In Phalen's series (4), the ratio of women to men was 3:1. Of these patients, 58% were between 40 and 60 years of age. The typical history is the gradual development of numbness and paresthesias in the median distribution of the hand (thumb, index finger, middle finger, and radial half of the ring finger). However, Fine and associates (5) reported 25 patient with carpal tunnel syndrome with pain or paresthesia exclusively or predominantly in a single digit. They attributed this to compression of a single fascicle. Phalen (4) observed that many of his patients complained of pain and numbness in the whole hand. He noted, however, that most of them reported the little finger to be spared after careful examination of their hands at night.

The most characteristic symptoms are nocturnal paresthesia and pain. These are most likely caused by the diminished return of blood from the limb during sleep because of hypotonia and lack of movement. Relief is commonly obtained by shaking the hand vigorously "to get the circulation going." Both flexion and extension of the wrists raise the pressure within the carpal tunnel (3). In addition, flexion forces the nerve against the flexor retinaculum. Sleeping with the wrists in the flexed position therefore might be a cause for symptoms at night. Driving, reading a newspaper, and sewing are also common precipitants.

Poorly localized deep aching wrist pain occurs frequently. Occasionally pain may also occur proximally in the forearm, elbow, and shoulder. In one series (6), proximal pain occurred in 57 of 90 limbs in 72 patients with carpal tunnel syndrome. Of the 49 patients in whom surgical correction was performed, 46 experienced relief of proximal symptoms.

Raynaud's phenomenon has been reported (7) to complicate carpal tunnel syndrome and even to antedate the characteristic neurologic symptoms. Phalen (8) believed

that the occurrence of Raynaud's phenomenon could be a result of the large sympathetic nerve supply carried by the median nerve. Dawson and associates (9), in their review of one series of 24 patients with carpal tunnel syndrome and Raynaud's phenomenon, noted that four patients had Raynaud's phenomenon in the feet as well and suggested that this group might have a higher incidence of systemic rheumatic disease. The incidence of Raynaud's phenomenon in carpal tunnel syndrome is low, and at least one study (9) suggests that the prognosis for the alleviation of vasospastic symptoms with carpal tunnel release is guarded.

The results of detailed neurologic examination in patients with carpal tunnel syndrome are probably best related to the duration of symptoms. The presence of objective sensory loss is not invariable despite the almost universal complaint of numbness. In Phalen's experience (4) from 1950 to 1970, nearly 70% of patients had decreased sensation in some part of the median distribution of the hand. In many of them this included only the tip of the middle finger. However, with widespread recognition of the syndrome, earlier diagnosis may be associated with a higher percentage of normal examinations even though the patient complains of symptoms in the median nerve distribution. Of Phalen's patients, 60% had Tinel's sign, a tingling sensation radiating out into the hand produced by tapping over the median nerve at the wrist. The wrist flexion or Phalen's test reproduced the symptoms in 80% of Phalen's patients. This maneuver entails unforced flexion of the wrist for 30–60 sec. In this position the median nerve is compressed between the proximal edge of the transverse carpal ligament and the adjacent flexor tendons and radius (4).

Motor signs in the form of thenar weakness or atrophy, particularly involving the abductor pollicis brevis, usually develop after sensory symptoms have been present for a period of time. Weakness is usually an indication of serious nerve compromise and almost always warrants surgical decompression.

Carpal tunnel syndrome must be distinguished most often from radiculopathy of the sixth and seventh cervical roots. Occasionally it must be distinguished from median nerve lesions at the elbow and rarely from spinal cord compression or cerebral lesions that cause sensory symptoms in the hand.

Pathology

The pathology leading to compression of the median nerve is varied but can be divided generally into three types: processes that involve the walls of the tunnel and thus decrease the space for its contents, factors that affect the contents of the tunnel directly, and idiopathic factors (3). The first group includes injuries to the wrist (e.g., dislocation of one of the carpal bones), hypertrophic arthropathy, ganglia of the carpal joints, and thickening of the flexor retinaculum. A small carpal tunnel may predispose the nerve to pressure and ischemia, particularly in occupations requiring repetitive wrist and hand movements. The second group, affecting the contents of the carpal tunnel, includes changes resulting from pregnancy, disorders of the tendon sheaths and bursae, hypertrophic neuropathies, and, rarely, lipomas.

In pregnancy, the increase in total body extracellular fluid probably results in soft tissue swelling within the canal. In most patients, this resolves after delivery (10). Carpal tunnel syndrome sometimes develops after delivery possibly because of the types of hand movements required in taking care of a baby (11).

Tenosynovitis of the flexor tendons and sheaths may occur in patients with rheumatoid arthritis. The tendons may also swell from a nonspecific tenosynovitis caused by occupational factors. In both instances, the intracanalicular space reserved for the median nerve may be decreased.

In gout, symptoms of carpal tunnel syndrome can result from deposits of urate along the median nerve and flexor tendons. With mild symptoms, medical management alone may be curative (12). Carpal tunnel syndrome may be the presenting symptom of amyloidosis, and staining of the removed tissue for amyloid fibrils at time of surgical decompression has been advocated (13).

Carpal tunnel syndrome had also been reported in association with both hypothyroidism and hyperthyroidism (14). In myxedematous patients, nerve compression is likely caused by thickening of the tendon sheaths by diffuse deposits of hyaluronic acid mucopolysaccharides. A similar process may also occur in patients with Graves' disease because localized myxedema occurs in a small number of these patients (14).

Median neuropathy in the carpal tunnel has been reported in patients with acromegaly and overactivity of the pituitary gland. In one series (15), successful treatment of the pituitary disorder abolished symptoms. In some patients, improvement was evident within weeks, suggesting that nerve entrapment was caused by edematous synovial tissue rather than osseous change. Persistence of symptoms was regarded as evidence for continued hypersomatotropism.

The placement of vascular shunts for hemodialysis has also been reported to cause carpal tunnel syndrome, probably by increasing hyperemia distal to the fistula (16).

Treatment

The treatment of carpal tunnel syndrome is successful in the majority of patients. Conservative measures are usually reserved for patients who have subjective sensory symptoms or reversible systemic conditions such as pregnancy or myxedema. Splinting the wrist is often effective in relieving pain in patients with mild symptoms. Local injection of steroids may provide relief but rarely prolong remission (4).

Most patients in whom conservative management fails are candidates for surgery. The majority of neurologists and surgeons would regard thenar weakness or atrophy as an absolute indication for surgical decompression at any stage. The success rate of surgery has depended on the duration of symptoms. In one series (17), a 97% success rate was obtained in patients with symptoms of less than 6 months' duration, but a failure rate of up to 25% was registered in patients with more prolonged complaints. Incomplete section of the flexor retinaculum is the most common cause for surgical failure.

ENTRAPMENTS OF THE PROXIMAL MEDIAN NERVE

Entrapments of the proximal median nerve are uncommon and usually occur near the elbow. When present, they commonly occur below the elbow in the region of the pronator teres muscle (pronator syndrome) or in the forearm (anterior interosseous nerve syndrome). Less commonly, the entrapment occurs above the elbow as a result of an anomalous band (the ligament of Struthers) running from the supracondylar process to the medial epicondyle (18).

Anterior Interosseous Nerve Syndrome

Anatomy

The anterior interosseous nerve is a pure motor branch of the median nerve arising 5–8 cm distal to the lateral epicondyle. It supplies the pronator quadratus, flexor pollicis longus, and flexor digitorum profundus muscles of digits two and three. It carries no fibers for cutaneous sensation but does carry proprioceptive and deep pain fibers from the wrist (19).

Clinical Features

Entrapment of the anterior interosseous nerve has been associated with the tendinous origins of the pronator teres, flexor digitorum profundus, and flexor digitorum sublimis muscles (20). Occupational stresses and strenuous exercise requiring repetitive elbow flexion and pronation can lead to compression of the nerve. Trauma to the nerve after intravenous cutdown in the anterior cubital fossa has also been reported (21).

Pain in the proximal forearm may herald the weakness, which has been characterized as a loss of dexterity in pinching. With pinching maneuvers, the index finger may remain hyperextended at the distal interphalangeal joint secondary to weakness of the flexor digitorum profundus muscle, and the thumb may assume a "straight" posture because of weakness of the flexor pollicis longus muscle (22). The intrinsic muscles of the hand may be affected when a median to ulnar crossover occurs originating from the anterior interosseous nerve (9). However, this is rare. Abduction of the thumb should be normal because the abductor pollicis brevis muscle is innervated by the parent median nerve.

Rupture of the tendons of the flexor pollicis longus or flexor digitorum profundus muscles (not uncommon in rheumatoid arthritis) must be distinguished from entrapment of the anterior interosseous nerve. The patient usually has a history of flexor tenosynovitis or locking of the thumb (9). Occasionally, idiopathic brachial plexitis can result in weakness in an anterior interosseous nerve distribution, sometimes in association with weakness in the shoulder girdle (23).

Treatment

The majority of patients with spontaneous anterior interosseous nerve palsy have a satisfactory return of function with conservative therapy (19). Surgical exploration may be indicated after 8–12 weeks if no improvement occurs.

Pronator Syndrome

Pronator syndrome may result from compression of the median nerve proximal to the branching of the anterior interosseous nerve. The three areas in which this occurs are beneath the lacertus fibrosus (bicipital aponeurosis), a thick fascial band extending from the biceps tendon to the forearm fascia; by a tendinous band in the substance of the pronator muscle; and under the fibrous arch of the flexor digitorum profundus.

Clinical Features

Typically, patients complain of an aching discomfort in the forearm, numbness in the thumb and index finger, and weakness in the hand. A notable finding at physical examination is tenderness over the proximal part of the pronator teres muscle that is aggravated by pronation of the forearm against resistance (24). Resisted pronation may also result in paresthesias in the distribution of the median nerve. A positive Tinel's sign is often present at the proximal edge of the pronator muscle.

Weakness of the pronator muscle can result if the entrapment is under the bicipital aponeurosis (25). Weakness in other muscles is variable depending on the degree of compression and can be absent. When present, weakness may involve long flexor muscles of the fingers and thumb and the abductor pollicis brevis muscle innervated by the median nerve. Usually, objective sensory loss is poorly defined (9).

Nerve conduction studies rarely show abnormalities localizing the lesion but are useful in excluding carpal tunnel syndrome (24). Needle EMG may be helpful in demonstrating signs of denervation in the forearm above the carpal tunnel but distal to the site of entrapment in the proximal forearm. In many patients, pronator syndrome is associated with activities causing muscular hypertrophy of the forearm. Acute trauma, elbow dislocation, compartment syndrome, and iatrogenic bleeding into the forearm can also cause compression (9). Surgical decompression may be necessary.

Entrapment at the Ligament of Struthers

Compression of the median nerve by the ligament of Struthers is rare and is usually associated with a supracondylar bone spur. Compression is even more unusual in the absence of a supracondylar bone spur (18).

Clinical Features

The symptoms in patients with entrapment at the ligament of Struthers are similar to those in patients with pronator syndrome, including severe pain near the elbow (18). Differentiation between the two syndromes may be aided by the finding of tenderness and pain above the elbow, which is sometimes at the site of bone spurs from which the ligament of Struthers arises. The signs and symptoms can be vague and nonspecific in both syndromes, and testing can be difficult because of pain. Radiography of the elbow demonstrating the bony spur above the lateral epicondyle may be helpful in diagnosis. Surgical excision of the ligament and the bony spur is usually curative.

ULNAR NERVE

ENTRAPMENT AND COMPRESSION OF THE ULNAR NERVE

The anatomic course of the ulnar nerve predisposes it to injury at the elbow and wrist. Compression of the ulnar nerve at the elbow can occur during anesthesia or periods of intoxication or coma. Compression can also occur in bedridden patients or in those who habitually lean on their elbows (26). Most entrapments of the ulnar nerve occur at the elbow as a consequence of degenerative arthritis with tardy ulnar palsy or compression within the cubital tunnel, as is discussed later.

The cubital tunnel is roofed by an aponeurotic band that bridges the two heads of the flexor carpi ulnaris muscle. The ulnar nerve passes under this band medial to the elbow joint, which forms the lateral wall of the tunnel. Cubital tunnel syndrome refers to compression of the ulnar nerve in this fibro-osseous canal.

The term *cubital tunnel syndrome* is currently reserved for ulnar nerve compression in the cubital tunnel not associated with degenerative arthritis of the elbow (27). However, the original report of cubital tunnel compression included two patients with classic tardy ulnar palsy (28), and it was suggested that scarring of the ligamentous joint tissue could cause nerve compression by thickening the floor of the tunnel.

Degenerative arthritis of the elbow resulting in chronic ulnar neuropathy has been termed *tardy ulnar palsy*. Tardy ulnar palsy classically appears years after a traumatic injury to the elbow. In Sunderland's (3) study of 14 patients, 10 experienced fracture from 5 to 30 years or more previously. In four patients, old fractures of the lateral epicondyle were evident. However, the original injury often could not be defined because of bony overgrowth and deformity. The lesion in tardy ulnar palsy results from a combination of friction, progressive interstitial neuritis, and tension across a deformed joint (3). Several of Sunderland's patients experienced a recent additional injury to the elbow or nerve. The symptoms of tardy ulnar palsy are usually progressive; however, several patients in Sunderland's series improved after they avoided excessive use of the arm (3).

Various patterns of motor and sensory loss can occur because the intraneural topography of the nerve is such that selected fiber bundles may be affected. Tingling and numbness of the medial half of the fourth finger and the entire fifth finger are usually the earliest indications of involvement of sensory fibers and were noted in each of Miller's nine patients (27). However, sensory loss is not invariable even in patients with advanced weakness. Pain uncommonly radiates into the field of the ulnar nerve, although it frequently accompanies the elbow disability (3). Of the nine patients, seven complained of pain that was variably characterized as steady, aching, or throbbing. The pain localized to the hand, forearm, shoulder, and elbow. Compression over the cubital tunnel reproduced the pain in six patients. Classically, in patients with advanced disease, atrophy of the ulnar intrinsic muscles occurs, as was noted in each of Miller's nine patients. This was most evident in the first dorsal interosseous muscle with relatively strong ulnar finger and wrist flexion.

No patient with cubital tunnel syndrome in Miller's series (27) had a history of elbow trauma or arthropathy. Several patients had occupations that required repetitive movements of the hands with the elbow in a flexed position. Bilateral symptoms were frequent, and occupational activity tended to worsen the symptoms.

Treatment

The cubital tunnel syndrome must be distinguished from tardy ulnar palsy. Decompression of the cubital tunnel is probably the procedure of choice in the former (29), and transposition of the ulnar nerve (a more complicated operation) is usually recommended for the latter (3). However, neither operation has been evaluated in a controlled fashion. The results of operation for tardy ulnar palsy are variable. An appreciable number of patients experience immediate or lasting improvements in pain and subjective symptoms (tingling and numbness). However, motor function often does not recover or is delayed (3).

In Miller's (27) patients with cubital tunnel syndrome, surgical exploration revealed the ulnar nerve to be compressed by a dense aponeurotic band at the cubital tunnel. At operation, the tunnel was observed with the elbow in 90° flexion and extension. In each instance, the nerve was tightly compressed by the aponeurosis in flexion. Most patients experienced improvement in strength and relief of pain subsequent to decompression of the tunnel.

Several investigators (26, 30) evaluating treatment of ulnar nerve lesions at the elbow have reported patients in whom a macroscopic abnormality was not demonstrated at the time of operation. These patients did not differ clinically in a clear-cut way from patients with the more definable causes of ulnar neuropathy. The cause of some of these patients' lesions may be external compression. Whether or not operation benefits patients in this subgroup is not known, although simple release was reported to be less effective than transposition (26, 30).

Most studies (26, 30, 31) of ulnar neuropathies at the elbow have shown that recovery from pain and weakness is more likely in younger patients without underlying neuropathy and in patients who have had symptoms for less than a year. In our experience and that of others (32), patients in whom compressive ulnar neuropathies develop concomitantly with a surgical procedure tend to fare poorly whether treated surgically or conservatively.

Entrapment and Compression of the Ulnar Nerve Below the Elbow

Ulnar nerve lesions below the elbow are uncommon. These occur at several sites. Compression within the forearm is rare and usually occurs in association with fracture, pressure from casts, or a closed compartment syndrome (9). The clinical picture is similar to that of compression at the wrist, although if the lesion is proximal to the dorsal sensory cutaneous branch, numbness over the dorsum of the hand results.

Damage to the dorsal sensory branch may result from blunt trauma or laceration. This branch splits from the parent trunk 6–8 cm proximal to the wrist, curves around the distal ulna, and supplies the dorsum of the hand and fourth and fifth digits. Painful dysesthesias can occur that resemble the quality of pain in lesions of the radial sensory nerve or lateral cutaneous nerve of the thigh.

Entrapment may occur at the wrist. As the dorsal cutaneous nerve exits proximally, sensory loss when present is confined to the palmar surface of the fingers of the fourth and fifth digits and the hypothenar eminence. To enter the hand, the nerve must travel through Guyon's canal, a fibro-osseous tunnel bounded by the transverse and volar carpal ligaments and the bony margins of the pisiform and hamate bones. Unlike the carpal tunnel, Guyon's canal does not contain tendons. Within the canal the nerve bifurcates into a superficial and a deep branch. The superficial branch supplies the palmaris brevis muscle and provides sensation to the hypothenar eminence and palmar surface of the fourth and fifth digits. The deep motor branch loops around the hook of the hamate and supplies the intrinsic muscles of the ulnar innervated hand.

Shea and McClain (33) described three variations in the clinical presentation of ulnar nerve lesions at the wrist. In their series, the symptoms and signs ranged from pure motor to pure sensory depending on where in the canal the nerve was compressed. The pure motor syndrome was most common, and isolated lesions of the superficial volar sensory branch were uncommon.

Lesions of the ulnar nerve at the wrist may be painless or may result in pain radiating to the digits and forearm. Dawson and associates (9) reported on six patients with these lesions occurring with Raynaud's phenomenon; the lesions probably resulted from concurrent thrombosis of the ulnar artery, which also travels through Guyon's canal. Ulnar neuropathy at the wrist has been reported to occur as a result of masses within Guyon's canal, such as ganglia; acute or chronic occupational trauma to the hypothenar eminence (9), such as in electricians (i.e., wire splicer's palsy), cyclists (34), or patients with walking frames (35); or acute laceration or fracture of the carpal bones.

RADIAL NERVE

Radial mononeuropathies can result from compression or entrapment above or below the elbow. Lesions of the proximal radial nerve are considered first.

ENTRAPMENT AND COMPRESSION OF THE HIGH RADIAL NERVE

Anatomy

The radial nerve is a continuation of the posterior cord of the brachial plexus. Branches to the long and medial heads of the triceps muscle arise in the axilla and brachioaxillary angle and run a relatively exposed and superficial course. In comparison, the remaining nerve trunk is more closely applied to the humerus in the spiral groove, explaining why weakness of the triceps muscle frequently results from crutch palsy but not humeral fractures or compressions distal to the axilla. The posterior cutaneous nerve of the forearm, like the branches to the triceps muscle, also lies more superficial and is not directly applied to the humerus. Thus, this nerve can also be spared in humeral fractures.

After winding around the posterior shaft of the humerus, the radial nerve pierces the intermuscular septum, leaving the spiral groove and the protective cover of the triceps muscle. As it continues subcutaneously around the supracondylar region, it is again susceptible to compression before running deep to the brachioradialis and brachialis muscles to the dorsum of the forearm (3).

Clinical Features

Compression of the radial nerve can result if another body lies on top of the arm for prolonged periods ("honeymooner's palsy"). The nerve can also be compressed in the axillary outlet by a crutch or the edge of a chair or bench. The latter types of compression occur most commonly during sleep or as a consequence of intoxication or anesthesia when warning sensations are not perceived. Radial nerve palsy above the elbow rarely results from nontraumatic compression. Compression from muscular effort (36), thickened epineurium (37), fibrous myopathy (38) (caused by drug injection), and tumor has been reported. However, most commonly the cause is traumatic, resulting from external compression or humeral fracture.

Treatment

The treatment of patients with high radial nerve palsy caused by traumatic compression is usually conservative. Patients with wrist-drop should have the wrist splinted in moderate extension to avoid joint stiffness and shortening of inactive muscles. The latent period to recovery depends on the level and type of injury. Patients with first degree nerve injuries that interrupt conduction but not axonal continuity begin to recover in 2–10 weeks. Patients with secondary nerve injuries that cause axonal degeneration may require 8–40 weeks for recovery (3).

Patients with third-degree nerve injuries that cause disruption of the connective tissue wall of the endoneural tube or complete severance of the nerve usually recover imperfectly if at all (3).

The treatment of compression of the radial nerve occurring in association with humeral fracture is controversial because both early exploration and observation have been advocated. The majority of patients recover spontaneously (3, 39). Some injuries occur after closed reduction and result from compression of the intact nerve by fracture fragments. In one study (39), these patients had a good prognosis after surgical exploration. Sunderland (3) recommends immediate nerve exploration for radial nerve injuries associated with complicated and open fractures or injuries resulting after closed reduction or both. This would avoid unnecessary surgery in patients in whom spontaneous recovery is likely to occur (simple nondisplaced fractures). Delayed surgical exploration is probably indicated if no recovery has occurred with conservative measures by 8 weeks.

COMPRESSION OF THE RADIAL NERVE AT OR BELOW THE ELBOW

Posterior Interosseous Nerve Syndrome

Anatomy

The posterior interosseous nerve forms at the level of the lateral humeral epicondyle where the radial nerve divides into deep and superficial divisions. It descends as a continuation of the deep branch under cover of the brachioradialis and extensor carpi radialis muscles anterior to the radiohumeral joint but lateral to the biceps tendon. It supplies both the extensor carpi radialis and supinator muscles before passing beneath the tendinous free edge of the supinator muscle, which forms an arch, the arcade of Frohse. Although some disagreement concerning its anatomy exists (21), the arcade is usually agreed to be the region of entrapment. It is dynamic in its proportions, narrowing when the wrist is supinated and extended (3). Distal to the supinator muscle, the nerve supplies the extensor carpi ulnaris muscle and extensor muscles of the fingers and thumb.

Clinical Features

Because the sensory branch of the radial nerve bifurcates just distal to the elbow (before the arcade), entrapment of the posterior interosseous nerve is purely motor and has no associated sensory loss or dysesthetic pain. The radial wrist extensor muscles are also spared because the point of entrapment is distal to their innervation. Thus, wrist-drop is not complete and wrist extension is performed with a radial predilection.

Lesions of the posterior interosseous nerve are rare. Some of these lesions are caused by trauma from fractures of the upper third of the radius or Monteggia's fractures (dislocation of the head of the radius and fracture of the ulna) (3). When not due to trauma, the syndrome usually presents over the course of several days to a week (9). The onset may be associated with pain and tenderness over the lateral epicondyle or in the proximal forearm, although pain is not a feature in many instances. Paralysis may be partial or sequentially involve only certain muscles. The wrist may be spared. For example, Dawson and associates (9) reported on three patients who also had rheumatoid arthritis in whom weakness began in the fourth and fifth fingers before progressing to involve the index finger, long finger, and thumb.

Nontraumatic posterior interosseous nerve compression may result from tumors (usually lipomas) (9, 40). In many instances, the tumor is palpable preoperatively (40). Radiography may also delineate a radiolucent mass. Decompression results in recovery when performed shortly after the onset of symptoms (9). Ganglion cysts and neurofibromas involving the posterior interosseous nerve have also been reported (41, 42). Rarely, rheumatoid synovitis may result in posterior interosseous nerve palsy. The thickened synovia can herniate beneath the supinator muscle, stretching and compressing the nerve.

Idiopathic posterior interosseous nerve syndrome is usually thought to result from compression by the arcade of Frohse, although other structures have been implicated (43). Repeated pronation, supination, and extension of the elbow joint can draw the edges of the arcade taut against the nerve (43). Alternatively, minor trauma can cause edema or synovitis that compresses the nerve against the arcade (9).

Treatment

If a mass cannot be demonstrated, operation should be delayed 8–12 weeks to see whether spontaneous recovery occurs. The nerve should be explored if weakness is progressive or nonresponsive to conservative measures (3, 9).

The association of posterior interosseous nerve syndrome with resistant tennis elbow is controversial. Although a subgroup of patients with resistant tennis elbow and forearm pain may have underlying posterior interosseous nerve entrapment, proving who does is difficult. It seems prudent to employ conservative measures in patients whose results of neurologic and EMG evaluation are normal.

Radial Sensory Neuropathy

Clinical Features

Superficial radial sensory neuropathy is usually a result of trauma. The quality of the pain is similar to entrapment of the lateral cutaneous nerve of the thigh (meralgia paresthetica) and is characterized by burning dysesthesia over the dorsoradial aspect of the hand (cheiralgia paresthetica).

The nerve lies freely between the tendons of the brachioradialis and extensor carpi radialis longus muscles and along the dorsoradial aspect of the radius unless the forearm is pronated, causing the tendons to cross (44). Pronation of the wrist, usually with flexion, can thus pinch the nerve and induce or aggravate symptoms. This movement, which also stretches the first dorsal compartment tendons, is the basis for the Finkelstein test used to diagnose De Quervain's extensor tenosynovitis. Thus, entrapment of the radial sensory nerve must be considered in the differential diagnosis of pain in the first dorsal compartment.

Radial sensory neuropathy can result from crush or twisting injuries to the forearm or compression by a tight watchband or handcuffs (45). Tight casts are a frequent cause. Damage to the nerve can also occur after De Quervain's tenosynovectomy, fracture of the radius, and cutdown for intravenous infusion (9, 46). In a series by Dellon and Mackinnon (44), 15% of patients had coexistent injury to the terminal branch of the posterior interosseous nerve, which innervates the dorsal wrist capsule, resulting in additional deep, aching, nonradiating pain.

Treatment

Conservative measures are usually effective in treating patients with radial sensory neuropathy. Removal of the offending compression often results in improvement within 6–8 weeks (9). Splinting and injection of hydrocortisone have been advocated as well as neurolysis and proximal nerve resection in patients with intractable pain.

THORACIC OUTLET SYNDROME

Thoracic outlet syndrome has been called "the most controversial entity encountered in the field of peripheral nerve disorders" (47). A number of different clinical entities are commonly grouped together under this heading. The term *thoracic outlet* refers to the area between the base of the neck and the axilla. Thoracic outlet syndrome refers to the symptoms resulting from compression of the subclavian artery or vein or brachial plexus in this region. It can be divided broadly into vascular and neurogenic types. Vascular thoracic outlet syndrome may be arterial or venous. Neurogenic thoracic outlet syndrome has been classified by Wilbourn (47) into four types: classical, true, or motor; atypical; droopy shoulder; and disputed. The need for a disputed category reflects the enormity of the controversy pertaining to this entity. Only the classic and disputed thoracic outlet syndromes are considered here.

Vascular Thoracic Outlet Syndromes

Arterial thoracic outlet syndrome can occur when the subclavian artery is repeatedly compressed or traumatized. The resultant symptoms are largely ischemic and are caused by anatomic changes in the artery. Intimal injury resulting in mural thrombosis and atheromatous degeneration can lead to arterial stenosis or the formation of emboli, jeopardizing the affected limb. Ulcerated fingertips or a cool, numb, pale hand with absent pulses can result (48, 49). Rarely, these emboli can travel retrograde to the carotid or vertebral arteries (48).

Venous thoracic outlet syndrome is caused by occlusion of the subclavian or axillary veins. It can also result from repeated compression. It is distinguishable from arterial thoracic outlet syndrome in that it results in a diffusely swollen, bluish arm and dilated veins over the chest and shoulder (47).

Numbness in vascular thoracic outlet syndrome is probably reflective of nerve ischemia and not nerve compression. Usually, the vascular and neurologic syndromes occur independently (50).

Neurogenic Thoracic Outlet Syndrome

Classic neurogenic thoracic outlet syndrome, although rare, is a well-defined entity. In England, Gilliatt (51) found only 20 patients with this syndrome over 15 years, and in this country, Wilbourn found 15 patients in approximately 9 years (47).

Clinical Features

The clinical, electromyographic, and radiographic features are characteristic (52). Wasting and weakness are usually marked in the thenar eminence, particularly in the median-innervated abductor pollicis brevis muscle. Most patients also experience weakness and wasting of the ulnar-innervated intrinsic muscles of the hand.

Pain and paresthesias commonly radiate to the inner aspect of the forearm. Sensory loss when present is over the inner side of the forearm and can involve the ulnar side of the hand and fingers (52). Sensory symptoms usually precede weakness. In a series by Gilliatt and associates (52) of nine patients, seven experienced pain as an initial symptom, either as an intermittent ache in the arm or forearm or diffuse pain in the limb.

The findings from EMG exclude the carpal tunnel syndrome (53). Median motor and sensory latencies across the wrist are normal, even though the pattern of wasting (thenar eminence) is suggestive of this diagnosis, and ulnar sensory potentials are typically diminished in amplitude. The characteristic radiographic abnormality is an elongated seventh cervical transverse process or rudimentary cervical rib.

Treatment

In the series by Gilliatt and associates (52), the compression was caused by a knife-like fibrous band that lifted and stretched the lower trunk of the plexus so that the nerve fibers from the thoracic outlet were angled sharply backward and downward to enter the axilla. The band extended from the tip of the abnormal cervical process or rib to the scalene tubercle on the first rib. Severing the band resulted in subjective improvement in most patients. However, improvement in strength and muscle wasting was usually minimal.

Although most patients with true thoracic outlet syndrome complain of pain in the arm before weakness develops in the hand, they clearly represent a minute subgroup of all patients with arm pain because classic thoracic outlet syndrome is uncommon. The number of operations performed for thoracic outlet syndrome is thus disconcerting. The majority are performed on patients without the objective neurologic findings or characteristic radiographic abnormalities previously discussed. Gilliatt (51), for example, referred only two patients with pain and paresthesias alone for operation over a 15-year period. Both patients had cervical ribs. Yet, the operation may still be a popular one in some centers, as illustrated by one large surgical series (54) in which operations were performed on patients without objective neurologic findings and with symptoms ranging from hemicranial headache to pseudoangina! Tragically, some experience serious injury to the brachial plexus or subclavian artery as a result of operation (55).

Whether thoracic outlet syndrome is as common as reported depends on whether one is a promoter of the disputed category as truly neurogenic. We agree with Wilbourn (47) that thoracic outlet syndrome

is a rare or nonexistent entity, usually erroneously diagnosed by physicians venturing out of their field of training and expertise, who are not recognizing carpal tunnel syndrome, cervical radiculopathy, anxiety-tension state, or "compensation disease." The end result is that patients are . . . subjected to needless and potentially harmful surgical procedures while being denied appropriate therapy.

MISCELLANEOUS ENTRAPMENTS OF THE ARM

AXILLARY NERVE

The axillary nerve is a branch of the posterior cord of the brachial plexus. Lesions of the axillary nerve are most often associated with injuries to the shoulder, for example, fractures of the surgical neck of the humerus (3). The nerve can also be stretched after inferior dislocation of the shoulder or when the arm is externally rotated and abducted. Paralysis of the deltoid is the most disabling consequence, limiting abduction of the arm. Cutaneous sensation over the outer aspect of the upper arm can be diminished or normal even with complete denervation of the deltoid (3).

SUPRASCAPULAR NEUROPATHY

Anatomy

The suprascapular nerve originates from the upper trunk of the brachial plexus where the fifth and sixth cervical roots join at Erb's point. It courses laterally deep to the trapezius and omohyoid muscles through the suprascapular notch, a U-shaped structure within the superior border of the scapula.

The suprascapular notch is bridged by the superior transverse scapular ligament, which inserts medially along the edge of the lateral border of the spine and laterally at the scapular neck or scapulohumeral joint capsule (56). The ligament provides an anatomic predisposition to entrapment (57). Shoulder movements that exert traction on the ligament can cause compression of the nerve where it passes through the notch (56).

Clinical Features

The primary symptom of suprascapular nerve entrapment is shoulder pain that is poorly localized but most severe at the posterior and lateral aspects of the shoulder (58). Thus, suprascapular neuropathy must be differentiated from rotator cuff injuries and subacromial bursitis, which can also result from vigorous physical activity involving the shoulder girdle. Physical examination can show weakness of the supraspinatus and infraspinatus muscles, which are abductors and external rotators of the shoulder. The suprascapular nerve has no cutaneous representation.

In addition to musculoskeletal conditions, entrapment of the suprascapular nerve must be distinguished from brachial plexitis and radiculopathy of the fifth or sixth cervical root, which can cause similar symptoms. Dawson and associates (9) cited four features that favor the diagnosis of suprascapular neuropathy: local pain or palpation of the suprascapular notch; relief of pain after anesthetic block of the nerve as it passes through the notch; increased pain from maneuvers that stretch and compress the nerve, such as swinging the arm forward across the chest; and abnormalities seen on EMG that are localized to the infraspinatus and supraspinatus muscles.

Suprascapular neuropathy can result from trauma to the shoulder from either injury to the nerve or damage to the transverse scapular ligament or surrounding tissue. It can also occur spontaneously or as a result of lipomas or ganglion cysts. Backpacking has also been implicated (57).

MUSCULOCUTANEOUS NERVE

Anatomy

The musculocutaneous nerve is a mixed nerve originating from the lateral cord of the brachial plexus at the lower border of the pectoralis minor muscle. It travels obliquely (downward and outward) between the brachialis and biceps muscles before emerging 2–5 cm above the elbow crease as the lateral cutaneous nerve of the forearm.

Clinical Features

The musculocutaneous nerve is rarely injured in isolation because it is deeply situated and well protected for much of its course. Because it is fixed at the coracobrachialis muscle, stretch injuries can result from violent extension of the forearm. Heavy exercise has also been reported as a cause of injury either from contractions of the coracobrachialis muscle or chronic pressure secondary to muscle hypertrophy (59). Lesions of the nerve in the arm can result in weakness of the biceps muscle and dysesthesias over the radial aspect of the forearm.

Injury to the sensory portion of the nerve at the elbow distal to its muscular branches can also occur, probably from compression by the lateral free edge of the biceps aponeurosis. Bassett and Nunley (60) reported on 11 patients in whom symptoms developed after repeated pronation and supination of the forearm (one man inserted 3000 screws in a weekend!) or after hyperextension and pronation of the arm (as might occur after a fall or from an improper tennis swing). Pain over the anterolateral aspect of the elbow was the presenting symptom in every patient. All patients had tenderness over the area where the musculocutaneous nerve exits from beneath the biceps tendon. Ten patients had sensory loss along the radial aspect of the volar part of the forearm, but only those with acute sensory loss had burning dysesthesias in this distribution (60). A majority of these patients required surgical decompression for relief.

Entrapment of the sensory division of the musculocutaneous nerve has been reported to occur spontaneously (9). Injury to the nerve can result from carrying a heavy handbag with the strap across the elbow crease (61). The nerve can also be injured by careless venipuncture where it is located beneath the cephalic and median cephalic veins (between the biceps and brachio-radialis muscles) (3).

SYNDROMES OF THE LONG THORACIC AND ACCESSORY NERVES

Scapular winging usually results from lesions of the long thoracic or accessory nerves.

Lesions of the Accessory Nerve

Anatomy

The accessory nerve arises from the upper cervical segments and travels cephalad through the foramen magnum before exiting the skull at the jugular foramen. In the neck, it becomes superficial just above the mid-point of the posterior border of the sternocleidomastoid muscle. It courses obliquely across the posterior triangle of the neck to the deep surface of the trapezius muscle to which it is attached (62).

Clinical Features

Accessory nerve palsy is associated with weakness of the trapezius muscle and variably with weakness of the sternocleidomastoid muscle. Most lesions develop after surgical procedures involving the posterior triangle of the neck, such as radical neck dissecttion or biopsy of a lymph node. The nerve can also be injured in sporting accidents. Rarely, accessory nerve palsy develops spontaneously without apparent cause (62). Injury to the accessory nerve results in shoulder pain and instability. The shoulder droops, and abduction of the arm is impaired. The scapula moves so that its superior angle is displaced farther from the midline than its inferior angle. Scapular winging is accentuated by flexion of the arm.

Lesions of the Long Thoracic Nerve

Anatomy

The long thoracic nerve is formed from the fifth, sixth, and seventh cervical roots. It courses posterior to the brachial plexus on the scalenus medius muscle over the outer border of the first rib and vertically down the thoracic wall to innervate the serratus anterior muscle. The nerve is attached to both the scalenus medius muscle above and the serratus anterior muscle below, making it susceptible to stretch injuries when the shoulder is depressed or the neck is flexed to the opposite side (3).

Clinical Features

In contradistinction to accessory nerve palsy, lesions of the long thoracic nerve cause minimal shoulder deformity at rest and more pronounced scapular winging with use. The inferior angle of the scapula becomes displaced farther from the midline and posterior chest wall than the superior angle. Scapular winging is accentuated by extension of the arm against resistance.

Compression of the nerve can occur during anesthesia if the patient is placed in the Trendelenburg position with poorly positioned shoulder rests that force the shoulder downward (3). Traction injuries can result from carrying heavy objects on the shoulder. Enlarged lymph nodes at the root of the neck and entrance to the axilla or their surgical removal can also result in nerve injury (3).

Lesions of the long thoracic nerve result in shoulder instability and weakness in raising the arm. The serratus muscle normally pulls the scapula forward and assists the trapezius muscle in rotating the scapula outward. Elevating the arm from a position of forward flexion or abduction is thus impaired (3). The weakness can be accompanied by shoulder pain radiating to the arm and neck.

Injuries to the long thoracic nerve can be accompanied by injuries to the brachial plexus or accessory nerve. Thus, winging of the scapula and weakness of the shoulder and arm can have more than one cause. Scapular winging can also result from paralysis of the dorsal scapular nerve to the rhomboid muscles and radiculopathy of the seventh cervical root (63).

LESIONS OF THE PERONEAL NERVE

The hallmark of peroneal nerve entrapment is footdrop caused by weakness of the tibialis anterior muscle. Weakness of ankle eversion is also usually apparent. The fibers of the peroneal nerve are among the nerves most commonly compressed in the leg. They clinically account for a distinct group, even in the upper thigh where they form a component of the sciatic nerve. Peroneal fibers split at the apex of the popliteal fossa where the sciatic nerve terminates into its peroneal and tibial divisions. The peroneal division courses laterally around the fibular head to enter a fibro-osseous tunnel bounded by the peroneus longus and fibula (9). The tibial fibers continue as a posterior tibial nerve. For reasons to be discussed, the peroneal division is often affected preferentially in proximal lesions of the sciatic nerve.

The fibers that make up the peroneal nerve are particularly vulnerable to focal lesions at the fibular head. Less often the peroneal components of the sciatic nerve are affected in the proximal thigh and clinically can mimic a primary lesion of the peroneal nerve at the knee. Compression of the peroneal nerve at the fibular head has a tendency to be neuropractic (caused by focal demyelination) (64), whereas lesions of the proximal sciatic nerve often have appreciable axonal loss.

At the fibular head the common peroneal nerve is particularly vulnerable to compression and penetrating injury because the nerve is only covered by skin and superficial fascia adjacent to the periosteum of the fibula (65). Inversion injuries of the ankle can cause damage to the peroneal nerve at the fibula head because the nerve is tethered proximally and has limited longitudinal mobility (66). Other causes of lesions of the peroneal nerve include infarction (64), pretibial myxedema (67), prolonged squatting (68), and tumors.

Prognosis depends on whether there is isolated conduction block due to focal demyelination or concomitant axonal injury present. Prolonged compression, such as that which occurs in someone chronically ill inadvertently crossing the knees or an intoxicated patient laying in one position, is usually associated with a good prognosis because focal demyelination is the major pathophysiologic mechanism. However, if axonal loss occurs, such as from penetrating trauma directly to the nerve, infarction, or sometimes with severe stretch injuries, prognosis for recovery can be one of a long and sometimes guarded course.

LESIONS OF THE SCIATIC NERVE

The sciatic nerve is most prone to injury at its exit in the pelvis at the sciatic notch. Although occasionally these lesions involve both the peroneal and tibial components, frequently a great portion of involvement affects the peroneal fibers. To the inexperienced observer this can mimic a lesion of the peroneal nerve at the fibular head. Predominant involvement of the peroneal fibers in lesions of the proximal sciatic nerve may be due to the presence of fewer and larger funiculi with less connective tissue packing in this portion of the sciatic nerve. It is also believed that the sciatic nerve is less tolerant of displacement because it is tethered at both sciatic notch and fibular head (64). In contrast, lesions of the midthigh usually compromise both peroneal and tibial function equally, probably because they tend to result from violent trauma, and in this position the fibers are equally vulnerable.

Damage to the sciatic nerve at the sciatic notch can result from fracture on dislocation of the hip, penetrating injuries, complications of hip surgery, prolonged pressure on the buttocks during various comatose states, and, rarely, spontaneous or anticoagulant-induced sciatic notch hematoma and primary or metastatic tumors, such as lymphomas.

Injuries caused by hip surgery or fracture are sometimes associated with a poor prognosis. Those arising during prolonged periods of coma can result in persistent disability. Stretch injuries can also occur at the time of operation, requiring utilization of the lithotomy posture. These injuries can also have persistent disabling sequelae. A poor prognosis is associated with axonal damage and inability of the nerve to regenerate over its great length to permit reinnervation. In contrast, if compression lesions mainly affect the myelin without axonal damage, as may be seen in pressure palsy or hip dislocations, the prognosis for full recovery is good, particularly in children (69).

SYNDROMES OF THE FEMORAL NERVE

ANATOMY

The femoral nerve is the largest branch of the lumbar plexus and forms in the abdomen in the substance of the psoas muscle. In the abdomen, it lies behind the ileocecal bowel on the right and sigmoid colon on the left. It innervates the psoas and iliacus muscles, coursing in the groove between them with the iliolumbar vessels before exiting the pelvis beneath the inguinal ligament to enter the thigh. Therefore, when these muscles are unaffected by a lesion to the femoral nerve, the lesion should be distal to the inguinal ligament.

In the thigh, the femoral nerve lies within the femoral triangle lateral to the artery. Several centimeters distal to the inguinal ligament it divides to supply the skin over the anterior thigh, the medial side of the knee, and the proximal part of the leg (via the saphenous nerve) and the innervation to the quadriceps and sartorius muscles (3). Lesions distal to the inguinal ligament can thus be partial because the femoral nerve breaks into numerous motor and sensory branches.

CLINICAL FEATURES

The femoral nerve is susceptible to open and closed injuries. Important causes of nontraumatic injury to the femoral nerve include hematoma and abscess of the iliacus muscle. The location of the nerve in the groove between the illiacus and psoas muscles makes it particularly vulnerable to an expanding mass in this area (43).

Hematomas usually occur as a consequence of anticoagulation or a clotting disorder, such as hemophilia (70). Characteristically, a large, sometimes painful globular swelling develops in the iliac fossa that in some instances extends into the groin. The hip can be flexed, abducted, and externally rotated to reduce tension on the nerve, which is stretched over the hematoma (70). The obturator nerve is classically spared. Treatment is controversial because complete recovery of nerve function has been reported even after large hemorrhage (71). However, with the availability of computed tomography to monitor lesion size a more precise assessment of the results of expectant treatment or surgical decompression may become available to guide management better.

Closed injuries can also occur as a complication of anesthesia. With the patient in the lithotomy position, the femoral nerve can be compressed under the inguinal ligament. Forced extension of the limb or hyperextension of the hip over the edge of a bed during coma can also injure the nerve, probably from undue stretch.

Open injuries to the femoral nerve can result from penetrating trauma, such as stab wound, or procedure involving catheterization of the femoral artery (3). They can also occur during the course of operation. Retraction injury, for example, has been attributed to forced lateral displacement of the psoas muscle (3).

SAPHENOUS NERVE

The saphenous nerve can be injured separately, resulting in pain down the medial aspect of the leg to the inner side of the foot or big toe. The point of emergence from the subsartorial fascia about 10 cm above the medial femoral epicondyle is its region of mechanical vulnerability. Entrapment here can mimic orthopedic causes of knee pain (72). Because the pain sometimes can be induced or aggravated by limb movement, it can also simulate intermittent claudication (73).

Isolated involvement of the prepatellar branch of the saphenous nerve can occur spontaneously or from trauma, for example, after medial meniscectomy. Stinging pain or an isolated spot of numbness below the knee can result. Tingling and a feeling like pins and needles can also occur when the knee is bent (74).

ENTRAPMENT OF THE LATERAL CUTANEOUS NERVE OF THE THIGH (MERALGIA PARESTHETICA)

ANATOMY

The nerve is derived from the second and third lumbar roots. In its intrapelvic course it penetrates the psoas muscle and travels obliquely across the iliac fossa to the anterosuperior iliac spine where it exits the pelvis beneath the inguinal ligament. It is particularly vulnerable to compression at the iliac spine where it passes between bone and the ligament and the attachment of the sartorius muscle (3).

CLINICAL FEATURES

The discomfort of meralgia paresthetica is variously described as burning, itching, pricking, or a feeling of coldness or numbness localized over the anterolateral aspect of the thigh. Hyperesthesia can also be present.

The syndrome has been associated with conditions that cause protuberant abdomens, such as pregnancy, obesity, and liver disease. It can also occur as a result of direct trauma, tight jeans, carrying a wallet in the front pocket, or standing at attention (75, 76). Presumably these conditions result in increased pressure on or stretch of the nerve.

Although meralgia paresthetica is usually benign, it rarely results from serious intrapelvic disease, such as retroperitoneal malignant tumor (77). Damage to the nerve can also occur as a result of abdominal surgery.

TREATMENT

Most patients with meralgia paresthetica recover spontaneously within weeks or months (3). Removal of sources of external compression is usually effective. Although local anesthetic block can be successful in providing symptomatic relief, this is rarely necessary be-

cause most patients cease to complain about the condition when reassured of its benign nature. Operation on the nerve, such as sectioning the nerve, is not recommended because of the risk of the development of painful neuromas that are worse than the meralgia itself (3). The role of neurectomy, decompression, or transposition has not been defined well for patients in whom conservative therapy fails.

ENTRAPMENT OF THE TIBIAL NERVE (TARSAL TUNNEL SYNDROME)

ANATOMY

The tarsal tunnel is located behind and inferior to the medial malleolus. It is bounded laterally by the bony tibia and medially by the flexor retinaculum (laciniate ligament). In addition to the tibial nerve, its contents include the tendons of the posterior tibial, flexor digitorum longus, and flexor hallucis longus muscles and the tibial artery and vein.

Within the tarsal tunnel or immediately distal to it, the tibial nerve divides into the medial and lateral plantar nerves. The calcaneal branch originates variably above or beneath the flexor retinaculum to supply the skin of the heel and calcaneus. The medial plantar division provides sensation to the plantar surface of the first, second, and third toes and the medial half of the fourth toe. It also supplies the abductor hallucis muscle. The lateral plantar nerve courses obliquely across the foot and supplies sensation to the lateral half of the fourth and fifth toes and innervation to the flexor digitorum brevis and abductor digiti minimi pedis muscles (78).

CLINICAL FEATURES

Foot pain and paresthesias are characteristic of tarsal tunnel syndrome and can be accompanied by sensory loss and Tinel's sign at the ankle (79). The pain is similar to that of carpal tunnel syndrome even to the extent that it occurs at night and can be accentuated or induced by prolonged standing or walking (9, 80). Weakness of the phalanges can also result, impairing the pushing off phase of walking (9). Although the tarsal tunnel syndrome has been likened to the carpal tunnel syndrome, the analogy falls short because tarsal tunnel syndrome is rarely a source of foot discomfort.

Tarsal tunnel syndrome must be distinguished from many other causes of pain in the foot, including painful peripheral neuropathies with which it may be associated. It also must be distinguished from entrapment of the medial plantar nerve in the foot, which has been reported to occur in joggers (81).

The most common cause of tarsal tunnel syndrome is trauma, such as fractures or dislocation of the ankle (9). Other possible precipitants include tenosynovitis; chronic thrombophlebitis; systemic diseases, such as gout, hyperlipidemia (82), hypothyroidism (83), and rheumatoid arthritis; and ganglion cysts.

TREATMENT

The treatment of patients with tarsal tunnel syndrome is initially conservative and may involve arch support, anti-inflammatory medication, or injection of steroids. Precipitating trauma should be removed. Sectioning the laciniate ligament frequently results in relief of symptoms when conservative therapy fails (9, 84).

REFERENCES

1. Gilliatt RW, Harrison MJG: Nerve compression and entrapment. In Asbury AK, Gilliatt RW (eds): *Peripheral Nerve Disorders: A Practical Approach.* Boston, Butterworth, 1984.
2. Carroll RE, Green DP: The significance of the palmar cutaneous nerve at the wrist. *Clin Orthop* 83:24–28, 1972.
3. Sunderland S: *Nerves and Nerve Injuries,* ed 2. New York, Churchill Livingstone, 1978.
4. Phalen GS: The carpal-tunnel syndrome: clinical evaluation of 598 hands. *Clin Orthop* 83:29–40, 1972.
5. Fin EJ, Wongjirad C, Agrawal S: Single-digit pain and paresthesia: a symptom of early carpal tunnel syndrome. *Ann Neurol* 16:150, 1984 (abstr P144).
6. Cherington M: Proximal pain in carpal tunnel syndrome. *Arch Surg* 108:69, 1974.
7. Serra G, Migliore A. Tugnoll V: Raynaud's phenomenon and entrapment neuropathies (letter). *Ann Neurol* 18:519, 1985.
8. Phalen GS: Reflections on 21 years' experience with the carpal-tunnel syndrome. *JAMA* 212:1365–1367, 1970.
9. Dawson DM, Hallett M, Millender LH: *Entrapment Neuropathies.* Boston, Little, Brown, 1983.
10. Massey EW: Carpal tunnel syndrome in pregnancy. *Obstet Gynecol Surv* 33:145–148, 1978.
11. Tobin SM: Carpal tunnel syndrome in pregnancy. *Am J Obstet Gynecol* 97:493–498, 1967.
12. Murphy F, Beetham WP Jr, Torgerson WR Jr: Carpal tunnel syndrome caused by tophaceous gout: report of two cases with review of the literature. *Lahey Clin Found Bull* 23:18–23, 1974.
13. Mahloudji M: Familial carpal-tunnel syndrome due to amyloidosis (letter). *Lancet* 1:1374, 1968.
14. Beard L, Kumar A, Estep HL: Bilateral carpal tunnel syndrome caused by Graves' disease. *Arch Intern Med* 145:345–346, 1985.
15. O'Duffy JD, Randall RV, MacCarty CS: Median neuropathy (carpal-tunnel syndrome) in acromegaly: a sign of endocrine overactivity. *Ann Intern Med* 78:379–383, 1973.
16. Holtmann B, Anderson CB: Carpal tunnel syndrome following vascular shunts for hemodialysis. *Arch Surg* 112:65–66, 1977.
17. Semple JC, Cargill AO: Carpal-tunnel syndrome: results of surgical decompression. *Lancet* 1:918–919, 1969.
18. Suranyl L: Median nerve compression by Struthers ligament. *J Neurol Neurosurg Psychiatry* 46:1047–1049, 1983.
19. Spinner M: The anterior interosseous-nerve syndrome. *J Bone Joint Surg* 52A:84–94, 1970.
20. Shahani BT: Median nerve entrapments at the elbow. In *1986 AAEE Course E: Entrapment Neuropathies,* Boston September 25, 1986. Rochester, MN, American Association of Electromyography and Electrodiagnosis, 1986, pp 11–12.
21. Fineili PF: Anterior interosseous nerve syndrome following cutdown catheterization. *Ann Neurol* 1:205–206, 1977.
22. Cherington M: Anterior interosseous nerve syndrome straight thumb sign (letter). *Neurology* 27:800–801, 1977.
23. Parsonage MJ, Turner JWA: Neuralgic amyotrophy: shoulder-girdle syndrome. *Lancet* 1:973–978, 1948.
24. Hartz CR, Linscheid RL, Gramse RR, et al: The pronator teres syndrome: compressive neuropathy of the median nerve. *J Bone Joint Surg* 63A:885–890, 1981.
25. Martinelli P, Gabellini AS, Poppi M, et al: Pronator syndrome due to thickened bicipital aponeurosis (letter). *J Neurol Neurosurg Psychiatry* 45:181–182, 1982.
26. Chan RC, Paine KEW, Varughese G: Ulnar neuropathy at the elbow: comparison of simple decompression and anterior transposition. *Neurosurgery* 7:545–550, 1980.
27. Miller RG: The cubital tunnel syndrome: diagnosis and precise localization. *Ann Neurol* 6:56–59, 1979.
28. Feindel W, Stratford J: Cubital tunnel compression in tardy ulnar palsy. *Can Med Assoc J* 78:351–353, 1958.
29. Miller RG, Hummel EE: The cubital tunnel syndrome: treatment with simple decompression. *Ann Neurol* 7:567–569, 1980.
30. Macnicol MF: The results of operation for ulnar neuritis. *J Bone Joint Surg* 61B:159–164, 1979.
31. Harrison MJG, Nurick S: Results of anterior transposition of the ulnar nerve for adult neuritis. *Br Med J* 1:27–29, 1970.
32. Miller RG, Camp PE: Postoperative ulnar neuropathy. *JAMA* 242:1636–1639, 1979.
33. Shea JD, McClain EJ: Ulnar-nerve compression syndromes at and below the wrist. *J Bone Joint Surg* 51A:1095–1103, 1969.
34. Noth J, Dietz V, Mauritz KH: Cyclist's palsy: neurological and EMG study in 4 cases with distal ulnar lesions. *J Neurol Sci* 47:111–116, 1980.
35. Reid RI, Ashby MA: Ulnar nerve palsy and walking frames. *Br Med J* 285:778, 1982.
36. Lotem M, Fried A, Levy M, et al: Radial palsy following muscular effort: a nerve compression syndrome possibly related to a fibrous arch of the lateral head of the triceps. *J Bone Joint Surg* 53B:500–506, 1971.
37. Stöhr M, Reill P: Chronic compression syndrome of the radial nerve above the elbow (letter). *Muscle Nerve* 3:446–447, 1980.
38. Kim LYS: Compression neuropathy of the radial nerve due to pentazocine-induced fibrous myopathy. *Arch Phys Med Rehabil* 68:49–50, 1987.
39. Shaw JL, Sakellarides H: Radial-nerve paralysis associated with fractures of the humerus. *J Bone Joint Surg* 49A:899–902, 1967.
40. Goldman S, Honet JC, Sobel R, et al: Posterior interosseous nerve palsy in the absence of trauma. *Arch Neurol* 21:35–441, 1969.
41. Bowen TL, Stone KH: Posterior interosseous nerve paralysis caused by a ganglion at the elbow. *J Bone Joint Surg* 48B:774–776, 1966.
42. Lallemand RC, Weller RO: Intraneural neurofibromas in-

volving the posterior interosseous nerve. *J Neurol Neurosurg Psychiatry* 36:991–996, 1973.

43. Carfi J, Dong MM: Posterior interosseous syndrome revisited. *Muscle Nerve* 8:499–502, 1985.

44. Dellon AI, Mackinnon SE: Radial sensory nerve entrapment. *Arch Neurol* 43:833–835, 1986.

45. Massey EW, Pleet AB: Handcuffs and cheiralgia paresthetica. *Neurology* 28:1312–1313, 1978.

46. Braidwood AS: Surgical radial neuropathy. *J Bone Joint Surg* 57B:380–383, 1975.

47. Wilbourn AJ: Thoracic outlet syndrome. In *1984 AAEE Course D: Controversy in Entrapment Neuropathies*, Kansas City, MO, September 20, 1984. Rochester, MN, American Association of Electromyography and Electrodiagnosis, 1984, pp 28–38.

48. Fields WS, Lemak NA, Ben-Menachem Y: Thoracic outlet syndrome: review and reference to stroke in a major league pitcher. *AJR* 146:809–814, 1986.

49. Judy KL, Heymann RL: Vascular complications of thoracic outlet syndrome. *Am J Surg* 123:521–531, 1972.

50. Gilliatt RW: Thoracic outlet syndromes. In Dyck PJ, Thomas PK, Lambert EH, Bunge R (eds): *Peripheral Neuropathy*, ed 2. Philadelphia, WB Saunders, 1984, vol 2, pp 1409–1417.

51. Gilliatt RW: Thoracic outlet compression syndrome (letter). *Br Med J* 1:1274–1275, 1976.

52. Gilliatt RW, Le Quesne PM, Logue V, et al: Wasting of the hand associated with a cervical rib or band. *J Neurol Neurosurg Psychiatry* 33:615–624, 1970.

53. Gilliatt RW, Willison RG, Dietz V et al: Peripheral nerve conduction in patients with a cervical rib and band. *Ann Neurol* 4:124–129, 1978.

54. Roos DB: The place for scalenectomy and first-rib resection in thoracic outlet syndrome. *Surgery* 92:1077–1085, 1982.

55. Cherington M, Happer I, Machanic B, et al: Surgery for thoracic outlet syndrome may be hazardous to your health. *Muscle Nerve* 9:632–634, 1986.

56. Aiello I, Serra G, Traina GC, et al: Entrapment of the suprascapular nerve at the spinoglenoid notch. *Ann Neurol* 12:314–316, 1983.

57. Hadley MN, Sonntag VKH, Pittman HW: Suprascapular nerve entrapment: a summary of seven cases. *J Neurosurg* 84:843–848, 1986.

58. Thompson WAL, Kopell HP: Peripheral entrapment neuropathies of the upper extremity. *N Engl J Med* 260:1261–1265, 1959.

59. Braddom RL, Wolfe C: Musculocutaneous nerve injury after heavy exercise. *Arch Phys Med Rehabil* 59:290–293, 1978.

60. Bassett FH III, Nunley JA: Compression of the musculocutaneous nerve at the elbow. *J Bone Joint Surg* 64A:1050–1052, 1982.

61. Hale BR: Handbag paraesthesia (letter). *Lancet* 2:470, 1978.

62. Eisen A, Bertrand G: Isolated accessory nerve palsy of spontaneous origin. *Arch Neurol* 27:496–502, 1972.

63. Makin GJV, Brown WF, Ebers GC: C7 Radiculopathy: importance of scapular winging in clinical diagnosis. *J Neurol Neurosurg Psychiatry* 49:640–644, 1986.

64. Wilbourn AJ: Peroneal mononeuropathies. In *1986 AAEE Course E: Entrapment Neuropathies*, Boston, September 25, 1986. Rochester, MN, American Association of Electromyography and Electrodiagnosis, 1986, pp 19–28.

65. Berry H, Richardson PM: Common peroneal palsy: a clinical and electrophysiological review. *J Neurol Neurosurg Psychiatry* 39:1162–1171, 1976.

66. Meals RA: Peroneal-nerve palsy complicating ankle sprain. *J Bone Joint Surg* 59A:966–968, 1977.

67. Siegler M, Refetoff S: Pretibial myxedema—a reversible cause of foot drop due to entrapment of the peroneal nerve. *N Engl J Med* 294:1383–1384, 1976.

68. Koller RL, Blank NK: Strawberry pickers' palsy. *Arch Neurol* 37:320, 1980.

69. Jones HR Jr, Gianturco L: Sciatic neuropathies in children: report of 9 cases. *Ann Neurol* 18:158, 1985 (abstr P157).

70. Nobel W, Marks SC Jr, Kubik S: The anatomical basis for femoral nerve palsy following iliacus hematoma. *J Neurosurg* 52:533–540, 1980.

71. Susens GP, Hendrickson CG, Mulder MJ, et al: Femoral nerve entrapment secondary to a heparin hematoma. *Ann Intern Med* 69:575–579, 1968.

72. Kopell HP, Thompson WAL: Knee pain due to saphenous-nerve entrapment. *N Engl J Med* 263:351–353, 1960.

73. Mozes M, Ouaknine G, Nathan H: Saphenous nerve entrapment simulating vascular disorder. *Surgery* 77:299–303, 1975.

74. Massey EW: Gonyalgia paresthetica (letter). *Muscle Nerve* 4:80–81, 1951.

75. Kaufman J, Canoso JJ: Progressive systemic sclerosis and meralgia paraesthetica (letter). *Ann Intern Med* 105:973, 1986.

76. Massey EW: Meralgia paresthetica: an unusual case. *JAMA* 237:1125–1126, 1977.

77. Flowers RS: Meralgia paresthetica: a clue to retroperitoneal malignant tumor. *Am J Surg* 116:89–92, 1968.

78. Kraft GH: Tarsal tunnel entrapment. In *1986 AAEE Course E: Entrapment Neuropathies*, Boston, September 25, 1986. Rochester, MN, American Association of Electromyography and Electrodiagnosis, 1986, pp 13–18.

79. Oh SJ, Sarala PK, Kuba T, et al: Tarsal tunnel syndrome: electrophysiological study. *Ann Neurol* 5:327–330, 1979.

80. DeLisa JA, Saeed MA: The tarsal tunnel syndrome. *Muscle Nerve* 6:664–670, 1983.

81. Oh SJ, Lee KW: Medial plantar neuropathy: a heretofore unrecognized mononeuropathy. *Ann Neurol* 20:135, 1986 (abstr P46).

82. Ruderman MI, Palmar RH, Olarte MR, et al: Tarsal tunnel syndrome caused by hyperlipidemia: reversal after plasmapheresis. *Arch Neurol* 40:124–125, 1983.

83. Schwartz MS, Macworth-Young CG, McKeran RO: The tarsal tunnel syndrome in hypothyroidism. *J Neurol Neurosurg Psychiatry* 46:440–442, 1983.

84. Kaplan PE, Kernahan WT: Tarsal tunnel syndrome. *J Bone Joint Surg* 63A:96–99, 1981.

CHAPTER 39

REFLEX SYMPATHETIC DYSTROPHY AND CAUSALGIA

NELSON HENDLER
SRINIVASA N. RAJA

CLINICAL SIGNS AND SYMPTOMS

Reflex sympathetic dystrophy (RSD) and causalgia are symptom complexes that evoke a great deal of confusion. Very often, physicians do not recognize that these are separate and distinct entities, and commonly assume that they are disorders of the same etiology, as well as responsive to the same treatment. Clinically, this has not proven accurate. RSD is a group of symptoms and clinical signs that usually follows a minor injury to a limb. In contradistinction, causalgia is usually associated with peripheral nerve injury, classically from a bullet wound or some other partial nerve damage. In a very fine review article, Payne clearly defined the distinction between causalgia and RSD (1). This has been further expanded by the International Association for the Study of Pain in a supplement edited by Harold Merskey in 1986 (2) (Table 39.1).

Clinically, one can make the distinction between the two disorders on the basis of not only signs and symptoms, but also response to treatment.

REFLEX SYMPATHETIC DYSTROPHY

Following the distinction drawn by Payne, one considers RSD as the result of minor trauma; inflammation following surgery, infection, or lacerations resulting in some degree of swelling in the affected limb; infarctions; degenerative joint disease; frostbite; and burns (1). One should add to this list the possibility of any compression, such as casting or swelling due to injury, that may cause prolonged pressure on peripheral nerves. Additionally, we have seen at least two or three cases per year of RSD brought about from arthroscopy. Unfortunately, no other reported cases appear in the literature, so this is really a clinical impression garnered from 15 years' experience working with RSD patients.

According to Schwartzman and McKellan, there seem to be three phases to RSD (3). Additionally, physicians should recognize that RSD is a symptom complex that is a cluster of symptoms and signs, and that patients do *not* present with all signs and symptoms during the course of their disease. In fact, very often, they may have only one or two of the signs and symptoms of the disorder.

As described by Payne and by Schwartzman and McKellan, the acute stage of RSD lasts several weeks, and is characterized by spontaneous pain, usually aching or burning, that follows the distribution of blood vessels or peripheral nerves. The acute stage may manifest as "hyperpathia" (this is described as a painful syndrome of overreaction to a stimulus or after-sensation following a stimulus) and may include hypesthesia or hyperesthesia (described as a decreased or an increased sensation to stimulation, respectively) or dysesthesia (described as an unpleasant abnormal sensation) (1, 3). Associated with these tactile sensations are usually a warm, dry, red skin or cold, blue, sweaty skin, with some swelling, and, surprisingly, increased hair and nail growth.

Additionally, the patient has dependent redness and reduced motion in the damaged extremity. This summarizes the acute stage of this disorder, which may last several weeks and may begin immediately or several days after the onset of the injury.

The second stage of RSD, beginning about 3–6 months after the injury, is called the dystrophic stage by Payne (1). During this stage, the patient experiences a burning type of pain, which radiates either above or below the site of the injury, and increased hypersensitivity or hyperalgesia (an exquisite sensitivity to touch or temperature—a most important distinction that is discussed later in the chapter). The patient has changes in the nails on occasion, as well as decreased hair growth. This seems to be a variable finding, and certainly is *not* a sine qua non of the diagnosis of RSD. Joints may become

Table 39.1.

Causalgia (1–4)

Definition	Burning pain, allodynia, and hyperpathia, usually in the hand or foot, after partial injury of a nerve or one of its major branches.
Site	In the region of the limb innervated by the damaged nerve.
Main Features	Onset usually immediately after partial nerve injury or, may be delayed for months. Causalgia of the radial nerve is very rare. The nerves most commonly involved are the median, the sciatic and tibial, and ulnar. Spontaneous pain. Pain described as constant, burning, exacerbated by light touch, stress, temperature change or movement of involved limb, visual and auditory stimuli, e.g., a sudden sound or bright light, emotional disturbances.
Associated Symptoms	Atrophy of skin appendages, secondary atrophic changes in bones, joints and muscles. Cool, reddish, clammy skin with excessive sweating. Sensory and motor loss in structure innervated by damaged portion of nerve.
Signs	Cool, reddish, clammy, sweaty skin with atrophy of skin appendages and deep structures in painful area.
Laboratory Findings	Galvanic skin responses and plethysmography reveal signs of sympathetic nervous system hyperactivity. Roentgenograms may show atrophy of bone.
Usual Course	If untreated, the majority of patients will have symptoms which persist indefinitely; spontaneous remission occurs.
Relief	In early stages of causalgia (first few months) sympathetic blockade plus vigorous physical therapy usually provides transient relief; repeated blocks usually lead to long-term relief. When a series of sympathetic blocks does not provide long-term relief, sympathectomy is indicated. Long-term persistence of symptoms reduces the likelihood of successful therapy.
Social and Physical Disabilities	Disuse atrophy of involved limb; complete disruption of normal daily activities by severe pain. Risk of suicide, drug abuse if untreated.
Pathology	Partial injury to major peripheral nerve; actual cause of pain is unknown. Peripheral central and sympathetic mechanisms involved in an unexplained way.
Essential Features	Burning pain and cutaneous hypersensitivity with signs of sympathetic hyperactivity in portion of limb innervated by partially injured nerve.

Reflex Sympathetic Dystrophy (1–4)

Definition	Continuous pain in a portion of an extremity after trauma which may include fracture but does not involve a major nerve, associated with sympathetic hyperactivity.
Site	Usually the distal extremity adjacent to a traumatized area.
System	Peripheral nervous system; possibly the central nervous system.
Main Features	The pain follows trauma (usually mild), not associated with significant nerve injury; the pain is described as burning, continuous, exacerbated by movement, cutaneous stimulation, or stress. Onset usually weeks after injury.
Associated Symptoms	Initially there is vaso-dilatation with increasing temperature, hyperhidrosis and edema. Hyperhidrosis and reduced sympathetic activity also occur. Atrophy of skin appendages, cool, red, clammy skin are variably present. Disuse atrophy of deep structures may progress to Sudeck's atrophy of bone. Aggravated by use of body part, relieved by immobilization. Sometimes follows a herniated intervertebral disc, spinal anesthesia, poliomyelitis, severe iliofemoral thrombosis or cardiac infarction. This may appear as the shoulder-hand syndrome. Later vasospastic symptoms become prominent with persistent coldness of the affected extremity, pallor or cyanosis, Raynaud's phenomenon, atrophy of the skin and nails and loss of hair, atrophy of soft tissues and stiffness of joints. Without therapy these symptoms may persist. It is not necessary for one patient to exhibit all symptoms together. An additional limb or limbs may be affected as well.
Signs	Variable; there may be florid sympathetic hyperactivity.
Laboratory Findings	In advanced cases, roentgenograms may show atrophy of bone.
Usual Course	Persists indefinitely if untreated; small incidence of spontaneous remission.
Relief	Sympathetic block and physical therapy; sympathectomy if long-term results not achieved with repeated blocks; may respond in early phases to high doses of corticosteroids, e.g., Prednisone 50 mg. daily.
Complications	Disuse atrophy of involved limb; suicide and drug abuse if untreated; sometimes spreads to contralateral limb.
Social and Physical Disability	Depression, inability to perform daily activities.
Pathology	Unknown.
Essential Features	Burning pain in distal extremity usually after minor injury without nerve damage.
Differential Diagnosis	Unrecognized local pathology (fracture, strain, sprain). Causalgia, post-traumatic vasospasm or thrombosis.

stiff, with decreased range of motion and possible thickening, associated with some degree of muscle wasting. Edema may be present, and with appropriate testing osteoporosis may be noted (1).

The third stage described by Payne is the atropic stage, which usually occurs 6 months or longer after the injury. According to Payne, the patient experiences pain, decreased skin temperature, trophic changes in the skin associated with a smooth glossy skin, stiff fixed joints associated with contractures, increased or decreased sweating in the affected extremity, and demineralization of the bone associated with wasted muscles and reduced strength (1).

Causalgia

Causalgia is usually associated with peripheral nerve injury and severe pain. According to Payne, pain occurring in causalgia follows an injury to a nerve trunk, usually a major proximal nerve branch, and is described as a persistent burning pain, but does not necessarily have to be burning in quality. It is unrelated to associated damage from surrounding tissue, and seems to be worsened by emotional or environmental stimuli. Most importantly, the pain seems to persist more than 5–6 weeks, which seems to be the length of time needed for surrounding tissue to recover from injury. Typically, the injury is due to damage by a bullet, a knife, sharpened rocks or parts propelled by a machine, or other such objects. When the injury is associated with a high-velocity missile, one must consider not only the actual damage to the tissue itself, but hydrostatic effects caused by shockwaves. When one takes into account the fact that the body is made up largely of water, it is easy to see how a high-velocity missile can cause damage not only to the actual tissue that has been penetrated by the missile, but also to surrounding tissue as a result of hydrostatically transmitted shock waves. If the reader desires additional information regarding the hydrostatic effects of high-velocity missiles, he or she is referred to a most amazing book entitled *Split Seconds* (4). Photographs in the book clearly illustrate the hydraulic effect in soft tissue caused by a bullet.

Typically, patients with causalgia report an onset of pain within several hours to a week after the injury, and describe the pain using words such as "stinging," "aching," "burning," or "tingling." Superimposed on the regular pain, patients may experience paroxysms of deep pain (1).

Long clearly made the distinction between causalgia and RSD (5). Causalgia is secondary to partial injury to major mixed nerves, caused by low- or high-velocity missiles, and manifests as trophic changes in the distribution of the nerve associated with extreme hypersensitivity. The pain is diffuse and burning, and true causalgia almost always responds to sympathectomy. Long suggested performing three or more sympathetic

blocks, sometimes every day for up to a week or longer, with the expectation that longer relief should follow each subsequent block. With positive responses to sympathetic blocks, he would suggest a sympathectomy (5). On the other hand, RSD usually follows a minor injury and does not involve a major nerve root (5). Frequently, the site of injury is the knee, ankles, or wrist, and the pain seems to get worse with cold but not with emotional upset, unlike causalgia. Demineralization of the bone occurs, with fibrosis of tendons and sheaths and spasm of the muscle. Dysesthesia suggests that there will be less success with sympathectomy.

Sympathetically Maintained Pain

This term has come into use in an effort to further define diagnostic accuracy, which would then allow better selection of treatment methods, and have some predictive value in terms of outcome. Raja and Hendler report clinical features of sympathetically maintained pain to be (1) spontaneous pain, (2) hyperalgesia to both mechanical and cooling stimuli, (3) soft tissue swelling, (4) vasomotor disturbances, (5) trophic skin changes, (6) diminished motor function, and (7) pain relief after sympathetic blockade (6). Using these criteria, one can have sympathetically maintained pain that could have features of either reflex sympathetic dystrophy or causalgia because either of these conditions could have features of sympathetically maintained pain.

Hendler originally described the use of oral phentolamine to treat reflex sympathetic dystrophy using the rationale that this drug was a postsynaptic alpha-1 blocker (7). Raja and his co-workers later described the use of intravenous phentolamine as a diagnostic test to confirm whether or not the pain a patient had was sympathetic in origin (i.e., "sympathetically maintained" (8). There is evidence that the mechanism of sympathetically maintained pain is present not only in reflex sympathetic dystrophy, but also in some cases of causalgia, however, because various authors have reported the benefit of sympathetic blocks in both disorders (5, 9, 10). Perhaps the best conceptual framework to use is one that takes into account both neurophysiology—that is, the presence or absence of major peripheral nerve injury documented by electromyography (EMG), nerve conduction velocities studies (NCV), and the sensory-evoked potential (SEP)—and response to pharmacologic intervention (i.e., response to IV phentolamine testing). A physician might consider six separate types of disorders, as shown in Table 39.2.

THEORY

With the above clinical descriptions in mind, one can then make an effort to define the various anatomic, neuroanatomic, and physiologic bases for these two disorders. Ghostine et al. have suggested multiple etiologies

Table 39.2.
Diagnostic Considerations

	Positive Response to Phentolamine IV	No response to Phentolamine IV	Partial Response to Phentolamine
EMG/nerve conduction velocity/somatosensory-evoked potential: *All negative*	Reflex sympathetic dystrophy Sympathetically maintained pain (SMP) SMP	Microvascular damage with swelling and mechanical hyperalgesia; Sympathetically independent pain (SIP)	Mixed injury
EMG/nerve conduction velocity/somatosensory-evoked potential: *at least one positive*	Causalgia; SMP	Neuroma or nerve entrapment at site of injury; SIP	Mixed injury

for causalgia (9). Various considerations include ephapse, in which there seems to be an erosion of the insulation between nerve fibers, allowing for short-circuiting between somatic afferent fibers and sympathetic efferent fibers, and experimentally produced neuromas, with resultant ephapses occurring both acutely and chronically between myelinated fibers. Because of the delay in developing the ephapses, which does not correspond to the clinical observations of a relatively rapid onset of RSD and causalgia, however, the theory of ephapses as the etiology of causalgia has fallen from favor (9). To replace this theory, the concept of nerve sprouts or free nerve endings that are sparsely myelinated seems feasible. Axonal sprouting has been noted to occur early after an injury, with a high frequency and without total axonal disruption. The possibility that causalgia is produced by these sparsely myelinated fibers is supported by evidence that the blood-nerve barrier, which is similar to the blood-brain barrier, has been destroyed in the injured nerve (9).

Perhaps the most comprehensive review of the neurophysiologic basis of RSD and causalgia has been advanced by Roberts (11). In his extensive review article, Roberts dealt with the neural mechanisms associated with pain of causalgia and RSD. He called these disorders *sympathetically maintained pain (SMP)*. His hypothesis regarding SMP is based on two assumptions: "(1) that a high rate of firing in spinal wide dynamic range (WDR) or multi-receptive neurons results in painful sensation and (2) that nociceptor response is associated with trauma which can produce long-term sensitization of the WDR neurons." Furthermore, his theory postulates that SMP is mediated by low-threshold, myelinated mechanoreceptors, and that these impulses, which carry messages to the brain, are the result of sympathetic fibers carrying messages from the spine and brain to act upon the receptors, or to act upon the fibers carrying messages to the brain (11). The most important part of this hypothesis is the fact that Roberts does not

postulate the need for nerve injury or for dystrophic tissue. Before one can more fully appreciate Roberts' theories, however, one has to explore the basic anatomy of the sympathetic chains.

Bennett at the National Institute of Health has advanced a brilliant theory that integrates clinical observations with basic neurophysiology (12). Bennett synthesizes three theories that show that damaged nerves, when they regenerate, have sprouts that are sensitive to norepinephrine; that they will discharge upon exposure to norepinephrine; that there is enough norepinephrine produced by sympathetic fibers to trigger firing of damaged nerves; that damaged nerves actually produce norepinephrine receptors at the damaged end; and that nociceptors (pain receptors) in intact nerves fire more in response to norepinephrine. "All of these mechanisms may be operating in the case of patient nerve damage due to physical trauma," he says, and "these events are likely to sensitize surviving afferent terminals, perhaps to the point of inducing an ongoing discharge. . ." (12). Bennett further differentiates between the type of injury: constriction or entrapment versus partial destruction of a major peripheral nerve (12). The former injury (constriction) does not seem to respond to sympathetic blocks 1–2 weeks after the injury, and this is attributed to the loss of noradrenergic vasomotor innervation, which takes several weeks to develop (12). The latter injury (partial nerve destruction) becomes painful within hours of the injury, remains painful for months, and responds to sympathetic blocks even months after the injury (12). Other researchers have expanded upon a purely neuron-mediated mechanism, and have suggested that autoimmune factors may be involved. Schwartzman's group, at Thomas Jefferson, found inflammatory skin lesions in the late stages of reflex sympathetic dystrophy, and attribute these lesions to a deposition of immune complexes in the skin (13). They feel the skin lesion supports the concept that cytokines and lymphokines such as interleukin-2 are produced as the result of the activation of complement, which in turn is excited by the progression of events beginning with local injury causing nerve growth factor release, which in turn activates sympathetic neurons, causing recruitment of neutrophils and monocytes, which in turn activate complement (13). Interestingly, interleukin-2 has been found to selectively stimulate sympathetic neurons, whereas nerve growth factor is produced in high concentrations after injury, which stimulates inflammation, which in turn activates complement (13). As research progresses, the various factors described above will need to be explored, with rigorous controls for (1) the type of lesion (crush versus cut), (2) the stage of the disease, correlating with anatomic and neurohumoral changes over time, and (3) the attempt to correlate the clinical symptoms with response to various treatments.

GROSS ANATOMY

The most startling finding, and one that flies in the face of commonly held beliefs, is a report by Kleiman in which sympathetic chains were found to have communication between them, in up to 80% of cases (14). This is an important finding, because this anatomic consideration is rarely, if ever, discussed in surgical textbooks or clinical papers. This finding also explains why some cases of RSD do not respond to sympathetic denervation, and why, paradoxical as it may seem, some cases do respond to contralateral blocks (i.e., if a patient has pain in the left leg, blocking the right lumbar sympathetic chain may produce relief). Additional anatomy has been described by Allen and Morety (15). When one traces the pathway of the sympathetic nerves, cell bodies are located in the lateral columns of the cervical, thoracic, and lumbar spinal cord. Cell bodies then give off axons, which form the preganglionic fibers of the sympathetic nervous system. From C7 to L2, these fibers are associated with the anterior spinal nerve roots, and leave the spinal cord in this pathway. They then separate from the nerve root and become the white rami communicantes, which then continue on to the paravertebral ganglia, which form a chain running from the skull to the coccyx. From the ganglia themselves postganglionic fibers run back to nerve roots, or become separate nerves supplying various organs. It is important to note that some ganglion cells are found in the anterior roots, as well as the white and gray rami (15). By the same token, some pre- and post-ganglionic fibers do not pass through sympathetic trunks, which again indicates that there is residual sympathetic innervation due to either normal variants or aberrant fibers that bypass the sympathetic trunk. This anatomic finding explains the failure of some ganglionectomies, and suggests that one might need to do anterior nerve root sections and preganglionic rami sectioning (Smithwick procedure) in patients in whom ganglionectomy has failed (15).

Cervical outflow, coming from the upper portion of the cervical chain, sends fibers to the pupils and the eyelids. These fibers radiate from the upper stellate ganglion, which also supplies various fibers in the head and face. The upper thoracic sympathetic chain receives preganglionic input from upper thoracic roots, and supplies the upper extremity through postganglionic fibers that pass through the brachial plexus (15). The lower extremities receive input from the T11–L3 nerve roots, forming ganglia, and from the lower two lumbar and upper sacral nerve roots, with gray rami (postganglionic) to the lumbosacral plexus (15).

MICROANATOMY

As described in the gross anatomy portion above, there are various sites along the sympathetic chain where damage can occur to a nerve. Additionally, there are several sites where chemical intervention is possible, notably at the synapses that occur along the sympathetic pathways. Additionally, the various fibers that carry sympathetic messages are important. It has been widely held that C-fibers, which are small unmyelinated fibers carrying sensory messages, are responsible for the transmission of pain. Some theories consider that SMP is mediated by activity in A-fibers, however, because C-fiber blockade fails to eliminate pain in patients with SMP (11). Therefore, one must start at the very beginning of the onset of pain—that is, the receptor itself—in order to fully understand SMP, RSD, and causalgia. Originally it was thought that nociceptor afferents (nerves that carry the message of pain from the periphery to the cord and the brain) were responsible for the continuous pain of SMP, RSD, and causalgia (11, 16, 17). In Roberts' paper, however, he adheres to a theory first advanced by Loh and Nathan (18) that indicates that low-threshold mechanoreceptors are responsible for SMP (11). Roberts takes this position because nociceptor afferents, which are typically considered unmyelinated C-fibers, do not have appropriate responses to sympathetic activity and, therefore, both practically and conceptually cannot be included as the receptors that mediate SMP. Roberts reported that mechanoreceptors do respond appropriately to both touch and sympathetic activity, however (11). For causalgia, others have proposed a neuroma formation as the cause of pain. Roberts believes that the sympathetic action of a neuroma is not capable of explaining why treatments that occur distal to the injury (in the form of either a nerve block or guanethidine infusion) are able to ameliorate causalgia, however; even so, Roberts used the summation theory, or convergence theory, to say that both the peripheral receptors (in this case, mechanoreceptors) that arise in the neuroma and those that arise in the skin itself are transmitting painful messages to the cord, and that distal blocks eliminate only the mechanoreceptors from the skin, which is not enough to trigger responses in the WDR neurons in the spinal cord. Additionally, the concept of a neuroma causing prolongation of causalgia-type pain does not fit the clinical observation that SMP may occur even in cases in which the nerve is not injured (11).

Ochoa advanced the theory that mechanical A-delta nociceptor endings become sensitized to multiple sensory inputs (19). This gives rise to the thermal hyperalgesia that is seen in RSD. On the other hand, Ochoa believes that there are abnormalities in distal nociceptor fibers that seem to have a low threshold. These low-threshold mechanoreceptors reside within large myelinated fibers, and are non–sympathetic dependent, because they transfer their information to nociceptor pathways proximal to the site of injury. These fibers may account for the mechanical hyperalgesia, manifesting as sensitivity to light touch. The above-mentioned receptors, which are the source of the hyperalgesia seen in RSD, are different than the burning pain receptors seen in causalgia. Ochoa believes that the burning pain of causalgia is mediated by unmyelinated C-fibers (19), whereas Payne believes that this pain is due to nerve stretch and axon disruptions (1). Another consideration is the fact that such pain may be mediated by nerve fascicles where all three types of C-fibers exist (19). Therefore, in summary, the current thinking seems to suggest that sparsely myelinated C-fibers carry the message of burning pain found in causalgia, whereas sparsely myelinated afferent fibers or the A-delta nociceptors may be responsible for pain in RSD.

SYNAPSES

Both synaptic considerations and axonal considerations have been raised as possible factors controlling both RSD and causalgia. Ephapses, or artificial synapses, have been demonstrated in normal peripheral nerves. The concept of synaptic factors in RSD and causalgia pain was first advanced by Granit et al. when they found that stimulating the motor root of a damaged mixed motor-sensory nerve also produced recordable electrical events in the sensory root (20). According to the review by Payne, the formation of ephapses after nerve injury may allow a short-circuiting or shunting of current from sympathetic fibers coming from the cord to the peripheral nerve into somatic fibers arising at the site of injury, carrying the message of pain back to the cord (1). Unfortunately, these cross-connections between fibers coming from the cord to the periphery, and conversely coming from the periphery to the cord, have been demonstrated in animal models, but not in humans (1). Another consideration is the possibility of an ectopic impulse resulting from alterations in calcium, sodium, and potassium channels (1). In effect, the damaged nerve becomes ''epileptic,'' and the spontaneous discharges from the sensory nerve may give rise to the ep-

isodic pain noted in some individuals. This could be due to lowered threshold or heightened mechanical sensitivity.

Neurosynaptic mediation of causalgia and RSD holds great promise for the future. When reviewing the synapses that are present within the sympathetic chain, it is apparent that these provide a potential site of mediation for sensory input. In order to understand synaptic mediation, one must review the anatomy of a synapse per se. Borrowing heavily from Roberts, one can define the functional neuroanatomy, and delineate the location of various synapses (11). First the trauma occurs, with receptors in the skin detecting various components of the trauma. Initially, the C-fiber nociceptors carry the message to the dorsal root ganglion, and thence back to the spinal cord neuron, where they synapse. After synapsing with the neuron in the spinal cord, these multiple neurons transmit information to the WDR neurons, which then send messages, via their axons, to the central nervous system or higher levels of the spinal cord. Using Roberts' model, additional light touch activates the mechanoreceptors, which travel in the A-fibers rather than in the C-fibers. Because the WDR neurons are already sensitized by the C-fibers nociceptors, they respond to what is usually subthreshold stimuli to the A-fiber mechanoreceptors. These mechanoreceptors travel in the A-fiber, reaching a neuron within the spinal cord, which again impinges on the WDR neuron, which in turn again sends messages up the spinal cord to the brain. Sympathetic fibers exist within the lateral portions of the thoracic cord, sending efferent messages to the sensory receptor. These efferent messages (i.e., messages traveling from the cord to the periphery, mainly to the sensory receptors) may occur in the absence of cutaneous stimulation. According to Roberts' theory, however, the sympathetic efferent activity requires no cutaneous stimulation, and is the cause of the SMP. In response to this efferent activity, the WDR neurons fire, again sending messages to the spinal cord and brain (11). The key to Roberts' theory is the fact that the WDR neurons in the spinal cord remain sensitized, and they will give a ''vigorous response to mechanical stimulation of A-fiber mechanoreceptors'' even after healing has occurred (11). In this schema, multiple synapses occur within the spinal cord, at the WDR neuron, and in the sympathetic ganglion. Therefore, synaptic regulation can occur at the spinal cord level or at the sympathetic ganglion level. When reviewing the actual synapse, one must conceptualize a presynaptic area wherein various chemicals are formulated, becoming neurosynaptic transmitters. The two synaptic transmitters that are of most interest to the study of RSD and causalgia are the indolamines, of which serotonin is an example, and the catecholamines, of which norepinephrine, epinephrine, dopa, and dopamine are examples. In the presynaptic area of the nerve, precursor substances are manufactured into neurosynaptic transmitters, which confer a degree of specificity on nerve transmission. L-Tryptophan becomes 5-hydroxytryptophan, which becomes 5-hydroxytryptamine (serotonin); dopa becomes dopamine, which can be converted to norepinephrine and epinephrine.

The specific type of the neurosynaptic transmitter determines whether or not it will occupy a specific postsynaptic receptor site. Biogenic amines, such as the indolamines and catecholamines, are constantly being formulated and broken down by monoamine oxidase. Thus, chemically, the presynaptic area may be described as an area of high flux, with formulation and degradation of the same chemical occurring in the relatively steady state. As electrical impulses travel down the axon, pore diameter changes, altering the permeability of the membrane and causing the release of neurosynaptic transmitters. These synaptic transmitters flow across a minute gap between nerves and occupy postsynaptic receptor sites. The gap, of course, is called the synapse. The postsynaptic receptor sites determine the strength and duration of the electrical impulse that the synapse propagates. This is done by the degree of specificity that the neurosynaptic transmitters have for a particular receptor site. It also depends on the affinity that a specific neurosynaptic transmitter has for a particular receptor site, and whether it is easily displaced or forms a tight bond. Almost all neurosynaptic transmitters have their activity ended by presynaptic reuptake, that is, the chemical that occupies the postsynaptic receptor site is then taken back into the presynaptic area. Acetylcholine is an exception, being degraded on the postsynaptic receptor site by acetylcholinesterase. Additionally, some small amount of degradation of biogenic amines occurs in the synapse itself by catechol-O-methyltransferase (COMT). It is thought that less than 5% of the chemical degradation of synaptic transmitters occurs in the synapse by COMT, and 95% of the degradation occurs presynaptically, by monoamine oxidase (MAO). Of course, there is constant rebuilding of the neurosynaptic transmitter presynaptically, creating the steady state mentioned earlier.

Obviously, there are multiple ways to modify the synapse. One can inhibit MAO, thereby enhancing the buildup of a monoamine neurosynaptic transmitter, such as the indolamines or the catecholamines. In fact, a class of drugs called MAO inhibitors do exactly that. By the same token, certain drugs can function as MAO exciters, which facilitate the degradation of biogenic amine neurosynaptic transmitters, such as the indolamines (serotonin) and the catecholamines (epinephrine, norepinephrine, dopamine, and dopa). Because the majority of the neurosynaptic transmitters have their activity ended by presynaptic reuptake, one can enhance the synaptic transmission by blocking presynaptic reuptake. This is how tricyclic antidepressants work. Conversely, one can diminish synaptic transmission by facilitation of presynaptic reuptake. Finally, one can work at the receptor end by using drugs that mimic the action of the presynaptic transmitters and occupy receptor sites, thereby triggering them as if the actual chemical had been released. By the same token, other drugs can be used that occupy the receptor sites but have no pharmacologic activity other than to inhibit the presynaptic transmitter from occupying the receptor site. For example, curare effects a total blockade of the acetylcholine receptor. In this sense, these drugs become inhibitors of neurosynaptic transmission. Receptor sites are found not only postsynaptically, but also presynaptically, very often for the same presynaptic neurosynaptic transmitter. As the number and sensitivity of these receptors change, so does the response to the neurosynaptic transmitter itself.

DIAGNOSIS OF CAUSALGIA

With the foregoing theoretical information, the clinical components of RSD and causalgia should be more readily differentiated by appropriate diagnostic studies.

According to both Raja and his co-workers and Payne, causalgia manifests as a burning pain, which is not a consistent finding of RSD (1, 21). Additionally, causalgia patients may experience paroxysms of pain, especially after stress, whether it be emotional or environmental. In an elegant study, Raja and his co-workers found that patients with causalgia rarely have cold hyperalgesia (two of nine), and they do not have heat hyperalgesia (none of nine). Additionally, these patients obtain no relief from sympathetic blocks. Raja et al. differentiated various types of hyperalgesia using sensory testing with either Von Frey hairs for touch, a drop of acetone for cold, or laser thermal stimulation for heat (21). Ochoa feels that causalgia is not always sympathetically mediated, and instead is mediated by unmyelinated C-fibers (19). Stretch injuries to the nerve or axon disruption of a major nerve branch is one explanation favored by Payne (1). Usually, the causalgia patient has a history of a nerve injury to a peripheral nerve, or surgery, that has damaged the proximal portion of the nerve trunk (1, 21). The causalgia may be related to damage of nerve fascicles where all three types of C-fibers exist (19).

TREATMENT OF CAUSALGIA

Various authors have reported that sympathetic blocks are or are not effective, with efficacy for sympathectomy being reported to be between 12 and 97% (1). No relief with sympathetic blocks was reported by Raja et al. (13). Payne has suggested that a dorsal root entry zone (DREZ) procedure may prove effective (1). Ghostine et al. have suggested the use of phenoxybenzamine (9). They reported 40 consecutive cases of causalgia, all of which involved nerve injuries from bullet or shrapnel wounds. The Ghostine group noted partial motor paralysis in the distribution of the damaged nerve in 70% of the cases. Over time these deficits resolved in many of the cases, however. They also noted vasomotor changes, usually severe vasodilatation and sweating and less often vasoconstriction (4). Rarely were trophic changes noted. The majority of the cases involved the sciatic nerve, median nerve, brachial plexus, cauda equina, and occipital nerve, in descending order. The treatment that Ghostine and his group used was phenoxybenzamine, which is a postsynaptic alpha 1–blocker and a presynaptic alpha 2–blocker. As mentioned earlier under the etiology of causalgia, nerve sprouts, which are one of the theoretical origins of this disorder, seem to be highly excitable upon the administration of norepinephrine, which can be reversed with alpha-blocking agents such as phentolamine but which are unaffected by beta-blocking agents (9). The dosage of the drug used by Ghostine et al. initially was 10 mg three times a day, although this varied from patient to patient. Eventually maximum dosages of 40–120 mg/day were reached, with treatment lasting 6–8 weeks. Common side effects were orthostatic hypotension in about 45% of the patients and reduced ejaculatory ability in about 8% of the patients. In some instances, treatment lasted as long as 16 weeks. It is important to note that the patients were all treated within 2–70 days after the onset of their injury, however.

In order for this treatment to be effective, it is most important that rapid diagnosis and institution of treatment occur. Another possibility for the pharmacologic treatment of causalgia would be the use of clonazepam, which has been reported by Bouckoms and Litman to be effective for "burning" pains (22).

Surgical sympathectomy has been recommended as a treatment for causalgia, after repetitive sympathetic blocks. Additionally, guanethidine, which is a ganglionic blocking agent, has proven effective in treating some forms of causalgia. Guanethidine must be used with caution, however, because it causes the release of norepinephrine prior to occupying the receptor sites itself, and the time course of the cessation of activity is variable. The fact that one may occlude an affected limb below the site of the causalgia and still achieve effective blocks with guanethidine suggests that its activity is not at the ganglion, but rather on the peripheral sensory nerves, which produces its effect on causalgia (10). Surgical intervention, in the form of surgical sympathectomy, has been used to treat causalgia with variable cure rates, ranging from 12 to 97% (1). The variability may be ascribed to lack of precision and diagnosis, with an overlap of RSD with causalgia, or RSD mistakenly diagnosed as causalgia; varying skills in performing blocks; collateral reinnervation of postganglionic sympathetic fibers; and a delay in performing a sympathectomy (1). For causalgia that is not responding to

sympathectomy, the possibility of a contralateral sympathectomy has been raised (14).

DIAGNOSIS OF REFLEX SYMPATHETIC DYSTROPHY

The clinical diagnosis of RSD is more complicated than that of causalgia. Some authors believe that there is a very definite set of criteria to establish the diagnosis, whereas other authors think that only several symptoms from a whole list of symptom complexes need be present to establish the diagnosis of RSD. Kozin and his coworkers have established the criteria for RSD as a patient presenting with pain and tenderness in an extremity associated with vasomotor instability (particular temperature or color changes) and generalized swelling in the same extremity (23). The second group of patients they consider are those with pain and tenderness associated with a vasomotor instability or swelling in an extremity; they call this group "probable RSD." This system lacks precision, however, because it does not take into account the particular type of pain that patients with RSD experience.

Raja and his co-workers define patients as having RSD if they have pain associated with signs of sympathetic hyperactivity (i.e., lower skin temperature, skin discoloration, increased sweating, and some trophic changes) and symptomatic relief after sympathetic blocks; they found that those with RSD also had thermal hyperalgesia either to cold or to heat (21). In contrast, their patients with causalgia did not experience thermal hyperalgesia to heat, and only two out of seven experienced hyperalgesia to cold. Both the causalgia and RSD patients experienced hyperalgesia to mechanical stimulation (21). On the other hand, Ochoa et al. found mechanical hyperalgesia, which they called *allodynia,* in their patients with RSD (19). Additionally, hypersensitivity to temperature was also found in patients with RSD, whether it be to heat or to cold (19, 21, 24).

One proposed mechanism for mechanical hypersensitivity is ectopic alpha-adrenergic chemosensitivity (25). Another consideration is a secondary abnormality in distal nociceptor fibers that escaped injury, or intact low-threshold mechanoreceptors with large myelinated fibers that are non–sympathetic dependent because of transfer of information to nociceptor pathways proximal to the site of injury (19). Additionally, Ochoa et al. advanced the concept of alpha-receptor sensitization, whereas others believe that the hypersensitivity of the mechanoreceptors could possibly be a central nervous system event (19, 24).

TREATMENT OF REFLEX SYMPATHETIC DYSTROPHY

Treatments for the mechanical hypersensitivity or hyperalgesia of RSD have been advanced by several authors, without clear-cut definition. One group of authors believes that sympathectomy may relieve mechanical hyperalgesia, whereas another group of authors reports that sympathectomy does not (19, 26). Another group has advanced the notion that nifedipine, a calcium channel–blocking agent, may prove effective (27). Finally, a group from South Africa suggested that low-dose naloxone, and possibly longer-acting naltrexone, may prove effective for reducing mechanical hyperalgesia, because of the existence of a hypergesic kappa system of opiate receptors (28). Again, the area of mechanical hyperalgesia is quite muddy, because all of the patients with either causalgia or RSD had mechanical hypersensitivity (21).

Thermal hypersensitivity to either heat or cold (hyperalgesia) has been reported by several groups (19, 21, 24). The mechanism behind the thermal hypersensitivity is not well elucidated, but one can clinically differentiate mechanical from thermal hypersensitivity by the use of a drop of acetone (21). Patients with RSD in the series studied by Raja et al. had hyperalgesia to cold (three of four, as tested by acetone drop) or to heat (four of five, as tested using a laser thermal stimulator) (21). Some patients had hypersensitivity and hyperalgesia to both heat and cold, but these patients did not have causalgia, but rather RSD. Of the group of patients with hyperalgesia to temperature change, six of six got relief with sympathetic blocks or sympathectomy (21). Other authors have reported that nifedipine is effective for treating hyperalgesia (27). Specifically, in 13 patients with pain having a burning character, dysesthesia, and cold intolerance, nifedipine beginning at 10 mg three times a day, and increasing to 30 mg three times a day, proved effective in 7 of 13 patients (27). Nifedipine is a calcium channel–blocking agent, and as such may work by dilating blood vessels and antagonizing the effects of norepinephrine on arterial and venous muscle (1). Also, nifedipine may interfere with ectopic impulse formation that occurs in regenerating nerves, by blocking calcium channel protein (1).

The dystrophic component of RSD is more difficult to delineate. Some authors have reported a diffuse or patchy bony demineralization (23), whereas others have reported frank osteoporosis late in the disorder (29). A number of authors have reported molted skin, again late in the disorder (1, 21, 23). Some authors have reported hair loss, yet again late in the disorder (21, 29). Vague terms such as *vasomotor instability* have also been reported, as well as trophic skin changes (23). The etiology for these components is not well-defined, but the consensus seems to be reduced blood flow to the various involved organs. A more precise diagnostic assessment was advanced by Holder and MacKinnon (30). They evaluated patients with RSD, which they defined as diffuse hand pain, diminished hand function, joint stiffness, and skin and soft tissue trophic changes with or without vasomotor instability. They also used three other control groups, including patients with diffuse

pain, focal pain, or vascular disease. Holder and MacKinnon found that 22 of the 23 patients who met their criteria for diagnosing RSD had positive delayed image bone scans, 12 of the 23 patients had positive blood pool images, and 10 of the 23 patients had positive radionuclide angiograms (30). Approximately half the patients with RSD had positive early phase bone scans, whereas almost all of the patients with RSD had positive delayed image bone scans (30).

This study compared favorably with work done by Kozin and his group. Kozin and his co-workers found that radiography is not a useful tool for diagnosing RSD (16). They did find that 83% of the patients with RSD had positive static (delayed) bone scans, however, whereas 69% of the patients had positive flow studies (23). Therefore, it is apparent that between 50 and 60% of patients with RSD will have positive early phase bone scans, but between 83 and 96% of patients will have positive delayed image bone scans (23, 30). Treatment for this component of RSD is difficult to assess. Kozin et al. reported that 90% of patients with a positive bone scan had good to excellent steroid response, beginning with steroids at the level of 60–80 mg/day and tapering them (23).

Schott has reported a variety of therapeutic modalities, including steroids, nonsteroidal anti-inflammatory drugs, alpha- and beta-blocking agents, griseofulvin, calcitonin, transcutaneous electrical nerve stimulation, physical therapy, sympathetic blocks, and intravenous guanethidine (29). None of these treatments has been studied in a systematized fashion, however.

Nail brittleness has been reported by Schlott (29) and Payne (1) late in the disorder. The etiology of this is not clear, nor is there any clear-cut treatment. Muscle spasm has been reported by a number of authors (5, 14, 29), again without a clear-cut mechanism describing the etiology (1). Interestingly, electromyography (EMG)–nerve conduction velocity studies seem to be relatively negative in RSD (31). The treatments that seemed most effective for muscle spasm were trigger point injections (1) and the use of baclofen (N.H. Hendler, unpublished observations). Baclofen is a GABA-minergic drug that centrally reduces muscle spasm. The inhibition of substance P may be implicated as part of its mechanism for reducing spasm and the pain associated with spasm (28). Soma and quinine have also been tried, with only limited success (N.H. Hendler, unpublished observations). Contractures, usually in the hand, have also been reported (1, 29). The etiology of this is unclear, but is probably related to disuse. Again, there is an absence of positive EMG–nerve conduction velocity studies (31), and the only treatment seems to be preventative, by the use of passive range-of-motion exercises and physical therapy.

Contralateral involvement has been reported by several authors (14, 29). The etiology for this, in approximately 80% of examined cadavers (14), is cross-communication between the sympathetic fibers and the sympathetic chains. Contralateral blocks and denervation have been recommended (14). Edema of the affected limb (1, 29), as well as swelling of a specific joint (23), have been reported. Again, the etiology is unclear. The diagnosis is established by measuring the proximal interphalangeal joint, which averages 12.9 mm larger in the affected hand than in the control hand (23). No treatment has been advanced for this, although nifedipine is suggested to be effective (27). We have observed some benefit from the use of spironolactone, or carbonic anhydrase inhibitors, but not on a consistent basis.

Lower skin temperature has been reported by a variety of authors (1, 7, 21), but it does not seem to be due to vasospasm (32). Reflex contraction due to altered activity within the afferent and efferent nerves is proposed as the etiology (32). Thermography is an excellent diagnostic tool to document the reduced skin temperature (7, 31). In fact, very often patients with RSD are diagnosed as having psychosomatic disorders, and thermography can be a most convincing diagnostic tool to confirm the otherwise subjective complaint (7).

Treatment for lower skin temperature associated with pain is best effected using regional sympathetic blocks employing reserpine (32). It is important to note that these reserpine blocks, or Bier blocks, are not effective for vasospasm, but specifically seem to function best for treating RSD (32). Therefore, vasospasm does not seem to be the etiologic mechanism for the coldness noted in the limb in RSD (32). Stiffness (1, 30) and tenderness (23) of the joints have been reported; again, the etiology is not clear (1). Very often, the involvement of the joint leads to misdiagnosis and confusion with other diseases that can affect the joint, notably infective arthritis, rheumatoid arthritis, Reiter's syndrome, systemic lupus erythematosus, and arthritides (23). In one series 71% of the patients with joint tenderness and stiffness had a poor response to stellate ganglion blocks (23). Steroids, notably prednisone (60–80 mg) for 2–4 days, then 40–60 mg for 2–4 days, and then 30–40 mg for 2–4 days, in four equally divided doses, were the initial therapy. Subsequently, the dose was rapidly tapered using a single morning dose of 40 mg, then 30 mg, 20 mg, 10 mg, and 5 mg over 2 or 3 days at each dose. Using this regimen, 82% of the patients with joint stiffness and tenderness obtained good or excellent relief (23).

An unusual complication of RSD is the appearance of pathologic fractures subsequent to minor trauma (N.H. Hendler, unpublished observations). In patients complaining of persistent pain in the limb that seems to be bony in origin, rather than part of the RSD, it would be imperative to obtain bone scanning to confirm the presence or absence of an undetected break. In our experience, one patient with long-standing RSD received a mi-

nor trauma (i.e., bumping her ankle while walking in a train) that resulted in a chronic intense worsening of pain in the heel. Radiographs of this area were within normal limits, but the pain persisted for several days after the event, and a bone scan was obtained. Only on bone scan did the break in the calcaneus appear, which had been totally missed by routine radiograph. Ninety-five percent of any breaks present will have a positive bone scan after 72 hours (33). Interestingly, after the fracture is healed, 90% of the bone scans have returned to normal 2 years from the date of the injury (33). Therefore, in patients with RSD who have minor injuries and complain of bony pain, it would be prudent to obtain a bone scan, and not rely on radiographs.

Payne has enumerated many attempted treatments for RSD (1). Unfortunately, there seems to be a lack of systematic investigation for these treatments, and most are based on clinical reports rather than on systematized trials. Reported pharmacologic interventions that may work for causalgia are the use of propranolol, a beta-blocking agent; prazosin, an alpha 1–adrenergic blocking agent; phenoxybenzamine, both an alpha 1– and an alpha 2–blocker; and guanethidine, a drug that produces a chemical "sympathectomy." Physical therapy has been advanced for the treatment of RSD, specifically to minimize muscle contractures and joint stiffness. It is never a definitive treatment, however, and should not be considered such. Electrical stimulation of the central nervous system, using either electrodes centrally implanted into the periaqueductal or periventricular gray or epidural stimulators, may prove effective, as might transcutaneous electrical nerve stimulation. Tricyclic antidepressants, nonsteroidal anti-inflammatory drugs, narcotics, and anticonvulsants have all been reported as treating some components of reflex sympathetic dystrophy, with varying degrees of success.

Surgical intervention is a treatment that is reserved until all other modalities of treatment have been attempted. In all cases, the criterion for surgical intervention would be repetitive successes with repeat sympathetic blocks. The most commonly employed surgical interventions are resection of the lower third of the stellate ganglion and resection of the upper two thoracic ganglia; however, some surgeons resect the second through fifth thoracic ganglia in an attempt to treat upper-extremity difficulties (15). There are four surgical approaches to upper extremity sympathectomies (15):

1. Above the clavicle (anterior cervical approach)
2. Posterior resection of the transverse processes of ribs 2 and 3, and proximal section of ribs 2 and 3
3. Anterior transpleural entry through the pectoralis muscle to the third intercostal space, pressing the lung, in order to reach the operative area
4. The axillary approach, which is through a transaxillary incision over the second intercostal space

Table 39.3.
Clinical Symptoms Associated with Causalgia and Reflex Sympathetic Dystrophy

Clinical Symptoms	Mechanism	Diagnostic Studies	Treatment
Causalgia			
a. Burning pain (1, 21)[a]	a. Unmyelinated C fibers (19)	a. Rarefly have cold hyperalgesia (2/7) or heat hyperalgesia (0/9) (21); do have mechanical hypersensitivity (21); use a drop of acetone and Von Frey hairs to test	a. Phenoxybenzamine (9) DREZ (1), Sympathectomy 12–97% effective (1), clonazepam (22)
b. Paroxysms of pain (1)	b. Nerve stretch and axon disruption (1)		
c. Partial motor paralysis (70%) (9)	c. Peripheral nerve injury, proximal nerve trunk (1, 21)	c. EMG/nerve conduction velocity studies	c. No relief with sympathetic blocks (21); β-blockers don't work (9)
d. Worse with stress (1)			
e. Vasomotor changes, but rare trophic change (9) (Ghostine, et al.)			
Reflex Sympathetic Dystrophy			
Hyperalgesia (allodynia)			
a. Mechanical—hypersensitivity to light touch (19)	a. Ectopic α-adrenergic chemosensitivity (25); sensitization of WDR neurons in the spinal cord (11); central nervous system mediated (24); intact low-threshold mechanoreceptor with A-delta afferents (19)	a. All patients have mechanical hypersensitivity; use Von Frey hairs to test (21)	a. Sympathectomy may relieve it (15, 19); sympathectomy did not relieve it (26); low-dose naltrexone may work (28); nifedipine? (27)
b. Thermal—hypersensitivity to either heat or cold (19, 21, 24)	b. No mechanism delineated	b. Patients have either cold hyperalgesia (3/4), and/or heat hyperalgesia (4/5); use a drop of acetone to test (21)	b. 6/6 got relief with sympathetic blocks or sympathectomy (21); nifedipine? (27)
Dystrophy			
a. Osteoporosis (29)	a. No mechanism delineated	a and b. X-ray did not correlate well with clinical symptoms, but bone scan did (69% abnormal flow images, 83% abnormal static images) (23) (also true for clinical features c, e, and l); if clinically had RSD, 22/23 had positive delay image bone scan (30)	a and b. Maybe calcitonin (29)
b. Diffuse or patchy bony demineralization (23)	b. No mechanism delineated		
c. Molted skin (1, 21, 23)	c. No mechanism delineated	c. Thermography (31, 7)	c. Prednisone, 60–80 mg to start (23)
d. Hair loss (21, 29)	d. No mechanism delineated	d. Clinical observation	d. Steroids (23, 29)
e. Vasomotor instability (23)	e. No mechanism delineated	e. History or longitudinal observation (23)	e. Sympathetic blocks (29); steroids (23)
f. Nail brittleness (1, 29)	f. No mechanism delineated	f. Clinical observation	f. Sympathetic blocks (29); steroids (23)
g. Muscle spasm (5, 14, 29)	g. No mechanism delineated	g. EMG biofeedback used as test (7)	g. Trigger point injections (1); baclofen (28)
h. Contractures (1, 29)	h. May be attributed to disuse	h. Longitudinal observation (29)	h. Physical therapy (29)
i. Contralateral involvement (14, 29)	i. Cross-communication between sympathetic chain in 80% of cadavers (14)	i. Effective contralateral block (14)	i. Contralateral sympathectomy (14)
j. Edema (1, 29)	j. No mechanism delineated	j. History and clinical observation	j. Nifedipine (27); spironolactone

Table 39.3.
(Continued)

Clinical Symptoms	Mechanism	Diagnostic Studies	Treatment
k. Lower skin temperature (1, 21, 31, 7)	k. Not vasospasm, but maybe an afferent and efferent reflex arc (32)	k. Thermography (31, 7)	k. Phentolamine (7); Bier block with reserpine (32); guanethidine i.v. (29); sympathetic blocks (21, 29)
i. Joint stiffness (1, 30) and tenderness (23)	i. No mechanism delineated	i. Proximal interphalangeal joint is 12.9 mm greater (average) in affected hand; rheumatoid and connective tissue blood studies (23)	i. Prednisone 60–80 mg to start, 82% not good or excellent relief (23)
m. Pathologic fractures (N. H. Hendler, unpublished data)	m. May be related to osteoporosis or patchy demineralization	m. 72 hours after a break 95% of bone scans are positive; 90% normal 2 years after break (33)	m. Proper casting
n. Pins and needles (7) and dysesthesias (1)	n. No mechanism delineated	n. History	n. Sympathectomy (7)

ªNumbers in parentheses are references.

Also a lumbar approach may be made through the external and internal obliques, and then the transversalis muscle, below the 12th rib, behind the kidney; others have suggested a thoracolumbar presacral neurectomy (15). Side effects of surgical approaches are postsympathectomy neuralgia, beginning 7–10 days after surgery, and a postsympathectomy dysesthesia that may last 2–14 weeks, and is described as continuous, severe, and worse at night. Anticonvulsants, such as diphenylhydantoin or carbamazepine, may be used to treat this (15). Dorsal root entry zone procedures, which produce lesions in the dorsal root interrupting the nociceptive pathways in the tract of Lissauer and in laminae I–V of the dorsal horn of the spinal cord, may prove to be an effective modality for treating causalgia for stretch injuries (1).

CONCLUSIONS

In summary, it is quite apparent that a great deal of confusion has arisen regarding the diagnosis of RSD and causalgia. This is evidenced by the lack of uniformity in clinical criteria for establishing the diagnosis. Because of this lack of uniformity, assessment of various articles detailing treatment of RSD and/or causalgia is difficult. What some clinicians take as symptoms of RSD are not always present in their entirety. Unfortunately, if one adheres rigorously to these criteria, proper diagnosis, and more importantly proper treatment, may be withheld. The various clinical symptoms that have been reported as associated with RSD and causalgia are shown in Table 39.3. We suggest that a patient be considered to have RSD if he or she has at least one type of hyperalgesia (either mechanical or thermal), lower skin temperature, and the sensation of pins and needles. At a

minimum, diagnostic studies that would facilitate the diagnosis of RSD would be thermography and bone scan. Clinical diagnostic studies that would prove important would be testing with a drop of acetone for cold hyperalgesia, and testing using Von Frey hairs for mechanical hyperalgesia. All patients suspected of having RSD should have at least three sympathetic blocks. After that, one should use various diagnostic and treatment techniques, depending on the patient's type of complaints.

For causalgia, one certainly should establish the diagnosis of burning pain as constantly present, in association with a partial peripheral nerve injury. Electromyographic nerve conduction velocity studies should be conducted to detect whether or not there is an associated nerve injury. Certainly, patients should receive sympathetic blocks and a trial with phenoxybenzamine.

Regardless of whether a patient has RSD or causalgia, one must be aware of the need to make a distinction between the two diagnoses, because the treatments vary. More importantly, if the patient has even a single symptom of RSD, a diagnostic assessment involving the above-recommended modalities would be warranted, and further diagnostic studies should be pursued if the diagnosis of RSD is not confirmed. Kozin and his co-workers clearly defined a number of overlapping conditions that may originally be misdiagnosed as RSD. Twenty-five percent of the patients who were found not to have RSD had peripheral neuropathy or trapped peripheral nerves, and half the patients misdiagnosed as having RSD had inflammatory arthritis (23). Therefore, laboratory studies, including erythrocyte sedimentation rate, antinuclear antibody, rheumatoid factor, and the like, should be conducted in patients thought to have

RSD but in whom the diagnosis is not complete. In any event, causalgia and RSD require clinical acumen to establish the diagnosis, and persistence in order to effect appropriate treatment. Aggressively pursuing all of the diagnostic studies available, as well as relying on clinical judgment, will provide better care for these patients.

REFERENCES

1. Payne R: Neuropathic pain syndromes, with special reference to causalgia and reflex sympathetic dystrophy. *Clin J Pain* 2:59–73, 1986.
2. Merskey H (ed) and the subcommittee on taxonomy, classification of chronic pain. *Pain (Suppl)* 3:28–29, 1986.
3. Schwartzman RS and McKellan TL: Reflex sympathetic dystrophy: A review. *Arch Neurol* 44:555–561, 1987.
4. Dalton S: *Split Seconds—The World of High Speed Photography.* Salem, NH, Salem House, 1984, pp 21, 28, 30, 31, 32, 34, 36.
5. Long DM: Pain of peripheral nerve injury. In Youmans J (ed): *Neurological Surgery, ed 2. Philadelphia, WB Saunders, 1982, vol 6, pp 3634–3643.*
6. *Raja SN, Hendler N: Sympathetically maintained pain. In Rogers M (ed): Current Practices in Anesthesiology. New York, Mosby Year Book, 1990.*
7. Hendler N, Uematsu S, Long D: Thermographic validating of physical complaints in "psychogenic pain" patients. *Psychosomatics* 23:282–287, 1982.
8. Raja SN, Treede RD, Davis RD, et al: Systemic alpha-adrenergic blockade with phentolamine: A diagnostic test for sympathetically maintained pain. *Anesthesiology* 74:691–698, 1991.
9. Ghostine SY, Comair YG, Turner DM, et al: Phenoxybenzamine in the treatment of causalgia (report of 40 cases). *J Neurosurg* 6:1263–1268, 1984.
10. Hannington-Kiff JG: Relief of causalgia in limbs by regional intravenous guanethidine. *Br Med J* 2:367–368, 1979.
11. Roberts WJ: A hypothesis on the physiological basis for causalgia and related pain. *Pain* 24:297–311, 1986.
12. Bennett GJ: The role of the sympathetic nervous system in painful peripheral neuropathy. *Pain* 45:221–223, 1991.
13. Webster GF, Schwartzman RS, Jacoby RL, Knobler RL, Uritto JT: Reflex sympathetic dystrophy: Occurence of inflammatory skin lesions with stages II and III disease. *Arch Dermatol* 127:1541–1544, 1991.
14. Kleinman A: Causalgia: Evidence of the existence of crossed sensory sympathetic fibers. *Am J Surg* 87:839–841, 1954.
15. Allen MB Jr, Morety WH: Sympathectomy. In Youmans J (ed): *Neurological Surgery, ed 2. Philadelphia, WB Saunders, 1982, vol 6, pp 3717–3726.*
16. Bonica JJ: Causalgia and other reflex sympathetic dystrophies. In Bonica JJ (ed): *Advances in Pain Research and Therapy.* New York, Raven Press, 1970, vol 3, pp 141–166.

17. Devo M, Janig W: Activation of myelinated afferents ending in a neuroma by stimulation of the sympathetic supply in a rat. *Neurosci Lett* 24:43–47, 1981.
18. Loh L, Nathan PW: Painful peripheral states and sympathetic blocks. *J Neurol Neurosurg Psychiatry* 41:664–671, 1978.
19. Ochoa J, Torebjorle E, Marchetti P, et al: Mechanisms of neuropathic pain: Cumulative observations, new experiments and further speculation. In Fields HL, Dubner R, Cervero F (eds): *Advances in Pain Research and Therapy.* New York, Raven Press, 1985, vol 9, pp 431–450.
20. Ganit R, Leksell L, Skoglund CR: Fiber interaction in injured or compressed region of the nerve. *Brain* 67:125–140, 1944.
21. Raja SN, Campbell JN, Meyer RA, et al: Sensory testing in patients with causalgia or reflex sympathetic dystrophy. Abstract presented at 6th Annual Meeting of American Pain Society, Washington DC, November 6–9, 1986.
22. Bouckoms AJ, Litman RE: Clonazepam in the treatment of neuralgic pain syndrome. *Psychosomatics* 26:933–936, 1985.
23. Kozin F, Ryan LM, Carerra GF, et al: The reflex sympathetic dystrophy syndrome (RSDS). *Am J Med* 70:23–30, 1981.
24. Meyer RA, Campbell JN, Raja SN: Peripheral neural mechanism of cutaneous hyperalgesia. In Fiel HL, Dubner R, Cevero F (eds): *Advances in Pain Research and Therapy.* New York, Raven Press, 1985, vol 9 pp 53–71.
25. Devor M: Nerve pathophysiology and mechanisms of pain in causalgia. *J Autonom Nerv Sys* 7:371–384, 1983.
26. Hoffert MI, Greenburg PP, Wolskee PJ, et al: Abnormal and collateral innervation of sympathetic and peripheral sensory fields associated with a case of causalgia. *Pain* 20:1–12, 1984.
27. Prough DS, McLeskey CH, Poehling GG, et al: Efficacy of oral nifedipine in the treatment of reflex sympathetic dystrophy. *Anesthesiology* 2:796–799, 1985.
28. Gillman MA, Lichtigfeld RJ: A pharmacological overview of opioid mechanisms mediating analgesia and hyperalgesia. *Neurol Res* 7:106–119, 1985.
29. Schott GD: Neurologic manifestation of bone and joint disease. In Ashbury AK, McKhann GM, McDonald WC, et al (eds): *Diseases of the Nervous System.* Philadelphia, WB Saunders, 1986, pp 1523–1537.
30. Holder LE, MacKinnon SE: Reflex sympathetic dystrophy in the hands: Clinical and scintigraphic criteria. *Radiology* 152:517–522, 1984.
31. Uematsu S, Hendler N, Hugerford D, et al: Thermography and electromyography in the differential diagnosis of chronic pain syndromes and reflex sympathetic dystrophy. *Electromyogr Clin Neurophysiol* 21:165–182, 1981.
32. Janoff KH, Phinney ES, Porter JM: Lumbar sympathectomy for lower extremity vasospasm. *Am J Surg* 150:147–152, 1985.
33. Matin P: The appearance of bone scans following fractures, including immediate and long-term studies. *J Nucl Med* 20:1227–1231, 1979.

CHAPTER 40
PHANTOM PAIN
PETER G. WILSON

PHANTOM PAIN is an interesting and exasperating phenomenon. To properly manage phantom pain we have to put it into a proper matrix. In this chapter we will give clinical examples of phantom pain, which will be followed by a description of various types of phantom pain and phantom sensation. At the present time we have no clear etiology for phantom pain—indeed it may be covered by a multitude of etiologies—but we will divide the possible mechanisms into (1) central neurologic, (2) peripheral neurologic, and (3) psychological. We will finally go on to look at the myriad of treatments using both our own ongoing study and those of others, which will include medical treatment, surgical treatments, pharmacologic treatments, psychologic treatments, and others.

CLINICAL VIGNETTES

The following three vignettes show patients at different time frames after the amputation. Some will deal with the difference in time and some will include a differentiation between phantom pain and phantom sensation. We will not deal with stump pain except in the area of differential diagnosis.

CASE 1

Roy, a 19-year-old boy, had been working unloading newspapers from a truck in the early morning when a drunken driver slammed him into the back of the delivery truck, leaving him on the ground, bleeding. An hour later, he was in the hospital. For the next 3 weeks, his leg was in traction with terrible pain, only moderately and intermittently controlled with pain medication, and there was a question as to whether an amputation would be necessary. One day he was told that he would have debridement of the area only to find on awakening that he had a below-the-knee amputation to which he responded with both rage and relief. A few days later, during house staff rounds, when questioned about pain he said that he did have some but it seemed to be a "strange place." This was not followed-up for a few

days until a nurse asked why, if he was in pain, he wasn't asking for pain medication, at which point he timidly mentioned that the pain was in the toes of the foot that he no longer had, and so—.

CASE 2

Anne, a 67-year-old widow, had a 10-year history of diabetes that had brought on peripheral vascular problems and that had caused increasing pain in her lower extremity over the past 2 years. She found herself walking less and less and, over the 6 months before coming into the hospital, less able to sleep at night, gradually ending up in a reclining chair where she was able to sleep for 3 or 4 hours on a good night. Life was becoming intolerable for both her and her family.

When she was finally admitted to the hospital, a large gangrenous area had formed on the sole of her foot, which was both smelly and painful. She was informed by her surgeon that they would be trying a bypass operation to which she readily agreed. A week later, it was obvious to the surgeons that the bypass was not working; it also was obvious to the patient, because the pain continued unabated even as she was given pain medication. She found herself getting rather droopy on the medication and rather resentful that the medical staff continued to talk to her about possible amputation. Four weeks after her admission to the hospital she was told that an amputation would be necessary, probably a below-the-knee amputation.

After the operation, she had numerous complications including infections and poor healing. She complained a lot of stump pain and needed large doses of pain medication every 3 hours. Because the surgeon felt that she was requesting too much medication, he arranged for a psychiatric evaluation, and Anne admitted to the psychiatrist that the pain was not so much in the stump, but in that "place where there isn't any leg." She was quite sure that she was crazy, in that if she mentioned this to the staff she would be "put away." On follow-up 2 weeks later, the phantom pain was less severe in that it no longer was a constant irritation, and would only bubble-up every 6–7 hours. She had also been taught by the staff to take some medication before the pain built up, so that in a 24-hour span she would actually need less of the medication.

Three months later on follow-up, she was complaining of occasional phantom pain with numerous phantom sensations during the day, and on 1-year follow-up, was commenting that she was having phantom pain about once a week, and phantom sensations every day. Five years after the operation, she was moving well with a prosthesis, was going through her daily activities roughly as she had before the onset of her crippling symptoms, and upon close questioning reported that she now had phantom pain lasting a number of minutes once every 2–3 weeks, and phantom sensations once a week.

Case 3

Kenneth was a 53-year-old self-employed man, married, with his sister-in-law also living in the apartment. A man who had traveled and lived in various parts of the world, he had suffered from periodic depressions from young adulthood to the present. Over the past 2 years, intermittent claudication of both legs had increased to the point where he could go no more than a half a block before he had to stop. He was no longer able to move about, and did most of his work at his desk and over the phone. His wife, who had always been careful about his diet and the care of both extremities, was horrified when he began developing ulcers on both lower extremities. Sympathectomy on both sides was done, but 4 months later it was obvious that this wasn't doing the job. Thrombotic episodes in both legs were followed by revascularization and the creation of new channels, but because of recurrent thrombotic episodes, this proved not fruitful. His surgeons began talking about possible amputation. He threatened suicide, so they talked less about it. Further bilateral thromboembolic episodes led to the necessity of quick amputations, and with his surgeon, wife, and sister-in-law insisting, Kenneth underwent bilateral above-the-knee amputations. After the operation, he screamed out in pain, and as a result was given massive amounts of Levo-dromoran and, because of severe depression, large doses of antidepressants. He had bilateral phantom pain and complained loudly about it being helped "only slightly" by the medication. Although he was sad, the depressive symptoms cleared, but the phantom pain remained intense and steady. He was given transcutaneous electrical nerve stimulation (TENS) treatment in the hope that this would decrease the need for medication, but this only helped for short stretches, right after the treatments. Three months later, on follow-up, the pain was nearly as intense as previously, and his wife reported that although he was getting around fairly well in his wheelchair, attempts to give him bilateral prostheses

had failed. Because the high dosage of Levo-dromoran was making him drowsy, he tried to take less of the medication, but unfortunately found that the pain was very, very bad. Hypnosis was attempted but he was a poor subject, so progressive relaxation and desensitization was tried and was also not successful. Another course of antidepressants was initiated, not because the symptoms of depression were so disabling, but in the hope that "it might help with the pain." Doses of up to 300 mg of nortriptyline did not help, either with mood or for pain. At the end of the year, he was still taking large doses of Levo-dromoran at times when the pain was "too bad," and he was still complaining of daily ongoing pain and poor sleep at night because of the pain. On a 4-year follow-up, the pain had decreased so that he was only having pain for a half hour once or twice a day.

THEORIES

Nearly all patients postamputation develop some kind of sensation in the area where the limb used to be. Jensen and Rasmussen best describe these under three primary headings: (1) kinesthetic sensations, (2) kinetic sensations, and (3) exteroceptive sensations (1). This covers everything from 1) positional sense, length, and volume of the amputated limb, (2) a sense on the part of the amputee that there is movement in the limb—"I moved my foot," (3) a pins and needles sensation or numbness in the amputated limb. The pain that is reported can be either in the stump or in the limb that is no longer there. It may be anything from a sharp knife-like pain that is infrequent to a continuous numbing pain that never leaves, day or night.

Although phenomenologically there is agreement about the nature of phantom limb pain, what causes the pain is not at all well understood. There are many theories concerning its etiology, which can be lumped into three groups: (1) central theories, (2) peripheral theories, and (3) psychological theories.

The central theories include Melzack's gate control theory, which centers around the idea of reverberating circuits and deals mostly with a rostral brain stem. According to Melzack and Loeser, it is the reticular activating system that exerts an inhibitory influence on the somatosensory projection system (2). With an amputation, many peripheral fibers are destroyed, the input is reduced, inhibition is decreased, and synchronous self-sustaining activity develops at all neuronal levels. Pain occurs when output from these self-sustaining neurons reaches the cortical level (3–5). Riddoch hypothesizes that a cortical representational body image develops over time as a result of peripheral input from all the senses (6). After amputation, this perception remains unaltered, and cortical cells independent of peripheral impulses are then responsible for the phantom phenomena. Others see the pain as due to a thalamic or subthalamic lesion; indeed, phantom pain shows some characteristics identical to those of thalamic pain. Unfortunately, none of the medullary or cerebral causes describe all or even most of the phantom pains, and it has never been possible to provoke pains by stimulating either the cortex or certain parts of the midbrain.

The peripheral theories hypothesize that the pain is caused by persistent sensation of the nerve endings in the stump (7). The amputee then feels that these sensations are assigned to the part of the body that was originally innervated by the severed nerves. Not infrequently, abscesses or scar tissues have been found to trigger the pain, but unfortunately the pain persists long after the injury has healed or after the scar tissue has been removed. Again, many questions are not answered by this peripheral theory, including the fact that amputees under 6 years old don't seem to have phantom pain (8), but more important that the pain does not follow the distribution of severed nerves.

Most people do not believe that psychological factors are the sole cause of phantom limb pain, but there are studies that seem to indicate that emotional factors are among the risk factors causing phantom pain. Many studies have looked at the personality structures of patients with phantom pain (9), and many risk factors have been found by various people to have an impact on the presence of pain. Unfortunately, none of these studies have been duplicated, although some, like those by Parkes (10), hold promise. In Parkes' study, the following were highly predictive of persistent phantom pain: (1) the appearance of stump or phantom pain within 3 weeks, (2) illness that had lasted longer than 1 year prior to the amputation and that persisted after surgery, (3) unemployment not due to pain, and (4) rigid and compulsively self-reliant personality types. The first three are measurable, the fourth difficult to measure. Others have looked closely at the concept of denial (11) or the denial of the loss of a body part (12). But here again there is a question of whether high denial or low denial is really very good.

TREATMENT

Before going on to the treatment, it is important to look at the time course of phantom limbs and phantom pain. Ambroïse Paré (13) first described phantom limb pain in 1551 and Weir Mitchell (14) in 1872 used the phrase "phantom limb." Most people will have phantom sensations; as a rule, if there are going to be changes, they will usually occur in the first 1–2 years after the amputation. It is a common phenomenon that "telescoping" occurs in that there seems to be a shrinkage of the phantom, meaning that the extremities seem to fade more and more into the stump. Frequently, at

the end of a year, telescoping is complete. The level of the amputation does not seem to have any influence on telescoping; as one patient put it, "as my toes got closer and closer to the top stump, they kept their size and I finally ended up feeling like the toes were right on top of the stump, same size." There are tremendous variations in the rate of diminishing of the phantom sensation (15, 16). Studies by Parkes (10) and Lunn (17) see a precipitous decrease of these sensations over a year's time. Everyone agrees though that the longer the phantom sensations and phantom pain last (18), the longer they are bound to stay and the greater the chances that they are going to be there permanently. In our own study, all 40 patients, on being questioned closely at the end of 7 years, reported phantom sensation, and 15% reported intermittent low level pains (19). It was of interest that even after years, the phantom limb experience did not conform to any peripheral nerve supply.

Many factors make a difrerence in the phantom sensation, especially in phantom pain. Rest, stump movement, heat or cold, or elevation of the stump will frequently relieve the pain, whereas psychopathology, hitting the stump, weather changes, and pain in other parts of the body will make the pain worse (1).

Because we don't know the etiology of phantom pain, treatment becomes a "pick and choose" kind of a situation. Sherman reported 68 treatment methods, of which he alleges 43 are successful (20–22). There are, however, a number of areas of agreement as to what will make for a better prognosis. At the top of the list is preoperative preparation, which should certainly include the warning to patients that phantom sensations are probable and phantom pain occasional. This preparation should also include evaluation of the patient's personality type, previous surgical experiences, and a thorough discussion of the meaning of the loss (23). Because the amputated member will have to be buried, there should be a discussion of the care and disposal of the part. The details of the surgical procedure should be left to what the patient wants to hear and not how little or how much the physicians wish to mention. Some patients are most interested in knowing all the details, whereas others will stop you after a number of sentences and say they have had enough. In either case the patient's wishes should be followed, unless there seems to be maladaptive denial. At this preoperative meeting, the rehabilitation program should be stressed, so that at a number of programs the prosthetician or the rehabilitation team come and talk to the patient. Postoperatively the patient should be allowed to mourn the loss, and counterproductive coping mechanisms using counterphobic and denial mechanisms should be looked for and addressed early. Some studies seem to indicate that early return to work and maximal use of prosthesis reduce the risk of developing phantom limb pain (19), and other studies seem to indicate that counseling of the family is helpful to the situation and may have an impact on phantom limb pain risk.

A second area of general agreement is that medical treatment and electrical stimulation should be tried before the surgical treatments are attempted.

Transcutaneous stimulation was used with good results in about half the patients by Thodon et al. in 1979 (24). Spinal cord stimulation and deep brain stimulation have been tried in a number of patients, sometimes with spectacular results (25, 26). Mundinger and Neumuller in 1981 used a combination of deep brain stimulation and transcutaneous stimulation, which worked in about half the patients (27). The reasons for using these electrostimulations are that they are nontraumatic and can be repeated. In a number of studies local anesthetics and nerve blocks have been useful, seeming to work for about one-third to one-half the patients (28, 29). Analgesics, especially salicylates, are frequently used but seem to be more useful in keeping the pain under some kind of control than eliminating it. Recently, propranalol (30) has been used with some success, and a number of studies have shown that carbamazepine (31, 32) is of great help. Various neuroleptics have been tried without much success, and the use of tricyclic antidepressants (33) as a help in chronic pain is well known.

This brings us to a discussion of pain and the philosophy of pain treatments. Perry has shown that doctors tend to undermedicate patients with pain, partly out of ignorance of pharmacokinetics, partly out of fear of addicting the patient, and sometimes as a way of differentiating themselves from the person in pain (34). No matter how we look at pain, it is real, and although it certainly has both objective and subjective components it is something that deserves treatment. This becomes especially important in phantom pain because the patient tends to see the pain as "crazy"—a viewpoint that not infrequently is shared by the surgical staff for their own reasons. Well-known studies by Twycross have shown that pain medication taken regularly and in adequate doses means that frequently patients will be taking less of the medication over a 24-hour period and that the effect will be greater (35). Fears of addicting patients have proven to be unfounded. This brings us directly to the point of narcotics and Jensen's excellent statement that "resistant pains are not to be accepted until narcotics have been tried" (1). He has found that the vast majority of patients can manage on a fixed morphine dose for many years without becoming addicted.

In surgical therapy both local and central procedures have been done. The peripheral surgical procedure includes the excision of neuromata (36), which seems to be most effective for stump pain. Even here the percentage of cures is small, and this procedure only useful when there are highly positive indications for the presence of neuromata. Unfortunately, this procedure is frequently used when the signs and symptoms of neuro-

mata are not that clear. Occasionally, more-extensive amputation has been tried to see if this will help with the phantom pain, but this is usually ineffective.

Rhizotomy used to be fairly popular (37), but is now nearly entirely abandoned. Cordotomy was fairly popular in the 1940s (38), but because a rather low number of patients improved, the treatment is not done frequently nowadays.

Sympathectomy was performed frequently in the 1950s, but at least three-quarters of the patients had recurrence of the pain within 6 months (39).

Midbrain lesions, thalamotomy, prefrontal lobotomies, and cortical ablations have been done in the past, probably out of frustration, and did not prove to be of much use.

The psychological treatments have proven to be of only limited use (40, 41). Relaxation techniques in our own group proved to help in the general wellbeing of the patient, but did not seem to help much with the pain. Biofeedback techniques have been reported as occasionally effective in individual patients (42), but have not be useful in large groups. Hypnosis was one of the treatments of choice in the 1950s and seemed to hold promise (43). It unfortunately does not seem to work over long periods and has been reported infrequently. Psychotherapy by itself was reported to be of limited help in the 1950s; again, there were indications that the treatment improved the general wellbeing of the patient, but it had little effect on the pain (44). Educational counseling used in conjunction with tricyclics frequently is of more use in chronic pain than intensive psychotherapy is. It is nevertheless important for patients to realize that they are understood and that the doctors feel that the pain is real. Work with the family should follow the same lines.

Physical therapy started early after the amputation seems to be of great use in keeping the phantom pain within limits (20), and there are studies that seem to indicate that early physical therapy may actually decrease the risk of the phantom pain. Ultrasonography, heat therapy, and peripheral stimulation have been reported as useful in certain individuals and certainly are safe enough to use. In many reports the pain seems to decrease over short stretches of time, and this is not to be sneezed at (45).

CONCLUSIONS

We are really at the beginning of studying these patients. It is hoped that more prospective studies like those of Parkes will be done in which researchers look at the patient thoroughly both physiologically and psychologically and, starting preoperatively, follow these people for many, many years. In our own study patients interviewed after 7 years reported occasionally having phantom sensations; some reported phantom pain (19).

It is crucial that we do not denigrate the pain, that we treat it with all the forces that we can marshal, going from one treatment to the other until (we hope) we hit something that works. With proper studies perhaps we will be able to match the patient with the appropriate treatment.

REFERENCES

1. Jensen TS, Rasmussen P: Amputation. In Wall P, Melzack R (eds): *Textbook of Pain.* New York, Churchill Livingston, 1984.
2. Melzack R, Loeser JD: Phantom body pain in paraplegics: Evidence for a central pattern generating mechanism for pain. *Pain* 4:195–210, 1978.
3. Jacobson L, Chabal C: A comparison of the effects of intrathecal fentanyl and lidocaine on established postamputation stump pain. *Pain* 2:137–141, 1990.
4. Naryshkin AG, Gurchin FA, Samo KA, et al: Pathogenesis of phantom limb syndrome and its treatment. *Vestnik Khirurgii Imeni I-I-Grekova* 144:50–53, 1989.
5. Sherman RA: Stump and phantom limb pain. *Neurol Clin* 7:249–264, 1989.
6. Riddoch G: Phantom limbs and body shape. *Brain* 44:197–222, 1941.
7. Livingston WK: *Pain Mechanism: A Physiologic Interpretation of Causalgia and Its Related States.* New York, Macmillan, 1994.
8. Simmel ML: The absence of phantoms for congenitally missing limbs. *Am J Psychol* 74:467–470, 1961.
9. Scott LE, et al: Preoperative predictors of postoperative pain. *Pain* 15:283–293, 1983.
10. Parkes CM: Factors determining the persistence of phantom pain in the amputee. *J Psychosom Res* 17:97–108, 1973.
11. Schilder P. *The Image and Appearance of the Human Body: Studies in the Constructive Energies of the Psyche.* London, Kegan Paul, 1935.
12. Zuk GH: The phantom limb: A proposed theory of unconscious origins. *J Nervous Mental Dis* 124:510–513, 1956.
13. Pare A: *The Works of That Famous Chirurgion, Ambrose Pare.* London, R. Cotes, 1649.
14. Mitchell SW: Phantom limbs. *Lippincott's Magazine of Popular Literature and Science* 8:563–569, 1871.
15. Setacci C, Di Massa A DeVito L, et al: Post-amputation pain in patients with vascular diseases: Clinical characteristics. *Angiologia* 41:194–196, 1989.
16. Orz R: Pain syndromes following amputation. Analysis of 100 affected patients with chronic stump and phantom pain. *Fortschritte Der Medizin* 108:53–56, 1990.
17. Lunn V: *Om Legemsbevidstheden.* Copenhagen, Munksgaard, 1948.
18. Sherman R, Sherman C: Prevalence and characteristics of chronic phantom limb pain among American veterans: Results of a trial survey. *Am J Phys Med* 62:227–238, 1983.
19. Wilson PG, Krebs MJS, Cohen DEI: Risk factors in amputation. *Vasc Surg* (in press).
20. Sherman RA, Sherman CJ, Gall N: A survey of current phantom limb pain treatment in the United States. *Pain* 8:85–89, 1980.
21. Sherman RA: Phantom pain: A lesson in the necessity for careful clinical research on chronic pain problems. *J Rehabil Res Dev* 25:7–10, 1988.
22. Sherman RA. The mystery of phantom pain: Growing evidence for psychophysiological mechanisms. *Biofeedback Self Regul* 14:267–280, 1989.
23. Langer E, Jania IL, Wolfer JA: Reduction of psychological stress in surgical patients. *J Exp Soc Psychol* 11:155–165, 1975.
24. Thoden U, Gruber RP, Krainick J-U, Huber-Muck L: Langzeitergebnisse transkutaner nervenstimulation bei chronish neurogenen schmerzzustanden. *Nervenarzt* 50:179–184, 1979.
25. Krainick J-U, Thoden U, Riechert T: Pain reduction in amputees by long-term spinal cord stimulation. *J Neurosurg* 52:346–350, 1980.
26. Hirano K, Yamashiro H, Maeda N, et al: A case of longstanding phantom limb pain: Complete relief of pain. *Masui-Japanese J Anesthesiol* 37:222–225, 1988.
27. Mundinger F, Neumuller H: Programmed transcutaneous (TNS) and central (DBS) stimulation for control of phantom limb pain and causalgia: A new method for treatment. In Siegfried J, Zimmermann M (eds): *Phantom and Stump Pain.* Berlin, Springer-Verlag, 1981, pp 167–178.
28. Sherman RA: Published treatments of phantom limb pain. *Am J Phys Med* 59:232–244, 1980.
29. Jacobson L: Relief of persistent postamputation stump and phantom limb pain with intrathecal fentanyl. *Pain* 37:317–322, 1989.
30. Marsland AR, Weekes JWN, Atkinson RL, Leong MG: Phantom limb pain: A case for beta blockers? *Pain* 12:295–297, 1982.
31. Doupe J, Cullen CH, Chance GQ: Post-traumatic pain and the causalgic syndrome. *J Neurol Neurosurg Psychiatry* 7:33–48, 1944.
32. Elliott F, Little A, Milbrandt W: Carbamazepine for phantom-limb phenomena. *N Engl J Med* 295:678, 1976.
33. Rogers AG: Use of amitriptyline (Elavil) for phantom limb pain in younger children. *J Pain Symptom Manag* 4:96, 1989.
34. Perry S: Undermedication for pain. *Psychiatr Ann* 14:960, 1984.
35. Twycross RG: Diseases of the central nervous system: Relief of terminal pain. *Br Med J* 4:212, 1975.
36. Baumgartner R, Riniker C: Surgical stump revision as a treatment of stump and phantom pains. Results of 100 cases. In Siegfried S, Zimmermann M (eds): *Phantom and Stump pain.* Berlin, Springer Verlag, 1981.
37. White J, Sweet W: *Pain and the Neurosurgeon: A Forty-Year Experience.* Springfield, IL, Charles C. Thomas, 1969.
38. Siegfried J, Cetinalp E: Neurosurgical treatment of phantom limb pain: A survey of methods. In Siegfried J, Zimmermann M (eds): *Phantom and Stump pain.* Berlin, Springer Verlag, 1981, pp 148–155.
39. Kallio KE: Permanency of results obtained by sympathetic surgery in the treatment of phantom pain. *Acta Orthop Scand* 19:391–397, 1950.
40. Sherman RA: Psychological factors influencing chronic phantom limb pain: An analysis of the literature. *Pain* 28:285–295, 1987.
41. Sherman RA: The relationship between situational stress

and phantom limb pain: Cross-lagged correlational data from six month pain logs. *J Psychosom Res* 34:71–77, 1990.

42. Sherman R: Case reports of treatment of phantom limb pain with a combination of electromyographic biofeedback and verbal relaxation techniques. *Biofeedback Self Regul 1*:353, 1976.

43. Siegel EF: Control of phantom limb pain by hypnosis. *Am J Clin Hypn* 21:285–286, 1979.

44. Postone N: Phantom limb pain. *Psychiatry Med* 17:57–70, 1987.

45. Katz J, Melzack R: Auricular transcutaneous electrical nerve stimulation (TENS) reduces phantom limb pain. *J Pain Symptom Manag* 6:73–83, 1991.

CHAPTER 41

POST-HERPETIC NEURALGIA
JOHN R. SATTERTHWAITE

Herpes zoster, or "shingles," is an infectious viral disease commonly encountered in primary medical practice. It is estimated that over 300,000 new cases occur each year in the United States (1). Most of these spontaneously resolve and require only symptomatic treatment during the acute illness. The acute infectious stage can usually be shortened with treatment by antiviral agents, which limit viral replication (2). Neuritic symptoms, resulting from incomplete but usually permanent sensory neural damage, can often be controlled or reduced by corticosteroids, analgesics, and nerve blocks. The lesions dry up and crust, and the pain usually resolves. Unfortunately, in a percentage of the population the lesions resolve but the pain persists and, in fact, often becomes more severe. This is especially true in the elderly, who have a higher incidence of experiencing excruciating, unrelenting pain long after the acute illness has resolved. This protracted painful syndrome is known as *post-herpetic neuralgia*, one of the most excruciatingly painful of the chronic pain syndromes.

Post-herpetic neuralgia has been called the most common cause of intractable, debilitating pain in the elderly (3). Its intensity and duration create such suffering that many consider suicide as a means of escaping its ravages. In fact, it has been said that post-herpetic neuralgia is the leading cause of suicide in chronic pain patients over the age of 70 (3). To appropriately manage these patients, a knowledge of the pathophysiology and epidemiology is essential in understanding the clinical course and treatment options in this disease.

ACUTE HERPES ZOSTER (SHINGLES)

Herpesvirus varicellae, commonly called *varicella-zoster virus*, is a DNA virus in the same group as herpes simplex, Epstein-Barr virus, and cytomegalovirus. The primary infection in nonimmune individuals is chickenpox. It is estimated that 95% of all children have been exposed to chickenpox by age 15 (4). As the chickenpox infection resolves, the virus enters the peripheral sensory nerve receptors and is transmitted via the sensory nerves to the dorsal root ganglia of the spinal nerves and extramedullary ganglia of the cranial nerves. Upon entry into the ganglia, the virus becomes dormant but retains its infectious capability (5). As a percentage of the viruses revert to an infectious state, they are quickly destroyed by the cellular immune system before clinical infection becomes evident. As long as the immune system remains intact, the reactivation of these viruses is blocked (6, 7).

Herpes zoster is a viral infection resulting from reactivation of the dormant varicella-zoster virus. Although the mechanism of reactivation is not entirely clear, it appears that a decrease in cellular-mediated immunity allows reactivation of the dormant virus in the dorsal root ganglia or extramedullary ganglia (8). As this reactivation progresses, immunity is stimulated by an active segment or segments sufficient to suppress other areas from activity but not enough to stop the initial reactivation. This likely explains the characteristic unilateral, segmental vesicular eruption that is seen most frequently (9). Reactivation of the virus is due to a fall in host cell–mediated immunity, which may be due to trauma, infection, chronic illness, acquired immunodeficiency syndrome (AIDS), malignancy, radiation therapy, chemotherapy, or immunosuppression therapy (10). Frequently there is no identifiable explanation for the decrease in immunity or cause for the reactivation.

Upon multiplication of the virus, it spreads within the ganglia, causing neuronal necrosis and inflammation characterized by intense lymphocytic infiltration, endothelial proliferation, focal hemorrhage, and ganglion sheath inflammation (6). As the infection continues, the virus subsequently enters the sensory nerve and is transported along the neuron to the nerve endings, where it is released. The virus then enters the corium and epidermal cells, where it multiplies, causing the characteristic cutaneous lesions to be formed (11).

On microscopic examination there is noted to be an intense necrotizing inflammation of the dorsal root, dorsal horn, and peripheral nerve axons with peripheral nerve demyelination and destruction of large-fiber neurons (11, 12). Examination of the skin lesions shows the characteristic intranuclear inclusion bodies, giant cell formation, epidermal cell edema, and inflammation of the corium (11).

Patients with AIDS and malignant neoplasms are most susceptible to herpes zoster. This is especially true of the lymphomas, and it is estimated that up to 25% of patients with Hodgkin's disease will develop herpes zoster (13). The occurrence of acute herpes zoster in a young, seemingly healthy individual may warrant further investigation of human immunodeficiency virus (HIV) risk factors and status. Wilkerson noted that the appearance of herpes zoster was frequently the first clinical manifestation of this disease (14). In one study of 48 patients presenting to a clinic with acute herpes zoster, 70% had HIV infection (15).

Herpes zoster is extremely uncommon in the young, healthy patient and much more common in the elderly, in whom the incidence is said to be in the range of 0.5–1.0% (5, 16). There is a natural, gradual decrease in cellular-mediated immunity as a person ages such that levels may decrease enough to allow reactivation (17). This may help to explain the increasing incidence with age. No seasonal variations or differences with regard to race, sex, or ethnic background have been reported (18). Persons who have never had chickenpox may develop the disease if exposed to an individual with acute herpes zoster vesicles, although it is extremely rare to develop herpes zoster solely from exposure to a patient with chickenpox.

CLINICAL MANIFESTATIONS

The pre-eruptive stage is usually characterized by fever, headache, lymphadenopathy, malaise, and progressively increasing pain with hyperesthesia and paresthesias over the involved dermatome for up to 14 days during the initial ganglionitis (19, 20). Occasional reports of a more protracted "preherpetic neuralgia" have been made with pain preceding the cutaneous eruptions by as much as 100 days (21). This may be related to long-term steroid therapy in these patients. The pre-eruptive stage is followed by erythematous dermatitis and subsequently by the characteristic maculopapular rash. This rash then evolves into clear fluid-filled vesicles over the next 72 hours. These vesicles can range from small isolated clumps to a confluent rash involving the entire dermatomal area in the form of a band; thus the name zoster or "girdle" (19). The locations of the eruptions of herpes zoster seem to correlate well with those of chickenpox (6) (Table 41.1). Eruptions are occasionally encountered outside the affected dermatome, but in less than 1% do they occur bilaterally (19). Contrary to the old belief, bilateral herpes zoster eruptions are obviously not a sign of impending death.

The entity *zoster sine herpete*, herpes zoster infection without the eruption, has been a topic of debate for

Table 41.1.
Average Distribution of Herpes Zoster Skin Lesions[a]

Distribution	Percentage
Cranial	15
(Ophthalmic division of the trigeminal nerve)	(10)
Cervical	12
Thoracic	55
Lumbar	14
Sacral	3
Generalized	1

[a]From Loeser JD: Postherpetic neuralgia: A review of pathophysiology and treatment. Presented at the Annual Meeting of the American Pain Society, Washington, D.C., November 8, 1986.

many years, particularly with regard to the actual existence of this entity. Pain without the cutaneous rash may represent an isolated viral ganglionitis with no peripheral spread, or possibly the eruption has been isolated and in small clusters and no lesions or residual scarring can be grossly detected.

Secondary infection is possible in acute herpes zoster; however, this is not that common and routine antibiotic therapy is not necessary, except in herpes zoster ophthalmicus, unless definite evidence of infection exists (22). Without treatment, and in the absence of superimposed bacterial infection, the vesicles progress to cloudy fluid-filled pustules, with eventual crusting and scab formation within 2–3 weeks and gradual resolution into irregular pink scars. These ultimately become the characteristic hypopigmented, anesthetic scars, which persist for many years.

Pain is slight or absent in children and young adults. Elderly patients seem to have more pain with the pre-eruptive and vesicular stages than the younger patients do. The pain is frequently described as aching, burning, shooting, stabbing, or soreness. Regardless of the extent of the eruptions, pain will most likely involve the entire sensory dermatome affected.

There is usually no visceral involvement with spinal nerve infection; however, lumbosacral herpes zoster can present as acute urinary retention, hemorrhagic cystitis, or constipation due to colorectal hypomobility (23).

There may also be a much greater incidence of motor involvement than has been previously realized (24, 25). If motor neurons in the anterior horn cells at the level of the infection become involved, muscular weakness or palsies can develop. Motor loss is not uncommon in cranial and cervical herpes zoster, but is less frequent in truncal zoster. The facial nerve is the most common site of clinically detectable motor involvement (18). Inflammation of the geniculate ganglion may lead to involvement of the external ear and ear canal or of the soft palate and to the loss of taste (Hunt's syndrome). This is often accompanied by seventh nerve paralysis.

The most serious complications exist with involvement of the trigeminal nerve. Ten to fifteen percent of reported cases of herpes zoster involve the ophthalmic division of the trigeminal nerve (26). It is the most commonly involved single nerve in herpes zoster, especially in older patients (10). In herpes zoster ophthalmicus, the sensory nucleus of the fifth cranial nerve, the meninges, trigeminal ganglion, and cerebral blood vessels may be affected. Most frequently the infection involves the supraorbital and supratrochlear branches of the frontal nerve, with vesicles occurring on the forehead and upper lid. This is accompanied by pain in the distribution of the nerves as well as headache and weakness of the periorbital and lid muscles. Vesicles are deep, and residual scarring of the lids is a common complication leading to impaired vision due to contractures. No ocular involvement is noted unless the nasociliary branch of the semilunar ganglion is affected (10). This occurs in 50% of patients with herpes zoster ophthalmicus and can lead to conjunctivitis, scleritis, iridocyclitis, extraocular muscle palsies, ptosis, and mydriasis, which can cause permanent damage to the cornea, sclera, or ciliary body (10). Involvement of the nasociliary branch can be determined by the presence of Hutchinson's sign, the presence of vesicles on the ipsilateral edge and tip of the nose.

Cutaneous and visceral dissemination are more common with herpes zoster ophthalmicus than with other forms of herpes zoster (10). Central nervous system (CNS) complications include Bell's palsy, encephalitis, myelitis, peripheral sensory neuropathy, and motor neuropathy (10). Such complications result from direct viral extension to the spinal cord, brainstem, or cavernous sinus and may occur prior to the appearance of the vesicular eruption. Aggressive treatment of ophthalmic herpes zoster is required in order to prevent these complications as well as later problems such as lid contractures, glaucoma, blindness, and post-herpetic neuralgia (10).

If the virus spreads along the posterior spinal nerve root, patients may also develop myelitis or meningitis.

Excessive pain, extensive dorsal horn inflammation, or involvement of the sympathetic ganglia may result in a secondary reflex sympathetic dystrophy, although this is thought by some to be rare.

The overall course of herpes zoster usually ranges from 10 days to 6 weeks. This also is age-related, with the younger patients healing faster.

COMPLICATIONS

Ocular complications of herpes zoster have been previously mentioned. Most complications of the disease occur during the eruptive stage and are related to the viral infection. Secondary bacterial infection may cause sepsis, fever, chills, and pyoderma. Neurologic sequelae include meningitis, myelitis, encephalomyelitis, paresis, and sensory and motor neuropathies with palsies or paralysis.

In immunocompromised patients, there is an increased incidence of dissemination as the viral infection spreads to adjacent dermatomal areas. As this progresses, fever and increasing debilitation may occur. With dissemination comes the associated threat of visceral involvement. The highest morbidity and mortality rates occur with visceral spread, and the gastrointestinal tract is a common site. Pericarditis, endocarditis, hepatitis, and encephalitis may also be seen. Less frequently, varicella pneumonia may occur in immunocompromised patients, and this diagnosis carries a high rate of morbidity and mortality (27). Prevention of dissemination or visceral complications should be considered and aggressive treatment carried out in severely immunocompromised patients, especially those with acquired immune deficiency and related disorders. In general, if the disease remains localized for 4–7 days, dissemination is much less likely (27).

DIAGNOSIS

In the initial stages prior to the eruptions, acute herpes zoster may frequently be misdiagnosed. More-common diagnoses such as herpes simplex, pleurisy, herniated intervertebral disks, cardiac disease, myalgias, costochondritis, cholecystitis, and other acute visceral illnesses are often suspected. Peripheral nerve blocks may frequently be helpful in differentiating herpes zoster pain from visceral pain. It is usually only when the eruption appears that the diagnosis is made with increased certainty.

Occasionally, rickettsial infections, impetigo, mycoplasmas, coxsackievirus, or a localized herpes simplex eruption may be confused with herpes zoster (19). Laboratory correlation is then necessary to differentiate the two diseases. Isolation of the virus from vesicles prior to crusting or demonstration of the antigen in vesicular fluid will greatly assist in the diagnosis. Other confirmatory tests include rising serum monoclonal antibody titers and positive Tzanck smear with demonstration of typical eosinophilic intranuclear inclusions, multinucleated giant cells, and "balloon degeneration" of epithelial cells in tissue biopsies or vesicle fluid (28).

Routine laboratory findings are usually normal with the exception of a slightly raised leukocyte count. In CNS infections, the cerebrospinal fluid (CSF) pressure and protein are slightly elevated and CSF sugar is normal. Mild pleocytosis may also be noted.

TREATMENT

Treatment of herpes zoster in the acute stage should be directed toward limiting the duration and spread of the viral infection, patient comfort, local skin care with prevention of secondary infection of the lesions, and prevention of post-herpetic neuralgia. Calamine lotion or Burow's solution applied topically offer local relief. Local care of the lesions with steroid creams and bandages also helps to decrease inflammation and discomfort.

ANALGESICS

Frequently, non-narcotic analgesics such as aspirin and acetaminophen are sufficient to control mild pain. Codeine-containing analgesics, propoxyphene, and oxycodone may be used for more-severe pain and suffice to control pain in most cases. Stool softeners should be used in the elderly to prevent narcotic-induced constipation.

Use of strongly addicting major narcotics should be avoided except in cases of severe pain uncontrolled by the above-mentioned drugs. Severe pain should also serve as a warning to the clinician that there is a strong potential for the development of post-herpetic neuralgia (22). Aggressive treatment with modalities thought to decrease the incidence of post-herpetic neuralgia should be considered in addition to analgesics.

Antibiotics

Although the cutaneous lesions may become secondarily infected, prophylactic antibiotics are generally not recommended (22). Systemics and topical antibiotics should be reserved for documented pyoderma or infection. When ocular involvement is present and corneal scarring is feared, prophylactic topical ophthalmic antibiotics should be considered (10).

Corticosteroids

Systemic corticosteroid therapy is currently the most common treatment for herpes zoster, but the use of corticosteroids is not without controversy (22). For some time, corticosteroids have been the primary weapon of physicians in treating acute herpes zoster. Numerous references may be found in the literature regarding the effectiveness of steroids in the treatment of acute herpes zoster and the possible preventative effect against post-herpetic neuralgia.

Elliot, in 1964, studied 20 patients over the age of 50 using a regimen of prednisone (60 mg/day for 1 week, 30 mg/day the next week, and 15 mg/day the third week). These patients were compared to a group of 10 untreated patients. All patients were experiencing severe pain. Average duration of pain in the treated patients was 3.5 days after treatment started, as compared to 3.5 *weeks* in the untreated group (29, 30).

Perhaps the most significant evidence of steroid effectiveness was in a study by Eaglstein et al. at the University of Miami in 1970 (31). This was the first age-controlled, double-blind study that showed the effectiveness of triamcinolone in the reduction of pain duration. Thirty-four patients over age 60 with severe pain were randomly assigned into two groups, one receiving

triamcinolone, the other lactose tablets. Study patients were dosed with triamcinolone (48 mg/day for 1 week, 24 mg/day the next week, then 16 mg/day the third week). Median duration of pain in the treated group was 6 weeks, compared with 10 weeks in the untreated group. Each group had one patient with pain lasting over 1 year. Skin healing and pain intensity were not affected.

In 1980, Keczkes and Basheer used 40 mg of prednisolone daily for 10 days, tapering the dose over the following 3 weeks in 40 patients over age 50 (32). They also noted faster relief of pain in the treated group by about one-half over a similar group treated with carbamazepine (400 mg/day). Although the results were statistically significant, the study was not blind and patients were hospitalized during the study. It does, however, help support the results of other studies with similar results.

A recent compilation of all controlled, randomized English-language studies comparing steroids with placebo in herpes zoster found that their use "significantly decreases the proportion of patients with post-herpetic neuralgic, but only (if used) early in the course of the natural evolution of this complication" (33).

Parenteral steroid use still remains controversial, with evidence supporting pain reduction and a lowered incidence of post-herpetic neuralgia on the one hand, and no significant reduction of post-herpetic neuralgia on the other.

Another use for steroids is topical application of steroid creams on the cutaneous lesions. This often helps decrease the local tissue reaction (10, 22). Topical steroids are used in herpes zoster ophthalmicus to reduce local cellulitis and inflammation in the eyelids to avoid scarring and resultant frozen upper lid (10). Systemic steroids may also be used for ophthalmic zoster as outlined above.

Subcutaneous infiltration of steroids has also been used to decrease pain and aid in healing of the lesions. This will be discussed later.

Concern has been expressed regarding the use of steroids and the risk of avascular necrosis of the femoral head or disseminated herpes zoster (34–38). Most studies have found no basis for this fear. Disseminated herpes zoster occurs commonly in patients with hematologic and other malignancies and has been seen to occur in up to 2% of otherwise normal patients (16). There is no evidence that this overall incidence is increased with short-term systemic steroids (38) as opposed to long-term corticosteroid therapy (39).

Antiviral Agents

With AIDS research taking the forefront these days, several new antiviral agents are being tried to combat this epidemic. As of this time, no evidence exists documenting their efficacy in treating herpes zoster infections. The mainstream antiviral agent in herpes zoster remains acyclovir. Therefore, patients with HIV infection undergoing antiviral therapy would still require concurrent treatment with a zoster-specific antiviral agent in the event of an acute herpes zoster infection.

Acyclovir

Perhaps the most effective, widely used treatment for acute herpes zoster is the antiviral drug acyclovir, which selectively inhibits viral DNA nucleotidyltransferase (10, 40, 41). Results from early studies have demonstrated a marked reduction in the time of viral shedding, skin healing, and partial pain reduction. In a 1979 study of 23 patients with malignancy and herpes zoster, Selby et al. showed a reduction in new lesion formation and systemic spread, with pain relief within 24 hours, using intravenous acyclovir at a dose of 5 mg/kg administered every 8 hours for 5 days (42). These findings were confirmed by the Collaborative Acyclovir Study Group, which showed faster symptomatic relief and prevention of lesion progression in a double-blind study of immunocompromised patients (43). Although the incidence of post-herpetic neuralgia was lower in the study group, this difference was not statistically significant. Intravenous acyclovir or vidarabine 10 mg/kg/day has been used in immunocompetent patients with similar effects. Early treatment (within 48 hours of rash onset or 4 days of pain onset) had a good effect on reduction of residual pain duration (44). Other evidence supports the ineffectiveness of acyclovir in the prevention of post-herpetic neuralgia (45). The drug in this case was well tolerated and without any adverse clinical side effects. In unusually severe or disseminated cases of herpes zoster, 30 mg/kg/day intravenously has been used in HIV patients (46).

In addition to its parenteral use, oral acyclovir continues to be evaluated in the treatment of herpes zoster. In a small study, oral acyclovir in a dose of 200 mg five times daily for 5 days showed rapid resolution of the rash if treatment was started within 24 hours of the initial eruption (47). Neither control nor study patients developed post-herpetic neuralgia.

Studies using 400 mg of acyclovir five times a day for 5 days (48), 600 mg five times a day for 10 days (49), and 800 mg five times a day for 7 days (50) and 10 days (51) showed that higher doses were more effective than were lower doses in shortening the period of viral shedding, accelerating time to crusting, reducing new lesion formation, and decreasing the intensity and duration of pain. The higher doses were relatively free of side effects.

One study using 800 mg five times a day for 10 days (51) showed a lower incidence of post-herpetic neuralgia than did a similar study using 800 mg five times a day for 7 days (50). This difference was felt to be due to the length of treatment, differences in pain criteria or, most

likely, age differences of the participants. The average age of patients in the 7-day study was 73 years, whereas the average age of patients in the 10-day study was 58 years.

Despite these differences, oral acyclovir now appears to be the first-line drug of choice for nonimmunocompromised ambulatory herpes zoster patients. Because of reports indicating a decrease in post-herpetic neuralgia, the high-dose, 10-day regimen is recommended in all patients, especially those at greater risk of developing post-herpetic neuralgia. Early implementation of acyclovir therapy (within 48–72 hours of onset of the initial eruption) appears to be the most effective treatment currently available. Other studies have also documented shortening of the acute viral illness with decrease in cutaneous or systemic spread (52–54). Although total mean analgesic consumption is reduced over 3–6 months following the acute illness, no direct evidence of prevention of post-herpetic neuralgia has been adequately documented.

Ganciclovir

Ganciclovir, a potent antiherpesvirus agent, has very little effect on varicella-zoster viruses (50).

Cytosine Arabinoside (ARA-C)

Cytosine arabinoside was one of the first antiviral agents studied in the management of acute herpes zoster (19). Conflicting results and frequent untoward side effects, especially persistent neurologic deficits, have caused this treatment to essentially be abandoned.

Adenine Arabinoside (ARA-A)

Adenine arabinoside (vidarabine) is incorporated into viral and host DNA and has been effective in treatment of immunocompromised patients. It was first reported in 1976 in a well-controlled study of immunocompromised patients (55). Rapid resolution of the disease, rapid cutaneous healing, and a decrease in pain duration and intensity were noted. Although the incidence of post-herpetic neuralgia was equal to that of the control group, duration of pain was shortened. Perhaps the best benefit of ARA-A is the lowered incidence of disseminated herpes zoster with early therapy (56). It is very effective in preventing visceral complications in hematologically compromised patients but relatively ineffective in treating them (56). Its use appears to be most beneficial in patients with disseminated herpes zoster, those with hematologic malignancies, or those who are otherwise immunocompromised (56). Treatment is most efficacious if begun within the first week following the eruption (10). Treatment is by 12-hour infusion over 5 days. There is some CNS, hepatic, and renal toxicity.

Idoxuridine

Topical idoxuridine, 40% in dimethyl sulfoxide (DMSO), has been reported to shorten pain duration and the acute vesicular stage in acute herpes zoster (35, 57). To be effective this is applied as a paste four times a day for the first 4 days following appearance of the vesicles. A double-blind study by Juel-Jensen et al. supports the claims of acute pain reduction and faster healing (37). DMSO is not easily available in the United States.

Topical idoxuridine has also been used in the treatment of ophthalmic herpes zoster (10). Again, this requires linen soaked in DMSO with 40% idoxuridine applied as above.

Systemic idoxuridine is associated with significant systemic toxicity.

Interferon

Interferon is a vital component of the body's normally functioning immune system. Early studies have shown high-dose therapy with interferon to be effective in decreasing local disease progression and systemic spread and diminishing the severity of post-herpetic neuralgia (58). Although its limited availability limits its usefulness, early consideration should be given to this therapy in severely immunocompromised patients and children with malignancies.

Zoster Immune Globulin

Zoster immune globulin has been shown to prevent varicella in susceptible individuals (59, 60). Its primary use has been in the prevention of varicella in children and immunocompromised patients exposed to chickenpox. There is no evidence that it is effective in altering the course of established herpes zoster (60) or in prevention of post-herpetic neuralgia (59).

Adenosine Monophosphate (AMP)

Adenosine monophosphate (AMP) is a natural cellular metabolite. Patients with herpes zoster have abnormally low levels of cyclic AMP in their serum (61). Several studies have been performed to evaluate the effectiveness of AMP on DNA virus infections (61–63). In a double-blind, age-controlled, crossover study using 100 mg of AMP injected intramuscularly every other day for 3 weeks, reduction of viral shedding and pain duration were demonstrated when compared to placebo treatment (2). Average pain duration was 3 weeks with no recurrence in 18–24 months of follow-up. Minimal side effects were noted.

Sklar reported having treated over 1000 shingles patients in over 14 years; no sequelae, side effects, return of rash, or persistent neuralgia have been noted (64).

Amantadine

In a double-blind, controlled study, amantadine was shown to shorten the duration of vesicle formation and severe pain, implying effectiveness on the incidence of post-herpetic neuralgia, but this was not defined (65, 66). Amantadine (200 mg/day for 28 days) has been considered effective in patients who are unable to take corticosteroids (67).

Other Antiviral Agents

In a brief clinical trial, cimetadine (300 mg by mouth four times daily) provided rapid relief of itching, pain, and crusting of the skin lesions in four patients with cancer (68). This was thought possibly to be due to the antipruritic effect of H_2 receptor antagonism, which may also inhibit suppressor T-cells, restoring the natural immune response (69–72). Pain relief and crusting of lesions were noted within 48 hours.

In in-vivo and in-vitro studies of cimetadine, 1200 mg/day, cimetadine shortened both the median interval until the first decrease in pain and the median interval until the complete resolution of pain, and promoted faster complete healing of skin lesions than did symptomatic treatment alone. Histamine receptor antagonism blocked excessive suppressor T-cell activity in patients with this immunoregulatory disorder who had the presence of cutaneous lesions less than 72 hours. Malignant disorders were excluded (73).

Thymidine analogs have some inhibitory effect on the varicella virus, and the antivaricella effects of other antiviral agents are under investigation.

ANTIDEPRESSANTS AND TRANQUILIZERS

Tricyclic antidepressants and phenothiazine tranquilizers are widely used substances in the therapy of severe pain due to acute herpes zoster as well as post-herpetic neuralgia. Although their serotonin effect may contribute to a central pain relief mechanism in acute herpes zoster, their antidepressant effect is also beneficial in this stage. The advent of newer antiviral agents with early pain relief may decrease the need to use these drugs in the acute phase. Their use may also be effective in patients who do not respond to other types of analgesics.

ANTICONVULSANTS

Anticonvulsants, primarily phenytoin and carbamazepine, are used to lessen the sharp, paroxysmal pains seen in both acute herpes zoster and post-herpetic neuralgia (74, 75). Their primary use is in post-herpetic pain, but they can be used in the acute infection if the paroxysmal pain does not respond to analgesics. They should be used cautiously because of the potential for blood dyscrasias.

NERVE BLOCKS

Nerve blocks have been used extensively in the treatment of pain in herpes zoster. Numerous attempts have been made to treat herpes zoster and prevent post-herpetic neuralgia using all forms of somatic and sympathetic nerve blocks (76).

Perhaps the most frequently used blocks involve local infiltration of the acute eruptions. This was described by

Epstein, who injected procaine with 0.2% triamcinolone subcutaneously in the areas of the eruptions and areas of pain and itching (77). He reported relief in almost 100% of the cases with a reduction in the incidence of post-herpetic neuralgia. Response was predictable and complications were minimal.

Peripheral somatic nerve blocks have been successful in temporary treatment of the acute pain; however, no evidence exists that they assist in avoiding post-herpetic neuralgia.

Because the acute inflammation is primarily located in the nerve roots, much work has been directed toward blocks in the nerve root area. The epidural route has been studied with much success in relieving the acute pain and shortening the duration of the infection (78). Perkins and Hanlon achieved excellent relief in patients with herpes zoster of less than 7 weeks' duration using epidural blocks (79). Pain was relieved, lesions dried up rapidly, and no development of post-herpetic neuralgia was noted. Fothergill et al. reported 113 patients, aged 14–93, who underwent epidural injections; immediate, permanent pain relief was achieved in 110 (80). Post-herpetic neuralgia developed in two of the three failures. In 192 patients over age 60, 12 (6.25%) developed post-herpetic neuralgia, which is less than the usual 50–60% (80). Immediate relief of pain and prevention of post-herpetic neuralgia was also noted in 100% of 113 patients with herpes zoster of less than 10 weeks' duration by Schreuder, who injected 8–12 ml of bupivacaine 0.25% with methylprednisolone (80 mg) epidurally (81). Although patients were injected with epidural local anesthetics combined with steroids, the additional effect of steroids has not been documented.

Much attention has been directed toward sympathetic blocks as an extremely effective method of treating acute herpes zoster (9, 82). Although the exact pathophysiology of pain in herpes zoster and post-herpetic neuralgia remains unknown, the role of the sympathetic nervous system is receiving more attention. Inflammation of the posterior root ganglia may increase sympathetic efferent activity, causing increased segmental vasoconstriction and increased pain (83, 84). Vasospasm and sympathetic sensitization of peripheral and central pain mechanisms may be relieved temporarily and possibly reversed by early sympathetic blockade. The earliest evidence of sympathetic blockade efficacy was noted in the 1930s when patients suffering from herpes zoster and reflex sympathetic dystrophy were administered sympathetic blocks for their reflex sympathetic dystrophy (9). It was noted that the herpes zoster eruptions in these patients dried and crusted within 2–3 days and their pain was immediately relieved. If these blocks were performed within the first 3 weeks of the eruption, there was rapid resolution of the acute illness and a decreased incidence of post-herpetic neuralgia (78, 82). In 1938, Rosenak pioneered the use of sympathetic blocks in acute herpes

zoster, noting rapid resolution of the eruptions and a decreased incidence of post-herpetic neuralgia (85). In 1969, Colding studied 300 patients who underwent sympathetic blocks during the acute stage, again noting pain relief and a reduction in the incidence of post-herpetic neuralgia (86). This was later reproduced in 483 patients (84).

Mani et al. studied sympathetic blocks and noted a decrease in the duration of the acute infection if blocks were performed within the first 4 weeks of onset (87). Riopelle et al., in 1984, noted brief and lasting relief with sympathetic blocks but no overall change in the incidence of post-herpetic neuralgia (88). They believed that this was related to the intensity of the acute pain. All patients studied who developed post-herpetic neuralgia had severe pain in the acute phase (88).

Trigeminal and ophthalmic herpes zoster appear to be especially amenable to treatment with sympathetic blocks (89, 90). Ipsilateral bupivacaine 0.25% stellate ganglion blocks within the first 3 weeks have been extremely successful in immediately stopping the pain, and the vesicular lesions crust within 48 hours (90, 91). Early use of stellate ganglion blocks should be considered in all patients with nasociliary ganglion involvement in an attempt to prevent ocular involvement and subsequent complications leading to vision loss (3). This has been duplicated in our own personal experience. When treatment is initiated after 3 weeks, the success rate drops rapidly (82, 91).

Stellate ganglion blocks can be used for facial, cervical, and thoracic lesions to T4. Below T4, the epidural route is preferred for sympathetic block because thoracolumbar paravertebral sympathetic blocks are difficult to perform and have more complications (82).

Interpleural local anesthetic administration for sympathetic blockade over several days had an "impressive therapeutic effect" with rapid resolution of the acute lesions. Seventeen of eighteen patients over age 50 did not develop post-herpetic neuralgia. This is a simple method of blocking somatic and sympathetic nerves to provide pain relief in the acute phase and perhaps lower the incidence of post-herpetic neuralgia (92).

POST-HERPETIC NEURALGIA: RELENTLESS PAIN FOLLOWING ACUTE HERPES ZOSTER

Severe pain during the acute eruptions and especially continuation of pain following resolution of the crusting stage of acute herpes zoster should raise the suspicion of post-herpetic neuralgia. There is evidence that the greater the severity of acute pain, the greater the likelihood of developing post-herpetic neuralgia (88). It is extremely rare for pain to subside and then recur following a period of complete pain remission (J.D. Loeser, personal communication).

The definition of post-herpetic neuralgia varies. Numerous references exist regarding the time frame required before the pain can be classified as post-herpetic neuralgia. These range from pain continuing after the crusting of the lesions (93) to pain lasting longer than 1–2 years following resolution of the acute disease (94). In general, the most common classification of post-herpetic neuralgia requires pain persistence for 4–8 weeks following resolution of the acute stage of herpes zoster (32).

The overall incidence of post-herpetic neuralgia is 18–35% of all herpes zoster patients (95, 96). Age is a major factor in the development of post-herpetic neuralgia and its duration. Herpes zoster is more common in the elderly, their pain is usually more intense with longer duration, and they are more likely to develop post-herpetic neuralgia (96–99). Post-herpetic neuralgia is rarely seen in patients under age 30 and even then usually spontaneously resolves within 1–2 weeks (8). The frequency of occurrence of post-herpetic neuralgia gradually increases to about 10% of all patients under age 50 and usually resolves spontaneously in less than a year. In patients over age 50 the likelihood of developing post-herpetic neuralgia increases dramatically; by age 60, 50% may develop the syndrome with a much lower incidence of spontaneous remission (100). Over age 70, the percentage is increased 1% per year (72). There is no difference in the incidence with regard to sex (101).

Post-herpetic neuralgia is more common following herpes zoster ophthalmicus than following truncal herpes zoster (18). Post-herpetic neuralgia is extremely common following herpes zoster in patients with diabetes mellitus (96, 102).

Spontaneous resolution of symptoms may be seen in 50% of patients within 3 months and in 80% within 1–5 years, although 2% of patients may experience pain for 5 years or more (14).

PATHOPHYSIOLOGY

Post-herpetic neuralgia is a form of deafferentation pain; however, its exact pathogenesis remains obscure (100). There appears to be a degeneration and dysfunction of both central and peripheral neural mechanisms. Although some autonomic characteristics are present, central and peripheral nervous system pathologic changes place post-herpetic neuralgia in the same category as other central/peripheral neurogenic pain syndromes. Patients with post-herpetic neuralgia show major sensory abnormalities mediated by both large- and small-diameter fibers similar to those seen in painful diabetic neuropathy (103). Microscopic examinations in acute herpes zoster patients have demonstrated destruction of peripheral endings, peripheral neural demyelination and axonal destruction, neuronal death in the sensory ganglion with secondary wallerian degeneration in the posterior columns, neural necrosis in areas of the anterior and posterior horn of the spinal cord, and

damage of the spinothalamic tract, thalamus, and sensory cortex. These areas are eventually replaced with areas of neural fibrosis. Although the damage may be extensive, the extent of neurologic damage does not correlate well with predicting the development of post-herpetic neuralgia (12). Pain in this acute phase is thought to be due to an inflammation of the dorsal root ganglion with abnormal dorsal horn discharges (32). In the chronic phase, fibrosis of the dorsal horn and ganglion may cause pain, and this is perpetuated by central mechanisms (32).

Somatosensory studies suggest that both central and peripheral nervous system degenerative changes are present in post-herpetic neuralgia causing sensory loss and pain, although the mechanism remains obscure (103). Several theories have been proposed over the years that attempt to explain the pain mechanisms of post-herpetic neuralgia. In 1959, Noordenbos demonstrated large-fiber demyelination and neural destruction in the peripheral nerve with resulting preponderance of small unmyelinated fibers (104). Intraneural edema and vasoconstriction resulting from the acute inflammation have been implicated in the destruction of these large peripheral fibers (3). Haas described a gate control mechanism of pain based on the destruction of large-fiber modulation in the peripheral nerve (105). He also noted that large-fiber regeneration was much slower than small-fiber regeneration was, and that regenerated large fibers were much smaller than their original size, thus leaving a proportionately larger number of small fibers. Pain carried to the CNS via small unmyelinated fibers is modulated at the cord level by input from large myelinated fibers. It is thought that this large fiber loss results in a loss of inhibitory input to the spinal cord (106). This leads to a relative increase in the sensitivity of small fibers to even light touch. This may help explain the prevalence of this syndrome in the elderly, because their neurophysiologic responses to injury are decreased (107) and they have proportionately fewer large fibers in peripheral nerves than their younger counterparts do (83). Many elderly patients also have small vessel disease that may increase the tendency toward peripheral neural ischemia, which may aggravate this destruction as well as slow recovery from peripheral neural ischemia and edema following the acute phase. Vasoconstriction and ischemia could also explain the efficacy of early sympathetic blocks in disease resolution.

Head and Campbell demonstrated pathologic changes and destruction in the dorsal horn of the spinal cord extending for several segments (108). Wall and Gutnick demonstrated spontaneous activity, increased sensitivity to mechanical stimulation, and increased sensitivity to alpha-adrenergic agonists and sympathetic efferents in experimental nerve transections (109). Chronically deafferentated second-order neurons respond indiscriminately to inputs from adjacent dermatomes. This reafferentation presumably involves activity in the wide-dynamic-range neurons. Recent investigations by Roberts and Foglesong support this and may help explain why the pain of herpes zoster can be lessened by sympathetic blocks (110). They have described peripheral sympathetic stimulation of mechanoreceptors, increasing their sensitivity to light touch. They have also detected this stimulation in wide-dynamic-range neurons in the dorsal horn area. Wide-dynamic-range neuron signals are coded as pain signals arising in the damaged dermatome (111). Spontaneous discharges following loss of peripheral input from this area have been detected (112, 113). These may be responsible for the hyperpathia and paroxysms of pain seen in post-herpetic neuralgia. It is conceivable that this hypersensitivity of peripheral and central transmitters combined with loss of normal large-fiber modulation acts in the production of the pain of post-herpetic neuralgia and the production of a central pain pathway.

As time progresses, the central processes proceed rostrally. Electrical changes have been detected in the midbrain, thalamus, and sensory cortex following peripheral deafferentation (114, 115). As this centralization progresses, pain becomes more resistant to conventional treatment and pain tolerance lessens.

Prolonged pain commonly causes anxiety and profound depression in post-herpetic patients, thereby further reducing endogenous pain control and increasing pain levels (116). Endogenous pain control mechanisms become more ineffective because they are cortically stimulated and negatively influenced by increasing emotional stress.

All of these factors must be considered when developing a treatment regimen.

Symptoms and Pain Characteristics

The pain of post-herpetic neuralgia is usually described as a continuous aching and burning with frequent paroxysms of sharp, shooting pains in a radicular pattern corresponding to the affected dermatome (18). Characteristically there are two discrete elements to post-herpetic pain. The first is a continual aching, burning superficial pain associated with hyperpathia and dysesthesia. This is dramatically increased by light touch. The second is a feeling of constricting tightness along the affected area associated with itching and a feeling of formication. These are accompanied by episodic lancinating pains shooting out in a radicular pattern corresponding to the affected dermatome (18). There is no definite urnal pattern to the occurrence of the hyperpathia and sharp pains, but frequently they are more severe at night, causing interruption of sleep. They can be spontaneous, but are most frequently associated with light touch, especially from clothing (117). Intensity varies but the pain is always present. There are no pain-free intervals. Some movements, light touch, and tem-

perature extremes will aggravate the pain. Often, there is an area in the affected dermatome that, when stimulated, will act as a trigger to the pain. This is usually in one of the hypopigmented areas of scarring. Examination will frequently show decreased sensation to pinprick but hypersensitivity to light touch. Pressure in this area does not increase the pain and, in fact, pressure applied in certain areas may reduce pain by counterirritation (118). Many patients have accidentally discovered this technique and will rub these areas constantly.

Classic physical findings include a unilateral, dermatomal, hypopigmented area of skin that is without sensation to pinprick but extremely painful to light touch (18). There is invariably sensory loss in one or more dermatomal areas in the affected area as well as allodynia (inappropriate sensitivity to tactile stimuli). Patients who develop post-herpetic neuralgia should have sensory changes in addition to pain; pain without sensory changes usually indicates other etiologies such as musculoskeletal problems (103). Virtually all patients have residual scarring with characteristic skin pigmentary changes. Areas of skin between these scars may be extremely hypersensitive. Patients complain of an inability to wear clothing and altered sleep patterns due to paroxysms of severe, sharp, shooting pain superimposed on a baseline continuous, dull, burning ache of varying intensity. They also complain of an associated tightness as if a constricting band was around the area.

Alterations in mood, personality, activity levels, and social interactions are common. Patients are frequently visibly depressed, teary-eyed, and, at times, desperate for even brief relief.

Treatment

There is no known, consistently reliable, preventative therapy or definitive treatment for permanent relief of established post-herpetic neuralgia (10, 101). Much debate exists over the optimal therapy of post-herpetic neuralgia in the literature. Every field of medicine has its own ideas of treatment protocols. Unfortunately, much of the literature evolved over the past 50 years lacks age control, double-blind design, and follow-up. Another problem with selected studies is determining whether relief is from treatment or the natural course of the disease in the specific patient. Spontaneous resolution of pain is possible during treatment, thereby causing false assumptions as to the efficacy of the involved treatment regimen. There are, however, studies that strongly suggest that the best treatment of post-herpetic neuralgia is early, aggressive treatment of acute herpes zoster infections (22). Shortening the duration of the acute viral phase combined with adequate pain relief may act to minimize the potential for post-herpetic sequelae (22). The primary goal in treating established post-herpetic neuralgia should be to afford the patient as much relief as possible until the disease runs its course. This can be as short as 6 months to 1 year and as long as 15–20 years (89).

Antiviral and Anti-Inflammatory Agents

Although these agents perform well in the treatment of acute herpes zoster and have been shown to aid in its prevention, antiviral and anti-inflammatory agents are of minimal benefit in established post-herpetic neuralgia (9). Persistent viral infection has been considered as a cause of post-herpetic neuralgia. In early neuralgia of less than 1 year's duration this may be a consideration. Treatment with acyclovir may prevent further ganglionic damage, although several studies have shown that without obvious evidence of ongoing infection or reinfection, use of antiviral agents in post-herpetic neuralgia is of minimal value (119, 120).

Analgesics

It has been felt that post-herpetic neuralgia often does not respond adequately to traditional narcotic analgesic agents (26, 118). The most frequently prescribed analgesics used in primary-care treatment of post-herpetic neuralgia are usually simple oral analgesics such as codeine-containing combinations, propoxyphene, and non-narcotic synthetic compounds. These are subsequently replaced with stronger narcotic medications. These analgesics may relieve a portion of the pain but are rarely effective in relieving the hyperpathia and dysesthesia (83). Controversy exists over the effectiveness of potent opioids in pain associated with central and peripheral nervous system damage (121). A study of oral codeine (120 mg) showed that this drug's effect did not differ from the analgesic effect of placebo (122).

In 19 patients with post-herpetic neuralgia, intravenous morphine and morphine with lidocaine gave good subjective pain relief, indicating some opioid responsiveness over the short term. Long-term use of controlled dose or scheduled narcotic management has not been adequately studied, but presumably some response may be seen, based on the short-term effects (121). Long-term use of narcotic analgesics for pain in post-herpetic neuralgia is to be discouraged because pain relief is incomplete, tachyphylaxis is common, and the risk of addiction is very real.

Propoxyphene appears to be very effective in the treatment of hyperpathic pain syndromes. A trial of propoxyphene may be beneficial. This should be given at regular 4-hour intervals, rather than as needed, because for best effect, constant blood levels must be obtained.

Antidepressants, Tranquilizers, and Anticonvulsants

Tricyclic antidepressants have been successfully used to treat post-herpetic neuralgia as well as other chronic painful syndromes, and pain relief is considered independent of the antidepressant effect (123). It is believed that tricyclics exert their pain-relieving effect by blocking reuptake of serotonin at serotonergic synapses, and

of norepinephrine in the descending pain-inhibitory pathways existing between the midpons and dorsal horn of the spinal cord (117, 124).

In 1965, Woodforde and associates reported that 11 of 14 patients receiving amitriptyline experienced good to complete pain relief within 2–4 weeks of oral therapy (125). In 1982, Watson and associates performed a double-blind, placebo-controlled crossover study using amitriptyline in post-herpetic neuralgia patients (123). Sixteen of twenty-four patients had good to excellent pain relief with a median dose of 75 mg/day. Serum concentrations were far below therapeutic levels for depression, and pain relief was not considered to be due to the antidepressant effect (123, 126). This is frequently observed in clinical practice, where high-dose tricyclics are relatively ineffective in relieving pain. Institution of therapy should be at low doses of 10–25 mg/day and gradually increased, and one must realize that it may take 2–4 weeks to detect any improvement (9). Drowsiness and dry mouth are frequent side effects and make bedtime administration more practical.

Desipramine is a tricyclic antidepressant that is a potent blocker of norepinephrine reuptake but not serotonin reuptake. It has very few anticholinergic and sedative side effects. In a randomized, double-blind crossover study of 26 post-herpetic neuralgia patients (median age 62, median pain duration 28.5 months), desipramine significantly relieved pain in 12 of 19 (63%) who completed the program. Pain relief was similar in depressed and nondepressed patients, indicating that pain relief was independent of mood elevation. Patients with severe burning pain and allodynia reported benefit. An average dose of 167 mg/day was used. It was felt that the norepinephrine reuptake–blocking effect of desipramine may mediate analgesia (127).

Antidepressants with norepinephrine reuptake–blocking effects (amitriptyline, desipramine, nortriptyline, and clomipramine) have each been shown to relieve neuropathic pain in clinical trials. Zimeldine, a pure serotonin reuptake blocker, does not, suggesting that serotonin reuptake blockade is not essential for tricyclic antidepressant–mediated analgesia. The conclusion of Kishore-Kumar et al. was that desipramine was a good alternative for patients who responded to tricyclic antidepressant analgesia but who were unable to tolerate sedative or anticholinergic side effects (127).

Perhaps the most effective analgesia can be obtained using combination therapy with tricyclic antidepressants and phenothiazine tranquilizers (128–130). In 1973, Taub reported an improved effectiveness of amitriptyline when combined with phenothiazines (perphenazine, fluphenazine, chlorprothixene, or thioridazine) (131). The exact analgesic mechanism of action of phenothiazines is not known. Perhaps it may be due to the dopamine antagonist effects, anxiolytic properties,

Table 41.2.
Some Recommended Doses

Propoxyphene Compound 65	One 3–4 times/day
Amitriptyline	25–75 mg/day
Nortriptyline	50–100 mg/day
Desipramine	50–200 mg/day in divided doses
Fluphenazine (Prolixin)	2–4 mg/day in divided doses
Clonazepam	1–3 mg/day in divided doses
Phenytoin	200–400 mg/day in divided doses
Carbamazepine	500–1000 mg/day in divided doses
Sodium valproate	200 mg 2–3 times/day
Mexiletine	100–300 mg t.i.d. with meals
Chlorprothixene (Taractan)	50 mg q6h for 5 days
Carbidopa-levodopa (Sinemet 25/100)	1 tablet 3 times/day increasing to a maximum of 6 tablets/ day
Baclofen (Lioresal)	5–15 mg 3 times/day
Nifedipine	30–90 mg/day in divided doses

potentiation of tricyclic effects, or some other mechanism (26).

Perhaps the most widely used and clinically most effective phenothiazine is fluphenazine (Prolixin). Initial doses in the range of 2–4 mg/day in combination with amitriptyline appear to be extremely effective in pain reduction. Because elderly patients are most prone to develop tardive dyskinesia, careful consideration should be taken in the use of fluphenazine in this population to avoid extrapyramidal side effects. These effects appear to be reversible when doses under 5–6 mg/day are used. Murphy stated that in 17 years of using the amitriptyline and fluphenazine combination, good pain relief was noted with no cases of tardive dyskinesia, provided medication use was properly monitored (132).

Tricyclic drugs have also been used in combination with anticonvulsants with good results (26). Anticonvulsants such as carbamazepine and phenytoin have been used in the treatment of other neuralgic disorders, such as tic douloureux. Anticonvulsants are thought to produce analgesia by raising the threshold for repetitive firing in first- and second-order neurons involved in nociception (117). Other studies suggest activation of pain-suppression pathways in the CNS (133).

Results using anticonvulsants alone have been limited, and combination therapy with tricyclics is recommended (26). Davis found that carbamazepine relieved only the lancinating pain and not the persistent burning ache (74). In a combination study, Hatangdi et al. administered carbamazepine (600–800 mg) or phenytoin (300–400 mg) with nortriptyline (50–100 mg) in divided doses to 34 patients (128). Of the original 34 patients, 30 (90%) had good to excellent pain relief. Pain relief with a bolus intravenous injection of 1–1.5 mg/kg lidocaine was used as a predictor of response to oral anticonvulsant therapy.

Raftery reported substantial relief with sodium valproate in combination with amitriptyline (75). Amitriptyline seemed to be most effective in reducing the burning and hyperpathia, whereas the sharp, shooting pain responded to sodium valproate.

Side effects of anticonvulsants are more serious and include bone marrow depression, hepatic dysfunction, ataxia, diplopia, confusion, vertigo, nausea, lymphadenopathy, and nystagmus. Combination therapy may also cause urinary retention.

Other Medical Therapies

Baclofen (Lioresal) is another medication that has been used in post-herpetic neuralgia (134). It is a muscle relaxant, antispastic drug that acts by inhibiting both monosynaptic and polysynaptic reflexes at the cord level. Gradual titration of dose to effect is recommended.

Chlorprothixene (Taractan) (135) and carbidopa-levodopa (Sinemet) (136) have also been used but are frequently ineffective if other medication regimens have failed (9).

Numerous other medical therapies have been tried over the years in an effort to effectively treat post-herpetic neuralgia. Oral and topical vitamin E, vitamin B_{12}, B complex, pimozide, ergot derivatives, vincristine iontophoresis, mephenesin, l-tryptophan, protamide, autologous blood transfusion, and even hypnosis all have proponents; however, there is minimal evidence at present to support any degree of improved effectiveness over the previously discussed therapies (18).

In my experience, amitriptyline and fluphenazine in combination with phenytoin or carbamazepine offer the best relief in patients who will respond to oral medication management (Table 41.2). An idealized protocol for management begins with amitriptyline (25–75 mg/day), usually administered at bedtime to take advantage of the sedative effect. Most patients complain of insomnia; tricyclics may help combat this problem. Two to three weeks of treatment are required to evaluate effectiveness of tricyclics in pain relief. If amitriptyline is ineffective alone, fluphenazine (2–4 mg/day in two to three divided doses) is added. Continued burning pain and hyperpathia may respond to gradual increases in amitriptyline over several weeks in increments of 25–50 mg/day either at bedtime or two divided doses (in the morning and at bedtime).

Consideration should be given to anticonvulsants if sharp, intermittent, lancinating pains continue. The effectiveness of anticonvulsants can be evaluated by short-term response to intravenous lidocaine (1.0–1.5 mg/kg administered in a bolus). If this is effective, phenytoin or carbamazepine should be started in the doses listed above.

This is an idealized protocol because most practitioners treating post-herpetic neuralgia begin those three medications simultaneously when the diagnosis is made in order to expedite treatment. Other protocols are available as well (Fig. 41.1). Early aggressive treatment is considered to be most beneficial in providing effective relief (22).

Topical Preparations

Capsaicin (trans-8-methyl-n-vanillyl-6-nonenamide) is a naturally occurring alkaloid found in chili peppers. It is available as a cream for topical application on the skin over the affected dermatomal distribution of post-herpetic pain in concentrations of 0.025% and 0.075%.

Noxious stimuli promote substance P release, which is felt to trigger hyperalgesia, inflammatory tissue responses, prostaglandin E_{-2} release, and the peripheral burning, itching, and hyperesthesia of post-herpetic neuralgia. Capsaicin is a neuroactive peptide that enhances release, prevents reuptake, and promotes depletion of substance P from type C and, to a lesser extent, type A-delta nerve fibers by inhibiting synthesis and reducing axonal transport of substance P to synaptic terminals. It is also theorized that capsaicin may elevate thresholds for release of substance P and other neurotransmitters (137).

Initial release of substance P is accompanied by an increase in burning and stinging with initial application of the cream, but this is transient and should resolve within 20–30 min of the initial application and should lessen as future applications are made. Application of the cream is necessary three to four times daily to produce and maintain pain relief. Less-frequent applications fail to produce total substance P depletion and inhibition, which will produce continued pain on application and reduced drug efficacy. Pain relief should occur within 14–28 days of proper use. With discontinuation of treatment, substance P stores return to normal and neural response returns accordingly.

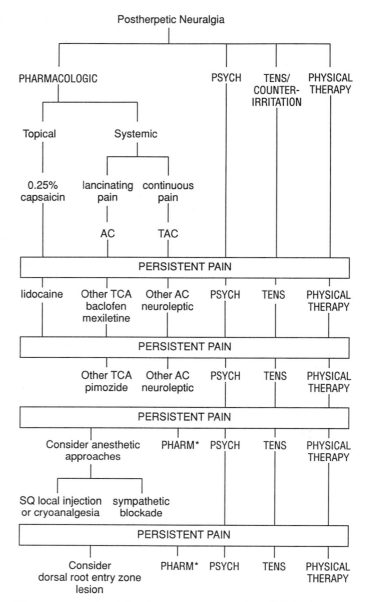

Figure 41.1. **Algorithm for management of established postherpetic neuralgia. Following comprehensive assessment, consideration should be given to use of multimodal approach, beginning with use of pharmacologic, neurostimulatory, psychological, and physiatric techniques. Persistent pain requires sequential drug trials and additional emphasis on psychological and physiatric interventions. Severe refractory pain may ultimately lead to consideration of invasive approaches. Management of patients with difficult disorders may be clarified through evaluation by specialists in a comprehensive multidisciplinary pain management setting. AC, anticonvulsant; TCA, tricyclic antidepressant; PHARM*, any pharmacologic agent that has proved even minimally efficacious should be continued. (From Galer BS, Portendy RK: Acute herpes and postherpetic neuralgia: Clinical features and management.** *Mt Sinai J Med* **58:257–266, 1991.)**

In a randomized, double-blind, vehicle-controlled study of 32 patients (age 54–90, median pain duration 3 years) who had poorly controlled post-herpetic neuralgia lasting 12 months or longer, capsaicin 0.075% was applied locally to painful areas three or four times daily for 6 weeks (138). Using a visual analog scale, results showed partial to complete relief from pain in nearly 80% of patients with chronic intractable post-herpetic neuralgia. These findings were consistent with a subsequent large multicenter trial of 143 patients who reported over 50% long-term improvement in pain (139).

Other topical agents have been tried, including topical lidocaine 5% (140), topical lidocaine 10% (141), EMLA cream (142), aspirin/chloroform (143), aspirin/vaseline (144), indomethacin stupe (145), and aspirin/diethyl ether (146).

The use of topical lidocaine 5% in 45% isopropyl alcohol, 10% glycerine, and 45% water applied under an occlusive dressing gave partial to complete relief of burning pain in 5 patients with repeated applications (140). EMLA cream is a mixture of lidocaine 2.5% base with 2.5% prilocaine emulsion.

Aspirin and nonsteroidal anti-inflammatory drug (NSAID) mixtures in multiple vehicles have shown anywhere from 40% to 90% temporary pain relief in acute and post-herpetic neuralgias when applied over the painful skin areas. Because of their simple application, relative safety, and low toxicity, these preparations may serve a useful role in the symptomatic treatment of acute herpes zoster as well as of post-herpetic neuralgia. Some evidence exists showing reduction in acute lesion healing time and a possible reduction in the occurrence of post-herpetic neuralgia, although controlled trials are needed to prove this.

Nerve Blocks

Nerve blocks are widely used in the management of post-herpetic neuralgia as diagnostic, prognostic, and therapeutic tools (88). The effectiveness of therapeutic nerve blocks in post-herpetic neuralgia appears related to the stage of the disease in which they are used. Early use of nerve blocks may give protracted relief by limiting input into damaged areas of the spinal cord, thus decreasing the potential for development of self-perpetuating central pain mechanisms. This may be especially true in the case of sympathetic blocks. As the syndrome becomes more established, however, nerve blocks become less effective because of centralization of pain-initiating mechanisms (147). Because of the complex pathologic changes in the nerve, spinal cord, and CNS, most relief is transient and the long-term therapeutic effectiveness of nerve blocks alone is minimal because of tachyphylaxis. Unlike acute herpes zoster, in which pain can be effectively managed by local or regional anesthetic blocks, the most beneficial effect in advanced post-herpetic neuralgia is usually temporary relief of severe pain, which allows the patient and physician time to begin other therapeutic measures.

Local Infiltration

Local subcutaneous infiltration of "hot spots" and trigger areas on the skin (areas of intense burning and itching that trigger intense pain when stimulated) appears to be an extremely popular technique. This technique is supported by Moya and associates in Miami (27). The affected areas are outlined and injected with 0.25% bupivacaine with 0.2% triamcinolone or 16 mg dexamethasone in 50 ml of 0.25% bupivacaine. This is injected subcutaneously once or twice a week for 3–4 weeks until relief is obtained. Good relief and low complication rates are cited advantages (27). Early use of this technique may afford prolonged relief and avoid further, more-aggressive therapy (27).

Peripheral Nerve Blocks

Because pain patterns are dermatomal, the most frequently used nerve blocks have been peripheral somatic blocks. These may help to decrease noxious input from damaged nerve fibers and provide transient relief; however, long-term relief is less likely. Repetitive intercostal or paravertebral blocks have been advocated to relieve pain and possibly offer a cure in selected cases. If performed early in the course of the disease process, a series of nerve blocks may provide relief while the syndrome runs its course, but whether the relief obtained is due to the block or to natural resolution of the disease is unknown.

Dorsal root selective nerve blocks are performed to evaluate the effectiveness of dorsal rhizotomy, surgical neurectomy, or chemical neurolysis in the treatment of the disease. Technical difficulty and complications prevent their general use as routine analgesic blocks.

Epidural Blocks

Because of the pathologic changes in the dorsal columns as well as in the peripheral nerves, much attention has been given to the role of epidural blocks in pain management (80, 101). Epidural steroid injections have been used for many years as a treatment modality for radicular pain. In a well-controlled study, Forrest obtained progressive relief of pain using a series of weekly epidural injections over 3 weeks using bupivacaine 0.5% with methylprednisolone 80–120 mg (148). Eighty-six percent of patients were pain-free after 6 months. This was verified with a 1-year follow-up. Perkins and Hanlon studied five patients with post-herpetic neuralgia using bupivacaine 0.25% and methylprednisolone administered epidurally (79). Only one injection was given per patient, and pain relief was reported as less than 50% in all patients. Epidural bupivacaine 0.25% with epinephrine can also provide temporary relief in severe pain (18).

Epidural and Spinal Opiates

Epidural and subarachnoid morphine have been used in the treatment of post-herpetic neuralgia with mixed results. Favorable results have occasionally surfaced, but experience is limited (9).

Sympathetic Blocks

With recent evidence further implicating the sympathetic nervous system in the propagation of post-herpetic neuralgia, sympathetic nerve blocks are becoming more popular in evaluation and treatment (9). Many claims have been made regarding the effectiveness of early sympathetic blocks in relieving post-herpetic pain. For example, Colding found that 50% of 67 patients treated with sympathetic blocks obtained pain relief or marked improvement in pain levels (84). Bonica obtained good relief in a series of paravertebral sympathetic blocks if pain duration was less than 2 months (149).

As mentioned earlier, sympathetic blocks in early herpes zoster have an impressive therapeutic effect, with rapid resolution of the acute illness and prevention of post-herpetic neuralgia. The use of sympathetic blocks early in the post-herpetic phase may also have an improved pain-relief potential. It has been our clinical experience and the experience of others that sympathetic blocks performed within the first 3–6 months of the syndrome's onset greatly improved chances for pain relief or at least diminution of pain to controllable levels. Milligan and Nash reported 77 cases of post-herpetic neuralgia with pain duration of 1 year or less (89). Seventy-five percent were improved and 40% were pain-free following stellate ganglion block. In patients with pain lasting over 1 year, only 44% were improved, with 22% pain-free. All but six patients were over age 60.

Perhaps sympathetic blocks prevent further changes in central pain perpetuation or decrease ongoing pain reflexes, or the response is just coincidence. No matter what the reason, the chances of decreasing future suffering in just one patient justifies the use of sympathetic blocks in all who may be at risk.

We have also clinically noted that recurrent pain following dorsal rhizotomy and peripheral neurectomy frequently responds favorably to sympathetic blocks. The mechanism of this pain relief is unclear at this time, and further study is necessary.

Interpleural Analgesia

Effective, long-lasting pain relief has been shown using infusions of bupivacaine 0.5% via percutaneous interpleural catheters. In a study of 26 patients with post-herpetic neuralgia (mean age 72.2, mean pain duration 3.15 years), pain reduction for 5–15 months was noted following daily infusions of bupivacaine 0.5% (30 ml) with 5 µg/ml epinephrine every 24 hours for 7–21 days.

Good relief was noted in within 20 min of the first injection. The best result were noted with deep pain; superficial burning pain was most resistant. The mechanism of action is thought to be blockade of the affected intercostal nerves as well as of the ipsilateral sympathetic chain (92).

Neuroablative Procedures

Sympathectomy (Chemical and Surgical)

Patients in whom sympathetic blocks have been temporarily effective may respond to oral sympatholytic medications. Regitine, phenoxybenzamine, and guanethadine are the most popular oral agents in the treatment of sympathetic dystrophy and may be tried in post-herpetic patients. Gradual titration of dosage is recommended to avoid hypotensive complications.

Recent information regarding the effectiveness of nifedipine in the management of sympathetic hyperactivity has led to increased use of this drug in reflex sympathetic dystrophy (150). I have used this medication in sympathetic dystrophy with good results. Although we have used it in a few post-herpetic patients, no definite information is yet available as to its overall efficacy in the management of post-herpetic pain.

Patients who respond consistently to sympathetic blocks but fail to maintain relief on medications and continue to have recurrence of pain may be candidates for surgical sympathectomy. Evidence of an effective and consistent response to several previous sympathetic blocks should be mandatory prior to this procedure.

Neurolytic Blocks

Neurolytic blocks have been performed in patients in whom prognostic peripheral or epidural blocks have provided significant pain relief (151). Ethyl alcohol 50%, absolute alcohol, or phenol 6% have been used for neurolysis. Duration of effect ranges from 2 months to 2 years.

Cryoanalgesia

Temporary neurolysis can be obtained using cold-induced lesions of the nerve under direct vision. The nerve is exposed under local anesthesia and frozen. In a small series of patients with trigeminal post-herpetic neuralgia, cryoanalgesia provided about 6 weeks' relief of pain (152). No long-term pain relief was noted.

Dorsal Rhizotomy

Peripheral neurolysis can also be accomplished by radiofrequency rhizotomy of the dorsal root ganglion (9). A prognostic local anesthetic block should be performed prior to rhizotomy. The results of rhizotomies and neurolysis in general have been gratifying with regard to short-term benefits, but long-term effectiveness varies (153). Most relief lasts less than 24 months, and in our experience many of these patients usually return with increasing hyperpathia, burning, and dysesthesia within 6–12 months of treatment. Further deafferentation and centralization of pain origination appear to be responsible for this recurrence of pain (154). Sympathetic stimulation of central pain pathways may also play a role in this recurrence; however, this most likely represents further cord destruction at the second-order neuron level in the dorsal horn (147).

Dorsal Root Entry Zone (DREZ) Lesions

Dorsal root entry zone lesions have been performed in post-herpetic patients in order to relieve long-standing pain (100). This surgical procedure involves radiofrequency destruction of the DREZ of the spinal cord, thereby destroying the damaged dorsal horn and also preventing pain transmission from the peripheral nerve (100). The ablation of second-order neurons in this area of the spinal cord stops the origination of pain from this area. Although initial results were quite promising, subsequent results and long-term follow-up have been less encouraging as to long-term pain relief, especially in patients with advanced post-herpetic neuralgia (D.E. Kennemore, personal communication). This is most likely due, again, to further centralization of the pain process.

Cordotomy

Percutaneous or open cordotomies interrupt ascending pain fibers in the spinothalamic tract. This procedure has occasionally been shown to result in significant pain relief when other modalities have failed (153).

Medullary Tractotomy

Medullary tractotomy divides pain fibers traveling from the orofacial region and replaces cordotomy in craniofacial post-herpetic neuralgia (9). As with cordotomy, tractotomy has the best success rate among surgical procedures for craniofacial pain. There is some risk involved with both procedures. Patients may also have return of their pain within 1–2 years of surgery (9).

Cingulumotomy and Frontal Lobotomy

These surgical procedures alter the central perception of pain but have not been proven particularly effective to date in relieving the pain of post-herpetic neuralgia (155, 156).

Counterirritation Techniques

Transcutaneous Electrical Nerve Stimulation (TENS)

Transcutaneous electrical nerve stimulation has been found to be somewhat effective in providing relief in some patients refractory to other types of treatment (106, 157). In our experience TENS has been effective in pain reduction when the unit is used after adequate skin desensitization. Use of TENS can increase pain if the skin is initially hyperpathic. We have found TENS to be most effective when applied following a series of epidural so-

matic/sympathetic blocks in conjunction with oral medications. Multiple electrode placements may be necessary for optimal relief.

Because of its ease of use, relative lack of side effects, and low cost, a TENS trial is certainly justified.

Dorsal Column and Thalamic Stimulation

A newer form of invasive counterirritation involves implantation of dorsal column or thalamic neural stimulators. These devices are implanted to block pain-conducting pathways and stimulate endorphin production (158). Evidence to date of the effectiveness of these procedures in the treatment or post-herpetic neuralgia is limited.

In a study of 15 patients undergoing epidural spinal cord stimulator placement, 10 patients reported 82.5% pain relief following trial stimulation. Long-term stimulation in these patients showed a slight decrease in relief but still greater than 50% relief. Although complete pain relief was not obtained, pain reduction was significant (159).

Ice Therapy

Local ice therapy and ethyl chloride spray have been used in an attempt to temporarily relieve pain. This is thought to potentiate activation of remaining large fibers, causing inhibition of pain transmission (9). Mechanical vibration and application of tight binders over the area have also been tried to increase large-fiber activity (9).

Acupuncture

Acupuncture has been tried in post-herpetic neuralgia and has been generally found to be of minimal therapeutic value. One well-controlled study concluded that acupuncture was of little or no benefit in this disease (160).

Ultrasonography

Ultrasonography has been used over the affected dermatome in the treatment of post-herpetic neuralgia with minimal success (161). In theory, application of peripheral neural stimulation will replace the large-fiber input into the spinal cord and "close the gate" to pain perception (106). In practice this has not been successful in long-term relief of pain (161).

Psychological Treatment

An especially important aspect in the treatment of post-herpetic neuralgia is psychological and emotional support. Chronic unrelenting pain is a major factor in the destruction of emotional stability. Severe depression is present in over 50% of patients suffering from post-herpetic neuralgia (27). Suicidal thoughts are common. Psychological support is extremely helpful in these patients. Drastic alterations in lifestyle, comfort level, and interpersonal relationships, with limitations to social activities, personal habits, and mobility, aggravate already elevated stress levels. Stress management, relaxation, and counseling can reduce anxiety and help the patient cope with the pain and lifestyle alteration. Behavior modification can prevent the establishment of chronic pain behavior states and allow the patient to adapt and lead a more productive life in spite of discomfort. Unless the chronic pain state is managed, organic treatment will be less successful when psychological stresses potentiate the suffering of the pain experience. Generalized physical deconditioning also accompanies periods of severe pain or illness, and a physical rehabilitation program should be incorporated into the psychological therapy in order to allow the patient to realize that many of his or her limitations are self-imposed.

CONCLUSIONS

Post-herpetic neuralgia is a severe, poorly understood syndrome that affects primarily elderly and debilitated individuals. Treatment of the established syndrome is extremely difficult and minimally successful. The best treatment for this problem appears to be early aggressive treatment of the acute herpes zoster infection, with special attention being paid to those individuals in the high-risk groups for developing post-herpetic neuralgia. Until we understand more about the pathophysiology of post-herpetic neuralgia, aggressive therapy of all herpes zoster patients is the only potential method of successfully treating post-herpetic neuralgia. Accurate predictions as to who will develop post-herpetic neuralgia are impossible. Prevention is the key to eradicating this most severe of chronic pain syndromes.

Should post-herpetic neuralgia occur, an integrated, interdisciplinary treatment regimen should be employed utilizing medical, psychological, and rehabilitation modalities concurrently to provide decreased pain and maximal patient support during the illness.

REFERENCES

1. Ragozzino MW, Melton LJ, Kurland LT, et al: Risk of cancer after herpes zoster. *N Engl J Med* 307:393, 1982.
2. Sklar SH, Blue WT, Alexander EJ, et al: Herpes zoster: The treatment and prevention of neuralgia with adenosine monophosphate. *JAMA* 253:1427–1430, 1985.
3. Winnie AP: Panel on herpes zoster. American Society of Regional Anesthesia 8th Annual Meeting Orlando, FL, March, 1983.
4. Dolin R, Reichman RC, Mazur MH, et al: Herpes zoster–varicella infection in immunosuppressed patients. *Ann Intern Med* 89:35, 1978.
5. Hope-Simpson RE: The nature of herpes zoster: A long term study and a new hypothesis. *Proc R Soc Med* 58:9–20, 1965.
6. Oxman MN: Herpes zoster. In Braude AI, Davis CE, Fierer J (eds): *Medical Microbiology and Infectious Diseases.* Philadelphia, WB Saunders, 1981, pp 1663–1671.
7. Ray CG: Chickenpox (varicella) and herpes zoster. In Petersderf RG, Adams RD, Braunwald E, et al (eds): *Harrison's Principles of Internal Medicine,* ed 10. New York, McGraw-Hill, 1983, pp 1121–1124.
8. Harnisch JP: Zoster in the elderly. Clinical, immunological, and therapeutic considerations. *J Am Geriatr Soc* 22:789–793, 1984.
9. Borowsky S, Shetter AG: Treatment of pain due to herpes zoster infection. *Arizona Med* 42(C1):16–19, 1985.
10. Liesegang TJ: Herpes zoster ophthalmicus. *Int Ophthalmol Clin* 25:77–96, 1985.
11. Ghatak NR, Zimmerman HM: Spinal ganglion in herpes zoster. *Arch Pathol* 95:411–415, 1973.
12. Zacks SI, Langfitt TW, Elliot FAL: Herpetic neuritis. A light and EM study. *Neurology* 14:744–750, 1964.
13. Schimpff S, Serpick A, Stoller B, et al: Varicella-zoster infection in patients with cancer. *Ann Intern Med* 76:241, 1972.
14. Wilkerson MG, Jordan WP, Kerkering TM: Herpes zoster as a sign of AIDS related complex. *Am Fam Phys* 36:232–235, 1987.
15. Friedman-Kien AE, Lafleur FL, Gendler E, et al: Herpes zoster: A possible early clinical sign for development of AIDS in high risk individuals. *J Am Acad Derm* 14:1023–1028, 1986.
16. Ragozzino MW, Melton LJ, Kurland LT, et al: Population-based study of herpes zoster and its sequelae. *Medicine (Baltimore)* 61:310–316, 1982.
17. Gershon AA, Steinberg SP: Antibody responses to varicella-zoster virus and the role of antibody in host defense. *Am J Med Sci* 282:12–17, 1981.
18. Loeser JD: Herpes zoster and postherpetic neuralgia. *Pain* 25:149–164, 1986.
19. Reuler JB, Chang MK: Herpes zoster: Epidemiology, clinical features, and management. *South Med J* 77:1149–1156, 1984.
20. Frengley JD: Herpes zoster—A challenge in management. *Primary Care* 8:715–731, 1981.
21. Gilden DH, Dueland AN, Cohrs R, Martin JR, Kleinschmidt-DeMasters BK, Mahalingam R: Preherpetic neuralgia. *Neurology* 41:1215–1218, 1991.
22. Dickinson JA: Should we treat herpes zoster with costicosteroid agents? *Med J Aust* 144:375–380, 1986.
23. Peto T: Shingles in general practice. *Practitioner* 333:398–403, 1989.
24. Thomas JE, Howard FM: Segmental zoster paresis—A disease profile. *Neurology* 22:459–466, 1972.
25. Malloy MG, Goodwill CJ: Herpes zoster and lower motor neurone paresis. *Rheumatol Rehabil* 18:170–173, 1979.
26. Thompson M, Bones M: Nontraditional analgesics for the management of postherpetic neuralgia. *Clin Pharm* 4:170–176, 1985.
27. Mayne GE, Brown M, Arnold P, Moya F: Pain of herpes zoster and postherpetic neuralgia. In Raj PP (ed): *Practical Management of Pain.* Chicago, Year Book, 1986, pp 345–361.
28. Veien N: Cytologic examination and viral and bacterial culture in herpes simplex, herpes zoster, and varicella. *Cutis* 22:61, 1978.
29. Elliot FA: Treatment of herpes zoster with high doses of prednisone. *Lancet* 2:610–611, 1964.

30. Elliot FA: Shingles. *Lancet* 2:170–171, 1968.
31. Eaglstein WH, Katz R, Brown JA: The effects of early corticosteroid therapy on the skin eruptions and pain of herpes zoster. *JAMA* 211:1681–1683, 1970.
32. Keczkes K, Basheer AM: Do corticosteroids prevent postherpetic neuralgia? *Br J Dermatol* 102:551–555, 1980.
33. Lycka BA: Postherpetic neuralgia and systemic corticosteroid therapy. *Intl J Dermatol* 29:523–527, 1990.
34. (Anonymous): Shingles: A belt of roses from hell [Editorial]. *Br Med J* 1:5, 1979.
35. Juel-Jensen BE: Herpes simplex and zoster. *Br Med J* 1:406–410, 1973.
36. (Anonymous): Disseminated herpes zoster [Editorial]. *JAMA* 188:749, 1964.
37. Juel-Jensen BE, MacCallum FO, McKenzie AMR, Pike MC: Treatment of zoster with idoxuridine in DMSO. Results of double-blind controlled trials. *Br Med J* 4:774–780, 1970.
38. Merselis JG, Kaye D, Hook EW: Disseminated herpes zoster: A report of 17 cases. *Arch Intern Med* 113:679–686, 1964.
39. Mazur MH, Dolin R: Herpes zoster at the N.I.H.: A 20 year experience. *Am J Med* 65:738–744, 1978.
40. Hirsch MS, Schooley RT: Treatment of herpes virus infections Part 1. *N Engl J Med* 309:963–970, 1984.
41. ADIS Editors and Consultants: Acyclovir. A review of its pharmacodynamic properties and therapeutic efficacy. *Curr Ther* 25:13–20, 1984.
42. Selby PJ, Powles RL, Jameson B, et al: Parenteral acyclovir therapy for herpes virus infections in man. *Lancet* 2:1267–1270, 1979.
43. Balfour HH Jr, Bean B, Laskin OL, Ambinder RF, Meyers JD, Wade JL, Zaia JA, Aepplie D, Kirk LE, Segretti AC, Keeney RE, and the Burroughs Wellcome Collaborative Acyclovir Study Group: Acyclovir halts progression of herpes zoster in immunosuppressed patients. *N Engl J Med* 308:1448–1453, 1983.
44. Klenerman P, Peto TEA, Luzzi GA, Juel-Jensen BE: Antiviral treatment and postherpetic neuralgia [Letter]. *Br Med J* 298:332, 1989.
45. Peterslund NA, Ipsen J, Schonheyder H, et al: Acyclovir in herpes zoster. *Lancet* 2:827–830, 1981.
46. Muma RD, Pollard RB: Therapeutics for HIV infection and associated illnesses. *Phys Asst* 16:21–30, 1992.
47. Finn R, Smith MA: Oral acyclovir for herpes zoster [Letter]. *Lancet* 2:575, 1984.
48. McKendrick MW, Case C, Burke C, et al: Oral acyclovir in herpes zoster. *J Antimicrob Chemother* 14:661–665, 1984.
49. Cobo LM, Foulks GN, Liesegang T, et al: Oral acyclovir in the treatment of acute herpes zoster ophthalmicus. *Ophthalmology* 93:763–770, 1986.
50. Wood MJ, Ogan PH, McKendrick MW, et al: Efficacy of oral acyclovir treatment in acute herpes zoster. *Am J Med* 85(Suppl 2A):79–83, 1988.
51. Huff JC, Bean B, Balfour HH Jr, et al: Therapy of herpes zoster with oral acyclovir. *Am J Med* 85(Suppl 2A):84–89, 1988.
52. Morton P, Thomson AN: Oral acyclovir in the treatment of herpes zoster in general practice. *N Z Med J* 102:93–95, 1989.
53. Freestone DS, Brigden WD: Acyclovir and post-herpetic neuralgia [Letter]. *Lancet* 335:1279, 1990.
54. McKendrick MW, McGill JI, Wood MJ: Lack of effect of acyclovir on postherpetic neuralgia. *Br Med J* 298:431, 1989.
55. Whitley RJ, Ch'ien LT, Dolin R, et al: Adenine arabinoside therapy for herpes zoster in the immunosuppressed. *N Engl J Med* 294:1193–1199, 1976.
56. Whitley RJ, Soong SJ, Donlin R, et al (NIAID Collaborative Antiviral Study Group): Early vidarabine therapy to control the complications of herpes zoster in immunosuppressed patients. *N Engl J Med* 307:971–975, 1982.
57. Dawber R: Idoxuridine in herpes zoster: Further evaluation of intermittant topical therapy. *Br Med J* 2:526–527, 1974.
58. Merigan TC, Rand KH, Pollard RB, et al: Human leukocyte interferon for the treatment of herpes zoster in patients with cancer. *N Engl J Med* 298:981–987, 1978.
59. Stevens DA, Merigan TC: Zoster immune globulin prophylaxis of disseminated zoster in compromised hosts. *Arch Intern Med* 140:52–54, 1980.
60. Groth KE, McCullough J, Markes SC, et al: Evaluation of zoster immune plasma—Treatment of cutaneous disseminated zoster in immunocompromised patients. *JAMA* 239:1877–1879, 1978.
61. Sklar SH, Wigand JS: Herpes zoster. *Br J Dermatol* 104:351–352, 1981.
62. Blue WT, Winland RG, Stobbs DG, et al: Effects of adenosine monophosphate on the reactivation of latent herpes simplex virus type-1 infections of mice. *Antimicrob Agents Chemother* 20:547–548, 1981.
63. Sklar SH, Buimovici-Klein E: Adenosine in the treatment of recurrent herpes labialis. *Oral Surg* 48:416–417, 1979.
64. Sklar SH: AMP for acute and postherpetic neuralgia. *Minn Med* 73:11–12, 1990.
65. Galbraith AW: Treatment of acute herpes zoster with amantadine hydrochloride. *Br Med J* 4:693–695, 1973.
66. Galbraith AW: Prevention of postherpetic neuralgia by amantadine hydrochloride. *Br J Clin Pract* 37:304–306, 1983.
67. Balfour RI, Bridenbaugh LD: Postherpetic neuralgia. *Bull Mason Clin* 33:17, 1979.
68. Mavlight GM, Talpaz M: Cimetadine for herpes zoster. *N Engl J Med* 310:318–319, 1984.
69. Talpaz M, Medina JE, Patt YZ, et al: The immune restorative effect of cimetadine administration in vivo on the local graft versus host reaction of cancer patients. *Clin Immunol Immunopathol* 24:155–160, 1982.
70. Rocklin RE, Breard J, Gupta S, Good RA, Melmon KL: Characterization of the human blood lymphocytes that produce a histamine-induced suppressor factor (HSF). *Cell Immunol* 51:226–237, 1980.
71. Jorizzo JL, Sams WM Jr, Jegasothy BV, Olansky AJ: Cimetadine as an immunomodulator: Chronic mucocutaneous candidiasis as a model. *Ann Intern Med* 92:192–195, 1980.
72. Weick JK, Donovan PB, Najean Y, et al: The use of cimetadine for the treatment of pruritis in polycythemia vera. *Arch Intern Med* 142:241–242, 1982.
73. Miller A, Harel D, Laor A, Lahat N: Cimetadine as an

immunomodulator in the treatment of herpes zoster. *J Neuroimmunol* 22:69–76, 1989.

74. Davis EH: Clinical trials of tegretol in trigeminal neuralgia. *Headache* 9:77–82, 1969.

75. Raftery H: The management of postherpetic pain using sodium valproate and amitriptyline. *J Irish Med Assoc* 72:399–401, 1979.

76. Lilley J-P, Su WP, Wang JK: Sensory and sympathetic nerve blocks for postherpetic neuralgia. *Reg Anesth* 11:165–167, 1986.

77. Epstein E: Triamcinolone-procaine in the treatment of zoster and post-zoster neuralgia. *Cal Med* 115:6–10, 1971.

78. Bauman J: Treatment of acute herpes zoster neuralgia by epidural injection or stellate ganglion block. *Anesthesiology* 51:223, 1979.

79. Perkins HM, Hanlon PR: Epidural injection of local anesthetic and steroids for the relief of pain secondary to herpes zoster. *Arch Surg* 113:253–254, 1978.

80. Fothergill WT, Ninaber V, Thick GC: A treatment of herpes zoster. *Practitioner* 229:747–749, 1985.

81. Schreuder M: Pain relief in herpes zoster. *S Afr Med J* 61:820–821, 1983.

82. Cousins MJ, Bridenbaugh PO: *Neural Blockade in Clinical Anesthesia and Management of Pain.* Philadelphia, JB Lippincott, 1980, pp 363, 632.

83. Lipton S: Postherpetic neuralgia. In Lipton S (ed): *Relief of Pain in Clinical Practice.* London, Blackwell Scientific, 1979, pp 231–248.

84. Colding A: Treatment of pain: Organization of a pain clinic. Treatment of acute herpes zoster. *Proc R Soc Med* 66:541–543, 1973.

85. Rosenak S: Procaine injection treatment of herpes zoster. *Lancet* 2:1056–1058, 1938.

86. Colding A: The effect of regional sympathetic blocks in the treatment of herpes zoster. *Acta Anaesthesiol Scand* 13:113–141, 1969.

87. Mani M, Keh L, Lee KN, Winnie AP, Salem R, Collins VS: Sympathetic blockade for herpes zoster. *Am Soc Anesthesiol San Francisco* 4:469, 1976.

88. Riopelle JM, Naraghi M, Grush KP: Chronic neuralgia incidence following local anesthetic therapy for herpes zoster. *Arch Dermatol* 120:747–750, 1984.

89. Milligan NS, Nash TP: Treatment of postherpetic neuralgia. A review of 77 consecutive cases. *Pain* 23:381–386, 1985.

90. Rosenak SS: Paravertebral block for the treatment of herpes zoster. *N Y State J Med* 56:2684–2687, 1956.

91. Winnie AP: The patient with herpetic neuralgia. In Moya F, Gion H (eds): *Postgraduate Seminar in Anesthesiology, Program Syllabus.* Miami Beach, 1983, pp 165–170.

92. Reiestad F, McIlvaine WB, Barnes M, Kvalheim L, Haroldstad P, Pelterson B: Interpleural analgesia in the treatment of severe thoracic postherpetic neuralgia. *Regional Anes* 15:113–117, 1990.

93. Oxman MN: Herpes zoster. In Braude AI, Davis CE, Fierer J (eds): *Medical Microbiology and Infectious Diseases.* Philadelphia, WB Saunders, 1981, pp 1663–1671.

94. Yardley DE, Schwartz RA, Adams HG: Herpes zoster. *Am Fam Physician* 28:138–144, 1983.

95. Kass EH, Aycock RR, Finland M: Clinical evaluation of aureomycin and chloramphenicol in herpes zoster. *N Engl J Med* 246:167–172, 1952.

96. Brown GR: Herpes zoster: Correlation of age, sex distribution, neuralgia and associated disorders. *South Med J* 69:576–578, 1976.

97. Burgoon CF Jr, Burgoon JS, Baldridge GD: The natural history of herpes zoster. *JAMA* 164:265–269, 1957.

98. DeMoragas JM, Kierland RR: The outcome of patients with herpes zoster. *Arch Dermatol* 75:193–196, 1957.

99. Rogers RS III, Tindall FP: Geriatric herpes zoster. *J Am Geriatr Soc* 19:495–504, 1971.

100. Friedman AH, Nashold BS, Ovelman-Levitt J: Dorsal root entry zone lesions for the treatment of postherpetic neuralgia. *J Neurosurg* 60:1258–1262, 1984.

101. Robinson PN, Fletcher N: Postherpetic neuralgia. *J R Coll Gen Pract* 36:24–28, 1986.

102. McCullouch DK, Fraser DM, Duncan LPJ: Shingles in diabetes mellitis. *Practitioner* 226:531–532, 1982.

103. Nurmikko T, Bowsher D: Somatosensory findings in postherpetic neuralgia. *J Neurol Neurosurg Psychiatry* 33:135–141, 1990.

104. Noordenbos W: *Pain. Problems Pertaining to the Transmission of Nerve Impulses Which Give Rise to Pain.* Preliminary Statement. Amsterdam, Elsevier, 1959, pp 6–10.

105. Haas LF: Postherpetic neuralgia, treatment and prevention. *Trans Ophthalmol Soc N Z* 29:133–136, 1977.

106. Nathan PW, Wall PD: Treatment of postherpetic neuralgia by prolonged electrical stimulation. *Br Med J* 3:645–647, 1974.

107. Price RW: Herpes zoster. An approach to systemic therapy. *Med Clin North Am* 66:1105–1118, 1982.

108. Head H, Campbell AW: The pathology of herpes zoster and its bearing on sensory localisation. *Brain* 3:353–523, 1900.

109. Wall PD, Gutnik M: Ongoing activity in peripheral nerves: The physiology and pharmacology of impulses originating from a neuroma. *Exp Neurol* 43:580–593, 1981.

110. Roberts WJ, Foglesong ME: Nociceptive spinal neurons responsive to sympathetically induced afferent activity. Presented at the Annual Meeting of the American Pain Society, Washington, D.C., 1986.

111. Melzack R, Loeser JD: Phantom body pain in paraplegics: Evidence for a central "pattern generating mechanism" for pain. *Pain* 4:195–210, 1973.

112. Loeser JD, Ward AA: Some effects of deafferentation on neurons of the cat spinal cord. *Arch Neurol* 17:629–636, 1976.

113. Loeser JD, Ward AA, White LE: Chronic deafferentation of the human cord neurons. *J Neurosurg* 29:48–50, 1968.

114. Devor M, Wall PD: Reorganization of spinal cord sensory map after peripheral nerve injury. *Nature* 276:75, 1978.

115. Wall PD, Eggerr MD: Formation of new connections in adult rat brain after partial deafferentation. *Nature* 235:542, 1971.

116. Casey KL: The neurophysiologic basis of pain. *Postgrad Med* 53:58–63, 1973.

117. Stein JM, Warfield GA: Herpes zoster and postherpetic neuralgia. *Hosp Pract* 17:96A–960, 1982.

118. Friedman AH, Nashold BS: Dorsal root entry zone lesions for the treatment of postherpetic neuralgia. *Neurosurgery* 15:969–970, 1984.

119. Klenerman P, Luzzi GA: Acyclovir and postherpetic neuralgia. *Biomed Pharmacother* 44:455–459, 1990.

120. Surman OS, Flynn T, Schooley RT, Baer L, Parker S, Hirsch MS, Davis LG: A double blind, placebo controlled study of oral acyclovir in postherpetic neuralgia. *Psychosomatics* 31:287–292, 1990.

121. Rowbotham MC, Reiener-Keller LA, Fields HL: Both intravenous lidocaine and morphine reduce the pain of post-herpetic neuralgia. *Neurology* 41:1024–1028, 1991.

122. Max MB, Schaffer SC, Culnane M, et al: Association of pain relief with drug side effects in postherpetic neuralgia: Single dose study of clonidine, codeine, ibuprofen, and placebo. *Clin Pharmacol Ther* 43:363–371, 1988.

123. Watson PC, Evans RJ, Reed K, et al: Amitriptyline vs placebo in postherpetic neuralgia. *Neurology* 32:671–673, 1982.

124. Lee R, Spencer PJJ: Antidepressants and pain: A review of the pharmacological data supporting the use of certain tricyclics in chronic pain. *J Int Med Res* 5(Suppl 1):146–156, 1977.

125. Woodforde JM, Duyer B, McEwen BW, et al: Treatment of postherpetic neuralgia. *Med J Aust* 2:869–872, 1965.

126. Watson CPN: Therapeutic window for amitriptyline analgesia. *Can Med Assoc J* 130:105–106, 1984.

127. Kishore-Kumar R, Max MB, Schaffer SC, Gaughan AM, Smoller B, Gracely RH, Dubner R: Desipramine relieves post-herpetic neuralgia. *Clin Pharm Ther* 47:305–312, 1990.

128. Hatangdi VS, Boas RA, Richards EG: Postherpetic neuralgia: Management with antiepileptics and tricyclic drugs. In Bonica JJ, Albe-Fessard D (eds): *Advances in Pain Research and Therapy*. New York, Raven Press, 1976, vol 1, pp 583–587.

129. Kocher R: Use of psychotropic drugs for the treatment of severe pain. In Bonica JJ, Albe-Fessard D (eds): *Advances in Pain Research and Therapy*. New York, Raven Press, 1976, vol 1, pp 579–582.

130. Taub A, Collins WR Jr: Observations on the treatment of denervation dysesthesia with psychotropic drugs: Postherpetic neuralgia, anesthesia dolorosa, peripheral neuropathy. In Bonica JJ (ed): *Advances in Neurology*. New York, Raven Press, 1974, vol 4, pp 309–315.

131. Taub AT: Relief of postherpetic neuralgia with psychotropic drugs. *J Neurosurg* 39:235–239, 1973.

132. Murphy TM: Fluphenazine and postherpetic neuralgia [Letter]. *JAMA* 263:2750, 1990.

133. Hitchcock E, Teixeira M: Anticonvulsant activation of pain suppressive systems. *Appl Neurophysiol* 45:582–593, 1982.

134. Steardo L, Leo A, Marano E: Efficacy of baclofen in trigeminal neuralgia and some other painful conditions. A clinical trial. *Eur Neurol* 23:51–55, 1984.

135. Nathan PW: Chlorprothixene (Taractan) in postherpetic neuralgia and other severe chronic pains. *Pain* 5:367–371, 1978.

136. Kernbaum S, Hauchecorne J: Administration of levodopa for relief of herpes pain. *JAMA* 246:132–134, 1981.

137. Brorson JR, Bleakman D, Miller RJ: Capsaicin reduces voltage-gated calcium currents in sensory neurons. *Neurology* 40(Suppl 1):232, 1990.

138. Bernstein JE, Korman NJ, Bickers DR, Dahl MV, Millikan LE: Topical capsaicin treatment of chronic postherpetic neuralgia. *J Am Acad Derm* 21:265–270, 1989.

139. Gen Derm Study 84-04/87-11. Gen Derm Corp., Lincolnshire, IL.

140. Kissin I, McDanal J, Xavier AV: Topical lidocaine for relief of superficial pain in postherpetic neuralgia. *Neurology* 39:1132–1133, 1989.

141. Rowbotham MC, Fields HL: Topical lidocaine reduces pain in postherpetic neuralgia. *Pain* 39:297–301, 1989.

142. Stow PJ, Glynn CJ, Minor B: EMLA cream in the treatment of postherpetic neuralgia. Efficacy and pharmacokinetic profile. *Pain* 39:301–305, 1989.

143. King RB: Concerning the management of pain associated with herpes zoster and postherpetic neuralgia. *Pain* 33:73–78, 1988.

144. Kassirer MR: King and Robert, Concerning the management of pain associated with herpes zoster and postherpetic neuralgia. *Pain* 35:368–369, 1988.

145. Morimoto M, Inamori K, Hyodo M: The effect of indomethacin stupe for postherpetic neuralgia—particularly in comparison with chloroform-aspirin solution. *Pain Suppl* 5:59, 1990.

146. deBenedittis GD, Besana F, Lorenzetti A: A new topical treatment for acute herpes neuralgia and postherpetic neuralgia: The aspirin/diethyl ether mixture. An open label study plus a double-blind controlled clinical trial. *Pain* 48:383–390, 1992.

147. Sweet WH: Deafferentation pain after posterior rhizotomy, trauma to a limb, and herpes zoster. *Neurosurgery* 15:928–932, 1984.

148. Forrest JB: Management of chronic dorsal root pain with epidural steroid. *Can Anaesth Soc J* 25:218–225, 1978.

149. Bonica JJ: Thoracic segmental and intercostal neuralgia. In Bonica JJ (ed): *The Management of Pain*. Philadelphia, Lea & Febiger, 1953, pp 861–867.

150. Prough DS, McLeskey CH, Poehling GP, Koman LA, Weeks DB, Whitworth T, Semble EL: Efficacy of oral nifedipine in the treatment of reflex sympathetic dystrophy. *Anesthesiology* 62:796–799, 1985.

151. Neuendorf TL: Epidural phenol in the treatment of postherpetic neuralgia. *J Am Osteopath Assoc* 86:75–77, 1986.

152. Barnard D, Lloyd J, Evans J: Cryoanalgesia in the management of chronic facial pain. *J Maxillofac Surg* 9:101–102, 1981.

153. White JC, Sweet WH: *Pain and the Neurosurgeon: A Forty-Year Experience*. Springfield, IL, Charles C Thomas, 1969, pp 380–386, 472, 477.

154. Denny-Brown D, Adams RD, Fitzgerald PJ: Pathologic features of herpes zoster: Note on "geniculate herpes." *Arch Neurol Psychiatry* 51:216–231, 1944.

155. Hitchcock ER, Schvarez JR: Stereotaxic trigeminal tractotomy for postherpetic facial pain. *J Neurosurg* 37:412–417, 1972.

156. Sugar O, Bucy PC: Postherpetic trigeminal neuralgia. *Arch Neurol Psychiatry* 65:131–145, 1951.

157. Lond D: Pain of peripheral nerve injury. In Youman JR (ed): *Neurological Surgery*. Philadelphia, WB Saunders, 1982, pp 3634–3643.

158. Mundinger F, Salamao JF: Deep brain stimulation in mesoencephalic lemniscus medialis for chronic pain. *Acta Neurochir Suppl* 30:245–258, 1980.

159. Meglio M, Cioni B, Prezioso A, Talamanti G: Spinal cord stimulation (SCS) in the treatment of postherpetic pain. *Acta Neurochirurg* 46(Suppl):65–66, 1989.

160. Lewith GT, Field J, Machin D: Acupuncture compared with placebo in postherpetic neuralgia. *Pain* 17:361–368, 1983.

161. Payne C: Ultrasound for postherpetic neuralgia. A study to investigate the results of treatment. *Physiotherapy* 70:96–97, 1974.

Chapter 42
Chronic Joint and Connective Tissue Pain
ROGER B. TRAYCOFF

Successful management of pain in patients with rheumatic diseases requires an awareness that pain is both an experience and a sensation. We observe pain behavior, not pain. The behavior may or may not be appropriate for the intensity of the nociceptive stimulus. It is affected by both past experience and environmental reinforcers. Failure to recognize the importance of these psychological factors may lead to inappropriate therapy. Treatment should be disease-, rather than symptom-oriented. Empiric therapy is seldom appropriate, often leading to suboptimal results.

The two major determinants of pain behavior are the intensity of the stimulus and the patient's interpretation of the meaning of the pain. When dealing with patients who have rheumatic diseases, the source of nociception is usually obvious. Physicians tend to focus on physical findings, being disease- rather than patient-oriented. The question of somatization is seldom raised, and the emotional component of pain behavior may not be considered.

To optimally manage patients with rheumatic diseases, one must understand the natural history of the disease untreated and the psychological and socioeconomic consequences of having a chronic debilitating illness. Patients are driven by both learned behavior and previous interaction with health care providers. The importance of the patient-physician relationship cannot be overemphasized. Patient satisfaction and compliance with therapy are affected by how they perceive their disease and their expectations regarding treatment and outcome.

Most failures in the management of pain due to rheumatic disease arise from (1) the physician's inability to make a correct diagnosis, (2) the physician's failure to educate the patient (3) the patient's noncompliance with therapeutic regimens, and (4) the physician's inappropriate use of analgesic drugs. Successful management of pain requires that physicians have an understanding of disease mechanisms, knowledge of drug pharmacoki-

netics and pharmacodynamics, and a sense of the patient's beliefs. More importantly, one must recognize the limitations of current treatments and the need for a conservative approach to management. It some instances, a physician may not have enough data to permit one to make rational choices regarding treatment. For example, it would be inappropriate to administer potentially toxic drugs to patients early in the course of their disease, when there is a high probability of spontaneous remission. Similarly, it would be incorrect to use symptom-directed therapy in patients with chronic progressive illnesses.

In the most basic construct, pain associated with rheumatic disease can be divided into (1) inflammatory or noninflammatory arthritis and (2) systemic or localized disease, based on pathophysiology. Treatment should be directed at the cause of the pain. Pain arising from inflammation should be treated with anti-inflammatory drugs rather than simple analgesics or opiates. Nonsteroidal anti-inflammatory drugs (NSAIDs) and the salicylates are prototypic drugs having both anti-inflammatory and analgesic properties. They are most effective in treating inflammation arising as a consequence of the release of prostaglandins and leukotrienes, however. In contrast, corticosteroids have no intrinsic analgesic properties. Relief of pain following treatment with corticosteroids is due to their anti-inflammatory effects. Disease-modifying agents such as gold compounds, penicillamine, and methotrexate have no intrinsic analgesic properties. Pain relief arises from suppression of inflammation through alteration of the underlying disease process.

NSAIDs are the mainstay of therapy of inflammatory joint disease, having both analgesic and anti-inflammatory properties. It appears that the NSAIDs are most effective in the presence of prostaglandin-mediated pain. For this reason, they are more correctly classified as anti-algesics than analgesics; NSAIDs act by raising the threshold for firing of free nerve endings. They do not alter neural transmission or the response to the nociceptive stimulus (1).

One's choice of simple analgesic is usually dictated by individual preference rather than differences among the various classes of drugs. There is little evidence to support the use of simple analgesics such as acetaminophen, codeine, or propoxyphene in the treatment of pain associated with synovitis. There are data, however, that show that acetaminophen is as effective as NSAIDs in the treatment of noninflammatory joint disease (2).

Using opiates to treat pain of rheumatic origin is inappropriate. Opiates can cause physical dependence and addiction. The short-term benefit of use is far outweighed by problems associated with physical dependence and loss of efficacy over time. Potent opiates such as morphine and meperidine are rarely used for treating rheumatic diseases except in the presence of major trauma. Even then, most musculoskeletal pain will respond to immobilization and therapy with anti-inflammatory drugs.

One must establish a doctor-patient relationship that promotes wellness and discourages dependency. In discussions with the patient, physicians should not be overly optimistic or pessimistic. Undue optimism will create unrealistic expectations, whereas excessive pessimism will cause patients to seek alternative care, often becoming prey to the purveyors of unproven remedies.

The major variables when treating pain are (1) the underlying disease process, (2) the patient's expectations regarding both outcome and response to therapy, and (3) the drugs available for use. Having a correct diagnosis is a prerequisite for providing effective care. Pain not associated with inflammation can be treated with either acetaminophen, low-dose salicylates, or NSAIDs. Psychotropic drugs such as benzodiazepines and tricyclic antidepressants are used as adjunctive therapy, recognizing that their effects are primarily symptom directed. Tricyclic antidepressants, used to treat depression and "fibrositis-like" symptoms, are particularly useful when treating patients with nonarticular rheumatism (3). Benzodiazepines such as diazepam should only be used for treating patients with "trait anxiety" (3). They are not appropriate for chronic use because of their potential to cause physical dependence. Drug-seeking behavior will increase rather than decrease pain behavior.

When treating patients with rheumatic diseases, the goals are to relieve pain, preserve function, and prevent joint destruction. Pain of inflammatory joint disease is best achieved by controlling inflammation. Educating and encouraging patients to participate in the treatment process will ensure compliance. Emphasis on wellness and promoting the concept of self-help are important adjuncts to pharmacotherapy. Referrals to allied health personnel such as physical therapists and occupational therapists, as well as use of arthritis support groups, should be incorporated into the treatment plan. Reliance on drug therapy alone should be discouraged because outcome may relate to variables other than pain control.

APPROACH TO DIAGNOSIS

The history and physical examination remain the cornerstones of the diagnostic process. Having a correct diagnosis is a prerequisite for optimal therapy. An empiric approach to management is seldom appropriate; it may lead to either over- or under-treatment. Therapy should be disease-specific as well as symptom-directed.

Being able to localize the anatomic source of pain is invaluable to the diagnostic process. One must determine whether the pain is articular, periarticular, muscular, or neurogenic in origin. The pain of rheumatic disease is most often articular in origin. It is characteristically associated with decreased and painful range of motion. Erythema and swelling are often seen when examining appendicular joints. Axial joints such as hips and shoulders seldom have clinical evidence of synovitis.

The absence of confirmatory physical findings does not preclude a physical basis for pain. The diagnosis of psychogenic pain is suggested by finding inconsistencies in either the history or the physical examination. Although psychogenic pain is rare, somatization with exaggerated pain behavior is not uncommon. Somatoform disorders and somatic pain can coexist. Pain is as much an experience as a sensation, being affected by learned behavior, environmental reinforcers, and secondary gain.

When it is difficult to distinguish articular from periarticular pain syndromes, the patient's response to intra-articular injection of local anesthetic can help define the anatomic source of pain. Failure to relieve pain with intra-articular injection of local anesthetic is evidence against the diagnosis of arthritis, assuming there is no coexistent extra-articular source for pain. When the response to intra-articular injection of local anesthetic is unclear, selective infiltration of extra-articular structures with local anesthetics can be of great diagnostic value, confirming or refuting the presence of tendinitis, bursitis, or enthesopathy.

It is also important to determine whether the patient's response to the nociceptive stimulus is appropriate. The patient's complaints should be taken at face value; pain is whatever the patient says it is. One must always remember that therapy should be disease- rather than symptom-directed, however. The goals are to decrease suffering and to treat the underlying disease process.

HISTORY AND PHYSICAL EXAMINATION

The medical history is the keystone of the diagnostic process. The history will suggest whether the disease is (1) systemic or regional, (2) acute or chronic, (3) inflammatory or noninflammatory, or (4) psychogenic in etiology. The patient's description of his or her pain is important. Articular and bursal pain are usually described as aching, cramping, or throbbing. Neuritic pain is characterized by numbness, tingling, or burning. The presence of hyperesthesia, dysesthesia, and allodynia suggests either deafferentation pain or reflex sympathetic dystrophy.

The relationship of pain to physical activity is also important. Pain that is present only with activity suggests a mechanical or vascular etiology. Pain present both with activity and at rest is often inflammatory. Pain that is worse at night or during periods of rest should suggest the possibility of tumor, infection, or neuropathy. Pain that is unrelated to position or activity and not responsive to therapy should suggest the possibility of deafferentation or psychogenic pain.

A systematic review of systems will provide a basis for distinguishing among the rheumatic diseases. A history of weight loss, photosensitivity, Raynaud's phenomenon, dermatitis, or polyserositis should suggest the diagnosis of systemic lupus erythematosus, or a variant. A history of ocular or genitourinary symptoms should suggest the diagnosis of Reiter's syndrome. A history of diarrhea or abdominal pain should raise the possibility of enteropathic or reactive arthritis. Complaints of back pain or stiffness not relieved by rest should suggest the diagnosis of spondyloarthropathy.

The physical examination can confirm and characterize abnormalities suggested by the history. It should be performed in a systematic and thorough manner. The examiner should look for joint swelling, articular tenderness, decreased range of joint motion, and deformities. Extra-articular manifestations of rheumatic diseases should be sought because of their diagnostic importance. Cutaneous involvement is a feature of psoriatic arthritis, Reiter's syndrome, systemic lupus erythematosus, and systemic vasculitis. Finding subcutaneous nodules should suggest the diagnoses of rheumatoid arthritis, rheumatic fever, or amyloidosis. Conjunctivitis and iritis are features of spondyloarthropathies such as Reiter's syndrome, ankylosing spondylitis, and enteropathic arthritis. Finding tophi is diagnostic of gout. Pitting of the nails is a sign of psoriatic arthritis, and clubbing a clue to hypertrophic osteoarthropathy. The presence of enthesopathy, tenosynovitis, or axial skeleton involvement should suggest the diagnosis of spondyloarthropathy. Decreased range of motion of the lumbar spine and decreased chest expansion are clues to ankylosing spondylitis.

LABORATORY ANALYSES

Laboratory studies should be used to confirm rather than make diagnoses. None of the available serologic tests for rheumatic diseases have perfect sensitivity or specificity. The basic laboratory evaluation should include an erythrocyte sedimentation rate (ESR), hemogram, urinalysis, and chemical profile or its equivalent. In general, an elevated ESR confirms the presence of an inflammatory process. Anemia is both a clue to systemic disease and a marker for chronicity. The finding of autoimmune hemolytic anemia suggests the diagnosis of systemic lupus erythematosus. Leukopenia and thrombocytopenia are features of systemic lupus erythematosus; their presence would be evidence against the diagnosis of rheumatoid arthritis, with the exception of Felty's syndrome. The finding of hypercalcemia in a patient with rheumatic complaints should suggest the diagnosis of hyperparathyroidism, and the possibility of pseudogout. Hyperuricemia, although not diagnostic of gout, is a helpful clue to urate arthropathy. The finding of proteinuria or hematuria on urinalysis should suggest the possibility of glomerulonephritis due to systemic lupus erythematosus or vasculitis. Nephrotic syndrome is also a characteristic feature of amyloidosis, especially when associated with an underlying lymphoproliferative disorder.

Serologic studies such as rheumatoid factors, antinuclear antibodies, tissue typing with human leukocyte antigens (HLAs), and serum complement levels may be helpful in the differential diagnosis of rheumatic diseases. Rheumatoid factors are markers for chronic antigenic stimulation. They are not a specific marker for rheumatoid arthritis, being found in other autoimmune diseases, including systemic lupus erythematosus, scleroderma, Sjögren's syndrome, polyarteritis nodosa, mixed connective tissue disease, and amyloidosis. Rheumatoid factors have also been identified in patients with chronic infections, patients with chronic liver disease, and in the elderly with no identifiable underlying disease process. The major value of the rheumatoid factor is its ability to distinguish rheumatoid arthritis and other connective tissue diseases from the spondyloarthropathies. The presence of a rheumatoid factor in the serum of patients presenting with rheumatic complaints makes the diagnosis of spondyloarthropathy unlikely.

Testing for antinuclear antibodies (ANAs) by indirect immunofluorescence is a useful screen for systemic lupus erythematosus; however, the ANA test lacks specificity. Antinuclear antibodies are found in sera of patients with scleroderma, mixed connective tissue disease, rheumatoid arthritis, and autoimmune liver disease. Antinuclear antibodies are often drug-induced, occurring in the absence of disease. A positive test for ANAs is not diagnostic of systemic lupus, but a negative result in a symptomatic patient is good evidence against the diagnosis. Patients whose test for ANAs is positive should have additional studies performed. Testing for antibodies against ribonucleoprotein (RNP), Smith antigen (Sm), and soluble cytoplasmic antigens (SSA and SSB) can be helpful.

Synovial fluid analysis has an important role in the diagnosis of arthropathies. Joint fluid should be routinely sent for white cell and differential counts, and for compensated polarized microscopy to screen for the presence of crystals. Gram's stain of the aspirate as well as culture and measurement of lactic acid levels in the synovial fluid should be ordered when infection is a consideration. Measurements of synovial fluid protein, glucose, and complement levels are of less value, often adding little to diagnostic process. Tissue typing for the presence of HLA-B27 is of little value as a screening test for the spondyloarthropathies. The high prevalence of HLA-B27 in the normal population limits its specificity. Up to 8% of the white population is HLA-B27–positive. The absence of HLA-B27 also has limited diagnostic value because a significant percentage of patients with spondyloarthropathies are HLA-B27–negative.

Measurements of serum complement levels have limited diagnostic value. In most rheumatic diseases, the serum complement levels are normal or elevated. The presence of hypocomplementemia may be a clue to the presence of immune complex disease. Usually one measures the total hemolytic complement level (CH_{50}), and the C3 and C4 component levels. A very low total hemolytic complement level is a marker for hereditary complement deficiencies. A low C3 level with a normal C4 level should suggest alternative pathway activation. A low C4 level with either a normal or low C3 level should suggest classic pathway activation as seen with immune complex disease.

DRUG THERAPY

SIMPLE ANALGESICS

Acetaminophen, dextropropoxyphene, and codeine are useful in the treatment of noninflammatory rheumatic pain; however, there is little evidence to support their use in treating inflammatory joint disease. They are often used empirically as single agents or in combination with other drugs. Acetaminophen is frequently used for treating mild to moderate pain. Codeine and propoxyphene are often reserved for treating patients with more-severe pain on the mistaken assumption that they are more effective analgesics. When used in recommended doses, they are no better analgesics than either aspirin or acetaminophen.

As a rule, codeine and propoxyphene should not be administered as single agents. Acetaminophen or aspirin combined with codeine or propoxyphene are the favored formulations. A combination of a peripheral acting drug with a central acting drug provides better analgesia than either agent used alone (5). Combining aspirin with acetaminophen or aspirin with an NSAID, however, is no more effective than using maximal recommended doses of each agent alone. Pain relief from combining NSAIDs is usually not additive, but the side effects appear to be increased in frequency and severity.

Acetaminophen, a central- and peripheral-acting analgesic, has an excellent efficacy–side effect profile (6). It is most often administered to patients who are intolerant of NSAIDs; it has been shown to be as effective as ibuprofen in the treatment of degenerative joint disease (2). Its role in the treatment of pain associated with inflammatory joint disease is less well defined. Intuitively, it would appear more reasonable to use an anti-inflammatory drug in this setting.

The major limitation of acetaminophen is its flat dose-response curve. In single-dose studies, increasing the dose of acetaminophen beyond 1000 mg provides no additional analgesia. Daily doses greater than 4000 mg have been associated with hepatotoxicity (7). Patients who chronically abuse alcohol appear to be at greatest risk for the development of hepatic necrosis.

Acetaminophen can be used in combination with codeine or propoxyphene to provide short-term analgesia. The major problems with using analgesic combinations containing opiate derivatives are the development of tolerance and physical dependence. Addiction is a real but most likely overstated risk.

SALICYLATES

For many years, salicylates have been the favored drug for treating inflammatory joint disease. Salicylates have anti-inflammatory, antipyretic, and analgesic properties. Although none of the newer NSAIDs have been shown to be superior to aspirin in the treatment of rheumatoid arthritis, the efficacy of aspirin for treating other inflammatory arthropathies is less clear. Aspirin may be less effective for treating patients with Reiter's syndrome or ankylosing spondylitis. The pain associated with gout and pseudogout also appears to respond better to NSAIDs than to salicylates.

Many formulations of salicylates are available (Table 42.1), yet aspirin remains the salicylate of choice in most instances. The major advantages of using nonaspirin salicylates are ease of administration, better patient tolerance, and fewer side effects. The major disadvantages are greater cost, less-flexible dosing schedules, and unpredictable absorption when administered orally.

Both the analgesic and the anti-inflammatory effects of aspirin have flat dose-response curves. Analgesic doses of aspirin range from 650 to 1000 mg; anti-inflammatory doses range from 3.5 to 5.0 g daily. A therapeutic blood level for anti-inflammatory effects is between 15 and 20 mg/dl.

Data are lacking on the relationship between analgesia and salicylate blood levels in the absence of inflammation. Pain relief in inflammatory joint disease is probably due to the anti-inflammatory rather than analgesic effects of salicylate. When treating pain with low doses of aspirin, it should be administered every 4 hours. As the dose is increased, the elimination half-life increases; hepatic enzymes become saturated. At higher doses, the

Table 42.1.
Salicylates Used in Treatment of Inflammatory Joint Disease

Drug	Dose (mg)	Daily Dose (mg)	Frequency
Aspirin	325	2500–5000	q.i.d.
Encaprin	325		b.i.d.
	500		
Easprin	975		q.i.d.
Cama	500		q.i.d.
Ascription	325		q.i.d.
Ecotrin	325		q.i.d.
Salts of salicylic acid			
Choline salicylate (Arthropan)	325	300–5000	q.i.d.
Choline magnesium trisalicylate (Trilisate)	500	3000	b.i.d.
Salicylsalicylic acid (Disalcid)	500, 750	3000	b.i.d.
Diflunisal (Dolobid)	500	1000	b.i.d.

aspirin can be administered as infrequently as every 8–12 hours (8). The exponential increase in salicylate blood levels seen with increasing dose means that small changes in doses can cause large changes in salicylate blood levels. Increasing the daily dose of aspirin by one or two tablets may result in toxicity. Tinnitus, although a useful marker for salicylate toxicity, may not be present in all cases. Therefore salicylate blood levels should be measured in children and the elderly.

There are few data to support the use of salicylates and NSAIDs concurrently. It does not appear that combining aspirin with an NSAID will increase efficacy. The side effects may be greater when used in combination. The lack of synergism may be related to altered pharmacokinetics. The significance of these interactions is unknown, however, Aspirin will decrease the absorption of fenoprofen and indomethacin.

The newer salicylates such as salicylate and choline magnesium trisalicylate have a better side effect profile than aspirin but have not been shown to be more efficacious. They appear to cause less gastric mucosal damage than aspirin and not to adversely affect platelet function. They are most often used in patients who are intolerant of NSAIDs because of gastric irritation or ulcer.

NONSTEROIDAL ANTI-INFLAMMATORY DRUGS

When treating rheumatoid arthritis, the choice between salicylates and NSAIDs is a matter of preference; none of the NSAIDs has been shown to be superior to aspirin in analgesic or anti-inflammatory effects (9). This may not be true for other rheumatic diseases, however. For example, aspirin is not very effective in treating crystal-induced synovitis and appears to be less effective than NSAIDs in the treatment of spondyloarthropathies.

The role of newer NSAIDs such as ketorolac in the treatment of rheumatic pain is undefined. There are few data to support its use in either osteoarthritis or inflammatory joint disease. Its side effect profile appears to be similar to that of other NSAIDs and therefore may add little to the treatment of pain associated with inflammatory joint disease.

A major limitation of NSAIDs is their flat dose-response curves; increasing the dose beyond the recommended level may not increase efficacy. This reflects the fact that they may act on only one component of the inflammatory response (i.e., inhibition of prostaglandin synthesis) (10).

NSAIDs appear to differ more in pharmacokinetics than in pharmacodynamics (Table 42.2). Drugs such as ibuprofen, fenoprofen, tolmetin, flubiprofen, and meclofenamate have short elimination half-lives, and must be administered every 6–8 hours. Sulindac, naproxen, and diclofenac have longer elimination half-lives and can be given twice a day. Piroxicam and nabumetone, having the longest elimination half-lifes, can be administered once daily.

Many of the side effects of treatment with NSAIDs relate to inhibition of prostaglandin synthesis (11). The side effect profiles of all NSAIDs are similar, and are dose-related. Nabumetone and meclofenamate may be exceptions. Nabumetone may have fewer gastrointestinal side effects because it is a pro-drug whose active metabolite has no enterohepatic recirculation. Meclofenamate is unique in having a greater tendency to cause diarrhea.

All NSAIDs are potentially ulcerogenic. The risk of ulcer formation appears to be directly related to dose and duration of therapy. Phenylbutazone and indomethacin are thought to be more ulcerogenic than other NSAIDs, which may relate to their potency as inhibitors of mucosal cyclo-oxygenase. The risk of gastric ulcer appears to be less with salicylate and nabumetone.

Table 42.2.
Pharmacokinetics of Nonsteroidal Anti-Inflammatory Drugs

Duration of Action	Recommended Daily Dose (mg)
Short-acting	
Etodolac (Lodine)	300–1200
Fenoprofen (Nalfon)	1200–2400
Ketorolac (Zoradol)	40–60
Kectoprofen (Orudis)	150–300
Ibuprofen (Motrin, Rufin)	1200–3200
Indomethacin (Indocin)	75–200
Tolmetin (Tolectin)	800–1600
Meclofenamate (Meclomen)	200–400
Nabumetone (Relafen)	1000–2000
Intermediate-acting	
Diclofenac (Voltaren)	150–300
Naproxen (Naprosyn)	730–1000
Sulindac (Clinoral)	300–600
Long-acting	
Piroxicam (Feldene)	10–20
Phenylbutazone (Butazolidin)	300–400

Table 42.3.
Corticosteroids Used in Treatment of Inflammatory Joint Disease

Duration of Action	Relative Potency	Equivalent Doses (mg)
Short-acting		
Hydrocortisone	1	20
Prednisone	4	5
Methylprednisolone	4	4
Intermediate-acting		
Triamcinolone	5	4
Long-acting		
Betamethasone	25	0.6
Dexamethasone	30	0.75

All of the NSAIDs have the potential for causing bronchospasm in salicylate-sensitive asthmatics. Those who wheeze when taking aspirin will tend to wheeze when given other NSAIDs. This may relate to inhibition of prostaglandin E (PGE), which acts as a bronchodilator. Fortunately, only a small percentage of patients appear to be aspirin-sensitive, and therefore NSAIDs can be used safely in many patients.

As a group, all of the NSAIDs appear to adversely affect renal function by decreasing prostaglandin-dependent renal blood flow. Indomethacin may have a greater potential for decreasing renal blood flow than other NSAIDs. The question of sulindac having the least effect on renal blood is in dispute (12). Patients with compromised renal function from either volume contraction or intrinsic renal disease are at greatest risk for the development of azotemia. Diabetics may develop hyperkalemia as a consequence of hyporeninemic hypoaldosteronism caused by inhibition of PGE synthesis. Renal impairment due to hypersensitivity reactions is less predictable. Immune-mediated nephropathy can be caused by any of the NSAIDs but is more commonly seen in patients treated with fenoprofen. Patients who develop edema while taking aspirin will usually be intolerant of other NSAIDs. Phenylbutazone is unique in that it promotes fluid retention by two different mechanisms: inhibition of prostaglandin synthesis and an aldosterone-like effect on renal tubules.

CORTICOSTEROIDS

Corticosteroids are potent anti-inflammatory agents, but have no intrinsic analgesic properties. They are only useful for treating pain associated with inflammation. Corticosteroids do not appear to prevent joint destruction or alter disease progression. When treating rheumatoid arthritis, they are most often used in conjunction with remittent drugs. Their ability to relieve pain is well established but the appropriateness of their long-term use is still debated.

The major risks associated with chronic use of corticosteroids are osteoporosis, avascular necrosis of bone, hypertension, glucose intolerance and cataract formation. There is no evidence that one class of corticosteroid is more efficacious or less toxic than another. Differences in side effects and efficacy relate more to differences in tissue half-life and potency than to mechanism of action. (Table 42.3) Dexamethasone, the most potent corticosteroid, has the longest elimination half-life and therefore the longest duration of action.

Many physicians prefer using short-acting corticosteroids such as prednisone and prednisolone. Shorter acting corticosteroids are favored because they may have less risk of suppressing the hypothalamic-pituitary-adrenal (HPA) axis. The side effects of corticosteroids appear to be dose-related. When using prednisone or its equivalent at doses less than doses of 7.5–10 mg/day, the side effects appear to be acceptable in most patients. There is also a relationship between side effects and duration of treatment. Alternate-day corticosteroid therapy may decrease the risk side effects, but is usually less effective than daily corticosteroid administration in suppressing inflammation and pain.

The major factor determining suppression of the HPA axis is the duration of exposure to corticosteroid. For this reason, single daily dose or alternate-day regimens are preferred. Multiple daily doses are more effective in decreasing inflammation, but are also more likely to cause HPA axis suppression. The advantage of less HPA axis suppression with daily single-dose therapy is lost when doses of prednisone or its equivalent exceed 15 mg/day.

The role of corticosteroids in the treatment of inflammatory joint disease is controversial. The question is whether the benefits outweigh the potential risks. Low-dose corticosteroids appear to have a role in the treatment of rheumatoid arthritis (13). The role of corticosteroids in the treatment of crystal-induced arthropathies and spondyloarthropathies is less well defined, however. Corticosteroids are rarely administered systemically in acute gout because their use may prolong an attack. NSAIDs and colchicine are more efficacious, being less subject to rebound attacks after discontinuation of therapy.

Some physicians believe that corticosteroids have no place in the treatment of the spondyloarthropathies. This may relate to the need to justify the use of corticosteroids in diseases wherein the probability of remission is high and the risks of joint destruction are low. The use of corticosteroids potentially exposes patients to undue risks. Nevertheless, corticosteroids are frequently used to treat patients with Reiter's syndrome and ankylosing spondylitis who fail to respond to treatment with NSAIDs.

Systemic lupus erythematosus is one of the few rheumatic diseases in which there is little controversy over the appropriateness of corticosteroid therapy. Questions relate more to dosage regimens than to appropriateness of therapy. Corticosteroids may be more effective than NSAIDs in treating pain due to pleuritis, pericarditis, and abdominal serositis. Most patients with arthritis can be successfully treated with salicylates when used in high doses.

Intra-articular corticosteroids are useful in treating acute flares of synovitis involving one to several joints. Their use often leads to rapid relief of pain and swelling, but the duration of relief is highly variable. When used infrequently, the risks appear to be low. Chronic use may be associated with progressive joint deterioration. It appears that the risk of joint damage is related more to the frequency of administration than to the agent used. Therefore, they should be used only in patients who receive substantial prolonged relief of pain following injection.

There is little controversy regarding the effectiveness of intra-articular corticosteroids in the treatment of inflammatory joint disease. Their efficacy in treating patients with osteoarthritis is controversial, however (14). Most of the patients who respond to intra-articular corticosteroid injections will have effusions or a history of joint stiffness similar to those of patients with rheumatoid arthritis. Patients with osteoarthritis who have no evidence of synovitis tend to respond less well, having little relief of pain following intra-articular injections.

Perhaps the most successful use of depot corticosteroids is in treating patients with bursitis or tenosynovitis. These patients typically have rapid relief of symptoms following injection. The risks of single injections of corticosteroids appear to be small. The major complications following injection are infection and fat atrophy. As with other therapies, excessive use increases the risk of side effects. When used too frequently, patients may become cushingoid from systemic absorption of corticosteroids.

OSTEOARTHRITIS

Osteoarthritis is a chronic articular disease characterized by degeneration of cartilage, sclerosis of subchondral bone, and osteophyte formation. It is not a single disease but rather an expression of a final common pathway leading to joint destruction. Most oligoarticular disease probably arises from trauma or developmental abnormalities.

Osteoarthritis is divided into primary and secondary forms based on the presence or absence of an identifiable cause. It can also be subdivided into oligoarticular and polyarticular on the basis of the number of joints involved. Oligoarticular osteoarthritis involves weight-bearing joints such as the hips and knees. It rarely affects the shoulder or elbow in the absence of trauma. Generalized osteoarthritis typically involves distal and proximal interphalangeal joints as well as large weight-bearing joints such as the hips and knees.

Primary osteoarthritis can be further subdivided into primary generalized osteoarthritis and erosive osteoarthritis. Secondary osteoarthritis is defined by disease associations. It may be secondary to trauma, developmental abnormalities, or metabolic disease. Among the metabolic diseases associated with osteoarthritis are diabetes mellitus, ochronosis, acromegaly, hypothyroidism, and Wilson's disease.

Most patients with osteoarthritis complain of pain and stiffness in the involved joints. Their pain is characteristically aggravated by activity and relieved by rest. Patients with osteoarthritis may also complain of stiffness and aching following immobilization, however. Typically, their stiffness is relieved by movement. Most of their pain occurs late in the day as a consequence of excessive use. The joint examination typically shows bony overgrowth at articular margins, decreased range of motion with crepitus, and the absence of synovitis. Signs of systemic disease are typically lacking.

The pain of osteoarthritis arises in both articular and periarticular structures. The pain-sensitive structures within the joint are (1) joint capsule, (2) articular fat pads, and (3) subchondral bone (15). Extra-articular sources for pain include ligaments, tendons, and bursae. Pain arising from chronic repetitive mechanical stress in muscle may also contribute to discomfort.

Early osteoarthritis is typically painless because articular cartilage is aneural. Radiographic changes may precede symptoms. Pain may arise from microfractures in subchondral bone and synovium. Subclinical inflammation, commonly seen in specimens of synovial membrane, suggests that synovitis may be a source of pain. The possibility that rest pain in osteoarthritis is due to intraosseous venous engorgement has also been raised (16).

TREATMENT

Treatment of osteoarthritis is directed at symptoms rather than the underlying disease process. There are no known cures. Therapy must be individualized to meet the needs of the patient. Types of therapy include (1) physical and occupational therapy, (2) drugs, and (3) surgery. Having an accurate diagnosis is a prerequisite for optimal care. The factors contributing to the pain behavior must be identified.

The goals of therapy are (1) to relieve pain, (2) to preserve function, and (3) to prevent joint destruction. Pain can be treated with simple analgesics such as acetaminophen or NSAIDs. Physical therapy has an adjunctive role. Reconstructive surgery is reserved for the most intractable cases.

Patients should understand both the nature and the prognosis of their disease. Patient education will help dispel potentially unrealistic expectations and do much to improve patient compliance. An educated patient is less likely to abuse medications or seek care from nontraditional practitioners.

Drug Therapy

Salicylates and NSAIDs have been the mainstay of therapy because of their analgesic and anti-inflammatory properties. In many cases, however, acetaminophen may be as effective as NSAIDs. Treatment is palliative; there is little evidence these drugs affect the underlying disease process.

Mild osteoarthritis is usually treated with simple analgesics such as acetaminophen or low-dose salicylates. Acetaminophen is administered orally in doses of 650 mg every 4–6 hours as needed. Aspirin is prescribed in analgesic doses of 2–3 g/day in divided doses. Patients with more-severe pain are often treated with aspirin or acetaminophen combined with either codeine or propoxyphene.

NSAIDs and high-dose salicylates are used for treating patients unresponsive to simple analgesics. They appear to be most effective in the presence of synovitis. Although there are few data suggesting that one NSAID is superior to another, indomethacin may be the exception. It may be more effective in treating the subset of patients with osteoarthritis who have coexistent crystal-induced synovitis. Patients having hydroxyapatite deposition disease or subclinical pyrophosphate ar-

thropathy may respond better to indomethacin than to salicylates.

Intra-Articular Corticosteroid Injections

Intra-articular corticosteroids are widely used for treating osteoarthritis; however, there is controversy over the appropriateness of their use. Data from controlled studies are contradictory; some studies show efficacy (17) whereas others show no benefit compared to placebo (18).

Questions regarding potential adverse effects on articular cartilage have also been raised (19). There are anecdotal reports of patients developing "Charcot-like" joints following repeated intra-articular injections of corticosteroids. Studies of the effects of corticosteroids on articular cartilage from animals are also contradictory. Intra-articular corticosteroids inhibit articular proteoglycan synthesis in rabbit, but not in primate cartilage. Taken together, these data indicate that intra-articular corticosteroids are useful in treating a subset of patients with osteoarthritis and that they have a significant potential for causing side effects when used inappropriately. Their use should be limited to patients who have not responded to either NSAIDs or high doses of salicylates. Intra-articular corticosteroids should not be administered more frequently than every 4 months and then only if the duration of benefit from the previous injection lasted more than 4 weeks. Short-term relief of pain does not justify the risks of repeated injections.

Physical Therapy

The major use of physical therapy is to correct postural abnormalities and to strengthen deconditioned muscles. Simple exercise programs such as walking can be helpful (20). Assistive devices such as canes, walkers, and crutches relieve pain by decreasing weight-bearing on symptomatic joints (21). Correction of structural abnormalities and weight reduction in the obese patient may be helpful. Application of heat and cold to symptomatic areas gives short-term relief, perhaps by decreasing muscle spasm.

RHEUMATOID ARTHRITIS

Rheumatoid arthritis, a chronic, polyarticular, multisystem disease, is distinguished from other rheumatic diseases by having symmetrical involvement of large and small joints of both upper and lower extremities. It is frequently associated with extra-articular manifestations such as subcutaneous nodules, serositis, pulmonary fibrosis, and vasculitis. Patients may be either seropositive or seronegative. Only 70% of patients have serum rheumatoid factor titers greater than 1:60. The prognosis is highly variable, and the course of individual patients is not predictable. The presence of subcutaneous nodules, high titers of rheumatoid factor, and the early appearance of joint erosion portend a poor prognosis and suggest the need for aggressive therapy.

The treatment of pain in rheumatoid arthritis is synonymous with suppression of inflammation; control of synovitis will result in control of pain. The pain of coexistent osteoarthritis is an exception. When pain is arising from nociceptors in subchondral bone, the pain will persist despite intensive use of anti-inflammatory drugs.

Many patients with rheumatoid arthritis have a fibrositis-like syndrome as well as pain associated with synovitis. Successful management of myofascial pain requires muscle-stretching exercises, trigger-point injections, and at times the use of tricyclic antidepressants. Corticosteroids and NSAIDs are not effective in treating these noninflammatory pain syndromes.

Successful management of pain requires an accurate localization of the pain generators. Extra-articular pain syndromes such as bursitis, tenosynovitis, enthesopathy, and entrapment neuropathies may coexist with arthritis. Failure to identify these sources of pain will lead to suboptimal results. The symptoms of nonarticular rheumatic complaints are often poorly responsive to treatment with NSAIDs and salicylates. Using potentially remittent drugs to treat "burned-out" rheumatoid disease or nonarticular rheumatic complaints would be inappropriate.

Drug Treatment

When treating rheumatoid arthritis, one must understand the natural history of the disease untreated. Patients with definite rheumatoid arthritis (nodular erosive disease) have persistence of symptoms. In contrast, patients with "probable" rheumatoid arthritis have a more variable course. These patients may have either spontaneous remissions, or persistence of symptoms without progression to joint destruction. At the outset, when the prognosis is in doubt, one should begin treatment with either salicylates or NSAIDs in maximally recommended doses. NSAIDs should be administered for at least 10–14 days before thinking of changing to another drug because it may take several weeks to obtain maximal effects. As a rule, if treatment with three consecutive NSAIDs does not provide adequate suppression of inflammation, it is unlikely that a fourth NSAID will be any more effective. Changing from one class of NSAIDs to another class of NSAIDs, although conceptually appealing, does not usually result in increased efficacy.

Before discontinuing treatment with an NSAID because of lack of benefit, one must confirm that the patient is taking the medication as prescribed. Compliance in taking medications is an important variable when assessing responses to treatment. One can confirm compliance by comparing the number of times a patient obtains refills of medication to the expected number of requests for refills.

When a patient has inadequate relief of pain or has had symptoms for more than 6–9 months, one should consider adding a remittent drug to the therapeutic regimen. One's choice of potentially remittent drug will vary depending on one's training and experience. Usually, either an antimalarial drug or chrysotherapy is considered as a first-line remittent agent. Auranofen, an oral gold compound, is often administered before treatment with parenteral gold or penicillamine because it is potentially less toxic (22). Remittent drugs are slow to act, requiring from 3 to 6 months before significant benefit is seen. The end point is having a decrease in inflammation, not just a decrease in pain.

Remittent drugs may have a significant placebo effect. Patients may claim improvement yet show no change in physical findings. Therefore, one needs to document a decrease in synovitis before committing a patient to a prolonged course of therapy. If no progress has been made after 3 months of therapy, one should change to another remittent drug.

Auranofin, a trialkylphosphine gold complex, can be administered orally. It has a lower frequency of mucocutaneous and renal toxicity than parenteral gold compounds. The major side effect of treatment is diarrhea. There is no correlation between auranofin blood levels and therapeutic efficacy (23). The usual dose is 3 mg given orally twice a day.

The use of gold compounds in the treatment of rheumatoid arthritis is controversial. Recent reports have questioned its value relative to toxicity. The issue is clouded by a lack of data from well-designed double-blind studies, however. Parenteral gold compounds include aurothioglucose and aurothiomalate (24). Both drugs have similar efficacy and potential toxicities. Aurothiomalate differs in causing a nitritoid reaction characterized by acute vasodilation and cutaneous flushing following intramuscular injection. The relationship between the dose of gold and efficacy is unclear. There is no difference in response when comparing the 10-mg weekly doses to the traditional 50-mg weekly dose. Doses higher than 50 mg/week appear to increase toxicity without conferring additional benefit. Parenteral gold is usually administered in doses of 25–50 mg weekly to a cumulative dose of 1000 mg. Patients are then placed on long-term maintenance therapy because most patients will have an exacerbation of arthritis following discontinuation of treatment.

The major toxicities of parenteral gold are mucocutaneous and renal. Patients frequently develop stomatitis or dermatitis, requiring cessation of therapy. Renal toxicity presents as proteinuria; the major risk is the development of nephrotic syndrome. Renal biopsy findings have been variable, ranging from a focal proliferative glomerulonephritis to membranous nephropathy.

Penicillamine is also used for treating rheumatoid arthritis unresponsive to NSAIDs (25). It is usually administered orally in doses of 375–1000 mg/day. Treatment is begun at doses of 125–250 mg daily and increased by 125 mg every 2–4 weeks. By gradually increasing the dose, the frequency of intolerance is significantly decreased. Major side effects are rash and loss of taste. Proteinuria is a common complication with a potential for progressing to nephrotic syndrome. Thrombocytopenia is also seen. Anemia and leukopenia are less frequently noted. Blood studies should be done at least every 2–4 weeks during the first 6 months of therapy, and then at least every 4–6 weeks thereafter. Side effects such as myasthenia gravis, Goodpasture's syndrome, breast gigantism, and lupus-like syndrome should be anticipated.

Azathioprine can also be used but may not be the drug of next choice because of its oncogenic potential (26). Nevertheless, it has been approved for use in the treatment of rheumatoid arthritis. Patients who smoke cigarettes or have a strong family history of cancer may not be good candidates for treatment because of their having a greater risk of developing a neoplasm while taking an immunosuppressant drug. The possibility of azathioprine playing a permissive role by impairing immune surveillance cannot be discounted.

Methotrexate has become one of the most widely used drugs for treating rheumatoid arthritis (27). It has been shown to be both safe and efficacious, having a favorable benefit–side effect profile. It is usually administered in doses ranging from 5 to 25 mg/week. The major side effects are stomatitis and gastrointestinal upset. Problems with abnormal liver function tests are common; however, the risk of hepatic fibrosis in this setting appears to be low. Patients with diabetes mellitus and alcoholics appear to have greater risks of liver toxicity following treatment with methotrexate. If there is a question about underlying liver disease, a percutaneous liver biopsy should be performed prior to beginning treatment. Patients having no risk factors may not need a liver biopsy at outset. The absence of abnormal liver function tests cannot be taken as evidence against the presence of hepatic damage. All patients should be biopsied after taking a cumulative dose of 2000–3000 mg, however.

Alkylating agents such as cyclophosphamide (28) and chlorambucil should be reserved for cases in which the indications for treatment are clear and incontrovertible. They are usually reserved for treating patients with life-threatening multisystem disease such as vasculitis.

There is no consensus on the use of corticosteroids in rheumatoid arthritis. They are usually given in low doses to treat patients who are candidates for remittent drugs, but not as first-line therapy. All patients taking corticosteroids should be placed on calcium supplements to prevent the development of osteoporosis; the exception is patients with absorptive hypercalcemia, who are at risk of nephrolithiasis.

Corticosteroids can be administered orally, parenterally, or intra-articularly. Prednisone, the most commonly used drug, is usually administered in doses of 5–7.5 mg daily. Split doses are more effective than single daily doses, but have a higher frequency of side effects. Depot corticosteroids are occasionally useful when one does not want to commit a patient to oral steroid therapy. Long-acting drugs such as triamcinolone acetonide can be used in doses of 30–60 mg intra-muscularly. Long-term use is associated with the development of a cushingoid habitus with all the complications of chronic corticosteroid use.

Corticosteroids are injected intra-articularly to treat oligoarticular flares of synovitis. The risk of damage to articular cartilage is most likely overstated. The risks of articular damage are minimal when injections are given no more frequently than every 4–6 months. The incidence of septic arthritis, when using a sterile no-touch technique, is approximately 1:20,000 injections. The joint should be aspirated prior to injection. If the joint fluid is not removed, the corticosteroid crystals may be sequestered in synovial fluid and not reach the site of inflammation. It is important to avoid over distending the joint during injection because excessive pressure will result in extravasation of drug into the subcutaneous tissue, increasing the risk of developing fat atrophy.

Antimalarials are useful in treating refractory synovitis (29). Controlled studies have confirmed their efficacy. Eye exams should be performed prior to beginning therapy and repeated every 4–6 months to identify subclinical retinopathy. Doses of chloroquine should not exceed 6 mg/kg/day; doses of hydroxychloroquine should not exceed 4 mg/kg/day. Doses should be decreased in patients with impaired renal function.

Physical Therapy

Physical therapy has a role in treating patients with rheumatoid arthritis (30). It provides short-term relief of symptoms both by promoting a sense of wellness and by helping to maintain function. There are few data to show that physical therapy has any effect on the progression of disease, however. Major problems with expense and poor patient compliance limit its use. Patients instructed by physical therapists seldom continue their exercises in an unsupervised setting. Nevertheless, the patient should be encouraged to see a therapist on a regular basis to prevent the development of contractures and damage to joints because of improper use.

"Step-Care" Approach

Rheumatoid arthritis is treated by a "step-care" approach whereby patients are given a series of potentially remittent drugs on a trial-and-error basis. Typically, patients will have taken a number of drugs to which there was an initial response but subsequent loss of efficacy. Drug-induced remissions may be lost following discontinuation of treatment; therefore, maintenance therapy is almost always indicated. The exceptions are methotrexate and the cytotoxic drugs, because of their potential for cumulative toxicity. Methotrexate has a risk of causing hepatic fibrosis and possibly interstitial pulmonary disease. Cyclophosphamide has the potential for causing hemorrhagic cystitis and carcinoma of the bladder.

CRYSTAL-INDUCED ARTHRITIS

Crystal-induced arthritis, in contrast to other forms of arthritis, has well-defined causes. The major effector cells are neutrophils rather than mononuclear cells. Treatment is limited to anti-inflammatory drugs and uric acid–lowering agents when appropriate. These arthritides lack systemic manifestations. There is no evidence that they respond to remittent drugs or benefit from immunosuppressive therapy.

Gout

Gout, perhaps the best understood of the crystal-induced diseases, arises as a consequence of hyperuricemia and crystal deposition. Monosodium urate crystals are the phlogistic agent. Treatment of acute attacks requires suppression of inflammation. Effective long-term treatment requires normalization of serum uric acid levels and depletion of the total body urate pools.

Pseudogout

Pseudogout, or calcium pyrophosphate dihydrate deposition disease (CPPD), is caused by deposition of calcium pyrophosphate dihydrate in articular cartilage. Acute attacks of arthritis arise from shedding of preformed crystals into joints, where they induce an inflammatory reaction similar to that seen with gout. Pseudogout can also present as pseudo-rheumatoid arthritis, pseudo-osteoarthritis, pseudo-neuropathic arthritis, and asymptomatic chondrocalcinosis. It can be idiopathic, familial, or associated with metabolic diseases such as hyperparathyroidism, hemochromatosis, hypothyroidism, ochronosis, or Wilson's disease. Treatment of calcium pyrophosphate dihydrate deposition disease is palliative because there is no known cure.

Hydroxyapatite Deposition Disease

Hydroxyapatite deposition disease is also pleomorphic. It can present as an acute inflammatory arthritis, a chronic painful degenerative arthropathy, or periarthritis. Periarticular disease includes bursitis, tendinitis, and tenosynovitis. Hydroxyapatite crystals have been implicated in the "Milwaukee shoulder" syndrome, a chronic degenerative arthritis of the shoulders characterized by degeneration of the rotator cuff, joint space narrowing, and the presence of microspheres containing hydroxyapatite crystals. These crystals have also been implicated in both the periarthritis and the destructive arthropathy seen in patients on chronic hemodialysis.

Treatment

In most instances, crystal-induced arthritis responds to NSAIDs (31). Phenylbutazone and indomethacin are perhaps the most effective agents. Other NSAIDs have also been reported to be efficacious, however. Doses of NSAIDs used for treating acute attacks of gout are generally 25% higher than the doses used for treating rheumatoid arthritis. Pain associated with crystal-induced synovitis responds poorly to simple analgesics, salicylates, and opiates. Relief can only be obtained by suppression of inflammation.

Colchicine is effective in the treatment of both acute gout and pseudogout when administered intravenously (32). The usual dose is 2 mg in 20 ml of saline administered over 20 min. Additional 1-mg doses can be given every 3–6 hours if needed, to a maximum of 4 mg/24 hours. Colchicine can also be administered orally in doses of 0.6 mg every 1–2 hours until a maximum of 12 tablets is given or side effects occur (33). Most patients obtain relief after two or three doses. Oral colchicine is not usually effective in the treatment of pseudogout.

The choice between an NSAID and colchicine is arbitrary because both regimens are effective. Intravenous colchicine is preferred by many physicians for the treatment of acute gout, whereas an NSAID is preferred for the treatment of pseudogout. Colchicine can be used to treat patients with a history of peptic ulcer disease because it has no ulcerogenic potential. It should be avoided in patients with intercurrent diarrheal disease, chronic renal insufficiency, or bone marrow dysfunction. Colchicine is primarily excreted by the kidneys and therefore tends to be retained in patients with impaired renal function. Accumulation may lead to suppression of marrow function with resultant anemia or leukopenia.

NSAIDs are usually effective and well tolerated. Indomethacin and phenylbutazone are often given because of their efficacy and a long history of use. Phenylbutazone can never be considered a drug of first choice, however, because agents with less significant risks are available. Indomethacin may be the NSAID of choice in treating acute attacks of gout or pseudogout.

Oral corticosteroids have a limited role in the treatment of crystal-induced arthritis. Systemic corticosteroid therapy will suppress an acute attack, but often there is an exacerbation of the arthritis upon discontinuation of therapy. This is in contrast to intra-articular corticosteroid injections, which are useful in treating monarticular arthritis unresponsive to either colchicine or NSAIDs.

Acute attacks of gout should not be treated with agents that lower the serum uric acid because of their risk of exacerbating an attack. In general, one should not lower the serum uric acid until the attack has completely subsided; then either allopurinol or a uricosuric drug can be given along with colchicine or an NSAID. Colchicine is usually given in a dose of 0.6 mg three times a day for 3–6 months as prophylaxis to prevent an exacerbation of arthritis while lowering the serum uric acid level (34).

The treatment of chronic gout requires continuous therapy to lower the uric acid. The goal is to reduce the total urate pool to normal. This can be done by using either allopurinol (35) or a uricosuric agent. Allopurinol is usually administered at doses of 200–300 mg daily. Divided doses of allopurinol are not required because of the long elimination half-life of oxypurinol, its active metabolite. On occasion, doses of 600–800 mg/day must be given to maintain a uric acid level below 7 mg/dl. Patients who are taking high doses of allopurinol or taking thiazide diuretics concurrently are at risk for developing the Stevens-Johnson syndrome or hepatotoxicity. Patients with impaired renal function may tend to accumulate the drug because of decreased renal clearance.

In most cases the choice between allopurinol and a uricosuric agent is a matter of preference. The exceptions are patients with a history of nephrolithiasis and patients who are over-excreters (those who excrete more than 1000 mg of uric acid per day on a regular diet). These patients should be treated with allopurinol rather than a uricosuric agent. Drugs enhancing renal excretion of uric acid have a risk for causing nephrolithiasis.

Probenecid and sulfinpyrazone are the commonly used uricosuric agents. Like allopurinol, they should not be given during an acute attack of gout. Probenecid is given in an initial dose of 250 mg/day, with the dose being gradually increased to 1.0–1.5 g/day, over 7–10 days (36). It must be administered in divided doses because of it having a short elimination half-life. Sulfinpyrazone is given at doses of 50 mg twice daily and gradually increased to 200–800 mg in divided doses (37). The uricosuric effects of both probenecid and sulfinpyrazone are blocked by salicylates. Sulfinpyrazone also has an effect on platelet function and on the metabolism of both warfarin and tolbutamide. Appropriate dose adjustments for these drugs should be made.

SPONDYLOARTHROPATHIES

The spondyloarthropathies include ankylosing spondylitis, Reiter's syndrome, psoriatic arthritis, and enteropathic arthritis. The diseases classified as spondyloarthropathies share features of enthesopathy, sacroiliitis, iritis, seronegativity (i.e., they lack rheumatoid factors), and an association with the histocompatibility antigen HLA-B27.

ANKYLOSING SPONDYLITIS

Ankylosing spondylitis is a chronic inflammatory disease that primarily involves the axial skeleton. It typically presents as back pain. The pain characteristically involves the low back or buttocks. The onset is often insidious without a history of antecedent trauma or a precipitating event. It is inflammatory in character, being associated with morning stiffness and improvement with activity. There may be an associated arthritis involving predominantly large joints such as the hips, shoulders, knees, and ankles. Involvement of the small joints of the hands and feet is less common. Small joint involvement is typically asymmetric. Enthesopathy is a characteristic feature of the disease. Patients may complain of chest pain due to involvement of costosternal and costochondral joints. Extra-articular manifestations such as iritis, conjunctivitis, and prostatitis are clues to the diagnosis. Late complications such as apical pulmonary fibrosis, aortic insufficiency, and cardiac conduction defects are uncommon.

REITER'S SYNDROME

Reiter's syndrome is defined by the triad of arthritis, conjunctivitis, and urethritis. There may be associated stomatitis, balanitis, keratoderma, prostatitis, or diarrhea. The arthritis typically involves the large weight-bearing joints of the lower extremities. Tenosynovitis and enthesopathy are common features of the disease. The presence of achilles tendinitis, plantar fasciitis, and costochondritis help distinguish incomplete Reiter's syndrome from rheumatoid arthritis. Extra-articular manifestations such as aortic insufficiency, pericarditis, and cardiac conduction defects are less commonly seen. Rarely one sees pleuritis or neurologic involvement with peripheral and cranial neuropathies.

PSORIATIC ARTHRITIS

Psoriatic arthritis is defined as a seronegative arthritis occurring in patients with psoriasis. Arthritis involving the distal interphalangeal joints and classic arthritis mutilans, although characteristic, is not the most common manifestation of the disease. Psoriatic arthritis typically presents as an asymmetric oligoarthritis. A small percentage of patients will have a rheumatoid arthritis–like pattern or will present with findings suggestive of ankylosing spondylitis. Extra-articular manifestations are uncommon. Conjunctivitis, iritis, and scleritis are seen in a minority of patients. Ocular involvement is strongly associated with sacroiliitis and the presence of the HLA-B27 histocompatibility antigen.

ENTEROPATHIC ARTHRITIS

Arthritis, a major manifestation of inflammatory bowel disease, is typically seen with Crohn's disease and ulcerative colitis, but is also a feature of Whipple's disease, intestinal bypass arthropathy, and reactive arthritis following enteric infections. These diseases are typically non-erosive and nondeforming. Enteropathic arthritis usually presents as an acute oligoarthritis predominantly involving the joints of the lower extremities. Upper-extremity involvement does occur, but is less frequent. There is an association between the presence of arthritis and activity of the inflammatory bowel disease. An association between spondylitis, iritis, and HLA-B27 is reported.

TREATMENT

As a group, the spondyloarthropathies are difficult to treat. With the exception of a subset of patients with psoriatic arthritis, there is no evidence that therapy with remittent drugs such as gold compounds is of any value. Therapy is limited to NSAIDs, physical therapy, and intra-articular corticosteroid injections. Remittent drugs such as antimalarials, gold compounds, and penicillamine have little value in treating patients with ankylosing spondylitis, Reiter's syndrome, or enteropathic arthritis. Physicians are less likely to treat these patients aggressively because the prognosis of the spondyloarthropathies is better than that of rheumatoid arthritis.

The choice of anti-inflammatory drug is empiric. Patients with spondyloarthropathies may respond better to treatment with NSAIDs than to salicylates. Phenylbutazone, one of the most effective drugs for treating spondyloarthropathies, is seldom the drug of first choice because of the potential for causing agranulocytosis or aplastic anemia.

With the exception of psoriatic arthritis, corticosteroids are seldom appropriate for treating the spondyloarthropathies. In psoriatic arthritis they are often used for treating the skin manifestations. Because the prognosis of the spondyloarthropathies appears to be more favorable than the prognosis in rheumatoid arthritis, physicians are reluctant to treat these patients with corticosteroids. There is no evidence that corticosteroids will prevent ankylosis or alter the progression of disease.

Therapy is usually begun with either aspirin or an NSAID. When aspirin is used, it should be administered in maximally tolerated doses. Therapeutic blood levels should be documented to confirm compliance. Aspirin should be given with meals and antacids to decrease the development of gastric erosions. Patients with a history of peptic ulcer disease may be given H_2 blockers at bed time to decrease HCl-induced gastric damage due to salicylates. If an NSAID is administered, it should be given in maximally recommended doses for at least 2–3 weeks before changing to another drug. The end point of therapy is suppression of inflammation as well as relief of pain.

Patients who may not respond to treatment with NSAIDs or salicylates may respond to treatment with cytotoxic drugs. Methotrexate and azathioprine are the most frequently used agents; however, data on their efficacy are lacking. There is no evidence that antibiotics have any role in the treatment of reactive arthritis due to venereal or enteropathic infection.

Some patients with psoriatic arthritis may respond to therapy with gold compounds. Others may be unresponsive, requiring treatment with cytotoxic agents. Methotrexate is the favored drug because it is effective in treating not only the arthritis, but the cutaneous manifestations as well. Only patients with chronic, potentially disabling disease should be considered for therapy.

Methotrexate is usually administered on a weekly rather than daily schedule. Doses range from 5 to 25 mg/week, with usual doses being from 5 to 7.5 mg/day. Methotrexate is absorbed well both orally and parenterally. The major factor determining toxicity is duration of exposure. Therefore, a single daily dose is to be preferred. Alternatively, the drug can be administered every 12 hours for three consecutive doses. Daily administration is associated with significant risk of toxicity. Patients with impaired renal function should not be given methotrexate because of the risk of accumulation. Patients taking aspirin are also at greater risk for toxicity. Potential drug interactions with probenecid and sulfonamides are important.

CONNECTIVE TISSUE DISEASES

The connective tissue diseases are a heterogeneous group that includes systemic lupus erythematosus, mixed connective tissue disease, progressive systemic sclerosis, and the systemic vasculitides. Pain most commonly arises from serositis and arthritis. Serositis manifests itself as pleuritis, pericarditis, and peritonitis. Patients complain of chest and abdominal pain.

Systemic lupus erythematosus (SLE) is a chronic, immunologically mediated multisystem disease characterized by the presence of multiple autoantibodies. It occurs most frequently in young women of childbearing age. Females are affected 7–10 times as often as males. The clinical manifestations of systemic lupus erythematosus are varied. Typically, patients will present with musculoskeletal complaints. They typically present with a polyarticular arthritis involving small joints of the hands, the wrists, and the knees. The arthritis is non-erosive but can be deforming, having an appearance similar to that of rheumatoid arthritis.

Patients may also have joint pain due to avascular necrosis of bone. This is usually seen in patients treated with corticosteroids. Patients complain of pain in the hips, knees, or shoulders. The pain of avascular necrosis generally does not respond to treatment with anti-inflammatory drugs.

Cardiopulmonary complaints are very common. Pleuritic pain can occur with or without effusions. Pericarditis, a common cardiac manifestation, occurs in approximately one-third of patients; patients complain of substernal chest pain that is typically aggravated by lying supine. Friction rubs are commonly heard, providing a clue to the diagnosis.

Patients with SLE may present with abdominal pain. The pain may be due to aseptic peritonitis or to mesenteric vasculitis. Ascites has been noted in up to 60% of patients who come to autopsy, suggesting that peritoneal involvement is more common than is clinically recognized. Mesenteric vasculitis with abdominal pain is uncommon, but may present as acute pancreatitis or ischemic bowel syndrome with perforation.

Sjögren's syndrome and mixed connective tissue disease have many features in common with systemic lupus erythematosus. Clinical manifestations are protean, involving almost every organ system. Patients may present with complaints of joint, chest, or abdominal pain.

The natural history of the connective tissue diseases is variable and unpredictable. The initial choice of therapy will depend on the severity of the illness and the organ system involvement. Pain arising from arthritis and serositis frequently responds to treatment with high-dose salicylates. The doses required to suppress articular inflammation range from 3.5 to 5.0 g daily. A few of these patients may develop salicylate-induced hepatitis, which usually subsides following discontinuation of the drug. In these cases, antimalarial drugs may be used to suppress the arthritis. Hydroxychloroquine is usually used in doses of 200–400 mg/day. The major risk is retinal damage with the potential for blindness. The risk of retinal damage is dose-related, and serious toxicity is rare if the patient is monitored appropriately.

Baseline eye exams should be done before beginning treatment and repeated every 4–6 months thereafter. NSAIDs drugs can also be used but are more likely than aspirin to cause side effects requiring discontinuation of therapy. Ibuprofen has been associated with central nervous system dysfunction and aseptic meningitis. NSAIDs have also been reported to cause significant impairment of renal function. This may range from a decrease in renal blood flow to acute renal failure due to interstitial nephritis.

Corticosteroids are indicated for the treatment of severe systemic manifestations of the disease. They are not usually needed for the treatment of either arthritis or serositis. If pain is unresponsive to treatment with either salicylates or NSAIDs, prednisone can be administered in doses of 5–10 mg/day as a single morning dose. Divided doses of corticosteroids, although potentially more effective, may suppress the HPA axis, causing obesity, hypertension, and glucose intolerance.

EXTRA-ARTICULAR PAIN SYNDROMES

Extra-articular pain syndromes can mimic arthritis. These include tendinitis, bursitis, and periarthritis. Recognition is imperative for optimal management. The periarthritis syndromes are characterized by enthesopathy. The character of the pain is variable but is generally described as aching, stabbing, or throbbing. The history, although suggestive, is often inconclusive. Diagnosis is made by physical examination and confirmed by infiltration block using local anesthetic. The local anesthetic should be infiltrated in the area of maximal tenderness. Assuming accurate placement, immediate relief of pain will confirm the diagnosis. Failure to relieve pain indicates either an incorrect diagnosis or improper injection technique. A depot corticosteroid can be mixed with the local anesthetic at the time of injection.

ROTATOR CUFF TENDINITIS AND SUBACROMIAL BURSITIS

Rotator cuff tendinitis, a common cause of shoulder pain, can be acute, subacute, or chronic. Characteristically, patients complain of pain in the deltoid area rather than the shoulder. Exacerbation of pain at night is characteristic. A painful arc is typically noted between 60° and 100° of abduction; other motions may be painful as well. The diagnosis is easily confirmed by injection of local anesthetic into the subdeltoid area using a lateral approach (33). Relief of pain and improved range of motion are observed immediately following injection.

BICIPITAL TENDINITIS

Patients with bicipital tendinitis frequently complain of pain in the area of the bicipital groove. The discomfort is reproduced by resisted supination of the hand with the elbow flexed. Marked tenderness is usually felt over the biceps tendon. Infiltration of the synovial sheath surrounding the biceps tendon with local anesthetic will result in immediate relief of pain (38). Many but not all patients respond to local injection of corticosteroid. Response to NSAIDs is less predictable.

LATERAL EPICONDYLITIS

Pain in lateral epicondylitis is localized to the dorsal aspect of the proximal forearm. Maximal tenderness is found over the insertion of the extensor muscles on the lateral epicondyle. Flexion and extension of the elbow is usually free and painless. Resisted extension of the wrist and resisted supination will exacerbate the pain. Patients are treated by splinting of the wrist, by local injections of corticosteroid, and less frequently by surgery. A small number of patients have entrapment of the deep radial nerve at the arcade of Frohse mimicking lateral epicondylitis. The differential diagnosis of entrapment neuropathy is confirmed by injection of local anesthetic, that is, conduction block of the deep radial nerve at the arcade of Frohse (39).

De Quervain's Tendinitis

In de Quervain's tendinitis there is tenderness over the radial styloid associated with inflammation of the abductor pollicis longus and extensor pollicis brevis tendons. The diagnosis is suggested by a positive Finkelstein's test (i.e., pain on lateral deviation of the wrist with the thumb adducted). It is often confused with superficial radial neuralgia and arthritis of the first carpal metacarpal joint. Patients are treated with NSAIDs, immobilization of the wrist and thumb, and local injection of corticosteroid. Those who do not respond to conservative therapy should be considered for surgical treatment (40).

Anserine Bursitis

Anserine bursitis is characterized by knee pain associated with tenderness localized to the insertions of the medial collateral ligament and the sartorius muscle on the medial aspect of the proximal tibia. The pain, arising in the distribution of the infrapatellar branch of the saphenous nerve, is felt just distal to the medial joint line and proximal leg. Anserine bursitis is best treated by injecting a mixture of corticosteroid and local anesthetic at the point of maximal tenderness; it tends to respond poorly to treatment with NSAIDs (41). Anserine bursitis is most commonly seen in women with genu varus deformities of the knee and often coexists with osteoarthritis of the knees.

Achilles Tendinitis

Pain in the heel associated with erythema and tenderness is diagnostic of Achilles tendinitis or retrocalcaneal bursitis. In most cases, inflammation is due to chronic trauma from ill-fitting shoes, but it can be a manifestation of an underlying spondyloarthropathy. Pain associated with trauma is usually short-lived and will respond to rest. Pain due to enthesopathy is persistent and usually requires treatment with NSAIDs or local injection of corticosteroid, however (42).

Polymyalgia Rheumatica

Polymyalgia rheumatica is a syndrome of diffuse proximal myalgias occurring in elderly patients (43). The onset can be acute or subacute. A subset of these patients will have giant cell arteritis. Another subset will have rheumatoid arthritis presenting with proximal joint involvement. The diagnosis of polymyalgia rheumatica is one of exclusion. Patients typically have a Westergren sedimentation rate of at least 50 mm/hour. Laboratory findings are nonspecific. The anemia of chronic disease, an elevated serum alkaline phosphatase level, and polyclonal hypergammaglobulinemia are frequently seen. Patients may have age-related antinuclear antibodies and rheumatoid factors but lack other serologic markers for autoimmune disease.

The diagnosis of giant cell arteritis is suggested by a patient having a history of headache, scalp tenderness, jaw claudication, or visual disturbance. In most cases the physical examination is normal. In a small percentage of patients, the temporal arteries will be tender and enlarged. The diagnosis is confirmed by temporal artery biopsy.

Treatment

The response to treatment with corticosteroids is also helpful diagnostically. Most patients with polymyalgia rheumatica will have a dramatic decrease in pain and stiffness within hours of beginning treatment with 7.5–10 mg of prednisone or its equivalent. Pseudopolymyalgia as seen in patients with rheumatoid arthritis will have a less impressive response to corticosteroids. Not having significant pain relief following treatment with low-dose prednisone should cause one to question the diagnosis of polymyalgia.

The term *polymyalgia rheumatica* is most likely a misnomer. There is little evidence that pain is of muscular origin. Muscle enzymes, electromyograms, and muscle biopsies are reported to be normal. Pain may arise from involvement of proximal joints such as shoulders and hips. The presence of synovitis is suggested by reports of increased uptake of radioisotopes in the shoulder region and by reports of an oligoarticular arthritis being present in many patients.

There is controversy over the need to use high doses of corticosteroid to treat patients with polymyalgia rheumatica who show no evidence of giant cell arteritis. Proponents of high-dose therapy argue that a negative biopsy does not rule out arteritis; therefore all patients should be treated as though they had the disease. Others argue that many patients with polymyalgia rheumatica do not have arteritis and that the use of high-dose corticosteroid therapy is unnecessary. Inappropriate use of corticosteroids in high doses will lead to increased morbidity and mortality from adverse effects of corticosteroids. In these cases, a negative temporal artery biopsy is reassuring.

The end point of treatment in polymyalgia rheumatica and giant cell arteritis is suppression of inflammation as evidenced by normalization of the erythrocyte sedimentation rate. These patients are usually given from 45 to 60 mg of prednisone daily for 1 month, followed by gradual tapering of the dose over 3–6 months while maintaining a normal erythrocyte sedimentation rate. Patients who have no evidence for arteritis can be treated symptomatically. In these cases, the end point of treatment is relief of pain. They are usually given from 7.5 to 10 mg of prednisone daily for control of symptoms, with tapering of the dose as tolerated. A small percentage of these patients will have subclinical arteritis; therefore, one should be prepared to increase the dose of corticosteroid when symptoms of vascular disease appear. Blindness is the major risk of inadequately treated giant cell arteritis. All patients should be given supplemental calcium to decrease the risk of corticosteroid-induced osteopenia. A minimum of 1000 mg of elemental calcium should be administered daily. The question of using vitamin D or its analogues to prevent loss of bone is still debated.

REFERENCES

1. Capetola RJ, Rosenthale ME, Dubinsky B, McGuire JL: Peripheral antialgesics—A review. *J Clin Pharmacol* 23:545–556, 1983.
2. Bradley JD, et al: Comparison of anti-inflammatory dose of ibuprofen and analgesic dose of ibuprofen and acetaminophen in the treatment of patients with osteoarthritis of the knee. *N Engl J Med* 325:87–91, 1991.
3. Rosenbaum JF: The drug treatment of anxiety. *N Engl J Med* 306:401–404, 1982.
4. Ward NG, Bloom VL, Friedel RD: The effectiveness of tricyclic antidepressants in the treatment of coexisting pain and depression. *Pain* 7:331–341, 1979.
5. Beaver WT: Combination analgesics. *Am J Med* 77:38–53, 1985.
6. Piletta P, et al: Central analgesic effect of acetaminophen but not of aspirin. *Clin Pharmacol Ther* 49:350–354, 1991.
7. Bonkowsky HL, Mudge GH, McMurtry RJ: Chronic hepatic inflammation and fibrosis due to low dose paracetamol. *Lancet* 1:1016–1018, 1978.
8. Levy G, Tsuchiva T: Salicylate accumulation kinetics in man. *N Engl J Med* 287:430–432, 1972.
9. Brooks PM, Day RO: Nonsteroidal anti-inflammatory drugs—Differences and similarities. *N Eng J Med* 324:1716–1725, 1991.
10. Ferreira SH: Peripheral analgesia: Mechanisms of the analgesic action of aspirin-like drugs and opiate antagonists. *Br J Clin Pharmacol* 10:2379–2455, 1980.
11. Blackshear JL, Napier JS, Davidman M, Stillman MI: Renal complications of nonsteroidal anti-inflammatory drugs: Identification and monitoring of those at risk. *Semin Arthritis Rheum* 14:163–175, 1985.
12. Swainson CP, Griffiths P: Acute and chronic effects of sulindac on renal function in chronic renal disease. *Clin Pharmacol Ther* 37:298–300, 1985.
13. Byron MA, Mowat AG: Corticosteroid prescribing in rheumatoid arthritis—The fiction and the fact. *Br J Rheum* 24:164–166, 1985.
14. Friedman DM, Moore MA: The efficacy of intraarticular corticosteroids for osteoarthritis of the knee. *Arthritis Rheum* 21:556–559, 1978.
15. Wyke B: The neurology of joints in osteoarthritis. *Ann Rheum Dis* 19:257–261, 1981.
16. Arnold CC, Lemper RK, Linderholm H: Intraosseous hypertension and pain in the knee. *J Bone Joint Surg [Br]* 57:360–363, 1975.
17. Hollander JL: Treatment of osteoarthritis of knee. *Arthritis Rheum* 3:564–569, 1960.
18. Wright V, et al: Intraarticular therapy in osteoarthritis: Comparison of hydrocortisone acetate and hydrocortisone tertiary butylacetate. *Ann Rheum Dis* 19:257, 1960.
19. Butler M, et al: A new model of osteoarthritis in rabbits.

III: Evaluation of antiarthrosic effects of selected drugs administered intraarticularly. *Arthritis Rheum* 26:1380, 1983.
20. Kovar PA, et al: Supervised fitness walking in patients with osteoarthritis of the knees. A randomized controlled trial. *Ann Intern Med* 116:529–534, 1992.
21. Felson DT, et al: Weight loss reduces the risk of symptomatic knee osteoarthritis in women: The Framingham study. *Ann Intern Med* 116:535–539, 1992.
22. Davis P, Harth M (eds): Proceedings—Therapeutic innovation in rheumatoid arthritis: Worldwide auranofin symposium. *J Rheum* 90(Suppl 8):1–209, 1982.
23. Champion GD, et al: Auranofin in rheumatoid arthritis. *J Rheum* 9(Suppl 8):137, 1982.
24. Cooperating Clinics Committee of the American Rheumatism Association: A controlled trial of gold salt therapy in rheumatoid arthritis. *Arthritis Rheum* 16:353–358, 1973.
25. Dixon A St J, et al: Synthetic D(-) penicillamine in rheumatoid arthritis. Double blind controlled study of a high and low dose regimen. *Ann Rheum Dis* 34:416–421, 1975.
26. Hunter T, et al: Azathioprine in rheumatoid arthritis: A long term follow up study. *Arthritis Rheum* 18:15–20, 1975.
27. Kremer JM, Lee JK: The safety and efficacy of the use of methotrexate in long term therapy of rheumatoid arthritis. *Arthritis Rheum* 29:822–831, 1986.
28. Cooperating Clinics Committee of the American Rheumatism Association: Controlled trial of cyclophosphamide in rheumatoid arthritis. *N Engl J Med* 283:883–889, 1970.
29. Adams EM, et al: Hydroxychloroquine in the treatment of rheumatoid arthritis. *Am J Med* 75:321–326, 1983.
30. Robinson HS, et al: Evaluation of a province-wide physical therapy monitoring service in an arthritis control program. *J Rheum* 7:387, 1980.
31. Kelly WN, Fox IH: Gout and related disorders of purine metabolism. In Kelly WM, Harris E, Ruddy S, Sledge C (eds): *Textbook of Rheumatology*, ed 2. Philadelphia, WB Saunders, 1985, pp 1382–1388.
32. Wallace SL: The treatment of the acute attack of gout. *Clin Rheum Dis* 3:133–143, 1977.
33. Wallace SL: Colchicine. *Semin Arthritis Rheum* 3:369, 1974.
34. Yu TF, Gutman AB: Efficacy of colchicine prophylaxis in gout. *Ann Intern Med* 35:179–192, 1961.
35. Brewis I: Single daily dose allopurinol. *Ann Rheum Dis* 34:256–259, 1975.
36. Yu TF: Milestones in the treatment of gout. *Am J Med* 56:676–685, 1974.
37. Emmerson BT: A comparison of uricosuric agents in gout with special reference to sulfinpyrazone. *Med J Aust* 1:839–844, 1963.
38. Cogen L, et al: Medical management of the painful shoulder. *Bull Rheum Dis* 32:88–92, 1982.
39. Goldie I: Epicondylitis lateralis humeroepicondyalgie or tennis elbow. *Acta Chir Scand Suppl* 339:1, 1964.
40. Muckart RD: Stenosing tendovaginitis of abductor policis longus and extensor pollicis brevis at the radial styloid (de Quervain's disease). *Clin Orthop* 33:201–207, 1964.
41. Larsson LG, Baum J: The syndrome of anserine bursitis. *Arthritis Rheum* 28:1062–1065, 1985.
42. Sheon RP, Moscowitz RW, Goldberg VM: *Soft Tissue Rheumatic Pain: Recognition, Management, Prevention*. Philadelphia, Lea & Febiger, 1982, pp 219–222.
43. Healy LA, et al: Polymyalgia rheumatica and giant cell arteritis. *Arthritis Rheum* 14:138–141, 1971.

CHAPTER 43

SINGLE-MUSCLE MYOFASCIAL PAIN SYNDROMES

DAVID G. SIMONS

THIS AND the next chapter together provide a solid basis for managing chronic myofascial pain syndromes (MPSs). Myofascial trigger points (TrPs) may occur in any skeletal muscle in response to strain by acute or chronic overload. Each of the body's approximately 500 skeletal muscles can develop TrPs that produce a referred pain pattern characteristic of that muscle. Each pattern becomes part of a single-muscle myofascial pain syndrome. Each single-muscle syndrome is responsive to appropriate treatment. To successfully deal with the multiple complex interwoven factors encountered in a chronic MPS, one should identify each single-muscle syndrome and every perpetuating factor, approaching them as discrete and soluble but interacting problems. The goal is to identify and treat the cause of the pain, not just the symptom of pain.

The process begins with the recognition of the composite single-muscle syndromes that together comprise the total myofascial pain picture as reported by the patient. This chapter first describes how to recognize an *acute* single-muscle syndrome due to TrPs. Next, it presents the distinctive characteristic pain patterns, stretch positions, and vapocoolant spray patterns of many of the common single-muscle syndromes throughout the body. The following chapter shows how this essential information is applied to manage a complex *chronic* MPS due to TrPs.

RECOGNITION OF A SINGLE-MUSCLE SYNDROME

Janet G. Travell is the pioneer responsible for first organizing these syndromes in a clinically useful way (1). Myofascial TrPs are equally common in men and women (2), and are a frequent source of musculoskeletal pain in children (3). One study reports a sample of 200 Air Force recruits without pain complaint who, by age 19, had developed points of tenderness that fit the current definition of latent TrPs in the shoulder-girdle musculature (2). Many of these TrPs referred pain on stim-

ulation. These latent TrPs tend to become active with the stresses of adult life and with the gradual deterioration of muscular function in time. Latent TrPs, although less irritable than active TrPs, at times may have any or all of the characteristics of active TrPs except the clinical complaint of pain. With chronicity, satellite TrPs tend to develop in muscles located in pain reference zones that exhibit true muscle spasm. Also with chronicity, secondary TrPs may develop in muscles in the same functional unit (4).

The diagnosis of MPS due to myofascial TrPs depends on eight clinical characteristics (4). All eight clinical features emphasize the fact that this is primarily an affliction of muscle:

1. History of the onset and its cause
2. Distribution of the pain
3. Restriction of motion
4. Mild, muscle-specific weakness
5. The focal tenderness of a TrP
6. The palpable taut band of muscle in which a TrP is located
7. A local twitch response to snapping palpation
8. Reproduction of the referred pain pattern on more sustained mechanical stimulation of the Trp

These first four characteristics are frequently very helpful, and the last four can be essential, for making the diagnosis.

HISTORY OF ONSET

By history, the onset of pain is often sudden and associated with a clearly remembered muscular strain, but the onset may be gradual, resulting from repetitive physical stress. The *distribution* of referred pain (or altered sensation) is more significant than the kind of pain. Pain referred from TrPs is usually described as dull, constant, and aching but may be described as shooting or stabbing, rarely as burning. Altered sensation is occasionally described as numbness and is substantiated by examination (5). Intensity is variable from hour to hour and from day to day. A newly activated TrP may spontaneously revert to a latent TrP. However, in the presence of serious perpetuating factors newly activated TrPs persist as chronically active or intermittently active, pain-producing TrPs. In addition, they are likely to multiply as satellite and secondary TrPs (4). Characteristically, pain symptoms are closely related to changes in the activity of or in the demands on the involved muscle.

DISTRIBUTION OF PAIN

Referred pain patterns are the key to identifying which muscle, or muscles, are most likely to be causing the myofascial pain. Examples in the next section show that each muscle has its own characteristic pain pattern (4). The sketchy pain drawings usually requested of patients are generally useless for identifying myofascial TrPs.

Accurately drawn referred pain patterns are the initial key to locating the TrPs. A *precise drawing* that includes the patient's complete pain distribution is essential. Each area of pain should be delineated by the patient with one *finger* on the body, and should be drawn by the examiner on an anatomically accurate body form, such as those designed for this purpose (4); the drawing is then corrected or confirmed by the patient. Leading questions are scrupulously avoided. The local tenderness *elicited* in response to pressure applied by the patient on a TrP must be carefully distinguished from the pain and tenderness *referred* to that area by a distant TrP. Patients often need help from the examiner to make these important distinctions.

When pain involves several parts of the body, it is important to number the pain areas in the sequence of their appearance, to distinguish between pains that occur at different times and to group together those that are experienced together in association with an activity or position. The known pain pattern of each muscle is then applied in reverse to identify the muscle or muscles that are most likely to be causing that piece of the patient's total pain picture. The importance of obtaining a complete and accurate pain drawing at the initial visit, as well as obtaining drawings that identify any changes at subsequent visits, cannot be overemphasized.

A myofascial TrP usually refers *tenderness* as well as pain to the zone of referred pain, which often confuses both the unwary examiner and the patient.

RESTRICTION OF MOTION

On examination, patients consistently have some painful limitation of the stretch range of motion. Passive lengthening of a muscle harboring TrPs causes pain when the muscle is forcibly stretched beyond its restricted range of motion. Also, strong voluntary contraction of an involved muscle, especially in the shortened position, is likely to be painful.

MUSCLE-SPECIFIC WEAKNESS

The involved muscle shows some degree of rachety weakness without atrophy. When carefully examined, it acts as if it is reflexly inhibited from maximal contraction.

FOCAL TENDERNESS

Exquisite focal tenderness of the TrP is identified by the jump sign—a vocalization by and withdrawal *of the patient*. This spot tenderness is an essential feature of both a TrP and a tender point (TeP).

Algometers are becoming widely used to quantify TrP and TeP sensitivity in clinical studies (6–10). Fischer designed a family of convenient spring-type pressure algometers (11–13) that are commercially available. Reeves and associates (14) have established the reliability of Fischer's pressure threshold meter (11). Jensen and associates developed and validated an electronic strain-gauge unit that is also being produced commercially (10). Schiffman and associates (15) have developed and tested an electronic strain-gauge unit with a blunt probe. When the probe is pressed across the TrP in a taut band, this unit simulates snapping palpation and returns considerable tactile feedback to the examiner. This algometer is especially well suited to the study of local twitch responses and should soon be commercially available.

PALPABLE TAUT MUSCLE BAND

The palpable band associated with a TrP is a dependable and totally objective finding. The TrP is the point of maximum tenderness along the course of a taut band in an involved muscle. The rope-like taut band (sometimes described more like a nodule) can be palpated if the muscle is sufficiently close to the skin. The tense fibers that comprise the palpable band are most easily distinguished from the normally relaxed fibers surrounding them by stretching the muscle gently just short of, or to the onset of, resistance. This degree of stretch maximizes the palpable differences in tension between taut and normal fibers.

LOCAL TWITCH RESPONSE

Firm snapping palpation across, or needle penetration into, an active TrP usually evokes a local twitch response of the fibers in the taut band. This response is an objective sign and has been observed only in response to abrupt mechanical stimulation of TrPs. It was recently studied electromyographically by Fricton and associates (16). This objective local twitch response is seen as a transient dimpling of the skin near the more distant tendinous attachment of the muscle or is felt as a transient contraction of only the fibers in the taut band, without contraction of the muscle fibers surrounding the taut band.

REPRODUCTION OF REFERRED PAIN

Mildly painful sustained pressure on an active TrP usually reproduces or increases the referred pain from that TrP, if the TrP is not already activated to maximum intensity. This confirms to both the patient and the examiner that this TrP is responsible for at least part of the patient's pain. In this way one can piece together the total pain distribution of patients with multiple TrPs that project multiple, often overlapping, single-muscle referred pain patterns. Each pattern contributes its own portion of the total pain distribution. It is noteworthy that sometimes a TrP may refer analgesia instead of pain (5).

SUMMARY

In summary, the first four of the above features are helpful in making a *clinical* diagnosis: the dependence of symptoms on muscular strain and muscular activity; the specificity of the referred pain and tenderness patterns initiated by each skeletal muscle; painful restriction of the stretch range of motion; and some weakness of involved muscles without atrophy.

The remaining four features are essential for making the diagnosis of myofascial TrPs for research purposes. Clinically, focal exquisite TrP tenderness is always present and a taut band is palpable whenever the muscle is accessible. The last two features, the local twitch response and the referred pain response, have been considered pathognomonic of TrPs (4). A possible exception would be if the pain can be referred from some TePs of fibromyalgia. These last two responses are most vigorous in the most active TrPs, but sometimes can be elicited from latent TrPs. An exquisitely tender TrP may be too sensitive for the patient to permit the application of sufficient pressure to elicit a local twitch response.

Only active TrPs are responsible for *clinical* pain complaints. Latent TrPs, although less irritable, may have any or all of the other characteristics of active TrPs, including local twitch responses and the reproduction of that TrPs referred pain pattern when the TrP is firmly compressed.

PATHOGENESIS OF TRIGGER POINTS

Although the pathogenesis of myofascial TrPs has not been fully documented, pathophysiologic mechanisms are well established that can account for the distinctive clinical characteristics of TrPs, and these mechanisms have been extensively discussed (17). The local tenderness of the TrP can be explained by sensitization of group III and/or group IV muscle afferents (18). Initiation of referred pain by the TrP is explicable by the same process of nerve sensitization. The central nervous system pathways of referred pain may depend on one or more of the four known mechanisms by which pain may be referred (17, 19).

The electrically silent palpable hardness of the taut band and its associated local twitch response are more difficult to explain. The same mechanism that causes the contraction without action potentials in McArdle's disease, if applicable locally at the TrP, could account for shortened muscle fibers. One possibility is that such a mechanism is sustained by an energy crisis locally in the muscle. This mechanism is substantiated by recent studies of "fibromyalgia" patients, many of whom had TrPs that referred pain (20). Studies have demonstrated reduced and disturbed oxygen tension (21), a deficit of high-energy phosphates with an excess of low-energy phosphates (22), and ragged red and moth-eaten fibers under light microscopy (23). The latter are found in muscles experiencing impaired metabolism.

ACUTE SINGLE-MUSCLE SYNDROMES

This section presents many of the common single-muscle syndromes found throughout the body. Every skeletal muscle has the potential to develop myofascial TrPs. The key to each syndrome is recognition of the referred pain pattern characteristic of that muscle. The syndromes are grouped according to the region of the body to which pain is referred. This referred pain is the pain for which the patient seeks relief. Detailed instructions in the principles of stretch and spray that apply to individual muscles are found in the next section.

HEAD AND NECK PAIN

A number of neck muscles, including the upper trapezius, sternocleidomastoid, splenii, and suboccipital muscles, refer pain strongly to the head. These muscles are often largely responsible for headache diagnosed as "tension" headache or "muscle tension" headache (24). Masticatory muscles frequently cause temporal, maxillary, and jaw pain, also earache and toothache; cutaneous facial muscles sometimes contribute to facial pain (4).

The masticatory muscles that are active during closure of the lower jaw include the masseter, temporalis, medial pterygoid, and upper division of the lateral pterygoid. The digastric and lower division of the lateral pterygoid muscles primarily open the jaw. The masseter and temporalis muscles are most likely to be responsible for ear pain, temporal headache, and hypersensitivity of the teeth to pressure, heat, and cold. Pain and tenderness referred to a normal tooth has resulted in the extraction of an innocent tooth when the myofascial origin of the pain was not identified. The lateral pterygoid muscle often is involved when pain and/or dysfunction include the temporomandibular joint.

The normal range of jaw opening is easily tested by the patient's ability to insert a tier of their first three knuckles of the nondominant hand between the incisor teeth (4). Masticatory muscles are most responsive to stretch-and-spray therapy when the patient is supine. When the patient is seated, the head should be tilted fully backward rather than upright to eliminate anti-gravity reflexes.

Upper and Lower Trapezius

The upper trapezius is probably the muscle that most commonly develops myofascial TrPs. Trigger points in the clavicular section project pain to the back of the neck and to the temporal region (Fig. 43.1A) (1, 25). Upper trapezius TrPs (black arrows) are likely to be activated and perpetuated by lack of support for the elbows when sitting; this happens much of the time when the person's upper arms are short in relation to torso height so that the elbows fail to reach the chair's armrests (4). Persistent avoidable elevation of the shoulders as a result of emotional tension commonly abuses this muscle.

For relief of upper trapezius TrPs, the patient should be seated and *relaxed*; the shoulder on the side to be stretched is anchored by the patient's grasping the chair seat or placing the hand under the thigh. The spray is applied (dashed arrows, Fig. 43.1A) upward from the acromion over the upper section of the trapezius muscle, including pain reference zones in the posterolateral aspect of the neck, behind the ear, and around to the temple and mandible. The muscle is placed in the maximum lengthened position by passively tilting the head and neck toward the side opposite the involved muscle with the face turned toward the side of the involved muscle. An effective home program of self-stretch has the supine patient place the head in the stretch position and gently but firmly add stretch tension exerted by the opposite hand.

The **lower trapezius** TrP (Fig. 43.1B) is usually found in the inferior margin of the lower trapezius muscle about where it crosses the vertebral border of the scapula. This TrP refers pain and tenderness to the upper trapezius muscle, generating satellite TrPs there. Such satellite TrPs rarely respond until the primary TrP, in the lower trapezius, is first inactivated.

The stream of vapocoolant spray is applied for TrPs in the lower trapezius muscle as shown by the dashed arrows in Figure 43.1B. Stretch is applied as indicated by the curved white arrow. The operator may pull the patient's elbow across the chest, lifting slightly to fully protract and elevate the scapula. Stretch is smoothly coordinated with unidirectional parallel sweeps of the spray. The patient should perform this same stretch as a self-stretch home exercise, preferably seated under a hot shower (4).

Sternocleidomastoid

The clavicular and sternal divisions of the sternocleidomastoid muscle present distinctively different pain patterns. The two divisions also refer different kinds of autonomic phenomena and differ in stretch positions.

Myofascial TrPs of the **clavicular division** refer pain *bilaterally* across the forehead. Referral across the midline is unusual for myofascial TrPs. Pain may also be referred deep in the ear, and close behind the ear (Fig. 43.1C) (4, 25). Postural instability, spatial disorientation, and dizziness may occur when the patient suddenly increases the tension in this muscle by flexing the neck, looking up, or turning over in bed.

A stream of vapocoolant is directed upward above the clavicle to cover the muscle, the occiput, and forehead (Fig. 43.1C). To stretch this division of the muscle, the patient anchors the hand under the chair seat or fixes the hand under the thigh. The operator cradles the patient's head against the operator's torso to provide head support. In this way, the patient relaxes and lets the operator gradually extend the head backward and side-bend it (Fig. 43.1C).

The **sternal division** refers pain to the occiput, to the vertex, to the cheek, around the eye, and to the throat (Fig. 43.1D). Its lowermost TrPs can refer pain downward over the sternum. Motor and autonomic concomitants are narrowing of the palpebral fissure, scleral injection, lacrimation, and coryza.

Following initial sweeps of spray, the sternal division is stretched by gently rotating the face to the same side and tipping the chin downward to the acromion. As this movement proceeds slowly, the spray is directed along the length of the muscle from the sternum to the mastoid process, including the back of the head (dashed arrows in Fig. 43.1D). Before the operator directs the sweeps immediately above the eye, the patient's eye is covered with an absorbent pad and the patient closes the eye tightly. Spray in the eye is fiercely painful for about 2 min but causes no permanent damage. Accidentally spraying the ear drum is also startling but painful only because of impact and cold.

Masseter and Temporalis

The superficial division of the masseter muscle refers pain to the face and upper or lower molar teeth (Fig. 43.1E), whereas TrPs in the temporalis muscle refer pain to any of the upper teeth and over the temporal bone and eyebrow in finger-like projections (Fig. 43.1F). Trigger points in the deep masseter may cause earache and ipsilateral tinnitus.

The masseter, temporalis, and medial pterygoid muscles may be stretched and sprayed together by combining the spray patterns (dashed arrows) of Figures 43.1E and F. The operator applies the spray over the lower jaw and continues in parallel sweeps upward behind the ear, then covering the cheek, temporal region, and eyebrow. For self-stretch, the supine patient places the fingers on the posterior molars and gently pulls downward, applying long axis distraction, and then pulls

HEAD AND NECK PAIN

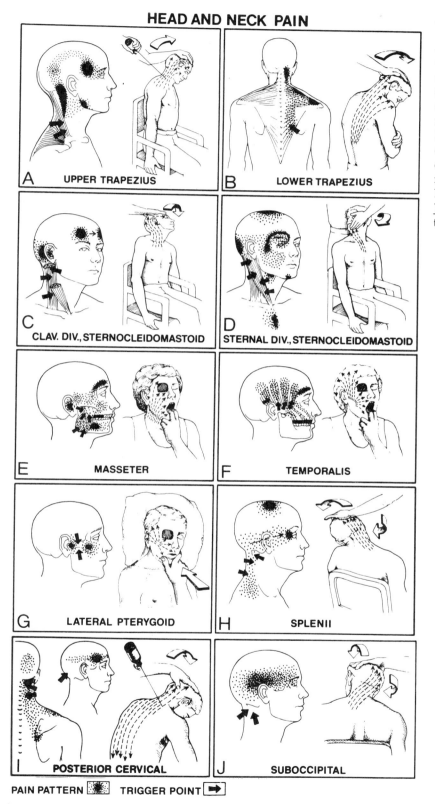

Figure 43.1. Location of TrPs (*solid black arrows*) and pain patterns (*solid black and black stipples*), stretch positions, and spray patterns (*dashed arrows*) for muscles that cause head and neck pain. The *curved white arrows* show the direction of pressure applied to passively stretch each muscle and the *dashed arrows* trace the path of parallel sweeps of vapocoolant spray to release the tension and permit stretch of each muscle. In *H*, the broken arrow in the pain pattern deep to the ear indicates pain deep in the head radiating to the back of the eye. (From Simons DG: Myofascial pain syndromes. In Basmajian JV, Kirby RL (eds): *Medical Rehabilitation.* Baltimore, Williams & Wilkins, 1984, pp 314, 315.)

A UPPER TRAPEZIUS

B LOWER TRAPEZIUS

C CLAV. DIV., STERNOCLEIDOMASTOID

D STERNAL DIV., STERNOCLEIDOMASTOID

E MASSETER

F TEMPORALIS

G LATERAL PTERYGOID

H SPLENII

I POSTERIOR CERVICAL

J SUBOCCIPITAL

PAIN PATTERN   TRIGGER POINT

slightly forward. To fully stretch the posterior temporalis fibers, the mandible also should be pulled to the opposite side.

Lateral Pterygoid

The lateral pterygoid (Fig. 43.1G) is difficult to stretch (4). It is inaccessible to ischemic compression. Alternate treatment techniques such as injection or ultrasound usually must be used.

Splenii

Myofascial TrPs in the splenius capitis and cervicis muscles refer deep-seated head pain, as in Figure 43.1H. Stretching these muscles requires combined head and neck flexion, sidebending of the head, and rotation of the face toward the opposite side, as illustrated. The patient's hand must anchor the torso, as for the upper trapezius. Relaxation during stretch and spray is facilitated for most muscles by having the patient slowly exhale with the eyes directed downward (26).

Posterior Cervical Muscles

Semispinalis cervicis and capitis TrPs refer pain to the occiput and to the temporal region (Fig. 43.1I). Multifidus TrPs are found deep in the paraspinal mass, often at the C5 and C6 levels; they refer pain to the suboccipital area and toward the scapula. These posterior cervical pain patterns are likely to appear together. Multifidus TrPs often initiate satellite TrPs in the suboccipital muscles.

For treatment of the posterior cervical muscles, the head and neck are flexed against the chest while bilateral parallel sweeps of spray are directed as in Figure 43.1I, starting at the base of the neck.

Suboccipital Muscles

The suboccipital muscles project pain inside the head and to the upper part of the face (Fig. 43.1J). They, the scalene, and the sternocleidomastoid muscles are commonly the cause of persistent whiplash symptoms following a rear-end collision. These muscles are responsive to stretch and spray, and to massage or pressure therapy (27). Injection of the lateral suboccipital muscles is not recommended because of TrP proximity to the external loop of the vertebral artery (4).

The stream of spray is applied as in Figure 43.1J. Stretch of the medial suboccipital muscles combines slight flexion of the head on the neck with rotation of the face to the opposite side (curved arrows, Figure 43.1J). To stretch the lateral suboccipital muscles, the head is flexed slightly and tilted on the neck toward the opposite side; only head movement on the cervical spine stretches these muscles.

SHOULDER AND UPPER EXTREMITY PAIN

Myofascial TrPs in some muscles of the neck, shoulder girdle, and upper extremity refer pain to the ipsilateral upper torso and upper extremity (Fig. 43.2). Persistent shoulder pain due to myofascial TrPs commonly follows trauma (28), such as a dislocated shoulder, fracture, or soft tissue injury in a fall (4).

Painful restriction of sidebending of the neck is likely to be caused by scalene and/or upper trapezius TrPs. The levator scapulae is more likely to restrict rotation than is the sternocleidomastoid muscle. Subscapularis TrPs often severely restrict abduction and external rotation of the arm at the shoulder. Moderate restriction of abduction may be caused by TrPs in the more vertical, lower sternal and abdominal fibers of the pectoralis major muscle or in the triceps brachii muscle. Myofascial TrPs in the long slack latissimus dorsi muscle minimally restrict forward flexion of the arm. Those in the infraspinatus, teres minor, and posterior deltoid muscles restrict internal rotation at the shoulder.

Scaleni

Any of the three scalene muscles can refer pain to the anterior, lateral, and posterior shoulder girdle regions and also down the length of the upper extremity to the index finger, skipping the elbow (Fig. 43.2A) (1, 29). Tension due to TrPs in the anterior and middle scalene muscles can also entrap the lower trunk of the brachial plexus, which often causes symptomatic neurapraxia of the ulnar nerve (4).

For relief, the jet stream of vapocoolant spray is directed downward over the scalene muscles and over their complete referred pain pattern, including the hand and upper back, while all of these muscles are passively lengthened by sidebending the head to the opposite side. The face position of Figure 43.2A places maximum stretch on the posterior scalene. Rotating the face toward the involved side emphasizes stretch of the anterior scalene muscle. Simple sidebending of the neck stretches chiefly the middle scalene. A self-stretch program and correction of mechanical perpetuating factors, such as paradoxical respiration (4), are usually necessary for sustained relief.

Levator Scapulae

A "stiff neck" syndrome with restricted rotation of the neck is commonly caused by active TrPs in the levator scapulae muscle (30). This muscle refers pain as in Figure 43.2B (4, 31).

The sweeps of spray extend downward, over the muscle and its referred pain pattern. The operator must simultaneously press the shoulder down and back to stabilize it and press the head forward and to the opposite side with one arm while applying sweeps of spray with the other hand (Fig. 43.2B). Instead, he or she may apply shoulder pressure and spray with one arm and assist stretch with the other. Full stretch combines flexion, sidebending, and rotation of the neck to the opposite side.

SHOULDER AND UPPER EXTREMITY PAIN

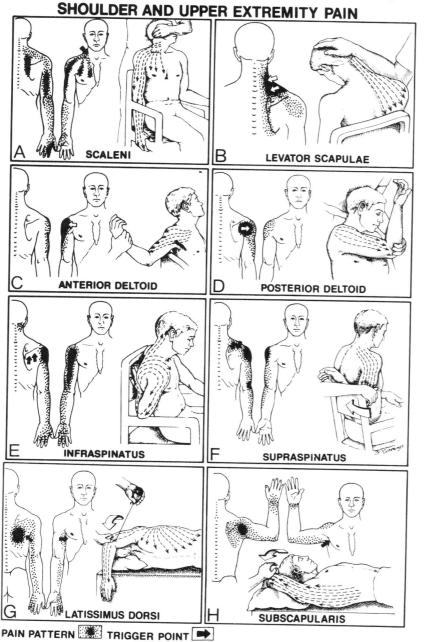

Figure 43.2. Location of TrPs (*short straight black*, or *white arrows*) and pain patterns (*solid black and stipples*), stretch positions, and spray patterns (*dashed arrows*) for eight muscles producing shoulder and upper extremity pain. The *curved white arrows* identify the direction(s) of pressure applied to stretch the muscle. The *dashed arrows* trace the impact of the stream of vapocoolant spray applied to release the muscular tension during stretch. (From Simons DG: Myofascial pain syndromes. In Basmajian JV, Kirby RL (eds): *Medical Rehabilitation.* Baltimore, Williams & Wilkins, 1984, pp 315–316.)

PAIN PATTERN ▓ TRIGGER POINT ➡

The neck must always be protected, particularly where there is hypermobility, loss of cervical lordosis, or cervical joint degeneration. When a levator stretch is needed, it is best done by stabilizing the head and neck and then moving the scapula downward and into lateral rotation.

Deltoid

The free borders of the anterior and posterior deltoid muscle are more common sites of TrPs than is the middle deltoid. Pain from deltoid TrPs, like pain from the gluteus maximus muscle, is referred locally (Fig. 43.2C and *D*).

Spray is directed distalward over the muscle and over its pain pattern (Fig. 43.2C and *D*). Maximum stretch of the anterior deltoid (Fig. 43.2C) requires both horizontal extension and external rotation of the arm. Stretch of the posterior deltoid (Fig. 43.2D) brings the elbow as far across the chest as possible. Additional stretch may be achieved by using internal rotation rather than the external rotation shown in Figure 43.2D.

Infraspinatus

The pain commonly referred from TrPs in the infraspinatus muscle is distinctive for its penetration deep into the shoulder joint (Fig. 43.2E) (31, 32).

The sweeps of spray follow the dashed arrows in Figure 43.2E. The seated patient reaches behind the back as high as possible toward the scapula and then leans back against the chair to relax. The arm is progressively repositioned passively until full range of motion is achieved.

Supraspinatus

The supraspinatus muscle usually projects pain and tenderness (Fig. 43.2F) to the middeltoid region and to the elbow, which the infraspinatus and scaleni patterns skip. Supraspinatus TrPs sometimes activate satellite TrPs in the deltoid muscle.

The spray path is shown as dashed arrows in Figure 43.2F and continues to the wrist. Full stretch is difficult to attain because the body obstructs pure adduction. The difficulty is circumvented by alternately adducting the arm behind and in front of the torso, as for the deltoid stretch.

Latissimus Dorsi

Myofascial TrPs in the long slack latissimus dorsi (Fig. 43.2G) are particularly troublesome to the patient because no positioning of the arm seems to relieve that pain. The TrPs causing the pain are easily overlooked. Referred pain from both the latissimus dorsi (Fig. 43.2G) and serratus posterior superior (see Fig. 43.4D) projects to the scapular area. The serratus posterior superior muscle refers pain more cephalad in relation to the scapula and deep into the chest. Pain into the chest is not characteristic of latissimus dorsi TrPs.

For the latissimus dorsi muscle, vapocoolant is applied from the TrP in the direction of referred pain to cover the entire muscle and its pain pattern, as in Figure 43.2G.

Full stretch can be attained seated, but patient relaxation is improved in the side-lying position and downward tilting of the pelvis is more easily achieved. Effective stretch of the latissimus dorsi (Fig. 43.2G) requires essentially the same arm position as for the subscapularis (Fig. 43.2H). Therefore, subscapularis TrPs may have to be released first to attain full stretch of the latissimus dorsi.

Subscapularis

Myofascial TrPs (black arrow in Fig. 43.2H) in the subscapularis muscle are often the key to a frozen shoulder syndrome. Active TrPs in this muscle severely restrict both abduction and external rotation of the arm (4, 33). This severe limitation of motion encourages TrPs in the other shoulder girdle muscles and leads to the frozen shoulder. Pain referred from the subscapularis concentrates on the back of the shoulder and frequently includes a "band" of pain and tenderness around the wrist.

Treatment begins with upsweeps of the spray that cover the side of the chest and axilla, as in Figure 43.2H. The sweeps include *all of the scapula*, especially its vertebral border, which is not shown in the figure. Sweeps

of spray are continued to include the wrist. Stretch employs gentle, progressive abduction and external rotation of the arm at the shoulder.

Biceps Brachii

Referred pain from biceps brachii TrPs radiates upward to the shoulder anteriorly and sometimes downward to the elbow (Fig. 43.3A). Bicipital tendinitis may sometimes be relieved by inactivation of TrPs in the long head of the biceps brachii.

The stream of vapocoolant is directed as in Figure 43.3A. The long head of the biceps brachii crosses two joints and for full stretch requires elbow extension, horizontal extension of the arm at the shoulder, and pronation of the forearm, as illustrated. The in-doorway stretch is strongly recommended for the patient's home program (4).

Brachialis

The brachialis muscle, remarkably, projects pain strongly to the base of the thumb (Fig. 43.3B). It is noteworthy that the supinator (Fig. 43.3D), brachioradialis (33), and adductor pollicis (33) muscles also refer pain and tenderness to the thumb area. The stream of spray is applied distally over the brachialis muscle and to cover the thumb and then cephalad over the biceps, which is its upper pain reference zone (4). The brachialis is stretched only by extension of the forearm at the elbow. Myofascial TrPs in the muscle are readily palpated by pushing the distal biceps aside, and they respond well to injection (Fig. 43.3B).

Triceps Brachii

Five TrP locations in the three heads of the triceps muscle refer individual pain patterns (4) that are combined in Figure 43.3C. Because the long head is a two-joint muscle, its TrPs restrict simultaneous flexion at the elbow and at the shoulder. The long head of the triceps is a commonly overlooked cause of shoulder dysfunction. The taut bands of the long head TrPs are readily identified by pincer palpation of its belly just above mid-arm adjacent to the humerus. The muscle is examined for taut bands by encircling the long head, inserting the tips of the finger and thumb between the muscle and the humerus. The taut bands are detected by rolling the muscle fibers between the fingertips (4).

The spray is applied in parallel sweeps (Fig. 43.3C). Full stretch requires simultaneous two-joint flexion as illustrated, a position seldom assumed in daily activity.

Supinator

Active TrPs in the supinator muscle are often responsible for "tennis elbow" or "epicondylitis." The supinator refers pain and tenderness to the lateral epicondyle and also to the dorsal web space of the thumb (Fig. 43.3D).

SHOULDER AND UPPER EXTREMITY PAIN (CONTINUED)

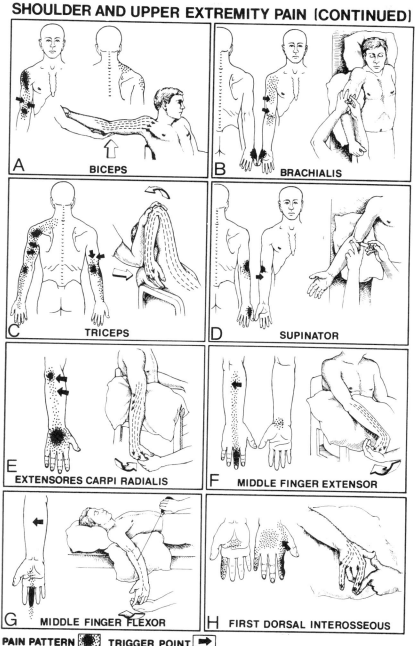

Figure 43.3. Location of TrPs (*short straight black arrows*) and pain patterns (*solid black and stipples*), stretch positions, and spray patterns (*dashed arrows*) for eight muscles responsible for shoulder and upper extremity pain. The *curved white arrows* identify the direction(s) of pressure applied to passively stretch the muscle. The *dashed arrows* trace the impact of parallel sweeps of vapocoolant spray applied to release the muscular tension during stretch. (From Simons DG: Myofascial pain syndromes. In Basmajian JV, Kirby RL (eds): *Medical Rehabilitation.* Baltimore, Williams & Wilkins, 1984, pp 316–317.)

PAIN PATTERN ▨ TRIGGER POINT ➡

The stream of vapocoolant is directed distalward over the muscle, then back and around to cover the lateral epicondyle and finally is continued distally over the dorsum of the forearm and thumb. Stretch requires combined extension at the elbow and pronation of the hand (4). Injection of the most common TrPs in the medial border of the muscle is illustrated in Figure 43.3D. The radial nerve should be avoided when injecting these TrPs (4). The extensor muscle mass on the dorsum of the forearm distal to the lateral epicondyle frequently also develops TrPs as part of the "tennis elbow" syndrome. These TrPs are readily identified by taut bands and local twitch responses.

Extensores Digitorum and Carpi Radialis

The hand and finger extensors that comprise the extensor muscle mass are strongly activated by a vigorous grip. Active TrPs in these muscles frequently cause the hand grip to be painful and measurably weakened; a cup or a glass may unexpectedly drop from the grasp. The extensor carpi radialis refers pain and tenderness to the lateral epicondyle and dorsum of the hand (Fig. 43.3E). Active TrPs in the finger extensors refer pain to the dorsal surface of the corresponding finger, as illustrated in Figure 43.3F.

The stream of spray is applied over the muscles and includes the wrist and fingers. Effective stretch of all of these muscles requires full flexion of the wrist and *fingers*, as illustrated.

Flexores Digitorum

The patterns of pain referred from the flexores digitorum sublimis and profundus are similar. Each section of these muscles refers pain to the corresponding finger; Figure 43.3G presents an example. Patients with TrPs in this muscle may describe the pain as extending to the tip of the finger, occasionally shooting beyond the tip.

Vapocoolant spray is applied distalward, as in Figure 43.3G. The wrist and fingers must be extended simultaneously for a full stretch.

Interossei of Hand

Myofascial TrPs of the interossei are relatively common. The dorsal interossei are readily palpable against the metacarpal bones. Interosseous TrPs refer pain along the side of the digit that corresponds to the distal attachment of that muscle. In addition, the first dorsal interosseous usually projects pain across the hand and into the little finger (Fig. 43.3H). In some patients interosseous TrPs are an important contributing cause of Heberden's nodes, which may be aborted early in their development by inactivation of the responsible interosseous TrPs.

The stream of vapocoolant spray is applied distalward with stretch by adduction of the index finger, as in Figure 43.3H. Frequently injection is required.

TRUNK AND BACK PAIN

Muscles of the chest and abdomen frequently exhibit misleading viscerosomatic and somatovisceral interactions. A viscerosomatic example is the development of satellite TrPs in the pectoralis major muscle in response to an acute myocardial infarction or to myocardial ischemia (4). Another example is the appearance of TrPs in the external oblique muscle of the abdomen secondary to pain referred into that region by gastrointestinal ulcer disease (34).

A somatovisceral example is the cardiac arrhythmia associated with the "arrhythmia TrP" in the right pectoralis major muscle (4).

Pectoralis Major and Minor

The pectoralis minor muscle and the more horizontal fibers of the sternal division of the pectoralis major muscle commonly refer pain that closely mimics cardiac ischemia (Fig. 43.4A) (4, 25). The lateral, nearly vertical lower fibers of the pectoralis major refer pain and *tenderness* to the breast (Fig. 43.4B), causing severe breast hypersensitivity that, in either sex, may render clothing contact intolerable.

For either of the pectoral muscles, vapocoolant is first directed upward and laterally over the muscle and its referred pain pattern as in Figure 43.4A and B.

Stretch is applied to the sternal division of the pectoralis major, as illustrated by the curved white arrow in Figure 43.4A, whereas stretch is applied to the pectoralis minor by retraction of the scapula with backward traction on the arm. The nearly vertical thoracic fibers along the lateral border of the pectoralis major are partially stretched by the intermediate position shown in Figure 43.4B. They are fully stretched by *full* flexion of the arm at the shoulder. This fully flexed position also stretches the anterior costal fibers of the latissimus dorsi. Therefore, when it, too, is tense, the latissimus dorsi also must be released, as in Figure 43.2G, to achieve full pectoralis range of motion.

For lasting inactivation of pectoralis TrPs, a head-forward, round-shouldered posture, which maintains the pectoral muscles in the shortened position, must be corrected. In the seated position this poor posture is spontaneously improved without muscle strain by use of a comfortable lumbar support, a towel roll or small pillow placed against the small of the back at waistline level (4). This ensures the maintenance of a full normal lumbar curve.

Serratus Anterior

Although the serratus anterior is not considered a respiratory muscle, its active TrPs restrict chest expansion and cause shortness of breath (4). Figure 43.4C portrays its referred pain pattern.

Vapocoolant is applied in radial sweeps (Fig. 43.4C) that should cover the lower half of the scapula. The serratus anterior may be stretched with the patient supine, as illustrated in Figure 43.4C, or comfortably seated in an armchair. Self-stretch is performed when seated by using the uninvolved arm to reach behind the torso and pull on the distal humerus of the involved side to strongly retract the scapula.

Serratus Posterior Superior

The enigmatic referred pain of the serratus posterior superior (Fig. 43.4D) is threateningly deep and frequently projects into and through the upper chest, suggesting visceral disease. Positioning of the arm often provides no relief. To palpate serratus posterior superior TrPs, the scapula must be fully protracted in order to uncover the lateral ends of the muscle (4). The tenderness of these TrPs is palpated through the trapezius and rhomboid muscles against the ribs. Some release of the muscle can be obtained by manual stretch, but stretch is frequently unsatisfactory. Trigger points in this muscle usually require ischemic compression or local injection, as illustrated in Figure 43.4D. When injecting, one should direct the needle nearly parallel to the skin surface and always toward a rib, not toward an intercostal space, to be sure of avoiding a pneumothorax.

Quadratus Lumborum

The quadratus lumborum muscle is one of the most common sources of musculoskeletal low back pain (25,

TRUNK AND BACK PAIN

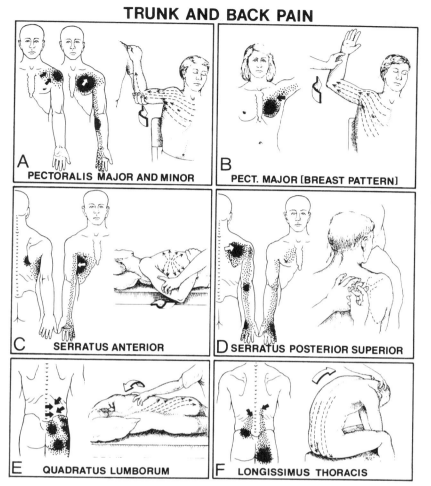

Figure 43.4. Location of TrPs (*short straight white* or *black arrows*) and pain patterns (*solid black and stipples*), stretch positions, and spray patterns (*dashed arrows*) for 10 muscles that cause trunk and back pain. The *curved white arrows* identify the direction(s) of pressure applied to stretch the muscle. The *dashed arrows* trace the impact of the stream of vapocoolant spray applied to release the muscular tension during stretch. (From Simons DG: Myofascial pain syndromes. In Basmajian JV, Kirby RL (eds): *Medical Rehabilitation*, Baltimore, Williams & Wilkins, 1984, pp 317–318.)

35, 36) and is commonly overlooked (37), partly because effective palpation requires unusual positioning of the patient. Active TrPs in the quadratus lumborum project pain to the sacroiliac joint, lower buttock, and lateral hip regions (Fig. 43.4E) (31, 35, 38). Satellite TrPs often generated in the posterior section of the gluteus minimus muscle cause a secondary sciatica-like pain pattern (see Fig. 43.5D) that further misleads the diagnostician. Bilateral quadratus lumborum TrPs are common and produce pain that extends bilaterally across the sacroiliac regions.

For precise examination of the quadratus lumborum muscle, the side-lying patient is positioned to open a space between the twelfth rib and the crest of the ilium. Space is provided by elevating the rib cage and tilting the pelvis downward on that side. The examination position is nearly the stretch position of Figure 43.4E, except that the upper leg lies behind the lower leg and the uppermost knee rests on the examining table (29, 35, 38).

The vapocoolant spray is directed distally to cover all of the lumbar area and buttock, emphasizing the sacral and sacroiliac joint region, especially when that region is reported as painful. Two stretch positions may be required (35). One is the leg-forward position shown in

Figure 43.4E, which tilts the pelvis away from the ribs and rotates it forward. The other is the leg-back position (29, 35), which places the upper leg behind the lower leg, reverses the rotation on the thoracolumbar region, and simultaneously lengthens the adjacent iliopsoas muscle. To release restricting tension in the latter muscle, spray is directed downward over the abdomen, close to the midline, and over the inguinal region and the inner thigh to completely cover the skin representation of the muscle and its pain reference zones (35, 38). The iliopsoas muscle can, itself, be an important source of referred pain (33, 36).

Injection of TrPs in the quadratus lumborum is effective, but requires careful technique and appreciation of the regional anatomy involved (29, 35).

Quadratus lumborum TrPs are usually perpetuated by a short leg and/or a small hemipelvis. Both are correctable by appropriate heel and butt lifts, which are often *essential* for lasting relief of this myofascial pain syndrome (4, 35, 38).

Thoracic and Lumbar Paraspinal Muscles (4, 38)

In the midthoracic region, the most medial paraspinal muscle, the spinalis, lies against the spinous processes.

Figure 43.4 **G–N.**

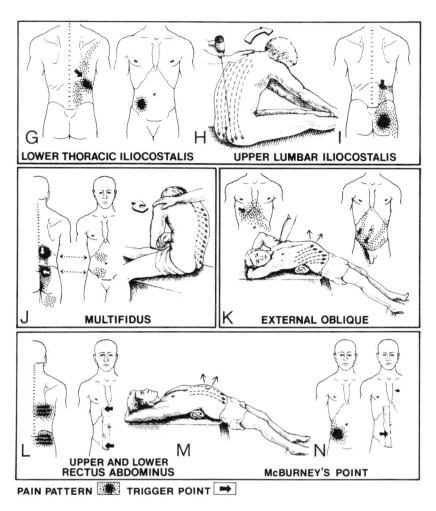

Next laterally is the superficial longissimus, one of the longest muscles in the body. It extends from the occiput to the sacrum. The superficial and most lateral paraspinal fibers, the iliocostalis, attach to the ribs. Bilaterally, the direction of the deeper paraspinal muscles, the multifidi and rotatores, presents an inverted "V" configuration; the deeper they lie the shorter they are, and the more diagonal is their course. The deepest, the rotatores, course between adjacent vertebrae at nearly a 45° angle. To adequately stretch these fibers one must often mobilize adjacent vertebrae by using a manual medicine technique, such as strongly rotating and flexing the spine simultaneously.

Taut bands and local twitch responses are easily identified in the longissimus fibers. These TrPs refer pain distally many segments removed, sometimes reaching the distal buttock (Fig. 43.4F).

Lower thoracic iliocostalis TrPs refer pain as in Figure 43.4G, whereas Figure 43.4I shows the pain pattern of upper lumbar iliocostalis TrPs. The multifidi refer pain locally (Fig. 43.4J). The rotatores frequently refer pain to the midline at the same segmental level. Generally, thoracolumbar paraspinal muscles refer pain caudalward (Fig. 43.4G), so that the spray is applied bilaterally

downward, including the buttocks (Fig. 43.4H). Multifidus TrPs respond to a shorter, more angulated unilateral spray pattern (Fig. 43.4J).

Stretch position for the longissimus is shown in Figure 43.4F, with the patient's feet on the floor and the legs spread apart far enough that the arms can dangle freely between them. The patient must allow the wrists and elbows to flex in a relaxed manner as the fingers encounter the floor. The parallel sweeps of spray should also cover the gluteus maximus muscle (Fig. 43.4F and I), because it is stretched by the full hip flexion. Relaxation and stretch of the iliocostalis may be augmented by rotating the patient's chest to the opposite side.

For stretch of the multifidi, full rotation is applied toward the involved side (Fig. 43.4J), preferably without flexion. Injection is often necessary for the deepest diagonal muscles. In the thoracic region the needle must be angled medially toward the spinous processes to avoid a pneumothorax.

Caution must be used in stretch of the lumbar paraspinals. Normal lumbar lordosis must not be compromised. If hypermobility is present, rhythmic stabilization exercise in the neutral position is preferable.

LOWER EXTREMITY PAIN

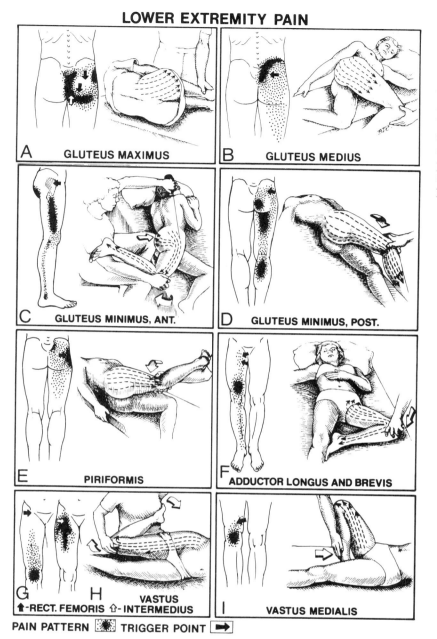

Figure 43.5. Location of TrPs (*short straight black* or *white arrows*) and pain patterns (*solid black and stipples*), stretch positions, and spray patterns (*dashed arrows*) for nine muscles responsible for lower extremity pain. The curved white arrows *identify the direction(s) of pressure applied to stretch a muscle. The dashed arrows* trace the impact of the stream of vapocoolant spray applied to release the muscular tension during stretch. (From Simons DG: Myofascial pain syndromes. In Basmajian JV, Kirby RL (eds): *Medical Rehabilitation.* Baltimore, Williams & Wilkins, 1984, pp 318–319.)

Abdominal Muscles

Myofascial TrPs in the abdominal external oblique muscle may refer pain locally, into adjacent areas, and sometimes across the midline (Fig. 43.4K), (4, 25, 39). Those TrPs close to the thoracic or pelvic attachment of the rectus abdominis muscle commonly refer pain *horizontally* across the back at nearly the same level as the TrP (Fig. 43.4L). A McBurney's point TrP in the rectus abdominis may convincingly simulate the pain and tenderness of appendicitis (Fig. 43.4N). Tensing the abdominal muscles by elevating both feet in the supine position easily permits differentiation of visceral from abdominal wall tenderness. This tensing of the abdominal muscles

augments TrP tenderness and protects the viscera from the pressure of palpation (40). If the patient has a suspected back problem that prevents this maneuver, he or she can, instead, strongly contract the abdominal muscles while supine by exerting downward extension of the upper limbs against resistance.

The spray pattern for TrPs in the rectus abdominis muscles is illustrated in Figure 43.4M. Stretch of the abdominal wall muscles is achieved by positioning the patient as in the same figure and having the patient protrude the abdomen by taking a deep breath and contracting the diaphragm while relaxing the abdominal wall muscles. The patient must not hold the breath (close the glottis). The rotation movement that should be added to stretch the external oblique muscle (Fig. 43.4*K*) is not required to stretch the rectus abdominis.

Lower Extremity Pain

Generally, TrPs in lower extremity muscles refer pain locally and/or distally. However, the adductor muscles also refer pain proximally. Since patients commonly identify gluteal pain as low back pain, gluteal muscle TrPs are likely to contribute to a "low back pain" complaint (39).

Gluteus Maximus

Like the deltoid muscle, gluteus maximus TrPs are easily palpated for taut bands and show vigorous local twitch responses. The gluteus maximus generates local referred pain that concentrates mainly over the sacrum and inferior surface of the buttock (Fig. 43.5*A*).

The patient is placed in the side-lying position for stretch and spray (Fig. 43.5*A*). The vapocoolant spray is directed distally, as illustrated, while the thigh is progressively flexed by bringing the knee toward the chest. Active gluteal TrPs are commonly associated with tight hamstring muscles; these would also need to be released by stretch and spray (see Fig. 43.6*C*) to achieve full range of hip motion and lasting relief.

Gluteus Medius

TrPs in the gluteus medius refer pain (Fig. 43.5*B*) along the crest of the ilium posteriorly and over the sacrum; pain may also extend across the buttock and over the upper thigh posteriorly.

The line of impact of the stream of vapocoolant spray extends from the crest of the ilium distalward over the upper *half of the thigh* as indicated in Figure 43.5*B*. For passive stretch, the thigh is flexed nearly 90° and progressively adducted as the spray is applied. Pulling backward on the anterior superior iliac spine augments the stretch. The Dudley J. Morton foot configuration, when present, is a perpetuating factor and should be corrected (4, 35, 39).

Gluteus Minimus

The anterior and posterior portions of the gluteus minimus project separate referred pain patterns. The anterior TrPs refer pain to the thigh laterally and also to the buttock, as in Figure 43.5*C*, whereas TrPs in the posterior part of the muscle refer pain to the lower extremity posteriorly, as in Figure 43.5*D*. This pattern suggests an S1 radiculopathy or "sciatica." Adding to the confusion, gluteus minimus TrPs may be perpetuated by an S1 radiculopathy.

Location of the sweeps of spray for release of TrPs in the anterior portion of the muscle and its stretch position are portrayed in Figure 43.5*C*. For TrPs in the posterior portion, they are shown in Figure 43.5*D*. In neither case is it necessary to fully bend the knee, but if the knee is

straight, hamstring tension may block full hip flexion. The gluteus maximus muscle is included in the posterior spray pattern to release restricting TrPs that it may harbor.

Piriformis

Active piriformis TrPs restrict both adduction and internal rotation of the thigh at the hip. Tenderness is elicited by external or rectal palpation (39). Figure 43.5*E* shows the piriformis referred pain pattern and the vapocoolant is directed as illustrated. For stretch, the thigh of the side-lying patient is flexed at the hip to nearly 90° and internally rotated as the knee is lowered gently to increase adduction at the hip, as depicted in Figure 43.5*E*. Gravity can be used to facilitate adduction by allowing the leg to hang over the edge of the treatment table. The gluteus maximus muscle also should be sprayed if it is blocking full range of movement.

Tension caused by taut bands due to TrPs in the piriformis muscle may entrap the peroneal part or all of the sciatic nerve, depending upon anatomic variations, as the nerve passes through instead of around the muscle (39).

Adductores Longus and Brevis

In addition to the pattern in Figure 43.5*F*, pain from either the long or short hip adductors may be referred upward throughout the groin (1, 33). Active TrPs in these muscles markedly restrict abduction of the thigh.

To inactivate TrPs in these muscles, sweeps of the vapocoolant that overlap in the midthigh are directed proximally as well as distally (Fig. 43.5*F*). As the spray is applied, the muscle is gradually lengthened by placing the patient in the position shown in Figure 43.5*F* and gently helping the knee downward toward the examining table (white arrow).

Quadriceps Femoris

Active TrPs in the rectus femoris muscle are usually located at the proximal end of the muscle near the solid black arrow in Figure 43.5*G*. They project pain to the front of the knee, as shown in the same figure.

Vastus intermedius TrPs are found in the area near the small white arrow in Figure 43.5*G*; they lie deeper and more distal than the rectus femoris TrP and refer pain intensely over the upper thigh anteriorly.

Vastus medialis TrPs refer pain (Figure 43.5*I*) to the anteromedial aspect of the knee and to the patellar area. When this muscle is suddenly overloaded, its TrPs may reflexly inhibit contraction without pain, giving rise to the buckling knee syndrome.

The TrPs found distally in the anterior portion of the **vastus lateralis** muscle (solid black arrow, Fig. 43.6*A*) are frequently multiple and difficult to eliminate; they refer pain intensely and extensively as shown in Figure 43.6*A*. The TrPs found more proximally in the posterior portion of the vastus lateralis are located near the small

LOWER EXTREMITY PAIN

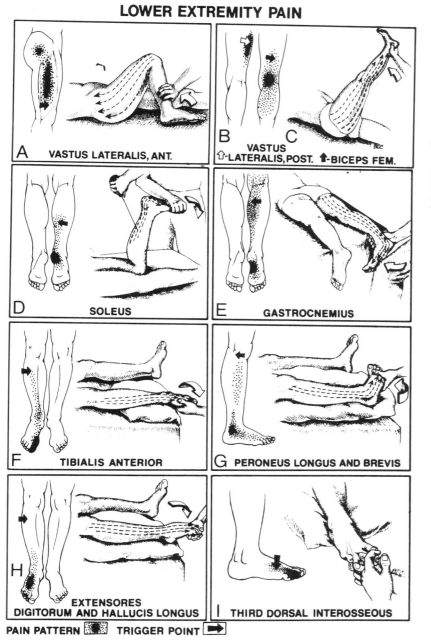

Figure 43.6. Location of TrPs (*short straight black* or *white arrows*) and pain patterns (*solid black and stipples*), stretch positions, and spray patterns (*dashed arrows*) for 10 muscles causing lower extremity pain. The *curved white arrows* identify the direction(s) of pressure applied to stretch the muscle. The *dashed arrows* trace the impact of the stream of vapocoolant spray applied to release the muscular tension during stretch. In *B*, both are right lower extremities. (From Simons DG: Myofascial pain syndromes. In Basmajian JV, Kirby RL (eds): *Medical Rehabilitation.* Baltimore, Williams & Wilkins, 1984, pp 319–320.)

white arrow on the right lower extremity shown at the left side of Figure 43.6*B*, and usually refer pain vertically in a local pattern.

To inactivate TrPs in the rectus femoris, the patient lies on the unaffected side, as in Figure 43.5*H*. The parallel sweeps of vapocoolant are directed distally, as illustrated, and the knee is flexed *while extending the hip.* For release of TrPs in the other three quadriceps muscles, the spray is applied distalward over each muscle as shown in Figure 43.5*H* and *I*. Knee flexion alone, regardless of hip position, stretches all three vasti, but not the rectus femoris.

Biceps Femoris

Pain is referred to the biceps femoris from TrPs that are located near the tip of the black arrow in Figure 43.6*B*. Release of hamstring tightness is most easily attained by initially directing the spray upward over the adductor magnus and inguinal region of the supine patient while horizontally abducting the thigh at the hip without raising the leg (not illustrated). The lower extremity is then elevated to bring the thigh directly from the abducted position to the 90° flexed position while the spray is applied over the true "hamstring" muscles in the pattern of Figure 43.6*C*.

Soleus

The TrPs in the soleus, a second-layer, single-joint muscle (Fig. 43.6*D*), cause referred heel pain and *tenderness* that frequently are mistaken for symptoms caused by a heel spur. Occasionally, TrPs in this muscle also project pain to the sacroiliac joint region on the same side, as illustrated elsewhere (35, 39).

The prone patient is positioned and vapocoolant is directed as in Figure 43.6*D*, over the entire muscle. Progressive downward dorsiflexion pressure is then applied firmly (curved white arrow) to the ball of the foot. Self-stretch of this muscle is accomplished by standing with the heel flat on the floor and progressively *bending the knee*. Self-stretch of the gastrocnemius is similar, but requires that the knee remain straight.

Gastrocnemius

Myofascial TrPs are usually found in the gastrocnemius, a superficial, two-joint muscle, in either the medial (Fig. 43.6*E*) or lateral (not shown) border of the muscle. The TrPs in either head refer pain essentially as seen in the same figure (31, 35). These TrPs render walking uphill especially painful and commonly cause nocturnal calf cramps.

For treatment, the patient lies prone with the knee straight and the foot dorsiflexed at the ankle, as in Figure 43.6*E*. The stream of spray is directed distally over all of the muscle and includes the foot, which is firmly dorsiflexed by the operator's knee in order to apply the necessary force in the direction of the curved white arrow in Figure 43.6*E*. As with all other muscles, the pressure applied should *NEVER* be painful, but applied only to the point of beginning discomfort.

The patient is taught how to self-stretch the gastrocnemius muscle by standing with the knee straight on the affected side and with the involved leg behind the other leg while shifting the pelvis and body forward. As the forward knee bends the ankle of the affected leg dorsiflexes with the rear knee fully extended. The *heel remains solidly on the floor*.

Tibialis Anterior

The tibialis anterior dorsiflexes and inverts the foot. Its TrPs (black arrow in Figure 43.6*F*) refer pain as illustrated, concentrating on the great toe (1, 31).

To release anterior tibial TrPs, the patient lies supine and spray is directed distalward over the muscle, as shown in Figure 43.6*F*. This muscle is passively lengthened by simultaneously plantar flexing and slowly everting the foot (white curved arrow, Fig. 43.6*F*).

Peroneus Longus and Brevis

The adjacent peroneus longus and brevis muscles have similar functions and essentially the same referred pain pattern. The TrPs in the peroneus longus (black arrow in Fig. 43.6*G*) are usually a few centimeters distal to the common peroneal nerve where it passes over the fibula beneath the peroneus longus muscle, just distal to the fibular head (1). Peroneus brevis TrPs are more distal, approximately midleg (35).

For both muscles, treatment begins with application of vapocoolant spray in the pattern shown in Figure 43.6*G*. The foot of the supine patient is plantar flexed and inverted (curved white arrow in Fig. 43.6*G*).

Tension caused by the taut bands of TrPs in the peroneus longus muscle can compress the deep peroneal nerve against the underlying fibula. This sometimes results in loss of sensation in the common peroneal nerve distribution with partial foot-drop weakness. When the TrPs are released, these symptoms, which are due to neurapraxia, resolve in minutes to days. This myofascial syndrome is perpetuated by the instability and stress of walking on the ''knife-edge'' of a long second metatarsal bone (D.J. Morton foot configuration) (4, 35).

Extensores Digitorum and Hallucis Longus

Active TrPs in the extensores digitorum and hallucis longus muscles, like those of the peroneal muscles, refer pain that includes the dorsum of the foot laterally (Fig. 43.6*H*). In addition, pain may extend further distally to the toes.

Vapocoolant is applied distalward in the pattern shown in Figure 43.6*H*; both muscles are stretched by simultaneously plantar flexing the foot and all toes.

Interossel of the Foot

As in the hand, foot interosseous TrPs are not rare. These TrPs, like those in the hand (4), refer pain distally to the side of the digit corresponding to the attachment of the involved muscle, as illustrated for the third dorsal interosseous in Figure 43.6*I*. These TrPs are commonly associated with the hammer toe that, if not too long-standing, can be alleviated by inactivating the corresponding interosseous TrPs. The taut bands and TrPs are exquisitely tender. They are readily palpable against the metatarsal bones and, therefore, easily injected (Fig. 43.6*I*). Stretch and spray alone may not be adequate therapy for these muscles.

Acknowledgment   The author gratefully acknowledges the thoughtful and meticulous review of the manuscript by Janet G. Travell, M.D. and Lois Statham Simons, R.P.T., M.S.

REFERENCES

1. Travell J, Rinzler SH: The myofascial genesis of pain. *Postrad Med* 11:425–434, 1952.
2. Sola AE, Rodenberger ML, Gettys BB: Incidence of hypersensitive areas in posterior shoulder muscles. *Am J Phys Med* 34:585–590, 1955.
3. Bates T, Grunwaldt E: Myofascial pain in childhood. *J Pediatr* 53:198–209, 1958.

4. Travell JG, Simons DG: *Myofascial Pain and Dysfunction: The Trigger Point Manual*. Baltimore, Williams & Wilkins, 1983.

5. Langs HM: Myofascial pain and analgesia. *Pain Suppl* 4:S297, 1987 (abstr 570).

6. Jaeger B, Reeves JL: Quantification of changes in myofascial trigger point sensitivity with the pressure algometer following passive stretch. *Pain* 27:203–210, 1986.

7. Crook J, Tunks E, Norman G, et al: A comparative study of tenderness thresholds in trigger points and non-trigger points in normal and fibromyalgia patients. *Pain Suppl* 4:S307, 1987 (abstr 509).

8. Scudds RA, McCain GA, Rollman GB, et al: Changes in pain responsiveness in fibrositis patients after successful treatment. *Pain Suppl* 4:S353, 1987 (abstr 677).

9. Tunks E, Norman G, Kalaher S, et al: Validity and reliability of the clinical use of a pressure algometer in the study of trigger points. *Pain Suppl* 4:S307, 1987 (abstr 590).

10. Jensen K, Andersen HO, Olesen J, et al: Pressure-pain threshold in human temporal region. Evaluation of a new pressure algometer. *Pain* 25:313–323, 1986.

11. Fischer AA: Pressure threshold meter: its use for quantification of tender spots. *Arch Phys Med Rehabil* 67:836–838, 1986.

12. Fischer AA: Pressure tolerance over muscles and bones in normal subjects. *Arch Phys Med Rehabil* 67:406–409, 1986.

13. Fischer AA: Tissue compliance meter for objective, quantitative documentation of soft tissue consistency and pathology. *Arch Phys Med Rehabil* 68:122–125, 1987.

14. Reeves JL, Jaeger B, Graff-Radford SB: Reliability of the pressure algometer as a measure of myofascial trigger point sensitivity. *Pain* 24:313–321, 1986.

15. Schiffman E, Fricton J, Haley D, et al: A pressure algometer for myofascial pain syndrome: reliability and validity. *Pain Suppl* 4:S291, 1987 (abstr 558).

16. Fricton JR, et al: Myofascial pain syndrome: electromyographic changes associated with local twitch response. *Arch Phys Med Rehabil* 66:314–317, 1985.

17. Simons DG: Myofascial pain syndrome due to trigger points. In Goodgold J (ed): *Rehabilitation Medicine*. St. Louis, CV Mosby, 1988 (in press).

18. Mense S, Schmidt RF: Muscle pain: which receptors are responsible for the transmission of noxious stimuli? In Rose FC (ed): *Physiological Aspects of Clinical Neurology*, Oxford, Blackwell Scientific Publications, 1977.

19. Institute of Medicine: *Pain and Disability: Clinical Behavioral and Public Policy Perspectives*. Washington DC, National Academy Press, 1987.

20. Bengtsson A, Henriksson K-G, Jorfeldt L, et al: Primary fibromyalgia—a clinical and laboratory study of 55 patients. *Scand J Rheumatol* 15:340–347, 1986.

21. Lund N, Bengtsson A, Thorborg P: Muscle tissue oxygen pressure in primary fibromyalgia. *Scand J Rheumatol* 15:165–173, 1986.

22. Bengtsson A, Henriksson K-G, Larsson J: Reduced high-energy phosphate levels in painful muscle in patients with primary fibromyalgia, *Arthritis Rheum* 29:817–821, 1986.

23. Bengtsson A, Henriksson K-G, Larsson J: Muscle biopsy in primary fibromyalgia. *Scand J Rheumatol* 15:1–6, 1986.

24. Graff-Radford SB, Reeves JL, Jaeger B: Management of chronic headache and neck pain: effectiveness of altering factors perpetuating myofascial pain. *Headache* 27:186–190, 1987.

25. Sola AE: Treatment of myofascial pain syndromes. In Benedatti C et al (eds): *Advances in Pain Research and Therapy*. New York, Raven Press, 1984, vol 7, pp 467–485.

26. Lewit K: Postisometric relaxation in combination with other methods of muscular facilitation and inhibition. *Manual Med* 1:101–104, 1986.

27. Rubin D: An approach to the management of myofascial trigger point syndromes. *Arch Phys Med Rehabil* 62:107–110, 1981.

28. Reynolds MD: Myofascial trigger points in persistent post-traumatic shoulder pain. *South Med J* 77:1277–1280, 1984.

29. Simons DG: Myofascial pain syndromes due to trigger points: 2. Treatment and single-muscle syndromes. *Manual Med* 1:72–77, 1985.

30. Travell J: Rapid relief of acute "stiff neck" by ethyl chloride spray. *J Am Med Wom Assoc* 4:89–95, 1949.

31. Sola AE: Trigger point therapy. In Roberts JR, Hedges JR (eds): *Clinical Procedures in Emergency Medicine*. Philadelphia, WB Saunders, 1985.

32. Reynolds MD: Myofascial trigger point syndromes in the practice of rheumatology. *Arch Phys Med Rehabil* 82:111–114, 1981.

33. Simons DG, Travell JG: Myofascial pain syndromes. Wall PD, Melzack R (eds): In *Textbook of Pain*. London, Churchill Livingstone, 1984, pp 263–276.

34. Melnick J: Trigger areas and refractory pain in duodenal ulcer. *NY State J Med* 57:1073–1076, 1957.

35. Travell JG, Simons DG: *Myofascial Pain and Dysfunction: The Trigger Point Manual, Vol. II*. Baltimore, Williams & Wilkins, in process, est. 1989.

36. Zohn DA: The quadratus lumborum: an unrecognized source of back pain, clinical and thermographic aspects. *Orthop Rev* 15:87–92, 1985.

37. Sola AE, Williams RL: Myofascial pain syndromes. *Neurology* 6:91–95, 1956.

38. Simons DG, Travell JG: Myofascial origins of low back pain. 2. Torso muscles. *Postgrad Med* 73:81–92, 1983.

39. Simons DG, Travell JG: Myofascial origins of low back pain. 3. Pelvic and lower extremity muscles. *Postgrad Med* 73:99–108, 1983.

40. Slocumb JC: Neurological factors in chronic pelvic pain: trigger points and the abdominal pelvic pain syndrome. *Am J Obstet Gynecol* 149:536–543, 1984.

CHAPTER 44

CHRONIC MYOFASCIAL PAIN SYNDROME

DAVID G. SIMONS
LOIS STATHAM SIMONS

THIS AND the preceding chapter provide a basis for managing the *chronic* myofascial pain syndrome (MPS). The goal is to eliminate the multiple *causes* of the pain rather than deal with it only as a symptom. The previous chapter summarized the identification and treatment of a single-muscle MPS due to trigger points (TrPs). Such a single syndrome can multiply by the addition of satellite and secondary TrPs that arise and persist because of perpetuating factors. A chronic MPS develops from these additional, but treatable, TrP syndromes. Management of this complex problem is simplified by resolving the total myofascial pain picture into its single-muscle components and by correcting the perpetuating factors. By identifying the myofascial syndromes muscle by muscle, one can recognize the pieces of the puzzle that comprise the total pain picture and proceed to manage each one individually.

This chapter first examines two kinds of perpetuating factors, systemic and mechanical. Then it reviews treatment techniques used to inactivate myofascial TrPs: stretch and spray, other physical methods, and injection with stretch. Next, it compares myofascial TrPs with two other closely interrelated but separate conditions, fibrositis/fibromyalgia and articular dysfunction. Finally, it summarizes how all of these issues are addressed in the care of a patient who has a chronic MPS due to TrPs.

Chronic pain that has not been attributable to an organic disease process is a major unsolved problem of the health care system in this country (1). This unsolved problem accounts for the popularity of pain management clinics that help the patient to *live with* his or her pain. Too often, the clinics do frustratingly little to teach the patient how to *relieve* the pain (1). Fields pointed out, "The most common persistent and disabling pains are those of musculoskeletal origin" (2), with which this chapter is concerned.

Many directors of chronic pain programs have come

to recognize two basic facts concerning their patients. First, few if any of these patients have only one condition that is responsible for their suffering. There are multiple *interacting* factors. Second, no two patients are alike. Thus, the success of a chronic pain program hinges on:

1. Identification of which of a multitude of sources are significant contributors to the suffering of the individual patient.
2. Estimation of the relative importance of the sources of suffering with an understanding of the interactions in the patient.
3. Effective therapy of the major causes applied in an order and combination that respects their interactions.

We have much to learn.

If the health care provider is to relieve the patient's chronic pain, that provider must address issues and apply therapeutic measures that were previously overlooked. A well-known disease like rheumatoid arthritis may be well managed, but the chronic myofascial TrPs may have been overlooked (3). Key answers must not have been part of conventional medical training; otherwise conventional medicine would have solved the problem.

Apparently, myofascial pain syndromes are a much more common cause of chronic pain than is generally appreciated. In a comprehensive pain center, myofascial TrPs were considered the primary cause of pain in 85% of the patients admitted to the program (4). In a dental clinic for patients with chronic head and neck pain, over half of the patients were found to have a primary diagnosis of myofascial pain syndrome (5). In a general practice of internal medicine, 10% of all patients, and 31% of those presenting with a pain complaint, had myofascial TrPs that were primarily responsible for their symptoms (6).

We owe Janet G. Travell, M.D., a great debt of gratitude for her clinical genius, research, and dedication that have established the diagnosis and management of myofascial pain. She published in 1952 the first compendium of individual pain patterns characteristic of the muscles most commonly responsible for myofascial pain throughout the body (7). This early work has been the key to understanding and managing acute single-muscle myofascial pain syndromes. Dr. Travell was the first to decipher the causal relationship between persistent myofascial TrPs that cause a chronic MPS and the multiple factors that perpetuate those TrPs. She clearly identified this relationship in 1976 (8) and described many perpetuating factors in detail in 1983 (9).

PERPETUATING FACTORS

Perpetuating factors act clinically like the missing link that converts an acute single-muscle syndrome into a chronic pain syndrome. These factors may be systemic or mechanical. Systemic factors are a frequent problem and they increase the irritability of the skeletal muscles throughout the body. Mechanical factors are equally ubiquitous and they overload and aggravate TrPs in specific muscles, depending on which muscle or muscles are overstressed (9).

In our experience, a patient with chronic pain due to myofascial TrPs nearly always has one, and often several, perpetuating factors that must be resolved before the myofascial components of the pain can be managed as single-muscle syndromes. Patients whose myofascial pain picture has remained essentially *static* for months or longer may not have serious perpetuating factors; specific myofascial local treatment can give these patients lasting relief. Patients in whom myofascial TrP symptoms have been *progressive* in time and who respond to treatment only temporarily, at best, consistently have perpetuating factors that must be resolved. Their primary TrPs generate satellite and secondary TrPs as previously described (9).

Generally, one stress activates a TrP and other factors perpetuate it. Prior to activation of a TrP, existing perpetuating factors usually cause negligible symptoms. For example, a leg length discrepancy of 6 mm (1/4″) may have caused no symptoms throughout most of a lifetime; however, when quadratus lumborum TrPs are activated by an accident or repetitive strain, the leg length difference becomes the perpetuator of the newly established TrPs. For lasting relief of the pain referred from the quadratus lumborum TrPs, the previously innocuous leg length discrepancy must be corrected.

The presence of significant perpetuating factors is confirmed by a poor response, or no response, to a trial of specific myofascial therapy applied to the muscle causing the myofascial pain. Although the initial response may be good, the symptoms soon return, sometimes in hours, more often in days. Lack of any response to the therapeutic trial may mean that treatment was applied to a latent TrP and not to the active TrP that was responsible for the pain. Occasionally, severe perpetuating factors render myofascial TrPs so extremely irritable that even gentle stretch and spray does not relieve the TrPs, and in fact may aggravate them.

SYSTEMIC FACTORS

Systemic perpetuating factors can aggravate TrPs in any muscle and increase the irritability of all skeletal muscles. These systemic factors render the muscles more vulnerable to the development of initial, secondary, and satellite TrPs (9). Major systemic factors include enzyme dysfunction because of nutritional inadequacy, metabolic and endocrine dysfunction, chronic infection or infestation, and psychological stress.

Correction of a significant perpetuating factor reduces irritability of the muscles. The patient has less pain. The responsiveness of the muscles to specific myofascial therapy improves.

Skeletal muscles are energy engines. They convert the energy stored in adenosine triphosphate (ATP) to mechanical movement. Understandably, *anything* that interferes with energy metabolism of the muscle tends to compromise this energy function and increase muscle irritability.

Enzyme Dysfunction and Nutritional Inadequacy

The nutritional inadequacies that most commonly are found to perpetuate myofascial TrPs are insufficient B-complex vitamins, particularly B_1, B_6, B_{12}, and folic acid. Other nutritional inadequacies that perpetuate TrPs are low serum levels of the electrolytes potassium or calcium and insufficiency of major minerals such as zinc, copper, iron, and essential trace minerals. The effect of prolonged inadequacies (low normal or marginal stores) of many of these nutrients is a relatively unexplored field of medicine.

A vitamin is an essential nutrient not synthesized by the body. It serves as a coenzyme to many apoenzymes that are supplied by the body. In the absence of the vitamin coenzyme, the metabolic step performed by that apoenzyme is blocked. The effect of this blockage depends on how critical to body chemistry are the functions served by that enzyme. A summary of the enzymatic functions of each of these vitamins has been reviewed in detail (9).

Vitamin *deficiency* is signaled by abnormally low laboratory values, often by the excretion of abnormal metabolites, and by characteristic symptoms ascribable to a lack of that vitamin. Vitamin *inadequacy* is identified by laboratory values in the lower quartile of the normal range. Abnormal metabolites may be demonstrable in the blood and urine. Laboratory values for vitamins in the lower range of normal are *not optimal* values. The

Table 44.1.
Distinctions Between Vitamin Deficiency and Vitamin Inadequacy

Vitamin Deficiency	Vitamin inadequacy
Subnormal laboratory values	Lower quartile and marginal laboratory values
Excretion of abnormal metabolites	Abnormal metabolites possible
Characteristic deficiency symptoms	Nonspecific or mild symptoms
Loss of function	Impaired function

usual basis for selecting laboratory control subjects does not screen out individuals with marginal insufficiency, including many who show chemical evidence of abnormal vitamin-dependent enzyme function (10). Laboratory values in the lower quartile of "normal" may be seriously suboptimal and are clinically responsible for increased irritability of the muscles. Clinically, correction of the inadequacy reduces muscle irritability and improves its responsiveness to therapy. Table 44.1 summarizes the clinical distinctions between a vitamin deficiency and a vitamin inadequacy.

Experience with patients shows that the lower these serum values are within the lower quartile of the "normal" range, the more likely it is that the inadequacy will perpetuate TrPs. Other than pain, vitamin inadequacies cause clinical complaints that are often subtle and nonspecific; mental and physical functions are suboptimal.

The prevalence of unrecognized vitamin *deficiency* is remarkably high, especially in hospital patients. Among 120 hospital patients, 88% had abnormally low levels in one or more of 11 vitamins (11). Despite this high prevalence, the history of dietary intake was inadequate in only 39%. More than half of the patients were low in two or more vitamins. Serum folate, which was the most common vitamin deficiency, was low in 45% of these patients. Symptoms of vitamin deficiency were clinically apparent in only 38% of them (11).

If vitamin *deficiency* can be this common, how much more common must be vitamin *inadequacy*? Well-controlled studies have yet to be conducted that answer this question definitively. If inadequacy is indeed common, and if such inadequacies perpetuate myofascial TrPs, then one would expect a large proportion of chronic myofascial pain patients to have vitamin inadequacy. In fact, over half of the patients referred to a myofascial pain clinic had vitamin B_{12} inadequacy, folate inadequacy, or both (D.G. Simons, unpublished data, 1987). Shealy (12) measured blood vitamin levels in 150 patients with chronic pain; he found that 80% of smokers and 35% of nonsmokers were deficient in vi-

tamin B_6. A *deficiency* of any of the four B vitamins is nearly always a serious perpetuator of myofascial TrPs; an *inadequacy* usually is a perpetuator. A recent study of inpatients with chronic pain (13) found insufficient blood levels of vitamins B_1, B_2, and folate. After pharmacologic supplementation with 12 vitamins for 12 days, the greatest pain relief was reported in those patients who registered the highest blood levels of vitamins B_1, B_6, B_{12}, and folic acid.

The common assumption that a well-balanced diet fully satisfies the metabolic need for a vitamin ignores loss of the vitamin during food preparation, impaired absorption, inadequate utilization, increased metabolic requirement, and increased excretion or destruction within the body (14). The wide variation in the requirements of individuals for essential nutrients, including vitamins, is well established (15). The official recommended dietary allowance (RDA) (16) is often considered the maximum amount anyone should need. That does not hold true for many chronic myofascial pain patients. As an extreme example, a few babies with a specific enzyme deficiency require megadose supplements of a vitamin coenzyme (e.g., B_{12}) for survival (17). These individuals have a severe congenital deficiency of an apoenzyme that requires that vitamin as its coenzyme. These congenital enzyme defects have been reviewed from the myofascial point of view (9). A minor degree of the same defect (poor genetic penetrance) could explain why some middle-aged patients gradually develop increased susceptibility to TrPs.

The Water-Soluble Vitamins

The B-complex vitamins and vitamin C are water soluble. They have remarkably low toxicity because an excess is quickly excreted in the urine; the safety of all of these water-soluble vitamins is not questioned at 10 times the recommended dietary allowance (18).

Thiamine. Inadequacy of thiamine (vitamin B_1) reveals its essential roles in nerve function and energy metabolism. Insufficiency causes increasingly severe loss of vibration sense at progressively more distal sites on the upper and lower extremities. The need for thiamine depends on the rate of energy expenditure. The daily RDA is 0.5 mg/1000 kcal of energy expenditure (16). Intact energy metabolism is essential to normal muscle function. The two life-threatening symptoms of severe thiamine deficiency are the disabling nervous system dysfunction of dry beriberi and the heart muscle failure with severe skeletal muscle weakness (19) of wet beriberi. Vitamin B_1 deficiency is well known in the alcoholic and heavy social drinker.

Pyridoxine. Remarkably so, pyridoxine (vitamin B_6) is a jack of all trades; it is an essential coenzyme for more than 60 apoenzymes in human metabolism. It is a metabolic necessity for the synthesis and degradation of numerous amino acids, including the methionine-to-cysteine pathway. It activates phosphorylase, which release glucose from glycogen. It is essential for the synthesis of many neurotransmitters, is required for normal cell reproduction, and is needed in the synthesis of at least 10 hormones (20).

Exactly which B_6-related enzyme dysfunctions increase the irritability of muscles is not yet clear. However, clinically, that irritability is relieved by correction of vitamin B_6 deficiency and inadequacy. Several drug classes increase the demand for vitamin B_6 and can easily cause inadequacy. These classes include antitubercular drugs, oral contraceptives, the chelating agent penicillamine, anticonvulsants, corticosteroids, and excessive alcohol consumption (20–23). Since laboratory testing for serum levels of vitamins B_1 and B_6 is so expensive and vitamin supplements are relatively inexpensive, when necessary, a pragmatic compromise is to prescribe a balanced B-complex supplement instead of measuring their values.

Both vitamins B_1 and B_6 are widely distributed in nature, but in relatively small amounts. Both are easily destroyed in food preparation. Vitamin B_1 (thiamine) is quickly leached out of food during washing and is destroyed in boiling. Likewise, pyridoxine suffers substantial losses during cooking and is quickly destroyed by ultraviolet light (sunlight) and oxidation (as when food is held on a steam table in a cafeteria).

Cobalamin and Folate. The strongly interacting pair cobalamin (vitamin B_{12}) and folate play an essential role in the synthesis of deoxyribonucleic acid (DNA) that is required for the maturation of erythrocytes and, therefore, for oxygen transport. Vitamin B_{12} is also essential to normal fat and carbohydrate metabolism, which maintains the integrity of the spinal cord and peripheral nervous system (17).

Deficiency of both vitamin B_{12} and folate characteristically causes megaloblastic anemia, but only vitamin B_{12} deficits produce catastrophic peripheral nervous system disease. When anemia that is caused by vitamin B_{12} deficiency is treated with folic acid (because blood values were not measured), the hematologic picture reverts to normal but neurologic deficits progress. Therefore, the Federal Drug Administration limits nonprescription folic acid preparations to the RDA value of $400 \, \mu g$/dose. Unfortunately, this approach compromises adequate supplementation of folate and does not adequately solve the problem addressed.

Both vitamins are critical for normal muscle function. Laboratory tests for serum vitamin B_{12} and folate are readily available. Therefore, chronic myofascial pain patients who respond poorly to treatment should be tested for both.

The serum level of both vitamin B_{12} and folate should be known before initiating treatment with either. Metabolic interdependence of folate and vitamin B_{12} results can precipitously lower the serum folate level, depleting what initially appeared to be an adequate reserve, and supplementation with only folic acid can deplete vitamin B_{12} reserves.

The amount of vitamin B_{12} in the diet is rarely deficient except in *strict* vegetarians. This vitamin is ordinarily synthesized only by bacteria (17). Daily ingestion of 3–5 μg of cobalamin is sufficient when absorption and metabolic utilization are normal. Dietary cobalamins and cyanocobalamin must be converted by the body to the only metabolically useful form, hydroxocobalamin. Some patients are seriously deficient in enzymes required to convert the other forms of cobalamin to the hydroxo-form; these patients respond only to supplements of hydroxocobalamin and not to cyanocobalamin.

On the other hand, folates are found in many foods, particularly leafy green vegetables (foliage), but at most in limited amounts. Compounding this scarcity, folates are largely destroyed by processing and cooking. Lack of folate is the most common vitamin deficiency and is especially frequent in elderly persons who eat institutional cafeteria-style meals.

Serum values in the lower quartile of normal for either vitamin should be supplemented to reach at least midnormal levels. An initial oral supplement of 2 mg of folic acid three times daily should elevate the folate level to midnormal range within 2–3 weeks. One milligram daily usually maintains this blood level. A daily 1-mg (1000-μg) oral supplement of vitamin B_{12} usually restores the serum level to midnormal within 4–6 weeks and maintains it there. Oral administration, if the vitamin is absorbed, avoids the necessity for injection. This dose is several hundred times the RDA, but totally innocuous, even if injected.

Ascorbic Acid. The importance of adequate stores of water-soluble ascorbic acid (vitamin C) to prevent ecchymoses in those patients receiving injection therapy has been reviewed (9). This vitamin is essential to normal muscle function and, when inadequacy is corrected, relieves postexercise soreness and stiffness. Large supplements of several grams a day cause no problems. Five hundred milligrams of timed-released vitamin C ingested daily usually provides an ample supply to prevent capillary fragility and to reduce postexercise soreness.

The Fat-Soluble Vitamins

The fat-soluble vitamins A, D, and E are well stored and can readily reach toxic levels. Above-normal serum vitamin A levels appear to be another source of increased muscular irritability. Therefore, chronic MPS patients taking a daily *total* (including dietary) of more than 10,000 IU of vitamin A should have their serum level tested. The National Academy of Science recommends physician supervision for ingestion of more than 10,000 I.U. daily (16).

Metabolic and Endocrine Dysfunction

Like the vitamin inadequacies discussed above, metabolic factors of gout, anemia, low electrolyte levels, and hypoglycemia increase muscle irritability and aggravate symptoms caused by TrPs; so do the endocrine disorders of hypometabolism and estrogen deficiency.

Since the monosodium urate crystals of gout are less soluble in the acidic media of injured tissues than in blood, they tend to deposit in areas of local injury or of metabolic distress such as TrPs. Chronic myofascial pain patients with a gouty diathesis often respond to treatment only when the hyperuricemia is under control. Generally, these patients respond better to injection than to stretch and spray. Vitamin C in relatively large amounts (1–4 g/day) is an effective uricosuric agent (24). The hyperirritability of myofascial TrPs subsides remarkably with uricosuric therapy in most patients with serum uric acid levels that are in the excessive, or even the high "normal," range.

Regardless of the cause for anemia, from the muscle's point of view the resultant hypoxia is a serious metabolic problem because the muscle depends on oxygen to sustain the oxidative metabolism that is essential for meeting its energy needs.

The presence of abnormally low electrolyte levels of ionized calcium and potassium can seriously disturb muscle function by increasing muscle irritability; these electrolytes play critical roles in the contractile mechanism. Serum ionized calcium, not merely total calcium, is the essential measure. Unfortunately, the total calcium found on the usual automated blood chemistry battery or profile correlates poorly with the level of serum ionized calcium (25).

The presence of hypoglycemia intensifies metabolic distress in muscles (26) and clearly aggravates myofascial TrPs. Therapy by stretch or injection is best deferred whenever patients are hypoglycemic. Treatment then is likely to aggravate rather than relieve the pain. A packet of powdered drinking gelatin in fruit juice provides a handy source of carbohydrate and enough protein to avoid subsequent hypoglycemia.

Evidence for hypometabolism (subclinical hypothyroidism) was reported in 13% of healthy elderly individuals (27) and is found in some treatment-refractory patients with pain due to myofascial TrPs. When inadequate metabolism is suspected, first, adequate serum folate and vitamin B_1 levels must be assured because these vitamin inadequacies can cause symptoms mimicking those of low thyroid function. Hypometabolism is a controversial diagnosis because the usual laboratory test results for thyroid function are low-normal, but still within "normal" limits in these patients. The patient often has marginally low L-triiodothyronine (T_3) uptake and low to midrange L-thyroxine (T_4) by radioimmunoassay (RIA). In these patients, low thyroid function is clearly revealed by a low basal metabolic rate (28) if the test is properly performed, or by a low basal body temperature (29), and by clinical symptoms of inadequate thyroid function. Thyroid insufficiency is confirmed therapeutically by the response to thyroid supplementation (28). When insufficiency is present, thyroid supplementation results in serum cholesterol decrease, basal metabolism or basal temperature normalization, decrease in irritability of the muscles, and return of normal energy and stamina (9, 30).

Basal temperature readings are obtained by having the patient place an ovulation thermometer in the axilla daily for 10 min in the morning before arising after sleep. The mean basal temperature over 3–4 days normally averages at least 36.1°C (97.0°F). The lower the basal temperature is under this value, the more vulnerable the patient is to hyperirritable TrPs in the muscles and often to depression. Usually, women who ovulate are at the basal (low point) of their cycle for only 3–5 days immediately following menses.

Thyroid supplementation should be avoided in patients with cardiac arrhythmias or myocardial disease that compromises cardiac reserve. Thyroid medication increases the load on the heart and also the requirements for vitamin B_1 and estrogen. It tends to increase blood pressure. Overmedication causes symptoms of hyperthyroidism. Adjustment of dosage in these patients depends primarily on the clinical responses to therapy. The site of metabolic dysfunction is apparently at the level of cellular utilization and is poorly reflected in serum levels of thyroid hormone.

Thyroid supplementation for those patients who meet the criteria described by Sonkin (28) remains controversial among endocrinologists, but it is of critical importance to those patients in whom this factor is a major perpetuator of disabling myofascial pain.

Chronic Infection and Infestations

Viral disease, bacterial infection, and parasitic infestation can also perpetuate TrPs.

During any systemic viral illness, including the common cold or attack of "flu," the irritability of myofascial TrPs is likely to increase markedly. One of the most common viral perpetuators is an outbreak of herpes simplex virus type 1; however, neither herpes simplex virus type 2 (genital herpes) nor herpes zoster is known to aggravate TrPs. Herpesvirus type 1 causes the common fever blister, aphthous mouth ulcer, canker sore, or cold sore. Isolated vesicles filled with clear fluid may also appear on the skin of the body or extremities. Lesions similar to those in the mouth have been reported in the esophagus. The symptoms of vomiting and diarrhea strongly implicate similar gastrointestinal involvement.

No drug is known to completely cure these infections of herpes simplex virus type 1, but a multipronged treatment approach can greatly reduce the frequency and severity of recurrences. A daily dose of 300–500 mg of niacinamide reinforces mucous membrane resistance. Three tablets (or 1 packet) of viable lactobacillus two or three times daily for at least a month helps to reestablish normal intestinal flora, which reduces the danger of an intestinal viral outbreak. Rubbing an antiviral ointment, such as Vira-A, into the skin or on mouth lesions three times daily accelerates their resolution.

Chronic bacterial infection tends to exacerbate muscle irritability. Persistent infection, such as an abscessed tooth, infected sinus, or chronic urinary tract infection, can perpetuate TrPs. Acute sinusitis may become chronic due to blockage caused by allergy. Normal erythrocyte sedimentation rate and C-reactive protein tests help to eliminate the possibility of chronic infection.

The danger of a parasitic infestation is of concern in travelers exposed to substandard sanitation and in active male homosexuals. The most common infestation was fish tapeworm, until pollution of fresh water greatly reduced fishing; next is giardiasis; and less common, but likely to be more serious, is amebiasis. The first two can seriously impair absorption of and consume vitamin B_{12}; amebae may produce myotoxins that are absorbed systemically. The diagnosis of infestation is investigated by stool examinations for occult blood, ova, and parasites on at least three samples. Serologic testing is available for amebiasis.

Post-Traumatic Hyperirritability Syndrome

The chronic myofascial pain perpetuated by the post-traumatic hyperirritability syndrome causes great suffering, is poorly understood, and is difficult to manage. This group of patients responds to strong sensory stimuli much differently than most patients. Patients with this syndrome have incurred a major impact to the body and/or head. The trauma characteristically has been an automobile accident or fall that was sufficiently severe to have disrupted consciousness and inflicted damage to the sensory pathways of the central nervous system. These patients experience constant pain that is augmented by normally inconsequential sensory stimuli, including a loud noise, vibration, prolonged physical activity, and emotional stress. The constant pain is also augmented by severe pain from other sources. An augmented state then persists and may take days or weeks to return slowly to the previous level of activation. During augmentation, the muscles exhibit an increased hyperirritability of TrPs.

After onset, coping with pain has suddenly become the focus of life for these patients, who previously had paid no special attention to pain. If they exceed their restricted limit of activity, they experience a marked increase in pain and fatigue that depletes their vital energy and severely limits their activity. Suppressing pain is exhausting to the patient.

Also, in patients with post-traumatic hyperirritability, augmentation of symptoms is associated with a marked increase in sensitivity to subsequent stimuli. Not only are they then in more pain, but they are more vulnerable to further activation by strong stimuli. This increased vulnerability of the sensory system also subsides slowly. Recovery to the previous degree of vulnerability may also take hours, days, or weeks depending on the intensity of the stimulus and the severity of the reaction to it. The inciting sensory input appears to modulate the excitability of the arousal system. These patients are vulnerable to major extension of their injury and intensification of their symptoms by additional trauma that to most people would be minor.

The most effective management approach found so far has been to inactivate all identifiable TrPs and to correct perpetuating factors. The patients must learn to pace themselves and stay within their stress tolerance. Elimination of stimuli that exacerbate symptoms is a prime goal. Occasionally, when necessary, the sensory system can be reset to baseline by pharmacologically suppressing central nervous system excitability through one night. To date, barbiturates have been most effective.

Psychological Stress

Recently a committee of the National Academy of Sciences agreed that among chronic pain patients malingering is rare, at most accounting for only a small percentage (1). Much difference of opinion is generated by the question: "Is the chronic pain an expression of the patient's psychological dysfunctions or is the pain driving the patient crazy?" If an organic cause of the pain is not obvious, it is tempting to conclude that the symptoms are psychogenic. This relieves the health care professional, but not the patient.

Patients who suffer a serious chronic MPS that is undiagnosed and untreated are strongly impacted psychologically. They are confronted with a severe inescapable pain of unknown origin and of uncertain prognosis that is devastating to their vocational, social, and private lives. Worst of all, family and physicians are questioning their psychological integrity until they begin to question their own sanity. The future is an ominous, impenetrable dark cloud. The ensuing depression aggravates the pain and reinforces uncertainty and a sense of hopelessness (1). The most important service one can render these patients is to recognize their treatable myofascial pain and to make an unambiguous diagnosis with a convincing demonstration and explanation of active TrPs. As patients learn self-treatment and self-management techniques they gain control of the pain; the pain no longer controls them and victimizes their lives.

Employment status is the most significant factor for predicting which patients in chronic pain rehabilitation programs will improve. Loss of employment is clearly a stronger perpetuating factor than ongoing litigation

Table 44.2.
Muscles Often Affected by Specific Mechanical Perpetuating Factors

Stress	Muscles	References
Anatomic variations		
Short leg and/or small hemipelvis	Quadratus lumborum	31, 32, 33 (Chap. 4)
	Iliopsoas	32, 33 (Chap. 5)
	Thoracolumbar paraspinals	9 (Chap. 48), 31
	Shoulder girdle and neck-righting	9 (Chaps. 7, 19, 20)
	Masticatory	9 (Chaps. 8–12)
Short upper arms or armrests too low	Levator scapulae	9 (Chap. 19)
	Upper trapezius	9 (Chap. 6)
	Scaleni	9 (Chap. 20)
	Rhomboids	9 (Chap. 27)
	Triceps brachii	9 (Chap. 32)
	Quadratus lumborum	33 (Chap. 4)
Long second metatarsal (D.J. Morton foot configuration)	Peroneus longus	9 (Chap. 4), 33 (Chap. 20)
	Vastus medialis	33 (Chap. 14)
	Gluteus medius	33 (Chap. 8)
Seated postural stress		
Hard smooth mat	Foot intrinsics	33 (Chaps. 26, 27)
Seat too high from floor	Hamstrings	33 (Chap. 16)
	Soleus	33 (Chap. 22)
Back unsupported	Quadratus lumborum	32, 33 (Chap. 4)
(no backrest contact, poor lumbar support, no	T-L paraspinals	
scapular contact)		9 (Chap. 48)
	Pectoralis major	9 (Chap. 42)
	Rhomboids	9 (Chap. 27)
Standing postural stress		
Head-forward posture	Pectoralis major	9 (Chap. 42)
	Rhomboids	9 (Chap. 27)
	Posterior cervicals	9 (Chap. 16)
Slanted running surface	Quadratus lumborum	32, 33 (Chap. 4)
	Scaleni	9 (Chap. 20)
	Sternocleidomastoid	9 (Chap. 7)
Vocational stress		
Shoulder elevation	Upper trapezius	9 (Chap. 6)
	Levator scapulae	9 (Chap. 19)
Arm elevation	Supraspinatus	9 (Chap. 21)
	Deltoid	9 (Chap. 28)
Hand supination	Supinator	9 (Chap. 36)
Grasp	Finger extensors	9 (Chap. 35)
	Finger flexors	9 (Chap. 38)
	Wrist extensors	9 (Chap. 34)
	Wrist flexors	9 (Chap. 38)

(1). When patients reorient their primary focus of attention from being productive members of society to becoming full-time pain patients, they develop a new self-image that shifts from function orientation to sickness orientation. Psychologically it is of utmost importance to preserve the patient's self-respect and function orientation through vocational activity.

MECHANICAL FACTORS

Systemic perpetuating factors may relate to any or all of the skeletal muscles. However, each mechanical perpetuating factor relates to specific muscles. The columns

in Table 44.2 identify specific perpetuating stresses and the muscle or muscle group that is most likely to be affected by that stress. Major mechanical factors include anatomic variations, seated and standing postural overload, and vocational stress.

Anatomic Variations

Two common and closely related anatomic variations are a short leg and/or a small hemipelvis (9). These variations often must be corrected by a heel lift, a butt lift, or both for lasting relief of low back (32) and sometimes head, neck, and shoulder pain due to myofascial TrPs.

To ensure appropriate correction, evaluation of these variations must be conducted with the patient in a functional standing or seated position. An effective technique for determining and making the required correction is described in detail (9).

The relatively common phenomenon of short upper arms is frequently an unrecognized perpetuator of TrPs in the shoulder elevator muscles. This anatomic variation is corrected by providing elbow rests or pads that modify the furniture to fit the individual (9).

The **long second metatarsal**, or D.J. Morton foot configuration, throws the foot off balance as a result of a knife-edge support during toe-off. This instability disturbs gait and overloads lower extremity muscles. The muscles most affected are primarily the peroneus longus and secondarily the vastus medialis and gluteus medius. This anatomic variation is compensated by inserting a toe pad under the head of the short first metatarsal bone to place the foot on a tripod base (9, 33).

Seated Postural Stress

This ubiquitous muscular stress may be induced by a small hemipelvis as noted above, by a hard smooth mat under an office chair, by a chair seat too high for heels to reach the floor, by lack of a firm back support, by lack of lumbar support, by low armrests, and by a persistent head-forward posture.

Use of **a hard smooth mat**, such as plexiglass, allows the office chair with free-rolling casters to glide whenever its occupant changes position or exerts the slightest pressure against the desk. Frequently, the intrinsic foot muscles and long toe flexors must try to grasp the slick surface; this repeated and prolonged but unconscious effort overloads and perpetuates TrPs in these muscles.

A **chair seat too high** for that individual's leg length leaves the heels dangling off the floor. This causes underthigh compression of the hamstrings and chronic shortening of the soleus muscle as the toes drop toward the floor. Both postural effects perpetuate TrPs in the corresponding muscles and can be avoided by providing a suitable footrest (book, pillow, or small footstool). A desk surface that is too high can be corrected by shortening the legs of the desk, or by elevating the seat height with appropriate adjustment of footrests.

A chair with **inadequate back support** may be the result of a poor seat design that renders the seat too long from front to back, that has a flat back that provides no lumbar support, that supplies no scapular contact, or that has a backrest with inadequate backward angulation. When the seat is too long from front to back, the backs of the knees are solidly engaged against the front of the seat, but the buttocks do not reach the backrest. The backrest should always be contoured to support a normal lumbar lordosis; otherwise, the patient must place a pillow or roll in the small of the back to provide this support. This lumbar support also helps to correct

the head-forward posture (9). This repositioning facilitates balancing the head over the shoulders with minimal muscular effort.

The **armrests** must provide solid elbow support. If their height is not adequate, the armrests should be elevated or padded to provide the needed support.

The troublesome **head-forward posture** is further relieved by placing the work or reading material on a slant board and, for those who require reading glasses, by tilting the *lenses* of the eyeglasses (9). Papers that are placed to one side require a crooked neck position that aggravates TrPs. Placing the work on a secretary's desk stand in front and nearly at eye level relieves this aggravation. Scapular contact with the backrest and backward angulation of the backrest help to carry the weight of the head and shoulders and to stabilize the spine, relieving the quadratus lumborum and paraspinal muscles.

The forward head position is a powerful mechanical perpetuator of TrPs, especially in some neck and shoulder-girdle muscles. This posture, with loss of the normal cervical lordosis, is also associated with a variety of painful cervical articular dysfunctions.

Standing Postural Stress

The head-forward posture that produces chronic muscular strains when standing is aggravated by shifting body weight backward onto the heels. Conversely, this posture is spontaneously improved and effortlessly held by shifting the center of gravity forward over the balls of the feet while emphasizing lumbar lordosis. This positioning allows the head to remain erect, balanced over the shoulders without muscle and joint strain. It elevates the chest and swings the scapulae backward to their normal resting position. This repositioning unloads the rhomboid muscles by relieving the persistent shortening of the pectoral muscles (9). This improved posture lessens the load on the posterior cervical muscles, which in the head-forward posture must support the weight of the head against the pull of gravity.

A slanted walking or running surface is common on the seashore or on a banked circular track. It produces the same effect as a short leg (9) and tilts the pelvis to one side. Contraction of the quadratus lumborum and/or paraspinal muscles must hold the spinal curvature that is required to compensate for the lateral tilt of the pelvis. This sustained contraction while on the feet causes a persistent overload that perpetuates TrPs in these muscles.

Vocational Stress

A work situation that encourages or requires sustained shoulder elevation commonly overloads the upper trapezius and levator scapulae muscles, which perpetuates their TrPs. Typists and other workers who must hold their hands in a sustained elevated position tend to persistently shrug their shoulders. For correction, the body should be raised or the work lowered.

Similarly, prolonged **arm abduction** overloads the supraspinatus and deltoid muscles. Suitable elbow support relieves the strain. The supraspinatus and upper trapezius muscles develop chronic myofascial syndromes when subjected to frequent repetitive movements that overload those muscles. When tested electromyographically, these painfully involved muscles had less endurance and more rapid onset of fatigue than nonpainful muscles. The authors (33) accounted for these findings by alteration in muscle metabolism due to ischemia.

Forceful or repetitive forearm supination with full extension at the elbow readily overloads the supinator muscle, as when playing tennis or turning a screwdriver (9). Full extension at the elbow eliminates the more forceful supinator function of the biceps brachii muscle. This repetitive motion with the forearm extended may activate TrPs in the supinator muscle, producing symptoms that frequently are labeled epicondylitis or tennis elbow. To decrease load on the supinator muscle, the forearm should be less than fully extended at the elbow when forcefully supinating the forearm.

Repeated or sustained strong grasp often activates TrPs of the finger extensors because these extensors function vigorously during grasp. The patient with TrPs of the finger extensors complains of a weak and painful grip. Items like a cup or glass are likely to slip unexpectedly out of the grasp, apparently due to unpredictable TrP-induced reflex inhibition of muscle contraction. The supinator muscle is frequently involved along with the wrist and finger extensors.

INACTIVATION OF TRIGGER POINTS

When the composite myofascial pain pattern of the patient with chronic MPS is analyzed into its component single-muscle syndromes, the TrPs responsible can then be managed, one muscle at a time, as single-muscle syndromes. This section presents the basic treatment principles applicable to most muscles. Details for individual muscles are summarized in the preceding chapter and described elsewhere (9, 32, 33).

In this section, first the principles of stretch and spray are summarized. Then, other physical methods such as postisometric relaxation, ischemic compression, and massage are noted. Finally, the technique of injection and stretch is reviewed.

STRETCH AND SPRAY

Treatment of an acute or chronic MPS by stretch and spray is one of the simplest, quickest, and least painful ways to inactivate the TrPs. Stretch and spray can be used alone or frequently is applied immediately after TrP injection. This postinjection application ensures in-

activation of any remaining TrPs in that muscle. Stretch and spray also is valuable for complex cases that involve many muscles in one or more regions of the body (35). Since muscles within one functional group interact strongly, stretch and spray permits release of several closely related muscles at one time.

The procedure of passive stretch and intermittent spray should cause little or no discomfort and should not excite reflex spasm. Complete voluntary relaxation while the muscle is lengthening is essential. The alarming cold stimulation produced by the vapocoolant spray on skin receptors over the muscle and its pain reference zone is needed to block reflex spasm and pain (8). The restoration of normal full stretch length of the muscle *inactivates* the TrP mechanism.

Vapocoolant spray is applied in one-directional parallel sweeps in a jet stream to the skin. When the skin is cold to the touch, rewarming should precede a repeat application of vapocoolant. Excessive cooling (frosting) of the skin and cooling of the underlying muscle should be *avoided*. Fluori-Methane (Gebauer Chemical Co., 9410 St. Catherine Ave., Cleveland, OH 44104) is more effective and much safer than ethyl chloride. Ethyl chloride is undesirably colder, is a potentially lethal general anesthetic, and is flammable and explosive. Fluori-Methane is none of these. Parallel sweeps of Fluori-Methane spray should be applied slowly at 10 cm (4 in)/sec. The spray pattern should cover the entire length of the muscle, progressing in the direction of and *including* the referred pain zone. The bottle is held about 45 cm (18 in) from the skin to allow the vapocoolant that starts at room temperature in the bottle to cool by evaporation before impacting the skin. The optimal angle of impact of the spray is about 30° (9).

To obtain the complete relaxation that is essential for effective passive stretch, the seated patient should be positioned comfortably with *all* limbs and the back and head well supported. The recumbent position is preferable, if it permits full stretch of the affected muscles. One or two sweeps of spray should precede the passive stretch to inhibit the pain and stretch reflexes. To take up any slack that develops while applying spray, the operator maintains gentle, smooth, *steady* tension on the muscle. He or she should carefully *avoid* force strong enough to produce pain and avoid any jerky or rapid rocking motions that could activate TrPs.

Treatment by stretch and spray is not complete until the skin has been rewarmed for several minutes by a moist hot pack or a wetproof heating pad. Then the patient should slowly execute several cycles of active range of motion through both the *fully shortened* and *fully lengthened* positions of the muscle group under treatment. Emphasis is placed on gently but surely reaching maximum range of motion in each direction. A more detailed description of the stretch and spray procedure is available (9).

One particularly effective way of facilitating relaxation is to ask the patient to slowly take a deep breath, and then gradually and completely to exhale through pursed lips. During this long, slow, and maximal exhalation, the muscles tend to relax and are more easily lengthened. Inhalation usually is facilitated by having the patient look up, and exhalation by having the patient look down toward the feet (36). The effects of simultaneously looking down and exhaling are additive in facilitating relaxation. The Lewit stretch technique (postisometric relaxation) (37), described below, may be combined with stretch and spray or used as an alternate method of lengthening the muscle.

OTHER PHYSICAL METHODS

Muscle lengthening can be achieved in several ways: by stretch and spray, as described above; by postisometric relaxation; by the use of reciprocal inhibition; by ischemic compression; and by deep friction massage. Additional modalities are sometimes used. Low-intensity ultrasound is valuable when applied directly to the TrP. This approach may be effective when the TrP is otherwise inaccessible. Some find electrical stimulation over the TrP helpful; high-voltage galvanic stimulation is reported to be effective in the hands of those accustomed to its use.

Postisometric Relaxation

The technique of alternating voluntary contraction with passive stretch for releasing tight muscles has been identified by many names. Physical therapists are likely to refer to this as contract-relax or rhythmic stabilization (38). Osteopathic physicians speak of muscle energy techniques (39).

Postisometric muscular relaxation as described by Lewit and Simons (37) is simple and effective. The effects are additive when it is combined with the stretch-and-spray technique. This stretch technique is routinely taught to patients as a home program of self-treatment for specific muscle syndromes. The muscle is gently lengthened to the onset of resistance (end of slack) and held there isometrically. For the next 3–7 sec, either the operator or the patient provides fixed resistance against which the patient contracts the muscle *gently* and *isometrically* at approximately 10% of maximal effort. While the *same position* is passively maintained, the patient "lets go" (relaxes the contracting muscle). Only after the patient has thoroughly relaxed is the muscle again *slowly, gently,* and passively lengthened, taking up all the slack that has developed. Gravity is used to provide the stretch force whenever possible. Elongation of the muscle should be painless. This contract-relax cycle may be repeated three to five times. Full release of tension usually occurs after the second or third cycle. Relaxation is facilitated by coordinating respiration (37) and eye

movements (36) as described above, under "Stretch and Spray."

Ischemic Compression

Ischemic compression, sometimes called "thumb therapy," is painful but noninvasive and effective (40). Pressure that directly compresses a peripheral nerve must be avoided. This technique may be applied either by the operator or as self-treatment by the patient. Constant pressure is applied directly to the taut band on the spot of greatest tenderness (the TrP) with a steady, moderately painful (tolerable) pressure. As the pain eases, the pressure is increased to maintain approximately the same level of discomfort. When the TrP is no longer painful (after 15 sec to 1 min of pressure) the pressure is released and full active range of motion performed. For the greatest effect, stretch and spray and then moist heat may be applied following ischemic compression.

Immediately after release, the blanching of the skin due to pressure is quickly replaced by a persistent reactive hyperemia. If the pressure produces a similar hyperemia at the TrP, the increased perfusion should contribute to recovery. The procedure is less painful, but takes longer, if the therapist applies less pressure repeatedly on successive days. Treatment is repeated until TrP tenderness is obliterated and the referred pain disappears.

Massage

Deep muscle massage (deep friction or stripping massage) is another way to inactivate TrPs in superficial muscles. This massage requires lubrication of the skin and the application of *firm* bilateral thumb pressure against the taut band while sliding the thumbs *slowly* progressively along its length. Fluid content of the band is "milked out" by the pressure between the thumbs. A sense of increased resistance and accumulation of fluid is experienced at the TrP. This procedure may be repeated several times until the tenderness and tautness of the palpable band are relieved and the TrP no longer refers pain. The slowly progressive "milking" action eliminates the sense of induration. This technique is effective but painful and is usually followed by local muscle soreness for a few days. In experimental studies, each massage treatment session caused a transient myoglobinemia until the abnormal tension and tenderness were relieved (41, 42).

INJECTION AND STRETCH

Injection of muscle TrPs is selected initially when the joint movement is mechanically blocked, as in the case of the coccygeus muscle, or when the muscles cannot be stretched fully, as in the case of the lateral pterygoid muscle (9). Injection is useful for releasing TrPs unresponsive to the foregoing noninvasive methods. Dry needling (9, 43) and isotonic saline injection (9, 44) also are effective; however, without a local anesthetic, dry needling is more painful. Isotonic saline for injection usually contains 0.9% of the preservative and local anesthetic benzy-alcohol. The flushing effect of the injected fluid on sensitizing agents may also be important. Reduction of local TrPs tenderness depends more on penetration of the TrP by the needle than on which substance, if any, is injected (44).

Needle penetration of the skin is less painful when the needle is inserted rapidly with a flick of the wrist after the antiseptic alcohol has dried. To make insertion painless the site may be chilled for 6–8 sec with a stream of Fluori-Methane spray applied in a figure-of-eight pattern. The needle is inserted in the crossover region of the spray pattern (9, 45). The skin is chilled just short of frosting; frosting causes an unnecessarily painful sting.

The essence of effective needle therapy is the mechanical disruption of the self-sustaining TrP mechanism. The critical role of penetrating the TrP with the needle was demonstrated experimentally (44). To do this required precise localization of the TrP before injection. The injection of 0.5% procaine in isotonic saline without epinephrine reduces the consistently severe and sometimes intolerable pain of TrP penetration. Importantly, the 0.5% concentration ameliorates the pain but preserves the tenderness to palpation of any remaining TrPs. Continuous injection of small amounts of procaine during needle insertion further reduces the sensory impact of needle contact with the TrP. The preservation of local TrP tenderness permits palpation for and detection of any TrPs that were missed, so that they, too, can be injected without withdrawing the needle, thereby avoiding additional shot penetrations.

The local analgesic effect of the 0.9% concentration of benzyl alcohol preservative permits the substitution of the saline for procaine injection in those few patients who are allergic to procaine. Lidocaine in 0.5% solution is less desirable than procaine but, if necessary, can be used. Long-acting local anesthetics such as bupivacaine should be avoided because they obliterate the tenderness of remaining TrPs and produce muscle necrosis, which is unnecessary. Necrosis is not caused by 0.5% procaine or lidocaine (46).

For injection, the patient should be recumbent, to prevent psychological syncope. When injecting muscles over the ribs, needle penetration between the ribs must be scrupulously avoided because it can easily cause a pneumothorax.

The first step in the injection of a tender TrP is to palpate its taut band between the fingers with the TrP localized accurately between the finger tips. The needle is then inserted precisely into the TrP (9). Needle contact with the TrP is confirmed by a jump response *of the patient* and/or a local twitch response *of the taut band* in the muscle. Probing with the needle should continue until such a response has been obtained or the region has been fully explored with the needle. Tenderness to palpation and the local twitch response can no longer be elicited following successful inactivation of a TrP. The tautness of the band may or may not disappear. Digital pressure is applied during and after injection to ensure hemostasis.

The injection is supplemented by a stretch-and-spray procedure and by a moist hot pack or pad to inactivate any remaining TrPs. The moist heat helps to minimize postinjection soreness that otherwise may last for 2–3 days. The patient should be alerted that aspirin or acetaminophen (Tylenol) relieves this soreness.

It is most important to conclude with several cycles of active range of motion that reach both the fully shortened and the fully stretched positions of the treated muscles, as described for stretch and spray. Repetition of this slow, but complete, range of movement helps greatly to reestablish normal function. The same stretching and range of motion exercises are routinely instituted as a home program. This home stretching program often makes a critical difference for maintaining the increased range of motion obtained by treatment.

CONFUSINGLY SIMILAR CONDITIONS

The pathophysiology of three of the most common, yet least recognized, causes of musculoskeletal pain has yet to be established. The three appear to be closely intertwined. They are myofascial TrPs (9); fibromyalgia (47–49); which was first called fibrositis (50–52); and articular dysfunction (53). To date, not one of the three has a reliable diagnostic laboratory or imaging test. Each diagnosis must be made by history and a directed physical examination. In each, the critical information would be missed on the usual history and routine physical examination. The examiner must know what questions to ask, what specific evidence to look for, and how to examine for each, and must take the time to look. The symptoms and findings that distinguish these three are based only on clinical experience. To be sure of any one of them, at this time, the examiner should be conversant with all three.

Investigators of one of these three conditions are very likely to include in their study a significant number of patients who are suffering from at least one of the other two conditions. In this event, their conclusions are as likely to be confusing as helpful. It now looks as if these three conditions have distinctively different causes, which can, and often do, produce confusingly similar clinical pictures. However, each of the three responds best to significantly different therapeutic approaches. Many patients doubtless have a combination of two or all of these conditions and, when treated for only one of them, respond poorly. Included in this circle of confusion are many additional diagnoses that also are likely to include patients with myofascial TrPs. A few of the most common of these additional diagnoses include nonarticular rheumatism (54), muscular rheumatism (55), osteochondrosis (56, 57), bursitis (9), tendinitis (9), and occipital neuralgia (58). For many others, see Simons (59, 60 (Table I)) and Reynolds (61).

MYOFASCIAL TRIGGER POINTS

A single-muscle syndrome due to myofascial TrPs starts with a focal disorder in one muscle as a result of acute or repeated overload stress. This condition is clearly myogenic, not psychogenic. However, this pain and tenderness are felt not at the TrP but at a distance. This referred pain, which appears in a characteristic pattern for each skeletal muscle (7, 9, 33, 60), seems inexplicable to practitioners unacquainted with these patterns. These TrPs may cause pain early in life (62) and occur with nearly equal frequency in men and women (63). A chronic MPS that proliferates over time due to systemic perpetuating factors is not so obviously myogenic; this chronic myofascial condition may look confusingly like fibrositis/fibromyalgia (64). Myofascial TrPs are distinguished clinically by eliciting referred pain and tenderness, by locating the palpable taut bands containing the TrP, and by demonstrating local twitch responses of the taut bands. When myofascial TrPs are recognized as an acute syndrome, and if there are no serious perpetuating factors, the pain is quickly and easily relieved.

FIBROSITIS/FIBROMYALGIA

It is increasingly clear that the second condition, fibrositis/fibromyalgia, is primarily a systemic disease that targets the muscles and the collagen of the dermal-epidermal junction (60). Fibrositis is characteristically a disease of women between 40 and 60 years of age. Less than 15% of fibrositis patients are men (52). In 1972, leading the recent resurgence of interest in fibrositis, Smythe (65) characterized fibrositis in terms of psychogenic rheumatism. Some still consider fibrositis or fibromyalgia as partly, if not predominantly, psychogenic (66–68). However, others recently have found no psychological difference compared with other chronic painful conditions (69). In 1977, Smythe and Moldofsky (51) redefined fibrositis as a nonrestorative sleep syndrome that was previously described by Moldofsky et al. (70). The redefined fibrositis was characterized by multiple diffuse tender points (TePs) at prescribed locations. In 1981, Smythe (71) updated this redefinition of fibrositis that, in essence, has been adopted by rheumatologists. This acceptance was confirmed at a recent symposium (72). Yunus and associates (49) in the following year renamed and modified Smythe's redefinition of fibrositis as primary fibromyalgia and increased the number of patients incorporated in the new term by reducing the number of TePs required to make the diagnosis. *Primary*

fibromyalgia is rapidly gaining recognition (48, 67, 72–75). It is less of a misnomer than the term *fibrositis*.

Smythe (76) now identifies essentially two different syndromes characterized by TePs in muscles: fibrositis, which he characterized as essentially a painful nonrestorative sleep syndrome with TePs; and another syndrome that causes referred pain. If Smythe's concept is correct—and there is rapidly accumulating evidence that these are two distinct conditions—one would expect to see a spectrum of patients. Those at one end would be pure fibrositis/fibromyalgia, those at the other end, pure MPS due to TrPs; a large group in the middle should have various proportions of both. Evidence for such a spectrum was observed by Bengtsson and associates (77).

The TePs of fibromyalgia patients have been distinguished from TrPs by identifying as TrPs those tender spots that caused referred pain when compressed (77). Other authors do not mention how they distinguish TrPs from TePs, if at all (49, 52, 74, 78). Both TrPs and TePs are always tender; TePs do not always (if ever) refer pain. Using only the referred pain criterion for TrPs, Bengtsson and associates (77), found that 35 of 55 primary fibromyalgia patients (64%) had both TePs and TrPs. Nine of the patients (16%) exhibited only TePs; 11 (20%) exhibited only TrPs. If only myofascial TrPs project referred pain and the fibromyalgic TePs do not, very likely this and possibly all fibromyalgia studies have included a mixed population of patients with both fibromyalgia and chronic MPS. On the other hand, if fibromyalgic TePs do refer pain, for experimental purposes it is essential that TrPs be unambiguously identified using other criteria. Myofascial TrPs can be unambiguously distinguished from TePs by their location in a palpable taut band and by the local twitch response of that band to snapping palpation.

Numerous investigators present evidence that fibromyalgia is a systemic disease involving both skin and muscle. Both Caro (79) and Bengtsson (73) have reported collagen changes at the dermal-epidermal junction characterized by abnormal deposition of immunoglobulin G (IgG). Bartels and Danneskiold-Samsøe (80) reported abnormal collagenous constrictions like rubber bands around muscle fibers in *nontender* muscles of fibrositis patients. Crook and associates (74) concluded that the abnormal muscle tenderness of fibromyalgia patients is much more widespread than only the prescribed spots of muscular tenderness. They confusingly called these tender spots TrPs (74). Others have reported clear indications of an energy crisis in nontender muscles of fibromyalgia patients (67, 73, 75, 81). These studies do not clarify which of these findings would or would not be found in patients with only myofascial TrPs. Only hypothesized mechanisms provide guidelines.

Current literature indicates that infrared thermography is useful for substantiating the common finding of circulatory disturbance in the skin associated with already diagnosed myofascial TrPs (82, 83). It is clear that thermography cannot at this time be used as a primary diagnostic tool (84). No studies are known to date that effectively distinguish the thermographic patterns of myofascial TrPs from those of TePs in fibrositis/fibromyalgia.

ARTICULAR DYSFUNCTION

The third condition, articular dysfunction, is marked by a loss of joint "play" and/or normal mobility (85). Karel Lewit (36, 86) emphasized that articular dysfunction, particularly in joints involving transitional vertebrae, causes musculoskeletal pain that is characteristically associated with tenderness and increased tension of specific muscles. These articular symptoms and dysfunctions are relieved by mobilization of the restricted joint and by restoration of normal range of motion in the associated muscles that can restrict motion of the joint.

James W. Fisk (87) also noted the importance of strong interactions between some joint dysfunctions and the muscles. Clinically, it is becoming increasingly clear that joint dysfunction can be a potent perpetuator of myofascial TrPs, if not the initial cause of some myofascial pain syndromes. The reverse is also true: the shortening and tension of muscles caused by myofascial TrPs can block mobilization or quickly undo its beneficial effects. Often, both conditions must be treated together for lasting relief.

An overlooked painful articular dysfunction of another kind is the recently reported *instability* of spondylolisthetic or retro-olisthetic lumbar vertebra (88). The painfulness is relieved by strengthening the deep spinal rotator muscles (O. Friberg, personal communication, 1987).

Radiculopathy is often associated with myofascial TrPs (9, 89) and osteochondrosis (56). However, the myofascial component may not abate simply with resolution of the neuropathy; additional specific myofascial therapy may be required to inactivate persistent TrPs.

MANAGEMENT APPROACH

This section explores how one can identify the multiple pieces that comprise the complex puzzle of a chronic MPS and emphasizes the importance of treating the whole patient, not just the TrPs.

First, this section provides guidelines for distinguishing acute and recurrent pain as compared with the suffering of chronic pain. A clear distinction is drawn between pain and suffering. Finally, the approach to management emphasizes resolution of the sources of the pain while eliminating factors that intensify the suffering.

ACUTE PAIN, RECURRENT PAIN, AND CHRONIC PAIN

The distinctions among acute versus recurrent pain versus chronic enigmatic pain are not always simple and clear-cut, as pointed out by Addison (90). The patient with acute pain usually recognizes a cause for the pain and expects it to be temporary. Recurrent acute pain is similar; the patient again expects relief within a reasonably short period of time.

Addison (90) characterized chronic enigmatic pain (his "chronic pain syndrome") as pain that:

1. Rarely serves a biologic function
2. Is associated with the development of chronic pain behaviors
3. Presents with a lack of pathophysiologic mechanisms to account for the pain and with a lack of physical findings that are diagnostic of a well-recognized organic disease

Obviously, disabling pain that persists, but that serves no discernible biologic function, will cause serious psychological difficulties and modify the patient's behavior. The failure to find an organic cause for the pain is, in many cases, a matter of overlooked diagnoses, which the preceding sections have detailed. In addition, there is no reason to assume that we already know all of the diseases that exist. We may not yet know how to recognize the organic cause of the patient's pain. That approach is far different from concluding decisively that the pain is due primarily to an aberration of the patient's psyche. The latter is true occasionally, but this conclusion should be reached *only* in the face of unambiguous, overwhelming evidence. To hastily reach this conclusion often does the patient a disastrous injustice (1).

A committee of the National Academy of Sciences concerned with chronic pain of enigmatic origin (1) concluded that identifying decrements in the patient's function at all levels was the most reliable means to verify serious chronic pain and suffering. The committee concluded that categorizing a patient as having "chronic pain syndrome" served no useful purpose. It obscured the need to better understand the diverse and multifactorial nature of enigmatic chronic pain.

Increasingly, a distinction is being drawn between the chronic pain per se and its affective dimension, suffering. Price and associates (91) underscored evidence that the relationship between measures of the sensory and affective dimensions in different types of clinical pain is powerfully influenced by the psychological context in which the pain is experienced. Since there is no objective measure of pain per se (1), one must accept the patient's description of his or her suffering at face value. The only appropriate question is why the patient experiences that degree of suffering. The suffering is caused by much more than pain sensation alone (91, 92). The clinical distinction between pain and suffering is blurred because patients tend to describe their suffering in terms of pain

Table 44.3.
Muscles Most Likely to Develop Trigger Points in 100 Consecutive Patients with Symptoms Related to a Single Motor Vehicle Accident (Driver and Passenger Data Combined)[a]

Muscle	Frequency of Involvement %	Most Likely Side[b]	Muscle	Frequency of Involvement %	Most Likely Side[b]
Deceleration (head on) (N = 16)			Acceleration-deceleration (rear end) (N = 52)		
Splenius capitis	94	B	Quadratus lumborum	79	R
Quadratus lumborum	81	R	Splenius capitis	77	L
Semispinalis capitis	75	L	Semispinalis capitis	62	L
Vastus medialis	69	B	Sternocleidomastoid	52	R
Infraspinatus	63	R	Infraspinatus	46	B
Sternocleidomastoid	56	B			
Levator scapulae	50	R			
Broadside from driver's side (N = 16)			Broadside from passenger's side (N = 16)		
Quadratus lumborum	81	B	Splenius capitis	75	R
Splenius capitis	69	L	Semispinalis capitis	69	B
Semispinalis capitis	63	L	Quadratus lumborum	63	R
Levator scapulae	56	L	Levator scapulae	44	R
Infraspinatus	50	L	Extensor digitorum	44	R

[a]Summarized from Baker BA: The muscle trigger: Evidence of overload injury. *J Neurol Orthop Med Surg* 7:35–43, 1986.
[b]Side on which the listed muscle was most likely to have developed active trigger points. All muscles showed some bilateral involvement. L = predominantly left side; R = predominantly right side; B = nearly equal bilateral involvement.

sensations. Unexplained persistence of the pain adds on psychological, social, behavioral, and vocational losses, all of which intensify suffering.

Causes of Chronic Enigmatic Pain

To identify organic causes of pain in a patient with chronic enigmatic pain one must discover overlooked diagnoses. When conducting the history and physical examination, one should be looking for clues that will identify each pain problem as primarily musculoskeletal, neurologic, cardiovascular, other viscerogenic, or, rarely, psychogenic. Musculoskeletal sources that are frequently overlooked are covered in this and the preceding chapter. The remaining known causes are covered in other chapters of this volume. Usually, much of the patient's pain is of myofascial origin, but some of it is not. The myofascial component is resolved into its single-muscle syndromes and each is dealt with as described previously. The remaining causes are corrected or managed by appropriate specialists.

The following analysis of which muscles developed myofascial TrPs as the result of motor vehicle accidents presents one example of the effect of major trauma on the muscles. Failure to inactivate the TrPs and to correct their perpetuating factors in the immediate postaccident period makes accidents a fertile source of chronic MPS. Baker (93) reported on 100 successive patients who had sought medical help for symptoms related to a single motor vehicle accident. He tallied the frequency of myofascial TrPs in 36 minutes for each of four directions of impact. Table 44.3 summarizes Baker's results; they identify which muscles are most likely to be involved in a patient who experienced an auto accident.

The following interpretation of Baker's data (93) is based on the fact that lengthening contractions are more likely to overload muscles than are shortening contractions (94, 95). His results show that in head-on collisions the head extensors were most likely to be overloaded. The impact of the head-on collision is often anticipated. These extensors could have been overloaded by resisting the anticipated forward movement of the head in response to initial deceleration. On the other hand, rear-end collisions are more likely to have taken the patient by surprise. The fact that the extensor muscles also most commonly developed TrPs in this reverse situation suggests that the muscles were overloaded chiefly when they attempted to resist forward head motion later during the subsequent deceleration phase as the car stopped.

Broadside impact would not always be anticipated. The impact usually produces an initial acceleration phase, followed very shortly by a rapid deceleration phase as the sideward motion stops. Although muscles on both sides of the body developed TrPs after broadside impacts, the muscles on the left were more likely to develop TrPs following impact from the left and muscles on the right were more likely to be involved following impact from the right (Table 44.3). The muscles most commonly involved were those that would be subjected to lengthening contraction during the subsequent deceleration, not during initial acceleration.

In the same paper, Baker (93) noted that extensor digitorum muscles of drivers, who have the steering wheel available for support, were more likely to develop TrPs than were the same muscles of passengers, with one exception. In head-on collisions where passengers would be likely to grasp the dashboard, they were as likely to develop extensor digitorum TrPs as were the drivers. Baker observed that in all of these patients, a number of muscles were free of TrPs: the biceps and triceps brachii, tibialis anterior, lateral gastrocnemius, lateral hamstrings, wrist and finger flexors, abdominals, and mid- and posterior deltoid.

Intensification of Suffering

A number of factors influence the suffering of patients with chronic pain. One of the most important is the patient's orientation. Suffering is ameliorated when the patient is function oriented and attention is focused on activities. Conversely, pain orientation intensifies the suffering. Because pain orientation affects the patient's responses so adversely, the reasons for pain orientation should be identified and addressed. The reasons are frequently multiple and have evolved from fear of the unknown cause of the pain and deep frustration with health care professionals for failing to explain and relieve the pain. This fear and frustration then lead to hopelessness and depression, loss of vocational activity, denigration of status in the family, and an escalating need for income. A patient with poor coping skills is quickly overwhelmed by this situation. Impoverishment of social life, waning of sexual activity, financial distress, development of pain and sickness behaviors, and iatrogenic drug addiction frequently follow. Each of these factors should be identified as such and appropriate corrective actions taken to begin the long hard climb back to function.

In many patients with chronic pain of enigmatic origin, a crucial factor is their fear of the future. They can find no satisfactory explanation for the cause of their pain and no one has been able to relieve it; therefore, they have no idea how rapidly or severely it will progress or how much more disabling it will become. Most important, it denies them any reason to plan for the future, which destroys hope. This situation understandably leads to frustration and anger, and the hopelessness often feeds a growing depression. Identification of the *cause* of the pain is the critical first step on the road to recovery.

Function Versus Pain Orientation

When patients have an outstanding lawsuit or pending application for disability, the question arises as to how great an impediment this is to their improvement. Frequently, finding an answer is as simple as asking these patients. One should find out what the remuneration expectations are and how critical the potential income is to their future. Frequently, expectations of remuneration are grossly inflated. Helping them to recognize reality can be tremendously beneficial in achieving functional orientation.

One should discuss candidly with the patient the fact that any improvement in his or her symptoms and function as a result of treatment will compromise the financial rewards of the suit. Some patients welcome a face-saving opportunity to forego treatment until the suit has been settled. After this conversation, it is much easier to discuss motivations openly and sympathetically.

Coping

Patients with inadequate or sick coping repertoires are frequently dependent on their pain symptoms to fill in the gaps. Poor coping skills may lead to unhealthy family relations, poor financial management, poor nutrition, and the like. By encouraging patients to verbalize and look for the stresses that aggravate their pain, it is possible to focus on improving those coping skills that will be of most immediate benefit.

FINDING PIECES OF THE PUZZLE

To resolve the enigma of chronic myofascial pain, one must identify the pieces of the puzzle that comprise the patient's *total* pain picture. All too frequently, patients receive fragmented health care in which each specialist focuses on one point of view or organ system, yet no one integrates the whole picture, including all aspects of the patient's functioning. When there are multiple interacting factors, someone needs to be concerned with all of them and their interactions to coordinate their management. Every patient should know clearly the name of the doctor whom the patient considers to be primarily responsible for his or her health care.

One effective approach to unraveling the complexities of a chronic MPS is to separately identify and number all of the patient's pain problems. A separate problem is distinguished by its own time and circumstances of onset, its own distribution of pain, and the tendency for that distribution of pain to become more severe or regress in response to a stress or remedy. When successive pain problems evolve one from another, one looks for perpetuating factors. When the pain problems have distinct independent origins, the problems more likely have unrelated causes that may or may not be influenced by perpetuating factors.

History

While conducting the history and physical examination, one needs to distinguish the organ system responsible for each pain problem. If the pain relates strongly to locomotor activity and body positioning, it is probably musculoskeletal in origin. In that case, the examiner should query and examine for the presence of myofascial TrPs, fibrositis/fibromyalgia, and articular dysfunction, separately or in combination.

To resolve difficult cases, the history should be comprehensive and detailed. All available past medical records, including a recent complete physical examination, should be reviewed. Of concern are past illnesses, hospitalizations, serious diseases, surgeries, accidents, injuries, and the organ system review. Gastrointestinal symptoms may be somatovisceral manifestations of abdominal wall TrPs (9, 96). A complete current history that explores all relevant issues is facilitated by a questionnaire (Fig. 44.1) that serves as a reminder and guide for more detailed questioning.

Concerning the major items in Figure 44.1, the vocational status is one of the most critical. Every effort should be made to maintain the individual in active em-

---

IDENTIFICATION:
Name _____ Date _____
SSN _____ Age _____ Sex _____
Home telephone_____

VOCATIONAL:
Occupation_____
      Right _____ or left _____ handed
I am still working __ or I last worked:
      _____ weeks ago
      _____ months ago
      _____ years ago
I stopped work because _____
_____
_____

PAIN:
Check pain in the following areas:
Right Left
_____ _____ Headache
_____ _____ Neck pain
_____ _____ Shoulder pain
_____ _____ Arms, forearms, & hands
_____ _____ Chest
_____ _____ Abdomen
_____ _____ Upper back
_____ _____ Mid and low back
_____ _____ Hips, buttocks, & groin
_____ _____ Legs and feet
* Please **PUT A STAR** in front of worst pain
  When did your pain first start?
_____ weeks _____ months _____ years ago
  How did pain start?
_____ suddenly _____ gradually
  Describe event that started the pain:
_____
_____
  How long have you had pain at the present level of severity?
      _____ weeks _____ months _____ years
  Pain is present: (mark one)
      _____ only during activity, or
      _____ sometimes at rest, or
      _____ all the time
  What do you think causes your pain?
_____
_____
  My typical pain level is _____
  (0 to 10, if 10 worst pain possible)
  Pain is increased by: _____
_____
_____
_____

I get relief by: _____
_____
_____
_____
I have pain ___ % of my waking hours.

DIET:
Typical breakfast: _____
_____
_____
Typical lunch: _____
_____
_____
Typical dinner: _____
_____
_____
I often eat: _____
__ red meat __ chicken __ fish
__ bread __ cereals __ cheese
__ yogurt
What vegetables: _____
_____
_____
What fruits: _____
_____
_____
How much milk per day? _____
How many cups of coffee and/or tea daily? _____
How many glasses/cans of other caffeine drinks? _____
  I snack on: _____
_____
  I avoid: _____
_____

SLEEP:
_____ I sleep well, no trouble
_____ I have occasional difficulty
_____ I have frequent difficulty
_____ I always have insomnia
I usually wake up feeling:
__ refreshed __ better __ as tired
as when I went to bed
  When I get up in the morning my muscles:
__ are no stiffer than usual
__ are stiff and take __ hours to
loosen up

Figure 44.1. **Patient Information Questionnaire.**

Sleep position:_____

_____

_____

_____

MEDICATIONS:
List *ALL* of the medications you take
or use either regularly or occasionally:
(include vitamins and home remedies)

_____

_____

_____

_____

_____

_____

_____

_____

_____

_____

_____

PREVIOUS TREATMENT FOR PAIN:
I have seen the following kind of
specialists and health care providers
concerning this pain problem (include
approximately when and results):

_____

_____

_____

_____

_____

_____

_____

_____

Exercise:
I get exercise by: (how often)

_____

_____

_____

Personal:
I smoke ___ packs per day. I don't
smoke ___
I do ___ do not ___ drink alcoholic
beverages
I am ___ married ___ single ___ separated
___ divorced ___ other
Sexually active? (problems ?)_____

_____

I live:
___ with my spouse and ___ family members
___ with a friend   ___ alone
I am ___ satisfied ___ dissatisfied with
this arrangement

Most of the time lately I feel:
(CHECK ONE WORD IN EACH COLUMN)
___ happy ___ anxious ___ worried ___ depressed
___ neutral ___ neutral ___ neutral ___ neutral
___ sad ___ relaxed ___ satisfied ___ enthusiastic

Disability benefits:
___ Receive compensation for_____
___ Have applied for (increased) benefits
___ No application pending
___ Have lawsuit pending

What are you unable to do because of
pain that you want to do? _____

_____

_____

_____

_____

_____

Figure 44.1. **continued**

ployment. The pain section helps to put the patient's pain in perspective. One must be sure to which pain the patient's answers apply. The patient's perception of what causes the pain influences strongly the response to treatment, especially compliance with self-stretch exercises. Some are seriously worried about cancer but are hesitant to mention it, unless asked. A convincing demonstration to the patient that the pain is of muscular origin, and reassurance that it is not caused by cancer, provides tremendous relief and helps greatly to refocus attention from pain to function. The dietary history helps to assess the likelihood of vitamin and other nutrient inadequacies, which are common perpetuating factors. Sleep disturbance, when secondary to myofascial TrPs, returns to normal with relief of the disrupting myofascial pain. Unrefreshing sleep is an important feature of fibrositis. A *COMPLETE* listing of all medications, vitamins, and remedies that the individual takes can give valuable insight into the medical care the individual is receiving. It clearly reveals medical condi-

tions that are currently under treatment and often reveals unnecessary drug clutter that may contribute to iatrogenic disease. The history of previous treatment provides valuable clues as to the cause of the pain by noting which therapies alleviated symptoms and which did not. Exercise is considered essential to optimal health in general and to unimpaired function of the musculoskeletal system in particular. Well-conditioned muscles are less vulnerable to myofascial TrPs. The personal section helps one to understand how much disruption in life-style and function the pain is causing and elucidates the emotional effects of the pain. The last question identifies the activities that are important to the patient and are disrupted by the pain. Useful goals for the treatment program come from this list.

The examiner next completes the pain drawing on a body form as described in the preceding chapter under the heading. "Recognition of a Single-Muscle Syndrome." The sequence of numbered pain problems is carefully correlated, problem by problem, with the past and current medical history. It is impressive how clearly many patients can distinguish among several pain problems with regard to the circumstances at onset, the distress each causes, and the relative degrees of threat they impose. When the patient indicates a pain level, the examiner must be sure to which pain problem it applies.

Throughout this history, the examiner attempts to sort out the contribution of organic disease and the contribution of learned and interactive pain behaviors. Patients with chronic pain characteristically suffer from a mixture of both. What is causing the patient's *pain*? What contributes to the patient's *suffering*?

PHYSICAL EXAMINATION

A minimal physical examination of the patient with pain problems that are primarily musculoskeletal should include hands-on examination of the muscles. Surprisingly, this critical step is too frequently overlooked. After a careful history, the physical examination substantiates suspected findings and resolves ambiguities. Techniques have been fully described to examine the patient for myofascial TrPs (9), for fibrositis/fibromyalgia (49, 71), and for articular dysfunction (53).

LABORATORY TESTS AND IMAGING

The following laboratory studies are routinely performed to help identify perpetuating factors in patients with a progressive MPS. The complete blood count screens for marginal anemia and for a macrocytosis that may reflect a vitamin B_{12} and/or folate inadequacy. An elevated erythrocyte sedimentation rate or C-reactive protein serves as a nonspecific warning of possible chronic infection. Normal values help to eliminate this possibility.

Chemistry Battery

The chemistry battery is most useful for detecting marginal hyperuricemia, low serum potassium or calcium (ionized calcium must be ordered separately and is more meaningful than total calcium), and elevated cholesterol that would relate to low thyroid function. A thyroid battery that includes T_4 and T_3 by RIA, T_3 uptake, T_4—resin T_3 uptake index, and thyroid-stimulating hormone helps to identify the commonly recognized thyroid deficiencies. The battery is indicated if clinical symptoms and signs of inadequate thyroid function are present.

Vitamin Studies

Serum vitamin B_{12} and/or folate values in the lower quartile of the normal laboratory values have been found to be perpetuators of myofascial TrPs in many patients. Vitamins B_1 and B_6 levels should also be obtained, if financially feasible. Plasma ascorbic acid should be determined if the clinical findings suggest low tissue reserves. Vitamin A should be tested if a total of more than 10,000 IU of vitamin A has been ingested daily for a period of time.

Imaging

Radiographs, computed tomography scans, and magnetic resonance imaging are rarely helpful for the identification of the three commonly overlooked musculoskeletal conditions. Imaging can be important for detecting perpetuating factors. Thermography is useful for documenting clinically diagnosed myofascial pain due to TrPs (84).

MANAGING THE PIECES

In patients with chronic MPS, one must balance therapy addressed to the origin of the pain with management of its psychological and behavioral complications. With both approaches, the focus of attention is directed toward function rather than pain.

Recovery from the complex interacting factors that comprise chronic pain is an incremental process. One can think of the patient as climbing up a ladder. Steps taken with one foot correspond to *resolution of causes of the pain*. Steps with the other foot represent *correction of factors that intensify* the *suffering*. For improvement of the patient as a whole, both feet must make stepwise progress.

APPROACH

The most effective first step usually is to select the most severe pain problem, or the major one that appears most likely to respond to treatment, and use it to test the therapeutic response in order to demonstrate to the patient the muscular origin of the pain. This is done: (a) by reproducing a myofascial referred pain pattern by pressing on the TrP, and (b) by immediate treatment that provides at least partial relief of the pain using specific myofascial therapy applied to the muscle. The operator makes sure that the patient understands the myofascial origin of the pain and understands that relief was provided by therapy that affected only the muscles and not the nerves or bones. To emphasize the muscular origin of the pain, the patient may be reminded of Dr. Janet Travell's quote, "Broken bones heal; injured muscles learn." By having patients note the exact positioning before and after stretch, they can see for themselves the increase in range of motion. Later, they can relate that increase in function to a corresponding reduction in pain.

Frequently, among patients suffering chronic pain, the origin of the pain is of more concern than the pain itself. Recognizing the muscular cause of the pain and learning how to relieve it themselves gives them control and is profoundly reassuring. Concurrently, the patient is screened for perpetuating factors; any mechanical factors that are apparent are corrected promptly, especially those that would perpetuate the specific pain syndrome selected for initial treatment.

With regard to the behavior issues, one starts correcting or neutralizing major reinforcers of pain or sick behavior. The spouse or significant other is often the key and should become involved in the treatment program. In the case of patients with a high proportion of sick or pain behavior, it may be wise to deal with the causes of the pain only on a prescheduled time-contingent basis.

This holistic approach is likely to require the coordinated efforts of a team of health care professionals. Many physical therapists have developed expertise in the specific manual myofascial treatment techniques and in the treatment of articular dysfunctions. Social workers and psychologists are experts at dealing with coping skills and remedial behavior. A physician must deal with the systemic perpetuating factors and administer TrP injections, if needed.

Continuing specific myofascial therapy (stretch-and-spray, injection, and other stretch techniques) is based on the response to previous therapy sessions. In patients with chronic myofascial pain, one must also locate and resolve perpetuating factors. For instance, correction of the commonly found forward head posture is essential. The patient comes to appreciate the fruitlessness of continued treatment until perpetuating factors are under control.

When a myofascial pain diagnosis has been established, complete failure of response to local treatment may be due to attention having been focused erroneously on a latent TrP instead of the active TrP responsible for the pain. It also is possible that the patient had several active TrPs that referred pain to the same area from different muscles and that not all of the active TrPs were inactivated.

It is essential that a detailed drawing of the pain under treatment be recorded at each visit so that changes in the referred pain pattern are clearly documented. Marked reduction in the pressure sensitivity of previously treated myofascial TrPs and disappearance of the corresponding pain pattern represents progress. The patient who is aware only of continuing residual pain may not appreciate the improvement. The recorded changes in the pain pattern assure both the patient and the clinician of the progress.

Many times, a previous pain reemerges because a less irritable TrP is now uncovered, like peeling off an outer layer of onion. Apparently, the central nervous system can attend to only a limited number of outstanding sources of pain at one time and a previously subliminal pain replaces that which was eliminated.

When the patient shows evidence of both myofascial TrPs and fibrositis/fibromyalgia, the myofascial TrPs are treated as such and the fibromyalgia is treated as outlined by Goldenberg (48). If the patient has a combination of myofascial TrPs and articular dysfunction,

generally progress is made by releasing the tight muscles. The joint is then mobilized, followed by inactivation of any remaining TrPs. Neither treatment by itself succeeds in many of the patients who suffer from both conditions.

DRUGS

Pain cocktails are used successfully to detoxify patients on excessive analgesic or narcotic medication. Tricyclic compounds, such as amitriptyline or doxepin hydrochloride, are most effective in relatively small doses, 50–75 mg at bedtime for improving sleep and reducing pain sensitivity. Primary antidepressant action requires larger doses. Sleep may also be improved by 50 mg of the soporific antihistiminic dimenhydrate (Dramamine) taken at bedtime. A nonsteroidal anti-inflammatory drug (NSAID) may be tried for temporary pain relief, but generally, when taken orally, they are of little or no help in relieving myofascial pain due to TrPs. The NSAID diclofenac, which is a prostaglandin antagonist, when injected in the TrP was more effective than lidocaine (97).

PATIENT EDUCATION

Characteristically, one muscular stress activates a TrP and a totally different factor, or factors, perpetuate it. The patient must understand this difference. Gradually, patients learn which of their muscles cause(s) a particular pain pattern and what movements overload those muscles, perpetuating the TrPs. These patients appreciate learning how to relieve the pain by self-stretch and how to avoid overloading the muscles. Patients must restructure their activities to avoid repetitive movement or sustained contraction that overloads and perpetuates TrPs in their muscles.

The patients are encouraged, whenever possible, to continue *what* they are doing by learning *how* to do it without overloading muscles. They learn to use, not abuse, their muscles. Correction of an anatomic or postural perpetuating factor frequently requires change of patient behavior; unless the patient fully understands the relationship between the pain and the perpetuating factor, he or she will soon revert to previous activity patterns and then wonder why the pain has returned.

INDUSTRIAL CASES

Although specific myofascial therapy appears to restore the muscle to its preinjury tolerance for stress in some patients, there is mounting evidence that in other patients inactivation of an active TrP leaves a latent TrP that is more vulnerable to reactivation than before injury. This poses a serious problem for many industrial cases where vocational rehabilitation is the critical issue. After inactivation of the TrPs, the patient is unable to do the same job in the same way that he or she did before. Often the gap between functional capacity and muscular demands of the job can be bridged by a combination of: (a) modifying the job to reduce muscle strain, (b) conditioning of the muscles with exercises to increase activity tolerance, and (c) regular performance of stretching exercises to minimize irritability of the TrPs.

Unemployed patients often can be transitioned back to employability through volunteer activities that place comparable demands on their muscles. This transition is now facilitated by work hardening and is practiced chiefly by occupational and sometimes by physical therapists.

The great tragedy is that often a complex chronic MPS could have been quickly and readily resolved initially, while still acute. If only it had been recognized and properly treated as myofascial, including correction of any perpetuating factors, much suffering and disability could have been averted.

Acknowledgments The senior author expresses an enormous debt of gratitude to Janet G. Travell, M.D., and to the fellow members on the Institute of Medicine Committee on Chronic Pain and Disability (1) for helping him to better understand chronic pain from the patient's point of view. The authors are deeply grateful to Dr. Travell for thoughtful review and constructive criticism of the manuscript and to Bernadette Jaeger, D.D.S., for her helpful suggestions.

REFERENCES

1. Institute of Medicine: *Pain and Disability: Clinical, Behavioral and Public Policy Perspectives.* Washington, DC, National Academy Press, 1987.
2. Fields HL: *Pain.* New York, McGraw-Hill, 1987, pp 209–214.
3. Reynolds MD: Myofascial trigger point syndromes in the practice of rheumatology. *Arch Phys Med Rehabil* 62:111–114, 1981.
4. Fishbain DA, Goldberg M, Meagher BR, et al: Male and female chronic pain patients categorized by DSM-III psychiatric diagnostic criteria. *Pain* 26:181–197, 1986.
5. Friction JR, Kroening R, Haley D, et al: Myofascial pain syndrome of the head and neck: a review of clinical characteristics of 164 patients. *Oral Surg* 60:615–623, 1985.
6. Skootsky S: Incidence of myofascial pain in an internal medical group practice. Presented at the Annual Meeting of the American Pain Society, Washington, DC, November 6–9, 1986.
7. Travell J, Rinzler SH: The myofascial genesis of pain. *Postgrad Med* 11:425–434, 1952.
8. Travell J: Myofascial trigger points: clinical view. In Bonica JJ, Albe-Fessard D (eds): *Advances in Pain Research and Therapy.* New York, Raven Press, 1976, vol 1, pp 919–926.
9. Travell JG, Simons DG: *Myofascial Pain and Dysfunction: The Trigger Point Manual, Vol I,* Baltimore, Williams & Wilkins, 1983.
10. Azuma J, Kishi T, Williams RH, et al: Apparent deficiency of vitamin B_6 in typical individuals who commonly serve

as normal controls. *Res Commun Chem Pathol Pharmacol* 14:343–348, 1976.
11. Baker H, Frank O: Vitamin status in metabolic upsets. *World Rev Nutr Diet* 9:124–160, 1968.
12. Shealy CN: Vitamin B_6 and other vitamin levels in chronic pain patients. *Clin J Pain* 2:203–204, 1987.
13. Siebert GK, Gerbershagen HU, Mäder, et al: Vitamin-status of inpatients with chronic cephalgia and effects of a 12 day-vitamin supplementation. *Pain* Suppl 4:S298, 1987 (abstr 572).
14. Wood B, Breen KJ: Clinical thiamine deficiency in Australia: the size of the problem and approaches to prevention. *Med J Aust* 1:461–462, 464, 1980.
15. Williams RJ: *Physicians Handbook of Nutritional Science.* Springfield, IL, Charles C Thomas, 1975, pp 48, 70–82.
16. National Research Council, Committee on Dietary Allowances: *Recommended Dietary Allowances,* ed. 9. Washington, DC, National Academy of Sciences, 1980.
17. Hillman RS: Vitamin B_{12}, folic acid, and the treatment of megaloblastic anemias. In Gilman AG, Goodman LS, Gilman A (eds): *The Pharmacological Basis of Therapeutics,* ed 6. New York, MacMillan, 1980, pp 1331–1346.
18. Danford DE, Munro HN: Water-soluble vitamins: the vitamin B complex and ascorbic acid. In Gilman AF, Goodman LS, Gilman A (eds): *The Pharmacological Basis of Therapeutics,* ed 6. New York, MacMillan, 1980, pp 1560–1582.
19. Neal RA, Sauberlich HE: Thiamin. In Goodhart ME, Shils ME (eds): *Modern Nutrition in Health and Disease,* ed 6. Philadelphia, Lea & Febiger, 1980, pp 191, 193–195.
20. Sauberlich HE, Canham JE: Vitamin B_6. In Goodhard RS, Shils ME (eds): *Modern Nutrition in Health and Disease,* ed 6. Philadelphia, Lea & Febiger, 1980, pp 219–225.
21. Rose DP: Oral contraceptives and vitamin B_6. In *Human Vitamin B_6 Requirements.* Washington, DC, National Academy of Sciences, 1978, pp 193–201.
22. Stead WW: Tuberculosis. In Wintrobe MM, Thorn GW, Adams RD, et al. (eds): *Harrison's Principles of Internal Medicine,* ed 7. New York, McGraw-Hill, 1974, p 867.
23. Theuer RC, Vitale JJ: Drug and nutrient interactions. In Schneider HA, Anderson CE, Coursin DB (eds): *Nutritional Support of Medical Practice.* New York, Harper & Row, 1977, pp 209, 300, 302.
24. Kelley WN: Gout and other disorders of purine metabolism. In Isselbacher KJ, Adams RD, Braunwald E (eds): *Harrison's Principles of Internal Medicine,* ed 9. New York, McGraw-Hill, 1980, pp 479–486.
25. Avioli LV: Calcium and phosphorus. In Goodhard RS, Shils ME (eds): *Modern Nutrition in Health and Disease,* ed 6. Philadelphia, Lea & Febiger, 1980, pp 298–305.
26. Lehninger AL: *Biochemistry.* New York, Worth, 1970, pp 383–550.
27. Cooper DS: Subclinical hypothyroidism. *JAMA* 258:246–247, 1987.
28. Sonkin LS: Endocrine disorders, locomotor and temporomandibular joint dysfunction. In Gelb HG (eds). *Clinical Management of Head, Neck and TMJ Pain and Dysfunction.* Philadelphia, WB Saunders, 1977, pp 140–180.
29. Barnes E: Basal temperature versus basal metabolism. *JAMA* 119:1072–1074, 1942.
30. Travell J: Identification of myofascial trigger point syn-

dromes: a case of atypical facial neuralgia. *Arch Phys Med Rehabil* 62:100–106, 1981.

31. Simons DG: Myofascial pain syndromes due to trigger points: 2. Treatment and single-muscle syndromes. *Manual Med* 1:72–77, 1985.
32. Simons DG, Travell JG: Myofascial origins of low back pain. 2. Torso muscles. *Postgrad Med* 73:81–92, 1983.
33. Travell JG, Simons DG: *Myofascial Pain and Dysfunction: The Trigger Point Manual, Vol II.* Baltimore, Williams & Wilkins, in process, est. 1989.
34. Hagberg M, Kvarnström S: Muscular endurance and electromyographic fatigue in myofascial shoulder pain. *Arch Phys Med Rehabil* 65:522–525, 1984.
35. Simons DG: Myofascial pain syndromes due to trigger points: 1. Principles, diagnosis, and perpetuating factors. *Manual Med* 1:67–71, 1985.
36. Lewit K: Postisometric relaxation in combination with other methods of muscular facilitation and inhibition. *Manual Med* 2:101–104, 1988.
37. Lewit K, Simons DG: Myofascial pain: relief by post-isometric relaxation. *Arch Phys Med Rehabil* 65:452–456, 1984.
38. Knott M, Voss DE: *Proprioceptive Neuromuscular Facilitation.* New York, Hoeber, 1968, pp 97–99.
39. Mitchell FL Jr, Moran PS, Pruzzo NA: *Evaluation and Treatment Manual of Osteopathic Muscle Energy Procedures.* Valley Park, MO, Mitchell, Moran and Pruzzo, Associates, 1979.
40. Simons DG: Myofascial pain syndromes. In Basmajian JV, Kirby RL (eds): *Medical Rehabilitation.* Baltimore, Williams & Wilkins, 1984, pp 209–215, 313–320.
41. Danneskiold-Samsøe B, Christiansen E, Anderson RB: Myofascial pain and the role of myoglobin. *Scand J Rheumatol* 15:154–178, 1986.
42. Danneskiold-Samsøe B, Christiansen E, Lund B, et al: Regional muscle tension and pain ("fibrositis"): effect of massage on myoglobin in plasma. *Scand J Rehabil Med* 15:17–20, 1983.
43. Lewit K: The needle effect in the relief of myofascial pain. *Pain* 6:83–90, 1979.
44. Jaeger B, Skootsky SA: Double blind, controlled study of different myofascial trigger point injection techniques. *Pain* Suppl 4:S292, 1987 (abstr 560).
45. Weeks VD, Travell J: How to give painless injections. In *AMA Scientific Exhibits.* New York, Grune & Stratton, 1957, pp 318–322.
46. Benoit PW, Belt WD: Some effects of local anesthetic agents on skeletal muscle. *Exp Neurol* 34:264–278, 1972.
47. Bennett RM: Fibromyalgia. *JAMA* 257:2802–2803, 1987.
48. Goldenberg DL: Fibromyalgia syndrome: an emerging but controversial condition. *JAMA* 257:2782–2787, 1987.
49. Yunus M, Masi AT, Calabro JJ, et al: Primary fibromyalgia. *Am Fam Physician* 25:115–121, 1982.
50. Campbell SM, Bennett RM: Fibrositis. *DM* 32(11):653–722, 1986.
51. Smythe HA, Moldofsky H: Two contributions to understanding of the "fibrositis" syndrome. *Bull Rheum Dis* 28:928–931, 1977.
52. Wolfe F: The clinical syndrome of fibrositis. *Am J Med* 81:(Suppl 3A):7–14, 1986.
53. Lewit K: *Manipulative Therapy in Rehabilitation of the Motor System.* Stoneham, MA, Butterworth, 1985.
54. Fassbender HG: Non-articular rheumatism. In *Pathology of Rheumatic Diseases.* New York, Springer-Verlag, 1975, pp 303–314.
55. Miehlke K, Schulze G: Der sogenannte Muskelrheumatismus. *Internist* 2:447–453, 1961.
56. Popelianskii Ialu, Bogdanov EI, Khabirov FA: [Algesic trigger zones of the gastrocnemius muscle in lumbar osteochondrosis (clinicopathomorphological and electromyographic analysis)] (Russian). *Zh Nevropatol Psikhiatr* 84:1055–1061, 1984.
57. Popelianskii Ialu, Zaslavskii ES, Veselovskii VP: [Medicosocial significance, etiology, pathogenesis, and diagnosis of nonarticular disease of soft tissues of the limbs and back] (Russian). *Vopr Revm* 3:38–43, 1976.
58. Graff-Radford SB, Reeve JL, Jaeger B: Myofascial pain may present clinically as occipital neuralgia. *Neurosurgery* 19:610–613, 1988.
59. Simons DG: Muscle pain syndromes—Parts I and II. *Am J Phys Med* 54:289–311, 1975; 55:15–42, 1976.
60. Simons DG: Myofascial pain syndrome due to trigger points. In Goodgold J (ed): *Rehabilitation Medicine.* St. Louis, CV Mosby, 1987 (in press).
61. Reynolds MD: The development of the concept of fibrositis. *J Hist Med Allied Sci* 38:5–35, 1983.
62. Bates T, Grunwaldt E: Myofascial pain in childhood. *J Pediatr* 53:198–209, 1958.
63. Sola AE, Rodenberger ML, Gettys BB: Incidence of hypersensitive areas in posterior shoulder muscles. *Am J Phys Med* 34:58–590, 1955.
64. Simons DG: Fibrositis/fibromyalgia: a form of myofascial trigger points? *Am J Med* 81(suppl 3A):93–98, 1986.
65. Smythe HA: Non-articular rheumatism and the fibrositis syndrome. In Hollander JL, McCarty DJ (eds): *Arthritis and Allied Conditions,* ed 8. Philadelphia, Lea & Febiger, 1972, pp 874–884.
66. Egle UT, Schwab R, Rudolf ML, et al: Illness behaviour and defense mechanisms of patients with psychogenic pain: rheumatoid arthritis and fibrositis syndrome. *Pain* Supl 4:S324, 1987 (abstr 624).
67. Henriksson KG, Bengtsson A, Larsson J, et al: Muscle pain with special reference to primary fibromyalgia (PF). *Pain* Suppl 4:S294, 1987 (abstr 564).
68. Landrø NI, Winnem M: Psychodiagnostic evaluation of patients with myofascial pain syndrome (fibrositis). *Pain* Suppl 4:S419, 1987 (abstr 808).
69. Clark S, Campbell SM, Forehand ME, et al: Clinical characteristics of fibrositis: II. A "blinded," controlled study using standard psychological tests. *Arthritis Rheum* 28:132–137, 1985.
70. Moldofsky H, Scarisbrick P, England R, et al: Musculoskeletal symptoms and Non-REM sleep disturbance in patients with "fibrositis syndrome" and health subjects. *Psychosom Med* 37:341–351, 1975.
71. Smythe HA: Fibrositis and other diffuse musculoskeletal syndromes. In Kelley WN, Harris ED Jr, Ruddy S (eds): *Textbook of Rheumatology.* Philadelphia, WB Saunders, 1981, vol 1, pp 485–493.
72. Bennett RM (ed): The fibrositis/fibromyalgia syndrome: current issues and prospectives. *Am J Med* 81(Suppl 3A):1–115, 1986.
73. Bengtsson A: Primary fibromyalgia: a clinical and labora-

tory study. Linköping: Linköping University Dissertations, No. 224, 1986.

74. Crook J, Tunks E, Norman G, et al: A comparative study of tenderness thresholds in trigger points and non-trigger points in normal and fibromyalgia patients. *Pain* suppl 4:S307, 1987, (abstr 509).

75. Lund N, Bengtsson A, Thorborg P: Muscle tissue oxygen pressure in primary fibromyalgia. *Scand J Rheumatol* 15:165–173, 1986.

76. Smythe H: Tender points: evolution of concepts of the fibrositis/fibromyalgia syndrome. *Am J Med* 81(suppl 3A):2–6, 1986.

77. Bengtsson A, Henriksson K-G, Jorfeldt L: Primary fibromyalgia, a clinical and laboratory study of 55 patients. *Scan J Rheumatol* 15:340–347, 1986.

78. Tunks E, Norman G, Kalaher S, et al: Validity and reliability of the clinical use of a pressure algometer in the study of trigger points. *Pain* suppl 4:S307, 1987 (abstr 590).

79. Caro XJ: Immunofluorescent detection of IgG at the dermal-epidermal junction in patients with apparent primary fibrositis syndrome. *Arthritis Rheum* 27:1174–1179, 1984.

80. Bartels EM, Danneskiold-Samsøe B: Histological abnormalities in muscle from patients with certain types of fibrositis. *Lancet* 1:755–757, 1986.

81. Bengtsson A, Henriksson K-G, Larsson J: Reduced high-energy phosphate levels in painful muscle in patients with primary fibromyalgia. *Arthritis Rheum* 29:817–821, 1986.

82. Fischer AA: Diagnosis and management of chronic pain in physical medicine and rehabilitation. In Ruskin AP (ed): *Current Therapy in Physiatry*. Philadelphia, WB Saunders, 1984, pp 131–134.

83. Fischer AA: Correlation between site of pain and "hot spots" on thermogram in lower body. *Postgrad Med Custom Communications*, March:99, 1986.

84. Simons DG: Myofascial pain syndromes: Where are we? Where are we going? *Arch Phys Med Rehabil* 69:207–212, 1988.

85. Mennel JM: *Joint Pain*. Boston, Little, Brown & Company, 1964.

86. Lewit K: Chain reactions in disturbed function of the motor system. *Manual Med* 3, 1987 (in press).

87. Fisk JW: *Medical Treatment of Neck and Back Pain*. Springfield, IL, Charles C Thomas, 1987, pp 65, 69.

88. Friberg O: Lumbar instability: a dynamic approach by traction-compression radiography. *Spine* 12:119–129, 1987.

89. Rubin D: An approach to the management of myofascial trigger point syndromes. *Arch Phys Med Rehabil* 62:107–110, 1981.

90. Addison RG: Chronic pain syndrome. *Am J Med* 77:54–58, 1984.

91. Price DD, Harkins SW, Baker C: Sensory-affective relationships among different types of clinical and experimental pain. *Pain* 28:297–307, 1987.

92. Melzack R: *The Puzzle of Pain*. New York, Basic Books, 1973, pp 22–24, 153–179.

93. Baker BA: The muscle trigger: evidence of overload injury. *J Neurol Orthop Med Surg* 7:35–43, 1986.

94. Evans WJ, Meredith CN, Cannon JG, et al: Metabolic changes following eccentric exercise in trained and untrained men. *J Appl Physiol* 61:1864–1868, 1986.

95. McCully KK, Faulkner JA: Injury to skeletal muscle fibers of mice following lengthening contractions. *J Appl Physiol* 59:119–126, 1985.

96. Melnick J: Trigger areas and refractory pain in duodenal ulcer. *NY State J Med* 57:1073–1076, 1957.

97. Frost A: Diclofenac versus lidocaine as injection therapy in myofascial pain. *Scan J Rheumatol* 15:153–156, 1986.

SELECTED TOPICS

CHAPTER 45

PAIN PROBLEMS IN PRIMARY CARE MEDICAL PRACTICE

CARLA RODGERS
TROY L. THOMPSON, II

MOST PATIENTS with acute or chronic pain initially seek out a primary care physician, such as a general practitioner, family physician, general internist, or obstetrician-gynecologist. Among the most common types of pain complaints in primary care practices are headaches, abdominal pains, and low back pain (1, 2). Pain complaints also make up a large percentage of primary care practices; in fact, persistent pain is the most common chief complaint bringing patients to see primary care practitioners.

Low back pain is especially common in those involved in work-related disability. Chronic low back pain is the most common reason given for repeated work absenteeism in the United States, and this condition alone accounts for almost 20 million physician visits annually in the United States. Compensation to those disabled with chronic low back pain accounted for approximately 40% of disability payments in California in one recent year. Headaches are estimated to account for another approximately 12 million physician visits per year (3–5). The differential diagnosis of lower back and spinal pain is discussed in Chapter 27, and pain caused by headache is discussed thoroughly in Chapters 19, 20, and 21.

NEUROANATOMY AND PHYSIOLOGY OF PAIN

What initiates the transmission of pain impulses and the exact pain pathway is not fully known. There are two types of peripheral nerve fibers associated with the transmission of pain: large myelinated A-fibers conducting impulses rapidly, and associated with sharp pain sensations; and small unmyelinated C-fibers, transmitting impulses more slowly, and associated with dull pain (6). The A-fibers may be more involved with acute traumatic pain and lead to spinal reflex withdrawal, if possible, of the traumatized part from the source of injury. The C-fibers appear to be more involved in chronic pain states. Substance P may be the primary neurotrans-

mitter of afferent receptors that initiate the pain pathway (7). Clearly, there appear to be neuroanatomic as well as psychological differences between acute and chronic pain (8, 9), which will be discussed more later.

The primary central nervous system (CNS) neuroanatomic pain pathway begins by pain stimuli traveling through fibers into the dorsal root zone of the spinal cord. Pain fibers then divide into ascending and descending branches that run in Lissauer's tract (the posterolateral fasciculus) of the spinal cord. The fibers are believed to fully leave this tract within two vertebral segments to synapse with posterior lower neurons. How they are affected at this level, or the exact connections and types of interneurons or other structures on which they impinge, is not fully known. It is believed, nevertheless, that alterations in pain stimuli may begin to occur at this level, perhaps involving T-cells or other neural systems, which will be discussed later. The pain stimuli then cross anterior to the central canal of the spinal cord in the anterior white commissure. They subsequently travel rostrally in the lateral spinothalamic tract. The limbic system (reticular formation), several thalamic nuclei, including the ventral posterolateral nucleus (VPL) of the thalamus, and the hypothalamus receive input from these pain fibers. The limbic system and the thalamic nuclei may be able to influence the transmission of pain stimuli at this level. The limbic system is closely related to a person's level of alertness and has been described as a modulator of cortical activity level. Pain fibers then relay pain impulses from the thalamus to the secondary somatic sensory area of the cerebrum. Some pain-stimulated fibers also go directly from the VPL nucleus to the primary somatic sensory area.

Pain stimuli may be modified by effects at the posterior horn or in the reticular formation by descending pathways from the cerebral cortex and other higher structures. Pain is not consciously perceived by the patient until the above impulses reach the thalamus. If cortical perception areas have been destroyed, pain may still be perceived if the thalamus has remained intact. Localization of the source of pain and the intensity of pain is perceived by the parietal cortex. Memory regions and cortical association areas also play a role in amplifying or diminishing reactions to pain stimuli. Memories or past experiences with a type of pain similar to the one currently being experienced may diminish or increase the patient's reaction to the pain, depending on whether those memories or experiences were benign or if significant psychological or physical trauma resulted.

Two basic types of pain sensation exist. The first is termed *fast pain*, which is reported as sharp or pricking and has little of an emotional component. The second type is *slow pain*, which is frequently reported as a burning sensation. Fast pain pathways appear to be more somatotopically arranged than slow pain pathways and allow fast pain to be sharply localized. Precise spatial or temporal information is not possible with slow pain, and slow pain seems to be much more influenced by emotional factors, possibly in the thalamic and hypothalamic regions.

The CNS, through as yet incompletely understood mechanisms, appears to have the ability to produce its own analgesia to some degree (10). The endorphins are compounds produced in the body and are a condensation of "endogenous morphine." The capacity of the body to produce its own analgesia and the effectiveness of this system varies greatly between individuals. It is possible that those who are responsive to biofeedback techniques or who have a marked placebo response may have a more effective endorphin system (11). Also, 30–40% of postsurgical patients report little or no pain and require little or no analgesics in the postoperative period. These might also be individuals with highly effective endorphin systems. Because approximately the same percentage of the population are also robust placebo responders, might the same people frequently be in both groups? Is it possible that some people can mobilize their endorphins in response to one situation and not another?

Opiate receptors appear to be highly concentrated in discrete areas of the brain, especially the periaqueductal and periventricular gray matter. Not surprisingly, the endorphin system seems to be concentrated in the same areas (12). It has also been found that naloxone, a commonly used opioid antagonist, may reverse the effects of placebo analgesia. This further suggests that placebos may be effective in part by activating the endogenous opioid systems (13).

Although the majority of patients have approximately the same threshold for pain perception, this threshold may be increased by almost half in most individuals, and even more in some, by several techniques or interventions. These techniques include acupuncture, biofeedback, relaxation techniques, hypnosis, and imagery training (11, 14, 15). A pleasant or euphoric mental state may also decrease pain perception. Likewise, if a person is preoccupied with some other event, such as an injury to a loved one, they may be inattentive to their own pain until the needs of the other have been addressed. Other modalities that decrease pain perception include analgesics and placebo (1, 16). Placebo can give significant relief to approximately one-third of patients with clearcut pain resulting from physiologic trauma. It is important for the physician to realize that a positive response to placebo does not rule out or decrease the possibility that a biomedical disorder underlines the pain. The exact mechanism of action of placebo is unclear. The belief of some persons that taking a medication will relieve their pain may lead them to be able to produce neurophysiologic changes that, in fact, result in pain relief. It is possible that these changes occur through effects of the cortex on lower CNS functions, or that a positive, upbeat mood increases endorphin levels.

The state of neurotransmitter systems not directly involved with pain transmission may still affect pain perception and tolerance. For example, depressed patients are usually much more responsive to painful stimuli. Because malfunctions of the noradrenergic and serotonergic systems have been associated with depression, alteration of those systems may make the patients more or less resilient to pain stimuli. For example, serotonergic neurons have been found to interact with the endorphin system. Most tricyclics act in part by increasing serotonin in the synaptic cleft, and this effect may relate to the relief that some pain patients experience (17). It is also possible that tricyclics may help pain patients by increasing the cortical inhibition of pain perception, in addition to their actions on catecholamines (6).

Because many of the neurotransmitter systems are inhibitory or facilitory of other systems in the brain, a change in one system might have multiple effects that could alter the person's perception or tolerance of pain. Malfunction of the dopamine system appears to be associated with schizophrenia, and some schizophrenic patients experience relatively little or no pain, even when significantly injured. Some anxious patients and those with panic disorders are exquisitely sensitive to painful stimuli. Disruption of gamma-amino butyric acid neurotransmitter systems are implicated in these disorders and may be related to this population's increased pain complaints.

Melzack and Wall proposed a "pain gate control" mechanism, which has been the subject of much attention and debate, in which they postulate a "gateway" cell in the spinal cord that might be opened or closed to allow or prevent pain stimuli from reaching higher levels in the CNS. If these hypothetical "gating" or transmitting neurons (or *T-cells*) are in the spinal cord, they could alter the number of pain stimuli reaching the level of the thalamus, resulting in altered pain perception. The substantia gelatinosa of the spinal cord is postulated to be the site of these T-cells (which are not the same as the T-cells of the immunologic system). The T-cells are also hypothesized to be affected by large peripheral afferent nerve fibers as well as by higher nervous system structures.

For severe and intractable chronic pain, nerve blocks and neurosurgical and neuroablative procedures have been used at virtually every level of the pain pathways previously described. Neurosurgical transection of the spinothalamic and spinoreticular formation pathways may initially relieve pain in up to 85% of selected patients (18). Unfortunately, a number of these patients have recurrence of painful sensations within a few months. It has been suggested that collateral pathways exist or develop in other than the anterolateral quadrant of the spinal cord (11, 13, 19). Nerve blocks, neuroablative techniques, and spinal surgery are discussed further in Chapters 6, 7, and 8, respectively.

Transcutaneous or dorsal column electrical stimulators have also been used to diminish pain perception. They operate on the principle of stimulating peripheral fibers that partially close or overload the gating cells (20). Pain impulses may be modulated by the relative activity of inhibitory A-fibers and facilitory C-fibers, as well as by descending influences from the brain (21, 22). Some dentists use "white noise" generators to decrease pain perception during dental procedures. Such machines presumably operate in a similar fashion but at the level of the cranial nerves. That is, sensory nerves are probably limited in the ability to conduct impulses, including pain. If some nonpainful stimuli bombards a nerve that is conducting painful stimuli, the various impulses will have to compete for the sensory nerves' capacity to transmit them. Therefore, the number of painful stimuli that would be transmitted would be reduced. It is not clear that a specific gating neuron, which has not been identified anatomically, would need to exist in this situation. If sensory nerves are being constantly bombarded with electrical stimuli, then they would perhaps be less responsive to other types of stimuli, including pain. Another possibility exists, however: if neurons were continually being bombarded, a hypersensitivity response might occur, particularly if the stimulation were stopped. This could lead to a small stimulus then producing an exaggerated response. Such a phenomenon might be analogous to that of kindling, in which a gradual buildup of predisposing factors leads to an otherwise minor event triggering a full seizure.

Another possible mechanism of action of transcutaneous stimulators may be stimulation of the patient's endorphin system. This hypothesis is supported by the fact that naloxone, an opioid antagonist, has been observed to reduce the effectiveness of transcutaneous electrical nerve stimulation treatment, especially of a high-frequency type (23). Neural stimulation techniques are discussed in further detail in Chapter 8.

The psychological significance that pain has for the individual clearly affects the perception and reaction to painful stimuli. The degree of pain experienced and the concomitant need for analgesia is often more strongly related to the psychological meaning of the injury and pain to the individual than to the actual amount of physiologic trauma present. Also, painful stimuli may have positive significance for some individuals. Beecher performed elegant research demonstrating these points (24). He found that many soldiers who sustained significant wounds in battle complained of little or no pain and refused morphine when it was offered; however, civilians experiencing similar wounds, often due to the same type of injury, complained of much more pain and requested more analgesia. Eighty percent of the civilians accepted analgesic medications, whereas only one-third of the soldiers accepted such treatment. Beecher speculated about the different responses between the two groups, focusing on the meaning the injuries had to each group. For the soldier, being alert and able to tolerate the pain without medication meant to him that he probably had a survivable wound, which would likely result in his being sent home. Being wounded might actually alleviate the anxiety associated with anticipation of more serious injury or death. Some soldiers have stuck an arm or leg out of their foxhole when they heard a shell coming in with the hope that they might sustain a minor shrapnel injury by doing so. Again, such an injury might be life-saving and, thereby, at least partially welcomed. Conversely, civilians usually do not have positive personal or social consequences accrue as a result of being wounded and seldom view these injuries as desirable. In his research, Pavlov was successful in training dogs to look forward to a minor wound or other traumatic stimuli if it was linked to being fed. Some individuals also learn to control others through self-mutilation, which is associated with pain. The wrist-cutter may learn that this act is a dramatic and sometimes effective way of gaining the attention of and controlling others.

Therefore, in summary, although it has been known for years that chronic pain is not a simple stimulus-response situation (25), the physician must continually remind himself of this fact when confronted with these difficult patients. The pain pathway may have appeared fairly straightforward in medical school; however, many psychosocial and physiologic factors are able to alter the perception of pain through mechanisms that are still incompletely understood. Another of the most useful concepts for the physician to remember when evaluating chronic pain patients is that their degree of disability is usually related to a combination of biopsychosocial factors (11, 26). Exceptions to this statement include the patient who has severe persistent pain due to a proven serious illness, such as metastatic cancer to bone, pancreatic carcinoma, and other similar conditions. These patients, while although complex to manage, present a different set of problems than patients with chronic pain for which no definitive diagnosis has been made, or whose pain complaints seem to greatly exceed the biomedical trauma that is evident.

ADAPTIVE NATURE OF PAIN

The physician may develop an automatic aversive response to chronic pain patients. These patients are often very difficult to diagnose because of the lengthy differential diagnosis to be considered for almost any chronic pain complaint. They are equally difficult to treat because of the wide variation in an individual's responses to pain and to pain treatment. The physician should bear in mind that the pain pathway is usually adaptive and essential to the health and well-being of organisms. Pain is often the earliest signal that an incipient disease process is occurring. The spread of illnesses such as cancer, or the existence of tissue damage with the possibility of further injury, can be signaled by pain, which may allow the physician to diagnose and treat a condition promptly.

The importance of pain sensation to the individual may be further appreciated by considering those people who have a congenital absence of pain (27). Pain as an early warning sign of trauma or illness is not recognized by these individuals, who therefore are prone to multiple physical injuries. Some patients with congenital absence of pain resort to self-injury, possibly because self-injury gives them some sense of control over trauma and out of frustration that they will be injured anyway. Also, one of the ways that individuals learn to distinguish themselves from the rest of the world is through pain sensation. Therefore, these individuals tend to not develop in a psychologically normal manner and have a distorted body image due to lack of such feedback.

SOCIOCULTURAL VARIABLES AFFECTING PAIN BEHAVIOR

Physicians often recognize that many patients who present with a variety of pain complaints are not seriously ill. In 75% of medical patients who presented with pain as their chief complaint in one study, no underlying organic pathology could be found (28). Individuals who are overly frightened of injury, illness, disability, or deformity may seek out a physician at the earliest development of even a minor pain. Concomitant psychiatric disorders in these patients include hypochondriasis, anxiety, and depression, all of which can contribute to increased pain sensitivity. Pain may actually be one symptom of an underlying psychiatric disorder (29). In milder cases, the physician may choose education and reassurance. The patient may require nothing

further if he or she can be assured that the pain will probably remain mild and be transient. Pain associated with more-severe psychiatric disorders will be discussed in another section.

An individual's unique response to painful stimuli is determined by a complex interaction of psychological, psychiatric, familial, social, cultural, and personality-related factors (16, 30, 31). These subjective, emotional, and largely unmeasurable factors affect the degree of pain perception and the number of pain complaints. This fact distinguishes chronic pain from other disorders that physicians treat. Another distinguishing factor is the lack of quantifiable pain-related laboratory data that can tell the physician about the degree of control or effectiveness of treatment. Some individuals may pay a great deal of attention to a small physical insult, whereas others may surprise the physician with the amount of illness or massive trauma they can tolerate. In part, this varied response may relate to sociocultural factors.

The close psychological and sociocultural associations between pain, guilt, and punishment may be better understood when it realized that the word "pain" has its origins in the Latin word *poene* and the Greek word *poine*, both of which mean "penalty" or "punishment." Illness and pain are often thought, at least unconsciously, to be inflicted on someone for wrongdoing. Some religions also believe that illness and pain are the direct consequence of a person's sins. As a result, their followers may believe that they deserve their illness and pain, and that a cure or analgesia might eliminate the punishment they deserve as a result of some real or imagined transgression or sin. In fact, paradoxically, they may feel that getting pain relief might make them deserve more pain and punishment. Some families and cultures still use physical pain as a means of punishment. Floggings or other methods of corporal punishment still exist in some countries as penalties for crimes, and some families still inflict pain by spankings or similar means to discipline their children (5, 6, 32). Different cultures, religions, family values, and psychodynamics will place varying degrees of emphasis on pain complaints (33). Patients of higher socioeconomic class are less likely to ascribe pain completely to physical rather than psychosocial causes than are patients of lower socioeconomic class (34). In his research at a large VA hospital, Zborowski identified four stereotypes of cultures as they relate to the pain-associated behaviors in these cultures (35). These stereotypes, specified in the next paragraph, should not be taken as literal guidelines, since because many individuals and families from the cultures discussed do not exhibit the stereotyped responses. Physicians need to remember, nevertheless, to review sociocultural as well as familial factors that can amplify or diminish pain response. The physician will be able to provide better care by remembering that the meanings of pain, illness, expected disability, and pain-related behaviors vary widely between cultures and even among families who are part of the same subculture (36).

The four stereotyped groups that Zborowski related to their pain responses were the Irish, Italian, Jewish, and "old American" ethnic groups. The Irish and "old American" subgroups appear to display more stoicism in the face of pain. Their families and culture seem to value minimal expression in the face of physical adversity and view crying or other emotional expressions as a sign of weakness.

There are clear potential risks and benefits of either extreme of emotional reaction. The extremely expressive subgroups may visit the doctor repeatedly with minor complaints, resulting in the physician wearying of them, especially if he or she does not understand these sociocultural factors. If the patient has a thick chart of negative findings, the physician may be less attentive and vigorous in the evaluation than when the patient presents with an easily identifiable medical disorder. This relative inattentiveness may be dangerous because the patient who has been labeled a "crock" or hypochondriac will obviously eventually die of some medical disorder (29, 37).

On the other hand, stoic subtypes also run some risks. Physicians are often themselves hardworking persons who deal with stress in their lives by redoubling their efforts and forging ahead; so physicians often identify with and, therefore, tend to like and admire this kind of patient. Consequently, it can be difficult for a physician to recognize this pattern of behavior as potentially maladaptive and pathologic. In fact, the physician may view the stoic as the ideal patient, whereas the emotionally expressive patient may be labeled as whining, whimpering, and one to be avoided. A vicious cycle may be established because the more the emotionally expressive patient and family are avoided, the more they tend to amplify the characteristics many physicians hate in an attempt to receive more attention from the physician.

Unfortunately, the emotionally constrained patient may not seek medical help until the illness has progressed significantly. He may continue to function with a chronic condition until literally unable to get to the doctor's office. Avoiding a visit to the doctor, the stoic may rationalize this avoidant behavior by feeling that he cannot really be sick; so not seeing a physician is magical protection from an illness and means the condition must be minor and transient. Sometimes, when literally no longer able to get up or having lost consciousness, such an emotionally constrained patient may be brought to the emergency room by family, friends, or an ambulance. Even then, it is striking that the stoic and the family and friends, who also of course tend to be stoics, may apologize for causing trouble for the physician and the emergency room staff and con-

tinue to deny or minimize a serious condition. While appearing self-reliant and almost overly independent, these patients may actually be terrified of illness and of needing to be dependent on anyone. By denying the possibility of either pain or death, they attempt to conquer their fear of both. They also fear passivity, and, once diagnosed as having an illness, often resolve to fight it to the end. They often use athletic or war metaphors while in treatment such as, "I'm going to show this thing who's boss," or ". . . defeat it." The patient may be described with pride as a fighter by family and friends. Another difficulty for stoics and their families is that they may not know when and where to let go or are unable to even do so. This inability to accept what they consider to be defeat can result in a great deal of time, money, and ensuing frustration seeking exotic cures and repeated evaluations by multiple medical experts or nonmedical "healers," sometimes including charlatans.

Crying in stoic individuals is usually viewed as a sign of weakness by both male and female stoics. It may be as unbearable for friends and family to watch (and hear about) the formerly "strong and proud" individual break down and cry as it is for that individual to have others see him or her cry. As a result, if pain becomes severe, stoic patients tend to withdraw rather than let others know their suffering.

Stoic patients are also more likely to request an operation than more emotionally expressive groups because stoics tend to view illness and injury more in mechanical terms and, therefore, to seek a mechanical cure. This is evident in their use of mechanical metaphors, such as "the old ticker isn't firing right so I need a new set of plugs put in," describing the need for a cardiac pacemaker and so forth.

The stoic may also wish to view the physician as completely self-reliant and in need of no additional help and may, therefore, be reluctant to accept the primary physician's recommendation of a consultation by a specialist. The more emotionally expressive groups may have the opposite response. They often seek opinions of several specialists and read medical literature to see if their physician is up on the latest treatment. The physician may feel insulted, become angry, and want to have even less to do with these patients and their families if he or she is not aware that emotional needs of these patients are being met by such behavior.

Some primary care physicians have had experiences wherein the chronically somatizing patient actually has complained less after developing a biomedical disorder, including such severe conditions as myocardial infarction or ruptured appendix, than with their chronic multiple, psychologically based physical complaints. Some of these patients will corroborate such observations. For example, a patient reported that a ruptured appendix and subsequent peritonitis were less painful and disabling than his usual abdominal distress, which was due to functional bowel syndrome.

APPROACH TO THE PAIN PATIENT

Chronic pain patients are probably the most challenging group for primary care physicians, as well as other types of physicians. Because virtually any biomedical and psychiatric disorder may present as, or be associated with, complaints of somatic discomfort and pain, the evaluation of chronic pain is complex (11). A pain complaint that is persistent or increasing, but whose source cannot be readily identified, may be very frightening to the physician as well as to the patient because many serious illnesses, such as cancer, may initially present with vague somatic discomfort. Such clinical situations present a dilemma to the primary care practitioner. Does one do the basics (i.e., history, physical examination, and routine laboratory studies) and then wait to see if the pain persists and becomes more specific? The risk is the possible progression of a potentially treatable disorder. The opposite course of action can also have adverse consequences of a different type. It would be expensive and time-consuming to thoroughly work-up each pain complaint presented to the primary care practitioner. In fact, if the average primary care physician sees about 50 patients per day, time constraints would make such work-ups impossible. One possibility is that after the initial evaluation that proves negative, the primary care physician could refer the patient to the specialist in the organ system or bodily region that seems most likely to be related to the pain's pathology. This process could also become expensive and time-consuming. If the first specialist then refers the patient to yet another specialist, and so on, an escalating spiral of cost, time, and diagnostic procedures may be set in motion, with each evaluation procedure also having associated morbidity.

The approach taken to chronic pain patients by most primary care physicians is an intermediate one. If the type of pain may be associated with severe pathophysiology, then the doctor usually promptly undertakes further diagnostic efforts to rule that possibility out. If the pain complaints appear to be benign in nature, however, most physicians take a "wait and see" approach. The most common management approaches in such clinical situations are appointments for reevaluation every 1–2 months and supportive and symptomatic therapies. The repeated observations by many primary care physicians that most patients' pain complaints will spontaneously improve and resolve over time, if they are followed, accounts for this approach. Allowing time to be the healer is often very effective for many benign and self-limited conditions, both biomedical and psychiatric. It is also much less of a financial burden for patients and third-party payers.

Most primary practitioners have also witnessed significant morbidity and mortality associated with vigorous diagnostic and therapeutic procedures. This is another reason that primary care physicians often initially adopt a conservative approach to pain symptoms. A clear example of this is the patient with persistent abdominal pain, who will doctor-shop until a physician is found who will perform exploratory surgery. A typical scenario is that the pain improves temporarily after surgery, though the surgery may not reveal any specific pathology. Previously, an appendectomy or cholecystectomy might have been performed "because we were in there anyway" or in the hope that some covert pathology in those tissues might be related to the pain complaints. After several weeks or months, unfortunately, the abdominal pain in such patients often returns, sometimes in a modified form, as if to convey to the physician the message "the last surgery did modify, so another surgery would probably help this pain as well." The well-intentioned surgeon, having spent many long years honing his skills, may decide to go back in and see if anything was overlooked and if something might be more evident since the previous surgery. If inexperienced with these type of patients, the surgeon may not realize that if nothing specific was found on the initial exploratory laparotomy, it is unlikely that another surgery will be useful if the only symptom is vague, persistent pain and if the pain is not typical of any known pathology. Recently, much surgical training has improved in educating surgeons to be more attuned to psychological factors involved with patients who repeatedly seek more and more surgery. The occasional anecdotal report of previously overlooked pathology and a treatment coup and cure on repeat surgery may be used to justify a follow-up attempt; therefore, some primary care physicians make a vigorous attempt to keep their chronic pain patients away from surgeons at all costs.

Some chronic pain patients are masterful in eliciting powerful rescue fantasies and wishes to be the brilliant hero in many physicians. Most primary care physicians do, nevertheless, realize that neurosurgical procedures can be effective for some chronic pain patients, and they consult with neurosurgeons, especially in a referral center that deals with a large number of chronic pain patients.

PERSONALITY AND SECONDARY GAIN FACTORS

Some forms of chronic pain and disability lead to financial secondary gain. This situation creates a tremendous bind, especially for the lower class and lower middle income individual. They may be able to receive as much, and on occasion more, compensation for continuing their disability as they could by working full-time at their usual occupation. If their financial compensation will be at least equal to that of them working, some individuals would understandably choose to have their time to themselves rather than working full-time, even though they are required to pay an occasional visit to the physician and the disability review board. A disturbing aspect of some disability compensation programs is that patients are viewed as either fully able to work or fully disabled. Some patients risk losing their disability payments completely if they work part-time, even though patients often do become somewhat rehabilitated and would be able to work part-time, and possibly gradually increase their workload. Increasing numbers of disability review agencies have become more enlightened with regard to this issue in recent years. They have come to realize that if they allow the patient to gradually increase a partial workload and gradually decrease disability payments proportionately, many individuals would prefer to work at least part-time rather than having nothing structured to do.

Some financial incentive may be included in this incremental approach that encourages the patient to engage in part-time work. The rigid either/or policy of some disability companies is much less efficacious in saving money and facilitating patient recovery. Flexible and gradual behavior-modification approaches have proven more effective, in improving patient functioning, quality of life, and reduce the amount of third-party payment (5). Chapters 53 and 54 cover the legal aspects of pain and Social Security disability and worker's compensation law.

Chronic pain may be related to and amplify psychological characteristics in some patients. Those developing specific psychiatric disorders as a response to the stress of chronic pain will be discussed later. The secondary gain that is associated with chronic pain can also take a variety of other forms. Some chronic pain patients reap interpersonal gains from their pain. For instance, they may receive more love and attention from friends and relatives because they are sick. Sometimes a patient wishes, either consciously or unconsciously, to remain ill in order to prevent a specific event, such as the breakup of a marriage or a child leaving home. This may be inadvertently confirmed by a spouse who may say, "I would leave him in a minute if he got well," or "I was getting ready to leave just before he became ill, but I couldn't live with myself if I left an ill man," or by similar types of comments made by others. Chronic illness and pain also give some patients a social purpose. They receive more attention and a degree of specialness and identification in a group as a result of their disability and illness. Examples include automobile license plates and other insignia granted to members of such groups. One purpose is to let others know that they should be viewed as distinguished, deserving of honor and some forms of special consideration.

A form of personal secondary gain may occur in which

chronic pain and illness will, seemingly paradoxically, be welcomed by individuals with certain kinds of personalities. If a person feels like a failure or is concerned that others view him in that way, then chronic pain provides a reasonable alternative to viewing oneself as a failure. One can say that had it not been for chronic disability and discomfort, one would have been a success as an athlete, employee, spouse, parent, and so forth. Some of these patients have referred to their pain as "an old friend" (38). The pain has become personified as a useful portion of their personality that can be called upon in time of need. Depending on the situation, pain may be used as a psychological crutch in various ways. Chapter 4 reviews psychological evaluation and testing of chronic pain patients.

Being alert for patients who have a combination of several of the psychosocial, familial, and cultural risk factors reviewed above may help the physician to know to try to intervene early, assertively, and comprehensively. The goal of early intervention is to avoid a vicious cycle from occurring; this cycle results in the establishment of a chronic pain syndrome, involving both patient and family. Early recognition of such patients is further discussed in Chapter 47.

DIAGNOSIS AND TREATMENT OF PAIN DISORDERS IN PRIMARY CARE

Because chronic pain patients tend to be complex and difficult to diagnose, the primary care physician understandably becomes frustrated when a specific diagnosis cannot be made and treatment does not seem to help. In such situations, the primary practitioner's frustrations may be revealed by terms used to describe the patient, such as "crock" (3, 6). When dealing with such taxing patients, the primary care physician is tempted to refer them to other physicians, especially to those interested in treating pain, including specialists at large pain centers. It is generally better for the patient, however, if his primary care physician is willing to oversee and coordinate his total health care efforts, even when outside consultation is indicated. If not, a loose confederation of subspecialists, who may not communicate well with one another, may each be attempting to take care of only one part of the problem. The situation is analogous to the story of the six blind men trying to describe the elephant, each only familiar with the part of the elephant he feels, but no one being able to put together the entire picture. If asked, such patients are often unable to say who their doctor is. Balint refers to this leaderless group effort at health care as a "collusion of anonymity." The patient does not, in fact, have a single identified physician (39).

The primary care physician, sometimes out of sheer frustration, may conclude that the patient's pain is all psychogenic. "It's all in your head and you'd better go see a psychiatrist," the doctor is tempted to, or sometimes actually, tells the patient. Because one can never be sure any pain is purely psychogenic, it is wise not to make such statements for medicolegal as well as humanistic reasons. An alternative is to tell the patient that the work-up has been negative so far, and, although this cannot be said with 100% certainty, it appears that the etiology is not life-threatening. The suggestion that the patient then see a psychiatrist may be explained as a method for the patient to learn how to better cope with the ongoing pain and adapt other aspects of his life to the pain, and that some psychiatric medications might help with secondary anxiety and depression due to the pain.

Table 45.1 lists the more common and persistent disorders that bring patients to see a primary care physician with pain complaints. It is important, however, to be aware that this table is far from inclusive because the patient with any medical condition that produces pain is likely to be initially evaluated by a primary care physician. The following are the seven key aspects of pain symptoms the physician should seek to learn:

1. Its quality and severity at onset
2. The exact location and if any migration occurs
3. If the quality of the pain fluctuates during the course of a painful episode
4. The typical duration and the course the pain follows
5. How the severity varies during its course
6. Any factors that alleviate or aggravate the pain or precipitate its onset
7. Any other signs or symptoms that may be associated with the pain

Many patients are willing to accept psychiatric consultation and referral if the primary physician indicates a willingness to continue to evaluate and follow the pain medically at regular intervals. A problem with a psychiatric referral often occurs when the primary physician says or implies that the patient only needs psychiatric treatment, and that the primary physician intends to withdraw from the case. Patients may rightly feel abandoned by such an attitude and approach. Furthermore, if a biomedical disorder is eventually discovered that may be associated with the pain, the referring physician can appear to have exercised poor judgment. In today's litigious atmosphere, a malpractice suit may ensue. At least 10% of pain patients who have been referred to specialized pain clinics for evaluation and treatment are found to have a covert biomedical disorder underlying their pain (3, 6).

The physician also needs to remember that there does not have to be either a biomedical or a psychosocial etiology for the pain exclusively. The patient can develop a biomedical disorder that produces pain even if the pain in a bodily region began as purely psychogenic. This situation is more likely if the chronic pain condition

Table 45.1.
Common Pain Disorders Seen by Primary Care Physicians[a]

Abdominal disorders
  Irritable (functional) bowel syndrome
  Peptic ulcer disease
Headache disorders
  Tension (muscle contraction) headaches
  Vascular (migraine or cluster) headaches
  Psychogenic
Ischemic disorders
  Angina pectoris
  Peripheral vascular disease (e.g., claudication)
Musculoskeletal disorders
  Low back pain
  Rheumatoid or other forms of arthritis
  Myofascial pain
Neoplastic disorders
  Direct invasion or compression of nerves
  Metastases causing invasion or compression of other
    structures
Neurologic disorders–nerve lesions
  Post-traumatic neuritis
  Causalgia
  Postoperative neuromas
  Amputation stump (phantom) pain
  Coccydynia
  Scar pain
  Nerve entrapments
  Postherpetic neuralgia—shingles
  Trigeminal neuralgia—tic douloureux
  Sympathetic dystrophy (e.g., shoulder-hand syndrome)
  Spastic states
  Thalamic pain
Psychiatric disorders
  Depression, atypical depression
  Hypochondriasis
  Anxiety, panic disorders
  Conversion symptoms
  Compensation neurosis
  Malingering
  Delusions due to psychosis (e.g., dementia, schizophrenia)
Other categories
  Temporomandibular joint (TMJ) syndrome (bruxism)
  Dental, nasal, sinusoidal, ophthalmologic, or otologic pain
  Gout
  Chronic pancreatitis

[a]Adapted from Boyd DB, Merskey H, Nielsen JS: The pain clinic: An approach to the problem of chronic pain. In Smith WL, Merskey H, Gross SC (eds): *Pain: Meaning and Management*. Jamaica, NY, SP Medical & Scientific Books, 1980, p 161: and from Thompson TL II: Headache. In Kaplan HI, Sadock BJ (eds): *Comprehensive Textbook of Psychiatry*, ed 4. Baltimore, Williams & Wilkins, 1985, p 1203.

has persisted for a number of years. If some degree of pain persists, a periodic physical reexamination is recommended, even if the patient has had a good response to psychiatric treatment in the past and the psychiatrist agreed that the pain was psychogenic.

Many patients, especially chronic pain patients, attempt to treat themselves before seeking medical help;

the latter decision usually occurs in conjunction with pain severity and disability, the length of time of the malady, and the failure of self-therapies. The primary physician should be aware of the likelihood of this situation. Over-the-counter drugs, alcohol, and many illicit drugs with actual or reputed analgesic properties are multibillion-dollar-per-year businesses. The physician needs to routinely ask about self-medication during the initial evaluation, and subsequently periodically review substance use or abuse, because patients are often reluctant or embarrassed to spontaneously discuss this behavior with the doctor.

Addiction must be treated if the patient is addicted to narcotic analgesics, before any other form of psychiatric treatment is attempted or at least before such treatments are likely to be effective. One should not add a second analgesic if an addicting level of the first analgesic has not been successful in relieving the pain.

Primary physicians also need to be alert for signs of withdrawal because many chronic pain patients have developed physical dependence on narcotic analgesics. Tapering the analgesics of these patients may need to be more protracted than tapering with other patients because sensitivity to pain may increase during the taper. Pain is also increased by the anxiety, agitation, and insomnia that often occur during a narcotic taper.

COMPREHENSIVE PAIN CENTERS

Pain clinics are discussed in Chapters 49–52; however, the primary care physician may wish to know some basic information about such clinics. There are approximately 20 centers that offer truly multidisciplinary evaluation and treatment (40), although there are hundreds of other advertised pain centers around the United States alone. Unfortunately, many of the latter centers use only one or two approaches, such as biofeedback or relaxation training. A number of major medical centers have excellent pain centers. To locate such centers, consider contacting university medical center faculty, especially in the departments of neurology, psychiatry, and anesthesia, because these faculty members tend to know where such centers exist regionally.

What should be offered at comprehensive pain centers? First, an initial evaluation of the patient should involve a work-up by a primary care physician, neurologist, and psychiatrist. Some centers involve other health care professionals such as psychologists and social workers. An anesthesiologist will be involved if nerve blocks are indicated, and a neurosurgeon will be involved if neuroablative procedures are indicated. In a university setting, multiple specialists may be involved, depending on site and type of pain. Some chronic pain patients benefit from physical medicine and rehabilitation (PM and R) services, which should

**Table 45.2.
Classification of Analgesics**[a]

Centrally active
  Narcotic agonists, naturally occurring
    Morphine
    Codeine
  Narcotic agonists, synthetic agents
    Diamorphine
    Diamophine
    Dihydrocodeine
    Meperidine
    Methadone
    Propoxyphene
  Narcotic partial agonists
    Nalorphine
    Penazocine
    Buprenorphine
    Butorphanol
    Cyclazocine
  Narcotic antagonists
    Naloxone
    Naltrexone
Peripherally active
  Nonsteroidal anti-inflammatory agents
    Salicylic acid derivatives
    Phenylalkanoic acid derivatives
    Pyrazolone derivatives
    Aniline derivatives
    Anthranililic acid derivatives

[a]From Chapman CR, Bonica JJ: *Chronic Pain.* Kalamazoo, Mi. The Upjohn Company, 1985, p 56, with permission from the publisher and authors.

not be overlooked. To help patients compensate for and lessen a number of musculoskeletal causes of pain, conditioning and exercise programs should be considered in treatment (41). Chapter 9 reviews the benefits of PM and R services for chronic pain patients in more detail.

ANALGESIC USE FOR CHRONIC PAIN

Although analgesic and anti-inflammatory medications are described more fully, and a number of special considerations in pharmacologic pain management are considered in Chapter 16, some aspects will be reviewed here. A number of other sources also discuss these issues in detail (42–45). Table 45.2 contains a basic classification of prescribed analgesic agents. An essential question to ask before prescribing any of these agents is whether you are dealing with "malignant" pain due to cancer or another serious biomedical condition that may require narcotic or other powerful analgesics, nerve blocks, and neuroablative procedures.

The reader is referred to Chapters 33–35 for more discussion of malignant pain. To manage patients with malignant pain, the physician should not hesitate to use large doses of narcotics if that is what is required. Patients with chronic "benign" pain should generally be prescribed non-narcotic analgesics. Other appropriate medications for benign pain include psychotropic agents, such as antidepressants, stimulants, and neuroleptics; psychotherapy patient education; and behavioral approaches (46).

A major factor in the underuse of narcotics, and probably of other CNS and emotion-altering drugs, is a strong societal stigma associated with their use. Regardless of the patient's clinical presentation, some lay people, and even physicians, believe only incompetent doctors prescribe large doses of these medications (47). There may be a concomitant underlying belief that if these doctors were better physicians their patients would not need these medications. Additionally, physician paranoia may also come into operation. That is, some physicians fear that if one of their patients does become physically dependent on such medication, the word will spread among their colleagues and the community that they are incompetent, negligent, and get their patients "hooked on dope." If habituation appears to be becoming a problem for a patient, the consequences may be attenuated by initiating a slow taper before discharge and obtaining prompt psychiatric and substance abuse consultation. Such ongoing prescribed analgesic dependence can almost always be avoided or short-circuited with an immediate treatment program. Additional guidelines for the use of narcotic analgesics in pain management are listed in Table 45.3.

The oncology patient with severe pain may need very large doses of narcotic to achieve pain control, and the physician should not hesitate to prescribe the dose required to relieve pain in this group of patients. Because their need is greater, they usually tolerate much larger doses than other patients. As the narcotic dose is steadily and carefully increased, a maintenance dosage can be arrived at that will allow the terminal patient to be relatively pain-free but alert. This clinical situation may ultimately be preferable to extensive nerve blocks and neurodestructive surgical procedures.

For a number of reasons, physicians are often reluctant to prescribe adequate doses of narcotics. The same reluctant attitude prevails when prescribing other CNS drugs, such as antidepressants and anxiolytics (6, 11, 27). A significant number of medical inpatients with bona fide medical etiologies for their pain, such as myocardial infarction, were consistently undermedicated with narcotic analgesics, according to a study by Marks and Sachar (48). Inadequate knowledge of pharmacology was one reason for inadequate medication. One-third of the physicians in this study overestimated the duration of action of meperidine, one-fourth exaggerated its potential for addiction in medical settings, and over three-fourths underestimated the likelihood of symptoms of withdrawal if the patient had been on meperidine for an extended period. Approximately 20% of

Table 45.3.
Guidelines for the Use of Narcotic Analgesics in Pain Management[a]

1. Start with a specific drug for a specific type of pain.
2. Know the pharmacology of the drug prescribed.
   a. Duration of the analgesic effect.
   b. Pharmacokinetic properties of the drug.
   c. Equianalgesic doses for the drug and its route of administration (see Tables 45.4 and 45.5).
3. Adjust the route of administration to the patient's needs.
4. Administer the analgesic on a regular basis after initial titration of the dose.
5. Use drug combinations to provide additive analgesia and reduce side effects [e.g., nonsteroidal anti-inflammatory drugs, antihistamine (hydroxyzine), amphetamine (Dexedrine)].
6. Avoid drug combinations that increase sedation without enhancing analgesia [e.g. benzodiazepine (diazepam) and phenothiazine (chlorpromazine)].
7. Anticipate and treat side effects.
   a. Sedation.
   b. Respiratory depression.
   c. Nausea and vomiting.
   d. Constipation.
8. Watch for the development of tolerance.
   a. Switch to an alternative narcotic analgesic.
   b. Start with one half the equianalgesic dose and titrate the dose for pain relief.
9. Prevent acute withdrawal.
   a. Taper drugs slowly.
   b. Use diluted doses of naloxone (0.4 mg in 10 ml of saline) to reverse respiratory depression in the physically dependent patient, and administer cautiously.
10. Do not use placebos to access the nature of pain.
11. Anticipate and manage complications.
    a. Overdose.
    b. Multifocal myocionus.
    c. Seizures.

[a]From Foley KM: The treatment of cancer pain. *N Engl J Med* 313:84–95, 1985: reprinted by permission.

physicians had unrealistic fears of causing addiction, even in terminal cancer patients. They would not give meperidine in adequate doses to such patients, and 14% wanted to discontinue analgesics and give placebos to these patients. One realization given was not wanting to addict the patient, which should not be as great a concern as out-of-control pain in terminally ill patients.

In treating most acute and mild to moderate pain, non-narcotic analgesics are very effective (Tables 45.2 and 45.4). Unless the pain is severe, and therefore dictates prompt and effective relief, as in pain from renal colic and cholecystitis, non-narcotic analgesics are the first-line drugs in almost all cases. In cases of severe pain, one would usually prescribe a narcotic (Table 45.5). Aspirin, at a dose of 650 mg, is one of the most efficacious oral analgesics. Even in relieving cancer pain, aspirin is as effective as a standard dose of codeine. Although

Table 45.4.
Oral Non-Narcotic and Narcotic Analgesics for Mild to Moderate Pain[a]

	Equianalgesic Dose (mg)[b]	Duration (hr)	Plasma Half-Life (hr)	Comments
Aspirin	650	4–6	3–5	Standard for non-narcotic comparisons; gastrointestinal and hematologic effects limit use in patients with cancer
Acetaminophen	650	4–6	1–4	Weak anti-inflammatory effects; safer than aspirin
Propoxyphene	65[c]	4–6	12	Biotransformed to potentially toxic metabolite norpropoxyphene; used in combination with non-narcotic analgesics
Codeine	32	4–6	3	Biotransformed to morphine; available in combination with non-narcotic analgesics
Meperidine	50	4–6	3–4	Biotransformed to active toxic metabolite normeperidine; associated with myoclonus and seizures
Pentazocine	30	4–6	2–3	Psychotomimetic effects with escalation of dose; available only in combination with naloxone, aspirin, or acetaminophen (US)

[a]From Foley KM: The treatment of cancer pain. *N Engl J Med* 313:84–95, 1985; reprinted by permission.
[b]Relative potency of drugs, as compared with that of aspirin, for mild to moderate pain.
[c]Some investigators have reported that a much larger dose (propoxyphene, 130 mg; codeine, 60 mg) is effective in patients with mild to moderate pain.

acetaminophen is sometimes substituted for aspirin, it has a lower therapeutic/toxic ratio. Because it is true that the earlier the intervention, the more effective the treatment (49), it may also be advisable in some cases to use other nonsteroidal anti-inflammatory agents, which are commonly used peripheral-acting agents. Although the nonsteroidal anti-inflammatory agents may possibly have some CNS effects, their primary mechanism of action is thought to be through the blocking of the conversion of arachidonic acid to prostaglandins (50).

Other, often more-expensive nonsteroidal anti-inflammatory agents have been used for their analgesic effects, but none of these agents seems to be more effective in pain relief than acetaminophen or aspirin. Many men and women do not eat three meals a day, but they should be counseled to do so when taking aspirin. They should also have a snack or glass of milk when taking additional doses. Aspirin should be prescribed at two or three 325-mg tablets with each meal; it should be emphasized that aspirin should be taken while patients are eating. If patients comply with such a regimen, they usually experience excellent analgesia with few side effects. Following these recommendations will often lessen the major adverse side effect of nonsteroidals, which is upper gastrointestinal irritation. The effect of aspirin on platelet aggregation is usually of little importance in most pain patients.

When prescribing narcotics, the physician must give a sufficient dose to provide adequate pain relief. In general, the optimal analgesic dose of morphine is 10 mg per 70 kg of body weight. Sixty-five percent of patients experience pain relief with this dose. Another 10% of patients experience relief at the increased dose of 15 mg,

but many begin to experience increased side effects at this higher dosage as well (81).

If there is persistent pain, opiates are most effective when an adequate dose is administered regularly and not on an "as needed" basis. If analgesics are given as needed, many patients will try to suffer through the pain and allow the pain to escalate to a more-severe degree before asking for analgesia. Some more stoic patients, discussed earlier, may never ask for analgesics, despite severe pain, and view asking for pain medication as a moral and personal defeat. If stoics succumb to the pain and admit they need medication, they may also lose face with their stoic family members and friends. Analgesics, therefore, should almost always be given on a regular schedule, based on the specific analgesic's duration of action, rather than waiting for a patient's request. Furthermore, regular analgesia will decrease anxiety and the fear and sensitivity to pain, leading the patient to ultimately use less medication to control the pain. Standing analgesia orders also dissociate experiencing pain from receiving pain relief. This dissociation is important in using contingency management and behavior modification approaches to pain control. These behavioral approaches teach the patient that he does not need to increase complaints about his suffering or disability to receive the attention and treatments that are needed (3, 6).

The physician may assume that a standard therapeutic dose of analgesic should be sufficient for all patients. This mistaken notion may lead them to label the non-responder a complainer and a potential addict. One of the most common errors in opiate prescribing is failure to evaluate the efficacy of the first dose and then adjust

Table 45.5.
Oral and Parenteral Narcotic Analgesics for Severe Pain[a]

	Route[b]	Equianalgesic Dose (mg)[c]	Duration (hr)	Plasma Half-Life (hr)	Comments
Narcotic agonists					
Morphine	IM	10	4–6	2–3.5	Standard for comparison; also available in slow-release tablets
	PO	60	4–7		
Codeine	IM	130	4–6	3	Biotransformed to morphine; useful as initial narcotic analgesic
	PO	200[d]	4–6		
Oxycodone	IM	15			Short acting; available alone or as five mg dose in combination with aspirin and acetaminophen
	PO	30	3–5	—	
Heroin	IM	5	4–5	0.5	Illegal in US; high solubility for parenteral administration
	PO	60	4–5		
Levorphanol (Levo- Dromoran)	IM	2	4–6	12–16	Good oral potency, requires careful titration in initial dosing because of drug accumulation
	PO	4	4–7		
Hydromorphone (Dilaudid)	IM	1.5	4–5	2–3	Available in high-potency injectable form (10mg/ml) for cachectic patients and as rectal suppositories; more soluble than morphine
	PO	7.5	4–6		
Oxymorphone (Numorphan)	IM	1	4–6	2–3	Available in parenteral and rectal-suppository forms only
	PR	10	4–6		
Meperidine (Demerol)	IM	75	4–5	3–4 Normeperidine 12–16	Contraindicated in patients with renal disease; accumulation of active toxic metabolite normeperidine produces central nervous system excitation
	PO	300[d]	4–6		
Methadone (Dolophine)	IM	10		15–30	Good oral potency; requires careful titration of the initial dose to avoid drug accumulation
	PO	20			
Mixed agonist-antagonist drugs					
Pentazocine (Talwin)	IM	60	4–6	2–3	Limited use for cancer pain; psychotomimetic effects with dose escalation; available only in combination with naloxone, aspirin, or acetaminophen; may precipitate withdrawal in physically dependent patients
	PO	180[a]	4–7		
Nalbuphine (Nubain)	IM	10	4–6	5	Not available orally; less severe psychotomimetic effects than pentazocine; may precipitate withdrawal in physically dependent patients
	PO	—			
Butorphanol (Stadol)	IM	2	4–6	2.5–3.5	Not available orally; produces psychotomimetic effects; may precipitate withdrawal in physically dependent patients
	PO	—			
Partial agonists					
Buprenorphine (Temgesic)	IM	0.4	4–6	?	Not available in US; no psychotomimetic effects; may precipitate withdrawal in tolerant patients
	SL	0.8	5–6		

[a]From Foley KM: The treatment of cancer pain. *N Engl J Med* 313:84–95, 1985; reprinted by permission.
[b]IM denotes intramuscular, PO = oral, PR = rectal, and SL = sublingual.
[c]Based on single-dose studies in which an intramuscular dose of each drug listed was compared with morphine to establish the relative potency. Oral doses are those recommended when changing from a parenteral to an oral route. For patients without prior narcotic exposure, the recommended oral starting dose is 30 mg for morphine, 5 mg for methadone, 2 mg for levorphanol, and 4 mg for hydromorphone.
[d]The recommended starting doses for these drugs are listed in Table 45.4.

accordingly. An effective dose of opiate given at appropriate intervals needs to be determined for each patient and then continued. Usually 2–3 mg of morphine sulfate or 15–25 mg of meperidine should be given intravenously every 20 min until analgesia is accomplished; this will indicate the dosage needed in a given interval.

The total dosage required to maintain pain relief of narcotic is usually less when opiates are given every 3–4 hours during the early postoperative period rather than PRN (52). Side effects may preclude full therapeutic doses, but often decreasing the dose will alleviate side effects and will still provide a significant amount of analgesia. Hypoventilation is usually not a problem with analgesic doses of narcotics, because pain results in respiratory stimulation, which counterbalances the respiratory depressant effect of these drugs (53).

Combining opiates and non-narcotic analgesics usually results in additive analgesic activity but with different side effects and usually less CNS depression. Combining the opiates with minor tranquilizers may potentiate the analgesic effect of the opiate. This potentiation can result in a lower dose required for analgesia, less respiratory depression, and decreased opiate-induced nausea and vomiting (54–57). Uses of tricyclic antidepressants related to pain symptoms include carotidynia, atypical facial pain, and migraine prophylaxis, possibly as a result of vasoconstrictive properties (58–60). Corticosteroids are useful in some pain patients for their anti-inflammatory and analgesic properties (61). Thus, opiates may be combined with other analgesics to enhance analgesic activity, reduce opiate dosage, counteract side effects of opiates, and improve tolerance.

PRIMARY CARE CHRONIC PAIN PATIENTS WITH PSYCHIATRIC DISORDERS

Psychiatric conditions may contribute to or result from chronic pain syndromes. Some of the most common of those psychiatric disorders are listed in Table 45.1. The term *pain shock* has been developed to describe the constellation of psychiatric distress symptoms that may develop in response to the emotional stress associated with ongoing pain. Physical sequelae can occur in response to these emotional stresses. Muscle atrophy and deconditioning with a concomitant worsening of certain types of pain develops in depressed, anxious, agitated patients and in patients who are chronically tired because of insomnia, which itself may be secondary to pain (3). Careful psychiatric evaluation, therefore, is recommended as early as is possible during the care of any chronic pain patient who is not responding to standard treatment approaches. A psychiatric consultant also may collaborate with the primary physician in the ongoing management of pain patients and their families (62, 63).

A group of chronic pain patients received a thorough psychiatric evaluation with the following results: 98% had an associated psychiatric disorder, including somatoform disorder (15%), psychological factors affecting physical condition (10%), adjustment disorders (8%), and several other disorders (2–4% each). Thirty-seven percent of these patients also had a personality disorder, including histrionic (30%), dependent (25%), borderline (15%), and narcissistic (10%), and one patient had each of several other types. Although some believe that most chronic pain patients do not fit into standard psychiatric diagnostic categories (64), this point is debatable. A wide range of psychiatric and personality disorders are associated with chronic pain symptoms (1, 65).

Research has been conducted with chronic pain patients using the Minnesota Multiphasic Personality Inventory (MMPI). Some of these studies have found chronic pain patients to have an increased rate of scoring in the "neurotic triad," which includes high scores on hysteria, hypochondriasis, and depression. Other pain patients have been found to have the "conversion V" pattern on the MMPI, which is created by high scores on the hysteria and hypochondriasis scales and a low score on depression (3). Whether these chronic pain patients would have had these patterns premorbidly and to what degree the patterns may have been created or amplified by the chronic pain is a critical factor to try to assess.

ALEXITHYMIA

Alexithymia is the inability to be aware of, and to verbalize, one's emotional state and includes a relatively concrete style of thinking. Chronic pain patients have been found to have a significant incidence (about 33%) of alexithymia. This may be one factor in geriatric patients' expressing emotional distress more often through somatic complaints (66), because older patients have also been found to be more alexithymic. Patients with a wide variety of psychosomatic-type disorders have an increased tendency to have alexithymic features. If these individuals cannot express their emotions verbally and through their actions, those emotional states are more likely to be expressed through somatic channels. Ongoing supportive management is often the best type of treatment for these individuals, who tend not to be psychologically minded and are generally not good counseling or psychotherapy candidates. Supportive therapy is often fairly successful with these patients and should not be minimized. Upon trying to make connections between obvious examples of psychosocial stress in a patient's life and an exacerbation of their symptoms with an alexithymic patient, a physician may be rewarded with a blank stare and denial of any problem, which can be infuriating to some physicians.

Patients with hypochondriasis often have alexithymic features. In fact, part of the patient's problem may be just that; he cannot perceive and correctly evaluate emotional factors in his life. A diagnostic clue that hypochondriasis or some other alexithymic-related disorder may be present is the anger the physician begins to feel at such patients, and the tendency to label these patients "crocks" or other pejorative terms (4, 37).

SOMATOFORM DISORDERS

The term *somatoform disorder* simply means that emotional distress is expressed through the form of a physical complaint. *Somatization disorder* is a general term frequently used to describe this group of patients. Another of the most common forms of somatoform disorders is hypochondriasis. A differential diagnostic point is that although patients with both somatization disorder and hypochondriasis may have multiple physical complaints that cannot be related to any biomedical disorders, patients with hypochondriasis often have a more pronounced fear of having a serious illness. The somatization disorder patient will not usually be as continually anxious and frightened as the hypochondriacal patient. They do not, however, have the classic *la belle* indifference of the hysterical patient with conversion symptoms. The chief complaint of hypochondriacal patients is their fear of multiple serious illnesses; whereas, the somatization disorder patient tends to have many physical complaints without the same degree of desperation.

Calm reassurance and the explicit statement that the physician is willing to follow the hypochondriacal patient is the best approach for the physician to take after a careful history, physical examination, and screening laboratory studies have been negative. Some physicians may complain that these patients do not respond to reassurance, but the form that reassurance takes may make a difference. The statement, "There is nothing wrong with you," is not reassuring to these patients, and it is also not accurate. There is something wrong with them: they have a somatoform disorder, such as hypochondriasis, and its consequences may be as real as most biomedical disorders.

Because the layman's knowledge and reaction to the diagnosis of hypochondriasis is usually that it means "There's nothing wrong with you," patients should not be told they have hypochondriasis per se. The physician should try not to get into a struggle with the patient to get them out of the sick role right away. The primary physician may need to give these patients some license to be at least a little sick and to somewhat adopt the "sick role" in their relationships. Actually, the physician does not have to "let" them do this; they have already done it. These patients are in the sick role and complaining of multiple somatic complaints because they emotionally need to do so; that is the best avenue that they have available in their personality traits repertoire to express their psychosocial distress. Reducing "doctor shopping," multiple subspecialty referrals, and going from health care agency to health care agency is a major goal of treatment of hypochondriacs. Managing the patient's covert emotional needs is the relevant challenge. Curing the patient of a physical malady is not. If the primary physician can back off from his own frustration and wish to confront the patient and instead form an ongoing supportive relationship with these difficult patients, that will usually be the best treatment for them. Paradoxically, if the physician can focus away from wishing to relieve the patient's physical complaints, those complaints usually will gradually lessen, most of the time.

Another descriptive term used for somatizing and hypochondriacal patients who present with pain as their primary symptom is *pain prone*; many other terms have been used, most of them not complimentary (67). Individuals with certain past experiences and personality traits are more susceptible to use pain repeatedly and in response to almost any stressor for underlying psychodynamic reasons. George Engel described these patients in depth and first used the term "pain prone" (68). Sternbach classified a subgroup of these patients as "lower back losers" (69); Szasz termed a similar group as *les hommes douloureux*, literally translated to "pain men" or "pain people" (70). A component of unconscious secondary gain is satisfied in some patients by having chronic pain. Over 50% of chronic pain patients, however, may not fit into criteria for a pain-prone disorder (64). Also, keep in mind that the secondary gain, paradoxically, may be punishment that they feel they deserve.

Also, paradoxically, pain may be related to feelings about success. Some individuals feel guilty, subconsciously if not consciously, about being successful in various aspects of their lives and feel they must balance this success with pain and suffering (32). An extreme example of the above groups are sadomasochistic individuals. These patients may even receive overt pleasure from suffering. These individuals may also feel they deserve to suffer and, therefore, pursue painful physical and emotional experiences on a chronically unhealthy and destructive path. Only when some of these individuals come to associate pain with certain types of pleasure, such as sexual activities, are these individuals able to feel the full extent of pleasure possible. Pain becomes a necessary antecedent to pleasure.

DEPRESSION

Depression predisposes to the development of chronic pain, and chronic pain frequently leads to and exacerbates depression (71). Also, pain may be a so-called *depressive equivalent* in some patients, usually an atypical form of depression in which pain may be their primary or only symptom. Such patients have an increased incidence of a personal and family history of depression (72). Onset of depression is frequently in young adulthood and middle age but may continue to increase in frequency with aging, especially if the elderly are prescribed antihypertensives and other CNS depressants. Depression in the elderly frequently is not accompanied by the usual vegetative symptoms of depression such as changes in appetite, weight, sleep, and energy level. The presentation of dementia symptoms may actually be due to depression, in which case the condition is termed *pseudodementia*. Depression that is not associated with depressed mood and vegetative signs is often termed *atypical*, and this presentation is more common in the elderly. Atypical depression symptoms often involve somatic complaints, including pain. Undiagnosed and ineffectively treated depression in the elderly may account in part for the reported increase in hypochondriasis in the elderly.

Although the use of psychotropic medications in pain management is the focus of Chapter 16, the topic will be discussed to some degree in this chapter, in part because primary care physicians are the specialists who most frequently use psychotropic drugs to treat pain patients as well as patients with the wide range of psychiatric conditions, doing so more often than do all mental health care professionals combined, including psychiatrists, psychologists, social workers, and other types of counselors (73).

Therefore, depression should be vigorously treated in any chronic pain patient known or suspected of having depression. This would include treatment with imipramine (150 mg/day) or its equivalent of another cyclic antidepressant for at least 4–6 weeks. Shorter trials, even though serum levels are within the therapeutic range, may be ineffective. Serum level determinations of imipramine, desipramine, and nortriptyline are useful in titrating and assuring that the dosage is in the therapeutic range, particularly if the patient has had no side effects at the current prescribed dose or is at or above a dosage that is usually therapeutic. If adverse side effects have been experienced, a serum level is also useful to ensure that the lowest dosage is being given that will lead to a serum level within the therapeutic range. In such cases, the side effects diminish while therapeutic effects are maintained at the lower dosage. Many potentially treatable depressions have persisted because physicians have been reluctant to increase the antidepressant dosage to an effective level, especially in elderly and medically debilitated patients. Many physicians have feared that antidepressants will cause cardiac arrhythmias. Tricyclics are safe for cardiac patients, however, except for a couple of months after myocardial infarction, and unless a conduction defect or persistent dangerous arrhythmia is present (74). Much more morbidity is seen in untreated depressed patients, especially those with chronic pain as well, than is seen with the careful use of tricyclics in the majority of cardiac patients (75).

Other alternatives to tricyclics currently exist. These include the atypical antidepressants, monoamine oxidase inhibitors (MAOIs) and electroconvulsive therapy (ECT) (76, 77). Fluoxetine (Prozac) is a relatively new antidepressant, which is not a tricyclic or an MAOI. It is primarily a serotonin reuptake inhibitor. The side effect profile includes nausea, anorexia, anxiety, and nervousness, but these usually subside within a week. Fluoxetine is much safer in overdose and does not cause the risk of ventricular arrhythmias as tricyclics do. Fluoxetine seems to be better tolerated generally by the elderly than tricyclics are (78). Fluoxetine, however, unlike tricyclics, does not appear to have any direct analgesic effects.

Psychostimulants have also been successfully used to treat some depressed pain patients. Dextroamphetamine may facilitate the response to morphine in some patients with acute pain (79), such as in postoperative pain, which is specifically discussed in Chapter 46. Prompt antidepressant effects may be seen in some patients with the use of methylphenidate; the dosage is titrated upward from 5 mg/day, generally not to exceed 30 mg/day. Hoping for an antidepressant effect, some patients in chronic pain may seek narcotics from the physician. Narcotics do not have antidepressant effects per se, so such behavior often leads to excessive narcotic use and dependence and also to poor results in treatment of the depression (80). It is important that any narcotic-seeking patient should be specifically evaluated for underlying depression, as well as other psychiatric disorders.

Schizophrenics and patients with other types of psychotic illnesses can develop pain as part of their presenting complaint. A psychotic individual will at times give bizarre and unrealistic explanations of what is causing the pain. Therefore, it is often useful to ask pain patients what they think is causing the pain; this will sometimes reveal a previously covert psychotic thought disorder. Nihilistic delusions relating to disease and decay may occur in psychotically depressed patients. For example, some may be convinced that they have cancer or some other potentially deforming, painful, and terminal illness. The fact, however, that a person has a known psychotic illness should not lead the treating physician to ignore and minimize pain complaints, especially if they are different than past complaints and of recent onset. Clearly, chronically psychotic individuals at some time in their lives are likely to develop pain due to a biomedical illness. Stories abound of psychotic individuals "ignoring" the pain of an acute myocardial infarction or other usually very painful conditions. Also, some stories exist of physicians who have overlooked or delayed diagnosis of a potentially initially curable medical condition until it became severe and incurable because they ascribe the pain solely to a known psychiatric disorder.

MUNCHAUSEN SYNDROME

The patient with Munchausen syndrome is often difficult to identify and equally or more difficult to treat. It is not possible to classify all patients with Munchausen syndrome as psychotic, although some probably are, at least in a partial and encapsulated sense. When treating the chronic pain patient, the physician may want to consider this possibility in the differential diagnosis, especially if the patient has had multiple diagnostic and exploratory procedures or has traveled to medical centers far and wide to be treated. Another diagnostic clue is that Munchausen patients often seem to enjoy giving their medical travelogue and regaling others at any opportunity about their medical odyssey.

Most chronic pain patients will accept the suggestion that they might benefit by obtaining psychiatric consultation, particularly if this suggestion is made without implying that the pain "is all in their head," or that they are "crazy," or that the primary physician wants to discontinue treating the patient. Another possible diagnostic clue to Munchausen patients is that they tend to react very negatively toward the suggestion that they see a psychiatrist. Even the mention of a psychiatrist may lead the Munchausen patient to leave a hospital promptly and against medical advice. Although Munchausen syndrome is often classified as a factitious disorder, it should not be regarded as consciously controlled malingering. The latter condition occurs more often with a drug addict or person desiring undeserved disability compensation. If repeated procedures and surgeries are performed, iatrogenic illness (e.g., due to adhesions) may be created, and thereby Munchausen syndrome can create a serious and potentially lethal disorder (81, 82).

POST-TRAUMATIC STRESS DISORDER

About 10% of patents receiving treatment at some pain clinics, especially veteran's hospitals, may have post-traumatic stress disorder (PTSD). These patients often have other psychiatric disorders as well, including depression, anxiety, and substance abuse (83). The veteran PTSD population must be carefully evaluated, because there may be a disability payment associated with having a chronic diagnosis—plus the veteran may also gain psychologically by being viewed as a soldier traumatized in a war.

HYSTERIA

Pain is one of the major presenting symptoms in certain patients with certain types of neuroses and personality disorders. Hysterical paralysis and pain is probably the most classic example, in which the patient develops symptoms that do not correspond to neurologic pathways (such as stocking and glove paralysis, anesthesia, and pain). Although other patients without hysterical traits, such as flamboyance and seductiveness, can develop conversion symptoms, hysterical patients are somewhat more likely to develop conversion disorders.

GRIEF

Grieving individuals may sometimes develop pain symptoms as part of their mourning process. Of course, such individuals should be medically evaluated, because there is an increased risk of morbidity and mortality during the acute grief process (84). The pain complaint may involve the part of the body they associate with the loved one and, sometimes, in which the illness

occurred that resulted in the death of the loved one. In other instances, the pain may occur in symbolically meaningful areas, such as the chest, representing a "broken heart" and "heartache."

BORDERLINE AND NARCISSISTIC PERSONALITY DISORDER

Patients with borderline and narcissistic personality disorders also are at increased risk for developing chronic pain syndromes (85, 86). The borderline patient may prefer to experience pain than to feel empty, hollow, and chronically bored. As a way of proving to themselves that they are alive, that they have boundaries, and that they are not empty, they may intentionally inflict pain upon themselves. Not only do they often slash their wrists but they may injure themselves in other ways to "feel real" or to bring themselves back to reality. Many Munchausen patients have borderline personality disorder or have some borderline features.

Common characteristics of narcissistic patients include intense involvement with their physical appearance and with the desired perfect bodily functioning, and intense fear of physical vulnerability, disability, and illness. They may present to the physician with what otherwise would appear to be small and inconsequential complaints, including minor pain, because they perceive illness to be such a threat to the physical attributes they prize. Their grandiosity is actually a psychological defense against feeling incredibly vulnerable, frightened, and inadequate.

THE DOCTOR AS AN ANALGESIC

Balint has given physicians a useful conceptualization, which may be especially helpful to primary physicians treating chronic pain patients (6, 39). He recommended that the physician view oneself as a "drug" being prescribed for the patient's well-being. A major asset and effective therapeutic force for physicians in treating pain can be the doctor-patient relationship. The physician may overlook the fact that for all of our technologic advances, the doctor-patient relationship is still one of the most powerful parts of our therapeutic armamentarium.

Increased use of technological devices may actually exacerbate a patient's chronic pain, but a good outcome almost always results from the "laying on of hands" and an appropriate "bedside" manner. The doctor patient relationship is still one of the most potent "drugs" in medical practice. Understanding the "pharmacology" of this powerful "drug," its side-effects and potential benefits, and how to determine its correct dosage and schedule of administration for various types of patients is key. Perhaps more than in other aspects of medical care, the doctor-patient relationship must be regularly utilized to its full therapeutic efficacy to be maximally effective in managing pain. Too much or too little "doctoring" may increase symptoms .

There are three basic models of the doctor-patient relationship. In the guidance-cooperation model, the doctor recommends an approach and the patient chooses to comply. In the mutual participation model the physician and patient together select the diagnostic and therapeutic approach for an illness. In the active-passive model, the physician assumes total responsibility (87). Whatever model is chosen, its utility hinges upon its appropriateness to the given clinical situation. The doctor's ability to gain the trust of the patient he or she hopes to help is key to successful treatment. The ideal doctor-patient relationship is one in which both the doctor and the patient can communicate freely about the patient's fears and wishes, as well as about medical facts. The doctor must listen not only to what the patient says but to what is being transmitted nonverbally. Also, what is the patient *not* saying? What is not being asked or talked about that would concern most individuals in this clinical situation? Problems in the doctor-patient relationship need to be diagnosed and managed, as consistently and carefully as treating the patient's medical problems, for optional patient care.

NONPHARMACOLOGIC MANAGEMENT CONSIDERATIONS

A conservative treatment approach is indicated if the patient is in the middle of a lawsuit, disability determination, divorce, or other situation that may be related to secondary gain for maintaining the pain symptoms. If the secondary gain associated with such situations is resolved, regardless of outcome, the physician may be able to evaluate the situation more clearly and treat it more effectively.

A person who is anxious is much more likely to be sensitive to any painful stimulus and to overreact to it. If a procedure is going to be performed, taking a few minutes to explain what will be done and answering questions the patient may have about it may greatly reduce patient's anxieties. The patient may be able to cooperate better if he knows what to anticipate during the procedure. Even a preoperative visit to the operating and recovery room, when they are not in use, may decrease anxiety when entering those settings later. Chapter 12 contains a more thorough discussion of cognitive and behavioral aspects of pain management.

Contingency management is also an important and sometimes overlooked approach in the treatment of chronic pain patients. A few comments of special relevance in this regard to primary care physicians are made here (11, 88). In Skinner's research with rats and pigeons, he discovered that almost any behavior could be increased or decreased in frequency if the rewards or punishments associated with that behavior were great

enough and repeated often enough. If a chronic pain patient receives more attention, money, or anything else that he values because he has chronic pain, it follows that his attitudes and behaviors associated with maintaining the chronic pain will increase. Similarly, if a patient is rewarded for displaying active, healthy, pain-free behaviors, those behaviors will be reinforced and increase in frequency. The more a person talks about his chronic pain and becomes preoccupied with this issue, the more his world will become centered around the pain and those who buy into that for their own psychological reasons. Healthy people will avoid such a person, so the preoccupied person becomes isolated or surrounded by those who are also preoccupied with their pain; a vicious and escalating psychosocial cycle may be thus created.

To break such a cycle, a contingency plan must be set up so the chronic pain patient receives more rewards for being active and trying to carry on a healthy lifestyle than for passivity and complaining. Spouses, family members, and employers may initially view such a plan as illogical and even cruel. Therefore, each of these groups of significant others should be counseled to reward the patient more for healthy behaviors and taught why they should ignore or give as little positive feedback as possible to pain-related behaviors and comments. Without the rewards for pain behavior, the patient may gradually become less focused on the pain and more involved in healthier aspects of his life—that is, a steadily building cycle toward health can also be set in motion and maintained.

REFERENCES

1. Hackett TP: The pain patient: Evaluation and treatment. In Hackett TP, Cassem NH (eds): *Massachusetts General Hospital Handbook of General Hospital Psychiatry.* St. Louis, CV Mosby, 1978, p 41.
2. Thompson TL II: Headache. In Kaplan HI, Sadock BJ (eds): *Comprehensive Textbook of Psychiatry,* ed 4. Baltimore, Williams & Wilkins, 1985, p 1203.
3. Thompson TL II: Chronic pain. In Kaplan HI, Sadock BJ (eds): *Comprehensive Textbook of Psychiatry,* ed 4. Baltimore, Williams & Wilkins, 1985, p. 1212.
4. Thompson TL II, Steele BF: The psychological aspects of pain. In Simons RC (ed): *Understanding Human Behavior in Health and Illness,* ed 3. Baltimore, Williams & Wilkins, 1985, p 60.
5. Long DM: The evaluation and treatment of low back pain. In Hendler NH, Long DM, Wise TN (eds): *Diagnosis and Treatment of Chronic Pain.* Littleton, MA, John Wright–PSG, 1982, p 31.
6. Luce JM, Thompson TL II, Getto CJ, et al: New concepts of chronic pain and their implications. *Hosp Pract* 14:113–123, 1979.
7. Von Euler US, Pernow B (eds): *Substance P.* New York, Raven Press, 1977.
8. Hendler NH: The four stages of pain. In Hendler NH,

Long DM, Wise TN (eds): *Diagnosis and Treatment of Chronic Pain.* Littleton MA, John Wright–PSG, 1982, p 1.

9. Foley KM, Posner JB: *Pain.* American Academy of Neurology Review Book. Minneapolis, American Academy of Neurology, 1978, p 199.

10. Snyder SH: Opiate receptors and internal opiates. *Sci Am* 236:44–56, 1977.

11. Reuler JB, Girard DE, Nardone DA: The chronic pain syndrome: Misconceptions and management. *Ann Intern Med* 93:588–596, 1980.

12. Pert A, Yaksh T: Sites of morphine induced analgesia in the primate brain: Relation to pain pathways. *Brain Res* 80:135–140, 1974.

13. Levine JD, Gordon NC, Fields HL: The mechanism of placebo analgesia. *Lancet* 2:654–657, 1978.

14. Melzack R: How acupuncture can block pain. In Weisenberg M (ed): *Pain: Clinical and Experimental Perspectives.* St. Louis, CV Mosby, 1975, p 251.

15. Hilgard ER, Hilgard VR: *Hypnosis in the Relief of Pain.* Los Altos, CA, William Kaufmann, 1975.

16. Strain JJ: The problem of pain. In Strain JJ (ed): *Psychological Care of the Medically Ill.* New York, Appleton-Century Crofts, 1975, p 93.

17. Lindsay PG, Wyckoff M: The depression-pain syndrome and its response to antidepressants. *Psychosomatics* 22:571–577, 1981.

18. Nathan PW: Results of antero-lateral cordotomy for pain in cancer. *J. Neurol Neurosurg Psychiatry* 26:353–362, 1963.

19. White JC, Sweet WH: *Pain, Its Mechanisms and Neurosurgical Control.* Springfield, IL, Charles C Thomas, 1955.

20. Campbell JN, Long DM: Transcutaneous electrical stimulation for pain: Efficacy and mechanism of action. In Hendler NH, Long DM, Wise TN (eds): *Diagnosis and Treatment of Chronic Pain.* Littleton, MA, John Wright–PSG, 1982, p 77.

21. Melzack R, Wall PD: Pain mechanisms: A new theory. *Science* 150:971–979, 1965.

22. Melzack R: *The Puzzle of Pain.* New York, Basic Books, 1973.

23. Proudfit HK, Anderson EG: Morphine analgesia: Blockade by raphe magnus lesions. *Brain Res* 98:612–618, 1975.

24. Beecher HK: Relationship of significance of wound to pain experience. *JAMA* 161:1609–1613, 1956.

25. Foley KM, Posner JB: *Pain.* American Academy of Neurology Review Book. Minneapolis, American Academy of Neurology, 1978, p 199.

26. Engel GL: The need for a new medical model: A challenge for biomedicine. *Science* 196:129–136, 1977.

27. Dubovsky SL, Groban SE: Congenital absence of sensation. *Psychoanal Study Child* 30:49–73, 1975.

28. Devine R, Merskey H: The description of the pain in psychiatric and general medical patients. *J. Psychosom Res* 9:311–316, 1965.

29. Rhine MW, Thompson TL II: Hypochondriasis. In Simons RC (ed): *Understanding Human Behavior in Health and Illness,* ed 3. Baltimore, Williams & Wilkins, 1985, p 73.

30. Wise TN: Pain–the most common psychosomatic problem. *Med Clin North Am* 61:771–780, 1977.

31. Webb WL Jr: Chronic pain. *Psychosomatics* 24:1053–1063, 1983.

32. Engel GL: Guilt, pain and success. *Psychosom Med* 24:37–48, 1962.

33. Weisenberg M, Kreindler ML, Schachat R, et al: Pain: Anxiety and attitudes in black, white and Puerto Rican patients. *Psychosom Med* 37:123–135, 1975.

34. Hollingshead AB, Hedlich FC: *Social Class and Mental Illness.* New York, John Wiley & Sons, 1958.

35. Zborowski M: *People in Pain.* Philadelphia, Jossey-Bass, 1969.

36. Smith WL, Merskey H, Gross SC (eds): *Pain: Meaning and Management.* Jamaica, NY, SP Medical & Scientific Books, 1980.

37. Lipsitt DR: Medical and psychological characteristics of "crocks." *Int J Psychiatry Med* 1:15–25, 1970.

38. Perman J: Pain as an old friend. *Lancet* 1:633–636, 1954.

39. Balint M: *The doctor, his patient and the illness,* ed 2. New York, International Universities Press, 1964, p 1.

40. Black RG: The clinical management of chronic pain. In Hendler NH, Long DM, Wise TN (eds): *Diagnosis and Treatment of Chronic Pain.* Littleton, MA, John Wright–PSG, 1982, p 211.

41. Reischer MA, Spindler HA: The use of physical medicine and rehabilitation in the management of pain. In Hendler NH, Long DM, Wise TN (eds): *Diagnosis and Treatment of Chronic Pain.* Littleton, MA, John Wright–PSG, 1982, p 235.

42. Halpern LM: Analgesic drugs in the management of pain. *Arch Surg* 112:861–869, 1977.

43. Stimmel B: *Pain, Analgesia and Addiction: The Pharmacological Treatment of Pain.* New York, Raven Press, 1983.

44. Brena SF, Chapman SL (eds): *Management of Patients with Chronic Pain:* Jamaica, NY, SP Medical & Scientific Books, 1983.

45. Fordyce WE, Brockway JO: Chronic pain and its management. In Usdin G. Lewis JM (eds): *Psychiatry in General Medical Practice.* New York, McGraw-Hill, 1979, p 353.

46. Merskey H, Hester RA: Treatment of chronic pain with psychotropic drugs. *Postgrad Med* 48:594–598, 1972.

47. Perry S: The undermedication for pain: A psychoanalytic perspective. *Bull Assoc Psychoanal Med* 22:77–94, 1983.

48. Marks RM, Sachar EJ: Undertreatment of medical inpatients with narcotic analgesics. *Ann Intern Med* 78:173–181, 1973.

49. Levine J: Pain and analgesia: The outlook for more rational treatment. *Ann Intern Med* 100:269–276, 1984.

50. Ferreira SH: Site of analgesic action of aspirin-like drugs and opioids. In Beers RF Jr, Basset EG (eds): *Mechanisms of Pain and Analgesic Compounds.* New York, Raven Press, 1979, p 309.

51. Lasagna L, Beecher HK: The optimal dose of morphine. *JAMA* 156:230–234, 1954.

52. Roe BB: Are postoperative narcotics necessary? *Arch Surg* 87:912–915, 1963.

53. Pflug AE, Murphy TM, Butler SH, et al: The effects of postoperative peridural analgesia on pulmonary therapy and pulmonary complications. *Anesthesiology* 41:8–17, 1974.

54. Keats AS, Telford J, Kurosu Y: "Potentiation" of meperidine by promethazine. *Anesthesiology* 22:34–41, 1961.

55. Moertel CG, Ahmann DL, Taylor WF, et al: A comparative evaluation of marketed analgesic drugs. *N Engl J Med* 286:813–815, 1972.

56. Moertel CG, Ahmann DL, Taylor WF, et al: Relief of pain by oral medications: A controlled evaluation of analgesic combinations. *JAMA* 299:55–59, 1974.

57. Bonica JJ: Fundamental considerations of chronic pain therapy. *Postgrad Med* 53:81–85, 1973.

58. Raskin NW, Prusiner S: Carotidynia. *Neurology* 27:43–46, 1977.

59. Moore DS, Nally FF: Atypical facial pain. *J Can Dent Assoc* 41:396–401, 1975.

60. Gomersall JD, Stuart H: Amitriptyline in migraine prophylaxis. *J Neurol Neurosurg Psychiatry* 36:684–690, 1973.

61. Regelson W, Butler JR, Schulz J, et al: Delta-nine tetrahydrocannabinol as an effective antidepressant and appetite stimulating agents in advanced cancer patients. In Braude MTC, Szara S (eds): *The Pharmacology of Marijuana.* New York, Raven Press, 1976, p 763.

62. DeVaul RA, Zisook S: Chronic pain: The psychiatrist's role. *Psychosomatics* 19:417–421, 1978.

63. Merskey H: The role of the psychiatrist in the investigation and treatment of pain. In Bonica J (ed): *Advances in Pain Research and Therapy.* New York, Raven Press, 1983, vol 5, p 249.

64. Bouckoms AJ: Recent developments in the classification of pain. *Psychosomatics* 26:637–645, 1985.

65. Reich J, Tupin JP, Abramovitz SI: Psychiatric diagnosis of chronic pain patients. *Am J. Psychiatry* 140:1495–1498, 1983.

66. Postone N: Alexithymia in chronic pain patients. *Gen Hosp Psychiatry* 8:163–167, 1986.

67. Blumer D, Heilbronn M: Chronic pain as a variant of depressive disease: The pain-prone disorder. *J. Nerv Ment Dis* 170:381–416, 1982.

68. Engel GL: "Psychogenic pain" and the pain-prone patient. *Am J Med* 26:899–918, 1959.

69. Sternbach RA: *Pain Patients.* New York, Academic Press, 1974.

70. Szasz T: *Pain and Pleasure.* New York, Basic Books, 1957.

71. Mersky H, Boyd D: Emotional adjustment and chronic pain. *Pain* 5:173–178, 1978.

72. Magni G, Bertolini C: Chronic pain as a depressive equivalent. *Postgrad Med* 73:79–85, 1983.

73. Regier DA, Goldberg ID, Taube CA: The de Facto US mental health services system: A public health perspective. *Arch Gen Psychiatry* 35:685–693, 1978.

74. Vieth RC, Raskin MA, Caldwell JH, et al: Cardiovascular effects of tricyclic antidepressants in depressed patients with heart disease. *N Engl J Med* 306:954–959, 1982.

75. Cahn J, Herold M: Pain and psychotropic drugs. In Soulairac A, Cahn J, Charpentier J (eds): *Pain.* New York, Academic Press, 1968, p 335.

76. Anthony M, Lance JW: Monoamine oxidase inhibition in the treatment of migraine. *Arch Neurol* 21:263, 1969.

77. Mandel MR: Electroconvulsive therapy for chronic pain associated with depression. *Am J Psychiatry* 132:632–636, 1975.

78. Feighner JP, Boyer WF, Meredith CK, et al: An overview of fluoxetine in geriatric depression. *Br J Psychiatry Suppl* 3:105–108, 1988.

79. Forrest WH Jr, Brown BW Jr, Brown CR, et al: Dextroamphetamine with morphine for the treatment of postoperative pain. *N Engl J Med* 296:712–715, 1977.

80. Halpern LM: Psychotropic drugs in the management of chronic pain. *Adv Neurol* 4:539–545, 1974.

81. Ford CV: The Munchausen syndrome: A report of 4 new cases and a review of psychodynamic considerations. *Int J Psychiatry Med* 4:31–45, 1973.

82. Spiro HR: Chronic factitious illness: Munchausen's syndrome. *Arch Gen Psychiatry* 18:569–579, 1968.

83. Benedikt RA, Kolb LC: Preliminary findings on chronic pain and post-traumatic stress disorder. *Am J Psychiatry* 143:908–910, 1986.

84. Parkes CM, Benjamin B, Fitzgerald RG: Broken heart: A statistical study of increased mortality among widowers. *Br Med J* 1:740–743, 1969.

85. Gross RJ, Doerr H, Caldioria D, et al: Borderline syndrome and incest in chronic pelvic pain patients. *Int J Psychiatry Med* 10:79–96, 1981.

86. Blazer DG: Narcissism and the development of chronic pain. *Int J Psychiatry Med* 10:69–71, 1981.

87. Szasz TS, Hollender MH: A contribution to the philosophy of medicine: The basic models of the doctor-patient relationship. *Arch Intern Med* 97:585–592, 1956.

88. Fordyce WE: An operant conditioning method for managing chronic pain. *Postgrad Med* 53:123–128, 1973.

CHAPTER 46

POSTOPERATIVE PAIN MANAGEMENT

THOMAS K. HENTHORN
TOM C. KREJCIE

THE SINGLE most important factor in managing patients who are experiencing acute pain is placing the emphasis on prevention: if pain can be effectively managed in the acute phase, the muscle guarding and dysfunction that may result tend to be avoided or at least reduced. Preventing progressive amplification of the pain cycle thereby permits the body's normal healing processes to occur without the encumbrances created by secondary pain factors.

Although there is always an overlap between pathophysiology and treatment for chronic and acute pain, the aim of this chapter is entirely concerned with the management of acute postoperative and post-traumatic pain.

The management of postoperative pain is generally overlooked once the "important" business of surgical diagnosis, operative procedure, and anesthetic management are settled. If the physician in charge does not assume an active role in the analgesic management of the patient, the role is relegated to the junior house staff (or routine orders) who in all likelihood are uninformed and unmotivated to devote much time and effort to what for them is just one aspect of postoperative management.

Finally, the emphasis of this chapter is on the description of the possible alternatives for therapy of adults. Although some of these same modes of therapy may be applied, in theory, to the pediatric population, there are a myriad of special considerations when dealing with children from the neonate to the teenager, and the reader is referred to McIlvaine's excellent review on this subject (1).

ANATOMY AND NEUROPHYSIOLOGY OF ACUTE PAIN

Noxious stimuli affect their high-threshold receptors in the skin, subcutaneous tissue, fascia, periosteum, blood vessels, and viscera. The resulting impulses from these nociceptors are known as *noxious* or *nociceptive* impulses at all points in their transmission prior to reaching the cortex of the conscious human. Nociceptive impulses will, when processed by the cerebral cortex, give rise to the perceptual-emotional experience called pain.

The primary afferent nociceptor is a bipolar neuron, with one pole being a centrally directed axon innervating the dorsal horn of the spinal cord and the other pole being a peripherally directed axon innervating the high threshold receptors. Inflammatory mediators such as prostaglandins, leukotrienes, purines, and indoleamines sensitize the nociceptor by lowering its threshold. Sensitization accounts for a major part of the pain experienced by patients after surgery. Opiate receptors are synthesized in the cell bodies of the nociceptors and are transported along the axons to both the central and peripheral terminals. The opioids that selectively activate the mu opiate receptors, by indirectly decreasing the production of cyclic adenosine monophosphate (AMP), an intracellular second messenger of nociceptor sensitization, raises the threshold of the terminal of the nociceptor, and thus decreases the perceived pain. The opioids also selectively activate delta and kappa opiate receptors to block the release of a variety of sensitizing agents, including prostanoids, from sympathetic postganglionic nerve terminals. Therefore, whereas the nonsteroidal anti-inflammatory drugs, or NSAIDs (cyclooxygenase inhibitors), selectively block the synthesis of prostaglandins, the opioids, by modulating cyclic AMP levels, can theoretically offer greater pain relief.

Transmission, or nociception, of these impulses originating in the nociceptors occurs via small A-delta and C-fibers to the spinal cord, where they synapse in the dorsal horn. The signal is then projected over multiple pathways of the neuroaxis (Fig. 46.1). Those to the anterolateral horn stimulate preganglionic neurons of the

600

AFFERENT PAIN PATHWAYS

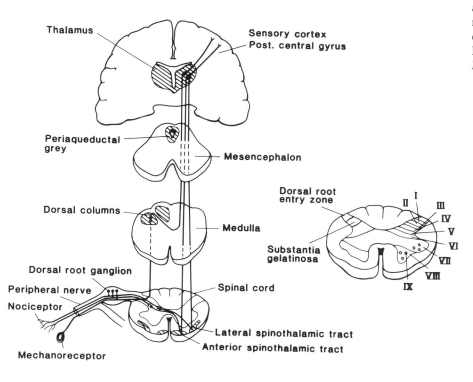

Figure 46.1. Afferent pain pathways and organization of dorsal horn laminae. (From Raj PP: Basic function and organization of the nervous system. In Raj PP (ed): *Practical Management of Pain.* Chicago, Year Book, 1986, p 56.)

sympathetic or parasympathetic systems, whereas transmission to the anterior horn stimulates somatic motor neurons. These are in addition to the traditional pain-transmitting spinothalamic tracts made up of axons of neurons located in various laminae of the dorsal horn.

The spinothalamic system is actually divided into the neospinothalamic tract and the paleospinothalamic tract. The rapidly conducting neospinothalamic tract has the capacity, via its discretely organized primary projection to the somatosensory cortex, to process discriminative information regarding the site, intensity, and duration of a stimulus, resulting in the perception of a sharp, well-localized pain. On the other hand, nociceptive impulses transmitted by the paleospinothalamic tract, composed of diffusely projecting fibers, provoke suprasegmental reflex responses affecting ventilation, circulation, and endocrine function. This multisynaptic system, unlike the neospinothalamic tract, lacks somatotropic organization, resulting in the slowly transmitted impulses perceived as poorly localized, dull, aching, and burning pain. The paleospinothalamic system may also provoke the powerful "fight or flight" mechanism.

MODULATION OF NOCICEPTION

This system of nociceptive transmission can be modulated at multiple points along its course, resulting in either amplification or inhibition of the signal. The release of intracellular substances into the extracellular space lowers the threshold of the local nociceptors. Furthermore, peripheral input into the dorsal horn is modulated by temperature, sympathetic function, blood flow, and the chemical environment, whereas modulation within the dorsal horn is affected by local, segmental, and suprasegmental influences.

Inhibition of nociception can result from the influence of supraspinal descending neural systems. One of the most powerful of these systems contains axons that make up the dorsolateral funiculus and receives signals that originate from neurons in the periaqueductal and periventricular gray matter. Stimulating this region of the midbrain produces a profound analgesia that can be blocked by naloxone.

Several recent publications provide evidence that opioids provide analgesia by action at peripheral sites (2, 3). These findings provide both new insight into the theories of nociception and modulation and new alternatives for pain therapy.

PATHOPHYSIOLOGY OF POSTOPERATIVE PAIN

Segmental responses are the result of nociceptive impulses being transmitted from the dorsal horn to the anterior horn or anterolateral horn and include skeletal muscle spasm, vasospasm, and a decrease in gastrointestinal and genitourinary tract activity. Skeletal muscle spasm initiates a vicious cycle of spasm leading to pain and more spasm. Pain resulting from a lowered nociceptor threshold is a direct consequence of vasospastic ischemia causing local tissue hypoxia, acidosis, and the

Table 46.1.
Stratification of Response to Nociceptive Impulses Following Intraabdominal Surgery[a]

I. Cortical responses
   A. Pain perception
   B. Psychodynamic mechanism—fear and anxiety
   C. Motivational
   D. Discriminative
   E. Overt voluntary motor activity/inactivity
II. Suprasegmental autonomic responses
   A. Endocrine (stress) response
   B. Alteration of ventilation
   C. Increased sympathetic tone with liberation of catecholamines and further increases in sympathetic tone
   D. Tachycardia → increased cardiac output
   E. Hypertension (as a result of C and D)
III. Segmental reflex responses
   A. Cutaneosomatic/somatosomatic responses
      1. Increased muscle spasm
      2. Ischemia
      3. Hyperhydrosis
   B. Cutaneovisceral/somatovisceral responses
      1. Bronchospasm
      2. Bronchiolar spasm
      3. Decreased gastrointestinal motility
         a. Distention
         b. Nausea
         c. Vomiting
      4. Decreased urinary function → oliguria
   C. Cutaneovascular responses → vasospasm
   D. Viscerocutaneous responses → results similar to A
   E. Viscerovisceral responses → results similar to B
IV. Local (microscopic) tissue responses
   A. Decreased circulation due to vasospasm and muscle spasm
      1. Decreased oxygen supply
      2. Decreased nutrient supply
      3. Retention of metabolites → lowered nociceptor threshold
      4. Cellular damage → liberation of pain substances
   B. Decreased lymphatic drainage → edema
   C. Muscle fatigue
   D. Inflammation

[a]Modified from Bonica JJ: Introduction, Pathophysiology of Pain. In *Current Concepts in Postoperative Pain*. New York, HP Publishing Co, 1978, p. 10.

production and retention of endogenous pain-producing metabolites. Incisional skin trauma initiates a cutaneovisceral reflex, which worsens the surgically induced dysfunction. An organized approach to the pathophysiologic responses to nociceptive impulses is presented in Table 46.1.

Hypoventilation and stimulation of the hypothalamic autonomic centers are categorized as suprasegmental responses to nociceptive impulses. Autonomic hyperactivity produces an increase in centrally mediated sympathetic tone and a resultant increase in cardiac output,

peripheral vascular resistance, and circulating catecholamines, which in turn further increase sympathetic tone.

The actual perception of pain, overt skeletal muscle activity, and emotional responses all result from cortical stimulation. Although skeletal muscle activity is actually manifested by voluntary or involuntary immobilization, the psychodynamic mechanisms that produce fear and anxiety probably facilitate transmission of the nociceptive impulses throughout the central nervous system (CNS). Consequently, these highly complex interactions produce the complex physiologic, behavioral, and affective responses that characterize the pathophysiology of acute pain. Appropriate and efficacious acute pain therapy involves early intervention in an effort to block the pain cycle and thereby decrease its sequelae.

PHARMACOLOGY OF SYSTEMIC ANALGESICS

The systemic administration of analgesic drugs is by far the most common means of treating postoperative pain (4). It is also the most likely mode of therapy to be inadequate for relief of this pain (4–6). The failure of these drugs almost always lies not with the properties of the drug itself, but with some aspect in the way it is prescribed or administered (5, 7). The effective use of these drugs can be realized only if their clinical pharmacology is understood by those practitioners making therapeutic decisions about pain therapy. Reliance on standard recipes or nursing procedure is no substitute for rational application of the pharmacokinetic and pharmacodynamic information that is increasingly being made available.

NARCOTICS

Opioid or narcotic analgesic agents are drugs that specifically bind with opiate receptors to produce any of a variety of effects. These effects include analgesia, respiratory depression, mood alteration, gastrointestinal immotility, miosis, and cardiovascular changes, especially increased venous capacitance. Opioids have been used for centuries to reduce surgically induced pain and anxiety. This remains the most common use for these drugs. Morphine was produced from opium early in the last century and has proven to be a highly efficacious analgesic for a variety of pain states. Although potency may vary, the opiates that have been introduced over the years, and continue to be introduced, have not exceeded the efficacy of morphine.

Drugs with efficacy equal to that of morphine are referred to as *pure narcotic agonists*, some of which are listed in Table 46.2. Narcotics with less efficacy are called *partial agonists* or *partial agonist-antagonists*, and these will be discussed later in this section.

Despite the availability of several narcotic agonists of proven efficacy in controlling pain, inadequate relief of postoperative pain remains a problem (4–7). The tradi-

Table 46.2.
Approximate Pharmacokinetic and Pharmacodynamic Values for Common Narcotic Agonists

Opiate Agonist	Approx. Dose Equiv. to 10 mg Morphine	Effective Plasma Conc. (ng/ml)	Volume of Distribution (liters/kg)	Clearance (liters/min)	Elimination Half-Life (hr)
Morphine	10 mg	21	4.0	0.8–1.5	2.5–4
Meperidine	100 mg	550	3.5	0.9	3–4
Fentanyl	100 μg	1–2	3.5	1.0	3–5
Alfentanil	500 μg	10–20	0.7	0.45	1.5–2.5
Methadone	10 mg	58	7.0	0.15	24–48

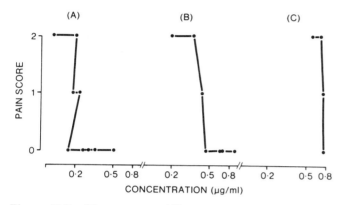

Figure 46.2. **Plasma meperidine concentration versus response data for three postoperative patients.** *Solid circles* **represent measured plasma meperidine concentrations and the corresponding pain score when the sample was obtained. Note the differences in concentration corresponding to vertical portion of the curves for each patient. These differences represent interindividual pharmacodynamic variation. (From Austin KL, Stapleton JV, Mather LE: Relationship between blood meperidine concentrations and analgesic response: A preliminary report.** *Anesthesiology* **53:460–466, 1980.)**

tional approach to postoperative pain relief has been to administer narcotics to patients by intermittent intramuscular injection. This approach is often inadequate for several reasons. The primary reason is that patients differ in their requirement for narcotics. In addition, there is a common tendency to overestimate the potency, duration of action, and addiction potential of these drugs. As a result, physician orders may be inadequate because either too small a dose or too long an interval between doses is prescribed (7).

In an attempt to allow for some variability in patient requirement, it is common to prescribe opiates for the relief of acute pain as "p.r.n." This comes from the Latin *pro re nata* (according as circumstances may require), but is sometimes seen as "per RN"—that is, when the nurse is convinced that there is a real need for a narcotic that outweighs the concerns for addiction potential or side effects (e.g., respiratory depression, sedation, constipa-

tion) and that this non-emergent request does not seriously interfere with completion of other important duties (7, 8). These concerns have been addressed. It has been repeatedly shown that dependence is a rare event, occurring in fewer than 0.1% of hospitalized patients (9–11). Regarding the concern for the side effects of opiates used for pain therapy, the observation has been made that this concern is "extravagant" and has "drastically" limited treatment on a scale that is unparalleled in medicine (12). Keats has addressed the logistical issue in a study in which it was shown that the amount of narcotic a patient received was directly proportional to the amount of nursing staff available to the patient (13).

Patients require differing dosages of opioids for a variety of reasons. The factors governing variability can be divided into two general categories: *pharmacokinetic* (differences in rate of absorption, tissue distribution, and elimination) and *pharmacodynamic* (differences in response to identical concentrations presented to the active tissue site or biophase).

Biophase concentrations, although rarely sampled, are generally considered to reflect blood or plasma concentrations, particularly during steady-state conditions. Most plasma concentration versus effect data for narcotic agonists have dealt with meperidine. Studies with other opioid agonists (morphine (14), fentanyl (15), alfentanil (16, 17), methadone (18), and ketobemidone (19)) have been consistent with the general pharmacologic principles that have been delineated with the meperidine model. Austin et al. examined plasma meperidine concentrations and pain scores at regular intervals during every-4-hour dosing with intramuscular meperidine (20). The data from three patients in Figure 46.2 illustrate some important findings. First, the concentration response curves are quite steep, with dramatic changes in pain score occurring over a narrow concentration range. Second, there is a fourfold difference in the plasma concentration required for complete pain relief between patients A and C. Patient B had an intermediate sensitivity to the drug. Studies by Tamsen et al., in which patients self-administered small intravenous doses of meperidine on demand, gave a similar

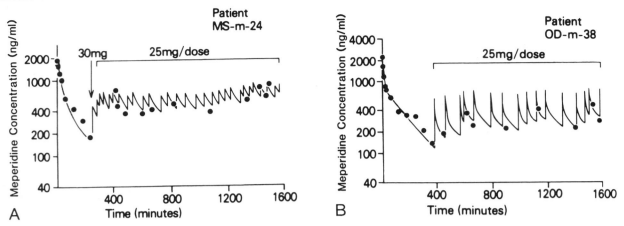

Figure 46.3A and B. Plasma concentrations of meperidine for two patients following a single dose (approximately 150 mg) for surgery and with 25-mg bolus-demand doses for PCA postoperatively. *Solid circles* represent measured plasma meperidine concentrations and *solid lines* are computer-generated estimates of the changes in plasma concentration with time. Note the increased demand frequency and higher "trough" levels of patient A. (Modified from Tamsen A, Hartvig P, Fogerland C, et al: Patient-controlled analgesic therapy: Part II. Individual analgesic demand and analgesic plasma concentrations of pethidine in postoperative pain. *Clin Pharmacokinet* 7:164–175, 1982).

picture, as shown in Figure 46.3 (21). Each patient tended to maintain plasma meperidine concentrations within a narrow range, suggesting that the concentration-response relationship is as steep as that demonstrated by Austin et al. (20). Additionally, the concentrations "selected" by patients could vary considerably. Thus, whereas intrasubject concentration variation should be expected to be small, intersubject variation should be expected to be large. Although traditional thought has ascribed large intersubject variability to a host of physical and psychosocial factors, recent evidence from Tamsen and co-workers has shown an inverse relationship between narcotic requirement and endorphin levels sampled from the cerebrospinal fluid of postoperative patients (22).

Pharmacokinetic variability can also account for differences in dosage requirement. Unfortunately, there are few studies that offer much guidance in making dosing adjustments for this type of variability. If the clinician is alert and expects these sources of variation, however, proper dose titration for a desired clinical effect is more likely.

The pharmacokinetics of absorption can be highly variable. The principle determinant of absorption from intramuscular injections is muscle blood flow. Several factors may cause the postsurgical patient to have diminished muscle blood flow. Such a decrease is particularly likely in patients who have suffered significant physiologic perturbations during their surgical procedure. Not only may these patients obtain subtherapeutic plasma concentrations because of poor absorption, but there is the danger that significant depression of sensorium and respiration may occur when muscle perfusion is restored and the narcotic depot is rapidly ab-

sorbed. Mather et al. have shown that absorption rates of meperidine have great interindividual variation following intramuscular injection, resulting in large differences in plasma concentrations and levels of pain relief (23). Similarly, oral absorption depends on splanchnic blood flow and gastric emptying, both of which may be adversely affected by the effects of surgery and anesthesia, especially when the insults are major. Significant liver dysfunction may lessen the first-pass metabolism, markedly increasing bioavailability. Such findings have led to the recommendation that oral meperidine doses be reduced in patients with cirrhosis (24).

Reductions in function of the major drug-clearing organs, the liver and kidney, may result in reduced drug clearance. Because of the relationship

$$Css = DR/Cle,$$

where steady-state plasma concentration (Css) is equal to the ratio of dosing rate (DR) to elimination clearance (Cle), one can see that higher drug concentrations will result if standard doses are given to patients with impaired clearing capacity.

All of the major narcotic agonists undergo extensive hepatic metabolism with minimal renal excretion of the parent drug. The two general categories of metabolism, the phase I oxidation and reduction reactions and the phase II conjugations, respond differently to hepatic insults. As a general rule, oxidative metabolic pathways are susceptible to functional impairment when hepatic disease is present. One should be alert to the possibility of reduced elimination clearance as well as reduced first-pass metabolism following oral administration when phase I metabolized drugs, such as fentanyl and meperidine, are given (24–26). On the other hand, glucuronidation pathways are more robust and seem to resist the influence of hepatic disease. Morphine, which undergoes glucuronidation, has normal clearance in cirrhotics (27).

Impaired renal function does not directly reduce the elimination clearance of the narcotic analgesics. The uremic state can, however, indirectly impair liver function and diminish hepatic metabolism. There is some evidence that morphine clearance is reduced in renal failure, perhaps by some indirect mechanism (28).

In the 72 hours during which acute postoperative pain management is a concern, it is unlikely that significant levels of metabolites of the narcotic analgesics could accumulate. Chronic administration of meperidine, however, can lead to the accumulation of its metabolite, normeperidine, which causes cerebral excitation leading to irritability and even seizures (29). The conjugated metabolites of morphine (morphine-3- and morphine-6-glucuronide) exceed the levels of the parent drug with chronic oral therapy (because of the lower clearance of these conjugates) and may be particularly high if the patient has renal failure and cannot excrete these water-soluble compounds (30). Morphine-3-glucuronide appears to be pharmacologically inert, and although morphine-6-glucuronide has analgesic effects in rats, it is uncertain whether or not this metabolite has any significant effect in humans (30).

OPIOID PARTIAL AGONISTS AND PARTIAL AGONIST-ANTAGONISTS

A variety of opioid drugs with limited agonist activity have been introduced in the past few decades. They have been touted as offering the advantage of similar analgesic efficacy as the opioid agonists but having a reduced potential for serious side effects such as addiction and respiratory depression. Because narcotic addiction is not an issue in the postoperative patient, one need not be influenced by claims of lower or absent addiction potential. The partial agonist-antagonists butorphanol, pentazocine, and nalbuphine and the partial agonist buprenorphine are the common analgesics available in parenteral form for postoperative pain therapy. In contrast to the pure agonists, these drugs have been shown to have a ceiling for respiratory-depressive effects (31, 32). They also demonstrate a ceiling in their analgesic potency, however (7, 33, 34). They are capable of antagonizing the analgesic (35), respiratory depressive (36), and electroencephalographic (EEG) effects (37) of pure narcotic agonists. A particularly cloudy clinical picture may result when a pure opioid agonist is given to a patient who has already received one of the mixed agonist-antagonists or vice versa. Although these drugs may have a place in the treatment of relatively minor pain that may follow some superficial or extremity op-

erations, we do not recommend their routine use for most surgical patients.

NONSTEROIDAL ANTI-INFLAMMATORY ANALGESICS

Since the introduction of aspirin in 1899, nonsteroidal anti-inflammatory drugs (NSAIDs) have been used to treat minor surgical pain. Although aspirin remains the standard to which others are compared, it is no longer the most common minor analgesic in surgical practice. Rather, the powerful opioid agonists are the drugs of choice for severe or even moderate postoperative pain, and the non-steroidal anti-inflammatory analgesics are generally relegated to oral administration following relatively minor procedures such as dental surgery or episiotomy. These agents have a plateau of analgesic efficacy and are effective only if the pain stimulus is not too strong (38). The NSAIDs are thought to act peripherally rather than centrally as the opioids do. By inhibiting the cyclo-oxygenase enzyme system they prevent the metabolism of arachidonic acid to its endoperoxide intermediates, which would then be converted to thromboxanes, prostacyclines, and prostaglandins. These interact with other local mediators to produce erythema, edema, and pain (Table 46.1). These local mediators of the peripheral nociceptors, whose production is blocked by NSAIDs, however, are not the only sensitizers to nociception (39). Much remains unknown about other antinociceptive mechanisms, but a central action and the possibility of other peripheral mechanisms have been suggested (38).

The number of operations performed on an outpatient basis has increased dramatically over the past few years and so, not surprisingly, has interest in these analgesics, because many of the newer anti-inflammatory analgesics have been demonstrated to have greater efficacy than aspirin and acetaminophen (38). Because it may be unacceptable in many situations to administer parenteral narcotics to postsurgical outpatients, it is expected that these anti-inflammatory analgesics will be used to an increasing degree for treating postoperative pain.

Ibuprofen (400 mg), indoprofen (200 mg), naproxen (400 mg), diflunisal (500 mg), and ketorolac (10 mg) (40) given orally all appear to have efficacy superior to that of aspirin (650 mg) or, in some cases, aspirin plus codeine in postsurgical patients (38). Ketorolac (30 or 90 mg) given intramuscularly has been shown to be as effective as morphine (12 mg) (41). Lysine acetyl salicylate by continuous intravenous infusion (1.8 g over 5 min followed by 1.8 g over 6 hours) was as effective as a continuous infusion of morphine (10 mg over 5 min followed by 10 mg over 6 hours) (42). Others argue from more recent evidence, however, that NSAIDs alone do not provide adequate analgesia for severe postoperative pain and that these agents need to be used with opioids in many cases (43). Combination therapy with opioids may offer the potential for additive or synergistic effects that may reduce the degree of postoperative pain to a greater degree than with either alone (44).

Because NSAIDs interfere with the initiation of pain in tissues by reducing the activation and sensitization of peripheral nociceptors and attenuate the inflammatory response seen after surgical trauma, the preoperative use of NSAIDs has been advocated (43). To date, however, very little evidence exists to substantiate this approach.

Alpha₂-Adrenergic Agonists

Through the experimental uses of alpha₂-adrenergic agonists and antagonists much new information is being learned about this neuro-endocrinologic system. This system goes far beyond the mediation of vascular tone. Of particular interest are their sedative, anxiolytic, and analgesic properties. These actions in combination or in some independent way reduce the requirement for potent volatile anesthetics (45). The mechanism of alpha₂-agonist–mediated analgesia is still speculative but probably involves descending medullospinal noradrenergic pathways that modulate spinal nociceptive processing (46). Alpha₂-adrenergic receptors are well placed on dorsal horn neurons to possibly inhibit the release of nociceptive neurotransmitters (47).

Information on the use of these agents is limited to fragmentary experimental data. However, the ability of clonidine to diminish shivering (48), nausea and vomiting (47), and cardiovascular instability (49) bodes well for the use of this or more-specific agents in this setting in the near future. When given after spinal fusion operations by continuous intravenous infusion (5 mg/kg over the first hour, followed by 0.3 mg/kg/hour), clonidine-treated patients required less morphine supplementation (50).

Clonidine has also been administered into the epidural space. Although Eisenach et al. have shown a significant analgesic effect lasting approximately 5 hours without sensory or motor block (51), work by Bonnet et al., in which similar results were obtained whether the clonidine dose was given epidurally or intramuscularly, raises questions about the site of action (52). Certainly, much work remains to be done before this class of drug can be recommended for routine use in the postoperative period.

Sedative Drugs Used as Adjuncts to Analgesics

A component of the discomfort of the postoperative period is often the attendant anxiety. This can often heighten the interpreted intensity of pain or the emotional reaction to it; thus an aggravating cycle, difficult to interrupt with analgesics alone, may ensue (53). Sedative drugs, although of no use for treating acute pain alone, may, in combination with an opioid, accomplish the desired goal of abating both the patient's pain and his focus on or anxiety concerning that pain. Drugs that

have been used in this way are promethazine 25–50 mg (54), hydroxyzine 25–100 mg (55), dextroamphetamine 5–10 mg (56), and benzodiazepines (diazepam 5–10 mg, oxazepam 15 mg, or midazolam 1–5 mg) (57). Promethazine, hydroxyzine (painful when given intramuscularly), and droperidol 1.25–2.5 mg are also antiemetics and may help counter the nausea that frequently accompanies opioid use (58). Although it is common practice to order some of these drugs in fixed combination with a narcotic analgesic, prudence would dictate their addition only when indicated. Most patients simply will not require these mood-altering drugs, whereas others may experience significant exaggeration of some of the side effects of concomitantly administered narcotics (sedation, respiratory depression).

METHODS OF SYSTEMIC ANALGESIC ADMINISTRATION

Selection of the appropriate systemic drug for a postoperative patient is important, but represents only the first step in the pharmacologic treatment of postoperative pain. The clinician must next decide how the drug will be given and how the effectiveness of the therapy will be assessed so that changes and adjustments can be made to suit a given patient. In deciding how the drug will be given one must consider both the route of administration and the dosing schedule.

Routes of Drug Administration

The route of drug delivery is often dictated by the drug formulations that are available or by patient considerations such as the availability of intravenous access or the ability of the patient to take medication orally. Most often the clinician chooses a particular approach in order to take advantage of the special properties that a route may offer. Understanding the pharmacokinetic properties associated with various routes of drug administration is essential to planning drug therapy and the interpretation of subsequent events.

Intravenous Drug Administration

To exert a systemic effect the drug must first reach the systemic circulation so that it may then be carried to the tissue sites of action. Understanding the fate of drugs given directly into the circulation is helpful in understanding the time course of events following other methods of systemic drug administration.

The fate or *disposition* of a drug injected intravenously involves the processes of *distribution* to body tissues and *clearance* by the organs of elimination. Drug distribution is governed by the laws of mass action, which drive blood and tissue concentrations toward an equilibrium. The physicochemical properties of drugs and the physiologic (i.e., tissue perfusion) state of the patient are both important factors in drug distribution. Highly lipid-soluble opioid analgesics, such as fentanyl, methadone, and meperidine, move across capillaries into and out of tissues rapidly, with the amount of blood flow to any particular tissue determining the extent and rate. The highly perfused tissue of the CNS equilibrates rapidly with the blood concentrations of these lipophilic drugs, so changes in the intensity of narcotic effects will quickly follow changes in plasma drug concentrations (16, 17). Following a rapid intravenous injection, concentrations in the blood and CNS will fall as distribution of drug continues to the large reservoir of less well perfused, pharmacologically inert tissues (e.g., skeletal muscle). The apparent size of the total tissue reservoir is termed the *volume of distribution*. This is usually only a theoretic volume and varies from drug to drug, depending on a variety of factors. Under most circumstances the process of distribution to this volume approaches completion in 0.5–1.5 hours. If drug concentrations fall below effective levels during this phase of disposition the pharmacologic effect dissipates. The termination of drug effect, therefore, is often a result of drug distribution, not drug elimination alone. Thus it is common to observe a duration of action of 0.5–1.0 hours following intravenous injection of a therapeutic dose of many drugs.

After distribution is complete, plasma drug concentrations continue to decrease, albeit more slowly, solely because of drug elimination. There are two terms used to describe the kinetics of elimination: *elimination half-life* and *elimination clearance*. Elimination clearance is expressed as volume per unit time and is a direct measure of the elimination processes. Its importance during drug therapy is expressed in the equation Css = DR/Cle, which shows that the eventual or steady-state plasma concentration (Css) is determined by the ratio of dosing rate (DR) (given intermittently or as an infusion) and elimination clearance (Cle).

Elimination half-life is the time required for the plasma drug concentration to decrease by one-half. This can be measured only after the drug distribution processes are complete. Half-life, which depends on the ratio of the distribution volume to elimination clearance, is often erroneously equated with duration of action, but it is only one of several factors that predict how long a drug may act.

Elimination half-life is, however, directly related to the time required to reach 90% of the eventual steady-state plasma concentrations for a drug given on a fixed schedule or by infusion. The time required to reach 90% of the eventual steady-state concentration can be calculated by multiplying the half-life by 3.3. Knowing this, one can predict that meperidine (half-life = 4 hours) given at 50 mg every 3 hours would approach a maximum steady-state concentration in about 13 hours (i.e., after four doses), whereas with methadone (half-life = 36 hours) given at 10 mg every 12 hours, a maximum steady-state would be approached in about 5 days (i.e., after 10 doses). This has important implications when

evaluating patients for analgesic efficacy and side effects after making dosage adjustments; maximum effect is approached in 3.3 half-lives.

The time to peak effect following a rapid intravenous injection or bolus infusion depends on the rate of rise of the CNS tissue concentration and the rate of decline of the plasma concentration, both of which are affected by the physicochemical properties of a drug (59). Fentanyl will reach a peak in 2–4 min following an intravenous bolus, compared with a peak effect for morphine, which occurs in 5–10 min. This time requirement is important clinically when one is titrating to an effect. With either patient-controlled or clinician-controlled administration, time must be allowed to observe the eventual effect of a dose before additional increments are given. This time can be shorter for lipophilic drugs such as fentanyl or meperidine, and may be as short as 1–2 min following an intravenous bolus of the new fentanyl congener, alfentanil (16, 59).

Gourlay and colleagues have elegantly made use of these pharmacokinetic principles in the treatment of postoperative pain with methadone (18). As shown in Table 46.2, methadone has a long elimination half-life (approximately 36 hours) because of its low clearance and large volume of distribution. Methadone is also lipid-soluble, allowing rapid plasma to brain equilibration. Effective doses given parenterally have generally resulted in short durations of action (60) despite the prolonged elimination half-life as plasma concentrations fall below effective levels during the distributive phase (i.e., before the terminal elimination phase). It is not feasible to give a dose that would result in an effective level after the distributive processes yield a pseudoequilibration of tissue concentrations so that the slow elimination phase could be exploited to produce a long-lasting effect. Such a dose would necessarily be large and initially result in high plasma concentrations that are associated with respiratory depression and excessive sedation. In the report by Gourlay et al., a relatively large methadone dose (20 mg intravenously) was given at the start of anesthesia. The patient's ventilation was then supported during the operation. The plasma methadone concentrations fell as a result of distribution during surgery so that by the time of arrival in the recovery room they were near effective levels. Smaller 5-mg doses were given incrementally in the recovery room so that the dose could be titrated to allow for individual variability (range: 1–3 doses). Because subsequent decreases in plasma methadone concentration were during the slow elimination phase, these investigators observed a mean duration of action of 21 hours.

Another means of providing prolonged action is by continuous infusion of a drug. Hug, in an editorial (61), called for increased efforts in defining the pharmacokinetics and pharmacodynamics of analgesics so that infusions could be rationally designed to maintain plasma

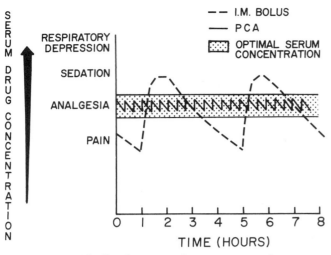

Figure 46.4. Idealized serum drug concentration versus time curves for intramuscular administration (*dashed line*) and intravenous PCA (*solid line*). The vertical axis includes measures for both narcotic concentration and effect. Note the relationship of the idealized concentration lines with optimal serum concentrations that avoid pain and sedation. (From Bennett RL, Griffen WO: Patient controlled analgesia. *Contemp Surg* 23:75–84, 1983.)

concentrations at an effective analgesic level while avoiding toxicity. As suggested in the foregoing equation, the critical pieces of information needed to devise an infusion are the target concentration (Css) and the elimination clearance (Cle). These variables, given for some narcotics in Table 46.2, when multiplied will yield the proper infusion rate (DR) for the average patient. Unfortunately, many postoperative patients are not average and, as discussed above in some detail, considerable variability in effective plasma concentration and elimination clearance should be expected. Nevertheless, in a very straightforward manner Duthie and colleagues gave a continuous fentanyl infusion of 100 μg/hour for 24 hours for postoperative analgesia and found it effective (15). Given an elimination clearance for fentanyl of 1.0 l/min (Table 46.2), one could predict a mean steady-state plasma concentration of 1.7 ng/ml; Duthie et al. found that the plasma concentrations in their 45 patients ranged between 1 and 3 ng/ml (15). Because steady state levels are not approached before 3.3 drug half-lives have elapsed, some provision for reaching these levels sooner (i.e., with a loading dose) must be made. In the study of Duthie et al. the anesthesia for surgery was narcotic (fentanyl) based, thus obviating the need for a loading scheme (15). When a narcotic has not been used during the course of anesthesia, loading should be accomplished with incremental intravenous bolus doses of the narcotic in the recovery room. Additionally, some feedback mechanism to ad-

just the infusion rate needs to be incorporated in the overall treatment plan.

Intramuscular Drug Administration

The process of intramuscular drug absorption is generally first-order. That is, a constant *fraction* of the remaining dose is absorbed at any given time. This results in a continuously diminishing amount of drug entering the circulation. Because absorption and tissue distribution take place concurrently, the result is a delayed and reduced peak plasma concentration despite absolute bioavailability that is usually equal to the intravenous route.

The resultant buffering of peak concentrations and effect has allowed larger, longer-acting doses to be given and has generally made the intramuscular route appear safer than the intravenous route. The rate of the absorption process depends on skeletal muscle blood flow, however. As previously mentioned, hypoperfusion of skeletal muscle is not a rare event in postsurgical patients. A reduced rate of absorption will delay the peak plasma concentration. It may be difficult to ascertain whether the reduced efficacy seen shortly after injection in an affected patient is due to poor absorption (pharmacokinetic factor) or decreased sensitivity (pharmacodynamic factor). The treatment for the former is allowing more time to elapse, whereas for the latter it is the administration of more drug. By administering more drug into a hypoperfused muscle, one runs the risk of observing a relative overdose if blood flow is suddenly restored, the absorption rate constant increases, and a much larger fraction of the drug remaining in the muscle reaches the circulation in a short time.

The merits of traditional intramuscular narcotic administration are mainly its low cost and simplicity. Almost by design, the plasma concentrations are not maintained constant, but swing widely between subtherapeutic (a requirement of most intermittent "p.r.n." regimens) and therapeutic and sometimes higher concentrations. Figure 46.4 graphically shows the time course of the plasma concentrations resulting from this mode of administration and the resultant toll in the time the patient must endure pain at one extreme and risk sedation and respiratory depression at the other.

In an attempt to mimic continuous infusions, regular timed intramuscular injections have been advocated in an attempt to avoid the unnecessary intervals of subtherapeutic plasma concentrations and the expense of infusion pumps. Welchew has shown that intramuscular morphine (10 mg) injections, every 4 hours gave pain scores and side effects (sedation and nausea) scores similar to those of on-demand fentanyl (62).

Subcutaneous Drug Administration

Because of the difficulties in maintaining intravenous catheters, particularly in outpatients, subcutaneously placed needles and catheters offer a reasonable alternative route for delivering drug either by continuous infusion (63) or by frequent intermittent bolus doses. As with intramuscular injections, absorption will delay the peak concentration and effect. A small 23- or 25-gauge needle can be placed subcutaneously, taped in place, and attached to the administration set of the delivery device. It is usually recommended that the needle be reinserted at a new site on a daily basis.

Oral Drug Administration

Oral administration is most often preferred because it is convenient, painless, and superficially appears to be nontechnical. Whenever feasible, patients and physicians will select this route. It is, however, fraught with technical difficulties that may jeopardize success. Therefore, alternative routes of administration when treating postoperative or other acute pain states are encouraged. Nevertheless, oral administration of analgesic drugs may be an acceptable choice following many types of operations.

Absorption from the gastrointestinal tract is far more complex than intramuscular or subcutaneous absorption, where tissue blood flow is the chief regulating influence. Because mucosal surface area is so important in determining the rate of absorption from the gastrointestinal tract, passage of the drug from the stomach to the duodenum, where there is a several-fold increase in mucosal surface area, drastically improves drug absorption. Delayed gastric emptying, as sometimes accompanies surgery or trauma, may limit the effectiveness of a dose of analgesic.

After gastric or intestinal absorption, drug is carried via the portal system to the liver, where metabolism may occur before the drug can gain access to the systemic circulation. This is called *first-pass metabolism*. It is significant for those drugs with moderate or high hepatic elimination clearance or extraction (i.e., hepatic clearance greater than about 300 ml/min). If normal adult liver blood flow is about 1500 ml/min, then a drug with a hepatic elimination clearance of 300 ml/min would have 20% of the dose lost on first pass; one with a clearance of 900 ml/min would lose 60%. Morphine, with a hepatic clearance of about 850 ml/min, loses a little over one-half of an oral dose to first-pass metabolism. Therefore, most patients will require about two to three times their usual intramuscular morphine dose when it is given orally (30). With some drugs, significant oral dose reductions are required in the presence of hepatic disease because the first-pass effect may be reduced, as discussed earlier (24).

As mentioned earlier in the chapter, because of the larger dose requirement made necessary by first-pass metabolism, oral administration will result in the production of a larger quantity of metabolites that may (e.g., meperidine [29]) or may not (e.g., morphine [30]) require clinical consideration.

Transdermal Drug Administration

Transdermal drug administration has proven to be a viable means of delivering many drugs including nitroglycerine, scopolamine, antihypertensives, and nicotine. As with other routes requiring absorption, this method requires a predictable blood flow at the dermal application site. Transdermal administration differs from other routes requiring absorption, however, in that the absorption process is not first-order (oral, subcutaneous, and intravenous absorption are), in which a constant fraction of the dose is absorbed at any given time, but is zero-order (like an intravenous infusion), in which a constant amount is delivered over any given time regardless of the amount remaining in the drug depot. When using the transdermal approach for narcotic administration, following application of a "drug patch," concentrations will begin an exponential rise toward a steady-state concentration. It will reach 90% of this steady state in 3.3 half-lives. Therefore, unless the anesthetic for the operation was narcotic-based and the patient already had significant narcotic plasma concentrations, it may be necessary to give a narcotic "loading" dose when starting transdermal treatment. Such transdermal dosage forms have been successfully used in postoperative pain management with fentanyl (64), but this mode of therapy is still controversial.

PATIENT-CONTROLLED ANALGESIA

Systemically administered narcotic analgesics, while frequently used in the treatment of acute postoperative pain, are not commonly used in a manner that can provide optimal analgesia. One factor responsible for inadequate analgesia is the interindividual variation in narcotic requirements. The minimum effective analgesic concentration (MEAC) in plasma is only one variable affecting the ability to obtain satisfactory postoperative analgesia in any given patient. MEAC can vary by 21% within a given patient over time and as much as eight times between patients (14, 19–23). For this reason alone, it is not surprising that "standard" orders for narcotic administration in the postoperative period will seldom provide optimal analgesia.

As mentioned above, the multiple factors affecting drug absorption rates or bioavailability can be circumvented by direct intravenous administration. Because of the rapid peak levels (and effect) obtained following intravenous bolus administration and the subsequent redistribution to terminate effect, however, it is usually not a practical use of available manpower to administer narcotic analgesics in this manner except in the setting of an intensive care unit or recovery room. Therefore, the combination of a machine controlling the intravenous administration of a narcotic either as an intermittent bolus or continuous infusion, or some combination of the two, while having the patient directly or indirectly altering the rate of administration, results in a highly successful modality for providing an optimal level of postoperative analgesia.

A method for providing intermittent demand-bolus administration is available and in current use. A method for providing a patient demand-based alteration in the administration rate of a continuous infusion is still under investigation. It is hoped that this latter mode of administration would further minimize both the peaks and troughs in plasma drug concentrations as well as the repeated and frequent patient intervention, particularly during intervals of sleep. With this technique, however, there is continued concern that the patient must be allowed to "surface" regularly so that the system continues to be patient-controlled rather than machine-controlled. If a high continuous administration rate were to be established, respiratory depression might occur during sleep or during periods of lesser stimulation. In fact, in the interest of safety, it may be best if some degree of pain is maintained. It has clearly been shown, in most patient-controlled analgesia (PCA) studies, that patients do not try to abolish all pain, but rather settle for a tolerable level of analgesia. Perhaps they are balancing all sensory inputs and selecting an acceptable level of comfort while minimizing distressful side effects.

The rational approach to PCA is based not only on the choice of the analgesic, but also on the route of administration, incremental dose, and concomitant therapy.

Route of Administration

The intravenous, intramuscular, sublingual, oral, rectal, and epidural routes have all been used in conjunction with investigating the efficacy of PCA. For intramuscular injection, a recommended approach is to sterilely place a plastic catheter in the nondominant deltoid muscle and connect this to an On-Demand Analgesia Computer (ODAC) (65). Using this technique, a lock-out period of 20 min was used to allow patient appreciation of one dose prior to permitting a repeat dose. We have no experience with this technique because intravenous access is commonly available in the postoperative setting and is the route of administration to be considered in the remainder of this section. *PCA via the oral route* is actually the proper terminology for analgesic therapy of the non-hospitalized patient and is most commonly used with non-narcotic analgesics (i.e., NSAIDs or acetaminophen).

Choice of Agents

Multiple drugs have been individually administered using a PCA technique. Most commonly employed have been the narcotic analgesics but NSAIDs have also been used. Most experience has been with morphine, but fentanyl (62), nalbuphine (66), buprenorphine (67), and meperidine (21) have been successfully used. Whereas a

**Table 46.3.
Suggested Patient-Controlled Analgesia (PCA) Orders**

1. No IM or IV narcotics, hypnotics, or sedatives shall be ordered or administered except by order of the Pain Control Service.
2. Syringe preparation for ____ ODAC device:
   Syringe size: _____ ml
   Analgesic: _____
   Drug volume: _____ ml
   Drug concentration: _____ ___ g/ml
3. Replace syringe as needed for up to 72 hr
4. PCA parameters:
   Demand dose: _____ ml
   Lockout interval: _____ min
   Dose limit (if relevant): _____ ml/ _____ hr
5. Droperidol (2.5 mg i.m. q 6 hr as needed) for nausea/vomiting
6. For inadequate analgesia, questions, problems, or desire to discontinue PCA prior to:
   Date _____
   Contact: _____
   Page # _____ Phone # _____

rapidly eliminated drug such as alfentanil might be useful in an ODAC designed to alter an infusion rate based on patient demand, a bolus-demand technique would be unacceptable to the patient because of the resulting frequent demand rate. Essentially any drug that is efficacious and can relieve pain in the clinical circumstances in which it is currently used, can probably be satisfactorily used in an ODAC for PCA.

Another unrecognized advantage of PCA is the ability to concomitantly administer a sedative/tranquilizer, anxiolytic, or antiemetic without the usual concern for adjusting the dose of the narcotic analgesic in an effort to prevent undue sedation or respiratory depression. As noted previously, a significant component of postoperative pain is either anxiety or a dose-limiting side-effect of the analgesic that precludes its optimal use by the patient. As seen in the example for postoperative orders (Table 46.3) we routinely make available droperidol as an effective antiemetic. This butyrophenone produces (in higher doses) a state of quiescence with reduced motor activity, reduced anxiety, and indifference to the surroundings. In addition to its antiemetic property, it exhibits mild alpha-blocking properties that may be beneficial, because not infrequently patients have some degree of elevated blood pressure in the early postoperative period. The usual concern with the use of such adjuncts is their unpredictable synergistic effect when combined with a narcotic analgesic, particularly with a drug such as droperidol, which may exert its effect for up to 6 hours. PCA gives the patient the ability to adapt to these changes and alter demand for the narcotic on an individual basis, however.

Loading

As discussed in the section on pharmacokinetics, the effect of a small intravenous bolus dose of drug will diminish rapidly. It is only with repeated doses over several hours that the tissues, to which the agent redistributes, reach equilibration so that with a diminishing concentration gradient the duration of effect of each bolus may be expected to increase. This fact, coupled with the notion that pain is *easier to prevent than to treat*, dictates that an initial dose, larger than the programmed demand dose, should be administered to *load* the patient when PCA therapy is first initiated. Although using intermittent bolus doses (1 mg every 10 min for morphine) may accomplish this goal, the patient might easily get frustrated during the first hour of self-administration. Although not as common, this same scenario may become apparent, to a lesser degree, after a period of sleep.

Lock-Out Interval

For any given drug, its chemical characteristics, pharmacokinetics, and pharmacodynamics will define the time of onset for a particular route of administration. An appropriate interval (10 min for morphine), during which a subsequent bolus dose will not be administered regardless of patient demand, must be selected to allow for patient appreciation of the effect of the previous dose prior to a repeat dose, thereby preventing an "overshoot" of both concentration and effect.

Bolus Demand-Dose

The bolus dose should be selected to give the patient a noticeable effect within the lock-out time, a reasonable duration of action, and yet avoid increasing the resultant concentration to a level that consistently produces unwanted side effects. The efficacy of PCA can be improved considerably by simply doubling the demand bolus dose of the narcotic. While dramatically decreasing the patient self-assessed pain score, the total drug requirement should increase only slightly. A recommended bolus dose for morphine would be 1–2 mg, whereas that for fentanyl would be approximately 10–30 μg.

Summary

Even after the successful execution of these pharmacologic details, individual counseling may be necessary to deal with patient attitudes. For example, some patients have a fear of taking opiates or of overdose; others desire someone else to take the active role for them. A complete summary of the PCA experience in the United States and Europe has been compiled by Harmer et al. (68). We recommend referring to this text prior to initiating this form of postoperative pain management.

INTRATHECAL AND EPIDURAL (NEURAXIAL) OPIOIDS

Quite soon after the demonstration of the "selective block" caused by opioid agonist effects at the spinal cord level, intrathecal and epidural administration of narcotic agonists for the treatment of chronic and acute pain states became almost commonplace. Narcotic agonists, such as morphine, were shown to have stereoselective binding at both pre- and post-synaptic receptors, mainly in the substantia gelatinosa of the dorsal horn of the spinal cord where nociception is modulated. Inhibition of neuronal cell excitation here produces the so-called "selective block" of pain conduction (69). Because spinal (intrathecal and epidural) administration of narcotics promised substantial theoretical advantages over similar administration of local anesthetic drugs (avoidance of motor, sensory, and autonomic block) or systemic administration of narcotic analgesics (longer duration, better analgesia, and avoidance, in most cases, of the central side effects of sedation and respiratory depression), this form of pain therapy gained almost overnight popularity.

Numerous early reports substantiated the efficacy of this approach for treating postoperative pain (70–72). Although the number of patients studied in these reports was sufficient to demonstrate efficacy, it was insufficient to accurately identify and assess risk. Case reports began to appear indicating that in a few rare cases slow cephalad transport of drug caused sedation and respiratory depression 8–15 hours after spinal administration (73, 74). Gustafsson et al. reported a nationwide survey in Sweden involving over 6000 cases in which spinal opiates had been used for treating postoperative pain (75). They estimated the incidence of ventilatory depression to be 0.25–0.40% and 4–7% when epidural and intrathecal morphine were used, respectively. They identified several risk factors, including advanced age (>70 years), large intrathecal doses (2–5 mg morphine), preoperative pulmonary compromise, concomitant administration of systemic narcotics, and use of morphine rather than meperidine as increasing the likelihood of encountering this serious side effect.

To better understand the risks and avoid side effects, more needs to be known about the fate of drugs injected intrathecally and epidurally. Despite recent research efforts, no pharmacokinetic model exists that can predict brain cerebrospinal fluid (CSF) concentrations and responses following spinal administration of drug. A framework for understanding the pharmacokinetic and pharmacodynamic events is realized when a basic physiologic model is referred to, however.

As shown in Figure 46.5, drug injected intrathecally will mix within the spinal subarachnoid CSF (the volume of which is approximately 30 ml). It will also diffuse into the spinal cord and meninges, be absorbed into the systemic circulation, and slowly travel rostrally with passive CSF flow (which is approximately 2.0 ml/min) (76). These processes are the mechanisms of spinal CSF clearance and may be considered to be in competition; the degree to which any one occurs largely depends on

Figure 46.5. Schematic of physiologic/ pharmacokinetic model used to describe the fate of drug $D°$ = un-ionized/lipo-philic and D^+ = ionized/hydrophilic forms) when deposited into the spinal cerebrospinal fluid (C.S.F.). Un-ionized form of drug is depicted interacting with receptors and nonspecific binding sites (*lined rectangles*) and being cleared from the C.S.F. through arachnoid granulations and by entering blood vessels to reach the systemic circulation. Ionized drug remains in the spinal C.S.F. and is cleared by passive bulk flow to the intercranial C.S.F. (From Cousins MJ, Mather LE: Intrathecal and epidural administration opioids. *Anesthesiology* 61:276–310, 1984.)

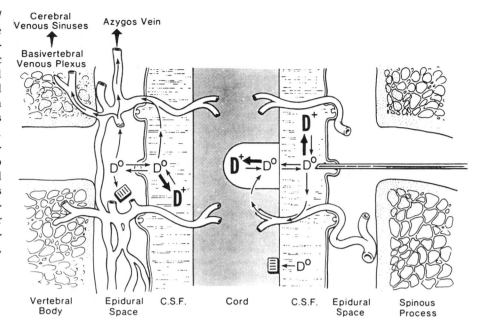

the physicochemical properties of the drug. Highly ionized, hydrophilic drugs such as morphine slowly diffuse into cord and meningeal tissue and will tend to be transported cephalad to the brain in the CSF, because uptake into the systemic circulation is also slow. Un-ionized, lipid-soluble drugs such as fentanyl, methadone, hydromorphone, and meperidine will rapidly diffuse into spinal cord and meningeal tissue and readily cross capillary membranes to reach the systemic circulation, leaving less drug in the CSF for passive, rostral transport, making respiratory depression unlikely as well as limiting the spread of analgesia. Morphine will thus have a longer duration of action, because its spinal CSF clearance is lower, being largely dependent on passive CSF transport, it tends to provide a larger area of analgesia, and it has a higher likelihood of exerting centrally mediated side effects than the more lipid-soluble drugs (76).

Drugs injected into the epidural space will have a fate similar to those injected intrathecally once the drug reaches the spinal subarachnoid space (presumably via arachnoid granulations in the dural cuff region and dural membrane penetration). Ability to enter the CSF also increases with an increase in lipid solubility, so that the more-lipophilic drugs will have a more-rapid onset of action. Conversely, clinical evidence indicates that for the more-hydrophilic morphine, onset of analgesia is slow, duration is prolonged, and the "band" of analgesia is widely distributed. This model and evidence imply that for hydrophilic narcotic agonists, it is the dose of the agent rather than the spinal level of epidural injection that determines the anatomic extent of the analgesia.

Although some drug enters the CSF, most drug in-

jected into the highly vascular epidural space is vigorously absorbed into the systemic circulation. The resulting opioid plasma concentrations are sufficient to produce opiate effects (77). The effects seen soon after epidural injection of opioids are probably wholly or partly a result of systemic, not spinal, action. Another theory put forth to explain early central effects of epidural narcotics purports that following absorption into the epidural venous plexus, under conditions of raised intrathoracic pressure, blood flow and drug could also be transported up the vertebral venous system directly to the brain, in addition to its normal entry into the inferior vena cava via the azygous vein (69).

Following epidural administration, redistribution, rather than systemic clearance, is probably more important in reducing plasma levels of these agents, which gain access to the systemic circulation and thus reduce the risk of respiratory depression. With the exception of a drug such as methadone (elimination clearance of only approximately 150 ml/min and plasma half-life of 36 hours), the ratio of the epidural dosing rate to plasma clearance will yield a low steady-state plasma concentration. For methadone the epidural dosing rate will result in relatively higher plasma concentrations at steady state, and because of the long half-life, accumulation to this level will not occur for several days.

Contraindications to subarachnoid or epidural narcotic administration include increased intracranial pressure, drug allergy, infection at the site of injection, and coagulopathy (a relative contraindication).

INTRATHECAL ADMINISTRATION OF NARCOTICS

Intrathecal morphine has been shown to reliably relieve postoperative pain for up to 24 hours following a single injection (76). Although doses have ranged as high as 20 mg, more-recent reports indicate that excellent analgesia for similar durations is obtained with doses in the range of 0.25–0.5 mg (72, 73). Because higher brain CSF concentrations should result and respiratory depression should be more likely with larger doses, it is recommended that the lower effective doses be used.

Despite the fact that subarachnoid administration is pharmacokinetically "cleaner" (i.e., the time and percentage of drug reaching the spinal CSF is precisely known and there is no significant systemic absorption), only in a minority of instances is this route of spinal opiate administration chosen (about 1.5% in the Swedish survey (75)); the remainder have used epidural injections. As will be discussed below, placement of an epidural catheter affords the advantage of dose titration to allow for interindividual variability as well as repeat doses without the increased risk that may accompany repeated needle placements or insertion of an indwelling intrathecal catheter. For operations in which a subarachnoid block is used, however, the addition of 0.25–0.5 mg of morphine to the local anesthetic was proven to be effective in providing about 24 hours of pain relief and did not appear to affect the local anesthetic block in any way (78, 79).

EPIDURAL ADMINISTRATION OF NARCOTICS

Choice of Agent

Various drugs have been used for postoperative epidural analgesia including local anesthetics, pure agonist narcotics, and the partial agonist and partial agonist-antagonist narcotics. Because many of these are experimental and not approved for epidural use, contain preservatives, or both, sufficient data are not yet available to properly evaluate their relative safety and efficacy. Preliminary evidence and experience to date suggests that the highly lipid-soluble agents may be preferable from a safety standpoint because rostral spread is limited (see earlier), but may not provide adequate thoracic analgesia when administered into the lumbar epidural space for this same reason. At this time either preservative-free morphine or hydromorphone seems to provide adequate postoperative analgesia for upper abdominal and thoracic surgery, whereas fentanyl or sufentanil provides safer (less respiratory depression) analgesia for lower abdominal and lower extremity pain.

Catheter Placement

Because of the increased technical difficulty and magnitude of complications related to placing and maintaining thoracic epidural catheters, placement of catheters into the epidural space higher than the lumbar level cannot be recommended for routine postoperative analgesia.

**Table 46.4.
Suggested Epidural Narcotic Orders**

1. Patient has epidural catheter for postoperative analgesia. Bolus of (e.g., fentanyl 100 μg qs to 10 ml NS) given at _____ (time).
2. Pharmacy to prepare _____ ml of _____ (drug) at a concentration of _____ mg/ml to run at an infusion rate of _____ ml/hr. Dose = _____ mg/hr.
3. No p.o./IM/IV narcotics, sedatives, or antiemetic medications without order from Pain Control Service.
4. Naloxone, 1 ampule of 0.4 mg at bedside at all times.
5. Maintain IV access while epidural infusion is in use.
6. Orders for nausea. (e.g., naloxone 0.1 mg IV—may be repeated q 10 min × 4 if needed; call Pain Control Service if ineffective)
7. Orders for pruritus. (e.g., same as above for nausea)
8. Orders to monitor respiratory rate. (e.g., apply vital sign monitor to patient and set respiratory rate alarm to 8/min; record respiratory rate q 1 hr)
9. Orders for respiratory depression. (e.g., for respiratory rate of 8/min or less, given naloxone 0.4 mg IV stat, then contact _____ ; For respiratory rate less than 12/min contact/ _____)
10. For inadequate analgesia, or questions/problems with the epidural catheter, contact _____ .

Routine Use

As opposed to transcutaneous electrical nerve stimulation (TENS) for somatic pain management, epidural narcotics are effective in relieving both somatic pain (orthopedic surgery) and visceral pain (thoracoabdominal surgery). Furthermore, there may exist a synergism between local anesthetic agents and narcotics that would make co-administration most efficacious. The relative merits of any of a number of methods of postoperative pain relief have yet to be elucidated. Even so, the use of an intravenous narcotic infusion or PCA, or regular intramuscular narcotic injections, can provide analgesia less invasively, require less technical skill, and possibly yield an equivalent or lower incidence of side effects or complications as compared to spinal opioid administration. Thus, the potential advantages of superior analgesia with spinal narcotics has to be justified in individual cases against the risks involved.

Taking all of this discussion into consideration and using the following guidelines, narcotic epidural analgesia has been found to be a very satisfactory method of postoperative pain management. A standardized form for orders prevents confusion and increases acceptance. An example of routine postoperative orders is reproduced in Table 46.4. A lumbar epidural catheter is placed either prior to or following the surgical procedure; the choice depends on logistical considerations, manpower and, obviously, whether or not the epidural catheter can or will be used to provide a component of the surgical anesthesia. One-half to one hour prior to the end of the surgical procedure, fentanyl (100 μg in 10 ml of saline) is injected into the catheter as a bolus and a continuous infusion of fentanyl (1250 μg in 125 ml of saline) at the rate of 0.5–1.0 μg/kg/hour is initiated. In the event of inadequate analgesia, noting the time to peak effect (up to 30 min), a repeat 100-μg bolus is given with an increase in the infusion rate up to a maximum of 1.5–2.0 μg/kg/hour (depending on patient comfort and respiratory rate). If there is any question that the catheter may be malpositioned, one can inject a bolus dose of an analgesic concentration of a local anesthetic agent (1–2% lidocaine). This maneuver will not only clarify the level of blockade, and likewise verify catheter position, but will also enable one to "catch up" with the patient's pain, which may be difficult to do with the narcotic alone (80). Among the advantages of this technique are that a continuous infusion decreases the incidence of tolerance and a lipophilic, rapid-onset drug decreases rostral CSF migration of drug. Because rostral spread is lessened, however, use of a lipophilic narcotic may not be as efficacious as the administration of a continuous epidural infusion of morphine following a thoracotomy. Finally, because of the continued concern regarding respiratory depression, appropriate patient surveillance must be provided (see below, "Side Effects of Neuraxial Opioids").

A comprehensive review of spinal opioids has been assembled by Cousins and Mather (76) and is recommended reading for those interested in pursuing this form of postoperative analgesia.

Tolerance

Tolerance is a problem often observed when spinal narcotics are used. Three separate methods can be used to combat the problem of tolerance. The first is alternating antinociceptive agents that are known to act on different systems (e.g., opioids vs. baclofen activation of a GABA system vs. ST-91, an alpha$_2$-adrenergic agonist). The second entails the continuous administration of the narcotic rather than intermittent exposure of the receptors to high concentrations from repeat bolus doses of the drug. The third reflects recent evidence that there are at least two populations of spinal opioid receptors, and that it might be possible to maintain spinal opioid analgesia for prolonged periods by alternating opioid agonists of different receptor characteristic as tolerance develops.

SIDE EFFECTS OF NEURAXIAL OPIOIDS

There are three groups of side effects or complications associated with the administration of epidural opioids aside from those related to the placement and extended use of an epidural catheter. These include, in order of increasing concern: (1) nausea/vomiting and pruritis, (2) urinary retention, (3) delayed diagnosis of a periop-

erative complication, and (4) sedation and respiratory depression.

Similar side effects are observed whether the opioids are injected into the intrathecal or the epidural spaces. In general the effects are seen more frequently and may be more severe when the intrathecal route is chosen (75). Most of what follows applies to both routes, but when significant differences occur, they will be mentioned.

Respiratory Depression

The complication of greatest concern is respiratory depression. Following epidural administration of narcotics, one may encounter acute and/or delayed respiratory depression, thus giving rise to the term *biphasic respiratory depression*. Because it is customary to carefully observe patients for the first 30–60 min following epidural injections, acute ventilatory depression occurring in a monitored patient, while of concern, does not command the attention and respect garnered by reports of respiratory depression or arrest occurring up to 12 hours later. As mentioned above, early respiratory depression can be explained on the basis of significant plasma narcotic levels occurring as a result of absorption into the systemic circulation from the epidural space. Because absorption from the CSF is slower and intrathecal doses are much smaller, early respiratory depression by this mechanism should not occur.

Delayed respiratory depression was reported following the use of intrathecal morphine (73, 74) in the same year, 1979, as the first report of its therapeutic use (81). These reports have been followed by many others. It appears that the opioid-naive surgical patient is at much greater risk than the more-tolerant cancer patient (82). With morphine, the onset of respiratory depression occurs 6–11 hours following injection and can last for up to 24 hours (76). It is generally responsive to naloxone, intravenous doses of 0.1–0.2 mg repeated every 2 min until attaining the desired effect, without sacrificing the spinal analgesic effect. Because the respiratory depression will last longer than the antagonism of the intravenous doses of naloxone, a continuous naloxone infusion should be started at a rate of 5 μg/kg/hour titrated to maintain eupnea, and continued for at least 24 hours.

When used for postoperative analgesia any of the following factors may contribute to the onset of delayed respiratory depression:

1. The concomitant administration of parenteral opioids other than those injected into the epidural space. This includes premedication or intraoperative administration as well as parenteral administration of narcotics after the analgesia provided by the epidural opioid has "worn off."
2. The residual effect of other centrally acting depressants administered during anesthesia.
3. An alteration or increase in drug transfer to the CNS via venous or CSF distribution. Increased intratho-

racic pressure from airway obstruction, grunting or positive pressure ventilation, and increased intra-abdominal pressure are all mechanisms by which rostral CSF flow may be augmented. These same pressure changes may cause epidural venous blood flow to be redirected through basivertebral veins to the brain.

4. Accidental dural puncture or delayed catheter migration through the dura would result in direct injection of a relative overdose (approximately 5–10 times) of the narcotic into the CSF.

5. Patient factors, such as advanced age and pulmonary insufficiency, have been found to increase risk.

Although the expected incidence of delayed respiratory depression can be made very low by attention to the predisposing factors, some provision for detecting its onset must be made. A controversy continues as to the level of monitoring required for a patient receiving spinal narcotics (i.e., Intensive Care Unit, monitored bed, or conventional postoperative care). Because the time course of respiratory depression is not well documented, disagreements about proper monitoring continue. Advocates of routine postoperative vigilance argue that the respiratory depression is not an acute occurrence but rather insidious and predictable, the gradual decrease in respiratory rate recorded every 30–60 min being easily noted. Others insist that the patient must be monitored in an intensive care setting. A large-scale study with an adequate number of patients clearly demonstrating the natural history of delayed respiratory depression/arrest is needed to resolve this debate. Accordingly, measures taken will vary from institution to institution and may even vary within an institution. Some have found devices that detect and measure respiratory rate to be useful, whereas others have relied on frequent observation. Regardless of the monitoring practice, nurses in units that care for these postoperative patients must be properly trained concerning the clinical course following spinal narcotic injections and instructed that naloxone and apparatus to artificially support ventilation should be readily available and used whenever decreased ventilatory rates or sedation are detected.

Delayed Diagnosis

Profound analgesia in the postoperative period does have its down side. Normally, a new onset of pain is the first indicator of a postoperative complication. If a pain control service is not aware of the possible surgical complications and strictly attempts to ablate all pain, the diagnosis of a postoperative complication may be unnecessarily delayed. A compartment syndrome of the lower leg may (83) or may not (84) be delayed by postoperative epidural analgesia. A delay in diagnosis can lead to a delay in appropriate therapy and permanent nerve damage.

Nausea and Vomiting

Nausea may be observed in 15–50% of cases of epidural narcotic administration and perhaps more frequently when narcotics are given intrathecally. Vomiting will occur in only about one-quarter of those patients reporting nausea. Onset of nausea and vomiting is noted to coincide with the onset of trigeminal analgesia approximately 6 hours after epidural or intrathecal injection and so, like respiratory depression, this side effect probably results from rostral migration of drug, in this case to the vomiting center and the chemoreceptor trigger zone.

The incidence appears to decrease with repeated doses and in chronic treatment of cancer patients. Systemic opioids and pain itself may cause nausea and vomiting in postoperative patients. Although nausea has also been reported after epidural fentanyl administration, the incidence, like that for respiratory depression, is much lower because of its lipophilicity and minimal central spread. Treatment of this side effect may be accomplished with naloxone or nalbuphine (85).

Urinary Retention

The incidence of urinary retention has been reported to be similar to that of nausea and vomiting, with 39% of postoperative patients requiring catheterization of the bladder in one study (86). Urinary retention, although not life-threatening, is a problem for patients not requiring urethral catheterization for other reasons. One hypothesis regarding the inability to void involves inhibition of acetylcholine release from efferent postganglionic neurons innervating the detrusor muscle, due to binding at opiate receptors. Hence, naloxone and/or bethanechol can relieve urinary retention in some subjects. Likewise, urinary retention subsides with subsequent exposures to the narcotics and is seen more often in volunteers than in postoperative surgical patients, and is rare in those with chronically treated cancer pain.

Pruritis

Pruritis may occur in 50–75% of postoperative patients given spinal opiates, although fewer than one-quarter of these may require treatment. Pruritis, although not apparently related to histamine release (it can even occur following fentanyl administration), is thought to be due to a widespread alteration in sensory modulation, particularly in regions of the upper cervical cord. Pruritis has been treated with promethazine and nalbuphine (85).

Summary

Pruritis, nausea, vomiting, and bladder dysfunction can all often subside with subsequent doses of the narcotic as an adaptation to the changes in sensation or the brain's tolerance to these side effects (much like that seen with respiratory depression). Although specific therapy, such as the administration of droperidol for nausea, may be effective, all side effects are antagonized by intravenous naloxone or nalbuphine without diminishing the analgesia provided by the spinal narcotic. Nalbuphine may cause increased sedation, however, especially in the aged. Furthermore, the incidence of all side effects, with the possible exception of urinary retention, can be diminished by the administration of highly lipid-soluble drugs such as fentanyl, thereby reducing the concentration of the agent presented via the CSF to the upper cord and brain.

Epidural Opioid/Local Anesthetic Combinations

One way of reducing the adverse effects of any agent is to reduce the dose. Lowering a dose to avoid side effects may also lead to less efficacious therapy, however. Therefore, an alternative approach that will maintain or enhance analgesia while lowering the incidence of opioid-induced adverse effects is the addition of a dilute solution of local anesthetic to the opioid for epidural administration (87). One combination that has found widespread use is fentanyl (10 μg/ml) and bupivacaine (1 mg/ml, 0.1%). The formulation used for a bolus/continuous infusion technique is fentanyl (1250 μg) in 25 ml 0.5% bupivacaine (125 mg) diluted with 75 ml of 0.9% normal saline (125 ml total volume). An initial bolus of 10 ml is given and followed immediately by an infusion of 0.5–1.5 ml/kg/hour as necessary. The addition of the local anesthetic, even at this low a concentration (0.1%), can elicit a sympathetic block. In the early postoperative period, especially in a poor-risk patient, this may increase the complexity of fluid management. Although some add the local anesthetic routinely when initiating postoperative epidural analgesia, others add it to the infusion only if side effects warrant a decrease in opioid dose or if pain is unresponsive to higher opioid doses alone.

PERIPHERAL NERVE BLOCKS

Intercostal Nerve Blocks

Intercostal nerve blocks have been useful for the treatment of postoperative pain in patients undergoing thoracotomies as well as for those having upper abdominal operations such as cholecystectomies. The major advantage is the relief of pain without the CNS side effects that may accompany systemically administered opioids. As discussed above, analgesia is important following these operations in order to permit satisfactory chest physiotherapy for clearing pulmonary secretions, and maintaining functional residual capacity. Kaplan et al. have shown that intercostal nerve blocks both significantly alleviate postoperative pain following thoracotomy and improve pulmonary function; these authors advocate their use whenever possible (88). Galway and co-workers also found good pain relief but did not show

any improvement in pulmonary function in the postoperative period (89). The major complication of intercostal block is symptomatic pneumothorax. Moore and Bridenbaugh have shown that the incidence is 1:1100 even with resident physicians performing the blocks (90). This is approximately the risk of clinically significant respiratory depression found with epidural opioid analgesia (91).

The 11 intercostal nerves and 1 subcostal nerve (beneath the 12th rib) are mixed motor and sensory and are formed from their respective spinal nerve roots and travel in the subcostal grooves with the intercostal arteries and veins. A collateral intercostal motor nerve splits from the main nerve and travels between the inner and innermost intercostal muscles along the lower margin of the intercostal space. Branches of the main intercostal nerve are given off that supply the skin over the lateral aspects of the thorax and abdomen. The upper six intercostal nerves pass anteriorly and end up as the anterior cutaneous branch that supplies the skin over the anterior chest and the parietal pleura, whereas the lower six do the same for the anterior abdomen and the parietal peritoneum as well as the abdominal muscles.

For treatment after abdominal procedures the patient is either placed in the prone or the lateral position (usually performed 7–9 cm lateral to the posterior midline). The injection must be made proximal to the origin of the lateral perforating branches that arise near the midaxillary line. This should be repeated at four or five interspaces if the wound is clearly unilateral and at matching contralateral interspaces if the wound extends to the midline.

With thoracotomies the surgeon can inject the local anesthetic solution under direct vision from within the chest. For adequate analgesia it is usually necessary to block four or five nerves at the level of the thoracotomy wound and two at the level of the drainage tube site.

Loder showed that the addition of dextran to a 1% lidocaine solution significantly extended the duration of anesthetic block (92). Kaplan et al. (88) demonstrated that this principle was applicable to intercostal blocks with 0.75% bupivacaine by addition of an equal volume of low-molecular-weight dextran-40. This mixture produced 36 hours of analgesia, whereas bupivacaine with saline produced a block lasting 12 hours. In the study of Galway and co-workers, in which poor results were obtained, both 0.5% bupivacaine and 1% lidocaine provided only about 3 hours of pain relief (89).

An anatomic study by Nunn and Slavin demonstrated that fluid injected into the intercostal space could easily spread superiorly and inferiorly behind the parietal pleura (93). In a case report O'Kelly and Garry used this information to give continuous analgesia to a patient with fractured ribs via an epidural catheter left in the intercostal space (94). They were able to provide analgesia from the fourth to the tenth segments with injections of 20 ml 0.5% bupivacaine. Similar spread of 20 ml of radiopaque fluid corroborates that the analgesia is a result of direct spread of the local anesthetic. Murphy went on to use the technique for postoperative pain relief following cholecystectomy and renal surgery (95). Restelli et al. have described a variation of this technique in which a catheter is inserted during thoracotomy (96).

Kvalheim and Reiestad described a novel intrapleural approach for blocking intercostal nerves for postoperative pain following cholecystectomy and renal and mammary operations (97). Their technique calls for insertion of a Touhy needle in an anesthetized patient lying in the lateral position. The insertion site is between the eighth and ninth ribs and the angle is about 45° (not perpendicular, as with Murphy's technique). After "walking off" the lower border of the upper rib and advancing the 3 mm into the intercostal space, the trocar is removed and a freely sliding glass syringe is attached to the needle. These are then advanced together until the parietal pleura is punctured; confirmation is achieved when the negative pleural pressure draws in the syringe's plunger. An epidural catheter can then be inserted 4–6 cm, and 20 ml 0.5% bupivacaine is injected to provide effective analgesia for 6–24 hours, at which time similar "top-up" doses can be given.

Concerns about this technique have been raised by Covino (98), suggesting that its wide acceptance should follow further research examining its mechanism, particularly concerning the nerves involved in providing analgesia, possible sympathetic and diaphragmatic effects, and further data about drug selection and dose.

BRACHIAL PLEXUS BLOCK

Selander has suggested that postoperative analgesia following upper extremity surgery be maintained with a brachial plexus sheath catheter for a continuous technique analogous to the continuous intercostal technique described above (99). This form of analgesia is particularly advantageous in that the accompanying sympathetic block, which can be maintained for several days, enhances graft survival.

A catheter can be threaded into the brachial plexus sheath from either the axillary, interscalene, or infraclavicular approaches. Improved success in gaining access to this space is associated with the use of the short bevel needle, which produces a "click" when this tissue plane is entered. Confidence is increased if one obtains a concomitant loss of resistance. A catheter can be inserted through the needle using a specially designed kit, or over the needle if standard intravenous catheters (at least 6.4 cm in length) are used.

SURGICAL WOUND PERFUSION

A recent report has shown that injection of 10 ml of 0.5% bupivacaine or saline directly into a drainage catheter (placed between the peritoneum and muscle layer

along the entire length of a Kocher subcostal incision for cholecystectomy) every 4 hours provides excellent pain relief (100). Though some patients experienced complete freedom from pain, they still suffered the usual fall in vital capacity. The fact that saline was as effective as bupivacaine in relieving pain and reducing narcotic requirement was explained in terms of the wound irrigation displacing humoral agents such as histamine and vasoactive peptides, which are thought to contribute to postoperative pain.

FIELD BLOCKS

Field blocks are often used to provide analgesia following relatively minor procedures such as inguinal herniorrhaphy and augmentation mammoplasty. The pain following such operations is generally the most intense during the first 8–12 hours. Injecting 0.25–0.5% bupivacaine with 1:200,000 or 1:400,000 epinephrine in a wide area, and down to the fascial plains to block the nerve branches supplying the area, can often produce significant analgesia for the first postoperative day and may obviate or reduce the need for other postoperative analgesic medications.

Field block for inguinal herniorrhaphy is made effective by injecting 20–30 ml of 0.5% bupivacaine with 1:200,000 epinephrine in a series of fan-like injections deep to the external oblique muscle in order to block the ilioinguinal and iliohypogastric nerves.

Another form of field block is the instillation of 40 ml of 0.25% bupivacaine into the intra-articular space following knee arthroscopy. This technique is also useful for outpatients.

Two recent publications provide evidence that the use of field blocks prior to incision affords excellent postoperative analgesia (101, 102). Both articles suggest that the prevention of the nociceptive impulses from reaching the CNS appears to be a key factor. Their hypothesis is that blockade of the surgical field suppresses the formation of the sustained hyperexcitable state in the CNS that is responsible for the maintenance of postoperative pain. This hypothesis, if true, supports the practice of injecting a local anesthetic into the site of the incision prior to most surgical procedures.

TRANSCUTANEOUS ELECTRICAL NERVE STIMULATION

Transcutaneous electrical nerve stimulation (TENS) is the practice of applying controlled low-voltage electrical pulses to the nervous system by passing electrical current through the skin. Initially, TENS was implemented as a screening procedure to assess the potential efficacy of dorsal column stimulators, placed surgically, in an effort to obtain relief of chronic pain. Although TENS was not successful as a screening tool, it was noted to provide a degree of local analgesia. Since that time TENS has become another treatment modality within the available armamentarium of a comprehensive program for chronic pain management (Chapter 12) while gaining a varying level of acceptability in the treatment of postoperative pain.

Applied Physiology

The physiology and pathophysiology of nociceptive impulse transmission, modulation, and perception has been described above. An explanation of TENS is but an extension of this neurophysiology.

The rationale for the use of electrical stimulation to produce analgesia is based on two separate mechanisms responsible for inhibition of nociception. The particular mechanism that applies might best be explained according to the type of electrical signal delivered to the affected region. In general, these two mechanisms are best explained as a neuromodulation technique based on the gate control theory of pain first described by Melzack and Wall (103). This theory postulates that large myelinated A-beta fiber activity inhibits nociceptive transmission ("closes the gate"), whereas activity in the smaller A-delta and C-fibers facilitates nociception ("opens the gate"). It has been demonstrated that large myelinated fibers have a low threshold for electrical stimulation. One form of TENS, involving the delivery of a series of impulses to and conducted by these large fibers, closes the spinal gate and thus the transmission of nociceptive impulses to the spinothalamic tract.

Cortical, and particularly midbrain, structures are the origins of descending fibers, which are part of an inhibitory neural system blocking transmission at several different levels in the CNS. The cortical origins of descending fibers further modulate the spinal gating mechanisms and account for cognitive processes influencing pain perception. The second mechanism thought to explain stimulation-produced analgesia (SPA) involves those inhibitory neurons which are part of a larger neural system that is selectively stimulated by morphine-like substances and blocked by the narcotic antagonist, naloxone. Opiate receptors have been identified in the substantia gelatinosa (laminae II and III of the dorsal horn) and the periaqueductal gray matter of the brain (Fig 46.1). The former is the proposed site of the spinal gating mechanism, and the latter is thought to be the origin and central control trigger for the descending anti-nociceptive fibers of the dorsolateral funiculus. It is therefore theorized that a second form of TENS results in SPA by effecting a release of endogenous morphine-like ligands in the brain.

In fact, these two separate mechanisms of action may play a part in the analgesic effects of TENS, which, as stated, depends on the type of stimulation delivered. For low-intensity, high-frequency stimuli (conventional TENS), the stimulation of the large myelinated A-beta fibers closes the gate to transmission of noxious impulses. This more-peripheral mechanism is not blocked by naloxone (104). As an alternative, high-intensity, low-frequency stimulation (acupuncture-like TENS) may cause release of endorphins that subsequently attach to receptors and thereby inhibit nociception. In fact, this second theory is consistent with the observations that TENS is not effective in patients with a history of prolonged narcotic use (105) and that other patients will respond to this high-intensity stimuli, administered for brief periods, with prolonged periods of pain relief.

Practical Considerations

Although TENS devices are manufactured and marketed by various companies, only recently have standards been developed for the manufacture and marketing of TENS units. The Neurosurgery Committee of the Association for the Advancement of Medical Instrumentation (AAMI) has established standards for labeling of the devices, electrical safety, and performance requirements as well as terminology.

Most stimulators produce either a symmetric or an asymmetric biphasic output in an effort to prevent iontophoresis or electrolysis (i.e., transfer of ions from the skin to the electrode and back). This biphasic current must be delivered equally in each phase of the wave, with the asymmetric wave being more comfortable for the patient. The frequency (given in pulses per second), the pulse width (in microseconds), and the pulse amplitude are the variables that, along with electrode placement, determine the mechanism of action and efficacy of this mode of therapy. The goal of selecting the optimal parameters for conventional (high-frequency) TENS is to specifically elicit recruitment of the large, densely myelinated afferent nerve fibers (as consistent with the aforementioned peripheral gate control theory of pain) to affect control of pain. Briefly, conventional TENS for postoperative analgesia is delivered through sterile pre-gelled electrodes applied to the skin approximately 1 cm away from the suture line. Initial parameters include a pulse width varying between 60 and 150 μsec with a stimulus frequency of 80–150 pulses/sec and an amplitude of 12–20 mA (that current which provides analgesia without muscle contractions). Initial settings at the low end of these ranges usually provides excellent clinical benefit. Conventional (high-frequency, low-amplitude) stimulation can provide rapid-onset, continuous analgesia for 48–72 hours.

Alternatively, there is acupuncture-like TENS which, because of the alleged stimulation of endogenous opiate release, does not require selective recruitment of afferent nerve fiber classes. Rather, results are only obtained with recruitment of motor fibers and the resultant visible muscle twitches. Therefore, stimulation parameters include a pulse width of 200–300 μsec at a rate of 1–4 pulses/sec. In this instance, as opposed to those parameters recommended for conventional TENS, amplitude is adjusted to produce visible muscle twitches within the tolerance levels of the patient. Whereas conventional

TENS has an immediate onset of analgesia, low-rate TENS does not produce immediate relief—the onset of analgesia may be delayed by as much as 30 min. Furthermore, the application of stimulation should be limited to no longer than about 45 min, to avoid residual muscle fatigue and concomitant soreness. The duration of analgesia usually persists for a prolonged period, as is consistent with the release and binding of a hormone rather than electrical events of the nervous system, which take place in seconds or milliseconds.

A hybrid of these two techniques is best described as *pulse-train* or *burst* TENS with, likewise, an effect and mechanistic explanation consistent with a combination of the two more widely used techniques just described. Parameters for pulse-train TENS include five pulses each of 200–300 μsec delivered over 100 msec at a frequency of one to four pulse-trains/sec and at an amplitude sufficient to produce visible muscle twitches. Because muscle twitches will occur at a lower current setting with this mode of delivery of the stimuli, pulse-train TENS will provide a more-comfortable sensation for the patient.

These types of therapy can easily be delivered by any one of many different TENS devices currently available. Several different options should be available on the particular device being employed, however. First, to deliver acupuncture-like TENS, the device must be capable of delivering rates as low as a single pulse per second. Likewise, the device must be capable of delivering one of various waveforms of adjustable width. Those generating spike waveform energy usually have external variables limited to pulse rate and amplitude. These types offer less flexibility and fewer applications. Although several different waveforms are available from various manufacturers, no one waveform has proven to be better than any other in TENS therapy. Constant-current rather than constant-voltage generators have several advantages, however. For any given waveform, one that is biphasic with a zero net DC current will reduce skin reaction and increase patient comfort. Finally, the more-advanced devices offer automatic variation in set parameters to minimize nerve adaptation or accommodation (more frequently seen with conventional TENS). By incorporating modulating features that automatically alter the frequency, pulse width, or delivered current amplitude within a preset range, these units restore effectiveness, increase tolerance to stronger stimuli, and delay accommodation. A book by Mannheimer and Lampe is an invaluable teaching resource and reference for the novice or expert wishing to pursue the use of this modality in the treatment of acute, primarily musculoskeletal pain (106). The use of TENS appears to offer a number of advantages in the treatment of acute pain because the problems of respiratory depression, sedation, orthostatic hypotension, drug reaction, drug delivery, and urinary retention can be avoided. However, although most articles claim that the use of TENS therapy decreases the amount of opioids used in comparison to a control (sham TENS therapy) group, others have failed to demonstrate any decrease (107).

CRYOANALGESIA

Cryotherapy is gaining increasing popularity in the management of chronic pain. This is primarily because of the recent introduction of cryotherapy needle probes and their attendant apparatus that allow this modality to be implemented using a percutaneous approach similar to that used for other major nerve blocks with local anesthetics or neurolytics. Earlier probes required direct visualization of the nerve and application of a relatively large probe. Although this method for producing analgesia was found to be efficacious for post-thoracotomy pain (108, 109), extension of this technique to other types of acute pain seems impractical. First, the nerve block has a duration (one to several months) greatly exceeding the usual duration of acute pain (48–72 hours). Second, the resulting nerve block is myocutaneous, or nondifferential, and will block motor function as well as sensory perception. Finally, the resolution of the block by nerve regeneration within an intact sheath may be accompanied by a prolonged period of hypasthesia. Maiwand et al. report their review (no control group) of cryoanalgesia after thoracotomy in 600 cases using an improved (Maiwand) probe and a shorter cryoexposure (110). Their favorable experience and their recommendations (no cryotherapy above the fifth intercostal nerve in women) provide further optimism for this technique. Clearly, further investigation of these techniques must be completed before cryoanalgesia will gain widespread application.

REFERENCES

1. McIlvaine WB: Perioperative pain management in children. *J Pain Symp Manag* 4:215–229, 1989.
2. Ferreira SH, Nakamura M: II-Prostaglandin hyperalgesia: The peripheral analgesic activity of morphine, enkephalins and opioid antagonists. *Prostaglandins* 18:191–200, 1979.
3. Stein C, Comisel K, Haimerl E, Yassouridis A, Lehrgerger K, Herz K, Peter K: Analgesic effect of intraarticular morphine after arthroscopic knee surgery. *N Engl J Med* 325:1123–1126, 1991.
4. Anonymous: Postoperative pain [Editorial]. *Br Med J* 2:517–518, 1978.
5. Utting JE, Smith JM: Postoperative analgesia. *Anaesthesia* 34:320–332, 1979.
6. Anonymous: Postoperative pain [Editorial]. *Br Med J* 2:664, 1976.
7. Mather LE: Pharmacokinetic and pharmacodynamic factors influencing the choice, dose and route of administration of opiates for acute pain. In Bullingham RES (ed): *Clinics in Anaesthesiology*, vol. 1, no. 1. London, WB Saunders, 1983, pp 17–40.

8. Weis OF, Sriwatanakul K, Alloza JL, et al: Attitudes of patients, housestaff, and nurses toward postoperative analgesic care. *Anesth Analg* 62:70–74, 1983.

9. Porter J, Jick H: Addiction in rare patients with narcotics [Letter]. *N Engl J Med* 302:123, 1980.

10. Miller RR: Clinical effects of parenteral narcotics in hospitalized patients. *J Clin Pharmacol* 20:165–171, 1980.

11. Marks RM, Sachar EJ: Undertreatment of medical inpatients with narcotic analgesics. *Ann Intern Med* 78:173–181, 1973.

12. Angell M: The quality of mercy [Editorial]. *N Engl J Med* 306:98–99, 1982.

13. Keats AS: Postoperative pain: Research and treatment. *J Chronic Dis* 4:72–83, 1956.

14. Dahlstrom B, Tamsen A, Paalzow L, et al: Patient-controlled analgesic therapy. Part IV: Pharmacokinetics and analgesic plasma concentrations of morphine. *Clin Pharmacokinet* 7:266–279, 1982.

15. Duthie DJR, McLaren AD, Nimmo WS: Pharmacokinetics of fentanyl during constant rate I.V. infusion for the relief of pain after surgery. *Br J Anaesth* 58:950–956, 1986.

16. Ausems ME, Hug CC Jr, Stanski DR, et al: Plasma concentrations of alfentanil required to supplement nitrous oxide anesthesia for general surgery. *Anesthesiology* 65:362–373, 1986.

17. Scott JC, Ponganis KV, Stanski DR: EEG quantitation of narcotic effect: The comparative pharmacodynamics of fentanyl and alfentanil. *Anesthesiology* 62:234–241, 1985.

18. Gourlay GK, Willis RJ, Wilson PR: Postoperative pain control with morphine: Influence of supplementary methadone doses and blood concentration-response relationships. *Anesthesiology* 61:19–26, 1984.

19. Tamsen A, Bondesson V, Dahlstrom B, et al: Patient-controlled analgesic therapy: Part III. Pharmacokinetics and analgesic plasma concentrations of ketobemidone. *Clin Pharmacokinet* 7:252–265, 1982.

20. Austin KL, Stapleton JV, Mather LE: Relationship between blood meperidine concentrations and analgesic response: A preliminary report. *Anesthesiology* 53:460–466, 1980.

21. Tamsen A, Hartvig P, Fagerlund C, et al: Patient-controlled analgesic therapy: Part II. Individual analgesic demand and analgesic plasma concentrations of pethidine in postoperative pain. *Clin Pharmacokinet* 7:164–175, 1982.

22. Tamsen A, Sakurada T, Wahlstrom A, et al: Postoperative demand for analgesics in relation to individual levels of endorphins and substance P in cerebrospinal fluid. *Pain* 13:171–183, 1982.

23. Mather LE, Lindop MJ, Tucker GT: Pethidine revisited: Plasma concentrations and effects after intramuscular injection. *Br J Anaesth* 47:1269–1275, 1975.

24. Neal EA, Meffin PJ, Gregory PG, et al: Enhanced bioavailability and decreased clearance of analgesics in patients with cirrhosis. *Gastroenterology* 77:96–102, 1979.

25. Klotz U, McHorse TS, Wilkinson GR, et al: The effect of cirrhosis on the disposition and elimination of meperidine in man. *Clin Pharmacol Ther* 16:667–675, 1974.

26. McHorse TS, Wilkinson GR, Schenker S: The effect of acute viral hepatitis in man on the disposition and elimination of meperidine. *Gastroenterology* 68:775–780, 1975.

27. Patawardhan RV, Johnson RF, Hoyumpa A, et al: Normal metabolism of morphine in cirrhosis. *Gastroenterology* 81:1006–1011, 1981.

28. Moore RA, Sear JW, Bullingham RES, et al: Morphine kinetics in renal failure. In Foley KM, Inturrisi CE (eds): *Advances in Pain Research and Therapy*, vol 8. New York, Raven Press, 1986, pp 65–72.

29. Inturrisi CE, Umans JG: Meperidine biotransformation and central nervous system toxicity in animals and humans. In Foley KM, Inturrisi CE (eds): *Advances in Pain Research and Therapy*, vol 8. New York, Raven Press, 1986, pp 143–153.

30. Sawe J: Morphine and its 3- and 6-glucuronides in plasma and urine during chronic oral administration in cancer patients. In Foley KM, Inturrisi CE (eds): *Advances in Pain Research and Therapy*, vol 8. New York, Raven Press, 1986, pp 45–55.

31. Nagashima H, Karamanian A, Malovany R, et al: Respiratory and circulatory effects of intravenous butorphanol and morphine. *Clin Pharmacol Ther* 19:738–745, 1976.

32. Romagnoli A, Keats AS: Ceiling effect for respiratory depression by nalbuphine. *Clin Pharmacol Ther* 27:478–485, 1980.

33. Murphy MR, Hug CC Jr: The enflurane sparing effect of morphine, butorphanol, and nalbuphine. *Anesthesiology* 57:489–492, 1982.

34. Kay B: On-demand nalbuphine for post-operative pain. *Anaesthetist* 32(Suppl):366–367, 1983.

35. Fragen RJ, Caldwell N: Acute intravenous premedication with nalbuphine. *Anesth Analg* 56:808–812, 1977.

36. Latasch L, Probst S, Dudziak R: Reversal by nalbuphine of respiratory depression caused by fentanyl. *Anesth Analg* 63:814–816, 1984.

37. Freye E, Hartung E, Segeth M: Nalbuphine reverses fentanyl-related EEG-changes in man. *Acta Anaesthesiol Belg* 35:25–36, 1984.

38. Cooper SA: New peripherally-acting oral analgesic agents. *Ann Rev Pharmacol Toxicol* 23:617–647, 1983.

39. Basbaum AI, Levine JD: Opiate analgesia: How central is a peripheral target? [Editorial]. *N Engl J Med* 325:1168–1169, 1991.

40. McQuay HJ, Poppleton P, Carroll D, et al: Ketorolac and acetaminophen for orthopedic postoperative pain. *Clin Pharmacol Ther* 39:89–93, 1986.

41. O'Hara DA, Fragen RJ, Kinzer M, et al: Ketorolac tromethamine as compared with morphine sulfate for treatment of postoperative pain. *Clin Pharmacol Ther* 41:556–561, 1987.

42. Jones RM, Cashman JN, Foster JMG, et al: Comparison of infusions of morphine and lysine acetyl salicylate for the relief of pain following thoracic surgery. *Br J Anaesth* 57:259–263, 1985.

43. Dahl JB, Kehlet H: Non-steroidal anti-inflammatory drugs: Rationale for use in severe postoperative pain. *Br J Anaesth* 66:703–712, 1991.

44. Sunshine A, Roure C, Olsen N, et al: Analgesic efficacy of two ibuprofen-codeine combinations for the treatment of postepesiotomy and postoperative pain. *Clin Pharmacol Ther* 42:374–380, 1987.

45. Bloor BC, Flacke WE: Reduction in halothane anesthetic requirement by clonidine, an alpha adrenergic agonist. *Anesth Analg* 61:741–745, 1982.

46. Fitzgerald M: Monoamines and descending control of nociception. *Trends Neurosci* 9:51–52, 1986.

47. Maze M, Tranquilli W: Alpha-2 adrenoceptor agonists: Defining the role in clinical anesthesia. *Anesthesiology* 74:581–605, 1991.

48. Goldfarb G, Ang ET, Debaene B, et al: Effect of clonidine on postoperative shivering in man: A double blind study. *Anesthesiology* 71:A649, 1989.

49. Quintin L, Roux C, Macquin I, et al: Clonidine blunts the endocrine and circulatory surge during recovery of aortic surgery. *Anesthesiology* 71:155, 1989.

50. Bernard JM, Lechevalier T, Pinaud M, et al: Postoperative analgesia by IV clonidine. *Anesthesiology* 71:154, 1989.

51. Eisenach JC, Lysak SZ, Viscomi CM: Epidural clonidine analgesia following surgery: Phase I. *Anesthesiology* 71:640–646, 1989.

52. Bonnet F, Boico O, Rostaing S, et al: Clonidine-induced analgesia in postoperative patients: Epidural versus intramuscular administration. *Anesthesiology* 72:423–427, 1990.

53. Beecher HK: Anxiety and pain [Editorial]. *JAMA* 209:1080, 1969.

54. Keeri-Szanto M: The mode of action of promethazine in potentiating narcotic drugs. *Br J Anaesth* 46:918–924, 1974.

55. Hupert C, Yacoub M, Turgeon LR: Effect of hydroxyzine on morphine analgesia for the treatment of postoperative pain. *Anesth Analg* 59:690–696, 1980.

56. Forrest WH, Brown BW, Brown CR, et al: Dextroamphetamine with morphine for the treatment of postoperative pain. *N Eng J Med* 296:712–715, 1977.

57. Yang JC, Clark WC, Ngai SH, et al: Analgesic action and pharmacokinetics of morphine and diazepam in man: An evaluation by sensory decision theory. *Anesthesiology* 51:495–502, 1979.

58. McKenzie R, Wadhwa RK, Lim Uy NT, et al: Antiemetic effectiveness of intramuscular hydroxyzine compared with intramuscular droperidol. *Anesth Analg* 60:783–788, 1981.

59. Hug CC Jr: Lipid solubility, pharmacokinetics, and the EEG: Are you better off today than you were four years ago? [Editorial]. *Anesthesiology* 62:221–225, 1985.

60. Beaver WT, Wallenstein SL, Houde RW, et al: A clinical comparison of the analgesic effects of methadone and morphine administered intramuscularly, and of orally and parenterally administered methadone. *Clin Pharmacol Ther* 8:415–426, 1967.

61. Hug CC Jr: Improving analgesic therapy [Editorial]. *Anesthesiology* 53:441–443, 1980.

62. Welchew EA: On-demand analgesia. *Anaesthesia* 38:19–25, 1983.

63. Goudie TA, Allen MWB, Lonsdale M, et al: Continuous subcutaneous infusion of morphine for postoperative pain relief. *Anaesthesia* 40:1086–1092, 1985.

64. Holley FO, van Steenis C: Transdermal administration of fentanyl for postoperative analgesia. *Anesthesiology* 65:548, 1986.

65. Harmer M, Slattery PJ, Rosen M, et al: Intramuscular on-demand analgesia: Double-blind controlled trial of pethidine, buprenorphine, morphine and meptazinol. *Br Med J* 286:680–682, 1983.

66. Lehmann KA, Tenbuhs B: Patient-controlled analgesia with nalbuphine, a new narcotic agonist-antagonist, for the treatment of postoperative pain. *Eur J Clin Pharmacol* 31:267–276, 1986.

67. Chakravarty K, Tucker W, Rosen M, et al: Comparison of buprenorphine and pethidine given intravenously on demand to relieve postoperative pain. *Br Med J* 2:895–897, 1979.

68. Harmer M, Rosen M, Vickers MD: *Patient-Controlled Analgesia*. Oxford, Blackwell Scientific Publication, 1985.

69. Yaksh TL: Spinal opiate analgesia: Characteristics and principles of action. *Pain* 11:293–346, 1981.

70. Graham JL, King R, McCaughey W: Postoperative pain relief using epidural morphine. *Anaesthesia* 35:158–160, 1980.

71. Mathews ET, Abrams LD: Intrathecal morphine in open heart surgery. *Lancet* 1:543, 1980.

72. Bromage PR, Camporesi EM, Chestnut D: Epidural narcotics for postoperative analgesia. *Anesth Analg* 59:473–480, 1980.

73. Glynn CJ, Mather LE, Cousins MJ, et al: Spinal narcotics and respiratory depression. *Lancet* 2:356–357, 1979.

74. Liolios A, Andersen FH: Selective spinal analgesia. *Lancet* 2:357, 1979.

75. Gustafsson LL, Shildt B, Jacobsen K: Adverse effects of extradural and intrathecal opiates: Report of a nationwide survey in Sweden. *Br J Anaesth* 54:479–486, 1982.

76. Cousins MJ, Mather LE: Intrathecal and epidural administration opioids. *Anesthesiology* 61:276–310, 1984.

77. Chauvin M, Samii K, Schermann JM, et al: Plasma pharmacokinetics of morphine after I.M., extradural and intrathecal administration. *Br J Anaesth* 54:843–847, 1981.

78. Katz J, Nelson W: Intrathecal morphine for postoperative pain relief. *Regional Anesthesia* 6:1–3, 1981.

79. Nordberg G, Hedner T, Mellstrand T, et al: Pharmacokinetic aspects of intrathecal morphine analgesia. *Anesthesiology* 60:448–454, 1984.

80. Chambers WA, Sinclair CJ, Scott DB: Extradural morphine for pain after surgery. *Br J Anaesth* 53:921–925, 1981.

81. Wang JK, Nauss LA, Thomas JE: Pain relief by intrathecally applied morphine in man. *Anesthesiology* 50:149–151, 1979.

82. Zenz M, Schappler-Scheele B, Neuhans R, et al: Longterm peridural morphine analgesia in cancer pain. *Lancet* 1:91, 1981.

83. Strecker WB, Wood MB, Bieber EJ: Compartment syndrome masked by epidural anesthesia for postoperative pain. *J Bone Joint Surg [Am]* 68:1447–1448, 1986.

84. Montgomery CJ, Ready LB: Epidural opioid analgesia does not obscure diagnosis of compartment syndrome resulting from prolonged lithotomy position. *Anesthesiology* 75:541–543, 1991.

85. Henderson SK, Cohen H: Nalbuphine augmentation of analgesia and reversal of side effects following epidural hydromorphone. *Anesthesiology* 65:216–218, 1986.

86. Lanz E, Theiss D, Riess W, et al: Epidural morphine for postoperative analgesia: A double-blind study. *Anesth Analg* 61:236–240, 1982.

87. Rucci FS, Cardamone M, Migliori P: Fentanyl and bupivacaine mixtures for extradural blockade. *Br J Anaesth* 57:275–84, 1985.

88. Kaplan JA, Miller ED, Gallagher EG: Postoperative analgesia for thoracotomy patients. *Anesth Analg* 54:773–777, 1975.

89. Galway JE, Caves PK, Dundee JW: Effect of intercostal nerve blockade during operation on lung function and the relief of pain following thoracotomy. *Br J Anaesth* 47:730–735, 1975.

90. Moore DC, Bridenbaugh LD: Intercostal nerve block in 4,333 patients. *Anesth Analg* 41:1–11, 1962.

91. Rawal N, Arner S, Gustafsson LL, et al: Present state of extradural and intrathecal opioid analgesia in Sweden. *Br J Anaesth* 59:791–799, 1987.

92. Loder RE: Local anesthetic solution with longer action. *Lancet* 2:346–347, 1960.

93. Nunn JF, Slavin G: Posterior intercostal nerve block for pain relief after cholecystectomy. *Br J Anaesth* 52:253–259, 1980.

94. O'Kelly E, Garry B: Continuous pain relief for multiple fractured ribs. *Br J Anaesth* 53:989–991, 1981.

95. Murphy DF: Intercostal nerve blockade for fractured ribs and postoperative analgesia: Description of a new technique. *Reg Anesth* 8:151–153, 1983.

96. Restelli L, Movilia P, Bossi L, et al: Management of pain after thoracotomy: A technique of multiple intercostal nerve blocks. *Anesthesiology* 61:353–354, 1984.

97. Kvalheim L, Reiestad F: Interpleural catheter in the management of postoperative pain. *Anesthesiology* 61:231, 1984.

98. Covino BG: Interpleural regional analgesia (Editorial). *Anesth Analg* 67:427–429, 1988.

99. Selander D: Catheter technique in axillary plexus block. *Acta Anaesth Scand* 21:324–329, 1977.

100. Thomas DFM, Lambert WG, Williams KL: The direct perfusion of surgical wounds with local anaesthetic solution: An approach to postoperative pain? *Ann R Coll Surg Engl* 65:226–229, 1983.

101. Tverskoy M, Cozacov C, Ayache M, Bradley EL, Kissin I: Postoperative pain after inguinal herniorrhaphy with different types of anesthesia. *Anesth Analg* 70:29–35, 1990.

102. Jebles J, Reilly J, Gutierrez J, Bradle EL, Kissin I: The effect of pre-incisional infiltration of tonsils with bupivacaine on the pain following tonsillectomy under general anesthesia. *Pain* 47:305, 1991.

103. Melzack R, Wall PD: Pain mechanisms, a new theory. *Science* 50:971–979, 1965.

104. Abram S, Reynolds A, Cusick J: Failure of naloxone to reverse analgesia from transcutaneous electrical stimulation in patients with chronic pain. *Anesth Analg* 60:81–84, 1981.

105. Solomon R, Viernstein M, Long D: Reduction of postoperative pain and narcotic use by transcutaneous electrical nerve stimulation. *Surgery* 87:142–146, 1981.

106. Galloway DJ, Boyle P, Burns HJG, Davidson PM, George WD: A clinical assessment of electroanalgesia following abdominal operations. *Surg Gynecol Obstet* 159:453–456, 1984.

107. Mannheimer JS, Lampe GN: *Clinical Transcutaneous Nerve Stimulation*. Philadelphia, FA Davis, 1984.

108. Katz J, Nelson W, Forest R, et al: Cryoanalgesia for postthoracotomy pain. *Lancet* 1:512–513, 1980.

109. Nelson KM, Vincent RG, Bourke RS, et al: Intraoperative intercostal nerve freezing to prevent post-thoracotomy pain. *Ann Thorac Surg* 18:280–285, 1974.

110. Miawand MO, Makey AR, Rees A: Cryoanalgesia after thoracotomy: Improvement of technique and review of 600 cases. *J Thorac Cardiovasc Surg* 92:291–295, 1986.

CHAPTER 47

EARLY RECOGNITION OF THE CHRONIC PAIN SYNDROME

MICHAEL HOUSTON
MARC HERTZMAN
ROSLYN RAKOFF
BRUCE SMOLLER

THE IDEAS of prevention and early intervention are among the cornerstones of public health work, under the names "primary" and "secondary prevention." They assume that disease is best prevented from happening altogether or, failing this possibility, detected as early in the course of illness as possible, and arrested or retarded. Prevention/early intervention (hereafter designated P/I, unless clearly one or the other is intended solely) contains a number of other propositions about our ability to intervene successfully, such as the following:

Without P/I the course of illness would be inevitably downhill, and/or

Even if the illness is self-limited, significant harm can occur while the course is being run, and this weakens the organism (patient) in harmful ways, which may make future episodes of illness more likely or more damaging. In other words, tissue damage may be cumulative.

The earlier detection occurs, the greater the likelihood that an illness can be arrested, reversed, or retarded in the rate of its progression.

We have the appropriate tools of detection available, or

We can effectively prevent a disease, whether or not we know its exact cause, or

An effective intervention to retard the rate of progress or ameliorate an illness exists.

P/I is likely to accomplish significantly more good than any harm of which it is capable.

The elaboration of this list of assumptions contained in the notion of P/I should be considered the public health advocate's Koch's postulates. That is, unless a reasonable minimal set of them is fulfilled, P/I may be worthless, or actually hazardous to one's health.

In this chapter we attempt to explore the idea of P/I as it may apply to pain, and especially the prevention of or early intervention in the chronic pain syndrome (CPS). For present purposes, CPS is used in its most widely accepted definition: unremitting experience of pain that persists more than 6 months, and that may not be consonant with the extent of the original injury or the anatomic distribution of the pain described. As this book amply documents, CPS is one of the main unconquered territories in medicine generally, and particularly in industrial and compensation forensic medicine.

One area, which when considered continues to serve as a limiting step in so far as it hinders the promotion of health in the individual, is the field of disability compensation and litigation. Although no one would attempt to argue that disabled CPS patients are not entitled to fair treatment in their attempts to regain health, evidence has accumulated that the present system for the provision of such entitlements and of health care can serve instead to foster and maintain a position of helplessness. We consider this complex subject from a perspective of what we hope would best serve the patient.

STATE OF THE ART

In 1989, when the first edition of this textbook was published, there was clearly ground for cynicism concerning the subject of P/I, particularly as it applies to CPS. To date little appears to have changed. Although treatment programs continue to proliferate, little evidence has accumulated that aggressive early identification of CPS or intervention is either possible or efficacious. This assessment emerges repeatedly from our review. New studies as well as the lack of studies, with rare exceptions, do not justify optimism. In fairness to the reader, however, we attempt to present as balanced a point of view as possible, in hopes that the material will stimulate readers to make up their own minds, perhaps by pursuing the evidence to its original sources, and not simply relying on our summary (but, we hope, thoughtful) judgments. After all, it is much easier to be a critic than it is to be a synthesizer.

We recognize that clinicians must function in a world where diagnostic and treatment decisions are made every day, without the luxury of scientific backing, or perhaps the resources or time to weigh them at each step of a treatment regimen. To the busy clinician we hope to offer some guide for the perplexed, although this is no substitute for continuing scholarship.

PRIMARY PREVENTION, EDUCATION, AND EFFECTIVENESS

Education, according to a despairing, waggish educator, is what we throw at a social problem when we do not have any solution to it. This somewhat irreverent quip may, in fact, aptly characterize much of education in socially significant health and mental health problems. The idea of education before the fact, of education to prevent recurrence or worsening of a problem, is seductively attractive, often in naive ways. For prevention education to have a chance of succeeding, however, a number of conditions have to apply.

For one, there must be some reason to think that there is really a body of knowledge that, if mastered, will shed genuine enlightenment on behavior. An example may be taken from the field of drug abuse prevention, which is analogous to CPS treatment. When drug abuse education was first instituted in secondary and elementary schools, the flair of interest in it quickly turned to dismay. Even where teachers were prepared to convey information about the physiology of drugs—information often better known to the student users than to the teachers—the teaching appeared to have little impact on students. At times it even had a negative impact: students who may not have previously been attracted to drugs, or who had limited their use, had possible new experiences brought to their attention.

How could this happen? Perhaps the idea of what constituted learning was somewhat narrowly conceptualized. For learning to change behavior, clearly more than the knowledge base must be affected. At a minimum, learning also includes motivations and behavioral responses. These, in turn, are conditioned by culture, previous experience, and social system influences.

The consequences of unidimensional thinking are, as one might expect, to handicap a program before it ever

begins. Thus, in the recent revival of concern and interest in doing something constructive about drug abuse, there seems to be greater thought about the impact of education programs on drug abuse.

Public service announcements are noble, and difficult to oppose but for their expense. Do they work, however? There are few data on the subject. A reasonable guess is that public service announcements and media advertisements may increase public consciousness. There is little reason to think that they convey even slightly complex information, however, or otherwise change behavior.

Of course, in P/I campaigns, the idea is to change public attitudes. How effective are they? Public images, as of popular figures, are notoriously fickle. On the other hand, given that attitudes are difficult to move and that fundamental switches in attitude are glacial, once attitudes begin to shift, their new formations are likely to last a long time. It is every nonprofit agency public affairs specialist's dream to be able to achieve such a shift. In fact, it rarely occurs.

In the classroom it is probably not unreasonable to be able to expect to demonstrate differences in information absorption on a short-term basis. Most assessments of educational programs are heavily weighted on short-term evaluations. Even getting children and adults to think in new ways can probably be considered a reasonable expectation in the short run from a P/I educational program.

This, however, begs the questions: how long-lasting is the effect, how widespread, and to what extent does it generalize to "real life" situations outside the classroom? These questions are much more difficult to address. Also, assuming that periodic reinforcement ("refresher courses") might maintain hard-won gains is risky at best.

There are very few readily available data on this subject when it comes to chronic pain. This is of some interest, in that there are at least two types of P/I education programs, and a third that appears to be gaining credibility. The first is that of industrial accident prevention publicity (e.g., "This is a hard hat area"), as well as more-formal didactic sessions and supervision for employees working in situations at risk. Elsewhere in this chapter we comment on the material that Strang has reviewed (1). It generally shows fairly limited benefits demonstrated to date for such programs, with no good fix on the cost/benefit ratio of mounting a campaign. In addition to these limitations, which seem somewhat more restrictive than some other types of health P/I efforts, we also note that there is little or no information available on the longer-term sustainability questions, the core evaluation issues on which the advisability of P/I as a positive course should be measured.

The second type of educational program is that embodied in so-called "back schools," which have shown a modest proliferation. Typically, they may be attached to a chronic pain clinic treatment operation, and may be prescribed as part of the rehabilitation program. Physical therapists (PTs) are the usual practitioners in them. The material is not just lectures and reading, although this may be part of the curriculum. Rather, PTs do what they know how to do best, which is to manipulate and demonstrate first passively, moving the patient's body, and soon actively, getting the patient to follow by small increments in doing motions themselves in the least hurtful ways.

This approach shows more promise. For one thing, it is literally "hands on." Theoretically, at least, it incorporates several different elements of behavioral learning theory from the outset. Learning is active, not just passive. There is an emotional component, not only in the physical aspects of touching, but also in the informal talking that surrounds the instructional, supervised exercise parts of the curriculum. If thoughtfully conceived and constructed, such back schools are coordinated with other aspects of the treatment program, so that the physicians, PTs, and others are making use of their mutual findings for the patient's benefit.

When we first examined the efficacy of this mode of therapy (see the first edition of this book), there was little empiric evidence that back schools had any lasting benefit. Recent studies have provided some cause for optimism. Follow-up at 1 year from a Swedish-type back school showed a decrease in analgesic use, an increase in strength and flexibility, and a decrease in pain (2). As is the case with many studies there were no differences between treatment and control groups with regard to duration of sick leave and missed work, raising the question of what other factors are at work. Indeed, the best predictor of a favorable outcome among the groups was not severity of pain or clinical measurements, but work satisfaction (3).

Lately the fashion in industrial prevention programs has swung toward the mounting of "wellness" programs. These vary substantially. What may distinguish them from other generations of corporate health plans, or industrial accident prevention and containment campaigns, are these two points:

1. They attempt to emphasize a variety of regular, health-promoting behaviors. These range from exercise and physical fitness training to "Smoke-enders" groups in the work place.
2. Wellness programs employ a range of therapies and, although they may incorporate some psychotherapy, they tend to use biofeedback, relaxation techniques, and even behavioral modification.

Much the same assessment could be made concerning data on the efficacy of wellness programs as was done about back schools several years ago. They are relatively new, although not so much so that study has been im-possible. Their promoters (fortunately) do seem to be at least somewhat more modest in public claims of their usefulness than some other P/I specialists have been. They are basically in the position of promoting approaches of uncertain efficacy and sustainability, however.

P/I WITH THE CPS-PRONE PATIENT

Although P/I is hard to study, and worthwhile studies in CPS are few and far between, there are several areas in which scientific work both is promising and offers some clinically practical applications. Probably the most energy has gone into the effort to identify which surgical patients will do well or poorly following surgery. A related but somewhat independent subject is consideration of psychological predispositions to postsurgical depression, and the persistence of psychologically linked symptoms.

The majority of work on surgical prediction is partially retrospective. That is, outcomes are rated on some scheme, usually combining measures of function (motor, social, and even work-related) with decrease in pain and other subjective symptoms. The basic strategy is to take general predictive measures, and see if they (more or less independently) correlate later with the treatment outcome assessments.

By far the most common instrument to use for this purpose is the Minnesota Multiphasic Personality Inventory (MMPI). It is unclear exactly why this should be a central measure, although perhaps it is simply because the MMPI is one of the most widely used and studied psychological screening instruments; and clinical psychologists, who tend to do such work for pain treatment programs, are well-versed in MMPI scoring and interpretation. The so-called classic pain triad on the MMPI consists of high scores on the Hysteria and Hypochondriasis scales and low Depression scale scores (4). The presence of this triad has not been shown to have significant predictive value, however, either alone or with other parameters, for the outcome of treatment. (For a negative critique of the limits of the MMPI in CPS measurement, see Hall. [5]) Moore et al. have suggested a revised view of the MMPI, in which some subvariables may make a contribution to prediction, although not the "pain triad" per se, which can be present or absent in patients responsive to therapy (6).

Murphy et al. studied the predictive validity of the MMPI and the Millon Behavioral Health Inventory (MBHI) in a sample of chronic pain patients (7). The MBHI was, according to the authors, "developed specifically with physically ill patients and medical-behavioral decision making issues in mind." In this study, over the course of a 1-year follow-up, neither the MMPI nor the MBHI was able to predict significantly subsequent pain-related behaviors. An important outcome of this study was that the psychologists who wrote the original consultations were more accurate than either the MMPI or the MBHI in predicting pain-related behaviors. Perhaps if *their* behavior could be modeled and captured, better progress would be made on prediction.

Until 1989 the MMPI had not been revised since its original publication in 1943. Over the years there have been serious concerns about the adequacy of the original sample, the use of obsolete and/or sexist language and references, and the exclusion of certain characteristics deemed important by test users. Although these revisions are important, there is little evidence to suggest the MMPI-2 will be any more significant for predictive value than the MMPI (8).

A variety of psychological instruments for assessing the degree of pain have been developed. Analogue scales are widely used and simple to apply, but are of little demonstrated value. Although these scales are expedient, 7–11% of patients are unable to complete them or find them confusing (9). The McGill Pain Inventory is the most widely accepted adjective checklist for descriptors of pain (10). Studies by Gracely and co-workers suggest that, with some modifications, the McGill Pain Inventory probably can be an item of measurement, at least in well-controlled studies—for example, of oral pain in dental surgery (11).

The problem with single variables, or small numbers of variables, is that they are likely to have limited predictive power. This should not be surprising, considering the large and usually uncontrollable number of factors that influence health and social interventions generally. The implication of this principle is that it makes sense to examine multiple measures any time the question of prediction is being examined. Another principle, which is often violated or ignored in practice, is that the prediction should be made in advance, and as specifically as possible in order to make the result strongly believable. Many social outcome studies are either retrospective cullings of small numbers of predictive variables from large numbers of measurements or claims of confirmation of hypotheses, when, in fact, the "predictor" variables have only been discovered after the fact, thus running the risk of rationalizing findings. Replications of findings, especially with truly comparable measurements, are also uncommon. All of this makes clinicians, and public policymakers, understandably jaundiced about the claims for the results.

One might well argue that expenditure of time and effort on structured interview schedules and the like becomes prohibitive in an evaluation. Most pain patients, however, do not necessarily have a heavy, crowded schedule in their day. Indeed, for many leisure is productive only of boredom, and the opportunity to concentrate more on their symptoms and pain. Thus, it is hardly an imposition, even in a busy practice, to take patients aside and sit them down—perhaps over several

Table 47.1.
Pain Diary

Hour	Activities	Medications	Pain Rating
1–7 AM	Sleep		
7–8	Chair-walk	Percocet	10
8–9	Bed		10
99–10	Bed		10
10–11	Chair		10
11–12 PM	Chair		10
12–1	Lunch	Percocet	10
1–3	Bed		10
3–5	Chair	Valium	10
5–6	Stand, make dinner		10
6–7	Chair	Tylenol-III	10
7–9	Bed		10
9–10	Chair	Sleeping pill	10
10–1 AM	Bed	Percocet	10

sessions, in order to avoid fatigue and the negative consequences of it upon responding—to complete comprehensive testing. In the final analysis, sitting down with the patient may prove to have the best predictive value (7).

Another device that has been found to be helpful is the use of diaries. Diaries have a respectable history in psychology, particularly in cognitive-behavioral and similar psychotherapies. They have the advantages of focusing the patient on rational, presumably healthy measures; they mobilize a patient's own inner resources; they are autogenic reinforcement measures; and they provide direct, or at least indirect (assuming they are completed diligently and honestly) measures of motivation. The pain diary is essentially "prescribing the symptoms," telling the patient to obsess about her symptoms when you already know she is doing exactly that.

So, why do it? In telling the patient to do more of what he is already doing, you are getting the patient to examine his own behavior. Also, at the same time you are obtaining important information about the patient.

Some examples of actual pain diaries are included in Tables 47.1 and 47.2. In the first (Table 47.1), the patient has been asked to indicate what he was doing during every waking hour, and in what position; the degree of his pain (on an analogue equivalent scale); and what medication he took. Some patterns are apparent even at a glance. Like most pain patients, he is automatically scoring his pain all "10's out of 10." The question is not whether his pain really varies less than this. With this kind of record, it should not be hard to achieve a noticeable (to the patient) reduction in scores, no matter what the intervention.

Another possible explanation of the value of the pain diary is the subtle use of "paradox." This is a behavioral

Table 47.2.
Pain Diary

Hour	Activities	Medications	Pain Rating
8–9 AM	Breakfast	Pill	10
9–10	Bed		10
10–11	Chair		9
11–12 PM	Bed		10
12–1	Lunch		10
1–3	Bed	Pill	10

psychotherapeutic technique borrowed from other quarters, which is most applicable when there is an implicit power struggle, usually passive-aggressive, between therapist and patient. It is quite analogous to forbidding a normal 2-year-old child to engage in some behavior: it often positively reenforces his actions. (For a more extensive review of paradox in therapy, see Dowd et al. [12].)

Still another pattern is the consumption of medication. Over the week, the patient is taking his medication irregularly, of a variety of types, and with no subjective, reported impact on his pain. Because the therapist is about to tell the patient that his pain medications are doing little good and possible harm, and should therefore be reduced or removed, the patient is reinforced in his own observations that the medicine is doing little to aid him in reducing pain. (The counterargument is, "But I'm afraid how much worse it would be if I stopped them." Of course, then "10" is not the correct score in the diary.)

In Table 47.2, a patient, now on a prescribed regimen of treatment, is recording the same items. Because the instructions are "Record exactly what you were doing during the last hour," the absence of information may be quite revealing. In this example, which is quite typical, one or only a few words are all that is typically recorded. The responses tend to be repetitive, and give little hint of the degree to which the patient may actually have engaged in activity. Looking at the diary, it would appear that she was hardly even leaving the bed to eat or go to the bathroom. By actual observation of inpatient pain treatment, patients substantially underestimate their actual movements, and consequently their functional capacity —just as they tend to underestimate the success of their outpatient treatment—compared to therapists' estimates. (This should be contrasted to general mental health treatment, in which exactly the opposite is the case: patients are consistently more optimistic than their caregivers.) It is also true that each patient's report in part reflects her (probably unconsciously) perceived self-interest, as well. Nonetheless, these findings make for constructive discussions with the patient.

Although it has not been studied for results, it probably makes sense to administer a systematic, although semi-structured, interview as part of the initial examination. By "semi-structured" we mean that the areas to be covered, and even the basic questions, are specified. However, the interviewer is allowed room to pursue other leads, get more detail, proceed in a different order, or do whatever is required in order to put the patient at ease initially. In other areas besides treatment of CPS, it is generally the case that semi-structured interviews have been shown to be somewhat superior to free-form interviews. The reasons include the likelihood of being complete and not forgetting important areas to cover, the opportunity to think through the wording of questions beforehand, and the enhancement of confidence that probes can be undertaken without going so far afield that the main areas will be neglected.

In Table 47.3 we present such an interview instrument. It is not our purpose here to belabor the assessment. (For more on this subject, see Chapters 6 and 25 in the 1989 edition). We wish to underscore, however, that the format encourages asking about areas that we have found that less experienced or even mature colleagues will sometimes shy away from, notably sexual functions, monetary affairs, and details of compensation and liti-

Table 47.3
Brief Pain Assessment Interview

Please tell me, what is the recent history of your pain? How did your pain begin? Tell me in detail what makes your pain worse? Better?
Describe the quality of your pain. (Probe.) What operations have you had?
Tell me in detail about your present medication; past medication:
For sleep? "Nerves"?
  Coffee, tea, colas? Beer, wine, hard liquor? Past drinking? Illegal drugs, including marijuana?
Describe your sleeping patterns in detail; eating pattern, any weight change. (Probe other depressive signs and symptoms.)
Tell me about others in your family. (Probe: marital difficulties and role changes; sexual problems; problems with children.)
Tell me about your other medical problems. (Probe: Tell me about your past. Probe: previous episodes of pain, mental health problems, alcohol and drug abuse.)
When was the last time you worked? (Probe: types of work, work history, physical requirements of jobs.)
Who is your attorney? (Probe: legal actions pending or past, disability or compensation actions.)
Now, tell me about how much of the following you can do, even though you may be greatly in pain:
  How far can you walk?
  How many pounds can you lift?
  What activities can you do around the house?
Please tell me what you expect from treatment.

gation. Elsewhere in this chapter we discuss the impact of such information, as well as incentives and disincentives for treatment.

Strang has discussed various aspects of primary, secondary, and tertiary prevention (1). As one might expect, tertiary prevention (treatment) takes up more text in the article than the other two combined. Strang does suggest both some clinical predictors that have proven unhelpful, and should therefore be avoided, and others that may yet yield some primary prevention value. Routine radiographs, especially of the lumbar spine, fall into the "no proven utility for prevention" category (although a case might still be made for liability protection in high-risk jobs). Pre-employment strength testing is one possible prevention: if the employee is straining near his limit to do the work, he probably should not be doing the job.

Education about lifting and fitness sounds like a good idea, but results have not been really well demonstrated to prevent back strain. Some effort has gone into mechanical aids and modification of work procedures for prevention. In terms of secondary prevention, Strang has drawn attention to the value of "an early and systematic case management program" as a claims limitation or prevention mechanism for insurers. Also, ergonomics may be useful in early impairment evaluation.

To these might be added certain key points about tertiary prevention. Often, patients could be returned to work if they were not required to do their old jobs, or were required only to do a fraction thereof. This is obviously an enormous problem for employers, who want to have able-bodied employees, and have them return to work. However, when the choice is paying—often for years—enormous sums of money for disability or finding less-strenuous work that these partially disabled employees can do, it may pay to try to be innovative. Certainly this has worked for some companies. It may be realistic self-interest for companies under the compulsion of further payments.

HISTORY AND EXAMINATION OF PATIENTS: PREVENTING CHRONICITY

CPS has long eluded attempts to codify those factors which can be deemed responsible for promoting chronicity and disability. Variables as diffuse as age, amount of compensation, educational level, use of psychotropic medications, number of surgeries, psychological adaptation, and previous work history have been cited in various retrospective and prospective studies as items in the history and physical examination that will lead to chronic disability. It may be ventured that a comprehensive set of predictors that would be useful to the clinician who wishes to intervene in the early stages of a CPS must cut across biologic, sociologic, and psychological antecedents to be of any use.

In any thoughtful history and physical, we look for the signs and symptoms that trigger the possibility that we are dealing with a syndrome that will become prolonged and dysfunctional. Factors that have been deemed to be correlated with long-term disability include the following:

1. Nonspecificity of diagnosis
2. Inconsistency on physical examination, but without a clear-cut psychiatric diagnosis of conversion reaction
3. History of maladaptive behavior
4. Concrete, magical thinking (e.g., "If the doctor could only find the right drug. . .")
5. Passive dependent personality
6. Poor work history, with multiple job changes over a short span
7. Somatically focused and alexithymic disposition (e.g., someone who has trouble putting feelings into words)
8. Resistance to conservative treatment
9. A protracted psychological course
10. A protracted physical course

Often the history is notable for disagreement among physicians. The patient stimulates disputes among doctors, and between himself and the caregivers. He expects cure, not palliation, and demands no less. The thick size and weight of a medical record are dramatic testimony to the degree of frustration and disagreement among the caregivers.

Complete examination of the patient suspected of having CPS, which may lead to long-term disability, must include an evaluation of all of the topics mentioned (13). A clear and concise formulation based on the answers is extremely difficult to synthesize, given the multimodal nature of the contributing factors. The extra effort at times suggests avenues of treatment that might otherwise remain obscured, however (14).

Early recognition and intervention into pain states also require a certain boldness on the part of the clinician in telling the patient that she is at risk for developing chronic pain. That tag carries with it at present the stigma of "weakness" or "differentness." Many physicians are surprised when patients themselves recognize that there is a growing difficulty in their ability to cope. The patients are reluctant to bring this to the attention of their physician for fear of being labeled "unusual."

For example, Mrs. C.L., who, after one laminectomy, was still disabled and complaining of low back pain, was anxious and depressed. It had been suggested to her by her physician that further surgery and a nuclear magnetic resonance scan were necessary to diagnose what must have been a residual surgery or new disk problem. When questioned closely, the patient herself recognized that further intervention was pointless. Her doctor, with the best of all intentions, had disabled her for work, cutting off a source of gratification this patient needed in an otherwise somewhat empty life. Mrs. C.L. recognized this, and declared not only her willingness, but her desire to return to work as soon as possible, understanding that the pain would remain whether she worked or not. It was only through the intervention of an independent examining physician that the patient was able to verbalize her antipathy toward the diagnosis of disability and to state with some certainty that she was ready to resume a functional life.

A careful history will determine whether the patient's symptoms fall into a psychiatric category that may be primary in producing them. There are only three syndromes that produce pain on a "purely" psychiatric basis. The first is *depression with somatization,* a common enough syndrome and one that must be recognized because the depression must be treated directly, rather than the pain per se. The second is *true conversion syndrome,* which is limited to those patients experiencing hysterical paralysis or blindness or paresis of an extremity. The third is *psychosis with delusions of pain,* a rare occurrence.

Later in this chapter we review more-recent thinking by clinicians who argue rather strongly that CPS itself might best be classified as a variant or subtype of depressive illness.

The clinician working up the chronic pain patient must be attuned to those psychiatric dilemmas that are "binding" great amounts of psychiatric problems into pain states. In contradistinction to the CPS patient, in whom psychological factors seem to be most important in promoting long-term disability, in the binding syndromes physical factors seem to be responsible for promoting and perpetuating mixed psychological/physical symptoms. An illustration will serve to differentiate binding syndromes from the early development of chronic disability syndromes.

Dorothy, a 62-year-old woman, developed phantom limb symptoms 7 years after a four-quarter amputation of her left arm. Lonely, unmarried, and working in an isolated fashion for a legal firm, the patient felt the fingers of her left, amputated arm helping her right arm in driving and sewing. After careful examination, it was determined that this phantom limb pain was in no way related to stump pain or neuromata and, indeed, had no demonstrable central pain representations. (Phantom limb usually recedes, distally to proximally, within a year following amputation.) The physical symptoms were perpetuating a depression that had existed for many years and kept Dorothy from being aware of feeling alone, rejected, and crippled. Subsequent treatment of her depression resulted in symptom amelioration after 6 weeks.

In contradistinction to the case of Dorothy, a CPS patient presented to a new physician with a 1-year history and a diagnosis of "chronic strain, refractory to all conservative therapies." The patient had had four jobs in the last 2 years. The family appeared oversolicitous and infantilizing. Passive, dependent features appeared in the patient's psychological testing and psychiatric evaluation. Perhaps most important, the transferential relationship with her previous doctor, who with all good intentions had emphasized her dysfunction, perpetuated this patient's disability. He had kept the patient off of work status. This served to reinforce the patient's disability, as did a solicitous family—all consonant with dependency needs in the patient (15).

In the first example of the binding syndrome, a clearly identifiable set of physical circumstances and a psychological syndrome combined to promote a serious depression, with pain syndromes a result of that depression. In the second example, an alexithymic, concrete patient, aided and abetted by overprotective family members and physician, was well on her way to developing a chronic syndrome. This same patient 5 years later might have had a rigid CPS. The factors picked up on an initial history and examination should have alerted those involved in the care of this patient to a potential long-term disability syndrome. Interventional steps needed to be taken immediately to prevent that syndrome from becoming fixed.

PHYSICAL EXAMINATION

Physical examination of the chronic pain patient involves different types of testing, depending on the locus of the syndrome. It is not true that nonanatomic pain distribution, hypersensitivity to examination, or a positive straight leg raising test while lying but not while sitting with the leg bent at 90° always indicates the presence of a CPS in the making. The presence of several such factors in combination with certain historic data, however, is highly suggestive of the potential development of CPS (16). This combination indicates that intervention should be begun immediately to prevent the encrustation of a simple injury with all the factors leading to an intractable CPS.

The presence of three such anomalous physical findings, in combination with three of the tagged historic features noted above, may be sufficient evidence for a diagnosis of incipient CPS, and vigorous steps should be called for at this stage. Early, consistent intervention by all physicians involved, based on the appropriate examinations, can lead to early termination of a progressively debilitating chronic syndrome.

The non–pain specialist can become quite adept at recognizing an incipient CPS (17). The red flags noted above should be considered potential harbingers of this most insidious of syndromes. A history of disability in the family, previous disability of the patient, or litigation for personal injury are particularly worrisome.

The goal is for early prevention of disability syndromes and adaptation to environmental adversity, which otherwise would tend to perpetuate obsessional concentration on pain. What should be done once the elements of a CPS have been detected? It is the responsibility of the assessing physician to demonstrate to the patient that a syndrome exists that is every bit as insidious as a purely physical chronic illness. Many patients will respond at least with acknowledgement and (later) acceptance, if the physician is forthright and open in explaining the peculiar set of circumstances that may lead to total dysfunction.

At the current state of knowledge, P/I in the clinic is limited. Laboratory techniques have been sought for years to aid in the early diagnosis of potential CPS. Endorphin levels, neuroamine transmitter levels, 3-methoxy-4 hydroxyphenylethyleneglycol levels, and many other tests have all been used to predict chronicity in early pain states. No consistently reliable indicators have generally been found for CPS. As noted above, the use of the MMPI and other psychological test variables has been inconclusive at best. In an extensive study by Moore et al., the MMPI, Profile of Mood States, Pain Severity Index, Sexual Functioning index, activity diaries, and MMPI subgrouping all were nonpredictive of differential treatment outcomes (6).

Patient Satisfaction Parameters

Sometimes patients are so angry, presumably in part because their basic dependency needs are not being met, or because paranoid ideation plays a significant role in their thinking, that they will seek another opinion. Indeed, the most frequently mentioned source of dissatisfaction among patients seeking treatment for low back pain is the failure to receive an adequate explanation for their pain (18).

Whether voiced or not this dissatisfaction leads the patient to searching out a second opinion and additional diagnostic tests. Sometimes patients will find physicians who concur that there are physical problems and enter into extensive therapy. This is a seduction, the promise to the patient of a pain-free existence through either surgery or medical therapy. It may be coupled with the physician's poorly articulated need to triumph where others have failed.

The outcome of such treatment is, too often, prolongation and worsening of the underlying CPS. Perhaps the best clue to a patients' dissatisfaction is the treating physician's own feelings of frustration. When such frustration is encountered it makes sense to inquire what thoughts the patient has regarding his pain. A detached yet sensitive inquiry along with gentle reassurance that the pain appears to be of a benign etiology may at times be enough to relieve the frustrations of both patient and physician. At a minimum, it will delay further harm.

CHRONIC BACK PAIN AS A PARADIGM OF P/I

One of the greatest difficulties faced by those who attempt to study and treat CPS is the simple fact that what is under investigation is not a single syndrome but a constellation of syndromes that has, we assume, a final common path. Generalization is, under these circumstances, quite risky, because there is no clear evidence that chronic pain resulting from, let us say, herpes zoster has any relation to the pain of rheumatoid arthritis; assuming such may limit both our theoretic and clinical understanding.

Still, the benefits of generalization are great in so far as a modality that has proven to be helpful in one area might by chance be therapeutic in another. With that in mind we will present a skeletal model of P/I as it might apply to chronic back pain, keeping in mind that our aim is always toward what is most practical.

Pain as a complaint or symptom is the number one reason for an individual to visit a physician, and back pain is the number one source of pain that patients report (19). Economically speaking, back pain, both acute and chronic, is the greatest source of lost work days, as well as Workers' Compensation and disability payments (20). These losses are primarily the result of work-related injuries suffered by young (under 45 years old), otherwise healthy individuals.

In terms of primary prevention we have already discussed the role that education, industrial accident prevention, employee screening, and wellness programs might play. All of these, from physical education programs in elementary and high schools to structured wellness programs as part of ongoing employee education, make sense and might result in a healthier population in general.

Given that every chronic pain patient was once an acute pain patient, primary care physicians find themselves in a position well suited for early and active interventions. Upon initial presentation the acute back pain patient is more likely to be young than old. He is more likely to be working in a position that requires heavy lifting or repetitive motions, or may work in a rather sedentary position such as at a keyboard or computer. Insofar as work satisfaction is one of the primary indications for both progression to disability and resistance to treatment, a patient's thoughts and feelings about her employment should be elicited early on as part of the initial history. Although a thorough physical examination is always indicated, we lean toward a conservative approach to further diagnostic evaluation and treatment. A short, monitored course of rest (not necessarily bed rest), muscle relaxants, and non-narcotic analgesics more often than not alleviate back pain in less than a few weeks.

One other intervention at this point would appear to make sense to the prevention-oriented physician: a structured back school, with appropriate attention to the modesty of its objectives. A brief course of back school allows for further diagnostic evaluation by a therapist trained in functional assessment, as well as a graded program designed to improve both muscle strength and flexibility.

Another benefit of referral to such a program would be to offer a message expressing both concern for the patient and, implicitly, that personal change is necessary in order to preserve health. A scheduled follow-up, either in person or by phone, further reinforces the physician's concern. Noncompliance at this stage of treatment or failure to comply with the referral would provide evidence of the patient's lack of motivation and would indicate the need for further investigation.

Further preventive interventions on a secondary level would be aimed at those patients with reoccurrence of back pain as well as those who continue to report pain and loss of function after conservative treatment. Additional attention needs to be focused here on recognizable causes of back pain other than musculoskeletal strain. Ruptured or prolapsed disks, spinal stenosis, spinal tumors, and infections are all uncommon, yet should not be overlooked. Adequate evaluation might include *selective* radiographs, computed tomography (CT), and magnetic resonance imaging (MRI) studies, as well as laboratory evaluations.

A comprehensive psychosocial evaluation is also indicated. This would include both a work-related history with specific attention to job performance and satisfaction, and a family history including a history of other members with disability and psychiatric illness, and more importantly an account of the current family structure and the changes that have occurred as a result of the patient's pain. It is not uncommon to find that the family has undergone a significant alteration in roles in a short amount of time.

Questions concerning past misfortunes and illness offer some clues as to the individual's coping mechanisms and strengths.

Attention should also be directed toward the patient's use of alcohol and drugs, because a significant number of patients with back pain may be abusing one or more substances.

This would also be the appropriate time to inquire whether the patient has begun Worker's Compensation or disability proceedings. Ongoing litigation is clearly a poor prognostic variable.

The clinician would best be served by inquiring into these areas in an open and direct manner, keeping confrontation to a minimum. The idea is to obtain a thorough history in order to identify areas that may need more attention rather than to give the impression that the pain is psychological in nature and hence "not real."

Some clinicians, considering their available time and comfort with exploring such matters, might opt for referral to a specialist in pain management. A complete evaluation by a pain specialist offers several advantages, the first of which is that it is most likely less expensive and safer than surgical intervention. There is evidence that a longer-term conservative treatment for disk disease is at least as effective as surgery (21). Confident primary care physicians may be comfortable directing their own multi-discipline treatment approach, in which case referral to a physical therapist and a psychiatric evaluation are indicated.

The area of pharmacology becomes quite important at this level of treatment—hence a considerable portion of this textbook is directed towards it. We will review only a few points. A physician needs to consider carefully the continued use of muscle relaxants, especially the benzodiazapines, given their potential for abuse and, perhaps more significantly, their tendency to worsen dramatically depressed states.

Some might be tempted to institute treatment with narcotic analgesics at this stage; given the severity of the patient's pain, their use might be indicated. A regularly scheduled regimen of pain medication, narcotic or otherwise, has been shown to be superior to PRN dosing. It offers the advantages of being easier to both titrate and monitor and of reducing the possibility of abuse. Pain diaries, as discussed earlier, become an important aspect of this work.

The efficacy of low-dose sensitive tricyclic antidepressants has long been known (22). They appear to work well in selected syndromes, both as a primary medication and as adjuvant therapy with other medication. The newer class of serotonergic antidepressants, including fluoxetine and sertraline, make sense theoretically, and are more tolerable to a number of patients. Thus far, however, there is little direct empiric evidence supporting their use.

The area of tertiary prevention and the treatment of CPS is largely the subject of this textbook. Still, a word might be said about two areas that receive less attention. The first of these is the area of Workers' Compensation, disability, and litigation, which we will address in a later section in this chapter. The other is the area of noncompliance, failure to respond, and relapse. Overall, even the most optimistic of the multi-modality pain programs present response rates of less than 50%, with an even smaller percentage of patients returning to work. Moreover, although some researchers have become adept at identifying which patients and factors contribute to success and failure, little effort appears to be directed at the sizable group of patients who predictably do not respond to treatment or who will relapse.

Interestingly, recent work at the University of Virginia has addressed the patient's beliefs and attitudes regarding pain and its treatment as a variable that predicts outcome (23). Because the cognitive therapies are aimed at altering such beliefs, it makes some sense to begin to explore the use of such interventions early on in the course of treatment.

PAIN CLASSIFICATION SYSTEMS

CPS CLASSIFICATION SCHEME

Recently a scheme for CPS was proposed and published (24). This system of nomenclature resembles the Diagnostic Statistics Model III, or DSM-III (and the DSM-III-R), in a number of major regards. Perhaps the construction of the CPS classification should not be surprising, considering the interest of at least some prominent psychiatrists in CPS, and the fact that the panel was chaired by Merskey, an English psychiatrist noted for his work on psychosocial aspects of pain.

A blue ribbon committee has taken up the banner of providing a classification scheme for pain syndromes, largely for chronic pain (24). The given impetus for devising such a system, according to Bonica (25), is that

> It is possible to define terms and develop a classification of pain syndromes which are acceptable to many, albeit not all readers and workers in the field; even if the adopted definitions and classification are not perfect, they are better than the tower of Babel conditions that currently exist; adoption of such classification does not mean that it is fixed for all time and cannot be modified as we acquire new knowledge; and the adoption of such taxonomy with the condition that it can be modified will encourage its use widely by those who may disagree with some part of the classification. This in fact has been the experience and chronology of such widely accepted classifications as those pertaining to heart disease, hypertension, diabetes, toxemia of pregnancy, psychiatric disorders, and a host of others. . .

In other words, according to Bonica, some explicit system, however faulty, is better than none at all. In particular, the CPS nomenclature uses a multiaxial system of classification for each diagnosis. The major component of the illness is along axis I, much as in DSM-III. The axes do differ somewhat from DSM-III in a number of ways, however.

Axis I categorizes the anatomic region in which the pain largely occurs (including a residual category, "More than three major sites"). Axis II catalogs the pain body system. Axis III is about duration, and axis IV, intensity (from time of onset). Axis V makes some statement about etiology. Axis V includes residual categories for "Dysfunctional (including psychophysiological)," "Unknown or other," and "Psychological origin." Axis V is an innovation, in that it offers several alternatives for diseases or pain of unknown cause, intertwined with psychosocial factors, be they cause or effects.

CRITIQUE

There are usually major advantages and disadvantages to any scheme. How does this particular classification scheme measure up to reasonable standards? In fact, is a faulty scheme really superior to none at all? Our tentative answer is a very qualified "yes," dependent mainly on the particular merits and drawbacks of the system proposed. On the other hand, the imposition of order where previously there had been loose threads or disagreements also brings with it potential disadvantages.

Merits

1. *It certainly attempts to be comprehensive.* The skeleton of this scheme is capable of accommodating new diseases, or shuffling up old, based on new data, thinking, or even fashion. It is already extensive and, although it is probably impossible even in principle to be sure whether a system is complete, this framework is at least thoughtful, and it is clear that a prodigious amount of work has gone into producing it. Whether one agrees with its premises or not, they are generally stated so clearly that at least there is basis for argument.

2. *The logic of the scheme is clear.* It is fundamentally organized around the existing (largely body system–based) coding system, although it often uses different diagnoses than the extant ICDA-IX, or uses words in unusual ways, to which most physicians and other practitioners may not be accustomed.

   Beyond axis I, however, the theoretical basis for the subcategories is less clear. It appears to be a division based on a series of parameters that describe pain. Thus, duration and so on are reified into axes. This is a subtle but important departure from DSM-III and DSM-III-R, wherein the first two (and most important) axes are psychiatric diagnoses, the third relates to other medical illnesses, and the remaining two are rating schemes.

   The proposed classification scheme also employs ratings, but each one of the axes appears to be anchored, at least for certain diagnoses, largely around the patient's self-reports of pain. On the one hand, this is not surprising, because this may be the state of the art in terms of our understanding of much of clinically relevant pain. On the other hand, it also draws attention to a severe limitation of this method: mainly, that in the absence of patient self-reports, there would be no classification scheme at all. Although the psychiatric nomenclature also depends heavily on patient self-reports, it accommodates other sources of information. It is not yet clear whether the pain classification is capable of being useful without overwhelming reliance on patient self-reports. Although a number of studies now document the reliability of behavioral observations in CPS, they prove nothing about their validity.

3. *It forces explicitness.* In general, this is probably a virtue, and it is the same one that "thinking models" generally serve. Most clinicians in practice operate on many assumptions that they have only partially articulated. Often various propositions that constitute motivations for purposive action-interventions are internally self-contradictory, even tautologic. Laying them out for others to see is perhaps the surest way to get feedback, some of it by way of agreement, and

some by way of counterattack by critics. In either event, the strengths and weaknesses of one's thinking will be elucidated.

4. *A system of classification is perforce an attempt to be relatively complete, comprehensive.* Therefore, it must have some logic to it. At the lowest level this would consist of the random assignment of corresponding numbers, although this is a simplistic example. Most systems in medicine consist of signs, symptoms, and historical items that appear to cluster together, have some diagnostic or prognostic value, or are associated with particular etiologic theories. In practice these items may be mingled beyond the ability of the reader to reconstruct the logic or relationships.

5. *If the logic of a system is coherent, and can be demonstrated to be tied to the real world (validation), then such schemes may reveal when hitherto unfound diseases ought to occur.* An analogy might be the periodic table of the elements. When this two-by-two matrix was first recognized for its fundamental properties in chemistry, it also became clear that certain elements ought to occur in nature, even though they had not been previously identified. In medicine, however, it is more difficult to think of clear examples that might fit this logic. Perhaps the closest we can come is the discovery of microorganisms without reference to disease, and the later linking of them to previously unknown illnesses (e.g., Serratia marcescens).

Drawbacks

1. *The pain classification definitely comes down heavily on the side of the severe illness.* As we have suggested above, this is an ominous development from the point of view of the student concerned about P/I. When do the various factors involved in a given diagnosis become important? The course of the illness, by definition, does not become clear except in retrospect. This makes empiric confirmation very difficult, because prospective study is possible only in high-risk populations. Although it should be possible to identify such populations, little such empiric work has actually been done. The data on predictions of surgical outcome, at their best, leave substantial groups of false-positives and false-negatives incorrectly classified. The authors of the present scheme have not, to our knowledge, printed a "concordance" that would clearly indicate which assertions are based on study, and which on "expert opinion."

2. *No system is "culture-free," or unbiased.* That is, although the stated purpose of a disease classification system may be to describe syndromes, illnesses, and diseases, without reference to etiology in which such is not clearly established, even a broad committee of clinicians and researchers must take some stands that at least imply their inclinations about theories of illness. In fact, as a practical matter, it is difficult to conceive of devising any system in medicine that does not carry rather substantial implications of bias about causality, and probably treatment as well.

3. *A classification may also (albeit unintentionally) empha-* size certain aspects of a problem and de-emphasize others. A common problem, for example, is that disease classification systems set up for elusive diseases, in which the tissue pathology is poorly defined or the categories overlap, may emphasize the most-severe cases. The worst cases usually have the most blatant signs and symptoms, and it is easier to obtain reliable agreement among clinicians who examine the patients.

For purposes of P/I, however, this type of classification may be problematic: the whole point of P/I is to develop ways of intervening as early on in the course of illness as possible. Also, the cutting points chosen for where diagnosis can be properly conferred are arbitrary. The pathology is on a spectrum that is more or less continuous from the mildest to the most severe forms of the disease. By contrast, a nomenclature assumes an "all-or-nothing" decision, in which a patient either has the illness or does not. This may be incompatible with the notion of attempting to increase sensitivity among clinicians to possible early forms of the illness.

It is, of course, possible to devise systems that specifically emphasize P/I. This presents the converse difficulty, but probably in more exaggerated form. If the utility is limited to P/I, or leans in this direction, most pathologic schemes are often ignored, or poorly understood in practice, including even the most universal (ICDA-IX); a system constructed for such a narrow purpose is unlikely to gain acceptance beyond the small number of secondary specialists who follow the field.

4. *A classification system may be inherently incorrect, unsatisfying, or even misleading.* The selection of a model does not ensure that it is the best available model, that it accurately reflects the real world (external validity question), that it is consensual, or that it is useful. The fact that an expert committee may have composed it does not mean that the entire field has a high degree of similar understanding of a particular problem. For instance, in constructing and revising the DSM-III, the American Psychiatric Association (APA) has had to resort to votes to settle what purport to be "scientific" questions (26). In addition, once a classification system is in place, it also may gain official credibility beyond its capabilities or its authors' intentions. It may become the official guide for purposes of insurance reimbursement, compensation, and even legal expertise on the subject. Laymen may presume that scientific standards underlie the work, when this may well not be the case.

What can be said, in sum, of this proposed classification system and its impact on P/I? On the balance, it does not necessarily augur well for future developments in this area. It appears to lean heavily in the direction of severe pathology, including psychopathology, possibly to the exclusion or at least de-emphasis of early identification. The authors are undoubtedly sincere in wishing to advance the search for causes and cures in CPS.

Indeed, the blue ribbon committee is filled with distinguished researchers. Why, then, this somewhat top-heavy pathologic presentation? Are there other classifications that could be used?

Psychiatrists have given increased attention in recent years to the assessment, treatment, and classification of pain. In DSM-II the connection between psychological and behavioral factors and medical conditions were found under the rubric of "pychophysiologic" disorders. This term was changed in DSM-III and in DSM-III-R to *psychologic factors affecting physical condition (PFAPC)*. It was believed that this category better "integrated psychological contributions to medical illness into a multiaxial diagnostic system" (27).

In fact, there is little to suggest that this terminology is any more successful than the DSM-II term. A DSM-IV work group has been charged both with studying disorders "often present at the interface between psychiatry and other medical disciplines" and to "bring greater specificity to the category of psychological subtypes to indicate the nature of the physiological factors" (28).

Much attention has also been given to pain as a variant of depression. Blumer and Heilbronn argued that the term "psychogenic pain" is vague and carries a stigma, and that patients with chronic pain are generally known to be depressed (29). Their studies "have led to the identification of a well defined psychobiological disorder with characteristic clinical, psychodynamic, biographic, and genetic features" (29), which they term *pain-prone disorder* and which is seen as a variant of depressive disease.

A concern with this, however, is that although similar symptoms are present in depression and in pain (e.g., insomnia, weight gain or loss, anhedonia, and lethargy), making pain a subtype of depression may minimize and "pathologize" the pain a person is experiencing. Although this maneuver emphasizes attention to psychological variables, it is also at odds with many patients' conceptions of their own illnesses.

In the last analysis, the value of a nomenclature is in the new work it generates. If a classification scheme stimulates thought and critical examination of the subject, then it will have been worthwhile, even were it eventually to be significantly modified or abandoned. We must await those studies—hoped to be forthcoming in the next few years—before passing judgement.

IMPACT OF COMPENSATION, DISABILITY, AND THE LAW ON PREVENTION AND EARLY INTERVENTION

One of the central issues around which debate rages on the subject of CPS is that of the potential disincentives offered by compensation and disability programs, public and private. It is clear that CPS in its various forms is one of the largest contributors to our annual health payments in both the public and private insurance sectors, and has been identified by Bonica and others as adding costs of billions of dollars per year to manufacturing and service industries (30). For this reason, among others, it is commonly and widely assumed that CPS is only a disincentive to improvement in symptoms, the compensation system working massively against motivation to improve in treatment.

A national Commission on Pain Evaluation of the Social Security Administration (SSA) wrestled mightily with this problem of how to deal with the potential disincentives of CPS (31). The Commission's report concluded that powerful disincentives exist in the SSA for patients to get better. By implication, the report is also an indictment of Workers' Compensation, and even private insurance systems, which generally fail to return people to work.

After more than a year and a half of testimony and review of the subject, the Commission, however, substantially failed to consider any testimony or significant evidence that might suggest the possibility that disincentives are less important than generally thought, or that judiciously constructed compensation and treatment systems can at least partially overcome them when the concern is CPS. Indeed, the systematic evidence on the side of the power of the disincentive turns out to be disturbingly inadequate. There are at least some arguments and studies on the opposite side of the question, and these are worthy of mention.

In the general case, the answer to the questions of how powerful incentives and disincentives are can be hinged on the character of the population being treated and studied, the nature of the incentives, and the timing of the interventions. Reviews of treatment outcome in chronic pain–specific treatment programs are relatively optimistic. These results are on selected populations. Although we do not detail these reviews extensively here, a number of comments about such studies are pertinent.

First, in general, the strength of the positive results from treatment is inversely proportional to the number and power of the outcome measures. For example, almost all studies report major reductions in unwanted medication use, often approaching zero, at least during the time of the treatment itself. When other measures, such as assessment of mobilization, are added, "success" rates typically drop from the 70% range to the below-50% range. Insurers and government are primarily interested in return to productive work, however. The figures in this area are typically quite discouraging, generally well below the 30% range. Those who are advocates of such programs argue that, without treatment, the figures would be closer to zero. This is a complex argument, which hinges on the believability of cost-benefit studies, because the cost of treatment is certainly significant. Occasional studies do, nevertheless, tend to be optimistic, even on this score.

Second, the nature of the incentives—what they are and how to quantify them—is a thorny and elusive area to try to understand. Carron has argued forcefully that the entire compensation-disability system is structured to militate against incentives to return to work (32). His analysis of secondary data suggests that many workers are close to their previous level of pay and perquisites in compensation, and are ill-advised to go back to work, because they might not actually come close to breaking even, or might even lose ground financially by doing so.

It is less clear that this analysis applies to the entire spectrum of disabled populations (as Carron would probably agree). The Pain Commission heard testimony from Social Security's Chief Statistician, Aaron Krute, Ph.D., about an in-house study of SSA-disabled lists. The data had many problems in terms of reliability, but this was partially balanced out by the large populations with which the government deals. It appeared that few of the disabled could reasonably qualify for an experiment to put them back to work, even though the numbers of the potentially totally disabled CPS population were large (perhaps upward of 10%).

In Social Security law, these people can only enter through a "back door" diagnosis at present, because chronic pain is not legally admissible as a diagnosis for purposes of this disability program. The reason for the small numbers who it appeared might qualify to be rehabilitated may have to do with the severe and pervasive nature of illness, poor education, low social status, and unskilled labor that go into the concoction that characterizes much of the SSA disability population. The Commission heard testimony that indicated the general failure of rehabilitation experiments of all kinds previously through SSA, generally attributable to the multiple handicaps that face most recipients of aid.

Moreover, a substantial number of cases that are adjudicated are overturned in court. One wonders whether the time, effort, and resources spent on such procedures could be better spent on compensation.

On the other hand, experiments in other countries may shed some light on what constitute reasonable incentives and motivational factors, even if the populations are not precisely comparable. In a Canadian study, Catchlove and Cohen dramatically reoriented the nature of their treatment program for CPS (33). They found that although they could not develop a cure-all, they could significantly improve their batting average for people going back to work. Basically, what they did was to announce to patients that they intended to get everyone back to work, and put teeth into this. Most patients and their families became vociferously angry, but a "working through" process generally occurred, and acceptance was manifested by greater effort put into the graded exercise program and vocationally directed rehabilitation.

Third, little is known about the timing of interventions, except that there is unanimity about the idea that sooner is better. The most widely accepted definition of CPS requires 6 months of pain without remission. Many industrial and other physicians believe that they can identify potential CPS victims within weeks of a reported accident on the job. Elsewhere in this chapter we mention the efforts to predict who make good surgical candidates. The present problem is more amorphous: predicting who will go on to develop chronic, unremitting pain, no matter what the intervention.

There may be an ethical dilemma here. At the present state of the art, identification of the pain-prone individual is fraught with peril and uncertainty at best. But even if this were not the case, would there be a problem? Let us assume that we could predict who would become a victim of CPS early on with a high degree of certainty, say, 95% of the time. Does that mean that 1 out of 20 patients should be incorrectly denied an operation that she wants? Should patients share in the risk and liability under such circumstances? —And only if they undergo an operation, and the operation fails? Besides, most such patients have few resources in the first place. What is the social obligation to CPS victims, and how broad is it?

The same potential ethical dilemma applies to early identification of CPS. The various designations for this syndrome are not neutral. They carry negative connotations of judgement about the patient, the patient's motivation, and even his or her character. Is the gain from early identification sufficient to warrant the epithets? At this state of the art—our ignorance—it is hard to make such a case convincingly.

How, then, can liability be limited within economically reasonable bounds? The answers to this question are basically political, and probably most closely influenced by the self-interest of the group responding. The insurance industry supports tough measures. Their assertion is that smart investigations can uncover dissembling and malingering, and that such measures, if adopted wholesale by government sanction, would go a long way toward containing spiraling costs and protecting the public interest. On the other hand, physicians expert in CPS who testified before the Pain Commission repeatedly asserted that malingering was rare, and could be detected relatively easily by examination. The insurance executives on the panel did not vigorously dispute this point, and it became a finding of the Commission.

Findings and fact, however, are not necessarily the same. We can detect little evidence that bears on this point one way or another. Is it really possible to distinguish clearly between malingering and limited effort at recovery? Or is it a continuum, wherein only the extremes can be defined satisfactorily? The latter seems more likely. Would it be possible to test this proposition, experimentally or statistically? The answer seems to be a qualified "yes."

Clinicians have turned there attention recently to the roles that disability and Worker's Compensation play in either delaying or sabotaging treatment (34). Ongoing litigation appears to interfere with a patient's ability to commit to treatment and rehabilitation earnestly. Another area of concern is the position of helplessness that physicians are cast into when they are left outside of the decision process, thereby separating treatment from what may be the primary motivation for treatment. The one slight hope that managed care interventions offer is the chance of linking these two again into an effective treatment course.

P/I AND LEGAL DISINCENTIVES

All of this brings us to the practical question of the circumstances under which P/I may or may not be possible in the face of legal disincentives, and how the likelihood of success can be maximized, even under adversity.

First, as a practical matter, the majority of patients who enter CPS treatment are under some kind of compensation disincentive, often one that compels their entry into the treatment. Given this fact, it is surprising that many are able to use the treatment to some advantage. In short, it pays to try.

Second, it probably clears the air to have as much in detail about the compensation aspects of a case up front as possible. If the patient is self-referred, or the issues have not been addressed directly, they should be so, and frankly, even over the telephone, before a potential patient is seen the first time (Table 47.3).

Third, caregivers need to be absolutely clear about the limits to which they are willing to go in rendering care in the face of disincentives. Self-interest is hardly sufficient rationalization for rendering care, especially extended, supportive care, if there is little reason to think it will help, or if the gain is prognosticated to be small and the cost large.

Fourth, in the initial interviews, certain questions help lead into frank discussions of compensation issues. When patients come for admission to the hospital, especially those who have "tickets of admission," say, to a psychiatry service (and CPS is one of them), they need to be questioned in a friendly but probing way. Our first question is sometimes, "Now, please tell me the name of your attorney." People without potential litigation rarely can name one. Next, details of cases determined or pending are relevant. The work history needs to be included in the preliminary history taking.

Fifth, if disability or compensation issues are raised by patients after treatment has already begun, the "treatment contract" should be renegotiated. When the patient has not been candid in the first place about his or her hidden motives for engaging the caregiver, it is not clear that the original contract is still in force.

Whether the professional is legally obligated to, for example, provide an opinion to an insurer or government agency, is murky at best. Certainly, it is a foolish patient who acts secretly to obtain such an opinion, because the therapist feels betrayed, lied to, and angry. Once the patient is engaged in treatment, however, it is also hard to ignore the professional's potential self-interest, which is to say, guaranteed payment.

One way around this dilemma is to insist that the treatment and the disability evaluation be performed by separate, unconnected professional parties. Ideally, this means that the evaluator has no stake in recommending treatment, or being optimistic about it. In practice, however, it is common (1) for such evaluators to honor the opinion of the treating physician, or (2) for companies to send patients for evaluations when they can guess the opinion in advance (thereby inviting litigation), or (3) for the insurer to insist on the treating physician's records, and refuse to accept another opinion. Moreover, the precedent at law is for the "patient's physician's" opinion to override the expert's.

For example, a 34-year-old statistical analyst was in pain, and claimed to be afraid of his work place. The treating psychiatrist instituted a behavioral desensitization program for return to work. Although this seemed to be working up to a point, as the patient actually took steps to get in the door of his workplace, he reported suicidal thoughts and actions behind the wheel of his car. Shortly after this, the patient's Workers' Compensation carrier contacted the psychiatrist, the first that the psychiatrist knew of the claim. After some discussion with his peers, the psychiatrist attempted to insist on an independent evaluation. The patient, the patient's wife, and the insurer together then began to pressure the treatment doctor to render an opinion. When he stood firm, the patient angrily left treatment, threatening suit—which, however, did not materialize.

Finally, limited hope should be offered to both carriers and patients about success rates for treatment of CPS in the face of continuing compensation issues. Insurers have become understandably cynical. Perhaps partly in response to this, the claims for success of treatment in CPS have become more and more extravagant and unreasonable. Treatment does have something to offer, but optimistic projections can only lead to dashed hopes and further cynicism.

REHABILITATION OF THE CPS PATIENT AND TERTIARY PREVENTION

Tertiary prevention involves recognition that illness has taken its toll, and yet measures of treatment may either prevent recurrence or at least lessen its impact. In some cases tertiary prevention is conceived of as retarding the inevitable progression of disease, or attempting to lessen pain and suffering. This, of course, is a tautology when speaking of CPS, because reported pain and suffering are central, and (by definition) not improving, or there would not be a tertiary problem. There is also the constant uphill task of working against the patient's (and often the family's and the doctor's) hopes that somehow a "cure" will be found, and hard work on rehabilitation will not be a necessity. Regrettably, the latter hopes often work strongly against optimal coping with the existing illness.

The heart of tertiary prevention is generally a behavioral approach. The theoretical as well as practical basis for this approach has generally been associated with Fordyce (35). It is not our purpose to detail this approach here, but to examine enough of its bases to comment on its P/I value and limitations. First of all, it assumes at least a modicum of cooperation and motivation on the part of the patient. It postulates that an incremental, goal-oriented system of rewards (and deterrents) will be additive, in a reasonable period.

The goal is to be as functional as possible, given that pain may persist or even worsen. In other words, it de-emphasizes the communications about pain and suffering, on the theory that they are counterproductive to functionality.

This approach has been reviewed in detail by Keefe (36) and by Linton (37). The main questions for present purposes have to do with the following considerations:

1. What is the evidence that behavioral change is sustained over time?
2. What is necessary in order to sustain gains from a behavioral modification approach, assuming that they do occur?
3. What are the costs in time and resources to optimize sustained functionality?

There are now some relatively long-term studies of outcome of treatment. Most CPS treatment programs have behavioral approaches at their core, although it is fair to say that most also take a variety of approaches simultaneously, and this makes it difficult to single out one for special consideration. In fact, it is generally true that multimodality treatment programs have generally been demonstrated to be the most consistently successful (38).

Perhaps the most difficult task is sustaining outpatient regimens that are roughly consistent with the intensive phase of treatment, be it originally inpatient or outpatient. Certain principles may have some practical value in bringing this about.

First, every effort needs to be made to concentrate care in one treatment coordinator's hands. Because the CPS patient is particularly prone to have multiple doctors, this concentration is essential. In some states Medicaid regulations have been adjusted to require patients to confine their visits to specified physicians and pharmacies. (Whether this is a civil rights matter is another consideration.)

Second, innovative and strenuous efforts may need to be undertaken in order to bring about this coordination. This is an example of how spouses and other family members may be essential in order to augment or correct communications between doctor and patient. Pharmacists may need to have detailed knowledge of the patients and their needs. Although there is much controversy about systems, such as the "prescription in triplicate" notion, CPS may be one area in which they are justified.

Third, at the present state of the art, if in doubt, a whole series of concurrent therapies should be directed at patients, including them as maintenance treatment after the intensive initial push. Although, as indicated earlier, the evidence for multimodality treatment is not so clear as one would like, the "grapeshot" approach to treatment can be justified on a number of grounds. Because our ability to predict who will respond to a given treatment is minimal, and we know that a group of CPS patients will respond to some treatment, all bases being covered may heighten the likelihood of success. Also, there is a tendency in practice to use those treatments that the caregiver knows how to render best. This is not better seen than in the liberal overuse of medications, at the expense of behavioral and cognitive treatments that may be quite important or even essential.

Fourth, because compliance is a notorious problem with outpatient treatments, any simple measures that will enhance the likelihood of following a treatment regimen have the promise of high payoff. A doctor's office can schedule telephone calls at intervals in order to provide a friendly reminder. Because intermittent reinforcement schedules tend to be more effective at maintaining established operant behavior, the calls should not be at regular, expectable intervals, but spaced out at close-enough intervals that compliance will not necessarily have strayed too far from prescription between calls. Postcards and newsletters, although less effective, are cheap and simple, and may have some value in this regard.

Other innovative devices should be employed without hesitation. For example, patients may continue their pain diaries at home, and have their entries checked at intervals by treaters.

Although devices as reinforcers have not been studied extensively, some are known to be effective in certain patients. The paradigm for this is the transcutaneous electrical nerve stimulation (TENS) unit. How TENS works—when it works—is not well established; recent studies suggest that it may be a placebo response (39). Even so, at least one function it serves is to remind the patient of the caregiver's expectations. The same thing may be true of programmable timers, which can be purchased inexpensively at radio discount stores and can sound an alarm at the appropriate intervals to remind the patient to carry out a particular set of tasks.

Fifth, visits to homes and work places may provide surprising diagnostic vignettes that require the caregiver to adjust her judgements of the patient's goodness of fit with her environment. Although it may be unrealistic for a doctor in practice to do this, there is now a cadre of enterprising vocational rehabilitation specialists, including public workers and private firms, who have particular interest in job and task analysis. Some are also experienced in negotiating job redefinition for workers who must be either returned to partial duty or retired at full pay.

Hertzman et al. have described an augmented operant/multimodality treatment process (40). The treatment is both educational and behavioral-psychological. The inducements to the families to assist are multiple. For one, family members are often at their wit's end as to how to help the patient who may be not merely noncontributory, but actually a tremendous drain on family resources of patience, affection, and even money. Dramatic role changes in families surrounding one person's becoming a CPS victim upset the family's equilibrium. A wife who was a homebody is forced to go out and become the principal wage earner, while a hitherto macho construction worker is forced to do housework. Often the children are caught in between them, and everyone suffers.

Certainly family participation in treatment seems to bode better for positive outcome. Although there are few systematic studies of the question, those that exist generally reflect the commonsense wisdom on the subject. Khatami and Rush studied the impact of family participation in a multimodality CPS treatment program (41). They were able to show strongly suggestive evidence that family work enhanced positive outcomes. Also, these effects were persistent at follow-up. Hertzman et al. obtained results that suggested the superiority of outcome when families participated in treatment (40). In this study, however, "preselection" may have caused families with positive risk factors to be chosen before the study started.

What is it about family participation that maximizes its usefulness? Many family members, usually inadvertently, are reinforcing pain. By observing the families directly, preferably even in a natural setting (e.g., at home), it may be determined that they are enabling the dysfunctional behavior to continue. The analogy to the "enabler" in the alcoholic family is possibly more than coincidental: alcohol and drug abuse are rife in these families, in both patients and relatives, and often precede the CPS (and may continue during it).

It is also the case that families are generally the best supporters that the CPS patient is going to have. Thus, if these family members can be bolstered in their own

most functional roles, it is often also of assistance to the patient. Of course, this is easy to assert, but not necessarily easy to do in practice. For instance, some research suggests that families in which spouses are in the most agreement about their analysis of the "pain problem" are also the most closed to changing it (42). Conversely, when marital (or other family) *dis*agreement exists about what the CPS patient should be doing, what roles family members should be assuming, and what treatment the patient should be getting are discordant, this may predict *greater* likelihood of willingness to change within the family.

Perhaps the most valuable piece of advice to the office clinician would be to take a healthy, skeptical attitude toward very optimistic or global claims to success in treatment. For example, flying in the face of most other opinion, one respected researcher suggested that the efficacy of multimodality treatment is poorly established, and that relaxation techniques have a much more solid body of evidence behind them (37). This is contrary to our reading of the scientific literature on the subject, and also to common sense.

Today much research is focused on isolating the value of particular treatment components, such as relaxation techniques. The state of the art of treatment outcome research remains crude, however, and the suggestion that single treatments with some demonstrated efficacy may be superior to "grapeshot" approaches confuses the value of selecting treatments for research purposes, and maximizing outcome by attempting a number of different strategies simultaneously, any combination of which may work.

REFERENCES

1. Strang JP: The chronic disability syndrome. In Aronoff GM (ed): *Evaluation and Treatment of Chronic Pain.* Baltimore, Urban & Schwarzenberg, 1985, pp 603–623.
2. Hurri H: The Swedish back school in chronic low back pain. *Scand J Rehab Med* 21:33–40, 1989.
3. Hurri H: The Swedish back school in chronic low back pain II. *Scand J Rehab Med* 21:41–44, 1989.
4. McCreary C, Turner J, Dawson E: The MMPI as a predictor of response to conservative treatment for low back pain. *J Clin Psychol* 35:278–284, 1976.
5. Hall W: Review: Psychological approaches to the evaluation of chronic pain patients. *Aust N Z J Psychiatry* 16:3–9, 1982.
6. Moore JE, Armentrout DP, Parker JC, Kivlahan DR: Empirically derived pain-patient MMPI subgroups, prediction of treatment outcome. *J Behav Med* 9:51–63, 1986.
7. Murphy JK, Sperr EV, Sperr SJ: Chronic pain: An investigaton of assessment instruments. *J Psychosom Res* 30:289–296, 1986.
8. Graham JR: *MMPI-2: Assessing Personality and Psychopatology.* New York, Oxford University Press, 1990.
9. Institute of Medicine: *Pain and Disability: Clinical, Behav-*

ioral, and Public Policy Perspectives. Washington, DC, National Academy Press, 1987, pp 215–216.

10. Melzack R: The McGill Pain Questionnaire: Major properties and scoring methods. *Pain* 1:277–299, 1975.

11. Gracely RH: Pain measurement in man. In Ng LKY, Bonica JJ (eds): *Pain, Discomfort and Humanitarian Care.* Amsterdam, Elsevier/North-Hollard, 1980, pp 111–138.

12. Dowd ET, Trutt SD: Paradoxical interventions in behavior modification. In Hersen M, Eisler RM, Miller PM (Eds): *Progress in Behavior Modification,* vol 23. London, Sage, 1988.

13. Reich J, Steward M, Tupin J, Rosenblatt RM: Prediction of responses to treatment in chronic pain patients. *J Clin Psychiatry* 46:425–427, 1985.

14. McCreary C, Turner J, Dawson E: Principal dimensions of the pain experience and psychological disturbance in chronic low back pain patients. *Pain* 11:85–92, 1981.

15. Feuerstein M, Sults S, Hocke M: Environmental stressors and chronic low back pain-life events, family and work environments. *Pain* 22:295–307, 1985.

16. Guck TP, Meilman PW, Skultety FM, Dowd ET: Prediction of long-term outcome of multidisciplinary pain treatment. *Arch Phys Med Rehabil* 67:293–296, 1986.

17. Chapman CR, Case KL, Dubner R, Foley KM, Gracely RH, Reading AE: Pain measurement: An overview. *Pain* 22:1–31, 1985.

18. Deyo RA, Dielh AK: Patient satisfaction with medical care for low-back pain. *Spine* 11:28–30, 1896.

19. Institute of Medicine: *Pain and Disability: Clinical, Behavioral, and Public Policy Perspectives.* Washington, DC, National Academy Press, 1987, pp 1–2.

20. Institute of Medicine: *Pain and Disability: Clinical, Behavioral, and Public Policy Perspectives.* Washington, DC, National Academy Press, 1987, pp 87–99.

21. Weber H: Lumbar disc herniation: A controlled perspective study with ten years of observation. *Spine* 8:131–140, 1983.

22. Ward NG: Tricyclic antidepressants for chronic low back pain. *Spine* 11:661–665, 1986.

23. Shutty MS, DeGood DE, Tuttle DH: Chronic pain patients' beliefs about their pain and treatment outcomes. *Arch Phys Med Rehabil* 71:128–132, 1990

24. International Association for the Study of Pain: Classification of chronic pain. *Pain Suppl* 3:3–226, 1986.

25. Bonica JJ, quoted in: Classification of chronic pain. *Pain Suppl* 3:3, 1986.

26. American Psychiatric Association: *Diagnostic and Statistical Manual of Mental Disorders,* ed 3. Washington, DC, American Psychiatric Association, 1980.

27. Stroudemire A, Hales RE: Psychological and behavioral factors affecting medical conditions and DSM-IV: An overview. *Psychosomatics* 32:5–13, 1991.

28. Frances A, et al: DSM-IV: Work in progress. *Am J Psychiatry* 147:1439–1448, 1990.

29. Blumer D, Heilbronn M: Chronic pain as a variant of depressive disease: The pain-prone disorder. *J Nervous Mental Dis* 170:381–394, 1982.

30. Bonica JJ: Importance of the problem. In Aronoff GM (ed): *Evaluation and Treatment of Chronic Pain.* Baltimore, Urban & Schwarzenberg, 1985, pp xxxi–xliv.

31. Social Security Administration: *Report of the Commission on the Evaluation of Pain.* Washington, DC, US Government Printing Office, 1986.

32. Carron H: Compensation aspects of low back claims. In Carron H, McLaughlin RE (eds): *Management of Low Back Pain.* Littleton, MA, John Wright-PSG, 1982, pp 17–26.

33. Catchlove R, Cohen K: Effects of directive return to work approach in the treatment of workman's compensation patients with chronic pain. *Pain* 14:181–191, 1982.

34. Talo S, Hendler N, Brodie J: Effects of active and completed litigation on treatment results: Workmen's compensation patients compared with other litigation patients. *J Occup Med* 31:265–269, 1989.

35. Fordyce W: *Behavioral Methods for Chronic Pain and Illness.* St. Louis, CV Mosby, 1976.

36. Keefe FJ: Behavioral assessment and treatment of chronic pain: Current status and future directions. *Psychology* 50:896–911, 1982.

37. Linton SJ: Behavioral remediation of chronic pain: A status report. *Pain* 24:125–141, 1986.

38. Hertzman MP: Pain as stress. In American Psychiatric Association: *Methods of Psychiatric Treatment.* Washington, DC, American Psychiatric Association, 1989.

39. Deyo RA, et al: A controlled trial of transcutaneous electrical nerve stimulation (TENS) and exercise for chronic low back pain. *N Engl J Med* 233:1627–1634, 1990.

40. Hertzman M, et al.: The family in chronic pain. *Psychiatric Forum* 14:24–36, 1989.

41. Khatami M, Rush AJ: A one-year follow-up of the multimodel treatment for chronic pain. *Pain* 14:45–52, 1982.

42. Bloch AR, Kremer EF, Gaylor M: Behavioral treatment of chronic pain: The spouse as a discriminative cue for pain behavior. *Pain* 9:243–252, 1980.

CHAPTER 48

ERGONOMIC CONDITIONS
IN THE WORKPLACE

MAHMOUD A. AYOUB

"ERGONOMICS," DERIVED from two Greek words *ergon* and *nomikos*, means literally the "laws of work." It seeks to design jobs, workplaces, and products for people to reduce physical discomfort, to enhance safety and well-being, and to improve job effectiveness and productivity—at home, on the road, and at work. Other labels are used to describe the field of ergonomics: human factors, human ergology, human performance, and the like. In the United States, *human factors* is the well-known and most heavily referenced label. "Ergonomics," however, is the label recognized and used worldwide. Biomechanics, work physiology, and man-machine systems are special areas of study within the field of ergonomics. For example, biomechanics is concerned with the interaction between people and their environments; it considers various aspects of energy exchange between people and the physical entities of the workplace: tools, seats, materials, and the like. It measures and assesses the internal and external forces generated by and acting upon the human body.

Ergonomics, as a discipline, is concerned with the design of jobs, workplace, and products, as well as employee selection and training. In this context, ergonomics is closely allied with industrial engineering, for both seek efficiency and productivity. The point of departure between the two is in the consideration given to human capabilities and limitations. While seeking high levels of productivity, ergonomics attempts to assure that job stresses (physical, physiologic, and psychological) can be tolerated by the human body and its systems. It minimizes job stress through design and integration (interfacing) of workplace hardware (e.g., seating, work surface), and elimination of motion elements and associated forces that might cause excessive muscular loading.

Ergonomics bases its principles and recommendations on knowledge and data taken from a wide cross-section of disciplines: engineering, physiology, anatomy, psychology, medicine, mathematics, and statistics. To this end, ergonomics offers a philosophy and approach for dealing with people's characteristics and limitations; it accepts people as they are, as individuals having various abilities that are neither constant nor completely measurable. It attempts to effect a match between people and their working environment, their products. In so doing, it considers the whole of the person: behavioral, physical, and physiologic attributes.

The key to a successful ergonomic effort lies in the integration of people's abilities and the demands of their environment (Fig. 48.1). Successful integration is achieved when people are not exposed to safety or health risks; when the job demands do not tax human work capacity, or can be met only by selected few individuals; when people are in control of their environment and machines; and when jobs promote the social interactions and well-being of those who perform them.

The literature of ergonomics contains numerous examples of how the interface between man and machine, if not controlled, can be hazardous to one's safety and health. In most instances, the interface may subject both man's anatomy and physiology to excessive and highly concentrated stresses and strains. Persistence of these stresses can lead to the occurrence of an array of health disorders and occupational diseases.

For example, the task in some occupations might force the individual to maintain an awkward posture during extended periods. Such awkward postures, when imposed (through faulty equipment design or workplace arrangement) over a number of years, are apt to deform the anatomic system of the human body and ultimately lead to permanent occupational deformities—a case that is not uncommon in dentistry. Furthermore, there is a correlation between diseases of the musculoskeletal system (muscles, tendons, joints, and bones) and work postures. For instance, static loading of the cervical vertebrae—a posture prone to the meat-packing industry—has been found to be conducive to lesions of the spine. After surveying many females (weavers, spinners, and

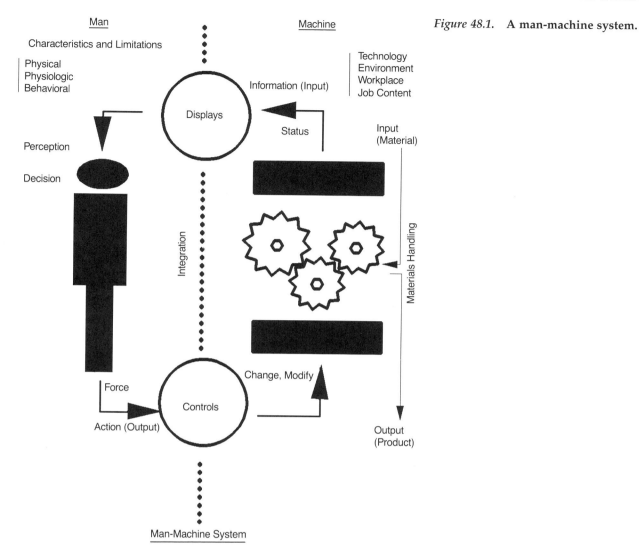

Figure 48.1. **A man-machine system.**

office clerks) of a silk spinning and weaving mill, it was concluded that most of the workers' complaints stemmed from static loading of the legs and feet. This static loading was aggravated by wearing unsuitable shoes. The problem was solved by providing the workers with specially designed shoes and allowing for periods of exercise. Many studies attribute to faulty postures the dissatisfaction and failure of workers to adapt to work on assembly lines.

APPROACH

The ergonomic approach to job design considers human capabilities, task demand, and workplace (equipment) characteristics. It attempts to determine the optimal (physical) interface between man and his machine—the interface that will protect the human structure from excessive stresses and strains without compromising productivity and efficiency. This optimal interface can be realized if industrial tasks are designed

so as to achieve maximum adjustments between human physiologic capacity and job demands.

AREAS OF STUDY

Biomechanics, the study of the body responses to the physical forces resulting from the use of hardware (tools, seats), manual handling, and maintaining various postures.

Work physiology, the measurement and categorization of human physiologic response to a given job situation and environment. Response measures such as oxygen consumption and heart rate are used as an indirect means of assessing stress and strain placed on the body. Also, human work capacity is established through measuring the responses under simulated conditions.

Skilled performance, assessment of the behavioral impact of job design on performance (quality and productivity) as well as on fatigue and boredom.

Safety and health studies of various approaches and techniques for hazard recognition, analysis, and control.

APPLICATIONS

Workplace design, specifying the physical characteristics of the hardware; integrating the various components to assure proper interface between people and their hardware.

Job design, specifying job content (type and number of tasks to be performed). The duration and schedule of rest breaks (periods) required to avoid overloading of individuals (fatigue); also included is job organization (sequencing of tasks and breaks).

Product design, specifying product physical characteristics (form, shape, dimensions, weight) and providing adequate instructions (warning) to assure safe use of the product. Assuring acceptable product quality for the intended use through design, material selection, manufacturing, marketing, and maintenance.

ERGONOMIC ANALYSIS

A worthwhile and trustworthy ergonomic design or assessment has to commence with the definition of the characteristics and attributes of the man-machine system under evaluation. Here, we would be interested in evaluating the strength or weakness of each of nine specific areas of ergonomic concern: management, job, workplace, machine, method, materials handling, environment, health care programs, and employee fitness and awareness. An ergonomic checklist (such as shown in Fig. 48.2) may be used for gathering data and documenting the observed conditions. In addition, employees should be interviewed concerning the demands of their jobs, and should complete an ''Ergo Snapshot'' (Fig. 48.3).

Following the initial survey, a set of objective data would be collected for the purpose of profiling job demands and the corresponding human responses (physical and physiologic).

ERGONOMIC DEFICIENCIES

Absence of ergonomics will bring inefficiency and pain to the workplace. An ergonomically deficient workplace will not cause immediate pain, because the human body has a great capacity for adapting to a poorly designed workplace or structured job. In time, however, the compounding effect of the job and workplace deficiencies will surpass the body's coping mechanisms, causing the inevitable—occupational disease, emotional scars, low productivity, and poor quality of work.

Ergonomic deficiencies are manifested by a number of well-defined and well-recognized symptoms: extreme posture, excessive force, concentration of stress, static loading, pain/discomfort, and high incidence of occupational diseases and disorders. The first four symptoms can be considered early warnings; the remaining two are the final outcome, occurring only when nothing is done to correct the existing deficiencies.

EXTREME POSTURE

This refers to alignment of body segments. Placing one or more body segments in an extreme position or out of alignment with other segments will produce extreme posture. Such posture places much strain on the body, including joints, tendons, and muscles. In most cases, extreme postures are the result of improper reach. Any reaches made with the arms fully extended and to points above shoulders or below the waist are typical causes of extreme postures. Another cause of extreme posture is improperly designed hand-held tools, products, and machine controls. For many of these either the object is too bulky to hold with ease or it is hard to get to without adapting an extreme posture, especially for the wrist and arm. In general, any posture (body alignment) that does not look right or that looks difficult to maintain can safely be labeled ''extreme.''

EXCESSIVE FORCE

Materials handling and use of hand and power tools require exertion of force. The force required will depend on the weight and bulk of the object handled or manipulated as well as on body posture. If any of these parameters is improper, a condition for exerting too much force develops.

CONCENTRATION OF STRESS

By definition, stress is a force divided by the area over which it is applied. For a given force, the larger the area, the less the stress; the opposite is also true. Putting it in the context of the human body, the fewer the muscles used to deliver force, the higher the stress placed on the body. Any task that utilizes few muscles or relatively weak muscles constitutes a troublesome concern and results in inefficient loading of the musculoskeletal system.

Repetitive jobs characterized by short and fast motions are prone to causing stress concentration. Miniature handtools or tools that tend to be buried within the palms are another example. As a rule, level of stress concentration is inversely related to the number of body segments engaged in the task motion/force application. That is, the fewer the segments, the higher the potential for stress concentration.

Time is an important consideration in developing stress concentration. That is, stress applied infrequently may not be as harmful as stress that dominates throughout the working day.

STATIC LOADING

This is a label given to a host of situations in which one or more body segments are kept motionless or allowed to change positions very infrequently. Static loading interferes with muscle/tendon functions, and if allowed to persist over time will eventually cause damage

ERGONOMIC CHECKLIST

ERGONOMIC STRESSORS

N	A	M	C	Extreme posture
N	A	M	C	Extreme reach
N	A	M	C	Static loading (frozen)
N	A	M	C	High force
N	A	M	C	Concentration of stress (few muscles)

POSSIBLE CAUSES

REMARKS

WORKPLACE

N	A	M	C	Seating
N	A	M	C	Work surface
N	A	M	C	Work space
N	A	M	C	Floor cover/ Footrest
N	A	M	C	Supplies

METHOD

N	A	M	C	Pace/pacing
N	A	M	C	Reach material
N	A	M	C	Data/Text Entry (R/L hand)
N	A	M	C	Support/holding of material
N	A	M	C	Handling Output (Prints)
N	A	M	C	Clothing (Protective)

MOUSE

N	A	M	C	Support
N	A	M	C	Size
N	A	M	C	Relative Motion

MONITOR

N	A	M	C	Orientation
N	A	M	C	Screen

MATERIAL HANDLING

N	A	M	C	Lifting (twisting)
N	A	M	C	Carrying
N	A	M	C	Pushing/ pulling

ENVIRONMENT

N	A	M	C	Noise
N	A	M	C	Vibration
N	A	M	C	Lighting
N	A	M	C	Climate

JOB

N	A	M	C	Number of tasks
N	A	M	C	Breaks
N	A	M	C	Standards
N	A	M	C	Shift work/ overtime

Fitness

N	A	M	C	Fit-for-job
N	A	M	C	Ergo Awareness?

N= no concern	M= marginal
A= acceptable	C= critical

Ayoub 1991

SYSTEM

- IBM - APPLE - OTHER,

WORKPLACE LAYOUT

show work surface, light sources, etc.

PRIMARY SOFTWARE

Y N	Desktop Publishing, specify	_____
Y N	Word Processing	_____
Y N	Graphics, specify	_____
Y N	CADs, specify	_____
Y N	Other	_____

ADD-ONS

1. SEAT	Y N TYPE/MODEL_____
2. STAND	Y N TYPE/MODEL_____
3. KEYBOARD	Y N TYPE/MODEL_____
4. MOUSE	Y N TYPE/MODEL_____
5. SCREEN	Y N TYPE/MODEL_____
6. MONITOR	Y N TYPE/MODEL_____
7. SYSTEM	Y N TYPE/MODEL_____
8. FOOTREST	Y N TYPE/MODEL_____
9. COPY STAND	Y N TYPE/MODEL_____
10. PRINTER	Y N TYPE/MODEL_____
11. OTHER	Y N TYPE/MODEL_____

Figure 48.2. Ergonomic checklist.

Date ————————————

ERGO SNAPSHOT

EMPLOYEE

Job ————————————

Shift ————————————

Supervisor ————————————

Area ————————————

Job tenure (years) ————————————

SYMPTOMS CHART

■ Place an X in any areas in which you may have symptoms

● For the marked areas, rank discomfort intensity using a scale from 1 to 5. Place the numbers on the diagram

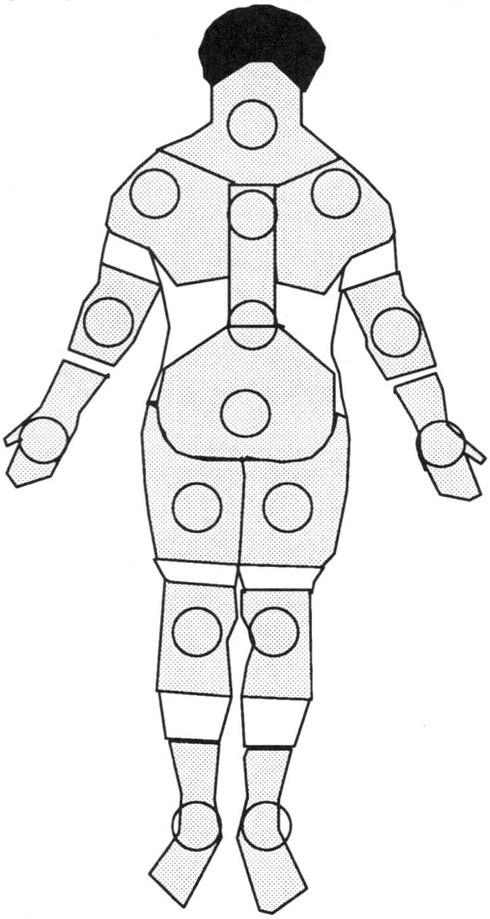

For the most severe discomfort, answer the following:

[1= slight discomfort ...... 5= very uncomfortable]

How often do you experience this discomfort?

☐ always, pain is constant
☐ occasionally
☐ only at rest
☐ only when active

How long has it been since you started to experience the discomfort?

☐ days
☐ weeks
☐ months
☐ years

How did the symptoms start?

☐ gradually, over time
☐ suddenly
☐ injury/ accident

What makes you feel better? specify:

————————————————
————————————————
————————————————

What makes you feel worse? specify:

————————————————
————————————————
————————————————

HOW DOES YOUR JOB MEASURE UP?

N	A	M	C	Workplace	seat, work surface, space, adjustability
N	A	M	C	Job Content	tasks, method, pace, breaks, standards
N	A	M	C	Machine/ Tools	controls, displays, maintenance/ weight, size, power
N	A	M	C	Materials Handling	weight, frequency, aids
N	A	M	C	Environment	temperature, ventilation, light, noise, vibration

N= no concern   M= marginal
A= acceptable   C= critical

AYOUB 1990

Figure 48.3.   ERGO snapshot.

to the body and the occurrence of cumulative trauma disorders. A comparable situation to static loading can be realized when the body performs repetitive and forceful motions with little or no chance for rest. In this case, although the body is kept in motion, speed and repetitiveness of the activity will make it equivalent to maintaining static posture.

Most situations of static loading can be attributed to method or to job designs, and a fair number can be attributed to workplace/machine interfacing with the individuals performing the tasks.

PAIN/DISCOMFORT

Frequent complaints of discomfort, fatigue, and outright pain are positive indications of the existence of ergonomic deficiencies. When the complaints increase in frequency or start to interfere with job performance, one can conclude that the need for ergonomic intervention is urgent. If management fails to recognize the meaning of the reported pain, the situation will worsen, setting the stage for the development of cumulative trauma disorders.

CUMULATIVE TRAUMA DISORDERS

When management lacks awareness of how its practices and policies are creating a deficient workplace, when it absolves itself from close monitoring of work practices, and when it does not share with the employees the responsibility of defining practical job standards, cumulative trauma disorders (CTDs) are a certain outcome. This may take a number of forms: sudden and unexpected increase in the number of reported cases of such disorders; increase in the number of employees out of work because of disability; high number of employees seeking treatment from the company medical department or from outside physicians; and an increasing rate of turnover or transfers from some jobs.

EARLY REPORTING OF PAIN

RECOGNITION

One must encourage early reporting of pain and discomfort in order to prevent a bad situation from getting worse. Indeed, employees should be advised to report the early symptoms of discomfort and pain.

Supervisors should do the following:

1. Listen to pain complaints
2. Respect what the employee reports (i.e., do not debate the source, severity, or legitimacy of the reported pain).
3. Review and improve the ergonomics of the workplace and job with the involved employees.

When an employee seeks help from his or her supervisor concerning on-the-job discomfort (pain), three steps are taken:

1. Treatment and counseling by the medical department
2. Improvement of workplace/job ergonomics
3. Retraining and close monitoring of the employee

PAIN RESPONSE

Following a CAD incident, the employee should be retrained to perform the job according to an ergonomically sound method. Emphasis should be on performance of tasks without assuming extreme postures or forceful exertions and unnecessary motions. The employee's supervisor, the engineering department, and the medical staff should work together in planning and developing the retraining program.

CUMULATIVE TRAUMA DISORDERS

Tendonitis, tenosynovitis, and carpal tunnel syndrome are new words in today's workplace, replacing more descriptive titles such as housemaid's knee, telegraphist's wrist, tennis elbow, golfer's shoulder, and baseball player's glass arm. Each describes a disorder characteristic of the occupation it typifies. The names given to the disorders, for the most part, refer to the nature of the soft tissues injured as well as to the anatomic sites of those tissues.

All names indicate an injury or disorder of the tendon and related anatomic structure (sheaths and nerves). Tendon injuries are found in labor-intensive industries (textiles, apparel), highly mechanized assembly-type industries (electronics), heavy industry, data processing, and jobs requiring the use of vibrating tools and awkward postures coupled with repetitive motions.

Cumulative trauma disorder (CTD) is the label used to define tendon- or nerve-related disorders resulting from repetitive motions (use), mechanical trauma (injury), and excessive forceful exertion. CTDs are seen often in three anatomic sites: neck and shoulder, hand and wrist, and low back. They may occur throughout the body, however.

To industry, CTDs mean low productivity, poor quality, and high medical and health maintenance costs. To the injured employee, the disorders spell pain, suffering, and low morale. In both cases, they are an undesirable outcome. Most states recognize CTDs as compensable work-related injuries/diseases. Current industry data show that a typical case would carry a cost tag of $5,000–$15,000, excluding indirect costs. Medical and legal costs constitute the major expense associated with CTDs. Such costs are expected to continue to increase. In recent years, the Occupational Safety and Health Administration (OSHA) has issued several well-publicized citations to various industries because of problems stemming from excessive cumulative trauma. Therefore, it is imperative that industry move toward the recognition and elimination of ergonomic deficiencies in the workplace. Ergonomics "done right, on time" would put a lid on the disorders.

PREVALENCE

CTDs are the final outcome in a long series of complaints of pain and discomfort. A survey of any manufacturing facility is likely to reveal a high percentage of the employees experiencing pain as a consequence of their jobs or activities. Complaints from as low as 20% to as high as 80% of the work force are to be expected.

Most estimates of CTD prevalence are considered underestimates because they are based on the late-stage or compensation cases. Higher prevalences are typically found between the two extreme conditions: pain and disability. Severe CTDs are basically rare events.

When early and mild cases of CTDs are considered, higher prevalence is likely to result. In a study that involved clinical assessment of approximately 2000 employees in five jobs across 14 plants, prevalence as high as 25% was observed. This high figure was the result of expanding the CTD criteria to include pain in early and mild cases, along with well-developed and advanced ones. This last category accounted for less than 5% of the employees at risk.

In the general population, the prevalence of the disorders is about even across the board. When there is a clear dominance by any specific disorder, then it is possible to recognize the role of some specific causal factors—those related to the job environment or to the characteristics of the individuals at risk.

The prevalence of these disorders among individuals in low socio-economic classes was rather high. Several explanations can be offered for this: (1) individuals in this class are typically employed in repetitive and stereotyped jobs, (2) because of their economic disadvantages, these individuals tend to maintain deficient diet along with little or no exercise, and (3) it is likely for the same individuals to experience frequent encounters with stress (at home or on the job).

One of the most troublesome CTDs has been carpal tunnel syndrome (CTS). Though infrequent in the general population (prevalence is considered less than 1%), several industrial studies have reported higher rates of CTS requiring surgery. A survey of over 1000 supermarket checkers showed that 62.5% of the participants had symptoms of CTS. Among Swedish meat packers, a rate of 56% was reported.

RATE OF OCCURRENCE

Management style, quality of supervision, and a host of behavioral factors play an important role in controlling the onset and spread of CTDs in a given plant. A workplace that fosters conflict either between management and employees or among employees may influence the prevalence and incidence rate of CTDs. Many industrial experiences support the contention that tendonitis cases seem to spread like a "rash," often developing without substantial forewarning.

Case studies show that a plant without a significant history of CTDs may suddenly experience an overwhelming and alarming incidence rate. Two plants similar in every respect (work method, performance standards, equipment, management) may exhibit quite different CTD histories. In most cases, the differences may be attributed to management practices and communication between management and employees.

CAUSES

CTDs are attributed to three types of factors: ergonomic, people, and management (1). The *ergonomic factor* focuses on the deficiencies in the man-machine interface at work. The *people factor* deals with the personal characteristics common to all CTD patients. A third cause less commonly discussed, but advocated here, examines the overall quality of working life—that is, the *management factor*.

ERGONOMIC FACTOR

From this perspective, CTD causality is assumed to be the direct consequence of deficient ergonomics involving the design of workplace, materials handling, tools, environment, machines, and job content. The link between the ergonomic deficiencies and the CTD development lies with the biomechanical interface. That is, the deficiencies create biomechanical stresses that may be expressed as a function of three parameters: extreme posture, high force, and task time and number of repetitions (frequency).

1. Extreme posture may be found in jobs in which workers are forced to maintain static (unchanging) positions or perform motions involving extreme and awkward (restrained or unnatural) reaches.
2. Excessive force results when high effort is applied. A comparable effect may result with moderate forces applied using small muscles repeatedly over time.
3. Time (frequency) becomes a concern when employees perform repetitious and stereotyped motions over very short task cycles.

High force comes about as either a single exertion of a damaging force or repetitive application of small force at a fast pace with inadequate rest breaks. The fitness of the person will have a moderating effect on the applied force. To an unfit person, the force exerted will increase the stress on the body many times, thus enhancing the potential for soft tissue injury.

Extreme posture with or without high force is likely to cause inflammation. Inflammation occurring in the course of repetitive motion will become chronic, for the body will not have adequate time to heel or repair itself. That is, the cause of inflammation will continue to be present.

The parameters (posture, force, time) are the equivalent of the measure of power in ordinary physical situations—that is, *force × distance / time.* Substituting Posture for distance, a measure of physical stress on the job can be written as:

Stress = Posture × Force × Frequency / Time

The higher the stress, the higher the risk for developing CTDs.

Workplace deficiencies manifested in extreme posture, high repetitions, and high force tend to accompany high CTD prevalence in certain jobs. In contrast, jobs free of or exhibiting less ergonomic deficiencies are likely to result in fewer cases of CTDs.

Deficiencies

Ergonomic deficiencies may be characterized by the two sources from which they arise.

Workplace

In this case there are inadequacies of the work station design, including its physical layout. Posture may be constrained by the components that make up the workplace: work surface, seat, work piece fixtures, and lighting. These components may be poorly designed, maintained, or improperly used. The failure to appropriately integrate all the workplace components may also cause posture problems.

Job

In this case there are limitations of the working posture governed by the work methods used for a particular task. These may be referred to as (1) the deficiencies manifested in the physical configuration of the equipment and work area, and (2) the deficiencies rooted in the job content (i.e., the tasks performed, their frequency and variety, the materials handled, and the tools used).

Performance Rates

High achievers and low achievers have the same probability of contracting CTDs because the amount of static loading will be the same for both. High achievers (exceeding the standard rate) end up with shorter work cycles and a higher number of work cycles per shift. Low achievers (falling below the standard) use a longer cycle coupled with proportionately fewer cycles per shift. Combining cycle time and total number of cycles per shift yields the exposure time during which static loading occurs. This time of static loading will be the same for those who fall below or exceed the standard by the same amount. Thus, low and high achievers following the same method are subject to the same risk of CTDs.

Environment

Noise, illumination, vibration, and cold can play a role in the causation of CTDs. Noise, considered a source of annoyance, may contribute to mental stress. Poor or inadequate levels of illumination causing visual strain (eye fatigue) may force the individual to assume and maintain a poor posture. For tasks requiring close visual contact, the contrast levels become extremely important. Poor contrast (white object on a white background) yields eye strain that forces the individual to concentrate more, resulting in mental and physiologic fatigue. Vibration contributes to the problem by acting as a direct physical stressor disturbing anatomic and physiologic characteristics of the soft tissues and by forcing an individual to develop and maintain awkward postures. A cold environment may affect the physiology of muscular actions, resulting in excessive physical loading.

PEOPLE FACTOR

Personal characteristics contribute to or enhance the development of CTDs. The attributes frequently cited follow.

Personal Attributes

Sex

It is primarily females who develop CTDs. As the literature explains, it may not be directly a function of "being female"; rather it is the types of jobs in which women are predominate. The biologic makeup of women does influence the development of these disorders. A high percentage of CTS cases are attributed to the hormonal changes resulting from use of oral contraceptives, pregnancy, menopause, and hysterectomies with bilateral oophorectomies.

Age

There is no significant age difference between CTD patients and workers as a whole. There is little or no evidence to support that age is a causative factor for CTD. The absence of a strong age influence demonstrates that job activities are a major causative factor.

Race

No conclusive findings regarding race and CTDs are available in the literature.

Geometry

Attempts have been made to link size of the wrist with the development of CTS. This is a point of controversy and disputed findings. For example, one published study suggests that the potential for CTS is high when the wrist is square. Other, equally persuasive studies show that wrist geometry has no significant effect on the development of CTDs.

Congenital Defects

Congenital soft tissue anomalies involving tendons, muscles, and joints have been shown to trigger CTDs, especially CTS.

Related Diseases

It has been ascertained that the presence of certain diseases may contribute to or potentiate the development of CTDs. Several systemic diseases related to circulation are believed to cause or exacerbate the development of CTDs—primarily CTS. Additionally, past injuries, traumatic conditions (such as bone architecture), and chronic trauma are present in a high number of CTD cases.

Summary

Although several attributes (age, sex, associated diseases) of CTD patients are identified, there exists no evidence that those patients differ from their non-injured co-workers. The personal attributes that "predispose" one to CTDs serve only to expedite the onset of the injury. Thus, they may serve no role in the actual CTD causation. Most of the injuries occur in the absence of those attributes.

Lifestyle and Environment

Unfit, overweight individuals have been found to experience CTDs more often than their physically fit counterparts. Similarly, obesity and cigarette smoking are both known to contribute to a variety of chronic diseases.

Diet

Deficient diet has been linked to many diseases, including those of the musculoskeletal system (e.g., arthritis). Living in a fast-paced and on-the-go society has its cost: deficient diet and loading on empty calories. Obesity is a major causative factor for several diseases: diabetes, hypertension, peripheral vascular disease, gout, and arthritis. An undesirable byproduct of obesity is the tendency of the individual to become inactive to the extent of leading to varicose veins. Obese individuals are the victim of emotional stress caused by discrimination on and off the job.

Vitamins

Often, the individual's diet may be acceptable in terms of the total caloric intake, but be deficient in vitamins B and C. Vitamin C is used by the body to build collagen and to aid in tissue regeneration. Vitamin B_6 deficiency may lead to depression, nerve irritation, and impairment of the immune system. Vitamin B_6 deficiency is one of the recognized causes of CTS. Evidence is presented to show that vitamin B_6 therapy is the treatment of choice (over surgery) for CTS.

Smoking

Smoking plays a considerable role in CTD development. Its effects on circulation and on the oxygen-carrying capacity of the blood are well established. Workers who develop CTDs are in large part smokers.

Fitness

Level of fitness seems to be the most critical factor in terms of CTD development. Many CTD cases show below-average scores for strength and flexibility. A sub-

stantial number (although not the majority) also exhibit below-average range of motion.

Stress

Stress from problems at home or conflict at work (arising from such factors as high job demands, unreasonable management expectations, and role ambiguity) can result in overloading the soft tissues to the extent of causing CTDs. Frequent and intense emotional reactions will cause damage to the body severe enough to produce a variety of painful disorders of the body. Migraine headaches, ulcers, numbness in the arms, heart problems, asthma, chronic constipation, and skin rashes are the outcome of chronic stress. These problems are neither imaginary nor "all in the head"; rather they occur because of real damage to the body. Although the damage is emotionally induced, it is as real and as painful as that resulting from physical causes. Personality types and emotional factors have strong influence on back pain.

Past Jobs

It can be assumed that many CTD patients previously worked in physically demanding jobs without the benefit of any ergonomic intervention measures, and that most of them held jobs in labor-intensive industries, such as manufacturing.

Time on the Job

The amount of time spent before the onset of injury varies considerably, from a few weeks to several years. This large difference in time to onset demonstrates that each individual is unique in his or her physical makeup (and in the possession of predisposing factors); this in turn determines the amount of time before job stressors cause CTDs.

Summary

In summary, several lifestyle factors seem to have some effect on the occurrence of CTDs. Cigarette smoking, below-average flexibility and strength, and lack of exercise and being overweight are primary contributors. Although these "fitness" variables do not show strong relationships with CTD patients, they cannot be ignored. Monitoring workers who are "unfit" may prove beneficial in CTD prevention. This also adds credence to the need for intervention in the form of fitness education or exercise programs.

The "CTD Person"

All the studies on personal attributes demonstrate that the individual's physical characteristics, as well as lifestyle, are in fact related to CTDs. From this we can profile the individual who is likely to experience a CTD. Such an individual could be described as follows:

A female over 40 years of age (perhaps postmenopausal) who is considerably overweight. She has had trouble with hypertension, diabetes mellitus, or other cardiovascular diseases. If employed, she works in a fast-paced, rigorously structured job requiring repetitious performance of stereotyped motions. Using only available data, however, we cannot determine which is the cause and which is the result, or which may serve to exacerbate the other's condition.

Clearly this is not the complete picture, and looking at personal attributes alone cannot provide us with a comprehensive view of CTD development.

Management Factor

Although personal factors explain some of the observed differences in CTD prevalence, health services and management practices exert their own influence.

Health Services

Medical facilities influence the presence or absence of effective means with which to cope with the problem. In most cases medical facilities, it is believed, can be considered the primary reason for the large difference in CTD prevalence among seemingly identical facilities.

Staff

Staff awareness is critical to the diagnosis and treatment of CTDs. In most cases, however, the in-house medical staff is unaware of ergonomics and the high risk of CTDs in the workplace.

Treatment Procedures

According to prevailing practice in industry, it is rather common not to take actions until a clear-cut diagnosis of the injury is reached. This delay is attributed to uncertainty as to the nature of the reported problem. Subsequent to the physician's diagnosis, case-tracking consists mainly of bookkeeping of days lost from work, restricted duty time, and job changes.

Once a diagnosis is made, the injured person returns to work in accordance with one of several options: the same job with full duty, the same job with restricted or light duty, a different job with full duty, or a different job with restricted duty. What happens to these workers after they return to work tells something about the likelihood of re-injury.

It is clear from many surveys that workers do not lose their jobs, nor do they spend much time in restricted (light work load) duty. Rather, they return to the same jobs that they held prior to the diagnosis of their injuries.

The problem with sending the worker back into the same job that may have caused the initial injury is simply re-injury. Further, the worker is most often put on restricted duty (whether or not it is the same job) while still recovering from injury.

Reports that cite common disorders associated with CTDs often list previous injury as a possible predisposing factor to more CTDs. Re-injury often occurs with CTDs.

It is acknowledged that finding appropriately different jobs for all injured workers (considering retraining and vacancy needs) is not always easy or feasible. The potential consequences seem severe enough to merit careful re-assignment of injured workers, however. Clearly the ability to place workers into substantially different jobs is impaired by unfamiliarity with job characteristics, a situation that is encountered at many medical facilities.

Quality of Working Life

The quality of working life is influenced by (1) communication, (2) presence of wellness and ergonomics awareness programs, and (3) the plant-wide work climate itself. These attributes (all functions of the organization) contribute to the overall (macro) ergonomic quality of the jobs.

Communication

The problems that arise from poor communication impair the quality of working life. Under such conditions, employees are reluctant to report problems that may relate to CTD development, such that early indications of the injuries (e.g., pain) go unreported. In those instances the problem is only identified when substantial damage has already been done. Additionally, impaired communication contributes to the overall stressfulness of the working environment, where an employee feels that he or she cannot get anyone to listen.

Plant-Wide Work Climate

Perhaps the factor impacting most on the quality of working life is the plant-wide organizational climate.

An atmosphere of acceptance toward worker's feedback regarding the job is important to encourage reporting of potential hazards. When workers recognize something to be a problem in their work area, they are more likely to report it if there is good communication with management. This is strongly influenced by how secure the job is. If one does not feel secure in the job, then one is less likely to report problems at work for fear of "rocking the boat." Thus, the hazards go unattended.

Early reporting of pain by workers, where encouraged by management, has significantly reduced incidence of CTDs. Workers who are uncertain about their job security may end up working in an overall atmosphere charged with conflict and mistrust.

Engineering Staff

Engineers play a secondary but important role in assuring the quality of working life. Their awareness of the implications of ergonomics in the design and maintenance of the workplace and jobs is equally relevant in minimizing job stressors. When successful, engineering interventions can play a large part in reducing CTDs.

Summary

Although these three resources (management, health services, engineering) in and of themselves seem to be important components, it is also important to consider the degree of interaction among them. Their cooperative efforts would seem to be effective in eradicating CTD from the work place. Unfortunately, quite often this is not the case. The professionals in these three areas are resistant to working outside their traditional roles.

ANATOMY OF A CASE OF CTD

January

Mrs. X is 44 years old. In her early twenties she was diagnosed as diabetic, and she has been on insulin ever since. She works at an incentive job in an electronic assembly plant. She has been with her company for approximately 6 years. She is slightly overweight and has been complaining about numbness in her right hand for about 3 months, which initially would come and go. Recently, however, her condition has worsened, and the numbness is present at all times. Her job performance has been affected. She is having much difficulty meeting the new production standard that was established a few months ago.

February

The plant nurse arranges for Mrs. X to see an orthopedic surgeon. Following detailed clinical examination and various tests, including nerve conduction, it is decided to perform a carpal tunnel release on the right wrist.

One Week Later

Following the operation, Mrs. X starts to feel better. The numbness in her hand is now gone. She and her doctor are quite pleased with the outcome. The doctor assures Mrs. X that it will not be long before she can go back to work.

Four Weeks Following the Operation

Mrs. X is back at work. She starts to feel some discomfort and occasional pain in the right wrist, the site of her old wound. She goes back to see the doctor. He recommends that she start wearing a wrist splint while at work.

Two Months Following the Operation

Mrs. X. is very concerned about her performance on the job. She is having a hard time meeting her production quota. The pain in her wrist is getting worse. She fears that the old problem will start all over again. She makes an appointment to see the doctor.

Three Months Following the Operation

Mrs. X is in pain; things are not going well for her. She has become very emotional about the whole thing. She has started to doubt the value of the operation. She blames the company and the job for all her problems. She is overcome with fears.

From the Doctor's Perspective

Mrs. X's case is extremely frustrating. Her wound healed satisfactorily. She has a good range of motion in her wrist. Her return to work was uneventful at the beginning. As she started trying to reach the target performance level for her job, however, things got worse. Her wrist started to hurt all over again. She has become very emotional. She talks about having the company to blame for all her troubles. It is quite difficult for me to advise her or to answer the questions she raises about her job and the responsibility of the company. There is nothing more to do for Mrs. X except to ask her to return to work. She qualifies for 5% permanent disability.

The End

Mrs. X does not return to work. Rather, she goes straight to see her attorneys. A suit is filed . . . well, the rest of the story should be familiar to everyone!

What Went Wrong?

Mrs. X's case is rather typical and is seen quite often in industry. The facts of the case are these:

1. Predisposed person assigned to unsuitable job.
2. Management failed to recognize the early warning signs of Mrs. X's condition: she experienced pain and numbness on and off for some time.
3. Following her surgery, no attempt was made to improve her workplace, method, or job content. That is, no effort was made to eliminate possible causative or aggravating factors that may retrigger the problem.
4. The doctor did not communicate to management what Mrs. X can or cannot do. Furthermore, the doctor did not attempt to learn much about Mrs. X's job demands.
5. From beginning to end, it is obvious that the involved parties (Mrs. X, management, and the doctor) did not communicate with each other. Mrs. X worked in pain for as long as she could tolerate it; management considered its job done when Mrs. X was sent to the doctor. The doctor's main concern was treatment of Mrs. X's condition—very little else mattered. The unhappy and emotional ending for Mrs. X was not warranted and certainly could have been avoided. Again, this shows the need to use ergonomics early in making a job fit a person with or without limitation.

STAGES

CTDs do not happen instantaneously or overnight; rather these disorders mark the end of a process that spans several stages of development. A person may go through four stages of pain prior to receiving a piece of paper from a physician designating the presence of a specific disorder such as tendonitis.

In Stage 1, the beginning, the person feels discomfort that usually disappears at the end of the day or with some extended rest. If the job and workplace characteristics are left unchanged, the discomfort will then turn into pain that is localized at some specific areas in the body such as the wrist or shoulder. Again, if nothing is done to address the root cause of this pain, it will become chronic. The pain then progresses to a point at which it starts to interfere with job performance.

During the second stage of pain, the person shows no specific signs such as warmth, tenderness, or redness. In many cases, the specificity of the cause of the pain may not be too apparent to the treating physician. More often than not, the situation is one of frustration for both the patient and the physician. Given time to run its full course, the pain will now be present along with some specific signs (Stage 3). The presence of such signs will help the physician in reaching a definitive diagnosis. At this point, Stage 4 is reached. To this end, standard clinical tests (such as Phalen's test for CTS) would yield reliable conclusions.

During the first two stages of the process, ergonomics can make its biggest contribution, and if done right, will eliminate the undesirable outcome—diagnosed cases. In contrast, if nothing is done about the early symptoms of pain, the condition will become progressively worse, changing from discomfort to a specific diagnosis.

TREATMENT

There are many prescribed courses of treatment for CTDs, from rest and taking some analgesics to surgery; from chiropractic manipulation to enrolling in pain centers; from physical therapy and exercise programs to behavioral counseling. Relaxation techniques, stress management, and biofeedback often help reduce tension and anxiety in chronic conditions.

All types of treatments have their place when it comes to dealing with CTDs. There are no guarantees of CTD treatment success with any one particular type. Many CTD cases were misdiagnosed, mistreated, or simply lost in the maze of pain clinics, therapy centers, or the "hush" offices of psychiatrists and psychologists. Therefore, the prudent course is prevention through the assurance of an ergonomically sound job.

Differential Diagnosis

Pain is a common symptom of many diseases and disorders that affect the body. Infection, tumors, injury, and systemic diseases are all producers of pain. And all share a common attribute—their origins are contained within the body. Accordingly, diagnosing the cause and prescribing an appropriate treatment are all but certain. This is not the case when it comes to disorders attributed to ergonomic stress. Factors such as posture, force, and time with a strong link to CTD causation may not be readily known to the treating physician. Absence of job data is likely to hamper the development of a timely and effective treatment.

Relief of Pain

Treatment consists of three parts:

1. Relief of pain and discomfort
2. Restoration of lost body functions through therapy
3. Protection against recurrence through improved job and workplace ergonomics

Perception

When in pain, we tend to fear the worst, expect ruin, and doubt a lasting cure. In sum, we work ourselves slowly toward anxiety and ultimately depression. All this complicates the situation and makes treatment difficult. Under certain conditions, some individuals may develop a pain personality in which it becomes more rewarding, either socially or financially, to stay with pain. Having the right expectation as defined by the treating physician and understood by the patient is the key to successful treatment.

The Culture of Medicine

Chronic pain continues to send the patient to see his or her doctor. Having no definitive resolution is a source of frustration for the physician who is accustomed to fast and short treatment courses. At some point, both the physician and the patient will become discouraged. The patient is then forced to seek other help or alternative medicine. Chronic cases are the orphans of American medicine.

Medication

Medication is often prescribed to relieve pain and discomfort. Drug therapies are often controversial; long-term drug therapies are never without some concomitant risk. Recommended drug remedies include analgesics, anti-inflammatory drugs, corticosteroids, muscle relaxants, local anesthetics, and vitamin B.

Splints

Splints or braces are used to ensure that the injured segment remains immobile (i.e., forced rest). Up to a point (no more than 4 weeks) such rest will be healthy.

Continuing rest by refraining from use or through restriction by splints may lead to loss of function or atrophy.

Although effective (if designed and fitted properly), splints can introduce new problems that include making job motions difficult and awkward. Exercise is a necessary adjunct to splinting to prevent stiffening of the affected joint.

Taping

Taping is supposed to increase joint integrity by maintaining the proper relationships between ligaments and tendons. Improper taping, however, can apply unnecessary pressure on the joint and its soft tissue to the extent of triggering inflammation.

Surgery

Surgery should be the treatment of last resort. Some CTDs respond well to surgery; others do not. Surgery should be only reserved for chronic and advanced cases. Even then, a second opinion should be sought. If symptoms are reported early, conservative treatment (through rest and medication) is likely to make surgery unnecessary.

Therapy

Therapy promotes constructive healing of the injured area. Muscles, tendons, and tissue will be returned to use gradually and carefully. This allows for faster healing and avoids stiffness and wasting of tissues following disuse. Therapy should commence within a day or two of injury. Other related approaches to therapy include the use of ultrasonography, cold treatment, heat treatment, diathermy, massage, manipulation, hydrotherapy, controlled laser systems, interferential currents, magnetic field therapy, and transcutaneous electric nerve stimulation (TENS).

Return to work

Following a CTD incident, the employee should be retrained to perform the job according to an ergonomically sound method. Emphasis should be on performance without assuming extreme postures or forceful exertions and unnecessary motions. Proper posture enhances movements and reduces the potential of joint and soft tissue injury. Optimal posture is possible only with adequate tissue flexibility, strength, and endurance.

The employee's supervisor, the engineering staff, and the medical staff should work together in planning and developing the retraining program.

Stretching

Tight muscles, tendons, and ligaments are injured easily and are likely to snap when subjected to sudden stress. Stretching reduces that risk by increasing blood supply to the tissues and by enhancing their elasticity. Stretching will make tissue more resistance to injury, sprain, or strain.

Ten to fifteen minutes of stretching before starting work is recommended. Frequent stretching throughout the working day is advised for repetitive jobs. "Pause stretching" is a label given to such exercises. It should be done slowly and for about a minute every hour or whenever possible. Fast or rapid stretching can cause more harm than help.

Wellness Program

Poor physical condition and obesity are closely associated with the development of CTDs (as well as job-related pain). It seems extremely important to provide some form of on-site exercise and conditioning program. Many companies offer after-work exercise classes.

Exercise

Exercise promotes the efficiency of both the cardiovascular and the muscular systems. It also enhances the action of the endocrine system (adrenal glands). Exercise improves the cardiovascular response to work, lowering heart rate and blood pressure while delivering adequate blood to the working muscles. It enhances the balanced development of tendons, ligaments, and muscles, leading to stronger and more-stable joints.

Physically fit individuals are capable of providing more steroids to minimize the effect of imposed stress and to aid in tissue healing. Exercise delays (and in some cases negates) some of the effects of the aging process by enhancing tissue nourishment and by making them stronger when they are subjected to stress and its byproducts.

CTD Control Program

A reliable and practical CTD control program would encompass (1) improvement and redesign of the workplace, materials handling, method, and job structure (2) education of employees and management, (3) monitoring employees at risk, and (4) rehabilitation (return-to-work programs).

Successful ergonomics means that a match between human work capacity and job demands has been effected. If this match is not achieved there will be manufacturing inefficiency, poor product quality, and pain at work. In almost all cases of ergonomic deficiencies, the causes or root cause can be isolated and profiled with certainty. Having the cause at hand, the next step is to develop and implement appropriate corrective measures to improve the ergonomic health of the workplace. To this end, a finite number of options are to be considered: (1) redesign the workplace, (2) restructure the job, (3) improve the method, (4) improve the materials handling and flow within and among work stations, and (5) increase employee fitness for work. A combination of several of these corrective measures is likely to be used to assure an effective and trustworthy solution.

ERGONOMIC TIPS

Ergonomic deficiencies can be eliminated through the diligent application of well-defined ergonomic principles and recommendations (2). There are many sources for such principles—textbooks, handbooks, and periodicals. In the mean time, for a start, the following design tips have proven their value in many industrial settings.

Avoid Extreme Reach

Integrate all workplace components and surfaces in order to have frequent task motions occurring in front of the body and between the hip (waist) and shoulders.

The optimal height would be within 1 inch of the elbows. Having adjustable work surface and seat (if one is used) will make the integration possible and effective.

AVOID EXCESSIVE FORCE

Reduce muscular exertions (forces) through minimizing weight handled, improving motion patterns, eliminating extreme joint motions (range of motion), avoiding awkward and maximum reaches, counter balancing and suspending tools, eliminating differential heights among product/component transfer points, using mechanical aids (e.g., powered conveyors, gravity feed devices) for moving products to and from the workplace, presorting and aligning work pieces (components), relaxing the fit tolerances for the assembly of components, and reducing pace or speed of motion (activity).

AVOID STATIC POSTURE

Job method should not impair circulation and should offer the muscles sufficient time to recover following exertions. Static loading can be eliminated through supporting body segments not involved in task motions. Seats and arm rests are examples of body supports. Use mechanical aids (jigs, special fixtures) for positioning and holding work pieces or components. Workplace should allow for flexible positioning of workpieces (adjustable height, angling, tilting, and rotation). Protective clothing should allow for freedom and ease of body movements and offer no impediment to circulation. Rest periods should be planned and scheduled to overcome any residual effects of static loading.

AVOID STRESS CONCENTRATION

Job activities should be shared by more than one muscle group. In so doing, static loading and excessive force may be eliminated as a byproduct. Use large-contact surfaces for hand-held tools. Use simultaneous arm motions. Change pinching to gripping, wrist motions to arm motions, and arm motions to shoulder motions. Eliminate pressure at points of contact between the body and the work surface, tools, machines, or any hard surface. For standing jobs, use cushioned floor support, modify job method to promote the use of "muscle pumps," especially in the lower extremity. Tightly fitted shoes and high heels (good examples of stress concentration) should be avoided.

AVOID FAULTY MAN-MACHINE INTERFACE

Machine controls should be designed according to the limiting values of human strength, body joint range of motion, and speed and accuracy of the required response. Identification, grouping, and the arrangement of controls and displays should conform to population norms and stereotypes. Eliminate the potential for ambiguous information feedback from the machine. Avoid

having the machine operator process complex pieces of data prior to making an appropriate response.

Display (visual or auditory) designs should take into consideration the potential user population, their skills and their degree of familiarity with equipment. Time, frequency of use, and the environment (noise, vibrating, light under which equipment will used) should also be considered.

AVOID EXTREMES OF THE ENVIRONMENT

Extreme environmental conditions are harmful because of the physiologic and stress responses they elicit from the body, as well as because of their potential for causing damage to the body tissues. Regardless of the type of the offending environment, from noise to vibration, from hot to cold temperatures, from brightly lit surfaces to high-intensity lights, the control strategies are the same. Basically, the following control options can be used separately or collectively:

1. Apply engineering changes and modifications to bring the level of the offending source to an acceptable level. Examples include the substitution of different material or energy sources, reducing the intensity (level) of the current source, and bypassing the source altogether through elimination or total enclosures.
2. Separate in space and time the offending source from the exposed individuals (receivers). Increasing distance from the source and shielding the receiver are examples of achieving the desired separation.
3. Eliminate any potential harm through limiting or minimizing the exposure of those working close to the offending source. The use of personal protective equipment is an example of this control strategy.

AVOID THE ONE-ELEMENT TASK, THE ONE-TASK JOB

The structure of many jobs in industry is based on the concept that efficiency results when employees are asked to perform singular activities or motions repeatedly throughout the work day. This is the rationale behind many of the assembly lines common to most manufacturing facilities. Years of research and field studies have shown the fallacy and harmful effects of the concept. Currently, the trend in industry is to have employees perform a cluster of tasks (jobs) either as individuals or as members of large teams. This shift in job structuring is known as *job enlargement* and/or *job enrichment*. Enlargement means that the job will encompass multiple tasks; enrichment means that employees will be entrusted with some control over the performance of their respective jobs.

AVOID PERFORMANCE STANDARDS THAT TARGET THE SUPERFIT

People should be fit for work. This fitness means possessing physical, physiologic, and psychologic abilities that exceed job demands. Ideally, job demands, as typified by established performance standards, should take into account individual differences. Differences due to age, sex, training, disease, and lifestyle play a significant role in defining the body response (strain) to a given demand level. When high demand levels cannot be lowered to accommodate the population at large, then pre-employment screening becomes inevitable. In such cases, job candidates have to be screened to establish a match between their abilities and the potential job openings. In any event, all screening tests should be developed in accordance with the EEOC guidelines and recommendations.

Avoid "Do's and Don't's" Training

Training of employees should go beyond the WHAT and the corresponding lists of Do's and Don't's. Although training in the WHAT is somewhat more efficient and in many cases economical, the employees are no better than the lists they memorized. For every rule it should not be difficult to name hundreds of exceptions. And in all likelihood, the exceptions will be the ones encountered in the workplace. It follows, therefore, that a better training strategy would be to teach the employees the *what* coupled with the *why*. Knowing the principle or the basis of given rules will allow the employees to deal with a variety of situations and conditions. In every case, they should be able to modify their performance to achieve the desired outcome. To this we may want to add the caution that no on-the-job-training should be used. Again, the harm that may result from unsupervised training would outweigh its expediency and cost many times.

Avoid Textbook Solutions

Textbook solutions may be nothing more than theoretical constructs and otherwise unproven proposals. Even when they have been successful, they may not be appropriate for a particular situation. The best advice is then to develop your own solutions—do not just buy answers, rather plan and test your solutions.

Any change or improvement in the workplace will be welcomed by a majority of those affected. Change always comes along with attention from management, the undeniable impact of a new thing, and real (or imagined) expectation for success. All of these factors tend to color the initial appraisal by employees. It would be prudent to plan for changes, to proceed carefully, and to objectively test any proposals prior to making the final decision.

It is also important to involve employees in the process of developing and implementing the changes. Sharing with the employees will undoubtedly tap a wealth of hands-on experience that may make a difference between success and failure. Many worthwhile improvement projects were doomed from the start because they were conceived, developed, and evaluated with little or no involvement from the employees—the ones who ultimately reap the benefits of our expertise, or pay a hefty price for our blunders. In other words, employees should not be the first to do and the last to know.

Ergonomic deficiencies are always accompanied with well-defined symptoms as discussed above. For almost all the symptoms, a proximate or triggering cause can be identified. For example, extreme or faulty posture is invariably the result of improper integration of the workplace and poor positioning of its operators. Table 48.1 provides some specific faulty postures and their respective proximate causes.

ERGONOMIC IMPROVEMENT SHOULD TARGET THE ROOT CAUSE

Treating the symptoms through dealing with the proximate cause may not lead to a lasting or perhaps significant improvement. Proximate causes are likely to be the byproduct of other deficiencies which may transcend several aspects of job content or workplace design (2, 3).

In searching for the root cause, the best approach is to critically examine the entire process, from start to finish, from receiving to shipping. As various workplaces and jobs are examined, the WHAT, WHY, HOW, and WHEN questions should be asked. At every point detail and evaluate what is being done, by whom, and why.

Consider the overall sequence and scheduling of various activities, tasks, and operations. In every case, consider the effect of rearranging, combining, simplifying, or perhaps eliminating some aspects of the workplace, the job, or the machine. Careful probing should help highlight the source of the observed deficiencies.

Quite often, the deficiencies may be attributed to one of three general classes of causes: (1) machine and tools, (2) materials handling within and among the workplaces, (3) job method and tasks making up the job assignment.

The following example illustrates the above points:

Example 1: Faulty Job Design

A manufacturer of large-scale electronic components delivers its products configured along with labels of included parts. Each label is a card that resembles a matrix whose entries are the codes for the different components that make up the customer's order (Fig. 48.4). The label is produced by a CAD (Computer Aided Design) system. The CAD operators receive from manufacturing a list of the parts that will be configured and shipped to the customer. Operators transfer the listing of component codes into matrix form using the CAD system. Up to this point the job is nothing more than a data entry task. Upon entering all the codes, the matrix is plotted by the system. The plot is then checked by the operator.

Table 48.1.
Faculty Sitting Posture and Its Possible Causes

Posture	Probable Cause
1. Head	
• Bent forward	• The operator cannot see the point of operation without bending head
• Tilted or rotated	• Direct or reflected glare
	• The seat is positioned incorrectly
2. Shoulders	
• Elevated/raised	• Work surface and/or some materials located too high
	• Seat too low
	• Some obstacles prevent operator from bringing the elbows down
	• Poor practice (habit)
• Sagged	• Operator seated too far from machine
3. Elbows	
• Elevated	• Materials located too high
	• Work surface too high
	• Backrest too wide, interferes with elbow movements
	• Some obstacles in workplace prevent ability to bring elbows down
	• Seat is too low
• Placed behind the shoulder	• Pick up materials from behind back
	• Poor practice
• Placed across the chest	• Materials located on poor side
	• Poor hand used to pick up material
	• Poor practice
• Elbow angle (flexion) is <90°	• Work surface too high
• Elbow angle is clearly more than 110°	• Work surface too low
	• Seat too high
	• Operator seated too far from machine
4. Hands	
• Located higher than elbow	• Work surface too high
	• Seat too low
	• Poor practice
• Located lower than elbow	• Work surface too low
	• Seat is too high
	• Poor practice
• Grasping, pinching or pressing forcefully	• Improper method
	• Poor tool
	• Soft material
5. Back	
• Bent forward	• (See "Head Bent Forward")
	• Poor practice
• Bent sideways or rotated	• (See "Head Tilted or Rotated")
	• Seat not positioned correctly toward machine
	• Poor practice
• Not in contact with the backrest	• Improper seat design
	• Improper backrest adjustment
	• Operator sits on front edge of seat
6. Thighs	
• Any weight on thighs	• Lack of convenient storage space
• Thighs pressed together	• Seat pan too narrow
	• Too much cushion on seat pan
	• Cushion too soft
	• Operator added makeshift cushion
• Seat edge presses thighs	• Seat too high
	• Seat pan has sharp front edge

Table 48.1. Continued
Faculty Sitting Posture and Its Possible Causes

Posture	Probable Cause
7. Knees	
• At different level	• Feet at different level
• Clearly higher than hip level	• Seat too low
	• Feet too high
• Angle is clearly more than 110°	• Operator seated too far from pedals
• Spread wide apart	• Lack of knee space under machine/table
8. Feet	
• Without support	• Lack of convenient footrest under machine/table
• At different levels	• Same as above
	• Pedals and footrest at different levels
9. General	
• The operator is sitting on front edge of seat	• Seat too far from machine
	• Operator added cushions to backrest
	• Poor practice
• The operator is sitting in skewed posture	• Seat not positioned correctly
	• Pedals not positioned correctly
	• Point of operation located too far to the right or to the left relative to the operator

If it looks okay, it is reduced to a standard size and shipped with the order.

To most CAD operators, the job was tedious and considered to be far below their skill level and training. Many complaints related to pain and general symptoms of fatigue were received from the operators.

To the field engineers, the labels had many errors: misplaced codes, wrong codes, incomplete information.

All the problems (operator's pain and field complaints) were attributed to a crowded workplace, improper lighting, and time pressure resulting from short job processing time.

To improve the situation, the obvious and expected recommendation was to improve workplace ergonomics: larger workplace, adequate work surface, adjustable seat, even illumination level and improved air circulation. All these changes would undoubtedly have a marked effect on the operators and their comfort as well as the quality of their work.

On reflection, however, one cannot avoid asking the question: have we really addressed the root cause of the problems recognized? The answer is a simple no! It is the job itself we should be concerned about, rather than the workplace. Manufacturing engineers produce component listings on their computers. These listings in turn are entered and printed in a special format by the CAD operators. The CAD treatment does not change or add anything new to the original data—that is, no value is

Figure 48.4. **Chart depicting CAD operator environment.**

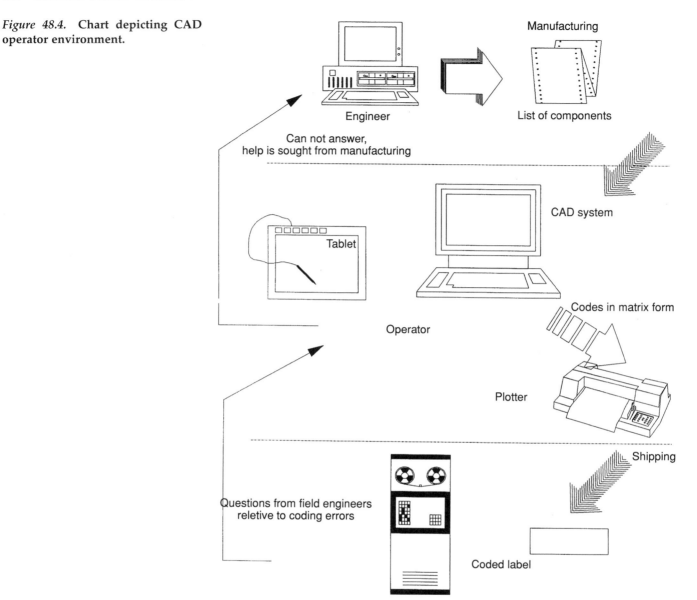

added. In other words, the CAD job is not required, for the engineers can format their output in the matrix form directly. This will eliminate errors in data entry, increase efficiency, and free the CAD operators to perform other jobs.

EXAMPLE 2: DO NOT IMPROVE AN OBSOLETE PROCESS

A tube-like product is made of several strips of rubber. The strips are laid on top of a drum with a diameter equal to that of the final tube (Fig. 48.5). Strips of different sizes (width and length) are then glued together to form the desired tube. A valve is also added to make the finished product. Throughout the tube building process, the operator is standing while using an assortment of rollers, brushes, and scissors. Preliminary ergonomic evaluation revealed that the operators spend more than 50% of their time using hand tools requiring exertion of

high force while maintaining extreme wrist postures (Fig. 48.6). A majority of the operators reported symptoms of pain, primarily in the wrist and low back. A few cases of CTS developed and required surgical treatments. The problem was attributed to the tools and the actual method used in building the tube. To address the problem, several improvement proposals were suggested. The proposals centered on (1) workplace modification to allow for using a sit/stand chair and for supporting the tools closer to the point of operation, and (2) redesign of tools to improve posture and reduce force. Successful implementation of these improvement proposals is likely to reduce the prospects of developing CTS. To some this would be considered a successful conclusion to a somewhat difficult problem—CTS. Considering the merit of the proposals and the state of the art in comparable processes, it was decided that tire-build-

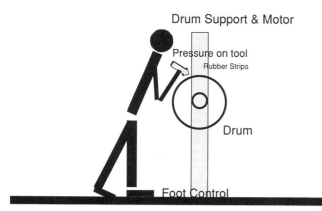

Figure 48.5. **Position of operator at drum rolling machine.**

Method Evaluation

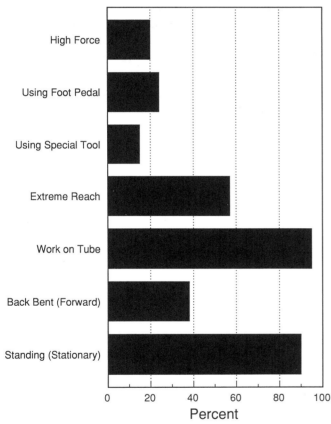

Figure 48.6. **Results of operators' reports.**

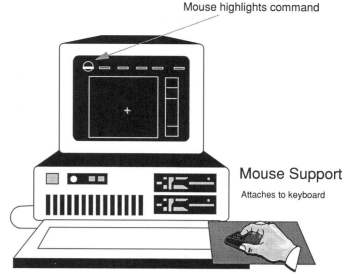

Figure 48.7. **Keyboard with mouse support attached.**

ing technology is readily adaptable for the product in question. Further, the new technology, being close to full automation, will totally eliminate the risk of developing CTS and concurrently improve productivity as well as quality. Cost analysis showed that the new system can pay for itself in less than 2 years.

EXAMPLE 3: DO NOT LIMIT IMPROVEMENTS TO THE OBVIOUS

The personal computer (PC) is unrivalled in its dominance in the office. It has become the sign of productiv-

ity and efficiency as well as independence. In the early days of the PC, the keyboard was the primary input device. Users of PCs labored for hours on their keyboards inputing commands and data in response to instructions from their software programs. As these programs started to pack in more power while offering more user-friendly features, the use of pointing devices became a necessity. Of all these devices, the mouse is the most widely used. The mouse, in a variety of sizes and shapes, complements the keyboard for input. And for some software applications, it has replaced the keyboard altogether.

Excessive use of the mouse has been linked with the development of CTS and other types of cumulative trauma disorder. We have encountered three cases in a small research office staffed with heavy users of PCs. The cases were initially attributed to the improper positioning of the mouse relative to the keyboard. To provide a remedy, a support for the mouse was added to the work surface (Fig. 48.7). The support, one of several commercially available models, did offer some improvement but failed to stop the persistent complaints from the users. This necessitated another examination of the problem, emphasizing the interaction between hardware and software (i.e., between the mouse and the computer program). The second evaluation determined that the design of the software program was at fault.

The three patients (one female and two males) used the mouse extensively to choose actions or commands by highlighting from a menu. Two of the cases were attributed to a specific graphics and charting program. The third case developed as a result of using a desktop publishing program. In every case, inputing data or making menu choices consisted of a series of mouse manipulations through several short moves.

When menu choices are numerous or packed closely together, mouse movements become short and are routinely made by wrist twisting and alternating from side to side. When these movements are rapid, the wrist becomes subjected to repeated cycles of acceleration to initiate the movement and almost immediately the wrist is decelerated to stop it at the desired command. The difficulty of the motion is amplified further when the PC monitor is small (e.g., 12 inches).

A menu with vertically stacked items is preferred over its horizontal equivalent, for it allows the wrist to remain straight while making most the selection with forward and backward hand/arm movements.

Therefore, it is a good advice to evaluate a software package in terms of its promised features as well as its mode of interface with the PC hardware, especially the mouse.

EXAMPLE 4: DO NOT IMPROVE THE SYMPTOM

A flashlight is manufactured overseas and shipped to the United States for packaging and distribution. Upon arrival at the United States facility, a sample of the lights are tested to assure the proper functioning of their on/off switches. If the switch fails to work on a certain number of units, the entire lot is rejected and sent to a special rework line for 100% inspection and repair, if needed. The rework line is simply a conveyor with a slow moving belt. Several operators, positioned on both sides of the belt, perform a sequence of operations. First the rejected light is taken apart (disassembled) by unscrewing the top from the body. Next the switch is checked out. If high resistance is encountered, a few drops of lubricant are injected over its base to minimize sliding friction. Following lubrication, the switch is retested. If it is satisfactory, the light is assembled without batteries and sent down the line for packaging and subsequently to shipping. Failure of the switch after repair will result in rejection of the light.

The rework line proved to be a source of pain for its operators. The intensive hand work (accompanying disassembly, reassembly, and switch repair) led to the development of several cases of CTS. A survey of the operators showed that 89% were experiencing pain and discomfort, and that most of them attributed their pain to working on the line (Fig. 48.8).

An ergonomic study was commissioned by the company with the express purpose of improving the line and bringing the CTS problem under control. Improving the line did not seem to be a difficult task. Indeed, with the help of the operators, several proposals were developed and their efficacy in addressing the observed deficiencies was assured. Before pursuing any of the slated improvements, however, the need for the rework line was put to question—why have a line to start with? If the light is manufactured and assembled correctly, rework would not be required. Several reasons were readily available to explain why it was difficult to con-

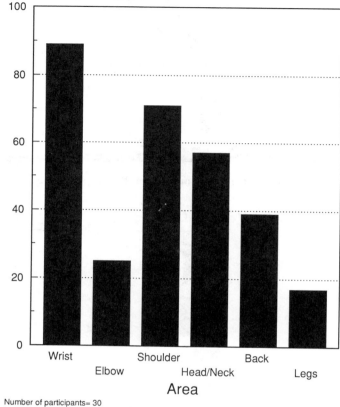

Where Does It Hurt?

Percent reporting pain

Number of participants= 30
Number submitting completed forms= 28

Figure 48.8. **Results of line-operator survey.**

trol product quality across two continents. In other words, management accepted poor quality as inevitable and responded by installing the rework line. Against conventional wisdom, it was decided to examine closely the basic design of the switch. This little side review revealed that the problem was with the switch all along. The switch block was designed with a slightly imperfect angle causing high resistance when pushed forward against its sliding arm. Any slight imperfection in forming the sliding arm added further to the difficulty of working the switch (i.e., it increased static friction). It follows, therefore, that the answer to the problem lies in the redesign of the switch and its contact angle with the sliding arm. The final recommendation was to eliminate the rework or "batch up" line and redesign the switch parts to minimize or eliminate static friction. In addition to switch redesign, recommendations were made to enhance the quality of the overseas manufacturing process.

ERGONOMIC IMPROVEMENT DOES NOT HAVE TO BE COSTLY

To achieve an ergonomically sound workplace does not mean a major investment and time-consuming

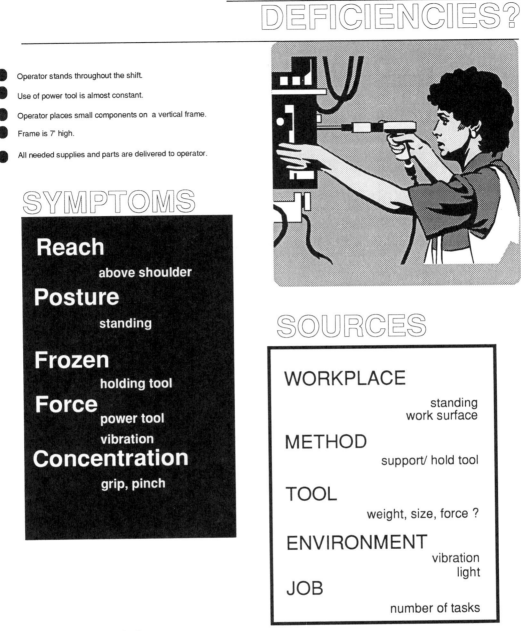

DEFICIENCIES?

- Operator stands throughout the shift.
- Use of power tool is almost constant.
- Operator places small components on a vertical frame.
- Frame is 7' high.
- All needed supplies and parts are delivered to operator.

SYMPTOMS

Reach
above shoulder
Posture
standing
Frozen
holding tool
Force
power tool
vibration
Concentration
grip, pinch

SOURCES

WORKPLACE
standing
work surface
METHOD
support/ hold tool
TOOL
weight, size, force ?
ENVIRONMENT
vibration
light
JOB
number of tasks

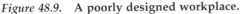

Figure 48.9.   **A poorly designed workplace.**

changes. Our experience confirms that a large percentage of ergonomic deficiencies can be attributed to poor integration of already existing workplace components or in not knowing how to take advantage of the features already in existence. An additional 20% of the deficiencies is the direct consequence of improperly designed workplace components. The correction of these can change the workplace to yield an ergonomics success story. The following are two examples.

EXAMPLE 5: IMPROPER MACHINE DESIGN

Consider the workplace given in Figure 48.9. As is clearly obvious, the posture of the operator is a sign of poor workplace ergonomics. Assuming that the desired ergonomic improvement is to eliminate this extreme posture, the decision becomes one of choosing between two alternatives: (1) replace the machine in question with a new one that exhibits recent advances in technology and, accordingly, would not require the observed reach and manipulation, or (2) eliminate the objectionable reach by simply elevating the operator closer to the controls. Alternative 1 presents a major and drastic departure from the existing practice. It will come about through a major investment in a new machine, job restructuring to accommodate the new machine, and retraining of operators to handle the advanced technology exhibited by the new machine. Summing up all these would make machine replacement a costly and perhaps infeasible alternative. In contrast, the second alternative is simple to implement—all that is required is to build a platform on which the operator can stand (Fig. 48.10). This can be refined further by adding a "stand/sit" seat to eliminate muscle fatigue. The platform can be made adjustable by using removable panels plus a base unit, allowing operators of different heights to maintain the same relative distance from the controls—in other words, an adjustable workplace.

Lesson Learned

The point of the above examples should be obvious— we should not rush to fancy, sophisticated remedies before taking a closer look at the existing situation. The answer we seek may be only a few inches away!

ERGONOMICS IS NOT ALWAYS 100% SUCCESSFUL

Sound job ergonomics is always equated with efficiency, product quality and, above all, well-being for employees. It follows that any ergonomic improvements in the workplace should yield instant success and acceptance among the employees. Unfortunately, our experience does not support this logical conclusion. It is safe to assume that any improvement project will, for one reason or another, be found unacceptable to some employees. The following is an example.

EXAMPLE 6: ACCEPTANCE OF ERGONOMICS

As a byproduct of an overall program to control (if not eliminate) a substantial risk of CTDs, a hosiery sewing job was targeted by management for improvements. Following an ergonomic review, several items were slated for change in the basic sewing workstation. The improvement list covered the seat, work surface, machine controls, materials handling, illumination, color, and contrast. Two new designs for the sewing workstation were proposed. We refer to them as workstations A and B. As with all ergonomic improvement projects, strong employee participation in all evaluation/testing was sought and encouraged. The two proposed workstations were placed on the floor in the sewing department for employee evaluation.

More than 40 operators took part in the evaluation of the two designs. Seventy percent of the sample preferred design A; only 50% preferred design B.

Following this initial evaluation, the best features in both designs (A and B) were integrated into one workstation that was tested by all the employees in the department. More than 86% of the employees judged the new workstation to be better than the existing one; 2% rated it worse ; 12% felt that the new station offered no appreciable improvement.

Not every change will be a welcome one from the start. Individual differences have to be addressed prior to

having the changes accepted. Our experience shows about 80% of those affected will accept the changes, if they are sound, without too much fuss. As for the other 20%, individual attention will be required. It should be the policy not to force any ergonomic changes on any of the employees. Rather, through "fine tuning" it should be possible to bring about an improvement that is satisfactory to the employee and, at the same time, is ergonomically sound.

Some resistance to change is natural and should be expected. In many cases, the unacceptance may be for genuine reasons, as when the selected improvement does not match certain individuals within the workplace. The problem can easily be resolved by "custom-tailoring" the change. On the other hand, occasionally some employees will not be happy with the change no matter what. Those employees can be easily recognized through the reasons they offer: "It will not work, my doctor says it is not for me, I am doing fine now, why change. . . ." All of these and many others can be considered symptoms of poor communication between those involved and management. Through personal counseling and education, most of those resisting the change can be won back.

INDUSTRY PRACTICE

A recent survey of industry indicated that workplace changes were suggested in more than 65% of improvement projects; making the workplace adjustable was the improvement of choice (Fig. 48.11). Job rotation and job redesign were the least advocated, recommended in no more than 17% of the cases.

RISK ASSESSMENT

Pain at work can be the byproduct of many sources; chief among them is improper ergonomics. This by no means negates or minimizes the contribution of other causative factors. Our ongoing research on this issue shows the strong and (statistically) significant contribution of two additional groups of factors: management and people (previously discussed).

In summary, pain on the job is likely to have ergonomic deficiencies as either the triggering or the aggravating cause. With ergonomic deficiencies, two additional contributors weigh heavily in the causation of pain: management and fitness.

Considering the role of these intervening factors, we would rewrite the basic CTD risk as follows:

$$\frac{\text{Force} \times \text{Posture} \times \text{Frequency}}{\text{Management} \times \text{Fitness} \times \text{Ergonomics}}$$

EXPERT SYSTEM FOR CTDs

An expert system for aiding in the detection of trauma-causing situations would ideally encompass the following:

Figure 48.10. **An adjustable platform greatly improves the workplace.**

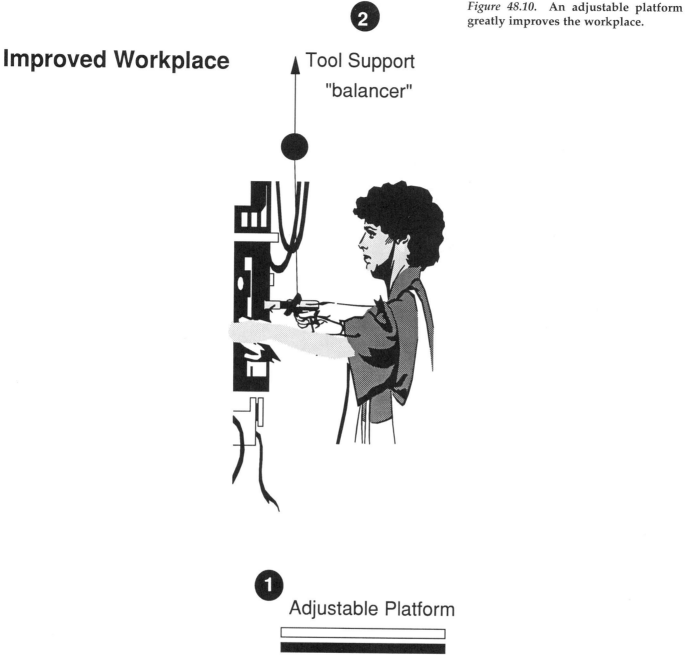

Improved Workplace

Tool Support
"balancer"

Adjustable Platform

1. The detection of ergonomic deficiencies in the workplace and the work method that could cause CTDs.
2. The prediction of possible disorders resulting from recognized deficiencies so that the seriousness of the situation can be assessed.
3. The interrelation of symptoms and deficiencies to a specific disorder so as to aid the treating physician in the diagnosis of specific disorders, and to link such disorders with specific ergonomic deficiencies.

The system, using artificial intelligence, would query the user about disease symptoms, workplace, and work method characteristics. Based on these responses and its knowledge domain, the system would then produce lists of possible disorders, relevant deficiencies, and suggestions for improvements (Fig. 48.12).

We developed a prototype of such a system using artificial intelligence. Artificial intelligence/expert systems are computer-based systems that make judgments and decisions of a complex nature similar to those rendered by an expert in a given field. They are used when the sheer magnitude of a problem involves an enormous amount of data for building the knowledge base of the system, coupled with the availability of few experts in the field. Such was the case concerning the many facets of CTDs and their causes.

Ergonomic Improvements

A Profile

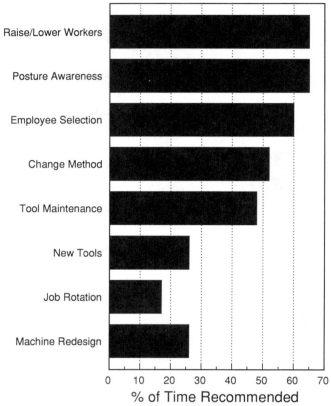

Figure 48.11. **Profile of industry recommendations for ergonomic improvements.**

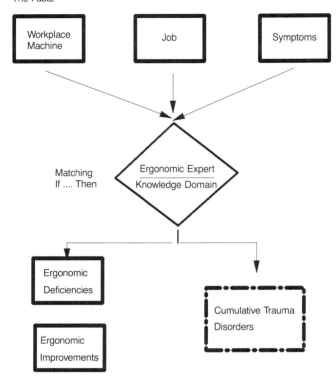

Figure 48.12. **A CTD expert system.**

Applications of expert systems already exist in several fields, ranging from agriculture to space technology, from engineering to medicine, from meteorology to information management, from electronics to law.

EXAMPLES

The intended uses and internal functioning of this prototype system can best be illustrated by considering three different application scenarios. All three scenarios deal with a female operator who assembles a variety of electronic parts. She performs her job sitting down. She is provided with a plastic chair that is fixed in height. The job method consists of reaching for parts placed in angled bins at eye level, and then attaching the parts at approximately shoulder level with a screwdriver to a board held in a vertical fixture (Fig. 48.13).

Scenario 1: Ergonomic Deficiencies

The plant industrial engineer decides to use the expert system to evaluate the deficiencies of the work station and the work method. Categories chosen to be evaluated are tools, seat, and work surface. Approximately 60 questions are asked by the expert system while searching for deficiencies. A condensed version of the session is presented below.

How many tasks or operations do you perform (type an integer)?	One
Is the cycle time of your task less than 1 min?	Yes
Is your task performed mostly with arm-hand motions?	Yes
Is your task equally shared by both arms? [Options = yes, left-dominated, right-dominated]	Right
Do you remain stationary during the entire task?	Yes
Do you follow the standard method for performing your task?	Yes
Is your tool a standard one?	Yes
Do you support your tool yourself while using it?	Yes
Does your tool pressure any part of your body?	Yes
Which body part receives the pressure?	Hand
Is your wrist extremely bent up or down during most of the processing?	Yes
Are your wrist motions accompanied by the use of twisting or force?	Yes
Is your elbow held up in the air when you use your tool?	Yes
Is your seat adjustable in height?	No
Do you have sufficient space for your legs and knees?	Yes
Do you usually sit forward on the front edge of your seat?	Yes
Is your work surface height adjustable?	No

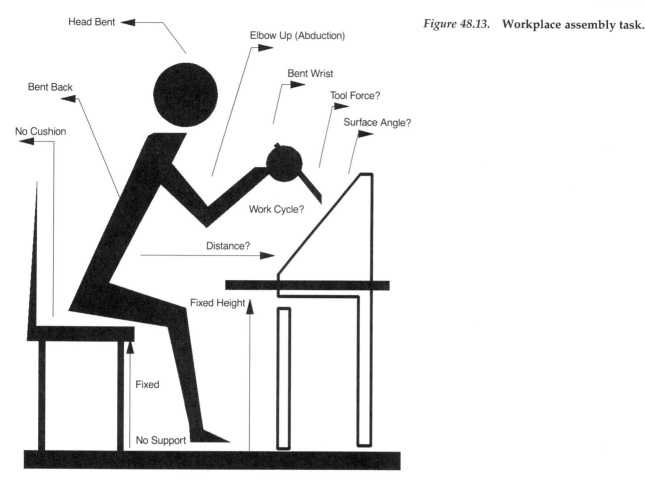

Figure 48.13. **Workplace assembly task.**

After asking the user the above questions, the system returns the following conclusion:

> I have determined that possible workplace deficiencies are:

Nonadjustable seat causing static loading on legs or lower back from not being able to change postures in chair; consider chair replacement with adjustable-type chair

Unadjustability of work surface height or angle causing possible eventual trauma to shoulder, head, lower back, or upper arms

> Possible work method deficiencies are:

Use of tool with extreme wrist deviation accompanied by use of force; suggest changing angle of tool so that wrist is kept straight

Standard tool is being used; investigate using tool more suitable for the job (possibly with ergonomically designed handle)

Short, concentrated task causing the likelihood of static loadings on muscles used; suggest enlarging job to include more tasks (such as obtaining materials—tasks having motions that would use a different set of muscles)

Scenario 2: Possible Disorders

If the above operator is actually experiencing aches and pains, or other symptoms, the operation of the system can be switched to the disease mode. If the operator states that her current pain areas involve the wrist and shoulder, the system will attempt to match symptoms to diseases by asking questions such as:

Is it true that symptoms = numbness and night-pain?	Yes
Is the affected trauma area stiff in the morning?	Yes
Can you make a strong fist?	No

Once all the questions have been answered, the system then concludes:

> *Possible diseases:*
> Carpal tunnel syndrome or pre-carpal tunnel nerve entrapment damage to the wrist and hand

Scenario 3: Potential Disorders

If the operator is not yet experiencing any symptoms, but wishes to receive an evaluation of possible diseases that may develop in the future, the system will first search for a body part that is being currently traumatized by work methods and/or the workplace. Once a body part has been matched with a workplace deficiency, possible diseases can be presented.

The preceding scenarios examining the same task from three different points of view show how the system data base is cross-linked among several categories. In other words, many of the queries are used in several categories with different rules. Accordingly, the expert system can take a minimal amount of information and apply it either to a disease or to work method/workplace deficiencies. This is how a CTD expert system incorporates the flexibility of a true expert into its program. The system, as presented and illustrated, can be considered a unique contribution to the field of artificial intelligence. Almost all medical expert systems in existence have dealt solely with matching symptoms with diseases in a diagnostic capacity. For instance, AI/Rheum diagnoses disorders of connective tissue rheumatology. Succeeding in relating symptoms not only with diseases but also with actual causal elements takes expert systems a step further into the realms of occupational preventive medicine and ergonomics.

CONCLUSIONS

Ergonomics alone is not the answer for dealing with pain at work. Instead, ergonomics should be incorporated in a comprehensive treatment that emphasizes improvement of the quality of working life through:

1. Workplace design
2. Job enlargement and enrichment
3. Employee selection and placement
4. Fitness and wellness enhancement
5. Communication and sharing between management and employees

Again, it is safe to say—and our industry experience supports this assertion—a workplace that is totally free from ergonomic deficiencies will not be free from pain.

REFERENCES

1. Burnett J, Ayoub MA: Cumulative trauma disorders: I. The problem, pain management, 2(4), 196–209, 1989.
2. ———. Cumulative trauma disorders: II. Assessment of risk pain Management, 2(5), 256–264.
3. Ayoub MA: Ergonomic deficiencies: I—Pain at work, *J Occup Med*, January 1989.
4. Ayoub MA: Ergonomic deficiencies: II—Probable causes, *J Occup Med*, February 1989.
5. Ayoub MA: Ergonomic deficiencies: III—The root cause and corrective measures, *J Occup Med*, March, 1989.
6. Ayoub MA, Wittels NE: Cumulative trauma disorders. *Int Rev Ergonom* 2:217–272, 1989.
7. Ayoub MA: *Ergonomics Digest*. Raleigh, NC, Ayoub & Associates, (PO Box 5702, Raleigh, NC), 1991.

ADDITIONAL READINGS

Ergonomics

Alexander DC, Pulat BM: Industrial Ergonomics: A Practitioner's Guide. Industrial Engineering & Management Press, Norcross, GA, 1985.

Drury C, Czaja S: Ergonomics in Manufacturing. Philadelphia, Taylor & Francis, 1987.

Ergonomics Group, Eastman Kodak, Ergonomic Design for People at Work, Volume II. New York, Van Nostrand Reinhold, 1986.

Grandjean E: Fitting the Task to the Man: An Ergonomic Approach. Philadelphia, Taylor & Francis, 1980.

Human Factors Section, Eastman Kodak. Ergonomic Design for People at Work. (Vol. I) (Lifetime Learning Publications, 1983.)

McCormick EJ, Sanders MS: Human Factors in Engineering and Designed 5. New York, McGraw-Hill, 1982.

Murrell KFH: Ergonomics: Man in His Working Environment. London, Chapman & Hall, 1965.

Shephard, Roy J. Men at Work: Applications of Ergonomics to Performance and Design. Springfield, IL, Charles C Thomas, 1974.

Singleton WT: Introduction to Ergonomics. Geneva World Health Organization, Geneva, 1972.

Singleton WT: Man-Machine Systems. Penguin, 1974, London. Biomechanics/Work Physiology.

Brouha L: Physiology in Industry ed 2. Elmsford NY, Pergamon Press, 1967.

Chaffin DB, Andersson G: Occupational Biomechanics. New York, John Wiley & Sons, 1984.

Ghista DN (ed): Human Body Dynamics. Oxford Clarendon Press, 1982.

Greenberg L, Chaffin DB: Workers and Their Tools. Midland, Michigan, Pendell Publishing Co., 1977.

Kroemer KHE, Kroemer HJ, and Kroemer-Elbert KE: Physiologic Bases of Human Factors/Ergonomics. Elsevier Science Publishers, 1986.

Pheasant S: Bodyspace: Anthropometry, Ergonomics and Design. Philadelphia, Taylor & Francis, 1986.

Ricci B: Physiological Basis of Human Performance. Philadelphia, Lea & Febiger, 1967.

Simonson E (ed): Physiology of Work Capacity and Fatigue. Springfield, IL, Charles C Thomas, 1971.

Singleton WT (ed): The Body at Work: Biological Ergonomics. Cambridge, England, Cambridge University Press, 1982.

Tichauer ER: The Biomechanical Basis of Ergonomics. New York, John Wiley & Sons, 1978.

Winter D: Biomechanics of Human Movement. New York, John Wiley & Sons, 1979.

Environment

Boyce PR: Human Factors in Lighting. New York, Macmillan, 1981.

Edholm OG, Bacharach AL (eds): The Physiology of Human Survival. New York, Academic Press, 1965.

Fanger PO: Thermal Comfort. New York, McGraw-Hill, 1973.

Hopkinson RG, Collins JB: The Ergonomics of Lighting. MacDonald & Co., 1970.

Horvath SM, Yousef MK (eds): Environmental Physiology: Aging, Heat, and Altitude. New York, Elsevier, 1981.

Huchingson RD: New Horizons for Human Factors in Design. New York, McGraw-Hill, 1981.

Oborne DJ, Gruneberg MM (eds): The Physical Environment at Work. New York, John Wiley & Sons, 1983.

Special Topics

Buckle P (ed): Musculoskeletal Disorders at Work. Philadelphia, Taylor & Francis, 1987.

Colquhoun WP, Rutenfranz J (eds): Studies of Shiftwork. Philadelphia, Taylor & Francis, 1980.

Grandjean E (ed): Sitting Posture. Philadelphia, Taylor & Francis, 1976.

Hockey R (ed): Stress & Fatigue in Human Performance. New York, John Wiley & Sons, 1983.

Ivergard T: Information Ergonomics. Kent England, Chartwell-Bratt Ltd., 1982.

Noro K (ed): Occupational Health and Safety in Automation and Robotics. Philadelphia, Taylor & Francis, 1987.

Polk EJ: Methods Analysis and Work Measurement. New York, McGraw-Hill, 1984.

Pope MH, Frymoyer JW, Andersson G (eds): Occupational Low Back Pain. New York, Praeger, 1984.

Salvendy G (ed): Handbook of Industrial Engineering. New York, John Wiley & Sons, 1982.

Sell RG, Shipley P (eds): Satisfactions in Work Design: Ergonomics and Other Approaches. Philadelphia, Taylor & Francis, 1979.

Sheridan TB, Ferrell WR: Man-Machine Systems. Cambridge, MA, The MIT Press, 1974.

Taylor W, Pelmear PC (eds): Vibration White Finger in Industry. New York, Academic Press, 1975.

Welford AT (ed): Man Under Stress. Philadelphia, Taylor & Francis, 1974.

Design

Clark TS, Corlett EN: The Ergonomics of Workspaces and Machines: A Design Manual. Philadelphia, Taylor & Francis, 1984.

Corlett EN, Richardson J (eds): Stress, Work Design and Productivity. New York, John Wiley & Sons, 1981.

Fallik F: Managing Organizational Change: Case Studies in Ergonomics Practice (Vol 3). Philadelphia, Taylor & Francis, 1987.

Flurscheim CH (ed): Industrial Design in Engineering. New York, Springer-Verlag, 1983.

Harker S, Eason K (eds): The Application of Information Technology: Case Studies in Ergonomics Practice (Vol 4). Philadelphia, Taylor & Francis, 1987.

Konz S: Work Design: Industrial Ergonomics ed 2. Columbus, OH, Grid Publishing, Inc., 1979.

Kvalseth TO (eds): Ergonomics of Workstation Design. Stoneham, MA, Butterworths, 1983.

Maule HG, Weiner JS (eds): Design for Work and Use: Case Studies in Ergonomics Practice (Vol 2). Philadelphia, Taylor & Francis, 1981.

Nadler G: Work Design: A Systems Concept. Homewood, IL, Richard D. Irwin, 1970.

VanCott HP, Kinkade RG (eds): Human Engineering Guide to Equipment Design. Washington, DC, US Government Printing Office, 1972.

Weiner JS, Maule HG (eds): Human Factors in Work, Design & Production: Case Studies in Ergonomics Practice (Vol 1). Philadelphia, Taylor & Francis, 1977.

Applications

Grandjean E: Ergonomics of the Home. Philadelphia, Taylor & Francis, 1978.

Grandjean E (ed): Ergonomics and Health in Modern Offices. Philadelphia, Taylor & Francis, 1984.

Grandjean E: Ergonomics in the Computerized Offices. Philadelphia, Taylor & Francis, 1987.

Grandjean E, Vigliani E (eds): Ergonomics Aspects of Visual Display Terminals. Philadelphia, Taylor & Francis, 1983.

Salvendy G, Smith MJ (eds): Machine Pacing and Occupational Stress. Philadelphia, Taylor & Francis, 1981.

Methods

Basmajian JV: Muscles Alive: Their Functions Revealed by Electromyography ed 4. Baltimore, Williams & Wilkins, 1979.

Chapanis A: Research Techniques in Human Engineering. Baltimore, Johns Hopkins Press, 1959.

Corlett EN, Wilson J (eds): The Ergonomics of Working Postures. Philadelphia, Taylor & Francis, 1986.

Corlett EN, Wilson J (eds): Methods in Applied Ergonomics. Philadelphia, Taylor & Francis, 1987.

Hashimoto K, Kogi K, Grandjean E: Methodology in Human Fatigue Assessment. Philadelphia, Taylor & Francis, 1971.

Meister D: Behavioral Analysis and Measurement Methods. New York, John Wiley & Sons, 1985.

Meister D: Human Factors Testing and Evaluation. New York, Elsevier Science Publishers, 1986.

Roebuck JA, Kroemer KHE, Thomson WG: Engineering Anthropometry Methods. New York, John Wiley & Sons, 1975.

Rohgmert W, Landau K: A New Technique for Job Analysis. Philadelphia, Taylor & Francis, 1983.

Singleton WT, Spurgeon P: Measurement of Human Resources. Philadelphia, Taylor & Francis, 1975.

Journals

American Industrial Hygiene Association Journal. Akron, OH American Industrial Hygiene Association (monthly)

Applied Ergonomics. Surrey England, IPC Science and Technology Press.

Behaviour and Information Technology. Philadelphia, Taylor & Francis (quarterly).

Ergonomics. Philadelphia, Taylor & Francis.

Ergonomics Abstracts. Philadelphia, Taylor & Francis (quarterly).

Human Factors. Santo Monica, CA, Human Factors Society (bimonthly).

IIE Transactions. Norcross, GA, Institute of Industrial Engineers (bimonthly).

International Journal of Industrial Ergonomics. New York, Elsevier (quarterly).

International Reviews of Ergonomics. Philadelphia, Taylor & Francis (annual).

Journal of Human Ergology. Tokyo, Japan (annually).

Journal of Occupational Medicine. Arlington Heights, IL, American Occupational Medical Association (monthly).

Work & Stress. Philadelphia, Taylor & Francis (quarterly).

Expert Systems/Artificial Intelligence

Andriole SJ (ed): Applications in Artificial Intelligence. Princeton, NJ, Petrocelli Books, Inc., 1985.

Waterman, DA: A Guide to Expert Systems. Boston, MA, Addison-Wesley, 1986.

Data

Diffrient N, et al: Human Scale 1/2/3, 4/5/6, 7/8/9. Cambridge, MA, MIT Press, 1978.

National Aeronautics and Space Administration: Anthropometric Source Book, Vol I, II, and III. NASA Reference Publication 1024. Washington, DC, Scientific and Technical Information Office, 1978.

National Aeronautics and Space Administration. Bioastronautics Data Book ed 2. Washington, DC, US Government Printing Office, 1973.

University of Surrey: Force Limits in Manual Work. Surrey, England, IPC Science and Technology Press, 1980.

Woodson WE: Human Factors Design Handbook. New York, McGraw-Hill, 1981.

CHAPTER 49

OFFICE AND HOSPITAL PAIN CONSULTATIONS

VICTOR C. LEE

PAIN PROBLEMS arise in the context of medical and surgical care. Physicians who diagnose and treat medical and surgical disorders must necessarily consider a patient's reporting of pain symptoms in order to formulate a diagnosis and a plan of intervention. This intervention must correct the pathophysiologic condition responsible for the pain, hence relieving the pain. This is the traditional model of medical practice which requires all physicians, and not just pain specialists, to understand pain symptoms and their underlying causes. Fortunately in most cases this medical model achieves its goals: pathophysiology is identified and with appropriate treatment there is indeed resolution of pain symptoms. Why, then, do we need pain consultants?

The pain consultant offers special expertise in the management of pain problems and the issues surrounding pain problems. Consultation with the pain specialist is required in the instances where merely identifying pathophysiology and instituting standard treatments fails to adequately deal with the pain experience and its impact on the patient. There are several well-appreciated scenarios in which this situation arises:

1. Pathophysiology is identified but is not reversible by standard treatments (e.g., pain of advanced malignancy, diabetic neuropathy, end-stage peripheral vascular disease, sickle-cell crises, acquired immunodeficiency syndrome [AIDS]), and persistent pain is a significant problem in spite of correct and appropriate medical care.
2. Pain is experienced acutely during institution of standard medical or surgical care (e.g., postsurgical pain). Although analgesics are prescribed, this pain may respond poorly to routine methods of analgesic administration. In the case of postsurgical care, inadequately treated pain can increase perioperative morbidity.
3. Pain persists in spite of (or because of) medical or surgical intervention (e.g., postlaminectomy back

pain, postsurgical sympathetic dystrophies, postamputation phantom pain). When the treating physician's interventions have failed to relieve the pain or have worsened the pain, he will often consult with a pain specialist.
4. Pain appears to exceed identifiable or understandable pathophysiology, and standard medical and surgical approaches are unable to offer any respite from chronic pain (e.g., chronic fibromyalgia, nonradicular back pain, refractory nonmigrainous headaches, abdominopelvic pain of indeterminate etiology). The primary treating physician may have little to offer this patient, and consults with a pain specialist.

The pain consultant plays an important role in assisting with the acute and chronic management of a pain experience that is otherwise inadequately controlled. The identification of physiologic and nonphysiologic factors important in sustaining severe pain, the institution of specialized interventions to supplement ongoing medical or surgical care, and the identification of a plan for managing chronic issues that may arise as a result of persistent pain are among the contributions made by the pain management specialist in the course of an office or hospital pain consultation.

MOST COMMON REASONS FOR INITIATING A PAIN CONSULTATION

OFFICE CONSULTATIONS

Pain Problems Typically Requiring Consultation

The pain specialist who is consulted in the outpatient setting is dealing in most cases with established chronic pain problems. The pain diagnoses in Table 49.1 comprise a typical mix of musculoskeletal and soft tissue pain, cephalgia, neuropathic pain, pain of malignancy, and other pain syndromes that are referred for consultation in a multidisciplinary pain management setting. Such patients are referred from a primary treating physician, whether he is in general medical practice or a

Table 49.1.
Most common diagnoses encountered at the University of Virginia Health Science Center Pain Management Center, 1991.

Diagnosis	ICD9 Code
Reflex sympathetic dystrophy	337.9
Kumbosacral radiculopathy	724.4
Extremity pain	729.5
Low back pain	724.2
Neuralgia/neuropathic pain	729.2
Herniated lumbar disk	722.10
Postlaminectomy syndrome	722.83
Musculoligamentous pain	728.9
Lumbosacral spinal stenosis	724.02
Lumbar strain/sprain	847.2
Fibrous myositis	728.2
Myalgia and myositis	729.1
Cervicalgia	723.1
Neuroma, lower extremity	355.8
Headache	784.0
Sacroiliac strain	846.1

specialty. The consultation is initiated because of pain issues for which the referring physician is inadequately equipped. This is not to supplant the role of the primary physician in diagnosing and treating pain. On the contrary, the primary treating physician is indispensable in assuring that a comprehensive and appropriate evaluation of the patient's pain disorder is initiated and appropriate medical care has been given. It is not generally the case, for example, that the pain specialist should be the one to diagnose a malignancy that the primary treating physician has failed to detect, although this may happen in rare instances (indeed, in some instances both primary physician and pain specialist miss a diagnosable medical condition such as malignancy or occult fracture).

How and When a Pain Consultation is Initiated

As "gate keeper" of medical resources, it becomes the role of the primary treating physician to determine at what point a particular patient's pain problem exceeds the conventional domain of medical diagnosis and treatment of identifiable pathophysiology. Only after conventional medical approaches have failed to resolve the pain disorder does the primary treating physician consult with the pain specialist, providing the pain consultant with as complete data as possible from his evaluation and treatment course.

On the other hand, care should be taken in not delaying a pain consultation, either. The pain experience may become unmanageable for the patient during the course of an appropriate medical work-up. For example, the use of analgesic medication may escalate inappro-

priately or the pain behaviors of a patient may become exaggerated during the medical evaluation, even before all the tests are completed. It is probably best to consult with a pain specialist earlier than later in these situations. A patient hospitalized acutely for evaluation of a severe pain disorder, for example, may be well served by a consultation with an acute pain service, even though the medical work-up is not yet completed. Certain pain behaviors may become entrenched in a patient's behavioral repertoire if allowed to go unaddressed for prolonged periods: successful intervention in a longstanding pain problem is probably more difficult to achieve.

It may also be prudent to consult with pain specialists prior to instituting treatments with irreversible consequences, such as back surgery or functional neurosurgery. The demise of the "low back loser" (1) has been well appreciated. Patients subjected relentlessly to repeated surgical procedures may be spared the downward spiral of pain and repeated surgery that only worsens the pain, if a pain consultation is obtained early in the process. Perhaps even the first operation may be avoided if it is found that objective pathophysiology contributes little or nothing to the patient's pain experience, and that psychosocial factors predominate (2).

Diagnostic and Therapeutic Nerve Blocks

Chapter 6 of this book is devoted to describing the role of diagnostic and therapeutic nerve blocks. The present discussion is not intended to duplicate that chapter, but merely acknowledges the emerging awareness in the medical and surgical community that nerve blocks have come to play a role in pain management. Consequently, a great number of referrals for pain consultation services often reflect the desire to have a certain patient either diagnosed or treated by a nerve block. Frequently the referring physician is most interested in having a nerve block administered in order to eradicate the patient's pain or in order to determine whether or not the patient's pain is "real."

The issue of "blockability" of a particular pain syndrome is a complex one. It is incumbent upon the pain specialist to define to the referring physician the proper role of nerve blocks in the care of the patient: whether or not a nerve block is indicated, whether or not it is expected to be of long-lasting therapeutic benefit, and whether or not it would provide any useful diagnostic or prognostic information. It should be pointed out that a particular pain syndrome may have multiple contributing elements: a given nerve block may or may not have the ability to alleviate all of the components of a given pain problem (e.g., a sympathetic nerve block may block either the burning pain or the allodynia, but not necessarily both of these elements of reflex sympathetic dystrophy [3], and may not block the accompanying myofascial pain or the joint pain elicited by physical therapy administered to a frozen shoulder).

In addition to multiple neurophysiologic components, a more global view of a particular pain problem may reveal that psychosocial and physical rehabilitation issues predominate, and that a focus on nerve blocks as a "curative" intervention may be improperly placed. Moreover, nerve blocks should probably be considered adjunctive rather than the primary mode of therapy (which would inappropriately link the success of pain management to the success of the block itself). With reflex sympathetic dystrophy, for example, appropriately administered physical therapy is often the key therapeutic intervention, with nerve blocks being administered largely for symptom control and to assist with the physical therapy (4). Finally, if any progress is to be made with patients suffering from chronic pain, it is important not to invalidate a patient's claim of pain: hence, nerve blocks should never be used as a "litmus test" to discriminate "real" pain from psychogenic or surreptitious pain.

Medication Issues

Frequently patients are referred for pain consultation after their primary treating physician has prescribed large doses of pain medication to no avail. The medications used (e.g., opioid medication, sedatives, and tranquilizers) engender long-term dependency issues and have frequently required escalating doses in order to stay the patient's complaints of inadequately relieved pain. It is certainly a highly desirable goal to have a patient's chronic pain managed without the use of dependency-producing medications, and a very important role of a pain consultation is to provide means of decreasing the need for such medications.

The use of opioid medication to treat chronic pain problems of nonmalignant origin is problematic for a number of reasons, not the least of which is controversy within the medical community itself (5). Opioids are of little or no use in certain types of chronic pain problems (6), and often some of the most serious issues generated by a chronic pain situation are best handled by psychological rather than pharmacologic intervention. The development of opioid tolerance, coupled with low efficacy of opiates for certain types of pain, often obliges the practitioner to escalate doses of narcotic medication. Patients who self-escalate their dosage may exhaust their prescriptions, necessitating inappropriate visits to emergency rooms or desperate phone calls to physicians at various hours of the day or night. Physicians facing this situation often consult with pain management specialists.

It is incumbent upon the specialty of pain management to educate our colleagues in the medical community not to overuse prescription medications. Chronic pain problems often are inappropriately managed by such medications. The minimal responsiveness of certain pain syndromes to opioid medication, the development of drug tolerance, drug dependence, chronic depression, and worsening pain all constitute a downward spiral that is often the patient's and the physician's worst nightmare. It is the hope of the pain management specialist to intervene early in the process of chronic pain and minimize or eliminate the use of opioid analgesics (e.g., by using nonaddictive adjunctive medication, or by invoking nonpharmacologic approaches such as counterstimulation techniques, biofeedback, and stretching exercises). But it is still fairly common to be consulted regarding a patient who has been receiving narcotic and sedative medications for years and whose referring physician has finally decided that he can no longer deal with the situation. It is then left to the pain management specialist to determine what approaches may be best used in reducing the patient's need and dependence on medication, to determine if drug detoxification is indicated and how it should be implemented, or if maintenance of certain medications is indicated. The answers are often not simple ones, and the pain specialist must be willing to take the time and effort to lead the patient as well as the referring physician through the complex issues that arise.

Back-to-Work and Disability Issues

Another frequently encountered question posed to the practitioner involved in the management of a chronic pain problem is "when will the patient be able to return to work?" It is a complex enough issue that embodies many separate questions:

1. To what extent is the patient's physical functioning limited by pathophysiology? —by pain? —by both?
2. Is improvement expected with treatment or rehabilitation? When is maximal improvement expected?
3. Will there be some residual functional impairment that would prevent the patient from resuming his original work duties?
4. If unable to resume his original duties, what sort of work can the patient be expected to perform?
5. When will a treatment course be completed, and what maintenance therapy may be needed after this?
6. If there is to be a permanent disability, what is the extent of this disability?

These questions are familiar enough to any practitioner who has worked with the on-the-job-injured patient, regardless of whether there is an ongoing pain problem. And yet they are often the most difficult questions to answer, particularly when there is a significant limitation imposed by pain alone, in absence of "hard" pathophysiology. An orthopedist referring a patient for a pain consultation may be unable to demonstrate an operable lesion or pathophysiology that would produce a quantifiable impairment, and yet requires an opinion from a pain specialist regarding the limitations imposed by pain itself on the patient. Although this is an area of medical determination fraught with ambiguity and inadequacy (7), increasing demands are being placed on the pain specialist to render an opinion regarding the impact of pain on the patient's ability to work. A pain consultant can expect to be confronted by such questions during the course of a clinical pain practice. Chapters 52–55 discuss the issues involved in assessing impairment in cases of worker's compensation.

HOSPITAL CONSULTATIONS

Chapter 51 discusses the organization and conduct of hospital-based inpatient chronic pain treatment programs. The present discussion will not duplicate this material, but rather deal with the issue of pain consultations that arise during the course of routine hospitalization. The patient may be suffering from pain that is directly related to his being hospitalized, or coincidental with the hospitalization. Hospital-based acute pain management services increase the availability of pain specialists who may assist with pain problems encountered in the hospital setting. The capability of responding to such problems in a timely fashion is also enhanced by such a service.

The management of acute pain problems in the hospital setting is best exemplified by the recent emphasis placed on the treatment of acute postoperative pain, motivating the 1992 release of the guidelines for acute pain management by the Agency for Health Care Policy and Research, Public Health Service, U.S. Department of Health and Human Services (8). The pain experienced following surgery often exceeds conventional analgesic regimens, in addition to posing special problems in certain situations (i.e., systemic narcotics administered to ventilator-dependent patients may delay or prevent weaning from mechanical ventilation). Consultation with specialists possessing expertise in managing pharmacologic techniques such as continuous narcotic infusions, patient-controlled analgesic regimens, perispinal opioid analgesia, and continuous local anesthetic infusions may be extremely beneficial for the surgical patient. Non-pharmacologic techniques such as transcutaneous electrical nerve stimulation (TENS), audio tape recordings of music or guided imagery for distraction or relaxation, and hypnotherapy may be applicable in selected cases. Chapter 46 discusses in greater depth the management of postoperative pain.

Besides postsurgical pain, a variety of other scenarios may prompt a hospital consultation for pain management services and may include examples such as the following: acute escalation of cancer pain, management of burn pain, trauma pain, pain of sickle cell crisis, pain of acute pancreatitis, and pain crises experienced during the work-up of acute musculoskeletal, abdominopelvic, or neurovascular pain of undetermined etiology. A hospitalized patient may require management of a concurrent chronic pain problem (e.g., low back pain, recurrent nonmigrainous headaches) during the course of hospitalization for an unrelated ailment. Occasionally, a narcotic-dependent patient may require special management during the course of hospitalization. Special advice regarding concurrent pharmacotherapy may be needed.

RESPONDING APPROPRIATELY TO A PAIN CONSULTATION

PROVIDING ANSWERS TO THE QUESTIONS

Responding adequately to a pain consultation demands an appreciation of what questions are being asked by the referring physician. It is important to appreciate the original course of diagnostic work-up and treatment of the patient; a mechanism for receiving this information from the referring physician is imperative. Professional acknowledgement of the referring physician's interventions is essential in a continuum of care. Although the consulted pain specialist may formulate an alternative hypothesis for the nature of the patient's pain complaints, the original questions raised by the consulting physician should be addressed in a satisfactory manner. For example, a patient referred for conservative management of lumbar radiculopathy may be found by the consulted pain specialist to be manifesting a myofascial pain syndrome. Perhaps a patient has been referred for evaluation of a suspected reflex sympathetic dystrophy; but the pain specialist instead determines that the patient's pain, although it may bear neuropathic features, is not a sympathetically maintained pain syndrome. Reasons for reformulating the working pain hypothesis, while discounting what may have been the referring physician's original hypothesis, must be detailed in a thorough and professional manner.

COMMUNICATING WITH THE PATIENT

Perhaps the most crucial element to successful intervention in a pain problem is communication with the patient. Often the greatest strides in pain intervention are made when the nature of the pain problem itself is delineated to the patient. In a highly technical and impersonal age of medical practice, the patient is most often left in the dark as to what is "wrong" with his body, why he continues to have pain, why little has been offered to him medically to take this pain away, why no more tests have been ordered, why he has been sent to specialists to no avail, and why he is even being referred to a "pain specialist." The primary referring physician may not have taken the time to discuss these issues with the patient.

First of all, the intentions of the referring physician should be explained to the patient, if this has not already been done (e.g., why did the doctor order or choose not to order a computed tomography [CT] scan?). The patient may already have perceptions, rightly or wrongly, verified or unverified, about what is causing his pain.

Table 49.2.
Primary Objectives of the Pain Control and Rehabilitation Institute of Georgia

1. Reduce the use and misuse of medication
2. Eliminate the use of optional health care services for primary pain complaint
3. Return to productive activity
4. Increase physical activities
5. Increase the patient's ability to manage pain and related problems
6. Decrease the intensity of subjective pain

Before a successful plan of intervention can be instituted, the patient must be convinced that a thorough and systematic evaluation of treatable pathophysiology has been conducted. He is unlikely to invest in a program of pain management if he feels that something about his body is still "wrong," that a pathologic process has been overlooked, and that all this business about "dealing with pain" is simply a diversion from getting the real problem "fixed." He is not likely to trust a pain consultant who is not in touch with all aspects of his original diagnostic workup (e.g., "Did you also get to see my x-rays, doctor?"). Effective communication to the patient concerning the development and rationale of his medical work-up, the nature of his pain problem, whether acute or chronic, the reasons for his consultation with a pain specialist, and the role of the pain specialist in his care constitute an essential beginning.

The nature of chronic pain is often the most difficult concept for a patient to grasp. On the one hand, he may become distrustful of a medical system that simply doesn't know how to fix his problem and feel that he has been "written off," or worse, is considered to have imaginary pain. On the other hand he may view the pain consultant as the ultimate rescuer who will devise a high-tech solution and completely eliminate the pain he has been carrying for years. The patient must be educated not only in the nature of chronic pain, but in the goals of pain management as well. Acceptance of his status as a "chronic pain patient" is frequently but not always the most difficult hurdle to overcome (indeed, some patients are relieved to have a physician finally tell them in an unambiguous way that there are no further medical or surgical interventions appropriate for their particular pain problem). Once acceptance by the patient is achieved, a set of realistic goals should be spelled out in great detail for the patient, such as decreasing medications, increasing activity, increasing tolerance for pain, and normalizing sleep patterns. Table 49.2 summarizes therapeutic goals embraced by the Pain Control and Rehabilitation Institute of Georgia (9). The pain specialist should never promise total elimination of pain unless he is prepared to guarantee such a result to the patient, or deal with the patient's disappointment when this promise is unfulfilled.

REASONS FOR UNSATISFACTORY PAIN CONSULTATIONS

The pain consultant does not practice his medicine in a vacuum; rather, he works within a network of primary and specialty physicians who rely on each other for effective management of particularly difficult cases. The multidisciplinary model of pain management, which is the current standard for comprehensive pain treatment, is built on the premise that no single specialist possesses all of the tools that may be necessary for the effective management of difficult cases of chronic pain. The "consultant" in pain medicine must necessarily rely on primary treating physicians for referrals into his practice, and must also have the appropriate resources for invoking treatments that may be outside of his own particular discipline (whether the pain consultant be a physiatrist, neurologist, psychologist, anesthesiologist, neurosurgeon, or other specialist). Such a consultant must know how to network effectively with his referral base as well as with allied disciplines in pain management in order to serve his patients well.

Whenever possible, the pain consultant should be in direct contact with the original primary physician. In a complex age of multiple specialty referrals, it is common for a patient to be passed along a chain of specialists until he finally arrives at the pain consultant's office. The primary treating physician may be unaware of the series of events and decisions that lead the patient to see the pain specialist. For one thing, the primary treating physician must be in agreement that the problem is indeed one of chronic pain. If not, the primary physician is certainly in a key position to "pull the plug" on what might otherwise be a positive therapeutic relationship between the patient and the pain specialist. It is imperative that the pain specialist establish a direct link with the primary doctor so that strategy and follow-up issues can be clarified for everybody, including the patient.

Ineffective networking probably accounts for many pain consultations that are perceived as unsatisfactory. Effective consultations require professional conduct at both ends of a consultative relationship, involving both referring physician and consulted pain specialist. The referring physician must be certain to provide complete and detailed information about his patient and the course of diagnosis and treatment, rather than sending a brief note having little more substance than "patient in pain, Dx and Rx" or a statement to the effect that "I've done all I can, now see what you can do to clear up this mess." Such consults are not likely to viewed as much more than a "dump."

Similarly, the pain consultant must not take such a stance with colleagues in allied disciplines of pain management whom he is likely to be consulting with (e.g., "None of my nerve blocks has worked, so now it is time for a psychological consult"). This type of serial referral of pain cases is likely to be ineffective and unsatisfactory because of its quasi-hierarchical nature and its lack of an interactive, or "interdisciplinary," structure. Such a serial, or hierarchical, referral structure is likely to bear the implicit message that the "most important" specialist takes the "first shot" at the patient, and that if he fails, the job falls to the "next most important" specialist in the hierarchy, until the final mop-up job is left with the least important team member.

A true interdisciplinary approach involves a parallel consultative structure incorporating the many specialties involved in the network of the pain management team. Each member in the team is consulted concomitantly, in a parallel fashion, rather than in a serial "trickle down" fashion. Each member must be consulted as a professional team member, and referrals should not be written in the manner that a prescription or doctor's order is written (e.g., "Rx: administer this type of physical therapy or that type of nerve block"). Each specialist should be consulted as to what specialized interventions unique to that particular discipline are deemed appropriate by that specialist. The overall strategy for managing a patient's pain problem must be planned by the team as a whole.

The pain consultant must also assure that specific questions raised by the consulting physician are answered in a satisfactory manner, as discussed in the previous sections. The consulting physician's original working hypothesis for the patient's pain problem must be acknowledged in a professional way, whether or not the pain specialist ultimately agrees with this hypothesis. It must also be worked out in advance what aspects of care will be handled by the consulted pain specialist and what matters will be directed back to the referring physician. Such issues include the following: who is responsible for medication prescriptions, who is responsible for taking the patient off his narcotics, who will order subsequent diagnostic studies or specialty referrals, and who is responsible for responding to the patient's worker's compensation and rehabilitation case workers. Many referring physicians are likely to expect that all of these matters would be taken care of by a pain consulting team, and indeed, well-organized pain consulting organizations are usually prepared to handle such issues. If not, the pain consultant should indicate up front what services are not going to be provided, such as drug detoxification (inpatient or outpatient) and the handling of worker's compensation issues, and what kind of follow-up responsibilities will be borne by the original referring physician.

Without effective communication regarding these matters, the patient is likely to "fall through the cracks," to be "left hanging," or to be "lost to follow-up." The pain consultant may begin to see fewer consultations directed to his practice. Inadequate communication be-

Table 49.3.
Pain Diagnoses by Location (Typically used as Primary Diagnoses)

Diagnosis	ICD9 Code
Head	784.0
Abdomen	789.0
Any extremity	729.5
Back	724.5
Chest	786.50
Face	784.0
Lumbar	724.2
Muscle	729.1
Neck	723.1
Thoracic	724.1
Sacrococcygeal	789.0
Shoulder	719.41

tween referring physician, pain consultant, and patient, as well as inadequate networking among the individual pain management disciplines, are likely to result in unsatisfactory pain management consultations.

PROVIDING SERVICE: CPT CODES AND WHAT THEY REPRESENT

In order to establish uniform guidelines for providing and billing for medical and surgical services, the American Medical Association has established the Current Procedural Terminology (CPT) handbook, which is by now familiar to most physicians. Medical reimbursement has become a quite complex science of its own, and changes in reimbursement practices occur in a yearly, if not monthly, fashion. The following section contains suggestions for how pain consultative services may be provided within the structure defined by the AMA's 1992 CPT codes (10).

The following section deals with services provided by a pain consultant, who is a specialist consulted by the primary physician. Services provided by a primary physician, namely, Office Visits, Hospital Care, and Critical Care, are not relevant here and therefore will not be discussed. The consultant services that are relevant to the pain consultant are termed Office Consultations and Hospital Consultations. Whenever consultations and procedures are performed, they must be rendered in conjunction with a medical diagnosis. Most medical reimbursement of services is based on standardized diagnostic terminology as provided by the ICD-9 listings (11); Tables 49.3 and 49.4 illustrate typical primary and secondary diagnoses used by pain consultants.

The crucial elements by Office and Hospital Consultations are History, Physical Exam, and Medical Decision Making, which are graded as to level of complexity by descriptors provided in the CPT handbook (Table

Table 49.4.
Pain Diagnoses by Presumed Etiology (typically used as secondary diagnoses)

Type of pain	ICD9 Code
Low Back Pain	
Lumbar strain/sprain	847.2
Sacroiliac strain/sprain	846.1
Arachnoiditis	322.9
Lumbar postlaminectomy syndrome	722.83
Lumbosacral spinal stenosis	724.02
Lumbar disk herniation	722.10
Lumbosacral radiculopathy	724.4
Spondylosis	715.18
Cervical Pain	
Cervical strain/sprain	847.0
Cervical radiculopathy	723.4
Postural neck pain	723.9
Herniated cervical disk	722.0
Cervical postlaminectomy syndrome	722.81
Neuropathic Pain Diagnoses	
Carpal tunnel syndrome	354.0
Causalgia	354.4
Reflex sympathetic dystrophy	337.9
Phantom limb syndrome	353.6
Intercostal neuralgia	354.8
Myofascial Pain Diagnoses	
Muscle pain	729.1
Fibrous myositis	728.2
Postural myositis	729.1
Muscle spasm	728.85

Table 49.5.
Office and Hospital Consultations and Their Corresponding CPT Codes

CPT Code	History Physical Exam	Medical Decision-Making Complexity	Suggested Times
New or Established Office Consultations			
99241	Problem-focused	Straightforward	15 min
99242	Expanded	Straightforward	30 min
99243	Detailed	Low complexity	40 min
99244	Comprehensive	Moderate complexity	60 min
99245	Comprehensive	High complexity	80 min
Initial Hospital Consultations			
99251	Problem-focused	Straightforward	20 min
99252	Expanded	Straightforward	40 min
99253	Detailed	Low complexity	55 min
99254	Comprehensive	Moderate complexity	80 min
99255	Comprehensive	High complexity	110 min

Refer to the AMA guidelines for Current Procedural Terminology for definitions of the above descriptors. All consultations should provide documentation of history-taking, physical examination, and medical decision-making. The suggested times are for reference only and should not be used as a basis for establishing level of consultation.

49.5). For a consultation to merit reimbursement, it must contain all three of these elements and provide adequate documentation of this. In the subsequent discussion, suggestions are provided for how to structure a pain consultation along these guidelines. These are suggestions only and not intended to be all-inclusive or exclusive of any tools that may be used by the great spectrum of clinician specialists who are pain consultants.

HISTORY

History-taking by a pain consultant should discuss elements of the pain complaint itself—precipitating events, exacerbating factors, sensory qualities of the pain (e.g., dull, sharp, burning, shooting), spatiotemporal aspects of the pain, and chronicity (including day-to-day variations). The patient should be asked about his medical work-up, what has or has not alleviated the pain, the impact of the pain on work and pleasure activities, social and family relations, and perhaps most importantly the patient's perception of his or her own pain problem. Based on how many of these elements are evaluated, the level of history-taking is rated as Problem-Focused, Expanded Problem-Focused, Detailed, and Comprehensive (Table 49.5). Most initial office con-

sultations should be conducted at the Detailed and Comprehensive levels, and most initial hospital consultations should be conducted at the Expanded Problem-Focused and Detailed levels. As mentioned previously, documentation must be provided.

EXAMINATION

Most examinations conducted by pain specialists focus initially on painful body regions; tenderness and limitations in range of motion and motor effort by pain; and alterations in the integument including edema, temperature, and trophic changes. Evaluation of trigger points is also included in such an examination (Problem Focused). The examination is expanded (Expanded Problem-Focused) when a neurologic exam is performed to evaluate sensory, motor, and reflex function. Pain syndromes producing perceived sensory alterations should prompt a "Detailed" sensory examination: qualities of sensation such as allodynia, mechanical and thermal hyperalgesia, and hyperpathia should be reported in addition to the basic sensory modalities of pinprick, thermal, vibratory, etc. The terminology used to describe pain-associated sensory alterations is defined in the International Association for the Study of Pain's published listing of pain terminology (12). Any report of headache, dizziness, altered special senses, or altered mentation should prompt an evaluation of the cranial nerves. Detailed kinetic and functional examinations, often involving specialized equipment, would probably fall under the category of "Comprehensive."

MEDICAL DECISION-MAKING

The clinician should probably take care to provide a level of decision-making that is commensurate with the amount of work put into his history and physical examination. The AMA descriptors of complexity of medical decision-making are Straightforward, Low Complexity, Moderate Complexity, and High Complexity. A recommendation of "continue present therapy and send patient back to me for follow-up in a month" is not likely to rate a very high level of medical decision-making, regardless of how many trigger points were examined or how many sensory modalities were tested.

The pain consultant's suggestions should, of course, incorporate a rationale and a plan of action based on a working pain hypothesis that would be presented in his "impressions" or "assessment" statement. This assessment should acknowledge that the referring physician has indeed performed a complete medical evaluation and provided correct medical care. Otherwise, if the pain consultant suspects that further work-up is needed, this should be made clear in his recommendations for further evaluations and diagnostic work-up. As stated before, pain consultants do occasionally find previously undetected pathology such as malignancy, thus reverting the case back to a traditional medical model at least until the pathology can be adequately worked up and correct treatment can be initiated.

The consultant's recommendations should address the patient's pharmacotherapy (e.g., continuing or discontinuing medications, instituting a different medical regimen). If pharmacologic adjuncts (e.g., antidepressants, anticonvulsants, skeletal muscle relaxants) are recommended, guidelines concerning medication selection, dosing, and projected duration of therapy should be provided. If the pain consultant disagrees with the use of narcotic or sedative-tranquilizer medications, this should be indicated, and the reasons provided. If a drug withdrawal program is advised, the consultant should provide detailed guidelines concerning how this should be done, and how pain escalation should be dealt with if this occurs during detoxification. If the pain consultant agrees that some level of drug maintenance is indicated, guidelines for this should also be provided.

The need for specialized interventions such as nerve blocks, stimulation techniques, physical therapy training and modalities, diet counseling, psychological counseling, and self-regulation techniques should be addressed if these are indicated (examples of CPT codes for some of these interventions appear in Table 49.6). The means for implementing such interventions should be described as well, if the consultant is not in a position to provide comprehensive services. Pain specialists are occasionally consulted regarding advisability of performing surgery, and a discussion and recommendations should be provided if this is the case. Finally, the consultant should provide some guidelines concerning

Table 49.6.
Examples of Procedural CPT Codes For Selected Services Provided By Pain Consultants

Procedure	CPT Code
Injection Procedures	
Trigger point injections	20550
Epidural block	62289
Other peripheral nerve block	64450
Physical Therapy Procedures	
Extreme testing	97720
Therapeutic exercise	97110
Functional activities	97114
TENS applications	64450
Psychological Services	
Psychological evaluation	90801
Psychotherapy 20–30 min	90843
Psychotherapy 45–50 min	90844
Psychotherapy 60–90 min	90841

follow-up care and what kind of response and long-term prognosis is projected, recognizing that this is fraught with some uncertainty and usually subject to change. Such guidelines should address such issues as ability to return to work, need for psychological or marital counseling, need for vocational rehabilitation, and the possibility of persistent functional impairment due to pain. Provision of most of the above elements in a pain consultation is likely to merit a level of "High Complexity" of medical decision-making, and anything less should be scaled down accordingly.

CONCLUSIONS

Pain consultative services are playing an increasingly important role in modern medical practice. Pain specialists provide special expertise in the management of patients for whom routine medical diagnosis and treatment (the traditional medical model) has failed to adequately deal with the experience of pain and the consequences of that pain. It is incumbent on the referring physician to still provide a thorough medical evaluation and appropriate medical care, but if the pain experience becomes unmanageable during the course of a medical work-up it is probably better to consult with a pain specialist sooner than later.

Most pain consultations present a number of recurring questions, beginning with querying the etiology of the pain (a working pain hypothesis) if that pain defies usual medical diagnostic approaches. Such pain problems can include acute as well as chronic pain problems, and the pain specialist is consulted regarding whether specialized pain interventions may help decrease the patient's pain experience, decrease his need for narcotic pain medications, or help restore him to a functioning existence. Although most office pain consultations will deal with chronic and subacute pain problems, hospital pain consultations deal in acute pain issues, such as traumatic and postsurgical pain, and with intercurrent chronic pain problems or medication issues.

Pain consultations should be provided within the context of a multispecialty, interdisciplinary practice network in order to assure that all pain issues can be adequately dealt with. The pain specialist should be able to review and acknowledge the patient's ongoing medical work-up and treatment and respond to specific questions raised by the referring physician. The consultation should be circumspect in its scope and specific with regard to the actual recommendations made. If interventions outside of the pain specialist's actual discipline or practice base are recommended, the consultant should provide specific instructions regarding the implementation of such interventions. Adequate communication should effectively link the pain consultant with the patient, referring physician, and associated pain specialists in the allied pain disciplines. The most common cause for unsatisfactory pain consultations is inadequate communication.

Pain consultative services can be structured within the AMA's CPT guidelines. Consultations must provide three elements: history, physical examination, and medical decision-making. Descriptors for level of detail or complexity of each of these elements are also found in these AMA guidelines. Reimbursement for different levels of consultative services will require adequate documentation of care in most cases.

REFERENCES

1. Sternbach RA, Wolf SR, Murphy RW, Akeson WH: Traits of pain patients: The low-back "loser." *Psychosomatics* 14:226–229, 1973.

2. Pondaag W, Oostdam EMM: Predicting the outcome of lumbar disc surgery by means of preoperative psychological testing. In: Bonica JJ, Liebeskind JC, Albe-Fessard DG (eds): *Advances in Pain Research and Therapy, vol 3.* New York: Raven Press, 1979, pp 713–717.

3. Lee VC: When sympathectomy fails to relieve causalgic burning pain. *Anesth Analg* 71:313–314, 1990.

4. Bonica JJ: Causalgia and other reflex sympathetic dystrophies. In: Bonica JJ (ed): *The Management of Pain, ed 2, vol 1.* Philadelphia: Lea & Febiger, 1990, pp 220–243.

5. Portenoy RK: Chronic opioid therapy in nonmalignant pain. *J Pain Symptom Mgmt* 5(Suppl 1):46–62, 1990.

6. Arner S, Meyerson BA: Lack of analgesic effect of opioids on neuropathic and idiopathic forms of pain. *Pain* 33:11–24, 1988.

7. Osterweis M, Kleinman A, Mechanic D (eds): *Pain and Disability: Clinical, Behavioral, and Public Policy Perspectives.* Washington, DC: National Acadamy Press, 1987, pp 211–231.

8. Acute Pain Management Guideline Panel: *Acute Pain Management: Operative or Medical Procedures and Trauma.* Rockville, MD: Agency for Health Care Policy and Research, Public Health Service, U.S. Dept. Health and Human Services, 1992.

9. Brena SF, Sanders SH: The business of pain management programs: How to plan and successfully operate a pain management facility. *APS Bull* 1:1–6, 1991.

10. Felts WR, AMA CPT Editorial Panel: *CPT 1992, Physician's Current Procedural Terminology, ed 4.* Chicago: American Medical Association, 1992.

11. Israel RA, ICD-9-CM Steering Committee, National Center for Health Statistics: *International Classification of Diseases, 9th Revision, Clinical Modification, revised edition.* Ann Arbor, MI: Commission on Professional and Hospital Activities, 1991.

12. Merskey H, International Association for the Study of Pain Subcommittee on Taxonomy: Classification of chronic pain, descriptions of chronic pain syndromes and definitions of pain terms. *Pain Suppl* 3:1–225, 1986.

CHAPTER 50

OUTPATIENT CHRONIC PAIN MANAGEMENT PROGRAMS

STANLEY CHAPMAN

CONSIDERING ITS prevalence, it is quite remarkable how little is known about chronic pain. Up until the 1960s, treatment options for patients with significant and unremitting pain were very limited. If patients persisted with pain complaints in the absence of medical findings, they often were labeled as malingerers, hysterics, or exaggerators. Often they were told to "live with it"; some were sent for psychiatric therapy, generally with little success. Paradoxically, the greatest advance in the understanding of pain in the last 30 years may be a realization of its complexity and of how little we know about it. No theory even begins to be sufficient in explaining the etiology of chronic pain, either from a medical or a psychological point of view. As pointed out in a carefully-prepared review article by Flor and Turk, the presence and severity of chronic pain among patients seen in pain centers is almost totally unrelated to medical findings (1).

This lack of correlation has led many individuals to espouse many alternative theories about chronic pain and its accompanying behaviors. The theory that such behaviors mainly are conditioned responses related to "secondary gains," such as disability money, drugs, relief from stress or responsibility, and sympathy from others, remains prevalent today. Among some who espouse this theory, there is the belief that this conditioning process occurs with little awareness on the part of the sufferer. Others express the belief (more often privately than in print) that many chronic pain sufferers merely are consciously exaggerating or fabricating their symptoms in order to achieve such gains. A careful reading of the research literature reveals that environmental reinforcers can greatly affect behaviors associated with chronic pain; such as inactivity, medication intake and verbal complaints; however, there is little or no evidence to support the idea that environmental rewards are important in the etiology of chronic pain or that chronic pain itself goes away with changes in those reinforcers.

Other psychological theories to explain the etiology of chronic pain may apply to some patients, but hardly have demonstrated anything approaching universal applicability. These theories have included suggestions that chronic pain is a response to prolonged stress, a form of depression masquerading as pain, or a response to a history of physical, sexual, or emotional abuse in childhood. A recent article by Gamsa compared 163 chronic pain sufferers with 81 control subjects on many measures of personal history, including parental bonding, depression, the quality of social relationships, work, and previous physical abuse, alcoholism, or drug abuse (2). Gamsa found that the presence of chronic pain generally was not associated with these variables, and suggested that emotional disturbance is more a consequence than a cause of chronic pain; however, it must be remembered that data from this study were based on patients' self-reported memories, the accuracy of which may be uncertain.

The realization that simplistic notions and beliefs cannot explain chronic pain represents an advance for research and for the assessment and treatment of patients. Researchers are recognizing that they need to refine their methodology, to look at selective subsamples of pain patients, and to evaluate many complex and interacting variables that may affect the expression and intensity of pain. Those who assess chronic pain are recognizing its complex and multidimensional nature and are being much more thorough and open to input from many disciplines. Similarly, chronic pain patients gradually are being treated with more respect for the legitimacy of their condition and problems rather than falling victim to a process of easy labeling. Unfortunately, this development has occurred only unevenly in the professional community and very sporadically among the lay public.

Well-structured interdisciplinary pain management programs are increasingly recognized as being necessary for chronic pain management. One can see evidence for this change in several developments, including the rapid growth of the American Pain Society as an interdisciplinary professional organization for expanding knowledge about pain; the explosion of journals and books that are designed for audiences of many disciplines; the development of specializations for chronic pain and/or behavioral medicine within many disciplines; and the increasing influence of accreditation standards for chronic pain management. Indeed, the number of centers accredited by the Commission on Accreditation of Rehabilitation Facilities (CARF) has increased each year since the first program at Emory University was accredited in 1983. As of June 2, 1993, there were 140 accredited programs, up from 38 in 1985. In addition, at least four states have mandated accreditation as a precondition for reimbursement for chronic pain management services through the states' Workers' Compensation systems. The CARF standards for accreditation clearly recognize chronic pain management as requiring specialized knowledge and an interdisciplinary approach (3). They include, as examples: provisions for specific training in chronic pain management for the medical director, regular involvement in the assessment and treatment of patients by a "core team" including the physician, psychologist/psychiatrist, physical therapist, and occupational therapist, and regular weekly team conferences to coordinate treatment among these and other disciplines.

Clearly, not all individuals with chronic pain are candidates for such an interdisciplinary approach. Professionals who see highly dysfunctional chronic pain patients often forget that there are millions of individuals with chronic pain problems in society who cope and function quite well and meaningfully with relatively little need for intensive treatment interventions; however, intensive interdisciplinary pain programs *are* often necessary for the many individuals with chronic pain who have ceased to function in a satisfying or adaptive way in many spheres of life. In a 1981 publication, Richard Morse coined the term "Disease of the D's" to describe such individuals (4), and included dysfunction, depression, dramatization of complaints, drug misuse, and disability as defining characteristics. One can add to this list several other related "D's," including a diversity of diffuse complaints, demoralization, disharmonious relationships, dependency on doctors, disuse of muscles associated with inactivity, and dollars and dollars of health care costs. The more of these D's that an individual has, the greater the likelihood that he or she will require an interdisciplinary approach in order to show functional improvement of these problems.

The structure of comprehensive chronic pain management programs has evolved and changed considerably since their inception. In the 1960s and early 1970s, most such programs consisted of costly inpatient treatment that would last anywhere from 3 to 6 weeks. Many of these programs were modeled closely after the program at the University of Washington espoused by Wilbert Fordyce in his pioneering text entitled *Behavioral Methods for Chronic Pain and Illness* (5). These programs used strict behavioral principles designed to replace pain behaviors (such as complaining, grimacing, staying inactive, and staying off work) with alternative health behaviors. Patients frequently were not allowed to talk about their pain and had to meet gradually more rigorous quotas for increasing physical activities and for tapering use of habit-forming medications to zero. The nature and length of treatment often were highly structured, if not predetermined. These programs demonstrated significant long-term success in meeting goals of medication reduction and reactivation, and a significant number of patients returned to work. Changes in levels of subjective pain intensity were modest, though many programs did not hold out subjective pain relief as a goal.

MODELS OF TREATMENT

The last 15 years have seen a growth of pain centers with very different structures and models. Many more patients with chronic pain participate in programs as outpatients, or stay in a motel or other unit outside the hospital. Treatment often is provided on a much less intensive basis, perhaps 1 or 2 days per week, rather than every day. This change has created some tension and disagreement regarding accreditation standards. Although the CARF still mandates that "a significant portion of the caseload attend a treatment at a frequency of 5 days per week for 5 hours per day" (3), there really has never been a clear definition of what the term "significant portion" really represents, leaving it up to the discretion of the survey team to decide if this standard is met successfully. Many outpatient approaches are far more flexible than the original inpatient programs, frequently offering a "menu" of a large number of different treatments that can be chosen to meet the differing needs of each patient.

Advantages and disadvantages exist for each model of treatment. Highly structured inpatient programs can be very powerful in their treatment effects because of the intensity of treatment and the control the staff has over the information and reinforcement received by the patient. A "therapeutic community" can be set up in which all interactions throughout the patient's day are structured to be part of the therapy process, and the patient can benefit from feedback regarding his or her behavior from other patients who are part of the community. The therapy team can supervise and aid the patient with many aspects of function on a daily basis, ranging from dressing and hygiene to social interactions and physical activities. The staff does not have to rely on the patient's self-report, but rather has the ability to observe behavior directly, and to take immediate corrective action to deal with any problem as it is occurring. Thus there is less opportunity for patients to provide lip service in support of rehabilitation, but not to engage in the behaviors necessary for its occurrence.

Another advantage of an inpatient approach is that the patient is taken out of the environment in which pain behaviors have developed. In some ways, the environment itself can have become a classically conditioned cue or stimulus for pain behavior; if so, a patient may be able to learn more-adaptive behaviors more easily in a "new" setting. In addition, an inpatient program may be absolutely necessary when the staff needs to have control over medications, either because of medical safety issues related to drug withdrawal or because the patient is so highly dependent on habit-forming substances that he or she cannot be relied on to withdraw such substances according to medical advice in an unsupervised setting.

Outpatient programs have substantial advantages of their own. One is greatly reduced cost; often the cost of an inpatient stay can be almost half the expense of an entire treatment program. In an outpatient setting, patients do not have to have their lives disrupted nearly as much. They can keep working if applicable, and they can maintain social and sexual relations. The staff has the advantage of getting feedback regarding how recommendations for behavioral change work out in the patient's natural setting. If treatments are spaced over a long period, the staff also can observe more easily the longer-term effects of interventions designed to reduce pain or increase function. It is much easier for staff to plan the termination of treatment, because visits can be made less and less frequent on a gradual basis as patients show improvement. In addition, the difficulty of transferring gains made in the hospital to the home environment is not present.

It also is much easier in an outpatient setting to individualize treatment and to make changes in the treatment plan as treatment continues. There is no requirement that in order to get paid a facility has to provide a certain number of hours of therapy whether the patient needs it or not. In addition, the staff does not have to be concerned with the possibility that patients will take on the identity of being very sick because they need to be hospitalized. Because of the flexibility of scheduling outpatient programs, patients frequently are exposed to a larger number of other patients dealing with chronic pain during their visits. This exposure can provide opportunities for modeling of patients who are being seen on a follow-up status or who may be much further along in reaching their treatment goals. It often is much easier for patients' families to be involved in outpatient approaches, because families can often accompany patients for their more-occasional visits.

There are few studies addressing the relative effectiveness of inpatient versus outpatient approaches for chronic pain management. In one study, patients had very similar types and hours of treatment regardless of whether they were inpatients or outpatients (6). Outpatients received their treatments primarily once a week for approximately 10 weeks, whereas inpatients were seen each weekday for 2 weeks. The main criterion for whether or not someone was assigned to be an inpatient or an outpatient was distance from the clinic, though other factors such as medication use and insurance approval did play some role; thus there was not truly random assignment of patients to inpatient versus outpatient treatment. Both at post-treatment and at 21-month follow-up, the inpatients and outpatients showed statistically equivalent improvements on all outcome measures, including subjective pain intensity, activity level, medication use, and return to work. The only variable on which they differed was on the total cost, which was much higher for inpatients. A more-recent controlled study by Peters and Large also showed similar post-treatment outcome data in patients undergoing a 4-week inpatient program and those undergoing a 9-week outpatient program for 2 hours per day (7). The authors looked at multiple physical, psychological, and behavioral outcome indices. Both the inpatient and the outpatient programs included interdisciplinary cognitive and behavioral treatments. Though this study did randomly assign patients to inpatient versus outpatient management, the number of treatment hours and the treatment personnel differed in the two programs.

In actuality, the key issue is not whether inpatient or outpatient approaches are superior, but rather what combination of treatments offered at what level of intensity and in what form are most effective for what types of chronic pain patients. Unfortunately, the research literature today provides us with very little guidance on this point. What is clear is that patients with high levels of pain behavior who show many aspects of the "Disease of the D's" are not likely to show functional improvement with medical interventions that do not address behavioral and emotional factors (8, 9). Such patients are likely to require intensive interaction that addresses physical, emotional, vocational, and social aspects of pain in a very systematic fashion. Requirements for excellence in such treatment are addressed in the following section.

CHARACTERISTICS OF EXCELLENCE IN CHRONIC PAIN MANAGEMENT PROGRAMS

CONSISTENT COMPREHENSIVE, INTERDISCIPLINARY, INDIVIDUALIZED CARE

A quality pain management program provides care that is interdisciplinary and comprehensive, with a well-structured, consistent, interdisciplinary team approach. Consistency is critical because so many patients with chronic pain have become confused and angered by the inconsistent messages heard previously about the etiology and treatment of their pain. Consistency requires evaluation by multiple members of the interdisciplinary team, who ascertain the likely contributors to the patient's dysfunction in the medical, behavioral, vocational, and social/environmental spheres. The team then needs to discuss and compare findings, consider the patient's goals, and formulate a treatment plan. The role and responsibilities of staff and patients in rehabilitation need to be specified and agreed on. Contingency contracts can be an effective vehicle for this purpose.

Interdisciplinary coordination is necessary because treatments often have the greatest power when they are offered contemporaneously and are interdependent. Many of the modalities offered at pain centers can mutually reinforce each other. For example, self-control methods for pain management such as relaxation can allow better success in drug withdrawal; injections for pain relief can allow more-vigorous physical therapy to be performed, and behavioral or pharmacologic interventions to enhance sleep can increase the success of daily self-control methods. To make everything work, the team must be more than a group of individuals from different disciplines, each of whom is seeing the patient. There must be constant communication among team members and mutual reinforcement of the overall goals. Team members must share a common philosophy of care, reinforce each other's role and communicate respect for each other's skills with the patient, and maintain awareness of what other team members are doing. Regular team conferences with all team members present are critical to maintain this treatment coordination.

Proper treatment coordination demands not only internal consistency, but also communication with outside parties involved with the patient's care. One frequently sees a tremendous waste of health care dollars and an undermining of the effectiveness of treatment from conflicting treatments involving physicians, chiropractors, or therapists who are not part of the pain center. Treatment programs need a coordinator who stays in touch with referral sources and outside treatment personnel; the time and cost of this coordination are miniscule compared with the consequences of failure to have it.

Specification of short-term and long-term goals and regular monitoring of progress toward these goals are critical. The goals that are set need to be specific, definable, and realistic. If anything has given pain centers a bad name among those who finance health care, it is continuing to see patients indefinitely with no documentation of goals or progress. When patients are not progressing toward goals, there is a need to explore the reasons and to intervene accordingly.

Treatment needs to be flexible and individualized as well as goal-oriented. Although it is easier to provide everyone with the same treatment regardless of diag-

nosis or individual needs, doing so is a prescription for failure. Programs sometimes provide treatment because the professional is there or because the machinery is there. Examples include giving physical therapy twice a day for 4 weeks to every patient regardless of need, or giving every patient biofeedback or hypnosis regardless of diagnosis or progress. Clearly, not every person has the same needs and not every individual progresses at the same rate. There is a need for a continuous redefining of goals and needs during team conferences.

Quality programs are aware of the costs and benefits of treatment and thus selective about whom they continue to treat. Early identification of the intractable patient is very important for cost containment. Categories of likely treatment failures include individuals who continue to look for a medical cure and never become oriented to a rehabilitation approach, those who persist in pain behaviors with no attempts to change despite interventions and education by the staff, and those who are so helpless and inadequate in coping with their problems that they are unable to learn from treatment suggestions. When it becomes clear that a patient cannot be helped in a program, it is the responsibility of the team to discuss the matter with the patient and to make appropriate referral or discharge arrangements.

Though programs need to constantly evaluate the appropriateness of treatment, they also must be careful about stereotyping patients too quickly. Professionals often do not realize how readily patients pick up on negative expectations or prejudices. There undoubtedly are many examples of patients being rejected because of their appearance, dress, social status, race, or educational level. It is clear from research to date that individual chronic pain patients are very different from each other, and that there is no such thing as a "typical pain personality" or a "typical Workers' Compensation patient."

One potentially harmful and commonly seen practice is to stereotype patients who may be having problems with certain aspects of treatment as being "not motivated." This labeling can be devastating, because it shuts off avenues of treatment that otherwise might be available. "Motivation" thus deserves a closer look. What motivation really refers to is the probability of engaging in a desired behavior. Borrowing somewhat from Thorndike, an early pioneer in psychology, I would like to suggest the following formula as describing this probability: $M = PS \times VR/E$, where M equals motivation, PS equals the probability of success in achieving a reward, VR equals the value of that reward, and E equals the effort required to obtain the reward. VR, in turn, can be expressed as the sum of the intrinsic value of a reward to the patient plus any external incentives provided. This formula basically states that individuals will be most likely to attempt something if they believe that they can achieve it, if achieving it is important to them, if someone provides them with an incentive, and if it requires minimal effort.

Looking at motivation in terms of its component parts can suggest particular avenues of intervention. Let us take the common example of a person assessed as not motivated to do physical therapy exercises. If that person's expectancy of success with physical therapy is low, the expectancy might change by having the person exposed to similar individuals who had gotten a lot better with physical therapy. The value of the reward might also need to be addressed. Increasing strength or range of motion may have limited meaning unless the patient understands that it will translate into much better ability to do tasks that are important to him or her. The value of doing it also might be enhanced if a reward system is put in place, such as by the spouse arranging a particular reward contingent on the successful completion of the daily physical therapy regimen. The effort to reach the reward might also need to be lessened in some cases, perhaps by reducing the strenuousness of the exercises or the number of repetitions or by teaching another way of doing them.

The comprehensiveness necessary for quality programs must exist in both the assessment and treatment phases. Diagnoses of patients' problems must follow careful evaluation that addresses the multiple areas of function affected by pain. Facile assumptions need to be avoided. (One of the most common is that a person's pain problem must be "psychological" because there is not physical evidence to justify it—an assumption based on the erroneous belief that one should be able to tell how much pain a person should have from medical testing results.) Assessment needs to include input not only from the patient, but also from important individuals in the patient's social and work environments. When interviewed separately, these individuals can corroborate the accuracy of patient self-report data (a major issue in outpatient treatment), and often can provide critical information not apparent from an interview with the patient. Frequent examples include problems with work performance, previous substance abuse issues, and important attitudes and expectations regarding treatment at a pain center. Employment of physicians who can thoroughly evaluate previous medical information, arrange whatever additional medical assessment needs to be performed, and then determine whatever restrictions (if any) need to be placed on activities also is critical for comprehensive assessment.

Treatment also needs to be comprehensive and to recognize the reality of a *chronic* condition. Ideally, a program has on staff enough professional resources to help with all the common problems and issues seen with chronic pain, including (as examples) work disability, sleep difficulties, inactivity, social and sexual dysfunction, and medical problems that arise. Recognition that the pain is chronic implies an avoidance of repeated treatment oriented toward temporary pain relief—unless such treatment fosters rehabilitation by allowing patients to improve their function.

FOSTERING PATIENT INDEPENDENCE

Every professional on the team (whether providing nerve blocks, physical therapy, or psychotherapy) needs to analyze the treatment he or she provides in terms of whether it is helping patients to be more dependent or to be more independent and functional. In order to be maximally independent, patients need to understand their condition thoroughly and how to manage it. Comprehensive patient education and the availability of staff to address patient questions and concerns thus are critical. Independent people have good stress management, assertion and communication skills, positive interactions with other people, and a high sense of self-efficacy and self-esteem. While these life skills and beliefs depend on experiences over a lifetime, quality treatment teaches and reinforces them along every step of the way. The atmosphere at quality programs thus needs to be positive and affirming, while challenging patients to improve their function despite the presence of pain. Many patients enter treatment with a tremendous sense of learned helplessness and need a lot of pushing and support to take the critical steps toward increasing function. The philosophy that patients can learn to live functional and satisfying lives despite the presence of pain must pervade every aspect of treatment.

VOCATIONAL REHABILITATION

Comprehensive vocational rehabilitation must be an integral part of a quality pain center. Failing to deal with issues related to return to work neglects one of the most important areas of people's lives that has been affected by pain. Employed individuals spend about one-fourth to one-third of their waking time at work, and work status is one of the most important factors in determining identity and self-esteem. In many cases, patients' sense of security and ability to make choices in life has been compromised not only by the presence of pain, but also by the loss of income associated with loss of work. Perhaps most importantly, work serves to make life more purposeful and meaningful. Evidence of the importance of this factor comes from observations of retirees who often feel a sense of aimlessness, and are particularly prone to depression. Moreover, work provides a social outlet and is a major source of friendships for many individuals.

Despite the importance of return to work, the reality is that there are obstacles for its achievement at every turn. The injured worker with chronic pain who contemplates returning to work often must overcome the demoralization and self-doubts that frequently accompany chronic illness and unemployment. Additional worries involve what the attitudes of peers and supervisors might be toward pain and limitations, the possibility of re-injury, and whether pain can be managed in the work setting. Though it is clear from the research literature that control over the pace of work is a critical variable for patients with medical limitations and pain, this control is rarely available.

Another obstacle for re-entry into the work force is that the injured worker may have to return to a rather unfamiliar job setting after prolonged absence or switch to a different kind of work. Doing so is likely to be stressful, particularly for the relatively unskilled individual who previously had been doing the same type of work for a long time. Prolonged inactivity and drug use may have resulted in reduced physical capacity and concentration, and thus can make working more difficult. The process of procuring work is difficult, particularly in today's environment in which prospective employers are fearful of escalating health insurance costs and cannot afford employees who may not be consistent in their carrying out of work tasks. Pain patients thus are faced often with the dilemma of discussing the health problems that they have had, with the risk of scaring prospective employers away, versus avoiding discussion of those problems and getting themselves into a situation where they have to fulfill work demands that are beyond their physical capabilities.

Obstacles from the standpoint of the employer include the possibility of increased health insurance costs, the risk of repeated injuries and absenteeism, and the costs of making special provisions to accommodate someone who has chronic pain or physical disabilities. Trying to arrange some kind of modified job schedule that would allow the worker some time to deal with acute flare-ups or engage in some self-management skills to prevent the exacerbation of pain can be economically or practically infeasible, particularly when other workers' completion of assignments is contingent upon getting certain tasks finished. Many injured workers lack the skill or education to assume job responsibilities that are more sedentary in nature, and sometimes unions have inflexible rules that prevent the employer from making special modifications in one individual's case. Special provisions may also run the risk of encouraging pain or illness behavior in other workers and in questions being raised (or lawsuits promulgated) regarding the fairness of different rules made for different employees.

Disability systems themselves often lack important provisions that would encourage return to work, such as provision for trial work periods or partial disability for lighter-duty or part-time work. The unpredictability of disability determination and the long waiting times involved are disincentives for return to work for an individual who is on disability.

A comprehensive interdisciplinary pain control center is in an ideal position to address disability issues associated with pain. Essential components of a pain and work

rehabilitation program include physicians who are specifically trained to assess impairment, disability, and functional capacity and who can specify what characteristics a work-place must have for the patient to be successful; physical and/or occupational therapists to deal specifically with physical and environmental obstacles related to return to work and to supervise a careful program that addresses these obstacles, which may include work simulation, design of the physical work environment, and supervision of regular practice of exercises designed to enhance physical capacity and conditioning; mental health specialists to assess and treat the fears, self-doubts, and other emotional and behavioral obstacles related to return to work; a vocational evaluator and/or counselor to assess the patient's skills and interests and guide him or her to feasible work solutions; and a team coordinator to work with insurance representatives, rehabilitation providers, prospective employers, and disability evaluators to communicate and implement the recommendations of the treatment team.

Though the responsibility of the staff to help is great, patients themselves must take most of the responsibility for their own vocational rehabilitation. Failures of patients to do so must be addressed immediately and clearly. Contingency contracts that clearly outline patient responsibilities often are necessary and beneficial. In order for there to be trust among all parties with a financial interest in the outcome, treatment facilities need to be regarded as fair—that is, neither as the agents of insurance companies by demanding that all patients return to work whether or not they are physically able, nor the agents of patients, by providing blanket certification of disability or by not holding patients responsible for their own role in rehabilitation.

FOLLOW-UP PLANNING

Quality programs must plan carefully for maintenance of behavioral changes over the long term. One study showed that 1 year after treatment only 18% of patients who had undergone comprehensive pain rehabilitation reported they were still doing daily all of the physical and occupational therapy and relaxation exercises that had been prescribed to them (10). Relapse prevention depends on many factors: a close and cooperative partnership with the treatment team so that patients feel that their problems will be heard and addressed as they occur following the end of treatment; gradual fading of treatment with appointments placed further and further apart as patients demonstrate increased independence in pain management, and the inclusion of the support system in follow-up planning. The family needs to know what behaviors to reinforce and suggest; the patient's physician needs to understand who will be handling medical care related to pain and what should happen if pain flares up; in Workers' Compensation cases, the insurance adjuster, rehabilitation provider and attorney

Table 50.1.
Patient Ratings at Post-Treatment Evaluation of the Helpfulness of Three Treatment Modalities

Modality	Number of Patients Treated	Rating (%)			
		Very Helpful	Somewhat Helpful	Not Helpful	Harmful
Physical therapy	221	60	35	5	0
Relaxation therapy	237	60	34	6	0
Sympathetic nerve blocks	222	22	45	31	0

all need to understand the follow-up plan, and the latter two need to be involved in efforts to return the patient to work.

Flare-ups also need to be planned for with the patient. Strategies for handling them may include the use of physical modalities of pain relief as well as cognitive strategies that address what the patient will say to himself or herself when a flare-up occurs. Left to their own devices, many patients will interpret a flare-up as meaning that the improvement that they had felt was not lasting or real, and they will therefore relapse into feelings of despair. If they are taught instead to see the flare-up as commonly expected, but controllable, then much of the fear and despair may be relieved.

PROGRAM EVALUATION

Quality programs need to develop meaningful ways to evaluate themselves on a regular basis. Indeed, meaningful program evaluation now is critical for accreditation of a chronic pain management program through the CARF. Standards mandate that each program evaluate itself in relation to its major goals on a regular basis, provide evaluation data to management, and then use those data to improve itself.

The development and implementation of a program evaluation system that works to create programmatic improvement are very difficult. Success depends on defining programmatic goals and on developing reliable and valid measures to determine success in reaching those goals. When goals are not reached successfully, ascertaining the reasons for failure can be an even more difficult task, and probably necessitates comparing one's data with those from other facilities with similar goals, programs, and patient populations. The CARF itself published a model program evaluation system that provides an outline of major objectives and methods of measurement common to pain management programs (11). The American Academy of Pain Medicine has established a committee to develop a highly specific and comprehensive system that can be duplicated at many centers.

As a CARF surveyor, I have noticed the following common problems of program evaluation systems: gathering of so much data that the time, expense, and cost of gathering it outweighs the benefit; using measures that are not reliable or valid (often because of their lack of specificity or objectivity), or that do not apply well to the chronic pain population, such as those designed for general rehabilitation populations; failure to provide sufficient data to explain outcomes, such as important diagnostic or demographic information; inappropriate periods of measurement, such as only post-treatment and not at follow-up, or so long after termination of treatment that results are likely to depend on too many factors independent from the treatment program provided; lack of standardized measures; and biased data gathering. Common examples of the latter would be having program evaluation data gathered by personnel actively involved in patient treatment, or failing to reassure patients that the program evaluation data they provide will not become part of their medical record.

PATIENT SATISFACTION MEASURES

Patient satisfaction with treatment is an aspect of program evaluation that now is required for CARF accreditation. The importance and practicality of such measures are reflected in their widespread use by profit-oriented businesses, which are willing to pay large sums of money to get customer input related to their products or services. Patient ratings of the perceived helpfulness of treatments have resulted in a reformulation and revamping of chronic pain management programs with which I have been associated. One example came from findings from a questionnaire in which patients were asked at post-treatment to rate each of a number of treatment modalities they had received as being "very helpful," "somewhat helpful," "not helpful," or "harmful." Results from over 200 patients revealed higher ratings for physical therapy and relaxation therapy (which consisted of only one session and suggestions for home practice with a tape) than for a series of lumbar sympathetic and/or stellate ganglion nerve blocks (Table 50.1). These results were startling to the medical director, who had expressed the belief that the nerve blocks were serving as a reward for rehabilitation efforts. This view was hard to maintain in the face of data that the reward was less positive to the patients than what they ostensibly were being

Table 50.2.
Mean Post-Treatment Helpfulness Ratings at Three Interdisciplinary Pain Management Centers

Treatment Modality	Center A (Outpatient)		Center B (Outpatient)		Center C (Inpatient)	
	Rating	N	Rating	N	Rating	(Ns = 17)
Medical						
Drug withdrawal	2.13	75	—	—	1.29	
Drug prescription	2.30	157	2.67	15	2.04	
Trigger point injection	2.14	162	0.75	8	1.60	
Sympathetic nerves	1.62	65	0.67	4	1.00	
Office visits	4.08	4	2.65	17	—	
Epidural steroid injection	—	—	0.33	9	—	
Psychological and medical						
Patient education	2.04	187	3.11	18	3.05	
Psychological						
Individual therapy	2.90	212	3.21	14	3.01	
Group therapy	2.15	132	4.00	17	3.67	
Relaxation therapy	2.53	224	2.78	18	3.69	
Biofeedback therapy	—	—	2.83	6	2.16	
Physical therapy						
Exercises	2.57	226	3.00	15	—	
Group Aerobics	—	—	3.00	19	2.59	
TENS	1.75	92	—	—	1.33	

rewarded for. As a result of these data, the physical therapy and relaxation programs were emphasized and strengthened further, and research was conducted to determine who was likely to benefit from the sympathetic nerve blocks. Several studies revealed that low levels of pain behavior were associated with better responses (8, 9). These data and increased medical testing to ensure the presence of sympathetic dysfunction resulted in much greater selectivity of injections and better cost-effectiveness of the program.

Patient satisfaction data are likely to be most relevant to a program when they can be compared with results from other programs in which similar kinds of patients are seen. I devised the "Treatment Helpfulness Questionnaire" as a standardized measure of perceived benefit of treatment. The concept and the method were very simple and were borrowed from previous work on visual analog scaling to measure subjective pain intensity. Horizontal 10-cm lines are drawn for each treatment modality with the following five headings centered at equal intervals above the lines: "Extremely Harmful," "Harmful," "Neutral," "Helpful," "Extremely Helpful." Vertical guidelines 1 cm apart along each horizontal line continuously reorient patients to the scale as they rate different treatment modalities down the page. Patients are instructed to make a mark along the lines to reflect the degree of helpfulness or harmfulness of each listed modality received. Each rating then is scored on a continuous scale ranging from −5 ("Extremely Harmful") to +5 ("Extremely Helpful"). The questionnaire

has been found to have excellent interscorer reliability (Pearsonian r = .979). Its test-retest reliability, as assessed with 19 patients and 152 sets of ratings repeated 1–5 hours apart, also was quite adequate (r = .856). The validity of the questionnaire is supported by findings of a significant association between helpfulness ratings for a given modality and the behavioral changes addressed by that modality, as measured at follow-up of 3–6 months. For example, significant correlations were found between standing/walking time and helpfulness ratings of physical therapy and of instructions to increase physical activity, as well as between self-ratings of ability to manage pain and related problems and ratings of the helpfulness of individual, group, and relaxation therapies. Though these kinds of findings are supportive of the utility of this patient satisfaction measure, it does need to be remembered that these correlations are based entirely on self-report data.

Table 50.2 presents mean post-treatment helpfulness ratings using the Treatment Helpfulness Questionnaire for patients at three major CARF-accredited comprehensive pain management programs. Center A was primarily an outpatient program with varying levels of treatment intensity depending on the individual needs of patients; Center B also provided outpatient treatment that included an intensive day treatment approach for many patients, and Center C provided an intense inpatient program lasting 3–4 weeks. These data revealed significant differences as well as similarities among the three centers. In general, psychological and educational

Table 50.3.
Mean Helpfulness Ratings at 3- to 6-Month FollowUp and Mean Cost of Treatment Modalities

Treatment Modality	Center A (Outpatient)			Center B (Outpatient)		
	Rating	Cost	N	Rating	Cost	N
Whole program	3.31	5982	8	2.92	6128	12
Medical						
Overall medical	3.00	4448	9	2.50	2800	12
Drug withdrawal	0.88	—	29	—	—	—
Drug prescription	2.19	—	67	2.80	—	11
Trigger point injection	2.07	638	79	0.29	617	7
Sympathetic nerve block	1.53	1661	44	0.00	4466	3
Epidural steroids	—	—	—	0.43	933	7
Office visits	2.62	984	9	2.67	201	11
Medical testing	2.95	2519	8	—	—	—
Work ability testing	2.31	459	7	—	—	—
Medical and Psychological						
Patient education	1.94	175	76	2.78	1043	9
Psychological						
Overall psychological	2.33	1311	9	3.64	2000	10
Individual therapy	2.30	791	95	3.16	512	7
Group therapy	1.91	144	70	3.09	624	11
Relaxation therapy	2.07	—	96	2.11	416	11
Biofeedback therapy	—	—	—	2.00	195	7
Physical therapy						
Overall physical therapy	2.17	765	103	1.82	1333	11
TENS	1.49	—	32	—	—	—

treatments ranked higher in patient satisfaction than did injections for pain relief. Findings that medical treatments tended to rank higher and group therapy and patient education to rank lower at Center A than at the other two centers were reflective of different emphases of treatment at the three centers.

Follow-up data from 3 to 6 months were available for both Center A and Center B, and included calculations of cost when those calculations were meaningful (Table 50.3). Some additions of treatment modalities to the Treatment Helpfulness Questionnaire allowed inclusion of data for some categories in Table 50.3 that were not presented in Table 50.2. Several interesting trends emerged. Overall, ratings tended to be lower at follow-up than at post-treatment, particularly for psychological, educational, and physical therapy approaches to pain management. Patients maintained ratings of a moderate helpfulness level for prescriptions of medications (generally antidepressants and nonsteroidal anti-inflammatory agents), whereas their ratings of the helpfulness of drug withdrawal (which was primarily withdrawal of narcotics) declined at Center A to near neutrality. There were some very striking differences between the two centers, with medical modalities generally continuing to be rated higher at Center A, and psychological and educational modalities to be rated higher

in Center B. When one looks at ratings of helpfulness in comparison to cost, the effectiveness of "cognitive" interventions such as office visits to the physician, patient education, and individual and group psychological therapy was underscored, whereas the cost-effectiveness of injections for pain relief seemed questionable, particularly at Center B.

These kinds of data have practical implications. One wonders if more-aggressive or different follow-up procedures would have helped to prevent some of the declines in ratings seen from post-treatment evaluation to follow-up, or if treatment at Center A could not be enhanced by modeling it after some of the successful psychological interventions (particularly group interventions) from Center B, and vice-versa for some medical interventions, such as trigger point injections. Inasmuch as significantly different mean ratings of the helpfulness of individual therapy were found among different psychologists at Center A, one also wonders if those with lower ratings could improve their ratings by observing and learning from those with higher ratings.

Another measure of patient satisfaction consists of comments patients are invited to make about a program post-treatment and at follow-up. A recent analysis of such free-flowing comments from 136 patients seen at a comprehensive pain center provided a different kind of insight regarding the effects of treatment. Though some patients had reported limited relief of pain with treatment, over 80% of their comments were positive. Three themes were prominent in the comments made: the importance of a positive and receptive treatment atmosphere (e.g., "everyone cared and took time and was enthusiastic that I could learn to cope with all the problems brought about by my pain"); the concept that pain could be managed if not changed (e.g., "I realized I could be a happy and worthwhile person even if I hurt"); and the importance of education (e.g., "understanding all the causes of my pain and having guidelines to teach me what I could do about it made a big difference"). Remarks about specific techniques and procedures were not prevalent in the comments.

GROUP APPROACHES

Patient comments and helpfulness data suggest how important group approaches can be in chronic pain management. Groups can provide an antidote to several "poisons" experienced by many chronic pain patients: isolation, hopelessness, low self-esteem, and feeling misunderstood. The ability to express these problems in a supportive environment seems to have a liberating or unblocking effect for many patients; however, the group must progress beyond a mere description of problems and frustrations to reinforcement for positive coping, enhanced function, and not letting oneself be defeated by the presence of pain and limitations.

For groups to be successful, good leadership from a therapist is critical. While encouraging patients to interact with each other, the leader must make sure that the group stays on relevant issues, that one person's problems do not dominate the group, and that no group member's needs are ignored or inappropriately punished. The leader also needs to make sure that groups do not deteriorate exclusively into a "Polyanna" group, in which there is no realistic working out of problems, or a complaint group that just simply reinforces negative emotions. A good group leader can foster a therapeutic process in which feedback and support are given by group members who are more experienced or skilled in pain management to those who are just starting or who are less skilled. Inasmuch as reaching out to help someone else can be as therapeutic for the provider of care as for the recipient of care, all can benefit from this process. This phenomenon suggests the importance of mixing in groups patients who are just starting with those who are well along in treatment.

Long-term support groups can be critical, because maintaining rehabilitation efforts in the absence of reinforcement can be difficult, lonely, and often discouraging. Many pain programs have support groups that meet at their center, either with or without professional supervision. The American Chronic Pain Association is an organization that supplies information, structure, and support for patients who wish to establish their own support groups. The Association has adopted 10 goals for patients to work toward or maintain, which are very much in harmony with the goals of most chronic pain management programs. These goals are based on the principles of acceptance, self-control, realistic goal setting, attention to emotions, relaxation, exercise, and adherence to the principles of gradual recovery and to the importance of reaching out for the support of others.

CONCLUSIONS

In summary, chronic pain patients are among the most difficult individuals to treat because of the breadth of their problems and the lack of scientific understanding of pain. To be effective, pain programs need to provide comprehensive, closely coordinated, and goal-oriented treatment in an interdisciplinary team approach. Staff at quality programs not only provide such treatment, but engage regularly in meaningful comparative program evaluation to continue to improve their responses to the complex needs of the patients they serve.

REFERENCES

1. Flor H, Turk DC: Etiological theories and treatments for chronic back pain. I. Somatic models and interventions. *Pain* 19:417–419, 1984.
2. Gamsa A: Is emotional disturbance a precipitator or a consequence of chronic pain? *Pain* 42:183–195, 1990.
3. Commission on Accreditation of Rehabilitation Facilities: *Standards Manual for Organizations Serving People with Disabilities.* Tucson, Author, 1991.
4. Morse RH: Pain and emotions. In Brena SF, Chapman SL (eds): *Management of Patients with Chronic Pain.* New York, SP Medical and Scientific Books, 1983, pp 47–54.
5. Fordyce WE: *Behavioral Methods for Chronic Pain and Illness.* St. Louis, Mosby, 1976.
6. Chapman SL, Brena SF, Bradford LA: Treatment outcome in a chronic pain rehabilitation program. *Pain* 11:255–268, 1981.
7. Peters JL, Large RG: A randomized control trial evaluating in and outpatient pain management programs. *Pain* 41:283–293, 1990.
8. Chapman SL, Brena SF: Learned helplessness and responses to nerve blocks in chronic low back pain patients. *Pain* 14:353–364, 1982.
9. Connolly GH, Sanders SH: Predicting low back pain patients' responses to lumbar sympathetic nerve blocks and interdisciplinary rehabilitation: The role of pretreatment overt pain behavior and cognitive coping strategies. *Pain* 44:139–146, 1991.
10. Lutz RW, Silbret M, Olshan N: Treatment outcome and compliance with therapeutic regimens: Long-term follow-up of a multidisciplinary pain program. *Pain* 17:301–308, 1983.
11. Commission on Accreditation of Rehabilitation Facilities: *Program Evaluation in Chronic Pain Programs.* Tucson, Author, 1987.

CHAPTER **51**

HOSPITAL-BASED INPATIENT TREATMENT PROGRAMS

RENEE STEELE ROSOMOFF
HUBERT L. ROSOMOFF

IT IS conceded that pain programs very often will take on the characteristics of the Program Director. This may bias a program toward a given discipline, but obviously does not preclude a multidisciplinary approach, despite the emphasis. In the same manner, programs may be influenced by the patient population that presents to the given center or clinic. The more complex, the more complicated, the more drug-dependent, to name a few characteristics, the more likely it is that a hospital-based program will be necessary. Aside from the medical necessity there are currently major issues concerning reimbursement for hospital-based programs. As such, validation of medical necessity becomes important, but rejection can occur and does quite frequently. Despite the most cogent arguments, reimbursement will still be denied.

We have found the following criteria to be the most powerful to support the request for hospitalization in a chronic pain patient. At least one of the following criteria must be present: one, the pain must be sharp, severe, and incapacitating, having a rapid onset with severe symptoms over a short course, even though this might be an acute exacerbation within a chronic condition. Two, the pain must be happening repeatedly at short intervals at least once every 8 hours or more. Three, it will be necessary to observe, evaluate, and specifically record observations about the patient's condition. These observations are necessary to the diagnosis or treatment of the patient's medical problem.

A second set of criteria may also be necessary: one, observation or treatment in a special care unit; two, a specific need for daily physician monitoring and full-time availability. This primarily refers to instances in which individuals have associated significant medical problems that require an acute care setting for diagnosis or treatment. In this setting, the patient may require acute treatment that refers to specific drug therapy, such as anticoagulants, psychopharmacologic agents, chemotherapy, anticonvulsants, and cardiac medications, which, during the initial phases of observation and treatment, require regulation of dosage. Furthermore, failure of nonsurgical intervention and conservative treatment at home must be fully documented, usually meaning previous treatment as an outpatient in physical medicine. To support the need for rehabilitation physical medicine in an acute setting, it may follow that the authorization will be restricted to the initial phases only, anywhere from 1 to 2 weeks. During this time, the patient must have documented rehabilitation potential and must demonstrate progress during therapy.

Another set of criteria refer to the severity of illness. Functional impairment of a body part may need to be demonstrated, as well as the need for medications that are changing in dosage and that need to be regulated no less than every 2 days. Radiologic studies may show pathology such as a herniated disk, but the decision may be made to attempt nonsurgical treatment, particularly in the acute setting. Treatments must require skilled physical therapy on a daily basis, and rehabilitation, evaluation, goal setting and management must be initiated within 24 hours of admission. Psychiatric criteria are those of a suicide attempt, suicidal ideation, or assaultive behavior. Disturbances such as seizures from withdrawal or toxic circumstances or impending loss of impulse control are other standards. Manic behavior, incapacitating anxiety or depression, severe incapacitation with obsessive thinking and/or compulsive behavior, and disabling paranoia are other conditions that may dictate hospitalization. The evaluation for drug tolerance and/or abuse, drug detoxification, and overdose are almost always acceptable for inpatient treatment.

Lastly, intensity of service must be documented with the administration of medications at least daily, intravenously or intramuscularly, or the regulation and monitoring of high-risk medication. The management of a noncompliant patient or a patient with potential medical complications also speaks to intensity, wherein comprehensive therapy planning requires close supervision because of concomitant medical conditions and the requirement of skilled around-the-clock observation, supervision, and/or treatment. When these criteria can be cited, hospitalization can be considered reasonable and necessary: when a diagnosis of a physical cause has been established, the usual methods of treatment have not been successful, and there is a significant loss of ability to function independently.

Most insurers accept that a hospital level pain rehabilitation program is one that employs a coordinated multidisciplinary team to deliver, in a controlled environment, a concentrated program designed to modify pain behavior through the treatment of the psychological, physical, and social aspects of pain. Such programs generally include diagnostic testing, skilled nursing, psychotherapy, structured progressive withdrawal from pain medications, and physical and occupational therapy to restore physical fitness including mobility, strength, and endurance to a maximal level within the constraints of a patient's physical disability. The use of mechanical devices and/or activities to relieve pain or modify a patient's reaction (such as massage, ice, hydrotherapy, nerve stimulation, systemic muscle relaxation training, and diversional activities) is acceptable. The nurse is a member of this team and has a responsibility to observe and assess, on a continuing basis, a patient's condition and response to the program as reflected by his or her actions while in the nursing unit and to assure that the atmosphere within the unit is not supportive of pain behavior. The day-to-day activities involve the carrying out of the program under the general supervision and, as needed, direct supervision of a physician. It is universally accepted that an inpatient program of 4 weeks' duration is required to modify or control pain. After this period, it would be expected that any additional rehabilitation services could be effectively provided on an outpatient basis. The first 7–10 days of such an inpatient program constitute, in effect, an evaluation period. If a patient is unable to adjust to the program within this period, it may be concluded that it is unlikely that the program will be effective, and the patient should be discharged from the program. Occasionally a program longer than 4 weeks may be required. In such a case, there should be documentation to substantiate that inpatient care beyond a 4-week period is reasonable and necessary.

PROGRAM DESCRIPTION

An inpatient treatment program should be multidisciplinary and designed to provide individualized, intensive, extensive, aggressive physical, behavioral, and avocational/vocational rehabilitation for persons with acute or chronic intractable pain whose level of function and productivity and whose lifestyle is moderately to severely impaired. Patients should have been judged to require observation and treatment in a hospital setting and on completion of a comprehensive multidisciplinary evaluation. The program should provide a safe, therapeutic environment with constant supervision for physically impaired, not totally independent, depressed, anxious, or otherwise disturbed or drug/alcohol-dependent patients who may or may not have underlying or associated medical problems that require observation and/or treatment.

PROGRAM GOALS AND OBJECTIVES

An inpatient program should be designed to physically recondition and restore the patient to a level of function that includes full range of motion, acceptable strength requirements, decreased pain level, and increased tolerances in preparation for transfer to an outpatient program or discharge home. The program should physically recondition and restore patients who require close nursing and medical inpatient supervision to full levels of function with minimal to no pain, with minimal to no limitations, and minimal to zero disability on discharge to the home. It should detoxify dependent patients from alcohol, narcotics, barbiturates, analgesics, and psychotropic medications and educate the patient to use alternative methods to alleviate pain. The patient should be able to self-administer any medication needed at the time of transfer or discharge to maintain health. Patients should be educated to manage pain episodes that may arise so they may be totally able to self-administer any modalities or exercises required in order to be discharged to a motel or home and be totally independent. The patient is expected to maintain his or her optimal weight to avoid exacerbation of pain due to excessive loading of the spine and hips. The need for assistive devices such as braces, corsets, canes, crutches, walkers, wheelchairs, and stimulators, which serve to perpetuate deconditioning and are counterproductive in the alleviation of pain, should be eliminated. Realignment of the spine and extremities to eliminate poor posture and maladaptive gait, which contribute to intractable pain and perpetuate the cycle, must be achieved. Stress management, relaxation, psychological support, and family counseling should be provided so the patient may be able to function appropriately in the outpatient setting or after return to his or her own environment. A positive behavioral change must be effected so the patient will be independent of the health care system and be in control of his or her situation. The patient must learn to substitute for inappropriate behavior and responses behavior that is appropriate to reduce pain-producing stress. Patients must come to understand self and be totally responsible for their actions and rehabilitation. The patient must regain confidence to return to employment without fear or anxiety and to perceive himself or herself as a well person. Constructive coping strategies must be developed to reduce stress, and biofeedback and relaxation techniques must be mastered to understand the relationship between muscle tension, anxiety, and pain in order to reduce stress and prevent re-injury. The program must alleviate and teach control of anxiety, depression, fear, anger, and interpersonal problems so the individual may function in an emotionally healthy manner, thereby maintaining the physical and mental gains made. Disability-oriented attitudes in the patient and family must be eliminated, and the patient's family must be educated to support wellness behavior and attitude. The patient must learn to relate to family and others appropriately; the patient's family must understand the patient's problem and abilities, as well as their role in his or her rehabilitative process, so that they may offer positive reinforcement and foster open communication within the family structure. The patient must learn to function at a high level and enjoy optimal wellness through training to instinctively use good body mechanics, pacing, and energy-saving techniques. The patient must be taught how to maintain rehabilitation gains and prevent re-injury without reliance on health care professionals, medication, and appliances. The program should enable the patient to participate in leisure activities, including active sports, in a safe and planned manner so that the patient may prevent injury or re-injury and enjoy a complete, well-rounded, and satisfying life. The program should restore the patient's capacity to return to previous employment, with minimal to no limitations or modifications to the work place, immediately upon discharge, including the patient's ability to physically, psychologically, and vocationally return to full-time employment, heavy labor not precluded, with confidence and with the ability to do the job in a safe manner. The patient must learn to overcome any obstacle that may interfere with return to employment through instructions in job-seeking skills, résumé writing, and application and interview techniques. Rehabilitation should allow the patient to return to previous employment or to a new work setting through the use of job simulation and functional restoration to full capacity based on a complete ergonomic and vocational analysis. The patient must learn to avoid situations that would contribute to a reoccurrence of the chronic pain cycle through knowledge of ergonomics and how to make simple adjustments to the home and workplace setting.

In summary, the overall goal is to interrupt the chronic pain cycle; to optimally rehabilitate the patient physically, behaviorally, avocationally/vocationally, and socially; and to teach responsibility, control, awareness of reinjury mechanisms, and total independence from drug use, appliances, and the health care system, thus enabling the patient to return to home, employment, and community as a fully rehabilitated, productive member of society.

PATIENT PROFILE

Our patient is one with a self-defeating background. He or she focuses on body cues and pain. The patient usually has a poor work history, poor interpersonal relationships, a low sense of self-esteem, poor skills, and little job satisfaction. The patient has never liked his or her job, blames the employer for his or her plight, and is angry with the insurance company. The family may have a previous history of low back pain, so their empathy makes them attentive to his or her needs and they assume his or her responsibilities at home. This frightened family is protective, angry, and supportive of disability.

The other contributors to this "loser" are the medical community, the attorney, the rehabilitation specialist, the insurance company, and the employer. The doctor has put the patient in bed with traction, passive therapy, pain medication, and muscle relaxants. He has been radiographed, imaged, myelogrammed, frightened by the results, and told that if he doesn't have an operation, he will be paralyzed and in a wheelchair. The insurance company joins with an uncaring attitude, supporting usually the least costly and, sometimes, the poorest kind of therapy, without questioning recommendations; thus operations mount one after another. The patient is punished if he or she either refuses the risky surgery or does have the operation and doesn't get better. The surgeon claims the surgery to be successful, so it is the patient who failed. The adjustor becomes hostile, delaying benefits, which compounds the anger and the now developing behavioral problems of the patient.

The employer remains basically uncaring. He or she doesn't bother to call the patient to inquire how he is. Actually, the employer may have wanted to be rid of that employee before all this started, and thus is happy. If an attorney is involved, he or she may tell the client to not trust, not cooperate, not communicate, not rehabilitate and, by all means, not go back to work.

The result is a patient with chronic pain, who is physically impaired, weak, drug-dependent, alcohol-dependent, hostile, untrusting, frightened, helpless, hopeless, and socially dependent, with sexual problems, anxiety, fear, anger, depression, no job, no future, totally disabled and potentially suicidal and homicidal. He or she has marital problems, has no motivation, and is disability-oriented. Everyone is angry. The patient is angry at himself or herself, the family, the boss, the employer, the physician, the lawyer, the insurance company, the disability system, and the law.

The patient believes that he or she is entitled to a handsome award for the disability and, of course, this is not forthcoming. She is fearful, and doesn't know if she will ever get better or can ever be productive again. The patient is afraid of re-injury and further loss of function, especially if frightened by the warnings of physicians. Most of all, the patient fears the loss of benefits if, somehow, he or she doesn't maintain this disabled pose. He or she is dependent on alcohol, narcotics, barbiturates, psychotropics, muscle relaxants, and often, street drugs. Our "poor me" patient appears not to be cooperative or well-motivated, is interested in secondary gain, and is full of self-pity. The real issues are fear and anger.

As one example, the University of Miami Comprehensive Pain and Rehabilitation Center has more than 100 personnel who are full-time at the Center and who are found in six divisions. Neurologic surgery is non-invasive but minds the nervous system. Physical medicine and rehabilitation directs the application of all physical medicine modalities and treatments. Nurses, trained in rehabilitation and behavior, monitor patient progress and serve as case managers. The behavioral division has both a psychiatrist and psychologists who are assigned as counselors to each patient and who administer biofeedback, behavioral modification, or other applicable techniques. A vocational rehabilitation division evaluates and directs job placement; and an ergonomics division simulates the job and adapts the patient and/or work site while computing daily achievement goals. Incidentally, orthopedics falls within the division of physical medicine and rehabilitation.

To enter the system, the patient must undergo multidisciplinary evaluation over a 3-day period. A problem-solving group attempts to identify the medical, behavioral, vocational, financial, social, and other significant problems of the patient. The approach is comprehensive and holistic. Patient selection criteria are broad. The patient must have the ability to understand and carry out instructions, must be compliant and cooperative, and must not have aggressive or disruptive behavior that would disturb the milieu. Patients with schizophrenia, manic-depression, or other major psychiatric disorders are not precluded as long as they are compensated for. Lastly, the patient, the family, and significant others such as the lawyer, the employer, and the insurer must accept the program. Worker compensation, liability cases, multiple surgeries, long histories of invalidism, or drug abuse are not exclusionary conditions.

The average program will last 4 weeks on an inpatient or outpatient basis or a combination thereof. Inpatient status is preferred for the difficult, complicated case, but it is not always feasible, as dictated by reimbursement status. It should be understood clearly that, in a tertiary referral center, few "simple" early primary cases are seen. We receive the most complex "court of last resort" salvage cases.

PHYSICAL MEDICINE AND REHABILITATION

Physical medicine has the goal of restoring body function to normal or to its closest equivalent. Because myofascial contracture is the common denominator in the low back disorders that we see, the first phase of management is muscle stretching and restoration of full range of motion in the joints of the hips, back, and lower extremities. This therapy includes gait retraining because of acquired maladaptive patterns, postural adjustment, proper use of effective modalities, elimination of adjunct equipment when possible, strength and endurance conditioning with instruction of body mechanics, prevention of re-injury, vocational or avocational requirements, sexual counseling and, lastly, a home maintenance program.

Modalities, when evaluated individually, may not show clear-cut evidence of effectiveness (1). They appear to be useful in combination, however, which unfortunately makes statistical evaluation more difficult. Nonetheless, scientific rationale exists for some. Ice application with lowering of temperature is known to decrease nerve conduction to the point of anesthesia, and inflammatory reaction is contained with a reduction of chronic changes (2, 3). To be effective, the body part must be packed in ice for periods in excess of 30 min. Heat does seem to soften muscle preparatory to stretching. An adjunct vapocoolant helps to block the stretch reflex and makes lengthening easier (4).

Traction is useful for certain specific indications. Conceptually, we apply traction to stretch muscle groups, not to distract the spine or to release nerve entrapment. We do not believe that distraction of the spine can be effected with the weights that are commonly used, and the principle of entrapment is not tenable. Therefore, traditional pelvic or leg traction is not employed. Gravity traction is applied for iliopsoas contractures in the patient with a spinal flexion deformity and/or failure to extend the back.

Auto-traction is an important technique that allows three-dimensional placement of the spine by rotating, flexing, or extending the unit as the patient imposes his or her own body force by pushing and pulling (5). The self-applied force of auto-traction will not exceed that which could be potentially injurious, but it will release tight paraspinal muscles. Auto-traction does not decompress the nerve root, as was the concept of its originators (6, 7).

Trigger-point desensitization is indicated. Liberal use of ice is the preferred method of treatment, but like the other modalities—ultrasonography, electrical stimulation, and neuroprobe—it is only an adjunct to stretching. Heat and massage also are used but, again, as adjunct treatment to enhance muscle lengthening and supple movement.

Transcutaneous electrical neural stimulation (TENS) is used infrequently and only with patients who are TENS responders and who can be assisted with a difficult detoxification for which TENS will give short-term relief as the drugs are withdrawn. TENS will not be given to the patient beyond this period; it has no role in long-term therapy. Conceptually, it is to be emphasized that we are aiming for resolution of the painful disorder by physical restitution, not by an attempt at distraction or at coping by "learning to live with pain."

Passive, then active ranging of motion is essential, especially about the hips and, in particular, the hip rotators. Hamstring lengthening is another mandate, because hamstring tightness will affect back movement. Full ranges of back motion are the ultimate goal, so flexion and extension exercises are instituted without prejudice for the proponents of either type. Both flexion and extension exercises are needed.

A full compendium of exercises is employed, as described in any standard physical therapy textbook, to establish full ranges of motion throughout the lower body with supple muscles and fluid movement. As this is being achieved, muscle strengthening and cardiovascular conditioning are added to the regimen with monitoring of those patients who have associated medical problems.

Movement therapy using musical input is an interesting adjunct, because patients with pain will often perform to music when seemingly they cannot move their bodies on command. When a specific muscle group is weak, functional electrical neuromuscular stimulation (FES) and muscle re-education are implemented (8). This technique can produce rapid and dramatic increases in muscle recruitment patterns and muscle strength; footdrop braces can be discarded.

Occupational and recreational therapy concentrate on body mechanics. Sitting, standing, walking, lifting, and driving tolerances are established and brought to normal levels of function. Pacing of activity is taught. Assistive equipment is used infrequently and only with specific indications. Energy-saving techniques are taught. Posture and gait are corrected; importantly, most patients are found to have poor posture and maladaptive gaits.

Activities of daily living are reviewed for home and work, looking for the proper use of body mechanics, with correction as needed. Driving evaluation is conducted and proper transfers are taught. Diversionary activities are reviewed and eye/hand/leg coordination and tolerances are established. Education and vocational goals are set and job simulation is begun.

Job simulation and work conditioning was another concept that we introduced to pain center management more than a decade ago. This is the ultimate goal of achievement for the working-age group, but it does not exclude students or elderly persons, who receive instruction for their needs. With respect to these problems, the occupational and physical therapists team with vocational counselors and ergonomists to develop the treatment plan.

VOCATIONAL REHABILITATION

Vocational rehabilitation counselors analyze factors of employment, such as age, educational level, work history, supervisory and peer relationships, job requirements, job skills, transferable skills, date and circumstances of injury, return to work since injury, and, most important, motivation and compliance. This type of program cannot be successful without the patient's full attention or effort. If the patient will not give both, he or she is not accepted. The vocational goal is full functional activity and return to previous employment. Retraining is recommended rarely. Even the heaviest physical capacities can be achieved in most patients.

BEHAVIORAL MANAGEMENT

Behavioral management is a key issue. Nearly 20% of Americans suffer from one or more emotional disorders, so the low back injury patient may be harboring such a problem. The psychiatric profile is inherited by the treatment team, insurer, and all others concerned. Our study of pain population patients found 62.5% to have anxiety disorders and 56.2% to have current depression (9). These conditions were co-mingled with other, less-prevalent disorders. Only 5.3% of 283 patients were found to have no psychiatric diagnosis. Further, this study questions the criteria for the diagnosis of psychogenic pain. Pure psychogenic pain is probably rare when presented as mental events giving rise to pain. Even so, all pain, as perceived by the patient, is real, regardless of cause. Most bodily pain is the result of a combination of factors (e.g., physical stimuli and mental events). Mental and emotional states may be due to circumstances of the moment, a background of past personal experiences with pain, or personality characteristics.

Behavioral analysis considers compliance, achievement level before injury, activity level after injury, functional capacities, anxiety, depression, personality disorders, marital status, role reversal, and family history. Psychological services offer biofeedback and relaxation training. Group and family therapy deal with social interactions, return to environment, employment, and disability versus wellness with an emphasis on function, not pain.

Individual counseling is given when needed, including sexual counseling. Every patient has an assigned counselor who monitors daily progress and reinforces the goal of physical restoration. Relaxation training includes coping approaches, muscle re-education, meditation and distraction, guided imagery, autosuggestion (especially to be used with physical activity), and tape supplements that enhance "live" therapy. Stress management is incorporated into the behavioral sessions.

Weekly family groups explore the goals of the patient with the spouse and/or other family members. How to respond to pain without fear is discussed. Communication is an important subject. The roles of the various family members are defined, both as to distribution and as to responsibility. Experiences and frustrations are shared. These sessions facilitate the return home to an environment that, it is hoped, will now foster wellness, not disability.

Biofeedback may be a pain control method, but we use it as a muscle tension/relaxation technique. Electromyographic biofeedback is used to regulate muscle tension, especially when an activity may, by past experience, have been pain-provoking. Reduction of muscle tension correlates well with reduction of pain (10).

Our psychologic assessment instrument is the Millon Behavioral Health Inventory Assessment. This instrument tests psychogenic attitudes, such as chronic tension, recent stress, premorbid pessimism, future despair, social alienation, and somatic anxiety. This instrument is not a predictor of outcome, nor should any other instrument, such as the Minnesota Multiphasic Personality Inventory (MMPI), be used for that purpose. We are trying to find out what the patient is like, so that the treating staff can interact with the individual in a manner that he or she is willing to accept. The patient has to be the partner in a rehabilitative process; otherwise, the effort will fail.

Lastly, the behavioral staff regulates detoxification from drugs. As stated earlier, this process is carried out rapidly while pursuing intense activation. Endorphin release will help ameliorate withdrawal, and symptoms are generally minimal. Most important of all, we do not teach people how to live or cope with their pain. We look for relief of pain. We attempt to reverse the somatic changes and, with behavioral modification, bring these patients back to equilibrium with their previous lifestyles.

ISSUE OF "OBJECTIVE FINDINGS"

A particular body of literature alleges that many patients suffering from chronic low back pain cannot be assigned a diagnosis conforming to a specific defined disease. The lack of "objective" physical findings in such patients has led to the designation of *chronic intractable benign pain* (11). This type of pain was thought to be a "central" phenomenon, which was made worse by sensory input. Poor adaptation made pain the focus of the patient's life. Patients so classified were often evaluated for behavioral abnormalities and often became candidates for the diagnosis of psychogenic pain. Presumably, no physical findings indicative of an organic dysfunction or pathologic process were present. Such a presumption is not supported by facts.

In a study that addressed this issue, 90 patients with back pain were isolated from a group of 283 mixed chronic pain patients who conformed to the diagnosis of chronic intractable benign pain (12). None had neurologic deficit; all radiologic studies were unremarkable. Almost all (97.6%) had tender/trigger points and multiple other non-neurologic abnormalities. Seven categories of abnormalities were identified: tender/trigger points, decreased range of motion, nondermatomal sensory abnormalities, contracted muscles, abnormal gait, miscellaneous physical signs, and decreased range of motion at the hips. Patients had an average of three of the seven categoric findings, led by myofascial syndromes and other soft tissue changes. Almost half (45.6%) had nondermatomal sensory changes; this condition is physiologic dysfunction, as cited earlier, not malingering or hysteria (13).

The investigators made the following conclusions:

1. Chronic intractable benign pain patients without "objective finding" can be shown regularly to have musculoskeletal disorders.
2. Myofascial syndromes are the source of nociception in these patients.
3. Criteria for the specific diagnosis of myofascial pain syndrome are demonstrable in 97.6% of the patients.
4. Multiple physical findings (average, 3.1) are usual.
5. The demonstrations of such physical findings invalidates the chronic intractable benign pain concept.
6. The DSM-III diagnosis of psychogenic pain is overstated, for which the criteria now need to be revised.

The investigators added an important comment: With respect to the nondermatomal sensory change, the decreased sensation is commonly "stocking" in distribution; but, often, the perception may appear to involve the lateral or medial foot. Careful examination, however, will demonstrate loss in only half of the dorsum of the foot, with escape of the plantar surface or vice versa. This condition looks more like a peripheral nerve alteration, consistent with possible sciatic entrapment, as might be seen with the gluteal or piriformis myofascial syndromes.

ERGONOMICS

About 11 years ago, industrial engineering and ergonomics were introduced to the Pain Center. We are learning much together, because ergonomics has much to teach us (14). Ergonomics studies the worker in his or her environment, trying to match the physical capabilities to the industrial task. This process may require designing and redesigning of the workplace and tools that are used. The goal is to condition the worker with regard to strength, posture, and flexibility while eliminating fatigability.

The engineers see the human body as a machine, working with levers and acting as a mechanical crane. Proper lifting dictates carrying the weight close to the body; the more bulky the weight, the more difficult it is to carry, and the less efficient the handling of materials. The objectives are human comfort, optimal efficiency of the man-machine system, safety and prevention, health, and work satisfaction. Work satisfaction is a very important issue.

Measuring outcome is a big problem. To account for psychophysical variants, a measure of back strength in back pain patients was developed called AME—acceptable maximum effort (15). This method is highly reliable and useful in determining treatment outcome. Reliability coefficients for all strength measurements are greater than 0.90.

The level of voluntary muscular effort beyond which the patient's level of pain becomes unacceptable is the principle. Patients are tested before, during, and after treatment. Back and leg strength may more than double in a 4-week treatment period, which is also true for composite strength. Human performance evaluations track overall strength, pace, reactions, hand steadiness, flexibility, level of cooperation, level of effort, ranges of motion, gait, posture, and pain level. The bottom line is to make the achievement level match or exceed the task demand.

The ergonomists also analyze the patient's anthropometric measurements, from which ideal layouts for chairs, desks, home furniture, work site equipment, and condition can be developed and printed out by computer. The pain program is a 6 day/week program for 4 weeks, with 10–12 hours of activity per day. Therapeutic time schedules allow the individual to have alternating but consecutive periods of major exertional and nonexertional activity.

By the time of discharge, patients may have achieved the best physical condition of their life. Usually, by 1 week, patients are ambulatory and independent in activities of daily living (ADL) with decreasing levels of pain. They are approaching full ranges of motion with increasing strength in 2–3 weeks. Relief of pain is not the endpoint; but, at the end of 4 weeks, sometimes 6 weeks, they have achieved full functional levels of activity. If a neurologic deficit has been present, motor strength may recover in 2–3 weeks, sensation in 2–3 months, and reflexes in 3 months. Complete pain relief is attained in one-third of patients at discharge; in the remainder, the pain usually dissipates over time or becomes controlled for functional comfort.

NURSING CARE

Nurses are cross-trained and play a vital and varied role in this hospital-based inpatient treatment program. They are involved in every aspect of the program from program direction, admission screening, case management, patient assessment and monitoring, counseling, education, coordination, medication and nutritional management, to discharge planning and follow-up, and are reinforcers of multidisciplinary team concepts and instructions.

COST-EFFECTIVENESS

Are pain programs cost-effective? We think they are (16). An average cost-benefit of $238,000 per patient was demonstrated in a study of 53 patients with industrial injuries (17). If only a 1% change in awards for social security disability were to be reversed over a 5-year period, this nation would save $900,000,000. That's truly cost effective.

CONCLUSIONS

The primary objective of the program described is restoration to full function. Other objectives include relief or decrease in pain with the abolition of pain medication, elimination of assistive devices, low or zero disability rating, job satisfaction with return to work and leisure activities without limitations, independence from the health care system, prevention of re-injury; and optimal wellness. The intense, multidisciplinary program described involves a full-time multidisciplinary staff, complete patient involvement, weight control, physical restoration and conditioning, home program maintenance, pacing, body mechanics, energy-saving techniques, re-injury prevention education, drug detoxification, behavioral elimination or control of pain, modification, biofeedback, relaxation, imagery, individual and group therapy, family therapy, assertiveness training, stress management, coping skills, vocational counseling, job planning/development/simulation, achievement of maximal function, immediate return to work at discharge, and follow-up care.

It is possible to return 86% of these patients to full function and work; they may have some residual pain, which should eventually remit. The 14% who "fail" are hardcore patients with major behavioral problems, although, to be fair, there are still unanswered questions to resolve. These people have problems that cannot be eliminated within the time we have to work with the patient. Lastly, these patients can be disturbed and dangerous, as evidenced by the headline of "A Former Patient Shoots, Kills, New York Neurosurgeon, Self, Wife" (18).

References

1. Deyo RA: Conservative therapy for low back pain: Distinguishing useful from useless therapy. *JAMS* 250:1057–1062, 1983.
2. Rosomoff HL: The effects of hypothermia on the physiology of the nervous system. *Surgery* 49:328–336, 1956.
3. Rosomoff HL, Clasen RA, Hartstock R, et al: Brain reaction to experimental injury after hypothermia. *Arch Neurol* 13:337–345, 1965.

4. Travell JG, Simons G: *Myofascial Pain and Dysfunction: The Trigger Point Manual.* Baltimore, Williams & Wilkins, 1983.

5. Larsson U, Choler U, Lidstrom A, et al: Auto-traction for treatment of lumbago-sciatica: A multicentre controlled investigation. *Acta Orthop Scand* 51:791–798, 1980.

6. Lind GAM: *Auto-Traction: Treatment of Low back Pain and Sciatica.* Sweden, Sturetryckeriet, 1974.

7. Natchev E: *A Manual on Auto-Traction Treatment for Low Back Pain.* Folksam Scientific Council Publ. B 171, 1984.

8. Abdel-Moty E, Khalil TM, Rosomoff RS, et al: Computerized electromyography in quantifying the effectiveness of functional electrical neuromuscular stimulation. In Asfour SS (ed): *Ergonomics/Human Factors IV.* New York, Elsevier, 1987, pp 1057–1065.

9. Fishbain DA, Goldberg M, Meagher R, et al: Male and female chronic pain patients categorized by DSM-III psychiatric diagnostic criteria. *Pain* 26:181–197, 1986.

10. Khalil T, Asfour SS, Waly SM, et al: Isometric exercise and biofeedback in strength training. In Asfour SS (ed): *Trends in Ergonomics/Human Factors IV.* New York, Elsevier, 1987, pp 1095–1101.

11. Crue BL, Pinsky JJ: An approach to chronic pain of non-malignant origin. *Postgrad Med J* 60:858–864, 1984.

12. Rosomoff HL, Fishbain D, Goldberg M, et al: Physical findings in patients with chronic intractable benign pain of the back and/or neck. *Pain* 37:279–287, 1989.

13. Wall P: The role of the substantia gelatinosa as a gate control. In Bonica JJ (ed): *Pain.* New York, Raven Press, 1980, pp 205–231.

14. Khalil TM, Asfour SS, Moty EA, et al: New horizons for ergonomics research in low back pain. In Eberts RE, Eberts CC (eds): *Trends in Ergonomics/Human Factors II.* New York, Elsevier, 1985, pp 591–598.

15. Khalil TM, Goldberg ML, Asfour SS, et al: Acceptable maximum effort (AME): A psychosocial measure of strength in back pain patients. *Spine* 12:372–376, 1987.

16. Steele R: Is the pain program cost effective? *Pain Suppl* 2:438, 1984.

17. Stieg RL, Williams RC, Timmermans-Williams G, et al: Cost benefits of interdisciplinary chronic pain treatment. *Clin J Pain* 1:189–193, 1985.

18. Pinckney D: A former patient shoots, kills, New York neurosurgeon, self, wife. *Am Med News* Mar 20, 1987.

CHAPTER 52

OCCUPATIONAL REHABILITATION TREATMENT PROGRAMS
LEONARD N. MATHESON

THE MOST devastating consequence of chronic pain is the loss of one's occupational role. Not only does the individual define himself in terms of his or her occupational role, but participation in an occupational role provides the individual with the financial resources to participate as a full member of society. Occupational rehabilitation provides the means by which the individual who is occupationally disabled because of chronic pain can return to participation in a previous or new occupational role and, thus, resume a position as a full-fledged member of society. Occupational rehabilitation is defined as a subset of rehabilitation that focuses on providing services to the adult who has suffered an industrial injury. These people, whom we will refer to as "injured workers," were employed at the time of injury and suffered injuries in the course and scope of their employment. A mix of the primary type of injury found in occupational rehabilitation treatment programs is presented in Figure 52.1.

Occupational rehabilitation treatment programs can be distinguished from other rehabilitation programs by their primary focus on returning the patient to the competitive work force. Rather than a focus on symptom reduction, increased physical capacity, improved skills, or other legitimate rehabilitation goals, the occupational rehabilitation treatment program focuses on returning an injured worker to his or her employer as a safe and productive member of the work force. Thus, there is a strong focus on restorative care rather than true rehabilitative care, although, as the field matures, rehabilitation in terms of developing the ability to avoid future illness and injury is gaining increased emphasis.

In addition to the benefit provided to injured workers, occupational rehabilitation is important to the employer. As part of the workers' compensation agreement under which the employer operates, the burden of financial responsibility for treatment of an industrial injury as well as indemnification from the employee's financial loss is on the employer's shoulders. The employer assumes this responsibility as part of a social contract that exempts the employer from tortious legal action. Indemnification for the employee's financial loss is controlled and is much less generous than would be the case if courts were allowed to adjudicate each case. In addition, both the employer and employee avoid the legal expenses in defending and prosecuting such matters. Although attorneys are involved in workers' compensation cases, their involvement is much more proscribed than in tort matters and has a strong bureaucratic flavor. Compensation for attorneys is limited in workers' compensation to one-quarter to one-third of the compensation available in tort lawsuits in most jurisdictions (1).

Employers' avoidance of unscheduled indemnification is so beneficial that workers' compensation insurance has been an important underpinning in the successful development of industrial economies. In recent years, however, the increase in health care expense that is part of the workers' compensation social contract has grown so rapidly that it has begun to impede industrial development in some jurisdictions. For example, in 1991 California experienced a net decline of manufacturing jobs based on an exodus of employers from the state to neighboring states and to Mexico. The single most important reason cited by employers for moving industrial plants out of California was the substantial increase in workers' compensation costs. During the prior decade, increases in indemnification did not keep pace with inflation whereas increases in health care were more than twice as steep as inflation. Workers' compensation costs for disability resulting from pain are not normally distributed because the person who is chronically disabled because of pain is exceptionally expensive to treat. Leavitt et al. found that 25% of the cases were responsible for 90% of the cost (1). Spengler et al. found that 10% of the back injuries at Boeing Aircraft were responsible for 79% of the cost (2). Additionally, Antonakes demonstrated a disproportionate increase in the cost of claims for pain-

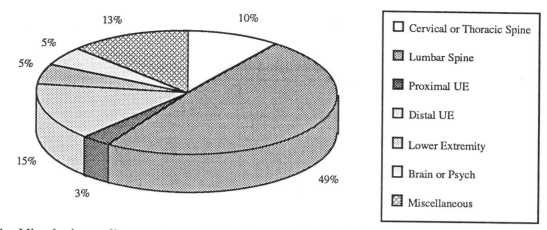

Figure 52.1. **Mix of primary diagnoses in one California occupational rehabilitation program.**

ful back injury relative to time since injury (3). The Quebec Task Force on Spinal Disorders confirmed that most industrial injuries do not result in long-term chronic disability (4). However, 7% of those individuals disabled because of back injury who remained out of work for 6 months or more accounted for 76% of the compensation cost paid for spinal disorders and 21.4% of the total compensation cost for all work injuries. Models that can predict the subsequent development of chronic disability point to the need for a full range of occupational rehabilitation treatment programs and lead to the expectation that some of the disproportionate costs can be avoided (5). Occupational rehabilitation, through successful treatment of injured workers who are disabled by pain, provides the means by which the employer can assist the injured worker to return to a previous or new occupational role and, thus, discharge the employer's liability.

HISTORICAL PERSPECTIVE

The origins of many of occupational rehabilitation's current concepts and techniques are found in the early 1900s. At that time, several societal trends culminated in a nationwide awakening to the rehabilitation needs of the disabled. Prior to this, care for the disabled usually took the form of custodial public support. This awakening was facilitated when World War I resulted in a large number of disabled veterans who returned home and wanted to lead economically productive lives. To return to the work place, these disabled citizens required more than medical care. Initially, occupational rehabilitation services were provided within the context of Veterans Administration hospitals and large private medical rehabilitation centers. In 1920, the passage of the United States Vocational Rehabilitation Act provided funds to assist disabled workers to return to work by retraining the disabled worker "around the disability." Public awareness soon expanded to include the even greater number of disabled civilians facing a sim-

ilar dilemma as the mechanization of American industry led to an increase in industrial accidents. It was apparent that injured workers needed retraining, sometimes to an entirely new occupation, in order to return to the workplace. Among the earliest efforts were programs in "Industrial Therapy" and the establishment of the "Curative Workshops." Industrial therapy was defined as "the prescribed use of activities inherent to the hospital operation, planned for the mutual benefit of patient and institution" (6). Various jobs within the institution were analyzed according to skill levels, physical and mental demands, and potential therapeutic benefits. The patient was assigned to work in keeping with his aptitudes, interests, experience, and therapeutic goals (7, 8). Treatment in the curative workshop was geared to restoration of the impaired body part to as normal function as possible, with return to work as the goal. Graded activities, often planned along the lines of the physical demands of the patient's original job, were used to improve function. Therapeutic activities were adapted so that "the muscles he has always used and must use again in his job are brought into play and restored to the patient's functional and economic needs" (9).

The "work evaluation" program in the 1940s at the Rochester Rehabilitation Center in New York represents another step in the conceptual development of occupational rehabilitation (10). This program was not only a treatment center to recondition a person for the return to work, but also was an evaluation center that supplied information for the identification of appropriate vocational goals. Individuals who had gained maximal physical restoration were admitted to the work evaluation program. In this program, they were presented with a variety of industrial jobs in work conditions that simulated the industrial environment. Over the course of several weeks, clients would learn to work at maximal efficiency to meet industrial standards. Performance was carefully observed and analyzed in terms of general worker traits (e.g., strength, tool handling, work habits, dexterity) to determine areas of employability.

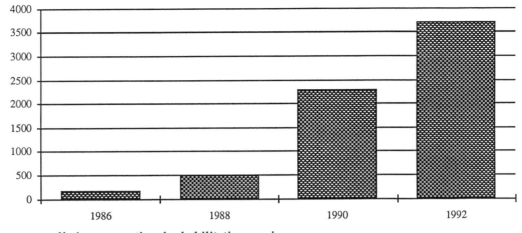

Figure 52.2. **Programs offering occupational rehabilitation services.**

Perhaps the best example of an early occupational rehabilitation program can be found in Wegg's description of the "work therapy" program at the May T. Morrison Center for Rehabilitation in San Francisco (11):

> This program consists of those activities which are simulations of actual on-the-job conditions which can be used both as an estimate of ability and as an exercise medium to develop work habits, confidence, increase physical and emotional tolerance, improve strength, range of motion, coordination, and dexterity. The familiar working situations promote good physiological effects. The clear treatment objectives provide motivation. The availability of the tools used in his trade allows the injured worker to begin developing the speed and skill he had attained during his employment. The occupational therapist is provided with an opportunity to grade activities as to length of time, resistances used, distances that weights are lifted and carried, positions of work, and so on.

In the late 1950s, many occupational rehabilitation programs were divided into "prevocational" and "vocational" services. In addition, there was movement toward using more-standardized vocational testing procedures. This led to the development of the profession of vocational evaluation. Vocational evaluation was seen as a comprehensive assessment process that used standardized work samples and psychometric tests to determine assets and limitations in the areas of work aptitudes, interests, temperaments, and skills. Prevocational programs, such as that developed at the Institute for the Crippled and Disabled in New York (12), helped prepare clients for the pressures and demands of vocational evaluation. The prevocational program was concerned with developing a client's work habits, work tolerances, coordination, and productive speed to levels acceptable for entry into vocational evaluation and eventual employment. The decision to undergo prevocational evaluation and training, begin vocational evaluation, or go directly into a job training program was

made by the rehabilitation team. This team often used information gained from structured "work tests" (13) or from "physical capacity evaluations" (14) developed and administered by occupational therapists.

In 1976, "Work Hardening" was introduced as a new occupational rehabilitation program model (15). Developed at Rancho Los Amigos in California, this model used functional capacity evaluation to identify the appropriate level of physical challenge to be presented to the injured worker in graded work simulations and structured physical conditioning tasks. The purpose of work hardening was to assist the injured worker to develop the work tolerances, habits, and attitudes that were necessary to return to and remain in the competitive workplace.

In recent years, occupational rehabilitation programs have flourished. Program growth has been experienced in the United States, Canada, Australia, Scandinavia, Europe, and Great Britain with differences between programs that reflect the differences in the workers' compensation laws in each jurisdiction (Fig. 52.2).

The mix of services in these occupational rehabilitation treatment programs has changed over recent years to reflect the increasing market demand for early intervention services. A survey of United States occupational rehabilitation programs in 1988 describes the mix of services at that time, depicted in Figure 52.3.

A follow-up survey of occupational rehabilitation programs in the United States in 1992 describes a mix of services that includes a substantial increase in work conditioning services with a concordant diminution of work hardening services, depicted in Figure 52.4.

OCCUPATIONAL REHABILITATION PROCESS

The occupational rehabilitation process can be considered in terms of the *Stage Model of Industrial Rehabilitation*, depicted in Figure 52.5. There are eight stages in the model.

1988 Survey

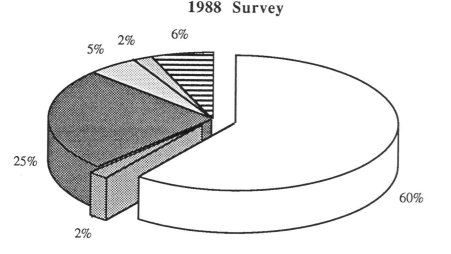

Figure 52.3.   **Mix of occupational rehabilitation services in typical program, 1988.**

1992 Survey

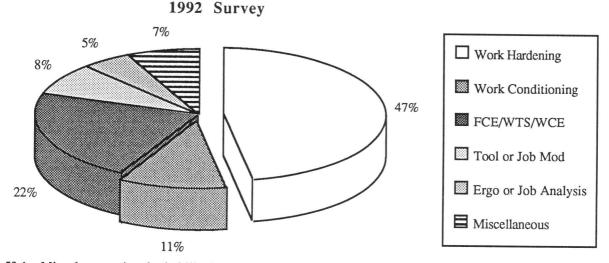

Figure 52.4.   **Mix of occupational rehabilitation services in typical program, 1992.**

The first stage in the process addresses the pathology that results from the injured worker's injury. In the second stage, as pathology has stabilized, impairment is evaluated and attempts are made to minimize the effects of pathology in terms of the loss of patency of the organ, joint, muscle, or bone. When these attempts are not fully successful, the process passes to the third stage, in which functional limitations are addressed. If the consequent functional limitations are sufficiently severe to impact the individual's usual and customary employment, the issue of occupational disability is addressed. Up through this stage, rehabilitative efforts are focused on returning the injured worker to his or her usual and customary employment. Injured workers exit the system if any stage provides successful treatment. If the individual's occupational disability is so severe that it challenges his or her ability to perform at any level in the competitive labor market, however, the process passes on to the fifth stage (Vocational Feasibility), in which the individual's work habits, attitudes, and residual vocational resources are addressed. If vocational feasibility cannot be established, the injured worker's case is settled and no further services are provided. If the injured worker is able to establish vocational feasibility, a new target occupation is identified at the sixth stage (Employability). After a new target occupation is identified, the injured worker continues in the system to the seventh stage, at which any mismatch between his abilities and the target occupation's demands are addressed. Finally, in order to achieve case resolution, the effect of the injury on the injured worker's earning capacity is estimated. In some cases, this estimation is done scientifically and takes into account many of the unique attributes of the injured worker. In most cases, however, this is handled bureaucratically with gross estimates based on a category of pathology or level of impairment.

STAGE MODEL OF INDUSTRIAL REHABILITATION		
STAGE	ISSUE ADDRESSED	MEASURED BY OR IN TERMS OF ...
ONE	PATHOLOGY	Studies of soft tissue, blood, and bone.
TWO	IMPAIRMENT	Anatomy, physiology, and psychology.
THREE	FUNCTIONAL LIMITATION	Reported symptoms and perceived limitations.
FOUR	OCCUPATIONAL DISABILITY	Occupational consequences of functional limitations.
FIVE	VOCATIONAL FEASIBILITY	Worker role consequences of disability.
SIX	EMPLOYABILITY	Useful resources; skills, knowledge, residual capacity.
SEVEN	VOCATIONAL HANDICAP	Ability to perform a particular job.
EIGHT	EARNING CAPACITY	Earned income over expected worklife.

Figure 52.5. **The industrial rehabilitation process.**

Occupational rehabilitation treatment programs address the issues that are presented at each stage in the process through the use of treatment techniques that reflect the industrial environment and the competitive demands of work. These include:

1. *Treatment context:* The development of a sense of vocational competence based on mastery of the work environment. Occupational rehabilitation usually involves the patient 5 days per week, following a normal work schedule.
2. *Environmental demands of work:* The physical environment within which integrated work hardening is conducted is of paramount importance (16). The industrial setting includes concrete floors, minimal temperature control, and substantial ambient noise. The office setting exposes the injured worker to professional-level office equipment including computer keyboards and video display terminals used at work desks much like the desk one would find at a typical place of employment. This necessitates the use of large facilities, usually away from the medical treatment facilities. A 1992 survey of United States occupational rehabilitation programs presents data that indicate that the more than half of the occupational rehabilitation programs require more than

3000 square feet of floor space, as depicted in Figure 52.6.
3. *Procedural demands of work:* In addition to simulating the physical and temporal structure of a work environment, the procedural structure of the program must simulate the work environment. The injured worker's day begins by selecting his time card from the time card rack, "punching in" on the time clock, and reviewing his clipboard on which his tasks for the "work day" are listed. The following behavioral demands (presented to the injured worker as "work rules") must be met:
   a. *Safety:* Follow rules and instructions, do not exceed work restrictions, use proper body mechanics.
   b. *Interpersonal behavior:* Accept supervisors' directions, get along with fellow workers.
   c. *Attendance:* Daily, Monday through Friday.
   d. *Workplace tolerance:* Start each morning on time. Take only scheduled breaks and return on time. Remain in the workplace for a full work day.
   e. *Productivity:* Work at the maximum pace that will allow next day attendance, completion of the scheduled workday, and sustained activity without an unscheduled break from work.

   These demands are consistent with the expectations of employers in the competitive labor market.
4. *Equipment:* Equipment used in occupational rehabilitation programs includes work simulation tasks and apparatus that are used for physical conditioning. The basic criteria are that all such equipment be safe, reliable, valid, practical, and useful. In terms of safety, occupational rehabilitation equipment must have a demand that is able to be measured and controlled by the professional and must be gradable in terms of duration, frequency, and load. That is, the task must be able to be increased along these gradients as the patient demonstrates the ability to tolerate increased load. In terms of reliability, the equipment used in occupational rehabilitation must have a demand that can be replicated, performance that can be measured, and a reasonable expectation that the patient's performance can be replicated. In terms of validity, the equipment must sample critical content of the target job's demands or the demands of a job cluster. The better the sampling of such critical job demands, the higher the validity. In terms of practicality, this equipment must have a daily cost (capital plus staff) that is reasonable. In terms of the usefulness or utility of the equipment, it must be able to bring about improvement in the target domain at whatever stage of the occupational rehabilitation process the patient is performing.

PROGRAM MODELS

Occupational rehabilitation program models can be considered in terms of the stage in the process that is the focus of treatment. Occupational rehabilitation treatment programs are differentiated in terms of the patient's post-injury status along the following continuum:

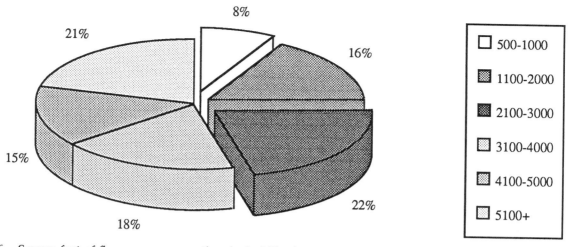

Figure 52.6. **Square feet of floor space, occupational rehabilitation programs, 1992.**

1. *Primary treatment:* To mediate pathology and limit impairment, primary intervention services are provided. These services include diagnosis, identification of pathogenesis, provision of short-term palliative relief, stabilization of an injured joint, muscle, or tendon, and development of a prognosis and preliminary return to work plan.
2. *Secondary Treatment:* Once pathology and impairment have stabilized, residual functional limitations can be evaluated and re-mediated. Remediation includes both physical reactivation and assistance to work around residual functional limitations that are permanent.
3. *Tertiary treatment:* If functional limitations preclude a return to usual and customary employment and/or secondary disability issues occur such as substance abuse, an affective disorder, or loss of worker role identification, tertiary care is provided.

Each of these models addresses the injured worker at subsequent stages in the occupational rehabilitation process with intervention strategies that are appropriate to that stage.

PRIMARY TREATMENT

The traditional approach to painful work injuries has been to recommend bed rest, mild analgesic and/or anti-inflammatory medication, and palliative physical therapy modalities. Apparently, this is an effective approach for the majority of injured workers. The Quebec Task Force on Spinal Disorders reported that 88% of all patients sustaining industrial injuries due to activity-related spinal disorders returned to work within 3 months, and an additional 5% returned to work within the next 3 months (4). Dixon found that almost 50% of painful industrial injuries improve in a week, and approximately 90% resolve within 1 month, regardless of treatment (17). Andersson et al. report that the recovery from low back pain to return to work is excellent, with more than 70% returning in 2–3 weeks

and 90% returning in 6 weeks (18). Deyo, however, reports that "only recently have actual clinical trials been conducted to test the efficacy of bed rest" (19). Deyo reports on a study in which he randomized 203 persons with back pain coming to a walk-in clinic into two groups, one receiving 2 days of bed rest and the other receiving 7 days of bed rest. Those receiving the 2-day recommendation missed almost half as much work as those receiving the 7-day recommendation, in spite of the fact that there were no other functional, physiologic, or psychophysical differences when the people were evaluated at 3 weeks or at 3 months after injury. Most people return to their usual employment activities prior to cessation of pain. Gilbert et al. compared a recommendation of 4 days bed rest to no bed rest and found that there were no differences in the degree of pain resolution (20). The bed rest group, however, required 42% more time to return to usual and customary activities than the no-bed-rest group. Fordyce et al. reported that recommendations for treatment or activity control that depended on cessation of pain resulted in more sick role behavior and in an increased level of impairment than when recommendations were made according to a fixed treatment schedule that was independent of the symptoms reported by the patient (21). Experience in rehabilitation of persons suffering from chronic disabling anginal pain (22) suggests that bed rest may be contraindicated beyond the length of time absolutely necessary to allow initial injury management. Traditional palliative measures of conservative care often produce a dependency on the therapist, physician, and the palliative measures themselves that is at cross purposes to the goal of returning the pain-disabled person to work. A treatment focus that is on remediation of pain rather than on return of function often results in protraction of off-work temporary disability status and increases the likelihood that the disability may become chronic. As a consequence, new models of conservative primary care have developed in recent years.

Active Conservative Care

Choler et al. (23) and Wiesel et al. (24) report on activity-oriented early intervention treatment protocols that achieve significant improvement in time off work and a substantial decrease in cost. Andersson and Frymoyer recommend avoidance of bed rest and continued ambulation for patients who are able to do so along with medication with aspirin or a nonsteroidal anti-inflammatory drugs (25). If pain is sufficiently severe, at-home structured bed rest is used with nonsteroidal anti-inflammatory medication. Muscle relaxants are rarely appropriate. Hot pack and cold pack treatment may be made available for use at the patient's discretion. After 2 days of bed rest, the patient is instructed to begin a program of short-distance walking several times a day, with gentle spinal flexion and extension. One week after the onset of symptoms, medical review may include radiographs if there has been no significant improvement or if sciatica is present. The patient is encouraged to return to work if sedentary or light work is available. If not, increased supervised activity may be appropriate to avoid cardiovascular deconditioning and musculoskeletal weakening. For the patient who is not improving at 1 week post injury but does not have any apparent pathology, enrollment in a physical therapy program designed to promote mobility is appropriate along with continued use of nonsteroidal anti-inflammatory medications. Narcotic medication is not recommended, nor are palliative physical therapy modalities. A heavy focus on muscle strengthening is also not recommended. The physician evaluates the patient on a weekly basis. After 4–6 weeks of this approach, a secondary treatment approach involving work hardening or a tertiary treatment approach involving functional restoration may be appropriate. A similar approach is used when sciatica is present, although the care is more gradual and protracted. As Andersson and Frymoyer report, ''Most patients with sciatica do not require surgery, however, and should be functional within 3 months'' (25).

Employer-Oriented Occupational Medicine

As the service delivery centerpiece of a community-based treatment facility, Matheson et al. describe the employer-oriented occupational medicine program (26). This program provides services through treatment staff who are familiar with the injured worker's work site and job duties. Familiarization is assured through on-site inspection by the treatment staff, supplemented by a job analysis library that is readily available and that staff are encouraged to use. In response to an injury, after the injured worker's pathology has been addressed and his or her impairment has been stabilized, the physician contacts the employer to learn whether or not temporary light-duty work is available. If available, the individual is returned to work immediately on a light-duty basis with concurrent treatment in the occupational medicine clinic to reduce swelling and maintain flexibility. If light-duty work is not available, the physician instructs the injured worker to return within 48–72 hours for a re-check. At re-check, the physician again inquires about the availability of light-duty work. Whether or not light-duty work is available, the injured worker begins active treatment, usually receiving services 3 days per week with a focus on maintaining flexibility and stamina. If light-duty work is available, the injured worker returns to work with time allowed for physical therapy treatment before or after the work day. Frequent communication from the physical therapist to the physician and employer ensures the earliest possible return to work.

Early-Intervention Counseling

Tessler reports on a primary care program that provides services to injured workers from the California Department of Corrections (27). In this program, a rehabilitation counselor meets with the injured worker at his or her home if the injured worker has not returned to work within 1 week of injury. The counselor provides detailed information on the rights and responsibilities of the injured worker in the workers' compensation system, with information tailored to the specific needs of the injured worker who is receiving the counseling. Additionally, the counselor works as a case coordinator to assure that appropriate treatment services are being provided and that the injured worker is satisfied with the level and type of care that is available. Problems that otherwise may not be identified are addressed before they are blown out of proportion. This model does not presuppose any particular medical treatment approach, instead relying on the services that normally would be available and assuring that they are provided in a timely and thoughtful manner. The results of this program have been dramatic.

Figure 52.7 demonstrates the results in terms of return to work, comparing the experience of injured workers at one prison whose personnel received the services with the experience of injured workers at the other prisons. Additionally, Figure 52.8 presents the comparison between treatment approaches in terms of the cost of the program. The additional cost for the early intervention case management is minimal compared to the savings that it facilitates.

Industrial Athletic Therapy

The injured worker as an industrial athlete is an idea that has been advanced by many in the field, including Mayer and Gatchel (28) and Mooney (29). The effect of sports medicine on the field of occupational rehabilitation has been considerable. Isernhagen reports on sev-

Return to Work Rates

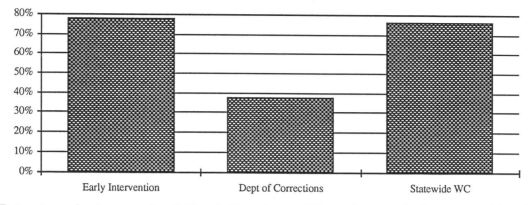

Figure 52.7. Return to work rate comparing California Department of Corrections standard program with early intervention program and statewide workers' compensation program.

Worker's Compensation Case Costs

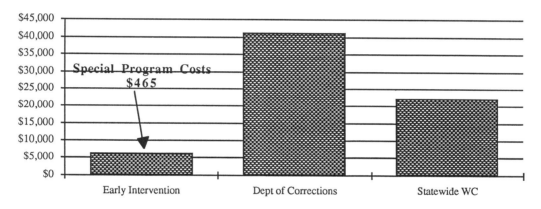

Figure 52.8. Program costs comparing California Department of Corrections standard program with early intervention program and statewide workers' compensation costs.

eral recent changes in the treatment of musculoskeletal injuries to avoid problems that result in occupational disability (30). This includes early intervention on an active basis to maintain range of motion and joint flexibility. Additionally, a shift has taken place from a focus on pain relief to functional improvement. Although traditionally the treatment for musculoskeletal injuries was focused on pain relief, the current emphasis in occupational rehabilitation is on increase in strength in spite of benign pain so that a return to full activity often takes place prior to cessation of pain.

In terms of the treatment for low back pain, De Rosa and Porterfield provide a model for conservative treatment that emphasizes early physical activation with services that usually are provided by physical therapists (31). These include the following:

1. Modification of pain or promotion of analgesia
2. Introduction of nondestructive forces to the injured

anatomic region to promote movement or increase physical activity
3. Enhance neuromuscular performance
4. Provide biomechanical counseling

McKenzie reports on an approach to treatment of low back pain that relies on postural change, exercises to promote stretching of shortened or contracted tissue that leads to dysfunction, and the application of local pressure to achieve proper anatomic alignment (32).

SECONDARY TREATMENT

Guided Reactivation

At the secondary intervention stage of occupational rehabilitation treatment, remediation of impairment is accomplished through aggressive physical reactivation guided by frequent functional evaluation. Termed "Guided Reactivation" by Mooney (29), the precepts of this model are well-supported in the literature on the pathophysiology of painful soft tissue injury. Improvement of physical tolerance is accomplished through physical conditioning. This not only provides the injured worker with a greater safety margin to prevent re-injury after returning to work, but it also has a tremendous impact on the worker's self-confidence and morale.

Often, an important part of the pain-disabled injured worker's problem has to do with his or her emotional orientation to pain. On admission, the injured worker is "disabled by pain" (a frequent self-description). Secondary intervention occupational rehabilitation programs are effective in improving work performance because they teach the pain-disabled injured worker to maintain work productivity in spite of symptoms. Injured workers frequently report no change in symptoms over the course of the occupational rehabilitation program while reporting a major improvement in productivity. "My symptoms are as bad as they were before but I can work now" is often heard as low-back-injured workers complete secondary intervention treatment programs (33, 34).

Work Conditioning

Isernhagen reports that physical therapists' functional restorative approach has become increasingly focused on specific return-to-work needs rather than addressing function on a more general basis (30). This has led to the development of work conditioning as a new occupational rehabilitation treatment model. Isernhagen defines work conditioning as follows (35):

> ... A work-relevant, intensive, goal-oriented treatment program specifically designed to restore an individual's systemic, neuromusculoskeletal function (strength endurance, movement, flexibility and motor control). The objective of the work conditioning program is to restore the client's *physical* health and function so the client can return to work or for the client to become physically reconditioned so vocational rehabilitation services can commence.

Isernhagen compares work conditioning with work hardening using the model depicted in Table 52.1.

The American Physical Therapy Association has developed formal guidelines for physical therapists to provide work conditioning services. It is expected that the American Occupational Therapy Association will develop similar guidelines for occupational therapists.

Work Hardening

In the mid-1970s work hardening as a treatment concept was developed at Rancho Los Amigos Hospital in Downey, California (15). This involved the use of graded work simulation as physical and emotional conditioning tasks in which the patient would be involved to achieve rehabilitation. Work hardening is a productivity-oriented treatment program that uses graded

Table 52.1.
Comparison of Work Conditioning and Work Hardening

Work Conditioning	Work Hardening
Generally follows acute care management, or in specific instances, the diagnostic process	Generally follows acute care management, or in specific instances, work conditioning
Requires work conditioning evaluation	Requires interdisciplinary evaluation
Single discipline model	Interdisciplinary model
Focuses on physical health and functional needs	Focuses on physical, psychosocial and vocational needs
Utilizes work relevant activities	Utilizes real or simulated work activities
Provided in multi-hour sessions (2–4 hours) available 5 days a week (2–8 weeks)	Provided in multi-hour sessions (4–8 hours) available 5 days a week (4–8 weeks)
Less costly	More costly

work simulations and specific functional conditioning tasks to do the following:

1. *Decrease secondary impairment.* Impairment is often magnified through disuse. Work hardening improves strength, flexibility, and endurance.
2. *Decrease functional limitations.* The client's style of work and the quality of his work behavior will often increase the functional decrement due to the impairment. Work hardening assists the client to learn efficient adaptive behaviors (36).
3. *Decrease disability.* Disability is the impact of functional impairment on the client's societal roles, among which work roles figure prominently. Work hardening assists the client to re-establish many of these roles. Improvement in these other areas generalizes to work roles and results in a concomitant decrease in work-related disability.
4. *Improve vocational feasibility.* Injured workers who become chronically disabled because of pain often develop habits and behaviors that conflict with the behaviors required to return to competitive employment. Occupational rehabilitation programs use as a frame of reference the work demands that employers place on workers in the competitive labor market. These are evaluated during the course of treatment through the use of the *Feasibility Evaluation Checklist*, depicted in Figure 52.9. The checklist includes 21 factors that have been identified as the most basic factors used to rate employees by employers in the competitive labor market. Matheson reported on a study of 462 consecutive patients admitted to an occupational rehabilitation program in which 35% who had not worked for 1 year or longer demonstrated feasibility

FEASIBILITY EVALUATION CHECKLIST

© 1992 Employment and Rehabilitation Institute of California

NAME: _____   RATER: _____

DATE: _____   PDC LEVELS TESTED: _____

	PRESENT FUNCTION				IMPROVEMENT POTENTIAL					PRESENT FUNCTION				IMPROVEMENT POTENTIAL			
	NOT EVALUATED	EMPLOYABLE COMPETITIVE	EMPLOYABLE SHELTERED	NOT EMPLOYABLE	HIGH	MODERATE	LOW	UNCERTAIN		NOT EVALUATED	EMPLOYABLE COMPETITIVE	EMPLOYABLE SHELTERED	NOT EMPLOYABLE	HIGH	MODERATE	LOW	UNCERTAIN
Section One - PRODUCTIVITY A. QUANTITY Evaluee's dependable demonstrated output.									B. USE OF PROPER BODY MECHANICS Evaluee's demonstrated consistency in the application of proper body mechanics to job tasks.								
B. QUALITY Evaluee's dependable demonstrated output of acceptable units.									C. WORK PLACE SAFETY 1. Audition 2. Vision 3. Sensation 4. Balance								
C. ATTENDANCE Evaluee's demonstrated consistency in reporting to place of work on assigned days.									D. USE OF PROTECTIVE BEHAVIOR Evaluee's demonstrated use of common sense in protecting himself/herself and other workers from danger.								
D. WORK-PLACE TOLERANCE Evaluee's demonstrated capacity to remain in the work-place on a dependable basis.									**Section Three -** **INTERPERSONAL BEHAVIOR** A. RESPONSE TO SUPERVISION Evaluee's demonstrated ability to appropriately:								
E. TIMELINESS Evaluee's demonstrated consistency in reporting to place of work on time, returning from breaks on time, and leaving place of work at appointed time.									1. Accept direction from a supervisor.								
F. INSTRUCTABILITY Evaluee's demonstrated ability to perceive, understand, and follow work instructions.									2. Adjust to different supervisors or supervisory styles. 3. Follow through with accepted directions								
G. MEMORY Evaluee's demonstrated ability to remember task instructions, work structure and safety rules.									B. RESPONSE TO FELLOW WORKERS Evaluee's demonstrated ability to work in concert with other workers addressing the same task.								
H. CONCENTRATION Evaluee's demonstrated ability to focus attention on the task to which he/she is assigned.									C. RESPONSE TO CHANGE Evaluee's demonstrated ability to adjust to changes in work routine, assignments, and conditions.								
Section Two - SAFETY A. ADHERENCE TO SAFETY RULES Evaluee's demonstrated adherence to industry safety rules.									D. GENERAL WORKER ATTITUDE Evaluee's demonstrated dedication to work and his/her role as a worker.								

Comments: _____

Figure 52.9.   **Feasibility Evaluation Checklist.**

problems that were sufficient to preclude return to work (37). Current and potential problems with vocational feasibility, including productivity, safety in the workplace, and interpersonal relations, are addressed in the work hardening program.

5. *Enhance employability.* Employability, the probability that the client will achieve employment, is directly related to the levels of the client's work tolerances (e.g., ability to lift, carry, stand) in comparison with other workers in the general labor market to which he or she must return. Work hardening identifies and develops these work tolerances.

6. *Decrease vocational handicap.* The match between the client and his job can be improved by increasing the client's level of function and by modifying the job's critical work demands. Work hardening involves both the client and the employer to address these issues as one unit.

Work Hardening Strategies

Work hardening results are achieved through the use of specific work-oriented treatment strategies. A few of the most important are the following:

1. *Functional capacity development:* The biomechanical, psychophysical, and metabolic-cardiovascular domains must be addressed in a coordinated fashion. In the psychophysical domain, functional capacity development depends to a large degree on the involvement of the injured worker in work simulation project tracks over several days. Project tracks are selected for the individual according to the appropriateness of the project in terms of the individual's goals. To the degree that the project is meaningful, involvement will lead to improved self-confidence. In the metabolic and cardiovascular domain, development of functional capacity begins with aerobic conditioning. In the biomechanical domain, work hardening focuses on the musculoskeletal system's ability to perform tasks that require strength and flexibility. Development of functional capacity is formally addressed each day in conditioning tasks. Validation of gains achieved as well as interpretation of the utility of these gains is obtained through serial functional testing.

2. *Symptom negotiation:* During the work hardening program, symptom control strategies are used to assist the individual with a painful disorder to learn that it is possible to "negotiate" with his or her symptoms and thereby improve functional capacity. Through the use of work pacing, proper body posture, and mechanics, and the substitution of productivity for symptoms as a method of self-assessment, symptoms become more predictable. The injured worker is more likely to learn to "work around" predictable symptoms than if the symptoms continue to be unpredictable.

3. *Work function theme development:* Work function themes are the rules (usually unstated and unconscious) that injured workers use to guide participation in work activities. Psychological variables that

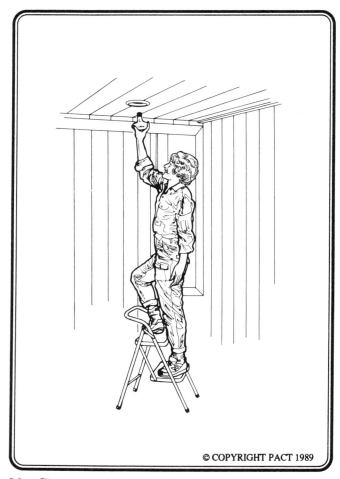

© COPYRIGHT PACT 1989

21. Change a light-bulb overhead.

Figure 52.10. **Sample test item,** *Spinal Function Sort.*

are centered around the perception of pain affect work performance and test performance in the injured worker (38). Clarification of the injured worker's work tolerances improves employability by allowing better definition of the jobs the injured worker is able to perform. One method for the identification of work function themes involves the use of the *Spinal Function Sort.* Figure 52.10 depicts a sample item from this instrument. The injured worker is asked to perform a subjective rating of the level at which he or she is able to perform 50 tasks that involve the spine to various degrees. A "rating of perceived capacity" score is obtained and compared to normative data. Additionally, this score is referenced to the United States Department of Labor's system for classifying the strength demands of work (39) to allow a link to be made between the injured worker's perception of his or her ability with a target job's demands.

4. *Serial functional testing:* In addition to providing the professional with information that can confirm the injured worker's progress, serial functional testing can have a therapeutic effect, if it is provided early. This effect has been described by Matheson and

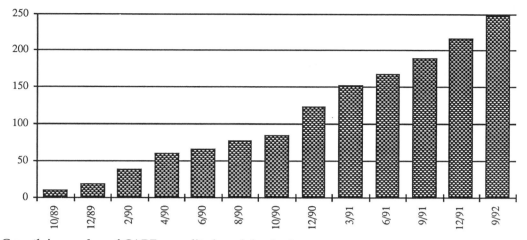

Figure 52.11. **Growth in number of CARF-accredited work hardening programs.**

Matheson (40). A significant interaction was found between chronicity of disability and the degree to which subjects improved as a consequence of one experience with functional capacity evaluation. Subjects who were within 90 days of injury had significant improvement in rating of perceived capacity that was not found with subjects who received functional testing more than 90 days post injury.

5. *Tool and job modification:* Tool and job modification is a necessary component of every work hardening program. As a primary course of action in a rehabilitation program, job modification has been shown to be both effective and inexpensive. Tool and job modifications occur in almost every job, whether or not the worker is disabled. Work hardening provides an opportunity to work with the injured worker in a "laboratory" setting. The work hardening environment, because it uses work simulation tasks with the injured worker on a daily basis for several days in a row, allows experimentation with different job and tool modifications so that by the time the injured worker goes out to the workplace, the job or tool modification has been fully tested and proven to be useful. A survey in California found that 81% of the job modifications that were used were either free or cost less than $500 (41). Another study of actual hardware costs found an average cost of $320; 34% of the recipients required less than $50 worth of modifications (42).

Work Hardening Program Accreditation

In 1988, the Commission on Accreditation of Rehabilitation Facilities (CARF) convened a National Advisory Committee composed of experts in the field of occupational rehabilitation to develop guidelines for accreditation of work hardening programs. This committee defined work hardening programs as

> . . . interdisciplinary in nature, which use conditioning tasks that are graded to progressively improve the biomechanical, neuromuscular, cardiovascular/metabolic and psychosocial functions of the individual in conjunc-

tion with real or simulated work activities. Work hardening provides a transition between acute care and return to work while addressing the issues of productivity, safety, physical tolerances, and worker behaviors. Work hardening is a highly structured, goal oriented, individualized treatment program designed to maximize the individual's ability to return to work." (43)

This definition and its attendant standards were placed in use for accreditation of rehabilitation facilities that offer work hardening as a treatment program. Based on additional feedback from the occupational rehabilitation programs that subsequently became accredited, a revision of these standards was developed by a second National Advisory Committee convened by CARF in 1991. The original definition was modified to include feedback from the accredited programs and the CARF surveyors who had applied the earlier standards to these programs:

> Work Hardening is a highly structured, goal-oriented, individualized treatment program designed to maximize the person's ability to return to work. Work Hardening Programs are interdisciplinary in nature with a capability of addressing the functional, physical, behavioral, and vocational needs of the person served. Work Hardening provides a transition between the initial injury management and return to work, while addressing the issues of productivity, safety, physical tolerances, and work behaviors. Work Hardening Programs use real or simulated work activities in a relevant work environment in conjunction with physical conditioning tasks. These activities are used to progressively improve the biomechanical, neuromuscular, cardiovascular/metabolic, behavioral, attitudinal, and vocational function of the person served. (44)

The CARF accreditation program was "market-driven" in that several state funding agencies, insurance carriers, and large self-insured employers requested that the CARF develop and provide standards to guide their actions in authorizing payment for occupational rehabilitation treatment services. Although concerns have been voiced about negative effects of the standards on small treatment programs (45), after the standards became available, growth in the number of accredited programs was rapid, greater than what had been found by the CARF in any of its other accreditation programs.

Work Hardening Program Outcome

In work hardening, several established programs have assessed outcome. Unfortunately, these programs have not used a uniform system for categorizing clients, program, services, or outcomes. Samples of outcome reports are presented below:

1. The Work Assessment and Rehabilitation Program at DCH Regional Medical Center in Tuscaloosa, Alabama, reports that its work hardening program has an "85% rate of success for . . . either returning to the same job or to return to the same industry with restricted physical demands" (46).
2. The Industrial Rehabilitation Program at Massachusetts General Hospital in Boston presents the following outcome data (47): Return to work, same job, same employer, 48%; Return to work, different job, same employer, 8%; Entry into a vocational training program, 4%; Medical management, 20%; Awaiting settlement, 8%; No information, 12%.
3. The Work Recovery Center at Piedmont Hospital in Atlanta, Georgia reports that "73.8% of the workers in the Workers' Compensation program have returned to work" (48). This program combines aspects of work conditioning, work hardening, and work recovery, using the ERGOS Work Simulator as its centerpiece.
4. The Work Hardening Program at the Irene Walter Johnson Institute at Washington University in St. Louis, Missouri, reports that 70% of patients who have completed the work hardening program have returned to work (49).
5. The Work Employment Rehabilitation Center at Loma Linda University in Southern California reports that of those who have entered the work hardening program, 55% have returned to usual and customary work, modified work, or a new job immediately after discharge (50). An additional 15% have entered the vocational rehabilitation program to receive training. Twenty-six percent of the patients from the work program returned for medical treatment.
6. The STEPS Rehabilitation Center program at Schwab Memorial Hospital in Chicago reports an 88% return-to-work rated as measured 30 days after discharge (51).
7. The PTS Program in Tacoma, Washington, affiliated with the University of Puget Sound, reports that 86% of its clients who have participated in the work hardening program have returned to work (52).
8. Niemeyer et al. describe a study conducted at the Employment and Rehabilitation Institute of California

that was based on 312 referrals for work hardening service (53). Approximately 15% of the people who were referred to the ERIC Work Hardening program were not accepted. Principal reasons for non-acceptance were of two types: need for pre-work hardening services such as basic physical therapy, occupational therapy, or drug detoxification; and mismatch between the type of work simulations needed by the person referred and those available in the program. Figure 52.12 indicates that approximately 68% of the people who entered the work hardening program were feasible for competitive employment at discharge. Most of those who completed the program were considered feasible for competitive employment. Figure 52.12 charts the follow-up of those people who, after leaving the work hardening program, began formal vocational rehabilitation programs. Approximately 12% were closed prior to plan implementation for various reasons, including declination of further services. Of those who completed the vocational rehabilitation program, 82% returned to work.

TERTIARY TREATMENT: FUNCTIONAL RESTORATION

Individuals who become chronically disabled because of a work-related injury present a unique set of characteristics that must be addressed by occupational rehabilitation treatment programs. Waddell et al. present a model of disability in which physical impairment accounts for approximately 40% of disability, and in which an additional 31% is due to psychological and/or behavioral factors (54). Waddell's "bio-psychosocial model" of treatment describes chronic disability as a consequence of several intertwining factors (55). In this view, disability is based on the injured worker's attitudes and beliefs and is learned. Feuerstein reports that "disability following an occupational musculoskeletal injury/illness is the consequence of a complex interaction of medical condition, physical capabilities, ergonomic demands, and a variety of psychosocial factors which . . . contribute to the exacerbation and maintenance of work disability" (56). Gatchel reports that "chronic pain patients develop specific psychological problems because of the failure of attempts to alleviate their pain that distinguish them from acute pain patients" (57). Sternbach et al. describe the use of MMPI profiles to discriminate between people who suffer from acute pain and those who suffer from chronic pain (58). Significant differences were found on scales that describe a neurotic preoccupation with bodily function, symptom reports and experiences, and depression. Matheson defines the "symptom magnification syndrome" and describes it as "a pervasive phenomenon that has tremendous impact on the ability of the health care system to deliver services . . ." (59). Moreno et al. describe research with pain-disabled injured workers and their response to a functional restoration program

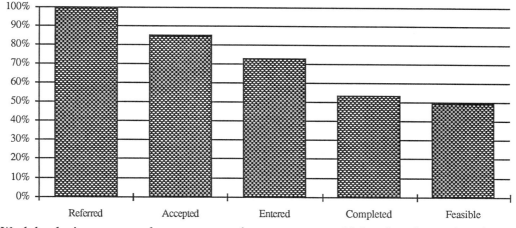

Figure 52.12. **Work hardening programs begun, expressed as a percentage of injured workers referred.**

(60). Although improvement was generally found, cognitive distortion was a useful factor to distinguish degree and area of improvement. Coste et al. found that 41% of their patients with nonspecific low back pain also had affective or anxiety disorders (61). Turk and Rudy present a multidimensional biobehavioral model of the relationship between pain and disability (62). In this model, the injured worker's "perceptions interact reciprocally with emotional factors, sensory phenomena, and behavioral responses" (62). Thus, an occupational rehabilitation treatment model must integrate the biomedical, psychosocial, and behavioral features presented by the patient to successfully ameliorate disability. Feuerstein and Thebarge present research that suggests that the multiple factors presented above may need to be supplemented by factors related to the employer (63). In a study that sought to discriminate between injured workers with pain who were working from those who were not working, variables such as job stress, supervisor support, and work pressure were found to be significant discriminant factors.

In addition to the psychological concomitants and sequelae of chronic pain disability, serious secondary physical impairment is also found. Mayer and Gatchel describe the effect of the "deconditioning syndrome" as a consequence of inactivity following a painful injury (28). This appears to be exacerbated by treatment approaches that rely solely on the injured worker's reports of symptoms to guide treatment. The deconditioning syndrome affects both the physiologic and psychologic components of the injured worker's disability on an intertwining basis. Disuse is initiated and maintained by the injured worker's symptom reports and leads to diminution of physical capacity which, in turn, leads to the perception by the injured worker that he or she is more significantly dysfunctional than would be expected, given the impairment. Reactivation of the injured worker, guided by frequent functional testing, impedes the development of the deconditioning syndrome.

However, the injured worker who is chronically disabled by pain and who suffers from the deconditioning syndrome requires a more aggressive and multifaceted treatment model.

Matheson et al. describe an interdisciplinary team approach to cardiac rehabilitation (22). The program is based on frequent functional evaluation beginning as early as 7–10 days after the cardiac event. These authors describe an interdisciplinary team as "a well-integrated, cohesive, multifaceted unit responsible for the holistic care of the patient . . . Each team member is responsible for patient care within his area of expertise and is responsible for the integration of his patient care input with those of the other team members" (22). This program also uses frequent functional evaluation to both establish safe performance limits and to monitor the patient's physical restoration. Additionally, "frequent evaluations offer the patient an opportunity to make gradual, realistic adjustments to his changing physical ability status" (22). This adjustment has important psychological consequences. The cardiac event, like the painful, disabling work injury, touches directly on the patient's self-concept and is a serious threat to his sense of self-worth. Ongoing evaluation gives the patient accurate information that he can use to resolve the physical abilities aspect of this "significance crisis."

Functional restoration is a tertiary treatment model developed by Mayer and colleagues at the P.R.I.D.E. center in Dallas, Texas. Functional restoration is used to resolve functional limitations of the permanently impaired worker so that he or she can resume a previous career path or find employment in a similar occupation. Functional restoration is defined as follows:

> . . . A medically-directed interdisciplinary *tertiary* treatment program, specific to spinal disorders in industrially-injured patients, designed to return patients to work, decrease dependence on the medical system, resolve impairment/disability disputes, and increase physical capacity to the highest functional level possible

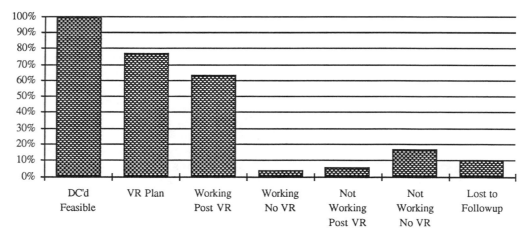

Figure 52.13. **Vocational rehabilitation (VR) outcome, expressed as a percentage of injured workers found feasible for competitive employment at time of discharge from work hardening program.**

to avoid recurrent injury after resumption of normal daily living activities. (64)

Gatchel et al. present eight critical elements that depict a functional restoration program (65). These are:

1. Formal, repeated modification of physical deficits to guide, individualize, and monitor physical training.
2. Psychological and socioeconomic assessment to guide, individualize, and monitor disability behavior-oriented interventions and outcomes.
3. Physical reconditioning of the injured functional unit.
4. Generic work simulation and whole-body training.
5. Multi-modal disability management program using cognitive behavioral approaches.
6. Psychopharmacologic interventions for detoxification and psychological management.
7. Interdisciplinary medically directed team approach with formal staffing, frequent team conferences, and low patient-to-staff ratios.
8. Ongoing outcome assessment utilizing standardized objective criteria.

Program Outcome

Mayer et al. reported an 81% success rate for individuals who had been disabled at the time of entry into the program for 17 months on average (66). Success was defined as employment at a 1-year follow-up. Mayer et al. reported an 87% success rate in terms of employment at a 2-year follow-up (67). In comparison, 41% of the nontreatment group was working at that point. Additionally, the control group demonstrated a five times higher rate of patient visits to help professionals, and about twice as many of the control-group patients had additional spinal surgery and/or unsettled workers' compensation litigation as compared to the treatment group.

Hazard et al. independently replicated the Mayer studies and found a return-to-work rate of 81% in the treatment group and 29% in the comparison group (68).

Both Mayer et al. and Hazard et al. had excellent follow-up rates for both the treatment group and the comparison group, achieving 90% follow-up at 1 year and 85% follow-up at 2 years.

Talo et al. report on a Finnish study that compared methods of categorization of patients who were randomly assigned to a functional reactivation or spa resort program (69). The functional activation program was based on the functional restoration model developed by Mayer and colleagues (66). A lower level of physical demand was placed on patients admitted to the spa resort program, utilizing one of three rehabilitation centers in Finland that are available for these services. Within-group changes were found at 12-month follow-up for both groups over several measures. These researchers found that results in the two programs were significantly affected by the characteristics of the patient and the interaction of these characteristics with the program's characteristics. They recommend the process of "subgrouping" in order to analyze treatment efficacy. Coste et al. also report the likelihood that there are specific differentiated subtypes to be found within groups of individuals disabled because of low back pain (70).

CONCLUSIONS

Occupational rehabilitation treatment programs have proliferated in recent years, in response to a growing need to control health care costs. Injured workers who are disabled because of pain have disproportionately expensive workers' compensation cases. Occupational rehabilitation helps to minimize this expense by providing treatment that:

1. Is focused on return to work as the primary treatment goal
2. Emphasizes the need to "negotiate" with pain while functional ability is developed rather than the need to eliminate pain before function can be restored

3. Utilizes functional testing to guide treatment and return to work decisions
4. Focuses treatment on specific areas of dysfunction that are pertinent to the occupational disability of the injured worker
5. Provides an interdisciplinary treatment team approach, the extent of which depends on the injured worker's needs

It is clear that occupational rehabilitation treatment programs are able to address problems experienced by the injured worker and his or her employer along the full spectrum of the occupational rehabilitation process. The efficacy of these programs is much less evident, however. Although attempts have been made to demonstrate efficacy using comparison group research methods (66–68), neither matched-control group studies nor randomly selected group studies have been undertaken. It must be pointed out that the absence of these studies is not simply a consequence of an absence of will on the part of the occupational rehabilitation treatment community. It is, in large part, due to the nature of the health care marketplace, which predominantly is funded by workers' compensation insurance carriers that are in a conflict-of-interest position with regard to program efficacy. For example, I was present at a meeting in a large rehabilitation hospital in the eastern United States with high-level executives from four large insurance companies. The purpose of the meeting was to design a study of the efficacy of work hardening using a matched control strategy. The insurance companies had been asked to provide information concerning control subjects to match in terms of gender, age, diagnosis, and severity of injury with injured workers who were admitted to a large work hardening program. This design would allow a comparison of the effect of treatment across a broad range of parameters. In addition to myself, several staff members from the hospital with excellent research credentials were present, as was the hospital administrator. The hospital intended to fund the project if the cooperation of the insurance carriers could be secured. The insurance carrier representatives were being asked merely for their assistance in identifying a control group. After considerable discussion, one of the insurance executives reported that "We really aren't that interested in formally establishing treatment efficacy. Our people out in the field tell us that work hardening is effective, and that's good enough for us." The other insurance executives concurred. With that, the meeting was adjourned and the project abandoned.

Occupational rehabilitation treatment programs are faced with both a risk and an opportunity in this set of circumstances. The risk is obvious and involves being caught up in wholesale cuts in health care expenditures. The cost of occupational rehabilitation treatment is easy to identify and, thus, easy to criticize. The opportunity for occupational rehabilitation treatment is much less obvious and is tied to the benefits provided by these programs. Retention of skilled and experienced employees, improvement in productivity in injured workers and in the work force in general, reduction in injury rates and re-injury rates, improvement in employee morale, and other factors that are difficult to measure are certainly results that occupational rehabilitation programs have the potential to bring to the industrial economy. Although there is no argument that occupational rehabilitation treatment programs are capable of providing such benefits, until efficacy studies are completed, occupational rehabilitation will grow at an unnecessarily slow rate and its contribution to a healthy economy will not be as great as the promise that it carries.

REFERENCES

1. Leavitt SS, Johnston TL, Beyer RD: The process of recovery: Patterns in industrial back injury. Part I: Costs and other quantitative measures of effort. *Indust Med Surg* 40:7–14, 1971.
2. Spengler DM, Bigos SJ, Martin NA, Zeh J, Fisher L, Nachemson A: Back injuries in industry: A retrospective study. I. Overview and cost analysis. *Spine* 11:241–245, 1986.
3. Antonakes JA: Claims costs of back pain. *Best's Review* September, 1981.
4. Spitzer WO: Quebec Task Force on Spinal Disorders. *Spine Eur Edition Suppl* 1:12(7S), 1987.
5. Gervais S, Dupuis G, Véronneau F, Bergeron Y, Millette D, Avard J: Predictive model to determine cost/benefit of early detection and intervention in occupational low back pain. *J Occup Med* 1:113–132, 1991.
6. Shalik H: *Introduction to Industrial Therapy.* Veterans Administration, Department of Physical Medicine and Rehabilitation, 1959.
7. Cooke D: Industrial therapy as applied in an occupational therapy department. *Occup Ther Rehabil* 6:39–42, 1937.
8. Wilson SC: Integration of occupational therapy and vocational rehabilitation. *Am J Occup Ther* 5:198–200, 216–217, 1951.
9. Gleave GM: The Delaware curative workshop. *Am J Occup Ther* 1:306–307, 1947.
10. Stevens AL: Work evaluation in rehabilitation. *Occup Ther Rehabil* 29:157–161, 1950.
11. Wegg L: The role of the occupational therapist in vocational rehabilitation. *Am J Occup Ther* 11:252–254, 1957.
12. Rosenberg R, Wellerson T: A structured pre-vocational program. *Am J Occup Ther* 14:57–60, 106, 1960.
13. Wegg L: The essentials of work evaluation. *Am J Occup Ther* 14:65–69, 79, 1960.
14. Reuss EE, Raws DE, Sundquist AF: Development of a physical capacities evaluation. *Am J Occup Ther* 12:1–14, 11958.
15. Matheson LN, Ogden LD, Violette K, Schultz K: Work hardening: Occupational therapy in industrial rehabilitation. *Am J Occup Ther* 39:314–321, 1985.

16. Ellexson MT. Environmental enhancements for work hardening. *Industr Rehabil Q* 1:14–15, 1988.

17. Dixon A: Progress and problems in back pain research. *Rheum Rehab* 12:165–174, 1973.

18. Andersson GBJ, Svensson H-O, Oden A: The intensity of work recovery in low back pain. *Spine* 8:880–884, 1983.

19. Deyo RA: Historic perspective on conservative treatments for acute back problems. In Mayer TG, Mooney V, Gatchel RJ (eds): *Contemporary Conservative Care for Painful Spinal Disorders.* Philadelphia, Lea & Febiger, 1991.

20. Gilbert JR, Taylor DW, Hildebrand A, Evans C: Clinical trial of common treatments for low back pain in family practice. *Br Med J* 291:791–794, 1985.

21. Fordyce WE, Brockway JA, Bergman JA, Spengler D: Acute back pain: A control-group comparison of behavioral vs. traditional management methods. *J Behav Med* 9:127–140, 1986.

22. Matheson LN, Selvester RH, Rice HE: The interdisciplinary team in cardiac rehabilitation. *Rehabil Lit* 36:366–376, 1975.

23. Chöler U, Larsson R, Nachemson A et al: *Back pain—Attempt at a structured treatment program for patients with low back pain* [in Swedish]. SPRI Report 188, Social Planerings-och Rational Isesingsinstitut Rapport, Stockholm, 1985.

24. Wiesel SW, Feffer HL, Rothman RH: Industrial low back pain: A prospective evaluation of a standardized diagnostic and treatment protocol. *Spine* 9:100, 1984.

25. Andersson GBJ, Frymoyer JW: Treatment of the acutely injured worker. In Pope MH, Andersson GBJ, Frymoyer JW, Chaffin DB (eds): *Occupational Low Back Pain: Assessment, Treatment and Prevention.* St. Louis, Mosby Year Book, 1991.

26. Matheson LN, Mooney VR, Jarvis G: Employer-based services: Dawn of a new age. *Indust Rehabil Q* 3, 1990.

27. Tessler S: Early intervention case management. In *Work Hardening: Applications in Case Management.* Videotape produced by American Rehabilitation Education Network. Pittsburgh, PA, 1990.

28. Mayer TG, Gatchel RJ: *Functional Restoration for Spinal Disorders: The Sports Medicine Approach.* Philadelphia: Lea & Febiger, 1988.

29. Mooney V: Guided reactivation: The industrial athlete in rehabilitation. In *Work Hardening: Applications in Case Management.* Videotape produced by American Rehabilitation Education Network. Pittsburgh, PA, 1990.

30. Isernhagen SJ: Physical therapy and occupational rehabilitation. *J Occup Rehabil* 1:71–82, 1991.

31. De Rosa CP, Porterfield JA: A physical therapy model for the treatment of low back pain. *Phys Ther* 72:261–272, 1992.

32. McKenzie R: A physical therapy perspective on acute spinal disorders. In Mayer TG, Mooney V, Gatchel RJ (eds): *Contemporary Conservative Care for Painful Spinal Disorders.* Philadelphia, Lea & Febiger, 1991.

33. Matheson LN: Integrated work hardening in vocational rehabilitation: An emerging model. *Vocational Eval Work Adjust Bull* 22:71–76, 1988.

34. Rainville J, Ahern DK, Phalen L, Childs LA, Sutherland R: The association of pain with physical activities in chronic low back pain. In Pope MH, Anderssoon GBJ, Frymoyer JW, Chaffin DB (eds): *Occupational Low Back Pain: Assessment, Treatment and Prevention.* St. Louis, Mosby Year Book, 1991.

35. Isernhagen SJ: Personal Communication, 1992.

36. Kornblau BL: Work hardening. In Tollison CD, Kriegel ML (eds): *Interdisciplinary Rehabilitation of Low Back Pain.* Baltimore, Williams & Wilkins, 1989.

37. Matheson LN: Vocational feasibility and its assessment. *Industrial Musculoskeletal Health,* University of Texas Health Science Center, Dallas, TX, September, 1988.

38. Papciak AS, Feuerstein M: Psychological factors affecting isokinetic trunk strength testing in patients with work-related chronic low back pain. *J Occup Rehabil* 1:95–104, 1991.

39. Matheson LN: *Work Capacity Evaluation: Systematic Approach to Industrial Rehabilitation.* Anaheim, CA: Employment and Rehabilitation Institute of California, 1986.

40. Matheson ML, Matheson LN: *Spinal Function Sort.* Performance Assessment and Capacity Testing. Mission Viejo, CA, 1989.

41. Collingnon F: The role of reasonable accommodation in employing disabled persons in private industry. In *Disability and the Labor Market: Economic Problems, Policies, and Programs.* New York, ILR Press, 1986.

42. Matheson LN: Prevention of disability-induced retirement. *Industr Rehabil Q* 1:1, 6–8, 1988.

43. Commission on Accreditation of Rehabilitation Facilities: Guidelines for work hardening programs. In *Standards Manual for Organizations Serving People with Disabilities.* Tucson, CARF, 1989.

44. Commission on Accreditation of Rehabilitation Facilities: Guidelines for work hardening programs. In *Standards Manual for Organizations Serving People with Disabilities.* Tucson, CARF, 1992.

45. Ellexson MT: The impact of CARF standards on the practice of work hardening. *Work* 1:69–72, 1990.

46. Fulper KE: Work assessment and rehabilitation program. In Ogden-Niemeyer L, Jacobs K (eds): *Work Hardening: State of the Art.* Thorofare, NJ, Slack, 1989.

47. Fortenbach M: The industrial rehabilitation program at the Massachusetts General Hospital. In Ogden-Niemeyer L, Jacobs K (eds): *Work Hardening: State of the Art.* Thorofare, NJ, Slack, 1989.

48. Brandon TL, Snyder L: Work recovery center Piedmont Hospital. In Ogden-Niemeyer L, Jacobs K (eds): *Work Hardening: State of the Art.* Thorofare, NJ, Slack, 1989.

49. Rhomberg S: Irene Walter Johnson Institute of Rehabilitation. In Ogden-Niemeyer L, Jacobs K (eds): *Work Hardening: State of the Art.* Thorofare, NJ, Slack, 1989.

50. Anzai D, Wright M: Freestanding work hardening programs affiliated with a hospital or rehabilitation facility. In Ogden-Niemeyer L, Jacobs K (eds): *Work Hardening: State of the Art.* Thorofare, NJ, Slack, 1989.

51. Ellexson M: S.T.E.P.S. Clinic Schwab Rehabilitation Center. In Ogden-Niemeyer L, Jacobs K (eds): *Work Hardening: State of the Art.* Thorofare, NJ, Slack, 1989.

52. Holmes MB, Mizoguchi JT: Professional services for the injured. In Ogden-Niemeyer L, Jacobs K (eds): *Work Hardening: State of the Art.* Thorofare, NJ, Slack, 1989.

53. Carlton RS, Niemeyer L: Employment and Rehabilitation Institute of California. In Ogden-Niemeyer L, Jacobs K (eds): *Work Hardening: State of the Art.* Thorofare, NJ, Slack, 1989.

54. Waddell G, Main CJ, Morris EW, Di Paola M, Gray ICM: Chronic low-back pain, Psychological distress, and illness behavior. *Spine* 9:209–213, 1984.

55. Waddel G: A new clinical model for the treatment of low-back pain. *Spine* 12:632–644, 1987.

56. Feuerstein M: A multidisciplinary approach to the prevention, evaluation, and management of work disability. *J Occup Rehabil* 1:5–12, 1991.

57. Gatchel RJ: Early development of physical and mental deconditioning in painful spinal disorders. In Mayer TG, Mooney V, Gatchel RJ (eds): *Contemporary Conservative Care for Painful Spinal Disorders*, 1991.

58. Sternbach RA, Wolf SR, Murphy RW, Akeson WH: Traits of pain patients: The low-back "loser". *Psychosomatics* 14:225–229, 1973.

59. Matheson L: Symptom magnification syndrome structured interview: Rationale and procedure. *J Occup Rehabil* 1:43–56, 1991.

60. Moreno R, Cunningham AC, Gatchel RJ, Mayer TG: Functional restoration for chronic low back pain: Changes in depression, cognitive distortion, and disability. *J Occup Rehabil* 1:207–216, 1991.

61. Coste J, Paolaggi JB, Spira A: Classification of nonspecific low back pain. I. Psychological involvement in low back pain: A clinical, descriptive approach. *Spine* 17:1028–1037, 1992a.

62. Turk DC, Rudy TE: Persistent pain and the injured workers: Integrating biomedical, psychosocial, and behavioral factors in assessment. *J Occup Rehabil* 1:159–180, 1991.

63. Feuerstein M, Thebarge RW: Perceptions of disability and occupational stress as discriminators of work disability in patients with chronic pain. *J Occup Rehabil* 1:185–196, 1991.

64. Mayer TG: Personal Communication, 1992.

65. Gatchel RJ, Mayer TG, Hazard RG, Rainville MD, Mooney V: Functional restoration: Pitfalls in evaluating efficacy [Editorial]. *Spine* 17:988–994, 1992.

66. Mayer TG, Gatchel RJ, Kishino N, Keeley J, Capra P, Mayer H, Barnett J, Mooney V: Objective assessment of spine function following industrial injury: A prospective study with comparison group and one-year follow-up. *Spine* 10:482–493, 1985.

67. Mayer TG, Gatchel RJ, Mayer H, Kishino ND, Keeley J, Mooney V: A prospective two-year study of functional restoration in industrial low back injury: An objective assessment procedure. *JAMA* 258:1763–1767, 1987.

68. Hazard RG, Fenwick JW, Kalisch SM, Redmond J, Reeves V, Reid S, Frymoyer JW: Functional restoration with behavioral support: A one-year prospective study of patients with chronic low-back pain. *Spine* 14:157–161, 1989.

69. Talo S, Rytökoshi U, Puukka P: Patient classification, a key to evaluate pain treatment: A psychological study in chronic low back pain patients. *Spine* 17:998–1011, 1992.

70. Coste J, Paolaggi JB, Spira A: Classification of nonspecific low back pain. II. Clinical diversity of organic forms. *Spine* 17:1028–1037, 1992b.

CHAPTER 53

LEGAL ASPECTS OF PAIN AND SOCIAL SECURITY DISABILITY

G. WAYNE McCALL

DISABILITY HAS been defined for the purpose of claims adjudication under the Social Security Act as an "inability to engage in any substantial gainful activity by reason of a medically determinable physical or mental impairment which can be expected to result in death or has lasted or can be expected to last for a continuous period of not less than 12 months" (1). The adjudication of claim for disability benefits under Title II (Social Security Disability benefits) and Title XVI (Supplemental Security Disability Income) of the Social Security Act is based upon the use of well-established, objectively demonstrable medical criteria described in the Listing of Impairments. Appendix to Subpart P of Regulations Number 4 and Subpart 1 of Regulations Number 16 of the Social Security Act. However, clear differences exist between what constitutes an "impairment" and what constitutes a "disability" within the context of the Social Security regulations, and it is within the interpretation of these differences that the Social Security Administration has placed considerable focus in the past several years.

The very definition of "disability" for Social Security purposes is based upon the claimant's ability (or inability) to "engage in substantial gainful activity," or to work. Thus, the adjudication of Social Security Act claims for disability is fundamentally a vocational issue rather than a medical one, according to Nadolsky (2). Nadolsky's position has been supported as far back as 1958, when the American Medical Association Committee on the Rating of Mental and Physical Impairment wrote in their "Guide to the Evaluation of Permanent Impairment, the Extremities and Back" that the determination of permanent impairment is purely a medical decision, and that whether or not a given impairment represented a disability was an administrative responsibility and function, rather than a medical one (3).

SEQUENTIAL EVALUATION PROCESS

The Social Security Administration (SSA) uses a process of "sequential evaluation" in determining eligibility for Title II and Title XVI disability benefits, and the first criterion of eligibility is a vocational, rather than a medical one, and involves determining whether a claimant is "engaging in substantial gainful activity," or working for a specific monetary amount in a specific period of time. These amounts may change from time to time based on changes in the national economy. Regardless of a claimant's medical or psychological status, he/she is not considered "disabled" for benefit purposes if he/she is working at a substantial gainful activity level.

If a claimant is not working, the next step in the sequential evaluation process is to determine whether the claimant has a "severe" impairment, or one that "has more than a minimal effect on the individual's ability to perform basic work activities" (4). Thus, a client's ability to work is the critical operational definition of disability, rather than the degree of medical impairment per se. In this step of the sequential evaluation process, the claimant's eligibility for benefits is presumed if functional restrictions in performing work-related activities are alleged by the claimant and supported by appropriate medical documentation. In the absence of medical support, however, a decision may be made that the claimant has a "slight" or "nonsevere" impairment. This step provides for the evaluation of the claimant's medical status to determine the extent to which objective medical findings support the alleged functional restrictions. This process uses the Listing of Impairments criteria referred to above and represents a statutory delineation of required medical signs, symptoms, and findings, broken down by body systems, that must be either "met" or "equaled" if an award is granted on a purely medical basis. If the criteria described in the Listing of Impairments are met or equaled, then the medical impairment becomes a legal definition of "disability," and an award is made based upon the statutory presumption that clients who "meet or equal" the Listings are incapable of engaging in substantial gainful activity.

The last step in the sequential evaluation process re-

712

quires the evaluation of the client's vocational prognosis to engage in work activity despite any functional restrictions that may be associated with his/her impairment or impairments. The determination of vocational prognosis is in itself a sequential process that requires evaluation of medical and psychological variables, along with evaluating the claimant's age, education, and prior work experience.

RESIDUAL FUNCTIONAL CAPACITY

The first step in determining the vocational prognosis of the client requires a medical determination of the client's residual functional capacity in terms of the work-related functions as described in the *Dictionary of Occupational Titles* (5), and at this point the objective determination of "disability" is based upon a physician's subjective interpretation of the impact of the claimant's medical impairments on his/her ability to perform work-related functions. The residual functional capacity assessment made by the physician requires evaluation of both exertional and nonexertional factors that may impact on the client's ability to work.

Evaluating Exertional Factors

The evaluation of functional capacity based on exertional factors involves the physician's evaluation of the claimant's ability to function in six physical demand areas under seven different kinds of working conditions, as described in Supplement 2 to the *Dictionary of Occupational Titles* (DOT, 3rd edition, 1968) (see Appendices 53.1 and 53.2).

In making judgments regarding a claimant's residual functional capacity, the factors of strength, exertional capabilities, and endurance must be considered. Review of the DOT Appendices suggests that a significant volume of data regarding vocational factors must be processed by the physician when making residual functional capacity judgments based on exertional factors alone, but the process may become more subjective when nonexertional factors are considered.

Evaluating Nonexertional Factors

Nonexertional factors include the claimant's cognitive capabilities to perform behaviors related to understanding and remembering instructions, responding appropriately to supervision in the workplace, and relating to coworkers and responding to customary work pressures in the work environment. It is in this area, where objective documentation is most often lacking, that the physician must make "educated guesses" based upon available psychological evaluation data or data from observations made in the workplace.

CONCEPT OF VOCATIONAL RELEVANCE

The concept of vocational relevance in establishing a vocational prognosis for a claimant is based upon not only the claimant's residual functional capacity but upon his/her age, educational background, and previous work history. This triad of factors is considered in the following general terms: (*a*) younger workers are presumed to be more employable than older workers, (*b*) skilled workers are presumed to be more employable than unskilled workers, and (*c*) claimants with higher education are presumed to be more employable than undereducated workers. Vocational relevance in establishing a vocational prognosis for the adjudication of SSA disability claims is further dependent upon the temporal concept of vocational recency and the concept of transferability of skills: (*a*) the longer a person is unable to work, the higher the probability that skill level will diminish, and (*b*) unskilled workers will remain unskilled workers regardless of time away from the job.

TRANSFERABILITY OF SKILLS

The sequential evaluation process for determining a vocational prognosis must consider whether the claimant possesses skills that will enable him/her to be more readily employable. Given two workers with the same residual functional capacity profile, a worker with transferable skills would have a better vocational prognosis than one who did not. The determination of a claimant's skills is based upon two variables defined in the DOT: general educational development level and specific vocational preparation time (see Appendix 53.3). As may be seen from these descriptions, the level of cognitive capability and general educational development level required for jobs described in the DOT has been well defined functionally in the reasoning, mathematical, and language spheres through the use of a 1 to 6 rating scale, and the specific vocational preparation time required to perform the job within industrially established norms is defined by a 1 to 9 rating scale.

The SSA has described in Section 404, Appendix 2 of the Social Security Regulations specific guidelines for the use of vocational factors in the adjudication of claims that evaluate a client's vocational prognosis by functional capacity level, based on the interrelationship between the vocational factors of age, education, and previous work experience. Each general vocational factor is divided into subcategories: age into specific age ranges; education into categories of illiteracy, limited or less education, and high school or more; and previous work experience into unskilled, semi-skilled, and skilled workers with transferable skills, and semiskilled and skilled workers without transferable skills. These subgroupings provide a structured mechanism for making vocational decisions and represent an attempt to objectify the decision-making process as it relates to the vocational arena.

OVERVIEW OF THE DISABILITY ADJUDICATION PROCESS

The process of sequentially evaluating medical, psychological, and vocational data provides an orderly process of disability claim adjudication in the Social Security system, and the statutory requirements of the law provide a mechanism for obtaining the necessary objective information to make an informed adjudication on a claim. The law also provides a mechanism of appeals if the claimant disagrees with the decision made on his/her claim. If a claim is denied initially, the claimant may ask that a reconsideration be made, and a reevaluation of the medical, psychological, and vocational evidence is performed by another disability adjudicator employed by the state agency performing the claims adjudication for the SSA. If the reconsideration results in a continued denial of benefits, the mechanism is available for the claimant to appeal his/her case to an administrative law judge.

SOCIAL SECURITY AND CHRONIC PAIN

The use of objectively demonstrable signs, symptoms, and medical findings as a basis for disability adjudication has served the intent of the law relatively well in problems related to acute medical conditions, but the law does not provide an objective mechanism for evaluating the chronic pain patient. Because the pain experience is a perception and because perceptions are not directly objectively quantifiable, pain was considered in the evaluation of disability only as a secondary factor associated with a medically determinable impairment. The SSA has had increasing numbers of court cases challenging this policy regarding the evaluation of pain since chronic pain sufferers often present with allegations of pain that are not consistent with medically determinable impairment(s). As a consequence of an increasing number of cases within the courts, the Social Security Disability Benefits Reform Act of 1984 (Public Law 98–460) directed the Secretary of Health and Human Services to appoint a Commission on the Evaluation of Pain to conduct a joint study with the National Academy of Sciences on the evaluation of pain as it pertains to claims adjudication under Titles II and XVI of the Social Security Act.

CLASSIFICATION OF CHRONIC PAIN PATIENTS

The Social Security Commission on the Evaluation of Chronic Pain recognized the pain experience as a multifaceted physical, mental, social, and behavioral process that may impact on the patient's behavior in all areas of his/her life, and recognized that chronic pain patients often experience similar behavioral consequences as they attempt to adjust to the perception of pain. The typical pain patient is one who develops a preoccupation with the pain that causes an increase in his/her use of the health care system, experiences a decrease in level of functional activity, has an increase in pain behavior as he/she becomes physiologically deconditioned, and has a decrease in vocational produc-

tivity with a correspondent decrease in ability to earn a living. The chronic pain patient syndrome represents a well-recognized symptom complex in which allegations of pain persist far beyond the expected healing time for an acute injury and most often are not supported by an objectively demonstrable medical etiology for said pain. Numerous psychological, social, and environmental factors have been demonstrated to affect the chronic pain experience (6, 7). The effects of chronic pain on economic considerations related to social disability systems are well described by Chapman and Brena (8).

The Commission defined four groups of chronic pain patients: (*a*) chronic pain, inability to cope, insufficiently documented impairment; (*b*) chronic pain, competent coping, insufficiently documented impairment; (*c*) chronic pain, inability to cope, sufficiently documented impairment; and (*d*) chronic pain, competent coping, sufficiently documented impairment. The Commission determined that groups *c* and *d* posed no problems in disability adjudication according to the current law, and recommended protocols for the evaluation of patients within groups *a* and *b*. The Commission specifically recommended interdisciplinary evaluation by appropriately trained medical, psychological, functional, social, and vocational specialists, and recommended the development of quantitative measurement of functional capacity and the establishment of rehabilitation goals within each disciplinary specialty. The Commission further recommended periodic reevaluation of the chronic pain patient as a measure of his/her compliance with the prescribed pain rehabilitation program and recommended vocational and avocational counseling to increase the patient's productivity level after completion of pain rehabilitation.

LEGAL IMPLICATIONS

The fact that the determination of disability for SSA purposes is an administrative function controlled by the statues within the Social Security law makes the Social Security disability adjudication essentially a legal decision based upon well-defined findings of fact. The recommendations of the Commission represent a positive advance in the SSA's perception of the need for interdisciplinary evaluation of chronic pain patients, and the need for regulatory criteria for establishing minimum standards for centers that provide these evaluations.

The utilization of psychometric evaluation tools, behavioral observation, and behavioral rating scales of pain behavior have been well described by numerous references in the literature and represent current advances in the sophistication of mechanisms for quantifying pain behavior. However, because of the differences between the medical determination of impairment and the legal determination of disability that follows, the critical operational definition that defines the differences between impairment and disability is the vocational prognosis for engaging in substantial gainful activity.

Brena, McCall, and Franco have addressed the need for standardized vocational evaluation protocols in the interdisciplinary evaluation of chronic pain patients and described the use of the vocational evaluation process and the data derived from same as a critical part of the objective documentation process (9). The use of vocational evaluation methodologies provides a common point of reference between the medical (impairment rating) professions and the administrative/legal (disability rating) professions, and the process of vocationally evaluating a patient affords the vocational evaluator an extended opportunity to observe the patient's level of motivation, endurance, attention span, concentration, and pain behavior, all of which assist in the developing of a functional diagnosis, which impacts directly on the resulting vocational prognosis.

The results of the vocational evaluation proper also yield important information relative to the establishment of a vocational prognosis if the claimant is prevented from returning to relevant past work by virtue of the functional restrictions placed upon him/her by the impairment rating physician. Botterbusch (10) gave an excellent overview and comparison of commercially available vocational evaluation systems, but the Career Evaluation System offers several advantages in evaluating patients impaired by chronic pain; a comprehensive vocational evaluation can be obtained in one extended session of 4–6 hr, which causes minimal disruption in the provision of therapeutic services; and the specific subtests yield a comprehensive profile of the patient's level of function in terms of nonverbal IQ and abstract reasoning, verbal and numerical aptitudes, and several measures of strength, reaction time, and visuospatial and perceptual-motor coordination. After computer processing of the raw data, including the functional restrictions imposed on the patient by the impairment rating physician, the resulting printout yields jobs within the patient's functional profile that the patient has demonstrated in evaluation to have the abilities to perform, and gives the pain treatment team valuable information with which to develop task-specific rehabilitation plans that are most cost-effective and oriented toward returning the pain-impaired patient back to vocational productivity.

The utilization of commercially available job-matching software is another technological advancement that has improved the provision of comprehensive vocational services in chronic pain rehabilitation centers. The Occupational Access System (OASYS) is but one example of job-matching software, but it has particular advantages in Social Security disability evaluations of vocational prognosis in pain centers because it allows for maximum flexibility in adjusting both worker traits and worker ability profiles across medical, vocational, aptitude, vo-

cational interest, and temperament variables. The resulting transferability of skills profile documents the presence (or absence) of jobs into which the pain patient could transfer within his/her medically established functional capacity, and offers the advantage of addressing the need for job modification strategies and on-the-job training. A recent overview by Botterbusch provides a detailed comparison of job-matching systems (11).

CONCLUSIONS

In summary, the adjudication of Social Security disability claims under Title II and Title XVI of the Social Security Act is based upon objectively demonstrable evidence of medical impairments that may or may not constitute a legal definition of disability. The recommendations of the Commission on the Evaluation of Pain support the need for comprehensive, multidisciplinary evaluation of chronic pain patients, including the provision of comprehensive vocational counseling and evaluation services. The necessary objective data base for closing the gap between impairment and disability exists within the vocational rehabilitation profession, whose standardized vocational evaluation and transferability of skills technologies can offer objective vocational prognoses that are cost-effective and time-efficient applications of the sequential evaluation process that will meet the needs of both the medical and legal professions.

Acknowledgment The editor wishes to acknowledge Benson Hecker, Ph.D., and Richard S. Vaughan, J.D., for reviewing this chapter and updating it from the previous edition.

REFERENCES

1. US Department of Health and Human Services, Social Security Administration, Office of Operational Policy and Procedures: *Social Security Regulations: Rules for Determining Disability and Blindness*, 4.04, 1505. SSA Pub. No. 64-014. Washington, DC, US Government Printing Office, 1981, p 2.
2. Nadolsky JM: Social security: in need of rehabilitation. *J Rehabil* 50:6–8, 1984.
3. AMA Council on Rating Mental and Physical Impairment: Guides to the evaluation of permanent impairment—the extremities and back. *JAMA* 166:1958.
4. US Department of Health and Human Services, Social Security Administration. Office of Operational Policy and Procedures: *Social Security Regulations: Rules for Determining Disability and Blindness*. 4.04, 1521. SSA Pub. No. 64-014. Washington, DC, US Government Printing Office, 1981, p 5.
5. US Department of Labor, Employment and Training Administration: *Dictionary of Occupational Titles*, ed 4. Washington, DC, US Government Printing Office, 1991.

6. Fordyce WE: *Behavioral Methods for Chronic Pain and Illness*. St. Louis, CV Mosby, 1976.

7. Brena SF, Chapman SL: The "learned pain syndrome": decoding a patient's signals. *Postgrad Med* 69:53–64, 1981.

8. Chapman SL, Brena SF: Pain and society. *Ann Behav Med* 7:21–23, 1985.

9. Brena SF, McCall GW, Franco AM: Functional diagnosis: vocational and disability evaluation. In Bonica JJ (ed): *The Management of Pain in Clinical Practice*, ed 2. (in press).

10. Botterbusch KF: *A Comparison of Commercial Evaluation Systems*. Menomonie, WI, University of Wisconsin–Stout, Material Development Center, 1987.

11. Botterbusch KF: *A Comparison of Computerized Job Matching Systems*. Menomonie, WI, University of Wisconsin–Stout, Material Development Center, 1987.

APPENDIX **53.1**

PHYSICAL DEMANDS

Physical demands are those physical activities required of a worker in a job.

The physical demands listed in this publication serve as a means of expressing both the physical requirements of the job and the physical capacities (specific physical traits) a worker must have to meet the requirements. For example, "seeing" is the name of a physical demand required by many jobs (perceiving by the sense of vision), and also the name of a specific capacity possessed by many people (having the power of sight). The worker must possess physical capacities at least in an amount equal to the physical demands made by the job.

THE FACTORS

1 LIFTING, CARRYING, PUSHING, AND/OR PULLING (STRENGTH)

These are the primary "strength" physical requirements, and, generally speaking, a person who engages in one of these activities can engage in all.

Specifically, each of these activities can be described as:

1. Lifting: Raising or lowering an object from one level to another (includes upward pulling).
2. Carrying: Transporting an object, usually holding it in the hands or arms or on the shoulder.
3. Pushing: Exerting force upon an object so that the object moves away from the force (includes slapping, striking, kicking, and treadle actions).
4. Pulling: Exerting force upon an object so that the object moves toward the force (includes jerking).

The five degrees of Physical Demands Factor No. 1 (Lifting, Carrying, Pushing, and/or Pulling), are as follows:

S Sedentary Work

Lifting 10 lbs. maximum and occasionally lifting and/or carrying such articles as dockets, ledgers, and small tools. Although a sedentary job is defined as one which involves sitting, a certain amount of walking and standing is often necessary in carrying out job duties. Jobs are sedentary if walking and standing are required only occasionally and other sedentary criteria are met.

L Light Work

Lifting 20 lbs. maximum with frequent lifting and/or carrying of objects weighing up to 10 lbs. Even though the weight lifted may be only a negligible amount, a job is in this category when it requires walking or standing to a significant degree, or when it involves sitting most of the time with a degree of pushing and pulling of arm and/or leg controls.

M Medium Work

Lifting 50 lbs. maximum with frequent lifting and/or carrying of objects weighing up to 25 lbs.

H Heavy Work

Lifting 100 lbs. maximum with frequent lifting and/or carrying of objects weighing up to 50 lbs.

V Very Heavy Work

Lifting objects in excess of 100 lbs. with frequent lifting and/or carrying of objects weighing 50 lbs. or more.

2 CLIMBING AND/OR BALANCING

1. Climbing: Ascending or descending ladders, stairs, scaffolding, ramps, poles, ropes, and the like, using the feet and legs and/or hands and arms.
2. Balancing: Maintaining body equilibrium to prevent falling when walking, standing, crouching, or running on narrow, slippery, or erratically moving sur-

faces; or maintaining body equilibrium when performing gymnastic feats.

3 Stooping, Kneeling, Crouching, and/or Crawling

1. Stooping: Bending the body downward and forward by bending the spine at the waist.
2. Kneeling: Bending the legs at the knees to come to rest on the knee or knees.
3. Crouching: Bending the body downward and forward by bending the legs and spine.
4. Crawling: Moving about on the hands and knees or hands and feet.

4 Reaching, Handling, Fingering, and/or Feeling

1. Reaching: Extending the hands and arms in any direction.
2. Handling: Seizing, holding, grasping, turning, or otherwise working with the hand or hands (fingering not involved).
3. Fingering: Picking, pinching, or otherwise working with the fingers primarily (rather than with the whole hand or arm as in handling).
4. Feeling: Perceiving such attributes of objects and materials as size, shape, temperature, or texture, by means of receptors in the skin, particularly those of the finger tips.

5 Talking and/or Hearing

1. Talking: Expressing or exchanging ideas by means of the spoken word.
2. Hearing: Perceiving the nature of sounds by the ear.

6 Seeing

Obtaining impressions through the eyes of the shape, size, distance, motion, color, or other characteristics of objects. The major visual functions are: (1) acuity, far and near, (2) depth perception, (3) field of vision, (4) accommodation, (5) color vision. The functions are defined as followed:

1. Acuity, far—clarity of vision at 20 feet or more. Acuity, near—clarity of vision at 20 inches or less.
2. Depth perception—three-dimensional vision. The ability to judge distance and space relationships so as to see objects where and as they actually are.
3. Field of vision—the area that can be seen up and down or to the right or left while the eyes are fixed on a given point.
4. Accommodation—adjustment of the lens of the eye to bring an object into sharp focus. This item is especially important when doing near-point work at varying distances from the eye.
5. Color vision—the ability to identify and distinguish colors.

Scale of General Education Development (GED)*

Level	Reasoning Development	Mathematical Development	Language Development
6	Apply principles of logical or scientific thinking to a wide range of intellectual and practical problems. Deal with nonverbal symbolism (formulas, scientific equations, graphs, musical notes, etc.) in its most difficult phases. Deal with a variety of abstract and concrete variables. Apprehend the most abstruse classes of concepts.	Advanced calculus: Work with limits, continuity, real number systems, mean value theorems, and implicit functions theorems. Modern Algebra: Apply fundamental concepts of theories of groups, rings, and fields. Work with differential equations, linear algebra, infinite series, advanced operations methods, and functions of real and complex variables. Statistics: Work with mathematical statistics, mathematical probability and applications, experimental design, statistical inference, and econometrics.	Reading: Read literature, book and play reviews, scientific and technical journals, abstracts, financial reports, and legal documents. Writing: Write novels, plays, editorials, journals, speeches, manuals, critiques, poetry, and songs. Speaking: Conversant in the theory, principles, and methods of effective and persuasive speaking, voice and diction, phonetics, and discussion and debate.
5	Apply principles of logical or scientific thinking to define problems, collect data, establish facts, and draw valid conclusions. Interpret an extensive variety of technical instructions in mathematical or diagrammatic form. Deal with several abstract and concrete variables.	Algebra: Work with exponents and logarithms, linear equations, quadratic equations, mathematical induction and binomial theorem, and permutations. Calculus: Apply concepts of analytic geometry, differentiations and integration of algebraic functions with applications.	Same as Level 6.

Scale of General Education Development (GED)* (Continued)

Level	Reasoning Development	Mathematical Development	Language Development
5	(Continued)	**Statistics:** Apply mathematical operations to frequency distributions, reliability and validity of tests, normal curve, analysis of variance, correlation techniques, chi-square application and sampling theory, and factor analysis.	
4	Apply principles of rational systems to solve practical problems and deal with a variety of concrete variables in situations where only limited standardization exists. Interpret a variety of instructions furnished in written, oral diagrammatic, or schedule form.	**Algebra:** Deal with system of real numbers; linear, quadratic, rational, exponential, logarithmic, angle and circular functions, and inverse functions; related algebraic solution of equations and inequalities; limits and continuity, and probability and statistical inference. **Geometry:** Deductive axiomatic geometry, plane and solid; and rectangular coordinates. **Shop Math:** Practical application of fractions, percentages, ratio and proportion, mensuration, logarithms, slide rule, practical algebra, geometric construction, and essentials of trigonometry.	**Reading:** Read novels, poems, newspapers, periodicals, journals, manuals, dictionaries, thesauruses, and encyclopedias. **Writing:** Prepare business letters, expositions, summaries, and reports, using prescribed format and conforming to all rules of punctuation, grammar, diction, and style. **Speaking:** Participate in panel discussions, dramatizations, and debates. Speak extemporaneously on a variety of subjects.
3	Apply commonsense understanding, to carry out instructions furnished in written, oral, or diagrammatic form. Deal with problems involving several concrete variables in or from standardized situations.	Compute discount, interest, profit and loss; commission, markup, and selling price; ratio and proportion, and percentage. Calculate surfaces, volumes, weights, and measures. **Algebra:** Calculate variables and formulas, monomials and polynomials, ratio and proportion variables; and squae roots and radicals. **Geometry:** Calculate plane and solid figures; circumference, area, and volume. Understand kinds of angles, and properties of pairs of angles.	**Reading:** Read a variety of novels, magazines, atlases, and encyclopedias. Read safety rules, instructions in the use and maintenance of shop tools and equipment, and methods and procedures in mechanical drawing and layout work. **Writing:** Write reports and essays with proper format, punctuation, spelling, and grammar, using all parts of speech. **Speaking:** Speak before an audience with poise, voice control, and confidence, using correct English and well-modulated voice.
2	Apply commonsense understanding to carry out detailed but uninvolved written or oral instructions. Deal with problems involving a few concrete variables in or from standardized situations.	Add, subtract, multiply, and divide all units of measure. Perform the four operations with like common and decimal fractions. Compute ratio, rate, and percent. Draw and interpret bar graphs. Perform arithmetic operations involving all American monetary units.	**Reading:** Passive vocabulary of 5,000–6,000 words. Read at rate of 190–215 words per minute. Read adventure stories and comic books, looking up unfamiliar words in dictionary for meaning, spelling, and pronunciation. Read instructions for assembling model cars and airplanes. **Writing:** Write compound and complex sentences, using cursive style, proper end punctuation, and employing adjectives and adverbs. **Speaking:** Speak clearly and distinctly with appropriate pauses and emphasis, correct pronunciation, variations in word order, using present, perfect, and future tenses.

Scale of General Education Development (GED)* (Continued)

Level	Reasoning Development	Mathematical Development	Language Development
1	Apply commonsense understanding to carry out simple one- and two-step instructions. Deal with standardized situations with occasional or no variables in or from these situations encountered on the job.	Add and subtract two digit numbers. Multiple and divide 10's and 100's by 2, 3, 4, 5. Perform the four basic arithmetic operations with coins as part of a dollar. Perform operations with units such as cup, pint, and quart; inch, foot, and yard; and ounce and pound.	Reading: Recognize meaning of 2,500 (two- or three-syllable) words. Read at rate of 95–120 words per minute. Compare similarities and differences between words and between series of numbers. Writing: Print simple sentences containing subject, verb, and object, and series of numbers, names, and addresses. Speaking: Speak simple sentences, using normal word order, and present and past tenses.

*From US Department of Labor, Employment and Training Administration: *Dictionary of Occupational Titles*, ed. 4. Washington, D.C., US Government Printing Office, 1991.

APPENDIX **53.2**

WORKING CONDITIONS

Working conditions are the physical surroundings of a worker in a specific job.

1 INSIDE, OUTSIDE, OR BOTH

I Inside: Protection from weather conditions but not necessarily from temperature changes.
O Outside: No effective protection from weather.
B Both: Inside and outside.

A job is considered "inside" if the worker spends approximately 75 percent or more of his time inside, and "outside" if he spends approximately 75 percent or more of his time outside. A job is considered "both" if the activities occur inside or outside in approximately equal amounts.

2 EXTREMES OF COLD PLUS TEMPERATURE CHANGES

1. Extremes of Cold: Temperature sufficiently low to cause marked bodily discomfort unless the worker is provided with exceptional protection.
2. Temperature Changes: Variations in temperature which are sufficiently marked and abrupt to cause noticeable bodily reactions.

3 EXTREMES OF HEAT PLUS TEMPERATURE CHANGES

1. Extremes of Heat: Temperature sufficiently high to cause marked bodily discomfort unless the worker is provided with exceptional protection.
2. Temperature Changes: Same as 2(2).

4 WET AND HUMID

1. Wet: Contact with water or other liquids.
2. Humid: Atmospheric condition with moisture content sufficiently high to cause marked bodily discomfort.

5 NOISE AND VIBRATION

Sufficient noise, either constant or intermittent, to cause marked distraction or possible injury to the sense of hearing, and/or sufficient vibration (production of an oscillating movement or strain on the body or its extremities from repeated motion or shock) to cause bodily harm if endured day after day.

6 HAZARDS

Situations in which the individual is exposed to the definite risk of bodily injury.

7 Fumes, Odors, Toxic Conditions, Dust, and Poor Ventilation

1. Fumes: Smoky or vaporous exhalations, usually odorous, thrown off as the result of combustion or chemical reaction.
2. Odors: Noxious smells, either toxic or nontoxic.
3. Toxic Conditions: Exposure to toxic dust, fumes, gases, vapors, mists, or liquids which cause general or localized disabling conditions as a result of inhalation or action on the skin.
4. Dust: Air filled with small particles of any kind, such as textile dust, flour, wood, leather, feathers, etc., and inorganic dust, including silica and asbestos, which make the workplace unpleasant or are the source of occupational diseases.
5. Poor Ventilation: Insufficient movement of air causing a feeling of suffocation: or exposure to drafts.

APPENDIX 53.3
TRAINING TIME

SPECIFIC VOCATIONAL PREPARATION (SVP)

Specific Vocational Preparation is defined as the amount of lapsed time required by a typical worker to learn the techniques, acquire the information, and develop the facility needed for average performance in a specific job-worker situation.

This training may be acquired in a school, work, military, institutional, or vocational environment. It does not include the orientation time required of a fully qualified worker to become accustomed to the special conditions of any new job. Specific vocational training includes: vocational education, apprenticeship training, in-plant training, on-the-job training, and essential experience in other jobs.

Specific vocational training includes training given in any of the following circumstances:

1. Vocational education (high school; commercial or shop training; technical school; art school; and that part of college training that is organized around a specific vocational objective);
2. Apprenticeship training (for apprenticeable jobs only);
3. In-plant training (organized classroom study provided by an employer);
4. On-the-job training (serving as learner or trainee on the job under the instruction of a qualified worker);
5. Essential experience in other jobs (serving in less responsible jobs that lead to the higher grade job or serving in other jobs that qualify).

The following is an explanation of the various levels of specific vocational preparation:

Level	Time
1	Short demonstration only
2	Anything beyond short demonstration up to and including 1 month
3	Over 1 month up to and including 3 months
4	Over 3 months up to and including 6 months
5	Over 6 months up to and including 1 year
6	Over 1 year up to and including 2 years
7	Over 2 years up to and including 4 years
8	Over 4 years up to and including 10 years
9	Over 10 years

Note: The levels of this scale are mutually exclusive and do not overlap.

GENERAL EDUCATIONAL DEVELOPMENT (GED)

General Educational Development embraces those aspects of education (formal and informal) that are required of the worker for satisfactory job performance. This is education of a general nature which does not have a recognized, fairly specific occupational objective. Ordinarily, such education is obtained in elementary school, high school, or college. However, it may be obtained from experience and self-study.

The GED Scale is composed of three divisions: Reasoning Development, Mathematical Development, and Language Development. The description of the various levels of language and mathematical development are based on the curricula taught in schools throughout the United States. An analysis of mathematics courses in school curricula reveals distinct levels of progression in the primary and secondary grades and in college. These levels of progression facilitated the selection and assignment of six levels of GED for the mathematical development scale.

However, though language courses follow a similar pattern of progression in primary and secondary school, particularly in learning and applying the principles of grammar, this pattern changes at the college level. The diversity of language courses offered at the college level precludes the establishment of distinct levels of language progression for these 4 years. Consequently, language development is limited to five defined levels of GED inasmuch as levels 5 and 6 share a common definition, even though they are distinct levels.

PHYSICAL DEMANDS—STRENGTH RATING (STRENGTH)

The Physical Demands Strength Rating reflects the estimated overall strength requirement of the job, expressed in terms of the letter corresponding to the particular strength rating. It represents the strength requirements that are considered to be important for average, successful work performance.

The strength rating is expressed by one of five terms: Sedentary, Light, Medium, Heavy, and Very Heavy. In order to determine the overall rating, an evaluation is made of the worker's involvement in the following activities:

1. Standing, Walking, Sitting
   Standing—Remaining on one's feet in an upright position at a work station without moving about.
   Walking—Moving about on foot.
   Sitting—Remaining in a seated position.
2. Lifting, Carrying, Pushing, Pulling
   Lifting—Raising or lowering an object from one level to another (includes upward pulling).
   Carrying—Transporting an object, usually holding it in the hands or arms, or on the shoulder.
   Pushing—Exerting force upon an object so that the object moves away from the force (includes slapping, striking, kicking, and treadle actions).
   Pulling—Exerting force upon an object so that the object moves toward the force (includes jerking).

Lifting, pushing, and pulling are evaluated in terms of both intensity and duration. Consideration is given to the weight handled, position of the worker's body, and the aid given by helpers or mechanical equipment. Carrying most often is evaluated in terms of duration, weight carried, and distance carried.

Estimating the strength factor rating for an occupation requires the exercise of care on the part of occupational analysis in evaluating the force and physical effort a worker must exert. For instance, if the worker is in a crouching position, it may be much more difficult to push an object than if pushed at waist height. Also, if the worker is required to lift and carry continuously or push and pull objects over long distances, the worker may exert as much physical effort as is required to similarly move objects twice as heavy, but less frequently and/or over shorter distances.

3. Controls

Controls entail the use of one or both arms or hands (hand/arm) and/or one or both feet or legs (foot/leg) to move controls on machinery or equipment. Controls include but are not limited to buttons, knobs, pedals, levers, and cranks.

Following are descriptions of the five terms in which the Strength Factor is expressed:

S—Sedentary Work Exerting up to 10 pounds of force occasionally (Occasionally: activity or condition exists up to 1/3 of the time) and/or a negligible amount of force frequently (Frequently: activity or condition exists from 1/3 to 2/3 of the time) to lift, carry, push, pull, or otherwise move objects, including the human body. Sedentary work involves sitting most of the time, but may involve walking or standing for brief periods of time. Jobs are sedentary if walking and standing are required only occasionally and all other sedentary criteria are met.

L—Light Work Exerting up to 20 pounds of force occasionally, and/or up to 10 pounds of force frequently, and/or a negligible amount of force constantly (Constantly: activity or condition exists 2/3 or more of the time) to move objects. Physical demand requirements are in excess of those for Sedentary Work. Even though the weight lifted may be only a negligible amount, a job should be rated Light Work: (1) when it requires walking or standing to a significant degree; or (2) when it requires sitting most of the time but entails pushing and/or pulling of arm or leg controls; and/or (3) when the job requires working at a production rate pace entailing the constant pushing and/or pulling of materials even though the weight of those materials is negligible. NOTE: The constant stress and strain of maintaining a production rate pace, especially in an industrial setting, can be and is physically demanding of a worker even though the amount of force exerted is negligible.

M—Medium Work Exerting 20 to 50 pounds of force occasionally, and/or 10 to 25 pounds of force frequently, and/or greater than negligible up to 10 pounds of force constantly to move objects. Physical Demand requirements are in excess of those for Light Work.

H—Heavy Work Exerting 50 to 100 pounds of force occasionally, and/or 25 to 50 pounds of force frequently, and/or 10 to 20 pounds of force constantly to move objects. Physical Demand requirements are in excess of those for Medium Work.

V—Very Heavy Work Exerting in excess of 100 pounds of force occasionally, and/or in excess of 50 pounds of force frequently, and/or in excess of 20 pounds of force constantly to move objects. Physical Demand requirements are in excess of those for Heavy Work.

CHAPTER 54

WORKERS' COMPENSATION
PENNY LOZON CROOK

Workers' compensation is, in the most general terms, a system of social legislation designed to protect workers from suffering undue financial hardship when they are unable to work as the result of an on-the-job injury. More specifically, workers' compensation is not a system, but a number of systems; there are separate workers' compensation laws in each state, the District of Columbia, and various U.S. territories. In addition, federal laws provide coverage for federal employees, and many maritime workers are covered under the federal Longshore and Harbor Workers Compensation Act. Despite the multiplicity of laws, however, they are for the most part sufficiently similar that we can, for the purposes of this chapter, discuss workers' compensation as though it were a single system, as first conceived by Larson (1).[a]

The definition of who is a covered worker varies from state to state. For the most part, however, the majority of "employees" are included in the system, while independent contractors are excluded. Certain classes of employees may also be excluded; some of the more prevalent exclusions are domestic employees, farm workers, executives and partners, and employees of very small employers (employers of fewer than the minimum number, e.g., two or five employees, are not required to have workers' compensation, although they may be able to affirmatively opt to be covered). In a few states, workers' compensation coverage is extended only to employees in "hazardous" occupations, but in those states the term "hazardous" is broadly defined. In most states, workers' compensation coverage is mandatory for all employers and employees who fit within the statutory definition.

As noted in the general definition, workers' compensation is designed to protect injured workers from un-

due financial hardship; it is not designed to totally replace lost income. Thus, under the most typical benefit scheme, a totally disabled worker will receive only two-thirds of his average weekly wage, subject to a state maximum benefit. Also, unlike tort systems, under which an injured person can collect for pain and suffering and other intangible injuries, the workers' compensation system is designed only to compensate injured workers for medical expenses and lost wages.

WORKERS' COMPENSATION VERSUS TORT-BASED SYSTEMS

As noted in the previous section, workers' compensation differs from the tort system in that the workers' recovery is limited to medical costs and compensation for lost wages and disability. Workers' compensation also differs from tort-based systems in another major way. Tort systems are designed to provide compensation (in the form of damages awards) from wrongdoers to those injured because of the wrongdoers' fault or negligence. Workers' compensation, however, is generally not concerned with questions of fault or negligence.[b] The only main focus is on work connection—that is, was this injury sufficiently related to the injured person's working conditions or duties.

To illustrate the differences between tort systems and workers' compensation, consider two simple "slip and fall" cases, in which Mr. Smith and Ms. Jones are hurt when they slip in a puddle of water on the floor and fall. In a tort system, whether Mr. Smith could recover from someone else for his injuries would depend on

---

[a]Dr. Arthur Larson first conceived of the idea of treating the 50-odd separate workers' compensation statutes in terms of their similarities in his 1952 treatise. The *Law of Workmen's Compensation*. During the ensuing 40 years, while that original 2-volume treatise has grown to 10 volumes, courts, compensation boards, and state legislatures have increasingly looked to Dr. Larson's wisdom in determining how issues should be handled.

[b]Fault considerations are a part of some workers' compensation statutes in the form of penalties to be assessed when the conduct of either the employer or the employee is particularly blameworthy. For instance, in many states an employee's compensation award may be reduced (and in some states, denied altogether) if his on-the-job accident was caused by his voluntary intoxication. Similarly, in many states an employee's award may be increased if the accident was caused by the employer's failure to follow state or federal safety rules. Since penalties are generally not favored in the law, both types of statutes are strictly construed and therefore of relatively little importance in the total workers' compensation scheme.

how the water got on the floor (for instance, he would be unlikely to recover anything if he had spilled the water himself); whether the owner of the building knew, or should have known, that the water was there and that Mr. Smith or persons like him were likely to be walking in that area (i.e., the owner probably has no duty to protect against the possibility that a trespasser would slip in the puddle); and whether Mr. Smith should have been able to see the water in time to avoid stepping in it. If all of these issues were resolved in Smith's favor, he could recover for his medical expenses in treating the injury, his past and future lost wages attributable to the injury, and his pain and suffering. In addition, his wife could recover for loss of consortium, that is, the diminution in value of his services to her as a result of the injury. The Smiths might also recover punitive damages if the judge or jury found that the defendant's conduct was especially blameworthy; for instance, if the puddle had been on the floor in an area heavily frequented by the public for a long time and the building's owner had deliberately refused to clean it up.

In contrast, if Ms. Jones had slipped in the puddle while she was working, questions of whose fault the accident was and who knew or did not know about the puddle would be generally irrelevant. The only issues would be whether her injuries were sufficiently work connected (under the formula discussed below) and whether those injuries kept her from working. Her recovery, however, would be limited to payment of her medical bills, payment of compensation benefits for the weeks she was unable to work, and, in most states, a "schedule award" for her presumptive future loss of wages if, after reaching the maximum medical recovery, it was determined that she had a residual permanent loss of function attributable to her injuries.

There are two more facets that should be noted in connection with these examples. First, if Ms. Jones' injury had occurred off the employer's premises—as, for instance, if she were a salesperson who slipped while calling on a customer—she could still bring tort action (a "third-party action") against the owner of the premises. That action would proceed just like Mr. Smith's action, except that Ms. Jones would be obliged to reimburse her employer out of her damages award for any workers' compensation benefits she received. Second, as to the employer, Ms. Jones does not have the option of suing or receiving workers' compensation; except in very limited circumstances not present in this example, workers' compensation is the exclusive means of collecting from the employer for an employee's injuries.

Injured workers are increasingly attempting to bring third-party actions so as to recover for intangible injuries such as pain and suffering and punitive damages. In addition to bringing actions against manufacturers and distributors of products involved in the injury, employees often attempt to sue their employers on the ground that their injuries were caused by the employer's "intentional" misconduct. Although most workers' compensation acts do indeed allow workers to sue the employer for "intentional" acts, these exceptions are generally applied strictly so as to allow actions only in cases of deliberate assaults on the employee and the like. In virtually every state, actions will not be allowed on the basis that the employer "intentionally" failed to furnish a safe place to work. [The problems involved in third-party actions occupy an entire volume in Larson's 10-volume treatise (ref. 1, vol. 2A).]

MEDICAL WITNESSES IN THE WORKERS' COMPENSATION SYSTEM

As the examples in the preceding section show, the workers' compensation system avoids much of the protracted litigation present in the tort system over issues of fault and damages. Thus, in the majority of workers' compensation cases, the system functions almost automatically; upon receipt of notice that an employee has been injured, the employer arranges for payment of his medical expenses and begins making weekly payments of the workers' compensation benefits to which the employee is entitled until he is able to return to work. Nevertheless, there remain many cases in which there is disagreement between the parties as to whether the employee has sustained a compensable injury and, if so, what benefits he is entitled to receive. Before discussing these issues more specifically, however, it will be helpful to understand the context in which the issues are decided and the role physicians can and do play in the process.

In most states, the initial determination on contested proceedings is a hearing before a hearing officer (often called a referee, an administrative law judge, or a deputy commissioner), a quasi-judicial employee of the state labor department. Because the procedure is an administrative-type hearing rather than a court trial, the rules of evidence may be less strictly applied than they would be in a court action. For instance, medical evidence may be admitted not only in the form of live testimony and sworn depositions, but also in the form of unsworn medical reports and letters. It should also be remembered that the hearing officers rarely have any medical training. Although a long-time hearing officer may have acquired familiarity with medical terminology, a relatively new hearing officer is unlikely to have such familiarity, nor is he likely to understand more esoteric terms and relationships.

And yet, the issues that are often contested are those of the causation of an injury and the extent and duration of a worker's disability. The proper resolution of both these issues often depends on expert medical evidence. This evidence must be properly introduced at the initial hearing on the claim, since, in most states, the hearing officer's determination will be affirmed in appeals to higher levels of the workers' compensation commission and the courts unless it is "clearly wrong." Although the terminology for this standard of review varies from state to state, the general rule is that the hearing officer's decision is presumed correct as long as it comports with any substantial evidence (see ref. 1, vol. 3, 80.20 *et seq.* for a collection of literally hundreds of cases that were affirmed on this ground). A hearing officer who accepts the credible testimony of one physician is not likely to be overruled merely because two or three physicians expressed an opposite view, particularly if the physician whose testimony was accepted actually treated the worker and the other physicians' evidence is based on merely reviewing the medical records.

Of course, the hearing officer stage is reached only in contested cases—those in which the worker and the employer (or more accurately in most cases, the employer's workers' compensation insurance carrier) disagree as to the cause of the injury or the extent of the disability. Most cases are disposed of simply on the basis of the reports given by the treating physician(s), and perhaps those of physicians who are called upon, by either party, to give a second opinion. Determinations in these cases are made by insurance adjusters.

Thus, whether or not a case is contested, medical evidence is often accorded great weight by persons who may be untrained in medical terminology. Therefore, a physician who is called upon to give a report in a compensation case must remember to be clear in explaining his diagnosis and prognosis, particularly in cases involving more unusual injuries and diseases. One should be prepared to explain an official diagnosis in layman's terms and to spell out in detail the causal relationship between the events of the job and the employee's current disability. When it comes to rating the degree of permanent partial disability sustained by a claimant, the physician should be aware that insurance companies and workers' compensation hearing officers expect to have ratings based on standard AMA Guidelines. If a chronic pain specialist believes that these Guidelines do not accurately reflect the true extent of the worker's disability because they do not take into account the degree of pain, he should be prepared to spell out clearly how and why his rating departs from the Guidelines. (The issue of chronic pain as a factor in disability is discussed more fully later.)

Another rule the physician should be aware of when reporting or testifying in a workers' compensation case is the "speculation and conjecture rule." Simply stated, this rule means that the workers' compensation commissions cannot legally make an award based on "maybes." Although hearing officers are rarely as unsophisticated as to expect medical testimony to be phrased in terms of certainty, they are nonetheless liable to find their decisions overturned if they accept testimony that is too equivocal. Thus the physician should be prepared to state his conclusions in as positive terms as possible. Instead of "I think" and "I feel," he should be prepared to express his opinions in terms of "reasonable medical probability" or percentages of probability if he can conscientiously do so.

THE COMPENSATION FORMULA

The workers' compensation system is designed to provide benefits only for work-related injuries; it is not designed to handle all disability of employed persons. Therefore, it is incumbent on a workers' compensation claimant to show that his injury comes within the state's statutory definition of work relatedness. The relevant wording of this definition varies from state to state, but it generally requires the employee to show that he has sustained "a personal injury by accident arising out of and in the course of employment." This requirement thus has several subparts, which may be broken down as follows:

1. A personal injury
2. An injury by accident
3. An injury that arises out of the employment
4. An injury sustained during the course of employment

For purposes of this chapter, we may safely dispense with the fourth requirement, that of course of employment, since the issues there rarely involve medical questions, but rather are confined to legal and factual issues, such as whether injuries sustained on a lunch or coffee break or while engaged in horseplay can be said to have happened during the course of employment (see ref. 1, vols. 1-1A, sects. 14.00–29.00). However, the other three parts of the formula often involve not only legal and factual questions, but also questions that can be resolved only through expert medical testimony.

Personal Injury

It may be difficult for a physician to understand why the requirement that an employee sustained a personal injury should be at all controversial, let alone one of the most controversial areas in current workers' compensation law. It must be recalled that the workers' compensation system was originally geared toward dealing with problems like that of an assembly line worker who loses a finger or breaks a leg in a fall. To a compensation board or commission used to dealing with clearly observable physical injuries like cuts and broken bones, the term *injury* may not seem to include mental or nervous "injuries." Yet employees do develop mental and nervous injuries as the result of events that happen at work. In fact, there are apparently an increasing number of employees whose work causes them to undergo emotional injuries; at least the number of reported cases in which such "injuries" appear is growing, and much controversy has been engendered as workers' compensation commissions and the courts that hear appeals from those commissions try to deal with the problems of emotional injuries.

In order to understand the scope of the controversy, it is helpful to use Larson's breakdown of the three categories of mental injuries (ref. 1, vol. 1B, sect. 42.21–42.25). These categories are:

1. *Physical-mental.* This includes all injuries in which a worker who first receives some sort of physical trauma to the body (e.g., a blow or a cut) becomes disabled from the psychic repercussions of that trauma.
2. *Mental-physical.* This category is comprised of cases in which the initial trauma is emotional—perhaps a sudden shock or fright or perhaps merely the cumulative effect of job stress—but the result is a clearly observable physical injury, such as a heart attack or bleeding ulcers.
3. *Mental-mental.* These are the cases in which there is no "visible" injury at either end of the equation (e.g., a disabling neurosis caused solely by stress).

The courts almost invariably find that cases in the first category are compensable, even where the initial trauma was slight. In fact, even in states with an express provision that mental injuries are compensable only if preceded by a physical impact, the courts have been quite resourceful in finding an initial physical trauma sufficient to satisfy the statute.

Cases in the second category have become increasingly prevalent in workers' compensation literature in recent years, particularly those cases involving stress-related heart attacks. In the heart attack cases, the issue of compensability almost always depends on the degree of stress involved. A claimant can rarely recover unless he can show some unusual degree or type of work-related stress that led up to the debilitating attack. (And his case will be strengthened greatly if some degree of abnormal physical exertion was also present.)

As might be expected, it is the last category, that of "mental-mental" injuries, that is the most controversial. Even within this category, a distinction must be made between cases in which the initial emotional stress was a sudden fright or shock and cases in which the causative factor was merely the gradual buildup of stress. Compensation is more or less routinely awarded in cases involving a sudden stimulus, as for instance a worker who suffers an emotional breakdown after seeing a friend or coworker killed on the job. It is much more difficult, however, for a worker to recover when his breakdown is attributable merely to the cumulative stresses of the job. Although there have been recent awards in such cases, the courts in these cases have stressed that awards in this category are permissible only if the worker can show greater than ordinary stress

leading up to the breakdown. There remains a very strong fear among courts and employers that allowing recovery for those debilitated by ordinary pressures and stress would turn the workers' compensation system into a general mental health insurance system that would favor those too emotionally "weak" to handle the normal pressures of life.

INJURY BY ACCIDENT

Because workers' compensation was not designed as insurance against the "wear and tear of ordinary life," most workers' compensation statutes protect only against "accidental" injuries. One obvious way that the accident requirement functions is to prevent recovery for deliberately self-inflicted injuries. This issue, which is currently usually handled by a specific statutory exclusion for intentional self-injuries, arises seldom and then usually only in the context of suicides. (As a general rule, suicide is noncompensable, but two major rules work so as to make many probable suicides compensable. First, there is a general civil law presumption that an unexplained death was not suicide, which, combined with the general rule that the workers' compensation acts are to be liberally construed in favor of the worker, serves to make the decision in many unexplained death cases one in favor of accident, rather than suicide. Second, most courts to have considered the issue have ruled that the suicide of a disabled worker is compensable if he was driven to commit the act by the pain caused by his work-related injury.)

Even though the self-injury question is of relatively little importance, there remain two primary areas of concern within the "by accident" requirement. The first, which is closely related to the preceding discussion of emotional injuries, is the unusualness requirement that has been read into the definition of an accidental injury. The second is the issue of disease as an accidental injury.

Unusualness Requirement

Even though workers' compensation is supposed to be a no-fault system, the historic requirement that an accident must have been unusual in order to satisfy the "by accident" definition reminds one of the "assumption of risk" doctrine in traditional tort law. The assumption of risk doctrine may be easily illustrated by imagining a professional boxer attempting to sue his opponent for his injuries. The assumption of risk rule dictates that he cannot recover; when he agreed to engage in the fight he voluntarily chose to assume the risk that he would be injured. A similar rationale was applied in early workers' compensation cases when courts denied recovery to workers whose injuries arose from the normal incidents of their employment—for example, a night watchman who suffered frostbite while making his rounds on a wintery night. Although the courts did not phrase their denials in terms of assumption of risk, their use of the "accident" terminology revealed the same reasoning as the assumption of risk doctrine. Common sense tells us that the boxer should anticipate the risk of being injured when he steps into the ring; common sense also tells us that a man who walks around checking doors all night in freezing temperatures should anticipate the risk of being frostbitten. Since the watchman, like the boxer, should have expected the result that actually occurred, the result was not unusual and thus was not a compensable "accident" under this reasoning.

Although the refusals to recognize the effects of exposure to the elements as accidents are now almost entirely a historic anomaly, the unusualness requirement has taken over another entire field of workers' compensation cases, those involving "breakage" of the body from the routine exertions of the job, particularly in cases involving heart and back injuries. The paradigmatic example of how these cases arise is that of a worker at the end of an assembly line whose job is to remove 40-pound boxes from the line and stack them on pallets. After months or years of routinely performing this task, he picks up a box and feels a sharp pain in his back or, perhaps more typically, goes home one night and wakes up with back pain. His physician reports that he has a lumbar strain or, perhaps, a herniated disk. Has he sustained an "accidental" injury?

The traditional answer to this question was no; there was no accident because nothing unusual occurred during the work. Although the result—the back injury— was unusual, the cause was not; the worker was simply doing his regular job. But in some instances, the courts found that there was an "accident" if there was anything unusual about the day's work—the boxes weighed 50 pounds, rather than the regular 40 pounds, or the worker had to carry them 2 feet further that day. In some instances, it might be held that there was a compensable accident if the worker felt a sudden pain on the line, but not if he simply awoke one morning with a back problem—that is, an injury was considered "accidental" only if the worker could point to a definite time and place where it occurred.

A moment's reflection will show that these distinctions are not only arbitrary but are also liable to draw false distinctions between workers with identically caused injuries. Thus, many jurisdictions are gradually coming to drop their artificial unusualness requirements in favor of a simpler test of medical causation: did this worker's exertion, whether or not unusual, in fact cause this injury? The process of change is, however, not only slow but uneven; a particular jurisdiction may require only proof of medical causation for heart injuries, but require a showing of unusual effort for back injuries, and retain elaborate rules on showing a definite time and place of injury for hernia cases. (see ref. 1, vol. 1A,

sects. 36.00–38.83 for a discussion of the "by accident" requirement and unusualness rules.)

Accident and Disease

The "by accident" requirement was originally thought to bar a workers' compensation recovery when the injury was due to a disease or allergy caused by exposure to conditions on the job, rather than to some sort of traumatic injury. However, recovery was generally allowed if the disease was a result of an initial trauma. Some cases also held the disease was compensable if it could be shown that the germs entered the body suddenly and unexpectedly, as where a tubercular coworker sneezed in the employee's face or where an employee was exposed to infection through an open cut or wound. Some occupational disease cases could also be brought within the accident requirement under the "repeated trauma" theory. This theory envisions each onslaught of germs or noxious particles as a small trauma—a "mini-accident"—and holds the resulting disease process compensable as the result of a series of accidents.

This sort of elaborate rationale is less frequently needed nowadays, since every state has some sort of occupational disease act, as part of, or as an adjunct to, its workers' compensation act. Difficulties may still arise, however, in states where the occupational disease statute is merely in the form of an exclusive schedule or list of covered occupational diseases.[c] In those states, it may be necessary to invoke the "repeated trauma theory" in order to attempt to fit an unlisted disease into the "accident" theory.

In states that do not have a schedule, or whose schedule is not exclusive, an occupational disease is usually defined as one "peculiar to" or "characteristic of" the type of employment, or at least one to which the employee had a greater exposure than that of the general public. Thus, an employee who seeks workers' compensation benefits for disability caused by a relatively common disease, such as pneumonia or hepatitis, must be prepared to show how the duties of his job exposed him to a greater risk of contracting this disease than he would have had in his everyday life. For example, in one Pennsylvania case, an employee was unable to convince either the commission or the reviewing court that distillery workers have a greater risk of developing alcoholism than does the general public. On the other

---

[c]The types of diseases included in these schedules are usually respiratory diseases, such as asbestosis and byssinosis, along with diseases caused by exposure to various heavy metals and toxic industrial chemicals. One major problem with both exclusive and nonexclusive schedules of covered diseases is the propensity of their drafters to include arbitrary time limits within the definitions. For instance, silicosis may be defined as a disease only if it results from exposure to certain forms of silica for a specified number of hours or workdays; or asbestosis may be defined as a covered disease only if it is diagnosed as such within a certain number of years after the employee's last on-the-job exposure to asbestos. These arbitrary limitations are criticized in Larson (ref. 1, vol. 1B, sect. 41.72).

hand, several recent cases have awarded workers' compensation benefits to assembly workers who developed tenosynovitis and/or carpal tunnel syndrome from the repetitive hand and arm movements required by their job, even though these diseases can also arise from nonoccupational causes (ref. 1, vol. 1B, sect. 41.00 *passim*).

INJURY "ARISING OUT OF" THE EMPLOYMENT

The "arising" requirement is a primary test for work connection of an injury. Like the course of employment test mentioned earlier, it has a strong factual and legal component. Among the legal-factual questions under the "arising" requirement are those dealing with positional or neutral risks—for instance, whether a worker who is injured by a sniper's bullet while on the job has sustained an injury arising out of the employment. One can argue that the worker was in no greater danger from the sniper than the members of the general public who were also in the area. On the other hand, however, one can argue in many cases that the general public had a choice over whether to be in that area, while the worker had no choice in the matter; the duties of his job required him to be in the "zone of danger." The latter view, which has been increasingly accepted by the courts, is the "positional risk" rule, under which risk is deemed to have arisen out of the employment if the worker's exposure to the risk was due to the fact that his employment required him to be in that place at that time. The positional risk rule is applied to a wide range of risks, not only to attacks by snipers and the like, but also to acts of God, such as tornados and lightning, as well as attacks by animals, such as bee stings, rat bites, and the like.[d]

In addition to these legal questions, the "arising" requirement also raises issues of medical causation, particularly in cases involving unexplained accidents, accidents arising from idiopathic causes, and the sequelae to on-the-job injuries.

Idiopathic and Unexplained Accidents

The controversy in both the unexplained accident and idiopathic causes cases centers around the rule that workers' compensation is not payable for an injury caused solely by the employee's own internal weakness. For instance, if a worker is disabled because high blood pressure (or low blood sugar, or any other idiopathic cause) causes him to collapse, the disability is not compensable merely because of the fortuity that the collapse happened while he was at work. However, even an idiopathically caused collapse may be compensable if the

severity of the injury was enhanced because of the work environment. Thus, compensation would probably be awarded if an employee who fainted from an idiopathic cause sustained serious injuries when he landed on a piece of machinery or fell to the ground from a scaffolding on which he was working.

In summary then, the general rule is this: an injury caused solely by idiopathic causes is not compensable but even an idiopathically caused injury is compensable if it was exacerbated by the employment. With this principle in mind, we can turn our attention to another "arising" issue; that of unexplained accidents. A fairly easy unexplained fall case would be one where a worker was found on the floor under the scaffold on which he was working, having sustained injuries consistent with a fall from the scaffold, but with no memory of how he happened to fall. This case presents a clear case for compensability since, as we have seen, the danger involved in working on the scaffold brings even an idiopathically caused fall within the "arising" rule. But the case becomes more difficult if there was no evidence that the worker was even on the scaffold and if his injuries are such that they may have been caused merely by the faint. Of course, unexplained accidents are not limited to falls; they also include unexplained deaths due to assaults and automobile accidents, as well as a variety of accidents in which the employee is unable or unavailable to explain what happened. Although the claimants in these cases are often aided by a presumption that the accident was work connected, the establishment (or refutal) of work connection can be aided greatly by medical "detective work." To the extent that the physician can clearly pinpoint (or rule out) an idiopathic cause, the legal conclusion as to whether the accident arose out of the employment is made much easier.

Consequences of Compensable Accidents

As a general rule, the natural and proximate consequences of a compensable job-related accident are also compensable, even though the seriousness of those consequences may be attributable to the employee's own preexisting weakness or disease. For example, if a worker sustains a minor cut, which would normally be expected to heal without incident, but, because of his preexisting diabetes, develops an infection that requires extensive treatment and/or surgery, the entire course of treatment and any resulting permanent impairment would normally be compensable. Likewise, depression or anxiety suffered by an employee as the result of the original accident or his inability to return to work is generally considered a compensable consequence, even if the employee had a preexisting tendency toward depression. Of course, in either case, the causal connection between the original injury and the consequences must be clearly established, usually through expert medical opinion.

---

[d]The "positional risk" rule, along with the other risk rules and their historic development, is discussed in Larson (ref. 1, vol. 1, sects. 6.00–12.20). The cases in those sections are among the most interesting in the workers' compensation field, including as they do issues such as assaults by jealous suitors and insane strangers, and buildings being attacked by all sorts of natural disasters, as well as the unexplained and idiopathic accidents discussed below.

If a worker's injury is exacerbated by medical malpractice or by a foreseeable accident flowing from the original injury—as, for instance, an automobile accident while the worker is on the way to his physician's office—the resulting exacerbation is generally compensable. (In these instances, the worker may also be able to maintain a tort action against the malpracticing physician or the driver of the car responsible for the accident. If so, the employer will be entitled to reimbursement from the worker's third-party recovery for the extra compensation he was required to pay because of the consequences caused by the third party.) Here again, however, the causal relationship between the original injury and the consequences must be established: the employer will not be held responsible if the employee sustains a new and independent injury while he is disabled—for instance, an injury in an automobile accident while on the way to his sister's house. In fact, if the new injury is to the same part of the body as the original work-connected injury, the commission, with the help of medical experts, will be faced with the nightmarish task of trying to establish when the original disability would have ceased had it not been for the intervening noncompensable injury.

There are two major exceptions to the general rule that a worker may recover for the natural consequences of an initial injury: no recovery is available for exacerbation due to the employee's own rash acts or to his unreasonable refusal of treatment. The "rash acts" exception is usually applied on a fairly straightforward and commonsense basis. For example, if an employee with an injured knee breaks his arm when the knee gives way and causes him to fall to the ground, the broken arm would probably be treated as a compensable consequence of the original knee injury if the fall occurred while he was walking sedately to his mailbox, but not if it happened while he was engaging in a foot race.

The other major exception to the compensable consequences rule is that for consequences attributable to the employee's unreasonable refusal of surgery or other treatment. Two of the contexts in which this issue frequently arises are weight reduction and surgery. The weight reduction cases usually involve employees with back or leg injuries whose physicians state that their disability would be lessened if they were to lose weight. The courts generally take a tolerant attitude toward these employees and will not deprive them of benefits if they have been making any reasonable efforts to lose weight.

The courts are also usually quite tolerant toward employees in the surgery cases, particularly in cases involving back surgery (spinal fusion or laminectomy). Apparently, for every medical witness who asserts that a spinal fusion will clear up the employee's back problems, one can find another equally reputable physician who will testify that the operation is as likely to make matters worse as it is to cure the problem. Since even the medical experts disagree as to the efficacy of the proposed surgery, the court is unlikely to find the employee is unreasonable in refusing to undergo the risks. On the other hand, if the employee has refused to undergo a relatively risk-free surgery (e.g., one that can be performed under local anesthetic), which has a great probability of success, his refusal is likely to be deemed unreasonable and the continuing consequences attributable to his refusal to undergo the surgery will not be compensable. Likewise, refusal to take prescribed medications or to cooperate with a physical therapy program will almost invariably be deemed unreasonable, since the benefits of the treatment will clearly outweigh the risks. The range of compensable consequences and the exceptions are covered in Larson (ref. 1, vol. 1, sect. 13.00 *et seq*).

BENEFITS

DISABILITY BENEFITS

As noted earlier, worker's compensation benefits are paid only during the period in which the employee is disabled from returning to work (and, in some instances, for presumed future disability). Simply put, the benefits are a fractional proportion (most commonly two-thirds) of the worker's loss in earning capacity attributable to the work-related injury. The details of how workers' compensation commissions calculate a worker's pre-and postinjury "average weekly wage" in order to determine the amount of his benefits are far too complicated for this chapter (see ref. 1, vol. 2, sect. 60.00 *et seq*). Suffice it to say that issues such as whether certain items should be included in the calculation are often fiercely litigated. In fact, in one case, the propriety of including certain contributions made to union benefit funds on a worker's behalf was contested all the way up to the Supreme Court of the United States.

The disability for which benefits are payable can be either temporary or permanent and either partial or total, leading to four "classes" of disability benefits:

1. Temporary partial
2. Temporary total
3. Permanent partial
4. Permanent total

Of these classes, temporary partial is a category that appears more often in theory than in practice—in fact, the author has never encountered a reported case in which the issue of temporary partial disability was a litigated issue.

Typically, an injured worker will go through a period of temporary total disability following an on-the-job injury. If this period is very short, he may not be entitled to disability benefits. For purposes of administrative convenience, many states impose a "waiting period" of, for example, 5 days during which no disability benefits are payable. If the worker is disabled for longer than the waiting period, benefits will be paid from the date of injury, but it is considered to be too much of a burden on the system to go through all the benefit computations when an employee misses only a few days or less of work as a result of an on-the-job injury.

Assuming that there was a period of temporary total disability, it will be determined at some point that the injured worker has attained the maximum medical improvement (MMI) that can be expected. Once MMI has been reached, a determination must be made, with the assistance of medical opinion, as to whether the worker has sustained any permanent impairment and, if so, the extent of that impairment. If it appears that the worker will be unable to return to work at any time in the foreseeable future, he will be classified as permanently and totally disabled and will be awarded benefits accordingly. In many states, this means that he will be entitled to receive his weekly benefit rate for the rest of his life or until circumstances change so that he can rejoin the workforce. However, in some states, even permanent total disability benefits are limited to a set time period of, for example, 400 weeks. Once that period has ended, the injured person will be totally without funds, unless he is able to qualify for some type of assistance such as welfare or Social Security disability. Also, in most states, the weekly benefit level determined at the outset of disability remains immutable throughout the period of disability—workers' compensation systems, unlike much other humanitarian legislation, rarely provide for cost-of-living adjustments.

If the worker is able to return to work, but has some residual physical disability attributable to the injury, he is likely to receive an award based on the state's "schedule" of injuries, combined with the medical ratings as to the degree of residual impairment. For instance, if the state's schedule provides that the loss of a leg is equal to 240 weeks of total disability, and the worker is rated as having impairment equivalent to a 15% loss of use of the leg, he would be given a permanent partial disability award equal to $.15 \times 240 \times$ his weekly benefit rate. Depending on the rules of the state, this award might be for 240 weeks of payments at 15% of his previous weekly benefit, 36 weeks of full benefits, or a lump sum payment of the whole amount.

The alert practitioner will have already noted two points in this process where medical opinion is not only necessary, but almost always indispensable—determining when the worker has reached MMI and "rating" the degree of permanent disability, which includes diagnosing whether residual impairment will cause permanent total or merely permanent partial disability. Detailed discussion of these two points is deferred to the next section, after we complete the discussion of the other types of benefits available to workers' compensation claimants.

DEATH BENEFITS

If a compensable accident causes a worker's death, his dependents will generally be entitled to death benefits. In most states, they need only establish that they fit within the statutory definition of dependents[a] and that the worker's death was causally connected to an injury that comes within the state's coverage formula. In a handful of states, however, the dependents' claim will be barred if the worker was not considerate enough to expire from his injuries within an arbitrary time period, such as 2 years after the date of the accident.

The weekly death benefit available to the dependents is usually the same as the worker would have received for permanent total disability. Benefits for dependent children usually terminate when they reach the age of majority, and benefits for dependent spouses are almost always stopped when they remarry. Benefits for other dependents (e.g., spouses who do not remarry, and dependent parents or siblings) may be limited to a set period, such as 400 weeks, or may last until their deaths.

MEDICAL BENEFITS

A worker who sustains a job-related injury is entitled to medical benefits, whether or not he is also entitled to disability benefits. Even if a worker misses no time from work because of his injury, he is entitled to have his medical treatment for the injury paid for by the employer. State statutes vary on whether it is the employee or the employer who has the right to choose the treating physician; some states compromise by providing that the employer may furnish the employee with a list of acceptable physicians and the employee must choose from among those listed. The commission will also generally provide procedures for change of physician, referrals to specialists, and the procuring of additional opinions in contested cases (ref. 1, vol. 2, sect. 61.00 *et seq*).

Medical benefits generally cover not only the cost of physicians, hospitals, and prescribed medications, but also nursing services, prostheses, and other medically necessary forms of treatment. The treatment costs awarded have, on occasion, included items such as the cost of day care for a mother with an injured back whose physician prescribed that she not lift her small child, and the cost of swimming lessons for another employee with

---

[a]Determining who are dependents can occasionally be quite complicated. It is not unheard of for a commission to be presented with the claims of two or more wives, each of whom contends she was never divorced from the deceased worker, along with children from both marriages, a handful of stepchildren, and, for good measure, one or two illegitimate children by a third woman. Or, in cases where the decedent left neither wives nor children, his parents, his grandparents, and his siblings may all present claims that they were actually dependent on his earnings. These issues are discussed in detail in Larson (ref. 1, vol. 2, sects. 62.00–63.00).

a back injury when his doctor prescribed swimming as therapy. Psychiatric treatment for injury-related depression is also included, under the compensable consequences rule.

An issue that has been addressed in several recent cases is the extent of medical benefits that can be awarded for purely palliative treatment. Many workers' compensation statutes are worded in terms of supplying medical treatment to "cure" the employee's condition. Under such statutes, questions arise, particularly in cases involving workers who are permanently and totally disabled as to whether the commission can order payment for treatment that merely relieves the claimant's pain, without effecting any change in the underlying condition. Most courts have been able to find a rationale that allows them to uphold such orders.

Rehabilitation Benefits

Nearly every state provides benefits for the costs of physical rehabilitation of injured workers; in fact, these costs may often be subsumed under the general medical benefits provisions. The majority of the states also have some sort of provision for vocational rehabilitation, although the availability of those rehabilitative services may be limited to those who would otherwise be considered permanently and totally disabled. The benefits available under these provisions are generally limited to furnishing the worker with "vocational training" (i.e., training in a trade or skilled labor field). College costs are almost invariably excluded, although some claimants have attempted to secure college training. In one recent case, a young man who had been injured on his summer job as a laborer sought to have that employer pay for the remainder of his college program as vocational retraining. Although the state supreme court correctly rejected his claim—since, after all, he was not really a laborer who needed retraining—it is the author's opinion that college training should not be foreclosed in all instances.

Vocational retraining benefits are often offered on a "carrot and stick" basis. The "carrot" in this instance is in the form of full payment for the costs of the training, in addition to the worker's normal disability benefit, and sometimes also an additional payment during the period of study. The stick takes the form of diminished weekly benefits for those who refuse to undergo training or make only minimal efforts to comply with their training programs.

Vocational rehabilitation benefits need not always be in the form of retraining. Benefits can also be directed toward reequipping the employee to perform his former job, as for instance by providing a specially designed work station to accommodate the employee's loss of physical function. Continued supervision and the ability to deal with changing conditions by the commission is indicated in these types of cases, however. If an employee who would otherwise be totally disabled is able to perform his old job with the help of special tools and the like, his disability benefits may be discontinued on the ground that he no longer has any loss in earning capacity. But if he loses that job as a result of economic conditions or other forces outside his control, he will again need the help of the workers' compensation system, either to again pay disability benefits or to help him find another job that is within his limitations.

DISABILITY, PAIN, AND THE CHRONIC PAIN SPECIALIST

Before discussing more specifically the role of the physician, and particularly that of the chronic pain specialist, in evaluating disability, we need a more exact definition of "disability" than we have used in preceding sections. Although we have spoken of disability as the employee's inability to return to the duties of his job, that definition is too narrow, because it would mean that an employee could be considered permanently and totally disabled merely because he could not perform his previous job, as for instance a typist who was perfectly healthy except for the loss of a finger. On the other hand, if we merely define disability as an inability to work, the definition becomes too broad; it is irrational to say that a skilled craftsman is not disabled because he is still able to do some kind of work, albeit as a dishwasher. Thus, disability in the workers' compensation sense can be defined as "inability, as the result of a work-connected injury, to perform or obtain work suitable to the claimant's qualifications and training" (ref. 1, vol. 1, sect. 57.00).

However, even that definition is somewhat ambiguous because it leaves open the question of what is the "inability to perform work": must the worker be physically unable to make the necessary muscle movements or can he be said to be unable to do the work if he can make those movements only in great pain? The answer, in most cases, lies somewhere between those two extremes: pain will generally be considered as a factor in assessing the extent of the worker's disability, but pain alone will rarely be considered disabling. As to where the line will be drawn in any given case, much will depend on the medical witnesses and on how well they can evaluate the worker's pain and its effect on his ability to perform his job and then "educate" the hearing officer, so that their evaluation will be properly understood.

In this respect, I would like to suggest that a primary duty of a pain specialist called upon to give an evaluation in a workers' compensation case is not only to evaluate the pain in relative terms but also to gain a clear understanding of the worker's job so that he can evaluate the pain in terms of the job duties. This suggestion is grounded in the author's own experience: A few years ago her husband sustained an accidental (although not work-related) cervical strain. The orthopedist who was treating him kept attempting to release him to return to work prematurely, in the belief that his continuing pain would not prevent him from working as an electrician. Those releases were apparently based on the physician's understanding of an electrician's job duties as installing lighting fixtures and switches and other light objects. He could not be made to understand that the patient was an industrial electrician, specializing in the installation of heavy pipes and metal trays that often weighed several hundred pounds and had to be carried a half-mile or more on the electrician's shoulders.

Similar misunderstandings could occur in almost any field of endeavor: leg pain that might not prevent a research physician or a trusts and estates attorney from working could render a busy clinician or a litigation attorney unable to perform normal duties. Thus, a full understanding of the worker's job duties would always seem to be indicated. Similarly, if it is contended that the employee is able to enter an alternative workfield, the duties of that field should be carefully considered in light of the worker's pain.

The pain specialist called upon to report or testify in a workers' compensation case should also remember that there is often a suspicion on the part of the employer that the injured worker is shirking and exaggerating his symptoms, particularly if there is no observable evidence of injury (i.e., "we can't see a thing on the x-ray"). In those cases, the specialist should be prepared to explain, and demonstrate if necessary, to the employer and the hearing officer how he can measure the pain. The more that the worker's pain can be objectified, the more likely it is to be believed. Of course, if the specialist has been called upon by the employer, an equally strong and objective showing should be made to demonstrate why the specialist believes that the worker's pain is nonexistent or less acute than the worker claims.

AMERICANS WITH DISABILITIES ACT

The Americans with Disabilities Act of 1990 (ADA) is the first comprehensive federal law designed to prohibit employment discrimination against the estimated 43 million Americans with physical or mental disabilities. Employment provisions of the act, which was signed into law on July 26, 1990, took effect in July of 1992 for employers with 25 or more workers and will take effect in July of 1994 for employers with 15 or more workers.

The ADA, which covers a broad area, mandates major changes in the way some companies and physicians assess the health status of applicants and employees. It also requires employers to make "reasonable accommodations" for disabled individuals who are otherwise qualified to perform the job, and it regulates medical records.

Although provisions of the ADA are already in effect, the full impact of this legislation will remain unknown until cases are settled in the court. The results of currently pending litigation should help more fully specify what procedures employers must follow in regard to interviewing, hiring, and employing handicapped workers.

Acknowledgments The author acknowledges with gratitude the support and encouragement of her husband, Jim, her daughter, Dawn, and her law partner, MaryEllen McDonald. A special thanks is due to the author's mother, Doris A. Lozon, who not only offered encouragement but also helped with the typing of the manuscript. Finally, the author cannot adequately express the gratitude that she personally owes to Dr. Arthur Larson, not only for encouraging her to write this chapter, but in teaching her, during the years she worked for and with him, this fascinating field of law.

Editors Acknowledgment The editor also wishes to acknowledge Alan R. Cochran, J.D., for reviewing this chapter and updating it from the previous edition.

REFERENCE

1. Larson A: *The Law of Workmen's Compensation.* New York, Mathew Bender & Co, 1952–1992.

CHAPTER 55

EVALUATION AND RATING OF PHYSICAL DISABILITY

SANFORD H. VERNICK
JULIE SAWYER
EDGAR MARIN
KAREN RUCKER

ONE ASPECT of medical practice that most physicians find troublesome is evaluation and rating of physical disability. Not only is it a time-consuming task, but it also carries heavy responsibilities. A physician's findings in a disability evaluation may determine whether someone will live in relative financial comfort or in near poverty.

Physicians in certain specialties, such as orthopedics, physiatry, neurology, and neurosurgery, are frequently asked to perform disability evaluations. Formal instruction in this subject, both during and after residency, has been minimal, however. In addition, much disagreement exists among physicians as to the specific evaluation and rating schedule to use when determining physical disability, and there are no clear guidelines or standardized measures that are uniformly accepted. In this country, most disability determinations are litigated, and because of the adversarial nature of these determinations some physicians try to evade the process altogether.

Musculoskeletal injury is the most common cause of work-related disability. This may stem from changes occurring in the American work force. The principal shift is away from a manufacturing-based to a service-based economy. In consequence, the hazards of exposure in heavy industry to black lung, pneumoconiosis, or silicosis are decreasing, whereas the hazards associated with office work involving repetitive motions are increasing.

In physical disability evaluation, standard terminology is needed. Otherwise, it is difficult to communicate findings and compare evaluations. Many organizations have provided definitions, and although not universally approved, the World Health Organization's (WHO) International Classification of Impairments, Disabilities, and Handicaps is frequently cited (1).

Impairment, according to the WHO, occurs at the organ level and represents "any loss or abnormality of psychological, physiological, or anatomical structure or function" (1).

Disability occurs at the person level and is "any restriction or lack (resulting from an impairment) of ability to perform an activity in the manner or within the range considered normal for a human being" (1).

Handicap occurs at the societal level and has been defined as "a disadvantage for a given individual resulting from an impairment or a disability that limits or prevents the fulfillment of a role that is normal (depending on age, sex, and social and cultural factors) for that individual" (1).

At the present time, most impairment and disability determination decisions are based on one of the three sources discussed in the next section.

IMPAIRMENT AND DISABILITY DETERMINATIONS

AMERICAN MEDICAL ASSOCIATION

The American Medical Association's *Guides to the Evaluation of Permanent Impairment* ("Guides") is one source (2). This is basically an impairment schedule, and deals with anatomic and physiologic losses rather than functional factors such as the ability to lift, bend, stand, and sit. Further, the Guides do not relate medical impairment to occupation or social responsibilities.

According to the Guides, *impairment* is an alteration of an individual's health status that is assessed by medical means, and *disability*, which is assessed by nonmedical means, is an alteration of an individual's capacity to meet personal, social, or occupational demands or statutory or regulatory requirements. An individual who is impaired is not necessarily disabled. Impairment gives rise to disability only when the medical condition limits the individual's capacity to meet the demands of life's activities. In general, a physician's evaluation of the patient should be understood to be a medical evaluation of health status. The physician does not determine industrial loss of use, economic loss, or any other type of loss giving rise to disability payments.

The "Guides" continues to espouse the principles that all impairments affect the individual as a whole and that all impairments should be expressed as impairments of the "whole person." This is done with the aid of a *Combined Values Chart*. Further, impairment should not be considered "permanent" until the clinical findings as determined over a period, usually 12 months, indicate that the medical condition is static and well-stabilized.

Chapter 3 of the Guides—The Extremities, Spine, and Pelvis—has been altered considerably from previous editions. The evaluation of the spine calls for using inclinometers rather than goniometers, thus making possible more accurate and reproducible results. Evaluation of the upper extremity has been revised in accordance with the methods adopted by the International Federation of Societies of the Hand and modified by the American Society for Surgery of the Hand.

Despite these revisions and modifications, the Guides has been criticized because it did not take into consideration chronic pain in the context of disability evaluation. In the foreword to the latest edition, it does address this issue. It says that "in recent years, the Institute of Medicine in Washington, DC and the Social Security Administration have conducted major reviews of chronic pain and its implications for impairment and disability. Both studies concluded that chronic pain should be considered in a more thorough and systematic fashion but that it was undesirable to add that subject as an impairment under the Social Security System" (2). This edition brings an appendix that summarizes the biopsychosocial issues that make it difficult to address "pain" in an impairment evaluation system.

Another criticism is that the Guides does not have a system to evaluate "function." In the section covering the hand and upper extremity, it says that the methods for evaluating impairments of the upper extremity may be considered anatomic, cosmetic, or functional. The physical evaluation is based on a detailed examination of the patient and the upper extremity and is necessary to determine the anatomic aspects of the impairment. The cosmetic evaluation concerns the patient's and society's reaction to the impairment or the results of surgical treatment. The functional evaluation is a measure of the individual's ability to perform activities of daily living or work. At present, the latter method has not been developed to the necessary level of exactness and reproducibility. Evaluation of anatomic impairment is considered to be the most dependable and reliable system and is the recommended method at this time (2).

Cumulative Trauma Disorder

If an impairment rating is being given for cumulative trauma disorders, it is suggested by the Guides that the evaluation take place after the individual has worked for 6–8 hours. This is an important statement, especially when electrodiagnosis is being performed for evaluation of carpal tunnel syndrome (CTS). CTS is the most common disorder among workers exposed to cumulative trauma. It is not uncommon that electrodiagnostic evaluation is negative in workers that have the symptoms of CTS when it is performed after several hours or days of rest.

SOCIAL SECURITY ADMINISTRATION

The Social Security and Supplemental Security Insurance program publishes a "Handbook" for physicians entitled *Disability Evaluation Under Social Security* (3). It states that "physicians provide medical evidence upon which impairment can be evaluated. The impact of the impairment on an individual's ability to work and the decision as to whether the impairment constitutes a disability is an administrative, not a medical decision. The physician is neither asked nor expected to make a decision as to whether his or her patient is disabled" (3).

It defines disability as "inability to engage in any substantial gainful activity by reason of a medically determinable physical or mental impairment which can be expected to last for a continuous period of not less than 12 months" (3).

To qualify for disability payments, an individual must have a medically determinable impairment. This means an impairment that is demonstrable anatomically, physiologically, or psychologically. Such abnormalities are medically determinable if they manifest themselves as signs or laboratory findings apart from symptoms. Abnormalities that manifest themselves only as symptoms are not medically determinable.

Pain may be an important factor in causing functional loss, but it must be associated with relevant abnormal signs or laboratory findings. Evaluations of musculoskeletal impairments should be supported where applicable by detailed description of the joints, including range of motion, condition of the musculature, sensory or reflex changes, circulatory deficits, and radiographic abnormalities.

This system is much more oriented to disease than to residuals of trauma. It is based principally on diagnosis supported by specific criteria of the history and physical examination and laboratory evaluation.

Many authors in the field of disability determination have emphasized the desirability of a system based on function. The Social Security Administration, as part of the disability determination process, usually asks the applicant's physician to fill out a form, which has a section on functional limitations. It requests an estimate of the length of time a patient can sit, stand, walk, as well as lifting capacities and postural considerations. This is the closest any system has come to a functional orientation.

Unfortunately, most physicians do not have the appropriate office equipment and setting to perform an evaluation of such kind. Furthermore, there is no financial incentive to perform these evaluations. The reimbursement for the physician's professional time to fill out the form is $10.00.

In practice, formal evaluation is not performed and the answers are extremely subjective. The "complainer" is rewarded and the "stoic" is punished.

AMERICAN ACADEMY OF ORTHOPAEDIC SURGEONS

The American Academy of Orthopaedic Surgeons has developed a *Manual for Orthopaedic Surgeons in Evaluating Permanent Physical Impairment* (4). In order to arrive at various levels of physical impairment, it takes into consideration anatomic lesions, physical signs, and subjective symptoms.

There is an urgent need to develop a methodology that accurately and adequately assesses what the patient can do and what work restrictions are recommended. Modern technology is developing instruments and equipment that promise to improve our capacity to evaluate physical performance independently of motivation.

With the advent of new technology, the most logical route to follow for medical impairment/disability determination is "functional capacity evaluation." This new field is developing very rapidly.

The evaluation of the disability and handicap is often time-consuming and considered unrewarding by many physicians. The problem is often hidden, and an inordinate amount of time must be spent to uncover it. An example is chronic neck pain.

Patients with this complaint often relate the onset to a motor vehicle accident in which they suffered flexion-extension injury ("whiplash" is the usual term for this problem); in many cases, however, the patient can relate no specific incidents to the onset of the pain. He or she will often say that it begins in the morning and gets worse as the day progresses. As with any chronic pain, the history is very important, beginning with the chief complaint, which is pain or loss of motion. One must be aware of and search for any intrinsic or extrinsic causes. Intrinsic causes involve the structure of the neck itself— vertebral bodies, disks, nerve roots, ligaments, blood vessels, and muscles. Extrinsic causes are only indirectly related to the cervical spine (e.g., tumors, infections, psychological impairments).

One must determine the type of pain. Is it sharp, burning, lancinating or paresthetic? Does it radiate, is there any dizziness, vertigo, or tinnitus? Does moving the head or arms make it worse? The answers to these questions will suggest an etiology. For example, pain that is constant and worse when lying often suggests a primary or metastatic tumor. Pain that is intermittent and increases with activity is probably a musculoskeletal problem. The patient's response to the pain is important. What actions are taken to relieve it? How does he or she sleep? Is the patient always tired? Are there any behavioral inconsistencies such as difficulty performing certain tasks at work, but no difficulties with other seemingly unrelated tasks such as shaving or showering and which involve complicated maneuvering of the cervical spine for someone with truly significant pain?

The past medical history, which often must be drawn out, may point to problems such as diabetes or cancer. Next the family history and social history should be evaluated. Is the patient married, divorced, or separated? Does he or she smoke or drink to excess? Are work or social relationships physically or psychologically stressful? The occupational history is essential. Is the patient satisfied from the point of view of employer support? Has return to work after injury been successful?

The physical exam follows and should consist of evaluation of range of motion of the cervical spine and upper extremities, asking the patient to actively flex, extend, and rotate the neck and move the upper extremities in their maximal range of flexion, extension, abduction, and adduction, as well as external and internal rotation. Watch for pain reaction, and document the end point of motion with a goniometer or inclinometer, and listen for crepitus. Next do manual muscle testing of the cervical spine and upper extremity myotomes and grade each muscle on the 1–5 scale or the trace-to-good scale. Next test sensation to pin prick and light touch. Nerve root pressure may cause loss of both. Reflex testing of C5, C6, and C7 is next. Diminution may suggest nerve root pressure at that level; hyperactivity may suggest a problem at a higher level.

This concludes the physical examination, and after evaluating any pertinent radiographic, magnetic resonance imaging (MRI), or laboratory results, evaluation and rating of any disability are required. Any inconsistencies between subjective and objective findings should suggest either conscious or unconscious malingering, and a psychological evaluation with MMPI should be sought.

REPORT AND RATING

The rating of the disability is just as difficult as the evaluation, and there are no clear guidelines or standards. Most insurance companies, lawyers, other third-party payers, however, require the use of the Guides. Users of the Guides know that it is a herculean task to decipher the strategies and calculations used to arrive at a rating. Even the title is not apropos, because it is disability and not impairment that demands rating.

The Guides first appeared in the *Journal of the American*

Medical Association in 1958. Between 1958 and 1970, 13 separate articles appeared on rating physical impairment. The Guides were first mentioned in workers' compensation literature in 1961. In 1971, an AMA committee produced the first *Guides to the Evaluation of Permanent Impairment*. It has since gone through three editions. In 1972, the National Commission of State Workman's Compensation Laws mandated the use of the Guides in workers' compensation cases.

It must be noted that the Guides do not relate impairment or disability to occupation or social responsibility. For example, the violinist with loss of a digit would receive the same medical impairment rating as a teacher with loss of the same digit. Further, in the Guides, pain/discomfort and loss of sensation is graded 0–100%, with 0% being no loss of sensation and no spontaneous or abnormal sensation and 100% being decreased sensation with pain that may prevent all activity. Although this grading system is an attempt to quantify pain, it is very subjective and dependent on the evaluator and the patient's compliance and understanding. We are all familiar with the patient that presents with severe and incapacitating pain without clinical evidence of sensory loss. Because all grade determinations require a loss of sensation, this patient would be difficult to grade. Secondly, pain and discomfort are used synonymously; therefore the distinction between mild pain and severe pain must be determined by the evaluator's subjective impression. The grading system for motor power in the Guides is similar to the grading system used in clinical practice. Spinal nerve root impairment is calculated from the sensory and motor grading systems of impairment relative to percentage of impairment of the involved extremity. The impairment of the upper extremity, for instance, is then factored into the percentage of impairment of the whole body. According to the *Guides*, each spinal root is rated a quarter of the maximal percentage of loss of function due to sensory deficits, pain, or discomfort; a maximal percentage loss of function due to loss of strength; and a maximal percentage of impairment of the upper extremity. For example, according to the Guides, for unilateral C5 spinal root impairment, maximal percentage loss of function due to sensory deficit, pain, or discomfort equals 5%, maximal percentage loss of function due to loss of strength is 30%, and maximal percentage impairment of the upper extremity is 0–34%. An example taken directly from the Guides is that of a 42-year-old right-handed man who fell 30 feet and landed on his upper back. He complained of neck pain radiating down his right arm. Examination revealed 20% sensory loss of the C5 area and 50% loss of strength of muscles innervated by C5. According to the Guides, impairment is calculated as follows:

1. 20% of 5% = 1% loss of function due to sensory deficits, pain, or discomfort.
2. 50% of 30% = 15% loss of function due to loss of strength.
3. 1% combined with 15% = 16% impairment of the right upper extremity
4. 16% impairment of the upper extremity = 10% impairment of the whole person

As one can imagine, this process can become quite complicated. In addition, how does one rate a patient with incapacitating pain, impaired cervical mobility due to the same, and no other discernable pathology? Our understanding of the pathology of pain is limited at this time, which is to say that all pain related to the neck, for instance, is not referable to a particular root pathology but may stem from ligamentous, musculoskeletal, or arthritic involvement and the like, all of which may be difficult to document with objectivity. In addition to these concerns, several other factors limit the usefulness of the Guides. First, the evaluation remains subject to observer error. Second, the quantification of pain still remains an enigma. Third, the Guides are not universally used or accepted and thus have limited applicability to the already controversial subject of disability evaluation.

To rectify these deficiencies and provide a more equitable rating system, we propose a restructuring of the methodology whereby disability is evaluated and rated using the functional capacity evaluation.

Disability is defined by the WHO as "any restriction or lack (resulting from an impairment) of ability to perform an activity in the manner or within the range considered normal for a human being" (1). In other words, disability is that function which the patient is "disabled" or unable to do in terms of his needs or desires.

Unfortunately, the definition of disability may vary depending on the administrative agency or organization making the determination. The Social Security Administration's test of disability, for example, is "that a person should be unable to engage in any substantial gainful activity by reason of any medically determinable, physical, or mental impairment which can be expected to result in death, which has lasted or can be expected to last for a continuous period of not less than 12 months" (3). The phrase "engaged in any substantial gainful activity" is the important one here. It seems to us that only a coma or persistent vegetative state would totally prevent someone from engaging in any substantial gainful activity. What really should be questioned and determined is what type of gainful employment the person can engage in. For example, a pianist who loses his little finger probably would be disabled from engaging in his occupation as a concert pianist. He could conceivably engage in the somewhat less demanding position of piano teacher, however. What we are really talking about, therefore, is a functional limitation that should be evaluated by means of the functional capacity evaluation.

A restriction or the lack of ability to perform an activity or function within the range considered normal for that person is described as functional limitation. Examples of functional limitation include the inability to lift over 20 pounds in an individual with lumbosacral disk disease, the inability to retain and follow a multistep direction in an individual with head trauma, inability to do stressful activities such as climbing stairs in a person with severe ischemic heart disease, or inability to function safely in the community in an individual with cognitive and affective changes due to closed head injury. Thus, functional limitations are manifestations of impairment that are evidenced in daily as well as occupational activities.

Functional capacity assessment can be defined as a measurement of function in which a series of tests and activities is used to address capabilities and limitations following an injury. These assessments have traditionally been used to document physical limitations in order to determine workers' compensation and to provide reimbursement during the rehabilitation process (5). Physicians initially used the concept of anatomic loss to determine the amount of disability (6). For example, if a person lost an eye he or she would receive 50% compensation; the worker losing both eyes would be compensated 100% (6). This method did not address how these injuries impacted daily living and vocational abilities, however. As mentioned earlier in the chapter, the Guides are currently used to rate physical impairment. The Guides, however, tend to place more importance on physical and laboratory findings instead of the clients' history, functional assessment, and pain behaviors (7). Another problem with the current rating system is the amount of variation that occurs between physicians. A study in California revealed that the disability ratings of "different independent medical examiners ranged from 0–70%" (7). In this chapter, another approach will be discussed to decrease the variability in disability ratings and enable the injured worker to return to competitive employment. The functional capacity assessment is primarily used as a liaison between health care professionals and the workplace (8). Further, it provides the rehabilitation team with vocational criteria in order to determine current capabilities and limitations (8). These evaluations are traditionally performed by an occupational therapist, physical therapist, or vocational evaluator. Depending on the facility, these assessments may be referred to as a functional capacity evaluation (FCE), physical capacities evaluation (PCE), work tolerance screen (WTS), work capacities evaluation (WCE), or work assessment (WA). These evaluations are administered in 1- and 2-day segments or as a week-long process. One-day assessments are often preferred by the referral source because of the cost factor and timeliness (6). These assessments are also easier to schedule and administer and decrease time of referral to testing. A 2-day assessment allows the therapist to document and make observations in relation to the activities and tasks performed on the first day. Finally, some therapists may occasionally administer a week-long evaluation. These are usually referred to as "tolerance tests" and are primarily performed with individuals who "have self-limiting behaviors" (6). Once these evaluations are completed, they help to answer a number of questions posed by the physician and the rest of the rehabilitation team. Some of these are defining the clients' physical ability to perform work activities, determining the need for further rehabilitation (work hardening), establishing guidelines to return to a modified job, matching the clients' current abilities to seek a different job, and compensating clients (9). Functional capacity evaluations will vary depending on the tests and assessments used and the physical area that is assessed. The U.S. Department of Labor suggests that there are 20 key areas to address during the evaluation:

1. Lifting
2. Standing
3. Walking
4. Sitting
5. Carrying
6. Pushing
7. Pulling
8. Climbing
9. Balancing
10. Stooping
11. Kneeling
12. Crouching
13. Crawling
14. Reaching
15. Fingering
16. Handling
17. Feeling
18. Talking
19. Hearing
20. Seeing

These demands assist the evaluator in determining what areas the client can physically perform in order to establish guidelines for return to work. These areas can be evaluated by using a variety of standardized tests, work samples, and clinical observations. Specific examples of these assessments will be discussed later in the chapter.

The first step in the evaluation process is the intake interview. The therapist should allow ample time to collect pertinent information as it relates to the client and the injury (i.e., medical history, current medications, previous surgery, specific therapies, date of injury, diagnosis, assistive devices, level of education, work experience, job description, and the client's goal statement). These are all important factors to consider prior to beginning the assessment and will provide insight into the client's overall adjustment to his or her injury.

For example, Mr. Sampson comes into the clinic with a diagnosis of chronic low back pain; he has been on medical leave for 2 years. The evaluator asks, "Mr. Sampson, what is your goal at this time?" He replies, "I can't really think of one right now, maybe to retire and go on disability." This type of interaction is indicative of a client who is probably not motivated to give maximal voluntary effort and who will be difficult to return to any type of competitive employment. It may also indicate the need for psychological support to provide counseling on ways to adjust to his or her injury. Some evaluators may also choose to administer a pain questionnaire to obtain information about the patient's pain tolerance and its impact on daily living activities. K.L. Blankenship has devised a standardized pain questionnaire to obtain information regarding the type of pain the client is experiencing, a numeric rating of pain and limitations of daily functioning due to pain (10). This information can be compared with physical performance areas in order to determine any inconsistencies between the two variables. These become critical factors in determining whether the individual can return to his or her previous job and also how much pain is related to the injury or to other psychological components. Once the interview is completed, the physical evaluation process begins.

A general functional capacities assessment includes tests of manual dexterity (fine and gross), endurance, lifting, posture/body mechanics, and pushing/pulling. A variety of standardized tests may be used to evaluate performance issues in relation to competitive employment. Many of these are used to obtain information on fine/gross motor manipulation, grip/pinch strength, maximal voluntary effort, and tolerance for working in different positions. Some of the commonly used instruments are the JAMAR hand dynamometer, pinch gauge, Baltimore Therapeutic Equipment Work Simulator (BTE), Purdue Pegboard Test, Minnesota Rate of Manipulation Test, and Valpar Whole Body Range of Motion Test. (This is just a small sample of available tests and should not be used exclusively to determine ability to return to work.) The examiner may supplement other work samples and standardized assessments depending on their theoretical background and test emphasis. The BTE work simulator consists of an "electronically controlled shaft" that can be adjusted to five different horizontal and vertical positions depending on the needed simulation. By attaching one of the many tools, the evaluator can adjust the resistance on a control panel to simulate a job task. The BTE can also be used to assess maximal voluntary effort. The test is administered in a standardized manner in which three repetitive trials are used (11). The evaluator is able to generate a computer printout that provides statistical information in reference to performance. This is based on the assumption that repeated trials within a short period will remain stable (11). It is also one way that the evaluator can obtain a numeric value in order to determine consistent performance. These results can then be compared with pain questionnaires and clinical observations to provide information on inconsistencies between performance and verbal responses. The hand dynamometer and pinch gauge also provide general strength information as compared to age norms. The JAMAR can also measure maximal voluntary effort using a rapidly alternating grip technique. The client is asked to perform repeated hand grips to measure consistent performance. The use of standardized manipulation tests serves a variety of purposes in evaluating overall abilities. Several of these were mentioned before, including the Purdue Pegboard Test, Minnesota Rate of Manipulation Test, and Valpar Whole Body Range of Motion Test. The Valpar Whole Body Range of Motion Test requires the client to transfer shapes on an upright board to different panels. Each transfer is timed separately and can be compared to competitive norms. Also the evaluator can observe the client's ability to work in a variety of positions including kneeling, crouching, stooping, and overhead. This is a challenging assessment, and it assists the evaluator in obtaining information regarding the client's endurance and perseverance to complete the task. The Minnesota Rate of Manipulation Test evaluates manual speed and dexterity (11). It consists of five subtests that require eye-hand coordination with unilateral and bilateral hand use. Clinical information can be obtained to include the client's tolerance for standing, repetitive reaching and fingering, and repetitive forearm supination and pronation. This assessment also has established norms based on individuals in the workplace. Finally, the Purdue Pegboard test assesses fine finger dexterity. It requires the client to place small pegs, washers, and cylinders into a hole within a restricted time span. It involves unilateral and bilateral hand use and assesses fine finger dexterity, sitting tolerance, and reaching. These tests are essential in that they allow the therapist to document observations related to the client's tolerance to work in different positions, impact of repetitive work on the injury, body alignment/mechanics, and pain behaviors. The client's pain behaviors will vary depending on the task and could include verbal complaints, body posturing, gesturing, and sighs (12).

There are three different lifts that are primarily assessed: floor to waist level, waist to shoulder, and shoulder to overhead. The evaluator determines the maximal amount of weight the client is able to lift using good body mechanics and alignment. This is a subjective measurement and requires close observation of the body mechanics used and resulting pain behaviors. Once these limits are established, the resulting work categories can be established. The U.S. Department of Labor (13) has defined the following work categories:

S—*sedentary work*: lifting up to 10 pounds on an occasional basis and negligible weight on a frequent basis.

L—*light work*: lifting up to 20 pounds on an occasional basis and up to 10 pounds on a frequent basis.

M—*medium work*: lifting up to 50 pounds on an occasional basis and up to 25 pounds on a frequent basis.

H—*heavy work*: lifting up to 100 pounds on an occasional basis and up to 50 pounds frequently.

VH—*very heavy*: lifting in excess of 100 pounds and/or frequent lifting of 50 pounds.

These guidelines allow the evaluator to communicate with the physician and employer as to specific lifting restrictions. For clarification purposes, occasional means performing these lifts 0–33% of the day. Frequent means performing 34–66% of the time. Constant means 67–100%, although these lifts are strongly discouraged because of an increase in cumulative trauma in industry.

Finally, the evaluator may choose to perform some type of endurance test in order to assess the client's ability to engage in simulated work tasks. Blankenship recommends that the client be engaged in simulated work activities over a period (10). The length of the endurance test will depend on the type of information needed, client's tolerance, and test emphasis. A 2-min work circuit is set up according to the type of activity to be tested. The evaluator sets up a circuit to closely simulate the worker's job tasks, and during the endurance section, blood pressure and pulse are frequently monitored to determine aerobic capacity. Although the client is encouraged to work continuously, he or she is not required to exceed the calculated maximal pulse (based on age and sex). The evaluator is able to observe and document work tolerance, body mechanics/alignment, and pain behaviors as they relate to specific job tasks. Again, this type of test is not always administered and will depend on each facility and the theoretical model used.

This chapter has focused a great deal on the history of determining disability and the lack of consistency of the current system. The challenge is now to use a different system based on the functional capacity test to determine disability and return the client to gainful employment. The functional capacity report can provide valuable information to the physician and employer regarding current capabilities and limitations; it is therefore proposed that physicians use a functional approach in determining disability instead of the AMA Guides. In order to effectively do this, the physician would need to acquire specific information from the FCE including lifting tolerances, overall endurance, standing and sitting limits, and ability to work in a variety of positions. The evaluator needs to provide a discussion on job tasks required and its impact on the injured worker. In order to obtain specific job information, descriptions can be obtained from the employer. If this information is not available, a job site visit/analysis should be done. The job analysis is important in that it provides areas of reasonable accommodation including work restrictions, job restructuring, job/site modifications, support services, and barrier removal (11). As mentioned previously, the analysis would assess areas of lifting, standing, walking, sitting, carrying, pushing, pulling, dexterity, etc. The evaluator would then combine the information from the functional capacity evaluation, job site/job description, and occupational resources in order to provide accurate information on the client's abilities and limitations. Frequently used resources include the *Dictionary of Occupational Titles, Classification of Jobs,* and *Guide to Job Analysis.* These provide valuable information related to physical demands, working conditions, skill level, aptitudes, materials handled, etc. (14). Once all the information is obtained, the evaluator compares the client's current abilities to the present job demands. For example, a school teacher incurs a work-related injury that results in an amputation of the fifth finger (dominant hand). Based on a job analysis, he or she wouldn't be significantly disabled from returning to her job as a school teacher. If this same injury occurred to a piano teacher, however, he or she would be considered permanently disabled. In the case of a low back injury, it would create greater clarification of job-specific tasks. An individual who is limited to lifting in the light work category may be 50% disabled if he is unable to perform half of the job tasks requiring lifting in excess of 20 pounds. In other words, the therapist would indicate which job tasks the client could presently perform and which jobs would need to be modified or deleted from the job description.

The assessment can provide additional recommendations in reference to return to work including job restructuring/modification, work hardening, and work evaluation/rehabilitation. The evaluator may then recommend a trial of work hardening to improve the clients' overall strength and endurance. If the worker "is able to perform 50% of the job tasks, then work hardening should be able to assist them in returning to work" (11). Typically, work hardening is a program lasting 4–6 weeks that uses simulated job tasks to assist in returning the injured worker back to the work force. The client engages in work-like activities for 5–8 hours a day (5 days a week). During this process, it is critical to maintain contact with the physician, rehabilitation specialist, and other team members to facilitate a smooth transition from work hardening to employment. Job restructuring or modification is another option that may be considered. Basically, job restructuring would not change the responsibilities of the job, but how the task is performed. Job modification would require changing or removing certain job duties and in most cases would require some cost to the employer (11). Occasionally, it will be determined that the worker is unable to return to his previous job, and a work evaluation may be indicated. A work evaluation will assess the client's abilities, aptitudes, interests, and specific job skills. It can also provide information regarding transferable skills into similar types of employment and ability for retraining.

Because of increased technology and awareness of disabilities, society is beginning to understand the importance of returning injured workers back to the work force.

The Americans with Disabilities Act (ADA) (15) was instituted to assist employers in handling disabled individuals, creating an even greater need for a more rational method of disability determination than now exists. This act "gives civil rights protection to individuals with disabilities that are like those provided to individuals on the basis of race, sex, national origin, and religion" (15). Further, it guarantees "equal opportunity for individuals with disabilities in employment, public accommodations, transportation, state and local government services, and telecommunications" (15).

The ADA addresses five major areas of access, including employment, public accommodations, transportation, state and local government operations, and telecommunications relay services. For the purposes of this chapter, the area of employment will primarily be addressed. The law states that employers who have 15 or more workers "may not discriminate against qualified individuals with disabilities" (15). Further, they must provide "reasonable accommodation" to qualified applicants unless it would cause "undue hardship" (15). Reasonable accommodation involves eliminating unnecessary barriers that may restrict employment and modifying or adjusting job tasks or the work environment. Matheson provides three types of reasonable accommodation, which are: "equal opportunity in the application process, enable the worker to perform essential functions of a job, and equal benefits and privileges of employment" (11). There continue to be numerous questions and speculations on the implication of the ADA, but it is felt that it will greatly influence injured workers in returning to work.

PRESENTING FINDINGS

The fundamentals of assessment have been discussed. A demonstration of how these findings would be presented to the referral source (e.g., physician, rehabilitation specialist, attorney) is now in order. Two types of information are important with regard to the client: (1) the clients' current (physical) functioning level and (2) how much the current injury impacts their return to work. The following case study is presented for clarification.

Case of Mr. Thomas

This 30-year-old man was involved in a truck accident that resulted in multiple contusions and abrasions. He was seen by Dr. X and given numerous diagnoses including cervical strain with chronic spasm, intramuscular hemorrhage, mild muscle strain of the right lower extremity, and abrasions throughout. At the time of the accident, he was driving a log truck and also worked as a bartender on a part-time basis. Dr. X referred him for

a functional capacity assessment and work hardening if indicated. His evaluation results were as follows:

Lifting:

> Floor to waist—unable to assess because of poor body mechanics
> Waist to shoulder—31.0 pounds
> Shoulder to overhead—21.0 pounds

Pushing/Pulling:

> 25.0 pounds

Grip Strength:

> Right   92.0 pounds (below average)
> Left   92.0 pounds (average)

Tip Pinch:

> Right   13.0 pounds (below average)
> Left   13.0 pounds (below average)

Key Pinch:

> Right   21.0 pounds (below average)
> Left   25.0 pounds (average)

Palmar Pinch:

> Right   21.0 pounds (below average)
> Left   21.0 pounds (below average)

Standing Tolerance:

> 15–30 min

Sitting Tolerance:

> 60 min

Climbing (stairs, ramp, grassy hill):

Client used a slow, reciprocating pattern when negotiating the stairs. He complained of increased leg and low back pain during these tasks.

Stooping:

Client was able to perform these activities with minimal difficulty. He noted increased tightness in the upper extremity and cervical region.

Kneeling and Crouching:

Client had great difficulty with these activities because of increased pain in his lower back and knees.

Reaching and Handling:

The Minnesota Rate of Manipulation test was given in order to determine the client's speed in working with his arms. When compared to older unemployed adults, the client scored below the 10th percentile for right placing and left placing. Below the 10th percentile is considered low performance. He scored in the average range for the placing and turning section.

Fingering:

The Purdue Pegboard test was given to assess fine finger manipulation. The client scored in the below-average range for right placing, left placing, bilateral hand use, and the assembly section.

Endurance Test:

A 30-min endurance test was given in order to assess the client's ability for continuous activity. A 2-min work circuit was set up according to the type of activity that the evaluator wanted to test. The client executed the endurance circuit with little complaint. He indicated that his pain rating was a 6 on a scale of 0–10 +. He rated the exertion factor of the test as a 13, indicating somewhat hard work. Mr. Thomas described his pain as generalized stiffness in the cervical region on the right side and in the lumbar region. He further noted a burning type of pain in the right leg and a throbbing sensation in his left knee.

Work Category

Based on the assessment results, this client is able to tolerate lifting in the light-to-medium work category. The light work category includes lifting up to 20 pounds on an occasional basis with a frequent lift of 10 pounds. The medium work category includes lifting up to 50 pounds on an occasional basis with a frequent lift of 20 pounds.

Test Consistency

A coefficiency of variation was performed on 16 tests for upper-extremity strength using the Baltimore Therapeutic Work Simulator. The client scored consistently on all 16 tests. Additionally, observations during testing and pain questionnaire responses were compared to assist in this therapist's determination of consistent performance. Responses on pain questionnaires and observations also supported consistent performance.

Results

Physical Demands	Job Demands	Client Abilities
Lifting	Light	Light to medium
Stooping	X	Limited
Kneeling	X	Limited
Crouching	X	Limited
Crawling	X	Limited
Reaching	X	Limited
Handling	X	X
Fingering	X	X
Feeling	X	X
Seeing	X	X
Environment:		
Inside/outside	X	X
Noise	X	X
Vibration	X	Not recommended

The physical demands of the job listed above are based on the *Dictionary of Occupational Titles* (13). Although this is a good reference, it does not provide other critical information of job tasks. For example, in measuring the amount of force needed to engage the clutch, or the amount of force it takes to turn the steering wheel, this reference can be adequately used in the initial process; however, it is recommended that a job site evaluation be obtained for more specific information. Based on the information presented, Mr. Thomas would be 50% disabled from returning to his former job. Another concern involves the type of lifting required for the job. Although he is able to lift in the light-to-medium work category, these lifts are occurring in the waist-to-shoulder range. Therefore, this does not account for lifting that may occur in the floor-to-waist level.

Recommendations for This Particular Client:

1. Client is unable to return to his previous job as a logging truck driver.
2. Client is suitable for light-to-medium work with restricted lifting in the waist-to-shoulder level.
3. It is not recommended that the client work in a situation that requires repetitive lifting.
4. A trial of 4–6 weeks of work hardening is recommended to improve overall endurance.
5. Referral for a work evaluation is recommended to address issues related to transferrable skills and possible retraining.
6. Referral to vocational rehabilitation is recommended to assist with job placement.

CONCLUSIONS

The functional capacity evaluation provides a new perspective on determining disability. It considers the patient's functional abilities as opposed to disability (or injured part). This method provides a more-accurate measure of a person's ability to return to gainful employment, and it allows for greater consistency in determining disability.

REFERENCES

1. World Health Organization: *International Classification of Impairments, Disabilities, and Handicaps.* Geneva, WHO, 1980.
2. American Medical Association: *Guides to the Evaluation of Permanent Impairment,* ed 3 (revised). Chicago, AMA, 1990.
3. *Disability Evaluation under Social Security: A Handbook for Physicians.* Washington, DC, US Department of Health, Education, and Welfare, 1979.
4. American Academy of Orthopaedic Surgeons: *Manual for Orthopaedic Surgeons in Evaluating Permanent Physical Impairment.* Chicago, American Academy of Orthopaedic Surgeons, 1988.

5. Frey WD, Netherton DR: Functional assessment: A new measure for disability. *Business Health*, June 31, 1988.

6. Miller M: Functional assessments: A vital component of work injury management. *Work* 1:6–10, 1991.

7. Rucker K, Metzler H, Wehman P, McKinley W, Zuelzer W, Rafii A: Pain literature and Social Security policy. *J Back Musculoskel Rehabil* 1:62–73, 1991.

8. Wickstrom R: Functional capacity testing. In Scheer SJ (ed): *Multidisciplinary Perspectives in Vocational Assessment of Impaired Workers*. Rockville, MD, Aspen Publication, 1990, pp 73–88.

9. Lechner D, Roth D, Straaton K: Functional capacity evaluation in work disability. *Work* 1:37–41, 1991.

10. Blankenship KL: *Industrial Rehabilitation* (procedure manual). Macon, GA, American Therapeutics, 1990.

11. Matheson LN: *Industrial Rehabilitation Resource Book*. Trabuco Canyon, CA, Performance Assessment and Capacity Testing, 1992.

12. Turk DC, Rudy TE, Stieg RL. The disability determination dilemma: Toward a multiaxial solution. *Pain* 34:217–229, 1988.

13. U.S. Department of Labor, Employment, and Training Administration: *Dictionary of Occupational Titles*, ed 4. Washington, DC, U.S. Government Printing Office, 1991.

14. Field JE, Field TF: *Classification of Jobs*, ed 3 (revised). Athens, GA, Elliott and Fitzpatrick, 1988.

15. U.S. Department of Justice: *The Americans with Disabilities Act* (brochure). Washington, DC, U.S. Government Printing Office, 1991.

CHAPTER 56
ASSESSMENT OF PSYCHOLOGICAL IMPAIRMENT AND DISABILITY

C. DAVID TOLLISON
DONALD W. HINNANT

DISABILITY IS, in general terms, a system of either social legislation or private insurance designed to protect individuals from suffering undue financial hardship when they are unable to work. Consequently, disability may result from physical, psychological, or a combination of physical and psychological disorders.

More specifically, disability is not a system, but a number of systems that include commercially available disability and wage protection insurance, personal injury liability, Social Security disability benefits (title II) and supplemental security income (title XVI), and workers' compensation insurance. Workers' compensation laws differ in each of the 50 states, the District of Columbia, and various U.S. territories. In addition, federal laws provide disability coverage for federal employees, and many maritime workers are covered under the federal Longshore and Harbor Workers' Compensation Act.

Despite the multiplicity of laws, jurisdictions, and workers' compensation versus tort-based versus social legislation systems, the determination of impairment/disability is sufficiently similar that we can, for the purposes of this chapter, discuss the clinical and administrative determination of psychological impairment/disability as if it were a single general system. Variances to this approach will be noted when applicable.

A basic premise underlying the determination of psychological functioning is the distinction between "impairment" and "disability." The definition of disability is based on an individual's ability (or inability) to engage in "substantial gainful activity," or to work (1). Thus, the adjudication of disability claims is fundamentally a vocational/administrative issue rather than a medical one (1). This position has been supported as far back as 1958, when the American Medical Association Committee on the Rating of Mental and Physical Impairment wrote in their *Guide to the Evaluation of Permanent Impairment, the Extremities and Back* that the de-

termination of impairment is purely a medical decision, and that whether or not a given impairment represented a disability was an administrative responsibility and function, rather than a medical one (2). Consequently, a physician or clinical psychologist is charged with a responsibility of determining and documenting "impairments," a term considered to be of medical parlance. "Disability," on the other hand, is generally considered a legal term and the determination of a ruling board, agency, court, or other authority. Therefore, an evaluating physician or clinical psychologist is responsible for determining the presence or absence of physical and/or psychological impairment that is subsequently considered in the nonmedical determination of whether an impairment constitutes a disability. The Social Security Administration, in fact, unequivocally states that "the physician is neither asked nor expected to make a decision as to whether the patient is disabled" (3). In this chapter we will focus on the determination of psychological impairment subsequent to physical injury and pain. Finally, the above paragraph notwithstanding, the terms "impairment" and "disability" may be occasionally used interchangeably, primarily as a result of the aforementioned confusion that exists in referenced literature.

PSYCHOLOGICAL IMPAIRMENT IN THE MEDICAL-LEGAL SYSTEM

There are numerous disability jurisdictions in the United States that oversee disability determination and monitor their own policies and procedures. Each jurisdiction has its own criteria for disability, as determined by administrative philosophy and policy, and there is considerable variation across jurisdictions. Likewise, the covered conditions, length and amount of payments, and review procedures also vary, as does the degree to which nonmedical factors (e.g., age, education, and social environment) are considered. For example, in certain situations, an individual may qualify for more than one form of disability compensation.

Despite the array of disability systems and the variability in criteria and structure, there appear to be two common factors across systems. The first is that physicians and clinical psychologists do not determine disability, although their findings are considered relevant. Health professionals may render a medical opinion in individual cases about the degree of impairment, treatment, and prognosis but, as previously mentioned, disability (work incapacity) remains an administrative or judicial determination following input from multiple sources (4). A second common thread across disability systems is the general recognition of two primary types of disability: physical and psychological.

Because the determination of psychological disability is based in part on the responsibility of physicians and clinical psychologists to provide specific information on impairment, we should have some familiarity with the procedures, regulations, and philosophy of the particular agency and the criteria for disability determination currently in use. However, because an analysis of every current disability system is far beyond the limitations of this chapter, we shall restrict our discussion to a relatively brief overview of three primary systems: (1) workers' compensation, (2) Social Security, and (3) personal injury.

WORKERS' COMPENSATION

Workers' compensation is a system of state and federal legislations designed to protect workers from suffering undue financial hardship when they are unable to work as the result of an on-the-job injury. The definition of who is a covered worker varies from state to state. For the most part, however, the majority of employees are included in the system whereas independent contractors and certain subclasses of employees may be excluded.

Workers' compensation is designed to protect injured workers from financial hardship but is not designed to totally replace lost income. Thus, under the most typical benefit scheme, a totally disabled worker will receive only two-thirds of his average weekly wage, subject to a state maximum benefit. Also, unlike tort systems, under which an injured person can collect for pain and suffering and other intangible injuries, the workers' compensation system is designed only to compensate injured workers for medical expenses and lost wages. Consequently, unlike tort systems, workers' compensation is generally not concerned with questions of fault or negligence. Thus, in the majority of workers' compensation cases, the system functions almost automatically: upon receipt of notice that an employee has been injured, the employer arranges for payment of his medical expenses and begins making weekly payments of

the workers' compensation benefits to which the employee is entitled until he is able to return to work. Nevertheless, there remain many cases in which there is disagreement between the parties as to whether the employee has sustained a compensable injury, and, if so, what benefits he is entitled to receive.

In most states, the initial determination on contested proceedings is a hearing before a hearing officer (often called a referee, administrative law judge, or a deputy commissioner), a quasi-judicial employee of the State Labor Department.

Because the procedure is an administrative-type hearing rather than a court trial, the rules of evidence may be less strictly applied than would be in a court action. For instance, medical evidence may be admitted not only in the form of live testimony and sworn depositions, but also in the form of unsworn medical reports and letters. Furthermore, it should be remembered that the hearing officers rarely have any medical training. Thus, whether or not a case is contested, medical evidence is often accorded great weight by persons who may be untrained in medical terminology. Therefore, a physician or clinical psychologist who is called upon to give a report in the compensation case must remember to be clear in explaining his diagnosis, impairment findings, and prognosis, particularly in cases involving more unusual injuries. The physician/clinical psychologist should be prepared to explain an official diagnosis in layman's terms and to spell out in detail the causal relationship between the events of the job-related injury and the employee's current impairment. With regard to a rating of the degree of permanent disability sustained by a claimant, the medical examiner should be aware that insurance companies and workers' compensation hearing officers expect to have ratings based on standard AMA Guidelines.

Workers' compensation benefits are paid during the period in which the employee is disabled from returning to work and, in some instances, for presumed future disability. The disability for which benefits are payable can be either temporary or permanent and either partial or total, leading to four classes of disability benefits: (1) temporary partial, (2) temporary total, (3) permanent partial, and (4) permanent total.

Assuming that there was a period of temporary total disability, it will be determined at some point that the injured worker has attained the maximum medical improvement (MMI) that can be expected. Once MMI has been reached, a determination must be made, with the assistance of medical/psychological opinion, as to whether the worker has sustained any permanent impairment and, if so, the extent of that impairment. If it appears that the worker will be unable to return to work at any time in the foreseeable future, he will be classified as permanently and totally disabled and will be awarded benefits accordingly. In many states, this means that he will be entitled to receive his weekly benefit rate for the remainder of his life or until circumstances change so that he can rejoin the workforce. In other states, however, even permanent total disability benefits are limited to a set period. Once that period has ended, the injured person will be without workers' compensation funds, unless he is able to qualify for other types of assistance such as Social Security disability.

If the worker is able to return to work, but has some residual physical or psychological disability attributable to the injury, he is likely to receive an award based on the state's "schedule" of injuries, combined with the medical/psychological ratings as to the degree of residual impairment.

At this point the reader will likely have noted two points in the above process at which medical/psychological opinion is not only necessary, but almost always indispensable—determining when the worker has reached MMI and "rating" the degree of permanent impairment, which includes diagnosing whether residual impairment will cause permanent total or merely permanent partial impairment.

SOCIAL SECURITY

Disability has been defined for the purpose of Social Security claims adjudication under the Social Security Act as an "inability to engage in any substantial gainful activity by reason of a medically determinable physical or mental impairment which can be expected to result in death or can be expected to last for a continuous period of not less than 12 months" (3). The adjudication of claim for disability benefits under Title II (Social Security Disability Benefits) and Title XVI (Supplemental Security Disability and Income) of the Social Security Act is based on the use of established medical criteria as described in the Listing of Impairments. As in other systems of disability determination, however, clear differences exist between what constitutes an "impairment" and what constitutes a "disability" within the context of the Social Security regulations, and it is on the interpretation of these differences that the Social Security Administration has placed considerable focus in the last several years.

The use of objectively demonstrable signs, symptoms, and medical findings at a disability adjudication has served the intent of the law relatively well in problems related to acute medical conditions, but the law does not provide an objective mechanism for evaluating the pain patient. Because the pain experience is a perception and because perceptions are not directly and objectively quantifiable, pain was considered in the evaluation of disability only as a secondary factor associated with a medically determinable impairment. The Social Security Administration has had increasing numbers of court cases challenging this policy regarding the evaluation of pain because chronic pain sufferers often present with allegations of pain that are not consistent with medically determinable impairment.

As a consequence of an increasing number of cases within the courts, the Social Security Disability Benefits Reform Act of 1984 (Public Law 98–460) directed the Secretary of Health and Human Services to appoint a Commission on the Evaluation of Chronic Pain to conduct a joint study with the National Academy of Sciences on the evaluation of pain as it pertains to claims adjudication under Titles II and XVI of the Social Security Act.

The Social Security Commission on the Evaluation of Chronic Pain recognized the pain experience as a multifaceted physical, mental, and behavioral process that may impact on the patient's behavior in all areas of his or her life and recognized that chronic pain patients often experience similar behavioral consequences as they attempt to adjust to the perception of pain. The Commission defined four groups of chronic pain patients: (1) chronic pain, inability to cope, insufficiently documented impairment; (2) chronic pain, competent coping, and insufficiently documented impairment; (3) chronic pain, inability to cope, sufficiently documented impairment; and (4) chronic pain, competent coping, sufficiently documented impairment. The Commission determined that groups 3 and 4 posed no problems in disability adjudication according to the current law, and recommended protocols for the evaluation of patients within groups one and two. The Commission specifically recommended interdisciplinary evaluation by appropriately trained medical, psychological, functional, social, and vocational specialists, and recommended the development of quantitative measurements of functional capacity and the establishment of rehabilitation goals within each disciplinary specialty. The Commission further recommended re-evaluation of the chronic pain patient as a measure of his or her compliance with the prescribed pain rehabilitation program and recommended vocational counseling to increase the patient's productivity level after completion of pain rehabilitation. A more-detailed examination of psychological impairment under Social Security will be outlined in a following section of this chapter.

PERSONAL INJURY

Anglo-Saxon law dictates, in legal parlance, a tort system for adjudication of personal injuries. Tort systems are designed to provide compensation (in the form of damages awards) from wrongdoers to those injured because of the wrongdoers' fault or negligence. Personal injury litigation allows the victim to sue for direct punitive damages as the result of wrongdoing, as well as for residual pain and suffering.

Crook illustrates the differences between tort systems and workers' compensation in consideration of two simple "slip and fall" cases, in which Mr. Smith and Mr.

Jones are hurt when they slip in a puddle of water on the floor and fall (5). In a tort system, whether Mr. Smith could recover from someone else for his injuries would depend on how the water got on the floor, whether the owner of the building knew or should have known that the water was there, whether Mr. Smith or persons like him were likely to be walking in that area, and whether Mr. Smith should have been able to see the water to avoid stepping in it. If all of these issues were resolved in Smith's favor, he could recover his medical expenses in treating the injury, his past and future lost wages attributable to the injury, and his pain and suffering. In addition, his wife could recover for loss of consortium, that is, the diminution in value of his services to her as a result of the injury. The Smiths might also recover punitive damages if the judge or jury found that the defendant's conduct was especially blameworthy; for instance, if the puddle had been on the floor in an area heavily frequented by the public for a long time and the building's owner had deliberately refused to clean it up.

In contrast, if Mr. Jones had slipped on the puddle while he was working, questions of whose fault the accident was and who knew or did not know about the puddle would be generally irrelevant. The only issues would be whether his injuries were sufficiently work-connected and whether those injuries kept him from working. His recovery, however, would be limited to payment of his medical bills, payment of compensation benefits for the weeks he was unable to work and, in most states, a schedule award for his presumptive loss of wages if, after reaching maximum medical recovery, it was determined that he had a residual permanent loss of function attributable to his injuries.

In general practice, personal injury litigation cases often rely heavily on the "pain and suffering" and other reactive psychological ramifications that may result from physical injuries received. Typically, such legal cases require that the physician/clinical psychologist testify as to the diagnosis, prognosis, and psychological impairment (temporary or permanent) resulting from the injury and attribute any reactive psychological dysfunction in a causal manner to an accident or injuries received. Such "injury" is not limited to physical tissue damage but may also be a "psychological injury." For example, a claimant is a passenger in an automobile driven by a friend. Because of the wrongdoing and fault of the driver of another automobile that strikes the car of the claimant passenger, the driver of the car in which the claimant was a passenger is killed. The claimant passenger may then bring a personal injury suit against the driver of the other car for psychological injuries received as the result of being pinned in the car and forced to watch the slow and gruesome death of the driver.

FACTORS INFLUENCING PSYCHOLOGICAL DISABILITY

It is generally accepted that a wide variety of psycho-socioeconomic factors influence psychological functioning. It is also true that a variety of factors affect psychological impairment and disability. A partial listing of these factors includes age, educational level, premorbid psychological functioning, social and environmental factors, and cultural influences (6). In the determination of psychological impairment, however, it is critical that the examiner differentiate individual personality and idiosyncratic factors from psychological symptoms associated with and reactive to some particular event or injury. Generally speaking, possible emotional conditions arising from significant illness or injury should be expected to present with relatively discrete and circumscribed symptoms, in addition to the requirement of being meaningful and logically associated with a substantive illness or injury. When the psychological course is protracted and the symptoms are generalized, individual personality composition factors are frequently found to be more contributory and of greater etiologic significance than any alleged physical trauma (7). Thus, in a general sense, it is reasonable to expect to determine more-generalized, nonspecific psychological dysfunction in individuals claiming disability from chronic disease and illness (e.g., cancer) and more-concrete and circumscribed emotional dysfunction in individuals claiming disability as a result of accidents and acute injuries. In addition to a variety of psychological conditions that may exist in reaction to pain, the literature suggests that victims may be conditioned or shaped into a role of psychological disability (8). In this section, we will briefly summarize a selected number of such conditioning factors as earlier outlined by Strang (7). Knowledge of these and other conditioning factors is important to the physician/clinical psychologist charged with the responsibility of determining psychological impairment.

Physician

Physicians commonly and inadvertently reinforce disability and development of chronic pain syndrome through mismanagement of the patient during the acute phase of pain and through the application of the acute pain medical model during the chronic phase of illness and injury. Fordyce and others have discussed techniques designed to prevent the development of chronic pain that are applicable in the acute stage of discomfort (9). Although the acute pain medical model works well in the great majority of medical situations, its application in the chronic phase of illness and injury can condition dependence, disability, dysfunction, and psychological impairment and disability.

Failure to Apply the Chronic Illness Model

Strang has reported that physicians often act in accordance with the acute illness model beyond its appropriateness (7).

Consequently, when patients enter a chronic phase, they may be encouraged to take it easy or may be told that they will be better in time, thus giving rise to the development of magical expectations. When they do not improve, patients frequently feel resentful, hopeless, and depressed. This inadvertent action on the part of physicians may well result in iatrogenically induced physical and psychological impairment.

Lack of Coordination of Consultants

Patients suffering a protracted period of pain generally are evaluated and treated by numerous physicians of varying specialities. Frequently a specialist provides information to the patient that may engender distrust or fear, which can increase the patient's potential for prolonged recovery or development of additional physical and psychological problems. For example, it is not uncommon for us to see patients who are frustrated and angry with their surgical outcome.

Often patients will be told that repeated test results were "normal," and because of continued symptoms the patients are suspicious of their treatment. A patient may be told by a specialist such as a radiologist that there are significant abnormalities, whereas the surgeon will consider these abnormalities to be insignificant. The development of distrust of physicians may lead to numerous consultations, and a search for "the right doctor." Unfortunately, the various findings are often not integrated into a coordinated treatment plan that encourages patients to become more responsible for recovery. The result of fragmented care is usually protracted disability.

Tendency of Physicians to Take Patients' Complaints at Face Value

Strang reports that physicians, in their desire to be helpful, often respond to repeated complaints of pain as presumptive evidence of some somatic lesion being the sole or main factor or of some new acute problem or slow-to-heal lesion (7). Patients seldom directly complain about vocational and related disabilities, focusing more on complaints of pain. Consequently, it is easy for physicians to overlook possible psychological factors in the overall symptoms.

Countertransference Issues

The attitudes and values of physicians and other health professionals are not always consistent with those of patients who do not work. Moreover, patients involved in litigation in related activities often have different goals, agendas, and influences than do treating physicians, thereby generating occasional tension in the physician-patient relationship. As a result, physicians who have difficulty managing reality-based or negative countertransference feelings may respond by offering repeated medical work-ups, diagnostics, and treatments, thus serving to shape the patient into a role of fear and dependence, and a conviction that all problems will ultimately be resolved with a unique diagnosis and therapeutic "magic bullet."

Collusion in the Disability Claims Process

It is not infrequent to encounter patients who are highly insistent about their inability to work. Physicians and health professionals may then be easily drawn into a collusion over the disability. There is often an unspoken agreement not to confront the reality of the disability itself that inhibits the formation of a working alliance and proper goal setting. If physicians feel responsible, for whatever reason, for the patient's failure to improve or return to work, they may lose objectivity and become over-involved in the disability process. In addition, if a physician is uncomfortable in confronting the patient with an obviously differing agenda (i.e., disability and return to work), the level of discomfort experienced by the physician may be resolved by avoiding confrontation and seeking relief through objective determination of functional impairment.

FAMILY

Fordyce has commented extensively on the role of family members as reinforcers of disability (9). Family systems are often altered with the emergence of mutually reinforcing hostile dependent relationships (7). Some spouses and family members remain gratifying and solicitous with hidden resentment, and others remove themselves, creating family networks characterized by isolation and decreased communication.

LAW

Individuals claiming disability retain certain rights to apply for compensation through existing disability sources as well as to redress unfavorable disability determinations through further administrative or judicial reviews or hearings. Ongoing litigation is common and may foster an adversarial climate between employees and employers or granting agencies. Our legal system is designed such that attorneys often receive contingency fees and, naturally, an attorney protecting the best interests of his client will attempt to present a level of disability deserving of the highest award or greatest length of compensation possible. Unfortunately, a return to productivity and employment, which is often clinically in the best interest of the patient, may undermine the disability process and claim. Attorneys, who are not clinically trained, may not appreciate the evidence that suggests that prolonged disability reinforces the very nature of the patient's difficulty and, in fact, the clinical well-being of the patient is not the responsibility

Table 56.1.
Impairment Due to Mental and Behavioral Disorders

Areas of Function	Class 1 No Impairment	Class 2 Mild Impairment	Class 3 Moderate Impairment	Class 4 Marked Impairment	Class 5 Extreme Impairment
Activities of daily living Social functioning Concentration Adaptation	No impairments noted	Impairment levels compatible with most useful function	Impairment levels compatible with some but not all useful function	Impairment levels significantly impede useful function	Impairment levels preclude useful function

or training of the attorney any more than legal representation of the patient in the disability process is the responsibility and training of the physician/clinical psychologist. Health providers notoriously are reluctant to confront the legal process and take the initiative in educating and conferring with attorneys. In our experience, the great majority of attorneys hold the long-term best interest of the patient as a priority and are both responsive and facilitating of clinical efforts to obtain maximum medical improvement if the clinician discusses the case with and works to educate the attorney and to clarify the clinical issues involved.

EMPLOYER AND ADMINISTRATIVE AGENCY

Light-duty employment is often difficult for employers and management to supervise and enforce. Employers frequently express concerns about workers taking advantage of "special" privileges that are also viewed as potentially disruptive to the work routine and morale of other workers. Furthermore, employers may face liability insurance considerations that may mitigate against the clinical need for injured employees to return to work in an early fashion. Unfortunately, even patients who are motivated to return to work often encounter a barrier in returning.

Consequently, patients occasionally perceive themselves as hopelessly caught in a system that does not care about them and, ultimately, the patient becomes frustrated and suspicious of the motivation of the employer. Obviously, as the relationship between the employer and employee becomes strained, the opportunity for resolution of the dilemma of returning the patient to productivity becomes diminished. Furthermore, such a situation results in a reinforcement of disability, and to make matters worse, the injured worker often develops a very strong sense of entitlement.

AMA GUIDELINES TO THE EVALUATION OF PERMANENT IMPAIRMENT

The American Medical Association publishes the *Guide for Rating Permanent Impairment* (third edition, 1990) (2). The chapter on diagnosing and evaluating

mental and behavioral disorders attempts to combine material taken from Social Security Administration regulations with the *American Psychiatric Association's Diagnostic and Statistical Manual of Mental Disorders—Revised*. Three major principles are considered central to assessing mental impairment. These are (1) diagnosis, (2) motivation for improvement, and (3) a longitudinal history, prior treatment, and attempts at rehabilitation. Table 1 in the manual describes the four primary areas of functioning and five classes of rating from no impairment to extreme impairment. Unfortunately, the AMA guidelines do not provide a clear method for making judgments about the percentage of impairment. The physician is required base the percentage on his evaluation and experience. This will of course create a great deal of confusion with regard to inter-rater reliability (Table 56.1). The third edition also includes an appendix entitled "Pain and Impairment."

Although this section attempts to define and explain acute and chronic pain, there are no guidelines for assigning an impairment rating. Fortunately the American Pain Society and the American Academy of Pain Medicine will be participating in the writing of a chapter for the next edition of the AMA's *Guide to the Evaluation of Permanent Impairment*. It is hoped that, in the future, acceptable improvements in assessment of pain and the degree of impairment will be forthcoming.

DISABILITY EVALUATION UNDER SOCIAL SECURITY

Psychological impairment/disability is recognized by a variety of disability agencies and sources, but probably none more readily or with greater complexity than in Social Security disability. The evaluation of Social Security disability on the basis of mental disorders requires the documentation of a medically determinable impairment as well as consideration of the degree of limitation such impairment may impose on the individual's ability to work and whether these limitations have lasted or are expected to last for a continuous period of at least 12 months. The listings for mental disorders under Social Security disability are arranged in eight diagnostic categories: (1) organic mental disorders, (2) schizophrenic, paranoid, and other psychotic disorders, (3) affective disorders, (4) mental retardation and autism, (5) anxiety-related disorders, (6) somatoform disorders, (7) personality disorders, and (8) substance addiction disorders. Each diagnostic category, except mental retardation and autism and substance addiction disorders, consists of a set of clinical findings (paragraph A criteria), one or more of which must be met, and which, if met, leads to a test of functional restrictions (paragraph B criteria), of which two or three must also be met. There are additional considerations (paragraph C criteria) in the categories of paranoid and other psychotic disorders and anxiety-related disorders.

The purpose of including the criteria in paragraph A of the listings for mental disorders is to medically substantiate the presence of a mental disorder. The purpose of including the criteria in paragraphs B and C is to describe those functional limitations associated with mental disorders that are incompatible with the ability to work. The restrictions listed in paragraphs B and C must be the result of the mental disorder that is manifested by the clinical findings outlined in paragraph A. The criteria included in paragraphs B and C of the listings for mental disorders have been chosen by the Social Security Administration because they represent functional areas deemed essential for work. An individual who is severely limited in these areas as the result of an impairment identified in paragraph A is presumed to be unable to work.

The existence of a medically determinable impairment of the required duration must be established by medical evidence consisting of clinical signs, symptoms, and/or laboratory or psychological testing findings. These findings may be intermittent or persistent, depending on the nature of the disorder. Clinical signs are medically demonstrable phenomena that reflect specific abnormalities of behavior, affect, thought, memory, orientation, or contact with reality. Social Security typically expects such an assessment to be performed by a psychiatrist or psychologist and documented by psychological testing. Symptoms are considered to be complaints presented by the individual. Signs and symptoms generally cluster together to constitute recognizable clinical syndromes (mental disorders). Both symptoms and signs that are part of any diagnosed mental disorder must be considered in evaluating severity.

In the Social Security evaluation of mental disorders, severity is assessed in terms of the functional limitations imposed by the psychological impairment (paragraph B).

In the following section we will outline four of the eight categories of mental disorders and impairments considered to constitute evidence for psychological disability by the Social Security Administration. The categories of Affective Disorders, Anxiety-Related Disorders, Somatoform Disorders, and Personality Disorders are the four categories most frequently encountered by professionals determining psychological impairment as a result of or in association with pain.

FOUR SOCIAL SECURITY ADMINISTRATION CATEGORIES OF MENTAL DISORDER

12.04 Affective Disorders

Affective disorders are characterized by a disturbance of mood, accompanied by a full or partial manic or depressive syndrome. Mood refers to a prolonged emotion that colors the whole psychic lift; it generally involves either depression or elation.

The required level of severity for these disorders is met when the requirements in both A and B are satisfied.

A. Medically documented persistence, either continuous or intermittent, of one of the following:
  1. Depressive syndrome characterized by at least four of the following:
     a. Anhedonia or pervasive loss of interest in almost all activities; or
     b. Appetite disturbance with change in weight; or
     c. Sleep disturbance; or
     d. Psychomotor agitation or retardation; or
     e. Decreased energy; or
     f. Feelings of guilt or worthlessness; or
     g. Difficulty concentrating or thinking; or
     h. Thoughts of suicide; or
     i. Hallucinations, delusions or paranoid thinking; or
  2. Manic syndrome characterized by at least three of the following:
     a. Hyperactivity; or
     b. Pressure of speech; or
     c. Flight of ideas; or
     d. Inflated self-esteem; or
     e. Decreased need for sleep; or
     f. Easy distractibility; or
     g. Involvement in activities that have a high probability of painful consequences that are not recognized; or
     h. Hallucinations, delusions or paranoid thinking; or
  3. Bipolar syndrome with a history of episodic periods manifested by the full symptomatic picture of both manic and depressive syndromes (and currently characterized by either or both syndromes);

AND

B. Resulting in at least two of the following:
  1. Marked restriction of activities of daily living; or
  2. Marked difficulties in maintaining social functioning; or
  3. Deficiencies of concentration, persistence, or pace resulting in frequent failure to complete

tasks in a timely manner (in work settings or elsewhere); or
4. Repeated episodes of deterioration or decompensation in work or work-like settings that cause the individual to withdraw from that situation or to experience exacerbation of signs and symptoms (which may include deterioration of adaptive behaviors).

12.06 Anxiety-Related Disorders

In these disorders anxiety is either the predominant disturbance or it is experienced if the individual attempts to master symptoms; for example, confronting the dreaded object or situation in a phobic disorder or resisting the obsessions or compulsions in obsessive-compulsive disorders.

The required level of severity for these disorders is met when the requirements in both A and B are satisfied, or when the requirements in both A and C are satisfied.

A. Medically documented findings of at least one of the following:
   1. Generalized persistent anxiety accompanied by three out of four of the following signs or symptoms:
      a. Motor tension; or
      b. Autonomic hyperactivity; or
      c. Apprehensive expectation; or
      d. Vigilance and scanning; or
   2. A persistent irrational fear of a specific object, activity, or situation that results in a compelling desire to avoid the dreaded object, activity, or situation; or
   3. Recurrent severe panic attacks manifested by a sudden unpredictable onset of intense apprehension, fear, terror, and sense of impending doom occurring on the average of at least once a week; or
   4. Recurrent obsessions or compulsions that are a source of marked distress; or
   5. Recurrent and intrusive recollections of a traumatic experience, which are a source of marked distress; and
B. Resulting in a least two of the following:
   1. Marked restriction of activities of daily living; or
   2. Marked difficulties in maintaining social functioning; or
   3. Deficiencies of concentration, persistence of pace resulting in frequent failure to complete tasks in a timely manner (in work settings or elsewhere); or
   4. Repeated episodes of deterioration or decompensation in work or work-like settings that cause the individual to withdraw from that situation or to experience exacerbation of signs and symptoms (which may include deterioration of adaptive behaviors); or
C. Resulting in complete inability to function independently outside the area of one's home.

12.07 Somatoform Disorders

Physical symptoms for which there are no demonstrable organic findings or known physiologic mechanisms are considered somatoform disorders.

The required level of severity for these disorders is met when the requirements in both A and B are satisfied.

A. Medically documented by evidence of one of the following:
   1. A history of multiple physical symptoms of several years' duration beginning before age 30, and that have caused the individual to take medicine frequently, see a physician often, and alter life patterns significantly; or
   2. Persistent nonorganic disturbance of one of the following:
      a. Vision; or
      b. Speech; or
      c. Hearing; or
      d. Use of a limb; or
      e. Movement and its control (e.g., coordination disturbance, psychogenic seizures, akinesia, dyskinesia); or
      f. Sensation (e.g., diminished or heightened).
   3. Unrealistic interpretation of physical signs or sensations associated with the preoccupation or belief that one has a serious disease or injury; and
B. Resulting in three of the following:
   1. Marked restriction of activities of daily living; or
   2. Marked difficulties in maintaining social functioning; or
   3. Deficiencies of concentration, persistence, or pace resulting in frequent failure to complete tasks in a timely manner (in work settings or elsewhere); or
   4. Repeated episodes of deterioration or decompensation in work or work-like settings that cause the individual to withdraw from that situation or to experience exacerbation of signs and symptoms (which may include deterioration of adaptive behaviors).

12.08 Personality Disorders

A personality disorder exists when personality traits are inflexible and maladaptive and cause either significant impairment in social or occupational functioning or subjective distress. Characteristic features are typical of the individual's long-term functioning and are not limited to discrete episodes of illness.

The required level of severity for these disorders is met when the requirements in both A and B are satisfied.

A. Deeply ingrained, maladaptive patterns of behavior associated with one of the following:
   1. Seclusiveness or autistic thinking; or
   2. Pathologically inappropriate suspiciousness or hostility; or

3. Oddities of thought, perception, speech, and behavior; or
4. Persistent disturbances of mood or affect; or
5. Pathologic dependence, passivity, or aggressivity; or
6. Intense and unstable interpersonal relationships and impulsive and damaging behavior;

AND

B. Resulting in three of the following:
1. Marked restriction of activities of daily living; or
2. Marked difficulties in maintaining social functioning; or
3. Deficiencies of concentration, persistence, or pace resulting in frequent failure to complete tasks in a timely manner (in work settings or elsewhere); or
4. Repeated episodes of deterioration or decompensation in work or work-like settings that cause the individual to withdraw from that situation or to experience exacerbation of signs and symptoms (which may include deterioration of adaptive behaviors).

NOSOLOGY: DIAGNOSTIC AND STATISTICAL MANUAL OF MENTAL DISORDERS

The determination of psychological impairment is predicated on the recognition of psychological disability either in combination with physical impairment/disability or as a distinct entity that does not require the determination of an organic or physical component. In the determination of psychological impairment following painful accidents or injuries, the busy clinician will likely encounter both.

To accurately communicate the determination of psychological impairment, a nosology that provides a common language is required. In determination of psychological functioning, this nosology is the *Diagnostic and Statistical Manual of Mental Disorders* (DSM), originally published in 1952.

The third edition of the DSM was published in 1980 by the American Psychiatric Association and revised (DSM III-R) in 1986 (10). Although developed for use with psychiatric and not pain patients, selected nomenclature in the DSM III-R is applicable to patients with chronic pain syndromes and includes both physical and psychological aspects of symptoms.

There has been extensive clinical research indicating the tendency for affective disorders or personality disorders to be present with intractable pain. The DSM III-R includes pain, either as a diagnostic criterion or concomitant symptom, in a number of diagnostic categories. The following section outlines these disorders, briefly discusses pain within the context of each disorder, and concludes with a discussion of depression as a proposed additional diagnostic disorder.

Diagnostic criteria from the DSM III-R are reprinted with permission of the American Psychiatric Association, whose cooperation is appreciated.

SOMATOFORM DISORDERS

The essential features of this group of disorders are physical symptoms suggesting physical disorders for which there are no demonstrable organic findings or known physiologic mechanisms, and for which there is positive evidence or a strong presumption that the symptoms are linked to psychological factors or conflicts. Although the symptoms of somatoform disorders are physical in nature, the specific pathophysiologic processes involved are not demonstrable or understandable by existing laboratory procedures and are conceptualized most clearly by means of psychological constructs. The production of symptoms by the patient is presumed to be unintentional.

Conversion Disorder

The essential feature of *conversion disorder* is an alteration or loss of physical functioning that suggests a physical disorder, but that instead is apparently an expression of a psychological conflict or need. The symptoms of the disturbance are not intentionally produced and, after appropriate investigation, cannot be explained by any physical disorder or known pathophysiologic mechanism.

Conversion disorder is not diagnosed when conversion symptoms are limited to pain (see "Somatoform Pain Disorder") but may be considered a diagnosis, in association with pain, to explain a concrete "physical" disorder generated by a psychological etiology.

For example, the most common and "classic" conversion symptoms are not pain but, rather, those that suggest neurologic disease, such as paralysis, seizures, coordination disturbance, akinesia, dyskinesia, blindness, anesthesia, and paresthesia.

The symptoms of conversion disorder usually develop in a setting of extreme psychological stress and appear suddenly. The effect of this disorder on a patient's life is usually marked and frequently impedes normal life activities.

Prolonged loss of function may produce serious complications, such as contractures or disuse atrophy. Antecedent physical disorders or severe psychological stress are generally considered predisposing factors.

The differential diagnosis of conversion disorder is sometimes difficult in that many physical disorders that present with vague, multiple somatic symptoms may, early in their course, be misdiagnosed as conversion symptoms. A diagnosis of conversion disorder is suggested if the symptoms are inconsistent with the actual known physical disorder—for example, anesthesia of the hand and arm following cervical trauma that conforms to the concept of the hand and arm rather than to the functional area served by a specific part of the ner-

Table 56.2.
Diagnostic Criteria: Conversion Disorder

A. A loss of, or alteration in, physical functioning suggesting a physical disorder.
B. Psychological factors are judged to be etiologically related to the symptoms because of a temporal relationship between a psychosocial stressor that is apparently related to a psychological conflict or need and initiation or exacerbation of the symptom.
C. The person is not conscious of intentionally producing the symptom.
D. The symptom is not a culturally sanctioned response pattern and cannot, after appropriate investigation, be explained by a known physical disorder.
E. The symptom is not limited to pain or to a disturbance in sexual functioning.

Specify single or recurrent episode.

Table 56.3.
Diagnostic Criteria: Hypochondriasis

A. Preoccupation with the fear of having, or the belief that one has, a serious disease, based on the person's interpretation of physical signs or sensations as evidence of physical illness.
B. Appropriate physical evaluation does not support the diagnosis of any physical disorder that can account for the physical signs or sensations or the person's unwarranted interpretation of them, and the symptoms in *A* are not just symptoms of panic attacks.
C. The fear of having, or belief that one has, a disease persists despite medical reassurance.
D. Duration of the disturbance is at least 6 months.
E. The belief in Part *A* is not of delusional intensity, as in *delusional disorder, somatic type* (i.e., the person can acknowledge the possibility that his or her fear of having, or belief that he or she has, a serious disease is unfounded).

vous system. Physical disorders in which psychological factors often play an important role should not be diagnosed as conversion disorder (Table 56.2).

Hypochondriasis

The essential feature of a diagnosis of *hypochondriasis* is preoccupation with a fear of having, or the belief that one has, a serious disease, based on the person's interpretation of physical signs or sensations as evidence of physical illness. A thorough physical examination does not support the diagnosis of any physical disorder that can account for the physical signs or sensations or for the person's unwarranted interpretation of them, although a coexisting physical disorder may be present. The unwarranted fear or belief of having a disease persists despite medical reassurance, but is not of delusional intensity, in that the person can acknowledge the possibility that he or she may be exaggerating the extent of the feared disease or that there may be no disease at all.

The preoccupation may be with bodily functions, such as heartbeat, sweating, or peristalsis, or with major physical abnormalities. In patients who have suffered trauma with residual pain and functional limitations, the presence of discomfort and physical signs, particularly radicular sensations, may be interpreted as having been caused by cancer or some other dreaded disease. The medical history is often presented by the patient in great detail and at length. "Doctor shopping" and deterioration in doctor-patient relationships, with frustration and anger on both sides, are common. Patients with this disorder often believe they are not getting proper care and that physicians have simply not found the true "cause" of their symptoms.

The most important differential diagnostic consideration in hypochondriasis is the presence of true organic disease, such as early stages of neurologic disorders, en-

docrine disorders, or neurologic disorders resulting from trauma. The presence of true organic disease does not rule out the possibility of coexisting hypochondriasis, however. In somatization disorder there tends to be preoccupation with symptoms rather than fear of having a specific disease or diseases. When the criteria for somatization disorders are met and the criteria for hypochondriasis are also met, however, both diagnoses should be given (Table 56.3).

Somatization Disorder

The essential features of *somatization disorders* are recurrent and multiple somatic complaints, usually of several years' duration, for which medical attention has been repeatedly sought, but that apparently are not due to any physical disorder. The disorder begins before the age of 30 and has a chronic but fluctuating course.

Complaints are often presented in a dramatic, vague, or exaggerated way, or are part of a complicated medical history in which many physical diagnoses have been considered. Patients frequently receive medical care from a number of physicians, sometimes simultaneously. Complaints invariably involve the following organic symptoms or types of symptoms: conversion or psuedoneurologic symptoms, gastrointestinal discomfort, cardiopulmonary symptoms, and pain.

In the diagnosis of somatization disorder, anxiety and depressed mood are often associated features. Because of constant consultation of doctors, numerous medical evaluations are undergone, both in and out of the hospital; there is frequently unwitting submission to unnecessary surgery. Furthermore, these patients run the risk of psychoactive substance abuse involving various prescribed medications.

The differential diagnosis of somatization disorder is,

again, sometimes difficult in that it is necessary to rule out physical disorders that present with vague, multiple, and confusing somatic symptoms such as myofascial, neurologic, and other types of symptoms. In conversion disorder one or more conversion symptoms occur in the absence of the full clinical picture of somatization disorder (Table 56.4).

Table 56.4.
Diagnostic Criteria: Somatization Disorder

A. A history of many physical complaints or a belief that one is sickly, beginning before the age of 30 and persisting for several years.
B. At least 13 symptoms from the list below. To count a symptom as significant, the following criteria must be met:
  1. No organic pathology or pathophysiologic mechanism (e.g., a physical disorder or the effects of injury, medication, drugs, or alcohol) to account for the symptom or, when there is related organic pathology, the complaint or resulting social or occupational impairment is grossly in excess of what would be expected from the physical findings.
  2. Symptom has not occurred only during a panic attack.
  3. Symptom has caused the person to take medication (other than over-the-counter pain medication), see a doctor, or alter lifestyle.

Symptom list:
  1. Vomiting (other than during pregnancy)
  2. Abdominal pain (other than during menstruating)
  3. Nausea (other than motion sickness)
  4. Bloating (gassy)
  5. Diarrhea
  6. Intolerance of (gets sick from) several different foods

Pain symptoms:
  7. Pain in extremities
  8. Back pain
  9. Joint pain
  10. Pain during urination
  11. Other pain (excluding headaches)

Cardiopulmonary symptoms:
  12. Shortness of breath when not exerting oneself
  13. Palpitations
  14. Chest pain
  15. Dizziness

Conversion or pseudoneurologic syptoms:
  16. Amnesia
  17. Difficulty swallowing
  18. Loss of voice
  19. Deafness
  20. Double vision
  21. Blurred vision
  22. Blindness
  23. Fainting or loss of consciousness
  24. Seizure or convulsion
  25. Trouble walking
  26. Paralysis or muscle weakness
  27. Urinary retention or difficulty urinating

Somatoform Pain Disorder

The essential feature of *somatoform pain disorder* is preoccupation with pain in the absence of adequate physical findings to account for the pain or its intensity. The pain symptom either is inconsistent with the anatomic distribution of the nervous system, or if it mimics a known disease entity, cannot, after extensive diagnostic examination, be adequately accounted for by organic pathology.

In some cases there may be evidence that psychological factors are etiologically involved in the pain, as when there is a clear temporal relationship between an environmental stimulus that is apparently related to a psychological conflict or need and initiation or exacerbation of the pain. In other cases the evidence may be the pain's permitting the person to avoid some activity that is noxious to him or her or to get support from the environment that otherwise might not be forthcoming. In still other cases, there may be no direct evidence of a etiologic role of psychological factors.

Somatoform pain disorder may be accompanied by other localized sensory or motor-function changes, such as paresthesias and muscle spasm. Characteristic are frequent visits to physicians to obtain relief despite medical reassurance, excessive use of analgesics without relief of the pain, requests for surgery, and assumption of the role of invalid. The patient usually refuses to consider the contribution of psychological factors to the pain. Symptoms of depression are frequent, and in many cases an associated diagnosis of major depression is warranted.

The complaint of pain in somatoform pain disorder usually appears suddenly, often following trauma, and increases in severity over weeks or months. Typically, the person has become incapacitated and has ceased to work. An invalid role is often assumed. The most serious complications are iatrogenic and include dependence on minor tranquilizers and narcotic analgesics and repeated, unsuccessful surgical interventions.

In approximately half of the cases of somatoform pain disorder the complaint of pain develops immediately following physical trauma. The dramatic presentation of organic pain, which may seem excessive to an observer because of minimal physical findings, is not sufficient for diagnosing this disorder (Table 56.5).

Undifferentiated Somatoform Disorder

Undifferentiated somatoform disorder is a category for clinical pictures that do not meet the full symptom picture of somatization disorder. There is either a single circumscribed symptom or, more commonly, multiple physical complaints, such as fatigue, loss of appetite, and nonspecific complaints of pain. As with somatization disorder, the symptoms are not explainable on the basis of demonstrable organic findings or a known pathophysiologic mechanism, and are apparently

Table 56.5.
Diagnostic Criteria: Somatoform Pain Disorder

A. Preoccupation with pain for at least 6 months.
B. Either (1) or (2):
  1. Appropriate evaluation uncovers no organic pathology or pathophysiologic mechanism (e.g., a physical disorder or the effects of injury) to account for the pain
  2. When there is related organic pathology, the complaint of pain or resulting social or occupational impairment is grossly in excess of what would be expected from the physical findings.

Table 56.6.
Diagnostic Criteria: Undifferentiated Somatoform Disorder

A. One or more physical complaints (e.g., fatigue, loss of appetite, gastrointestinal or urinary complaints).
B. Either (1) or (2):
  1. Appropriate evaluation uncovers no organic pathology or pathophysiologic mechanism (e.g., a physical disorder or the effects of injury, medication, drugs, or alcohol) to account for the physical complaints
  2. When there is related organic pathology, the physical complaints or resulting social or occupational impairment is grossly in excess of what would be expected from the physical findings.
C. Duration of the disturbance is at least 6 months.
D. Occurrence not exclusively during the course of another somatoform disorder, a sexual dysfunction, a mood disorder, an anxiety disorder, a sleep disorder, or a psychotic disorder.

Table 56.7.
Diagnostic Criteria: Psychological Factors Affecting Physical Condition

A. Psychologically meaningful environmental stimuli are temporarily related to the initiation or exacerbation of a specific physical condition or disorder (recorded on Axis III).
B. The physical condition involves either demonstrable organic pathology (e.g., rheumatoid arthritis) or a known pathophysiologic process (e.g., migraine headache).
C. The condition does not meet the criteria for a somatoform disorder.

linked to psychological factors. The diagnosis is not made if the disturbance is of less than 6 months' duration or if it occurs only during the course of another somatoform disorder such as somatoform pain disorder. Anxiety and depressed mood are commonly encountered, and functional impairment is generally less than that determined in somatization disorder (Table 56.6).

PSYCHOLOGICAL FACTORS AFFECTING PHYSICAL CONDITION

The category of *psychological factors affecting physical condition* can apply to any physical condition to which psychological factors are judged to be contributory. It may be used to describe disorders that in the past have been referred to as either "psychosomatic" or "psychophysiologic."

Common examples of physical conditions for which this category may be appropriate include, but are not limited to, tension headache, migraine headache, headache following cervical trauma, sacroiliac pain, rheumatoid arthritis, and gastric or duodenal ulcer. This category should not be used in cases of conversion disorder or other somatoform disorders, which are regarded as disturbances in which the specific pathophysiologic process involved in the disorder is not demonstrable by existing standard laboratory procedures and which are conceptualized by psychological constructs only (Table 56.7).

MALINGERING

Malingering is considered a subset of the major diagnostic category termed *codes for conditions not attributable to a mental disorder that are a focus of attention or treatment* in the DSM III-R (10). The essential feature of malingering is intentional production of false or grossly exaggerated physical or psychological symptoms, motivated by external incentives such as avoiding work, obtaining financial compensation, evading criminal prosecution, and obtaining drugs.

According to the DSM III-R malingering should be strongly suspected if any combination of the following is noted:

1. Medicolegal context of presentation (e.g., the person's being referred by his or her attorney to the physician for examination);
2. Marked discrepancy between the person's claimed stress or disability and the objective findings;
3. Lack of cooperation during the diagnostic evaluation and in complying with the prescribed treatment regimen;
4. The presence of antisocial personality disorder.

Malingering is differentiated from conversion and other somatic disorders by the intentional production of symptoms and by the obvious, external incentives. The person who is malingering is much less likely to present his or her symptoms in the context of emotional conflict,

Table 56.8.
Diagnostic Criteria: Psychoactive Substance Abuse

A. A maladaptive pattern of psychoactive substance use indicated by at least one of the following:
  1. Continued use despite knowledge of having a persistent or recurrent social, occupational, psychological, or physical problem that is caused or exacerbated by use of the psychoactive substance
  2. Recurrent use in situations in which use is physically hazardous (e.g., driving while intoxicated)
B. Some symptoms of the disturbance have persisted for at least 1 month, or have occurred repeatedly over a longer period.
C. The criteria for psychoactive substance dependence have not been met for this substance.

and the presenting symptoms are less likely to be symbolically related to an underlying emotional conflict.

Although the physician/clinical psychologist examiner may occasionally encounter a malingerer in the course of determining psychological impairment, it has been our experience that such a disorder is generally uncommon and, when encountered, is usually presented by individuals with limited intellectual sophistication that results in symptoms and behaviors generating a nonchallenging and uncomplicated diagnosis of malingering.

Psychoactive Substance Abuse

Psychoactive substance abuse is a residual category for noting maladaptive patterns of psychoactive substance use that have never met the criteria for dependence for that particular class of substance. The maladaptive pattern of use is indicated by either (1) continued use of the psychoactive substance despite knowledge of having a persistent or recurrent social, occupational, psychological, or physical problem that is caused or exacerbated by the use of the substance or (2) recurrent use of the substance in situations when use is physically hazardous (10). The diagnosis is made only if some symptoms of the disturbance have persisted for at least 1 month or have occurred repeatedly over a longer period. The diagnosis is most likely to be applicable to patients who have only recently started taking psychoactive substances and, therefore, are less likely to be in danger of marked physiologic withdrawal or withdrawal symptoms (Table 56.8).

Organic Mental Syndromes and Disorders

It is accepted that head injury, occasionally associated with painful cervical trauma, may result in *organic mental syndromes and disorders*. Consistent with the orientation of this chapter, however, we shall not address psychological impairment resulting from neuropsychological sequelae.

Post-Traumatic Stress Disorder

The essential feature of this disorder is the development of characteristic symptoms following a psychologically distressing event that is outside the range of usual human experience. The stressor producing this syndrome would be markedly distressing to almost anyone, and is usually experienced with intense fear, terror, and helplessness. The characteristic symptoms involve re-experiencing the traumatic event, avoidance of stimuli associated with the event or numbing of general responsiveness, and increased arousal. The diagnosis is not made if the disturbance lasts less than 1 month.

The most common traumata involve either a serious threat to one's life or physical integrity; a serious threat or harm to one's children, spouse, or other close relatives and friends; sudden destruction of one's home or community; or witnessing the serious injury or death of another person as the result of an accident or physical violence. The trauma may be experienced alone or in the company of groups of people. Stressors producing this disorder include natural disasters (e.g., earthquakes), accidental disasters, (e.g., car accidents with serious physical injury), or deliberately caused disasters (e.g., bombings). Sometimes there is a concomitant physical component of the trauma, which may even involve direct damage to the central nervous system (e.g., head injury). The disorder is apparently more severe and longer-lasting when the stressor is of human design.

Symptoms characteristic of post-traumatic stress disorder are often intensified or precipitated when the person is exposed to situations or activities that resemble or symbolize the original trauma. Symptoms of depression and anxiety are common and, in some instances, may be sufficiently severe to be diagnosed as an anxiety or depressive disorder. Furthermore, there may be symptoms of an organic mental disorder, such as failing memory, difficulty in concentrating, emotional lability, headache, and vertigo. Symptoms usually appear immediately or soon after the trauma. Impairment may be either mild or severe and may affect nearly every aspect of life (Table 56.9).

During the preparation of this chapter, the American Psychiatric Association was proceeding with development of a revised DSM-4. Fortunately, the DSM-4 will contain a new category entitled *Pain Disorders*, with acute and chronic pain classified into the following subgroups:

1. Pain related to psychological factors
2. Pain related to another mental disorder
3. Pain related to a nonpsychiatric medical condition
4. Pain related to both a nonpsychiatric medical condition and psychological factors
5. Pain not otherwise specified

Although this classification system is an improvement

Table 56.9.
Diagnostic Criteria: Post-Traumatic Stress Disorder

A. The person has experienced an event that is outside the range of usual human experience and that would be markedly distressing to almost anyone (e.g., serious threat to one's life or physical integrity; serious threat or harm to one's children, spouse, or other close relatives and friends; sudden destruction of one's home or community; or witnessing the serious injury or death of another person as the result of an accident or physical violence).

B. The traumatic event is persistently re-experienced in at least one of the following ways:
   1. Recurrent and intrusive distressing recollections of the event (in young children, repetitive play in which themes or aspects of the trauma are expressed)
   2. Recurrent distressing dreams of the event
   3. Sudden acting or feeling as if the traumatic event were recurring (includes a sense of reliving the experience, illusions, hallucinations, and dissociative [flashback] episodes, even those that occur upon awakening or when intoxicated)
   4. Intense psychological distress at exposure to events that symbolize or resemble an aspect of the traumatic event, including anniversaries of the trauma

C. Persistent avoidance of stimuli associated with the trauma or numbing of general responsiveness (not present before the trauma), as indicated by at least three of the following:
   1. Efforts to avoid thoughts or feelings associated with the trauma
   2. Efforts to avoid activities or situations that arouse recollections of the trauma
   3. Inability to recall an important aspect of the trauma (psychogenic amnesia)
   4. Markedly diminished interest in significant activities (in young children, loss of recently acquired developmental skills such as toilet training or language skills)
   5. Feeling of detachment or estrangement from others
   6. Restricted range of affect (e.g., unable to have loving feelings)
   7. Sense of foreshortened future (e.g., does not expect to have a career, marriage, children, or long life)

D. Persistent symptoms of increased arousal (not present before the trauma), as indicated by at least two of the following:
   1. Difficulty falling or staying asleep
   2. Irritability or outbursts of anger
   3. Difficulty concentrating
   4. Hypervigilance
   5. Exaggerated startle response
   6. Physiologic reactivity upon exposure to events that symbolize or resemble an aspect of the traumatic event (e.g., a woman who was raped in an elevator breaks out in a sweat when entering any elevator)

E. Duration of the disturbance (symptoms in *B*, *C*, and *D*) of at least 1 month.

over prior diagnostic categories, there is still an emphasis on the psychiatric view of pain disorders, and in our opinion, the classifications are too broad. Nevertheless, this new addition will complement the classification of pain without the direct assumption that pain has a primary psychiatric etiology.

DEPRESSION AS AN ADDITIONAL DIAGNOSTIC CATEGORY

Aronoff originally reviewed the use of the DSM III in the diagnosis of chronic pain states and found it incomplete in not providing a category for *depression* (as distinct from its listing under Affective Disorders) (11). It is our opinion that the same criticism may be leveled against the DSM III-R.

Depression is the most common emotional disorder determined in patients with chronic pain syndromes (12). Yet this diagnosis is omitted in the DSM III-R's diagnostic categories associated with pain. Although the relationship between chronic pain and depression is often complex, the clinician must be prepared to encounter depression as a concomitant feature of intractable pain and consider this diagnosis in determination of psychological impairment.

Aronoff reports that it is incumbent upon the clinician to recognize and distinguish functional from organic causes of depressive symptoms (11). These may range from dementing processes, some of which may not be reversible, to the most readily reversible organic causes of depression and dementia such as toxic states, endocrine or other metabolic disorders, and normal pressure hydrocephalus. The experienced clinician has likely encountered severely depressed patients presenting with memory disturbance and concentration deficits, superficially representing a pseudodementia that tends to disappear once the depression improves. In addition to clinical evaluation and routine psychological testing, it may be necessary to perform a complete neuropsychological evaluation in patients presenting complex diagnostic pictures, particularly following painful cervical trauma. Although the presence of depression in association with pain is often thought to be reactive to pain, suffering, and alteration in lifestyle, it is not at all uncommon to evaluate patients whose depression preceded the pain or in whom the pain-depression relationship is unclear.

There is growing evidence that depression lowers pain tolerance, increases analgesic requirements, and in a variety of other ways adds to the debilitating effects of pain (13). In the determination of psychological impairment, these symptoms can have significant impact on residual psychological functioning. Patients in pain often suffer from the vegetative signs of depression, including insomnia, appetite fluctuations, diminished libido, excessive use of alcohol or narcotic and sedative-hypnotic medications, and loss of interest in outside activities—all residual signs of psychological impair-

Table 56.10.
Clinical Features of Chronic Pain with Depression

A. Depression may be reactive to pain or may precede pain.
B. The patient suffers from the symptoms of depression in DSM-III:
  1. Poor appetite or significant weight loss (when not dieting) or increased appetite or significant weight gain
  2. Insomnia or hypersomnia
  3. Psychomotor agitation or retardation
  4. Loss of interest in or enjoyment of sex
  5. Social withdrawal
  6. Feelings of unworthiness, self-reproach, or excessive inappropriate guilt
  7. Recurrent thoughts of death, suicidal ideation, wishes to be dead, or suicide attempt
  8. Fearfulness or crying
C. The patient often denies psychological causes of depression and attributes depressive symptoms to pain.
D. Primary defenses are most often somatization, denial, and repression.
E. There is a decreased pain threshold.
F. There is a tenuous support system.
G. Depression is frequently associated with somatic preoccupation and hypochondriasis.
H. Depression is often associated with pain-prone disorder.
I. There is an increased family incidence of pain, depression, and disability.

ment. Although patients usually attribute these problems to pain rather than to depression, the clinician must carefully investigate the causal relationship that exists and determine depression as a psychological impairment if it exists in reaction to pain. Once the pain/depression/insomnia cycle is established, it becomes self-perpetuating and requires active intervention.

Aronoff lists a number of clinical features of chronic pain with depression that are worthy of consideration by the clinician faced with the responsibility of determining psychological impairment (11). It is hoped that future revisions of the DSM will include the diagnostic category of depression in categories associated with pain (Table 56.10).

CONCLUSIONS

Psychological impairment and resulting disability, which often occur in association with pain, will probably continue to be a controversial topic among health professionals for years to come. Historically, our litigious society has intentionally or unintentionally complicated the combination of physical and psychological consequences following injury. It is becoming common practice, however, for many health professionals who evaluate and treat accident victims to secure a multidis-

ciplinary evaluation. There is a growing establishment of pain treatment centers that are specifically designed for the evaluation of the pain patient suffering associated psychological symptoms. Such a comprehensive center may provide a thorough evaluation, including reports from medicine, psychology, psychiatry, physical therapy, and vocational rehabilitation, that collectively addresses the patient's total sphere of functioning.

Early recognition of psychological as well as physical aspects of pain may lead to proper early intervention strategies and prevention of chronicity.

Acknowledgements Portions of this chapter appeared in *Painful Cervical Trauma* (edited by Tollison CD and Satterthwaite JR, published by Williams & Wilkins in Baltimore, 1992. Reprinted with permission of Williams & Wilkins).

REFERENCES

1. Nadolsky JM: Social security: In need of rehabilitation. *J Rehabil* 50:6–8, 1984.
2. AMA Council on Rating Mental and Physical Impairment: Guides to the evaluation of permanent impairment—The extremities and back. *JAMA* 169:1990.
3. United States Department of Health and Human Services, Social Security Administration: *Disability Evaluation Under Social Security*, SSA Pub. No. 64–039. Washington, D.C., U.S. Government Printing Office, May, 1992, pp 68–75.
4. Ziporyn T: Disability evaluation: A fledgling science? *JAMA* 250:873, 1983.
5. Crook PL: Workers' compensation. In Tollison CD: *Handbook of Chronic Pain Management*. Baltimore, Williams & Wilkins, 1989.
6. Sternbach R: *Pain Patients: Traits and Treatment*. Academic Press, New York, 1974.
7. Strang JP: The chronic disability syndrome. In Aronoff GM: *Evaluation and Treatment of Chronic Pain*. Baltimore, Urban & Schwarzenberg, 1985.
8. Tollison CD: Diagnosing and managing chronic pain syndrome. *J S Carolina Med Assoc* Sept:449–452, 1984.
9. Fordyce WE: *Behavioral Methods for Chronic Pain and Illness*. St. Louis, CV Mosby, 1976.
10. American Psychiatric Association: *Diagnostic and Statistical Manual of Mental Disorders*, ed 3—Revised. Washington, D.C., American Psychiatric Association, 1987.
11. Aronoff GM: Psychological aspects of nonmalignant chronic pain: A new nosology. In Aronoff GM: *Evaluation and Treatment of Chronic Pain*. Baltimore, Urban & Schwarzenberg, 1985.
12. Tollison CD, Kriegel ML: Selected tricyclic antidepressants in the management of chronic benign pain. *South Med J* May:562–564, 1988.
13. Tollison CD, Kriegel ML, Satterthwaite JR: Comprehensive treatment of acute and chronic low back pain: A clinical outcome comparison. *Orthop Rev* 1:59–64, 1989.

INDEX

Page numbers followed by "t" denote tables; those followed by "f" denote figures

A-delta fibers, 11, 600
  in opioid action, 157
  specific for nociception, 307
  in teeth, 310
A-delta nociceptor endings, 489
A-fibers, 11, 581, 583
  nociceptor, 308
  in reflex sympathetic dystrophy and causalgia, 488
A vitamin
  inadequacy of, 559
  serum level of, 573
Abdominal muscle pain, 551–552
Aberrant movement subluxation, 98
Ablative neurosurgery, 447–451. *See also* Neuroablative techniques
Abscess, periodontal, 290
Accessory nerve lesions, 479
Accidents
  compensable, 727–728
  compensation formula for injury of, 725–727
  idiopathic and unexplained, 727
Acetaminophen
  in children, 217
  for chronic pain, 590–591
  dosing of by age and weight, 217t
  for malignancy pain, 422–423
  for osteoarthritis, 530
  for rheumatic disease, 526
Acetylsalicylic acid
  development of, 165
  in pain production, 166
Achilles reflex, 99
  absence of, 100
Achilles tendinitis, 537
Acquired immunodeficiency syndrome (AIDS), 504
Active conservative care, 700
Activities of daily living, 690
Activity diary, 630
Acupuncture, 117–120, 582
  in opiate detoxification, 229t
  in pain pathway modulation, 425–426
  for post-herpetic neuralgia, 517
  problems with, 118
  success rate with, 118–119
  in surgical analgesia, 119–120
Acupuncture points, 117
Acyclovir, 507
Adaptive Copers, 144
Adductores brevis muscle pain, 552
Adductores longus muscle pain, 552
Adenine arabinoside (ARA-A), 507
Adenoid cystic carcinoma, 291
Adenomyosis, 403

Adenosine monophosphate, 508
Adenosine triphosphate, storage of, 557
Adjunctive treatment techniques, 108–124
Adjuvant drugs, malignancy, 423–424
Adrenergic blockers, detoxification protocol for, 235
Affective disorders, 748–749
Affective disturbance assessment, 26
Afferent fibers
  pain, 11
  T5-T10, 12
  visceral, blockade of, 59–60
Afferent nociceptors, 600
Afferent pain pathways, 601f
Aging
  pain and, 219
  physiologic and pharmacokinetic changes with, 220, 221t
Alcohol
  headache and, 241
  incidence of abuse and dependence on, 233–234
  in neurolysis, 426–427
  withdrawal detoxification protocols for, 234–235
  withdrawal signs of, 234
Alcohol block, celiac plexus, 451
Alcoholism, malnutrition with, 465
Alexithymia, 593
Alkaloids, 254–255
Alkylating agents, 532
Allergy, 241
Allodynia, 491
Allopurinol, 534
Alpha$_2$-adrenergic agonists, 606
Alpha-adrenergic blockers, detoxification protocol for, 235
Alpha-conducting fibers, 11
Alpha-receptor sensitization, 491
Alprazolam (Xanax), 207
Amantadine, 508
Amebiasis, 261
American Academy of Orthopaedic Surgeons, *Manual for Orthopaedic Surgeons in Evaluating Permanent Physical Impairment*, 734
American Academy of Pain Medicine (AAPM) survey, 142–143
American Chronic Pain Association, patient support by, 685
American Medical Association
  disability and impairment guidelines of, 732–733
  permanent impairment evaluation guidelines of, 747
American Physical Therapy Association guidelines, 702
Americans with Disabilities Act, 731, 739

Amitriptyline
  for acute pain, 182
  with analgesics, 189
  for arthritic disorders, 188
  depressive symptoms with, 186
  for headache, 186
  for low back pain, 187
  mechanism of action of, 189
  for migraine, 186, 258
  for mixed chronic pain, 188
  for neurologic disorders, 182–185
  for peripheral neuropathy, 467
  for post-herpetic neuralgia, 300–301, 512, 513–514
  selection of, 199–200
Amnesia, hypnotic, 111
Amphetamines
  mechanism of action of, 197–199
  for pain, 197
Amygdalectomy, 71
Amyloidosis, 465
Amyotrophic lateral sclerosis, 339
  cervical spine and, 342
  spinal degeneration with, 334
Analgesia
  acupuncture, 119–120
  interpleural, for post-herpetic neuralgia, 516
  patient-controlled, 425, 609–611
  placebo, 120–124
  stimulation-produced, 618
    mechanisms of, 75–76
Analgesics, 155. *See also* Narcotics; Opioids; specific drugs
  agonist-antagonist, 160–161
  for back pain, 631
  for cancer pain, 433
  for chronic pain, 589–593, 631
  classification of, 589t
  clinical use of, 157–158
  continuous infusion of, 607–608
  doctor as, 596–597
  guidelines for selection of, 161–162
  headache with, 241
  for herpes zoster, 506–508
  history of, 155
  intramuscular, 608
  intravenous administration of, 606–608
  lithium interaction with, 204
  for malignancy pain, 421–423
  for migraine, 256
  minimum effective concentration of (MEAC), 609
  narcotic, in children, 217, 218t
  neuroleptics interaction with, 205
  nonnarcotic, 162–163
    interaction with neuroleptics, 205
  NSAIDs as, 167–168
  opioid, 155–162
  opioid receptors and, 155–157
  oral, 609
  for post-herpetic neuralgia, 512
  pure agonist, 158–160
  for rheumatic disease, 526

Analgesics—*continued*
route of administration of, 606–609
subcutaneous, 608–609
systemic
administration methods for, 606–611
pharmacology of, 602–606
transdermal, 609
tricyclic antidepressants as adjuncts to, 188–189
Anatomic variations, 562–563
Anesthesia, neuralgia, 321
Anesthetics
local, with epidural opioids, 616
in nerve block, 52
Angina pectoris, referred, 313
Ankle
fracture or dislocation of, 481–482
jerk, change in, 362
Ankylosing spondylitis, 534
of cervical spine, 371
corticosteroids for, 529
neck pain with, 344
thoracic pain with, 372
treatment of, 535
Annular fibers, 387
Annulus, 386–387
Annulus fibrosis, 369–370
Anserine bursitis, 537
Anterior interosseous nerve syndrome, 472–473
Anterior tarsal tunnel syndrome, 46
Anterolisthesis subluxation, 97
Antianxiety drugs
drug therapy outcomes of, 194–197
for pain, 194–197
in pain syndrome treatment, 206–209
treatment outcome for, 196t
Antibiotics, 506
Anticonvulsants
analgesic effects of, 163
with antidepressants, 201
for herpes zoster, 508
for malignancy pain, 424
for migraine, 259
for post-herpetic neuralgia, 513, 514
Antidepressants
commonly used, 201t
cyclic, 181–182
in depressed pain patients, 202, 595
detoxification protocol for, 235
drug therapy outcomes of, 181–191
for headache in children, 263
for herpes zoster, 508
for malignancy pain, 424
mechanism of action of, 189
for migraine, 258
new, 188
in nondepressed pain patients, 201
for post-herpetic neuralgia, 512
for tension headache, 262
tricyclic, 524
for acute pain, 182
in children, 217–218
for chronic pain, 182–189
interactions of, 199
pretreatment evaluation for, 199
properties and side effects of, 199
selection of, 199–200
treatment techniques with, 200–202
Antiemetics, 256

Antiglycemic therapy, 464–465
Antihistamines, 424
Anti-inflammatory agents, 512; *See also*
Nonsteroidal anti–inflammatory drugs
Antimalarials, 532
Antinuclear antibody test, 525
Anti-panic agents, 233
Antipsychotics, 192–193t
Antiviral agents
for herpes zoster, 506–508
for post-herpetic neuralgia, 512
Anxiety
assessment of, 26
benzodiazepines for, 208–209
management of, 597
postoperative, 207
Anxiety-related disorders, 749
Aphthous, recurrent, 291
Aplastic anemia, with carbamazepine therapy, 295
Apoenzymes, 557, 558
Appendix, pain from, 12
Aquatic exercises, advanced, 397–398
Aquatic rehabilitation
background of, 386
contraindications for, 389t
lumbar spine, 386–398
program of, 393–397
Aquatic stabilization exercises, 396t
Arachidonic acid
cascade, 378
metabolism products of, 165–166
Arachnoiditis, 380
Arachnoidopathy, 380
Archimedes, 389
Arm abduction, prolonged, 564
Armrests, 563
Arteries, thalamus, 70–71
Arthritis. *See also* Osteoarthritis
crystal-induced, 533–534
enteropathic, 534–535
gouty, 342
inflammatory and noninflammatory, 523
NSAIDs for, 165
psoriatic, 534, 535
rheumatoid, 343–344, 530–533
of temporomandibular joint, 317
traumatic, 317
tricyclic antidepressants for, 188
Arthropathies
hip joint, 373–376
painful, 369–376
sacroiliac joint, 369, 373
spinal, 369–373
Arthroplasty, hip, 375–376
Arthroscopy, temporomandibular joint, 316–317
Arthrosis, thoracic, 372
Articular dysfunction, 568
with myofascial trigger points, 574
Aspirin
for cancer pain, 194
for chronic pain, 590–591
development of, 165
for post-herpetic neuralgia, 515
for rheumatic disease, 526–527
for spondyloarthropathies, 535

Aspirin-type drugs, 422–423
Association bundles, long, 16
Atenolol, 235
Atlantoaxial joint, 332
instability of, 370
Atlanto-occipital joint, 331–332
Atrophy
with immobilization, 106
of injured muscle, 92
with musculoskeletal pain, 88
Attention diversion techniques, 441
Augmented operant/multimodality treatment process, 638
Auranofin, 531
Auriculotemporal nerve damage, 325
Aurothioglucose, 531
Aurothiomalate, 531
Auto-traction, 689
Autogenic relaxation, 113, 272
for cancer pain, 441
Autonomic nervous system
nerve blockade of, 58–60
pelvic pain with disorder of, 407
Axillary nerve entrapment, 478
Azathioprine
for rheumatoid arthritis, 532
for spondyloarthropathies, 535

B-complex vitamins, inadequacy of, 558–559
B fibers, 11
B$_{12}$ vitamin
deficiency of, 465
inadequacy of, 559
serum level of, 573
Babinski's reflex, 337
Back
inadequate support of, 563
physical examination of, 357–358
tenderness of, 358
Back pain
active vs. inactive therapy for, 329–330
benzodiazepines and hydroxyzine for, 195–197
consultation for, 668
low
chronic, 581
differential diagnosis of, 347–368
with myofascial syndromes, 548–552
prevention/early intervention in, 630–631
referred, 353
spinal manipulation for, 96–106
spinal surgery for, 328–330
uncomplicated, 99
uncomplicated chronic, 99
Back schools, 624–625
for chronic pain prevention, 630–631
Back-to-work issues, 669–670
Baclofen (Lioresal), 173
dosage of, 174
for migraine, 259
for post-herpetic neuralgia, 513
for post-traumatic headache, 263
for reflex sympathetic dystrophy, 492
side effects of, 174
for trigeminal neuralgia, 281, 295
Bacterial infections
chronic, 261

with herpes zoster, 505
Bacterial septicemia, cervical spine, 371
Balancing, 716
Baltimore Therapeutic Equipment Work Simulator (BTE), 737
Barbiturates
  detoxification protocols for, 229–235
  for pain, 195
Basilar artery migraine, 246
Beck Depression Inventory, 26
Bed rest, contraindication to, 699
Behavioral approaches
  in cancer pain treatment, 442
  in tertiary prevention, 637
Behavioral assessment guidelines, 22–24
Behavioral assessment of pain questionnaire (BAP), 28
Behavioral data collection, 22–24
Behavioral management, in inpatient program, 690–691
Behavioral Methods for Chronic Pain and Illness (Fordyce), 677
Behavioral/physical assessment, 24
Behavioral psychotherapeutic techniques, 626–627
Bellergal, 259
Benign mucous membrane pemphigoid, 291
Benzedrine, 197
Benzodiazepines
  in alcohol withdrawal detoxification, 234–235
  as analgesic adjunct, 606
  for anxiety, 208–209
  for chronic pain, 195–197
  detoxification protocols for, 231–235
  interactions of, 207
  mechanism of action of, 197
  as muscle relaxant, 173
  for pain, 194–195
  physical dependence on, 229–230
  pretreatment evaluation for, 207
  properties and side effects of, 206–207
  selection of, 207
  treatment technique with
    for acute pain, 207–208
    for chronic pain, 208–209
  withdrawal from, 231
Benzoin tincture, 324
Beta-blockers
  detoxification protocol for, 235
  for headache in children, 263
  for migraine, 257
Beta-endorphins, 156
  hypnoanalgesia and, 111–112
  in peripheral nerve endings, 157
Biceps
  reflex testing of, 98–99
  stretch reflex, absence of, 45
Biceps brachii muscle pain, 546
Biceps femoris muscle pain, 553
Bicipital tendinitis, 536
Binding syndrome, 629
Biofeedback, 112–113, 582
  in behavioral management, 691
  for cancer pain, 441
  in chronic pain treatment, 144
  electromyographic, 28, 273–274, 441

forms of, 273
  for headache pain, 273–275
  long-term effects of, 277
  for migraine, 186
Biofeedback-assisted relaxation, 28
Biomechanical fault, 96
Biomechanics, 640, 641
Blistex, 324
Blockage, definition of, 96
Blubourethral glands, 412
Body
  alignment of, 642
  ergonomics of, 691–692
Body roll, 395
Bolus demand-dose, 611
Bone
  demineralization of, 486
  intrinsic pathology of, 335
  orofacial infections of, 289
  pathologic fracture of, 460
  radiation palliation of pain in, 459–460
Bony injury, cervical spine, 343
Borderline personality disorder, 596
Bowstring sign, 358–360
Brachial plexus
  avulsion of
    deafferentation pain in, 62
    mechanism of, 64f
  block of, 617
  malignant invasion of, 460
Brachialis muscle pain, 546
Brachioradialis reflex
  anatomy of, 333
  nerve root responsible for, 99
Bracing, for cervical spine tumors, 340
Bradykinin, 166
Brain. *See also* Cerebral cortex
  abscess of, headache with, 249
  electrical stimulation of, 452
  lesions of for cancer pain, 450–451
  metastases to, 460–461
  tumor of, 249
Brainstem, pain systems of, 13–15
Breast cancer, brachial plexus infiltration in, 448
Breathing technique, 114–115
Brief pain assessment interview, 627–628
Brief Pain Inventory, 436
Bright pain, 11
Brompton's mixture, 197
Bruxism, 287, 318
Buck's fascia, 410
Bulbous urethra, 410
Buoyancy, 389–390
  center of, 389–390
Bupivacaine (Marcaine, Sensorcaine)
  for herpes zoster, 509
  in nerve blockage, 52
  for post-herpetic neuralgia, 515
  for post-traumatic neuralgia, 321
Buprenorphine, 160
  in patient-controlled analgesia, 610
  substitution/detoxification protocol of, 227t
Burning feet, 465
Burning mouth syndrome, 291, 323–324

Bursitis
  anserine, 537
  corticosteroids for, 529
  subacromial, 536
Buspirone, 233
Butorphanol, 161
  pharmacology of, 605
Butyrophenones, 194

C1-C2 instability, 370
C-fibers, 11, 581, 583, 600
  in causalgia, 490
  nociceptor, 308
  in reflex sympathetic dystrophy, 488–489
  stimulation of, 117–118
  unmyelinated, 157
C-polymodal nociceptors, 157
C7 radiculopathy, 41
C8 radiculopathy, 41
C vitamin
  inadequacy of, 558–559
  uricosuric effect of, 560
Caffeine
  mechanism of action of, 198
  for pain, 197
Calamine lotion, 505–506
Calcium antagonists
  for cluster headache, 261
  for migraine, 258
Calcium channel blockers, 258
Calcium pyrophosphate dihydrate deposition disease (CPPD), 533
Calcium supplement, 538
Cancer
  coping strategies for, 435
  neurologic evaluation of, 419–420
  oral, 291
  pain of
    assessment of, 433–438
    complications of, 436
    factors affecting report of, 437–438
    incidence and severity of, 431
    meaning of, 432–433
    neuroleptics for, 194
    neurosurgical treatment of, 447–452
    precipitators of, 434–435
    psychological treatment of, 431, 438–444
    radiation therapy for, 454–461
    severity ratings of, 432
  pain syndromes associated with, 420t
  physical evaluation of, 419–421
  physical treatment of, 421–428
  radiation therapy for, 455
  in terminal stages, 439
  testicular, 415
Cancer mentality, 407
Capsaicin, 162
  for post-herpetic neuralgia, 514
Capsaicin cream, 467
Capsular stretching, manual, 92
Carbamazepine (Tegretol)
  in alcohol withdrawal detoxification, 235
  analgesic effect of, 163
  for atypical facial pain, 300
  in benzodiazepine detoxification, 233
  for geniculate neuralgia, 299
  for glossopharyngeal neuralgia, 285, 299
  for lithium nonresponse, 204

Carbamazepine—*continued*
for migraine, 259
for post-herpetic neuralgia, 513
for post-traumatic headache, 263
side effects of, 295
for trigeminal neuralgia, 281, 294–295
Carbidopa-levodopa (Sinemet)
for lithium nonresponse, 204
for post-herpetic neuralgia, 513
Carbon monoxide poisoning, 241
Carcinoma
neuropathy with, 466
orofacial, 302
penile, 416
Cardiac rehabilitation, interdisciplinary, 707
Cardiopulmonary conditions, 86
Cardiovascular disorders, 354
Career Evaluation System, 715
Carisoprodol
action of, 174
dosage of, 174
as muscle relaxant, 173
side effects of, 175
Carotidynia, 300
Carpal tunnel syndrome, 42–43, 378, 470–471
clinical features of, 471
pathology of, 471–472
prevalence of, 646
treatment of, 472
Carpi radialis muscle pain, 547–548
Carprofen, 168–169
Carrying, 716
Catechol-O-methyltransferase, 490
Catheter
lumbar epidural, 613
placement for narcotic administration, 613
Cauda equina syndrome, 360
Caudal medulla, 14
Causalgia, 12
clinical signs and symptoms of, 464–495t, 485t, 486
diagnostic considerations for, 487t
with neuromas, 314
syndrome of, 380
theory of, 486–488
Causalgia minor, 58
Celiac ganglion block, 59–60
Celiac plexus, alcohol block of, 451
Central nervous system
lithium effects on, 203
pain pathways of, 309f
in pain transmission, 581
Central nervous system stimulants
for acute and chronic pain, 197
drug therapy outcomes of, 197–199
interactions of, 209
mechanism of action of, 197–199
for pain syndromes, 209
properties and side effects of, 209
treatment outcome of, 198t
Central spine spondylosis, 248–249
Cephalgia, benign orgasmic, 247
Cephalic vasomotor feedback, 273, 275
Ceramide trihexosidase deficiency, 466
Cerebellopontine angle tumor, 281

Cerebral cortex
pain impulse to, 15–16
in pain perception, 16
Cerebrospinal fluid
blocking of, 241
clearance mechanisms of, 611–612
elevated pressure of, 249
Cervical cordotomy, 71
Cervical muscle pain, posterior, 544
Cervical nerve roots, 333
blockade of, 55
pain with disorders of, 336
Cervical outflow, 488
Cervical pain syndromes, 338–343
differential diagnosis and management of, 331–346
manipulation for, 101
Cervical spine
anatomy and biomechanics of, 332–333
arthropathy, 370–371
management of, 371–372
referred pain in, 372
benign or malignant lesion of, 371
clinical examination of, 335–337
diagnostic studies of, 337–338
hyperextension of, 371
inflammatory disease of, 371
medical history of, 335
pathology of, 334–335
stiffness of, 370–371
strain/sprain injuries of, 101
traction of, 372
traumatic injuries to, 342–343, 371
tumors of, 339–340
Cervical spondylosis, 324
Cervicoencephalic syndrome, 27
Cheiralgia paresthetica, 44
Chemical hypophysectomy, 71–72
Chemical neurolysis, 426–427
Chemical sympathectomy, 516
Chemistry battery, 573
Chemotherapy, 340
Chickenpox infection, 69, 503
Children
dosage in, 216
drug interactions in, 218
drug selection for, 216–217
headache treatment of, 262–263
pain assessment in, 31–32
pain questionnaire for, 33f
pharmacologic pain management in, 215–219
Children's Comprehensive Pain Questionnaire (CCPQ), 32
Chinese pain philosophy, 117–120
Chlorambucil, 532
Chlordiazepoxide (Librium), 207
for acute pain, 208
in alcohol withdrawal detoxification, 234
for headache, 195
for pain, 194
Chlorphenesin, 175
Chlorphenesin carbamate (Maolate), 295
Chlorpromazine (Thorazine)
analgesic activity of, 191
for cancer pain, 194
for cluster headache, 261
for headache, 263
interaction with neuroleptics, 205

for migraine, 256
Chlorprothixene (Taractan), 512, 513
Chlorzoxazone, 175
Choline magnesium trisalicylate, 527
Chondrosarcoma, maxillary, 289
Chronic enigmatic pain, 568
causes of, 569–570
Chronic intractable benign pain syndrome (CIBPS), 383t, 691
Chronic pain, 306–307. *See also* Chronic pain syndrome
affective dimension of, 568–569
alternative theories of, 676
analgesics for, 589–593
anxiety with, 208–209
assessment instruments for, 21t
behavioral and emotional factors in, 19–20
behavioral and observational assessment of, 22–24
of benign origin, 447
in children, 31–32, 215–219
classification of, 7–10, 714
cognitive-behavioral assessment of, 136, 141–144, 149
cognitive-behavioral treatment of, 144–149
cognitive component of, 5–6
components of, 4–6
in elderly, 30–31, 219–222
hypnosis in, 109–112
joint and connective tissue, 523–538
legal implications of, 714–715
of malignant origin, 447
monoamine oxidase inhibitors for, 203
nerve blocks in management of, 51–52
neural stimulation techniques for, 74–82
outpatient management programs for, 676–685
predictors of conservative treatment of, 29–30
predisposing central factors to, 381t
with psychiatric disorders, 593–597
psychological assessment in, 19–20
psychosomatic, 377
psychotherapy for, 383
radiation palliation of, 454–461
Social Security and, 714–715
taxonomy of patients with, 143–144
Chronic pain specialist, 730–731
Chronic pain syndrome
characteristics of, 568
classification scheme for, 632
critique of, 632–634
early recognition of, 623–638
education campaigns for, 624–625
groups in, 144
history and examination in, 628–630
mixed, 188
rehabilitation and tertiary prevention of, 636–638
Ciguatera, 339
Cimetadine, 508
Cingulate gyrus activity, 310
Cingulotomy, 450–451
for thalamic pain, 71
Cingulumotomy, 517
Classification types, 7–8
Claudicant leg pain, 355t
Climbing, 716

Clinical Analysis Questionnaire (CAQ), 29

Clinical medicine, classification systems in, 8–9

Clinical symptom complex, 89, 90

Clomipramine (Anafranil), 186

Clonazepam (Clonopin)
in benzodiazepine detoxification, 233t
for pain, 194
for trigeminal neuralgia, 208, 295

Clonidine (Catapres)
in alcohol withdrawal detoxification, 235
for cancer pain, 451
for migraine, 259
in opiate detoxification, 226–228, 229t, 230t
pharmacology of, 606

Clorazepate (Tranxene), 207

Cluster analysis, 143–144

Cluster headache, 240, 247–248
chronic, 247, 259
distinguishing features of, 248t
episodic, 259
etiology of, 247
treatment of, 259–260
preventive, 260–261
symptomatic, 260
trigger factors in, 247
variant, 247–248
with vascular dysfunction, 300
warning signs of, 241

Cobalamin, 559

Cocaine, 197

Codeine, 159
in children, 217
interaction with MAOIs, 202–203
for post-herpetic neuralgia, 512
for rheumatic disease, 526

Cognitive assessment, 26–27

Cognitive Behavior Therapy Package (CBTP), 443

Cognitive-behavioral approach
assumptions of, 138–139
to chronic pain assessment, 141–144
chronic pain concepts in, 136–140
to chronic pain treatment, 144–149
components of, 147–149
interdisciplinary team in, 145–147
objectives of, 139–140

Cognitive Error Questionnaire, 26

Cognitive restructuring, 441–442

Cognitive Strategies Questionnaire, 29

Cognitive techniques
for cancer pain, 441–442
for headache pain, 275–276

Colchicine, 533

Collagen disease
of cervical spine, 371
orofacial pain with, 325

Collagen fiber, growth and realignment of, 88

Colle's fascia, 412

Colloid cysts, 241

Collusion, 746

Colon cancer, 461

Colostomy, 157

Commission on Accreditation of Rehabilitation Facilities (CARF), 18
standards of, 677, 682–684

work hardening programs of, 705–706

Commission on Pain Evaluation of the Social Security Administration, 634–636

Commissural myelotomy, 449

Communication
with patient, 670–671
skills of in cognitive-behavioral approach, 140

Compensation
for chronic back pain, 581, 630
for disability, 586–587
formula for, 724–728
impact on prevention/early intervention, 634–636
in tort-based system, 722–723
Workers' Compensation and, 722–731;
See also Workers' Compensation

Complex repetitive discharges, 38

Compliance, 690

Comprehensive pain centers, 589

Comprehensive treatment programs, cancer, 442–443

Comprehensiveness, 678–680

Compression neuropathy
definition of, 470
of median nerve, 470–473
of radial nerve, 475–476
of ulnar nerve, 473–475

Computed tomography
in assessing low back pain, 347
cervical spine, 337, 343
of head, 243
for mechanical low back pain, 365–366

Computer operator
environment of, 655–656
repetitive movements of, 657–658

Conceptualization-translation, 443

Conditioning principles, 105

Condyloma acuminata, 416

Condylomata, 417

Connective tissue disease, 535–536
treatment of, 536

Conservative treatment, predictors of, 29–30

Consistency, 678–680

Contingency contracts, 681

Contingency management, 597

Contingent reinforcers, 442

Conversion disorder, 750–751

Conversion state, headache with, 270

Conversion syndrome, 629

Conversion V pattern, 593

Coping skills, 570

Coping strategies
for cancer pain, 435, 441–442
plans for, 149

Cordotomy
anterolateral, 449–450
for phantom pain, 500
for post-herpetic neuralgia, 517

Corgard. See Nadolol (Corgard)

Corona radiata, 16

Corpus luteum cyst, 404

Corpus spongiosum, 410

Corticosensory evoked potentials, 28

Corticosteroids

for chronic pain, 593
for connective tissue disease, 536
for crystal-induced arthritis, 533
depot, 529
for herpes zoster, 506
for inflammatory vascular disease, 300
intra-articular, 529, 530
for polymyalgia rheumatica, 538
for rheumatic disease, 528–529
for rheumatoid arthritis, 532
for spondyloarthropathies, 535

Corticothalamic fibers, 15

Cost-effectiveness, of inpatient programs, 692

Costen's theory, 318

Costovertebral-costransverse subluxation, 98

Counseling, 690–691
early intervention, 700

Counterirritation techniques, 517

Countertransference, 746

Cox, James C., manipulation technique of, 102

Cracked tooth syndrome, 290, 323

Crane breathing, 397f

Cranial nerves, 239
eleventh, 332
ninth, 284–285
in orofacial nociception, 308
seventh, 284
sympathetic, 12

Cranial neuritides, 249–250

Cranial tissues, pain sensitivity of, 240t

Craniofacial pain, musculoskeletal origin, 286–289

Crawling, 718

Crepitus, 288
of temporomandibular joint, 320

Crossover kick, 93

Crouching, 718

Crying, 585

Cryoanalgesia, 619
for post-herpetic neuralgia, 516

Crystal-induced arthritis, 533
treatment of, 533–534

CTDs. See Cumulative trauma disorders

Cubital tunnel syndrome, 43, 473–474

Cue-controlled relaxation, 272

Cultural stereotypes, 584–585

Cumulative trauma disorders, 645
anatomy of case of, 650
causes of, 646
control program for, 652
engineering intervention for, 649
ergonomic factor in, 646–647
expert system for detecting, 660–664
impairment rating for, 733
management factor in, 649–650
people factors in, 647–649
prevalence of, 646
rate of occurrence of, 646
stages of, 650–651
treatment of, 651–652

Current Procedural Terminology (CPT) codes, 672–675

Cyclo-oxygenase enzyme inhibition, 166

Cyclobenzaprine, 176
tricyclic-like, 173

Cyclophosphamide, 300
  for rheumatoid arthritis, 532
Cyproheptadine (Periactin)
  for cluster headache, 261
  for migraine, 259
Cystoscopy, 413
Cysts, ovarian, 403–404
Cytosine arabinoside (ARA-C), 507

D vitamin
  inadequacy of, 559
  for polymyalgia rheumatica, 538
Danazol (Danocrine)
  for endometriosis, 405
  for migraine, 264
De Quervain's syndrome, 44
De Quervain's tendinitis, 537
Deafferentation pain
  with cancer, 420
  chemical hypophysectomy for, 71–72
  dental, 314
  diagnosis of, 62
  facial, DREZ lesions for, 450
  neurosurgical treatment of, 62–72
  with paraplegia, 65–66
  post-herpetic, 67–70
  with spinal root avulsion, 63–65
  syringomelia and, 66–67
  in thalamic syndrome, 70–71
  treated by thalamic electrode
    placement, 79
Death benefits, 729
Deconditioning syndrome, 707
Deep brain stimulation, 79–80
  electrode system for, 78f
Deep-heating modalities, 85
Degenerative cascade, 387
Degenerative joint disease,
  temporomandibular, 317
Delayed diagnosis, 615
Delirium, alcohol withdrawal, 234
Delta receptors, 156
  stimulation of, 157
Deltoid muscle pain, 545
Delusional state, headache with, 270
Dementia, drug-induced in elderly, 222
Demyelinating neuropathies, 463
Denervation, facet joint, 60
Denovilliers' fascia, 410
Dental pain, 306–308
  pathologies of, 314–326
  physiologic background of, 308–314
  temporomandibular dysfunction and,
    314–320
Dentin, 311–312
  sensitivity theories for, 311–312
Dephenylmethane derivatives, 194–195
Depression, 594–595
  assessment of, 26
  atypical, 594–595
  chronic pain with, 755–756
  cyclical, cluster headache and, 261
  definition of, 182
  as diagnostic category, 755–756
  headache and, 241, 261
  patterns of, 243t
  with somatization, 629
  tricyclic antidepressants with, 202

Depressive equivalent, 594
Dermatomes, 11–12
  involved in shingles, 69
Descending pathways, 17
Descending spinal tracks, 18
Desipramine (Norpramin, Pertofrane)
  for acute pain, 182, 200–201
  for low back pain, 188
  for post-herpetic neuralgia, 185, 512
  selection of, 199–200
Dexamethasone, 529
Dexedrine, 197
Dextroamphetamine
  as analgesic adjunct, 606
  for depression, 595
  for malignancy pain, 424
Dextromethorphan, 202
Dezocine, 161
DHE
  for cluster headache, 260, 261
  for headache, 263
Diabetes
  mononeuropathy of, 355
  neuropathy of, 467
  peripheral neuropathy in, 464–465
  relaxation training with, 116
*Diagnostic and Statistical Manual of Mental
  Disorders*, 750–756
  revised edition of, 182
Diagnostic Statistics Model III, chronic pain
  classification of, 632–634
Diagnostic technology, 18
Diamond Headache Clinic study, 244
Diazepam (Valium), 176–177, 207
  for acute pain, 195, 207–208
  in alcohol withdrawal detoxification, 234
  for back pain, 196–197
  in benzodiazepine detoxification, 233t
  for chronic pain, 195
  depressive symptoms with, 186
  dosage of, 177
  for headache, 186
  for pain, 194
  side effects of, 177
Diclofenac, 169
  for myofascial pain syndrome, 574
  for rheumatic disease, 527
Dictionary of Occupational Title, 737, 740
Diffuse idiopathic skeletal hyperostosis, 344
Diflunisal, 605–606
Diltiazem (Cardizem), 258
Dimenhydrinate (Dramamine), 574
Diphenhydramine derivative, 178
Diphenylhydantoin, 281
Direct diminution, 439–440
Direct observation, 22
Disability
  adjudication process of, 713–714
  benefits for, 728–729
  with chronic low back pain, 581
  collusion in claims of, 746
  compensation for, 586–587, 630
  decreased, 702
  definition of, 4, 86, 742
  determination of, 732–734
  evaluation and rating of, 732–740
  exaggerated, 351–353
  issues of, 669–670

  legal aspects of, 712–721
  nonorganic, 349, 353t
  pain in, 86–87
  physical, 732–740
  presenting findings on, 739–740
  preventing long-term, 628–629
  prevention/early intervention impact on,
    634–636
  psychological, 742–756
  report and rating of, 734–739
  vocational relevance of, 713
Disability Evaluation Under Social Security,
  733–734
Disability specialist, 730–731
Disabled patient, 144
Discomfort, ergonomic analysis of, 645
Disease
  accident and, 726–727
  definition of, 86
Disk degeneration, 387
Diskectomy, 373
Displacement suggestions, cancer pain, 440
Dissociation, 440
Distraction, 441
Distress and risk assessment method, 26
Dopamine system, 582–583
Dorsal column stimulation, 517
Dorsal rhizotomy, 516–517
Dorsal root entry zone, physiology and
  neuroanatomy of, 62–63; *See also* DREZ
  operation
Dorsal root ganglia, 11–12
Dorsal root ganglionopathy, 466
Dorsal root selective nerve blocks, 515
Do's and don't's training, 654
Dosage
  of acetaminophen, 217
  in children, 216
  in elderly, 220–221
Doxepin (Sinequan, Adapin)
  for acute pain, 182
  with analgesics, 189
  for atypical facial pain, 187
  for migraine, 258
  for mixed chronic pain, 188
  in opiate detoxification, 228
  selection of, 199–200
DREZ. *See* Dorsal root entry zone; DREZ
  operation
DREZ caudalis electrode, 68
DREZ operation
  for cancer pain, 450
  for causalgia, 490–491
  in cord medulla, 69f
  overall results of, 71f
  in paraplegia, 65–66
  for post-herpetic neuralgia, 517
  for post-herpetic pain, 68–70
  for spinal root avulsion, 63–65
  for syringomyelia, 67
  in traumatic paraplegia, 65–66
Drop attacks, 241
Droperidol, 606
Drug detoxification, 691
Drug detoxification protocols
  hyponosedative, 229–235
  miscellaneous, 235
  for opiates, 224–229

Drug interactions. *See also* specific agents
in children, 218
in elderly, 220–221
Dundee group, 191
Dynorphin, 156
in opioid action, 157
Dysesthesias, 62
in peripheral neuropathy, 463
Dysesthetic chronic pain, 382
Dysfunctional patient, 144
Dysmenorrhea, 402–403
with endometriosis, 405
Dyspareunia, 407
Dystonia, 205

E vitamin, inadequacy of, 559
Eagle's syndrome, 301, 325–326
Ear, lesions of, 289–290
Earache, 313
Early intervention, 623. *See also*
Prevention/early intervention
counseling in, 700
Ectopic impulse, 489
Ectopic pregnancy, 402
Education
in cognitive-behavioral treatment, 147
for phantom pain, 500
in primary prevention, 624–625
Educational skills training programs,
cancer pain, 442
Efferents, visceral, blockade of, 58–59
Ehlers-Danlos syndrome, 325
Elavil. *See* Amitryptyline
Elbow, degenerative arthritis of, 473–474
Elderly
altered pain perception in, 215
dementia in, 222
dosage in, 220–221
drug interactions in, 220–221
excretion of medications in, 220
homeostasis in, 220
overprescribing in, 215
pain assessment in, 30–31
pharmacokinetics in, 220
pharmacologic pain management in,
219–222
polypharmacy in, 221, 222
unpredictable drug effects in, 222
Electrical stimulation. *See also* Electrical
stimulation devices; Transcutaneous
electrical nerve stimulation
analgesic mechanisms of, 75–76
of brain, 452
for chronic pain, 583
considerations in patient management
with, 76
deep brain, 79–80
of peripheral nerves, 74–75
spinal cord, 76–79, 452
Electrical stimulation devices
failure of, 79–80
implanted, 80–81
increasing use of, 74
indications for implant of, 76
Electroconvulsive therapy, 595
Electrodiagnostic examination, 46–47
Electrodiagnostic studies, 36–47
clinical applications of, 40–46

for mechanical low back pain, 367
Electrolytes, low levels of, 560
Electromyographic biofeedback, 28, 273,
274
in cancer pain treatment, 441
Electromyography, 36–37
of cervical spine, 338
insertional activity in, 37
for mechanical low back pain, 367
of resting muscle, 37–38
of voluntary muscle contraction, 38
Electrophysiologic testing, cervical spine,
338
EMG. *See* Electromyography
Emotional constraint, 585
Emotional state, 5
Employability enhancement, 704
Employer-oriented occupational medicine,
700
Employers, psychological disability and,
747
Endep. *See* Amitriptyline
Endocrine dysfunction, 560
Endometriosis, 404–405
internal, 403
Endorphins, 156–157, 582
activation of, 378–379
in drug detoxification, 691
hypnoanalgesia and, 111–112
Enkephalin, 118, 156
in opioid action, 157
in orofacial analgesic systems, 312
Enteropathic arthritis, 534–535
Entrapment neuropathy, 463–467
of arm, 478–479
definition of, 470
of femoral nerve, 480–481
of lateral cutaneous nerve of thigh, 481
of median nerve, 470–473
of peroneal nerve, 479–480
of radial nerve, 475–476
of saphenous nerve, 481
of sciatic nerve, 480
of tibial nerve, 481–482
of ulnar nerve, 473–475
Entrapment syndromes, 383
electrodiagnosis of, 42–46
Environment, extremes of, 653
Environmental stimulation techniques, 441
Enzymes, dysfunction of, 557–559
Ependymoma, 339
Epicondylitis, lateral, 536
Epicritic pain, 11
Epididymis, 411
pain from, 415
Epididymo-orchitis, 416
Epidural nerve block, 54
for post-herpetic neuralgia, 515
Epidural venography, 367–368
Epileptogenic foci, development of, 314
Epinephrine, 52
Episilon receptors, 156
Equipment, occupational rehabilitation, 698
Ergo Snapshot, 642, 644f
Ergonomic checklist, 643f
Ergonomics

analysis, 642
applications of, 642
approach of, 641
areas of study in, 641
cumulative trauma disorders and, 645–
654
deficiencies of, 642–645, 662–663
definition of, 640
detecting deficiencies of, 661
effectiveness of, 660
expert system for detecting cumulative
trauma disorders, 660–664
improvements in workplace, 654–658
cost of, 658–660
industry recommendations for, 662f
in inpatient treatment programs, 691–692
principles of, 640
in risk assessment, 660
Ergonovine maleate (Ergotrate), 257
Ergot alkaloids
for migraine, 257–258
rebound headaches with, 241
Ergotamine, adverse effects of, 255
Ergotamine tartrate
inhalant or rectal forms of, 264
for migraine, 254–255
Ergotism, 255
ERIC Work Hardening program, 706
Ernest's syndrome, 326
Erythrocyte sedimentation rate (ESR), 525
Ethanol. *See* Alcohol
Ethmoid sinus infection, 289
Ethyl chloride spray, 517
Etodolac, 169, 170
Evaluation and Treatment of Chronic Pain, 383
Evoked potentials
in pain assessment, 28
somatosensory, 40
Exaggeration reaction, with back pain, 349
description of, 351–353
Exercise
in aquatic lumbar spine rehabilitation,
393–397
for cumulative trauma disorder, 652
for musculoskeletal function, 572
physiatric prescriptions for, 85
in rehabilitation, 690
Extension subluxation, 97
Extensor digitorum muscle
pain of, 547–548, 554
trigger points of, 569–570
Extensor hallucis longus weakness, 362
Exteroceptive sensations, 498
Extra-articular pain syndromes, 536–537
treatment of, 537–538
Extracranial surgery, 321
Extrapyramidal symptoms, 205
Extremities, physical examination of, 358–
360; *See also* Lower extremities; Upper
extremities
Eye movement abnormalities, 79

F wave, 39–40
Fabry's disease, 466
Facet degeneration, 387
Facet joint
block and denervation of, 60
block of, 366–367

Facet joint—*continued*
  neurolysis in denervation of, 53
Facet syndrome, 60
Facial pain, atypical, 250, 283, 291
  neurosurgical treatment of, 299–300
  tricyclic antidepressants for, 187
Facial sensation, anatomical organization
  of, 67–68
Failed back syndrome, 328
  causes of, 329
  spinal cord stimulation for, 76, 77
Family
  in chronic pain treatment, 146
  in psychological disability, 746
  in rehabilitation and pain prevention
    program, 638
  therapy for, 690
Fasciculation potentials, 37–38
Fatigue, headache and, 241
Feasibility Evaluation Checklist, 702, 703f
Feedback, negative, 117–118
Feeling, 718
Female genital tract, 401
  pain etiologies of, 401–407
Femoral nerve
  anatomy of, 480
  entrapment of, electrodiagnosis of, 45
  stretch of, 360
  syndromes of, 480–481
Fenamic acids, 170
Fenoprofen, 527
Fentanyl, 160
  intravenous, 606–607
  in patient-controlled analgesia, 610
Fentanyl/bupivacain formulation, 616
Fibrillation potentials, 37
Fibroids, 403
Fibromyalgia, 541, 567–568
  tricyclic antidepressants for, 188
Fibrositis, 567–568
Fibrositis/fibromyalgia, with myofascial
  trigger points, 574
Field blocks, 617
Fight or flight mechanism, 601
Financial incentives, 586–587
Fingering, 718
Finklestein's test, positive, 44
Fisk, James W., 568
Fitness education, 628
Five Axis Pain Taxonomy, 8–9
Fixation
  definition of, 96
  of vertebral motion, 98
Flexion-subluxation, 97
Flexor hallucis longus weakness, 362
Flexores digitorum pain, 548
Flubiprofen, 527
Fluori-Methane technique, 319
Fluoroscope, 53
Fluoroscopy, 54, 55
Fluoxetine (Prozac), 188
  for depression, 595
  efficacy of, 186
  for migraine, 258
Fluphenazine (Prolixin)
  for chronic pain, 206

for headache, 194
for post-herpetic neuralgia, 301, 512, 513–
  514
Flurbiprofen, 168–169
Focal tenderness, in single-muscle
  myofascial syndromes, 540
Folate, inadequacy of, 559
Folic acid deficiency, 324
Follicle-stimulation hormone, 403
Follicular cysts, 403
Follow-up planning, 681–682
Foot, pain in, 554
Foraminal encroachment subluxation, 98
Force
  excessive, 642
    avoidance of, 653
  high, 646
Fordyce, Wilbert, 677
  gate control model of, 136–137
Forearm supination, forceful or repetitive,
  564
Forrestier's disease, 344
Fossa navicularis, 410
Fractionation, 111
Fractures
  with bone metastases, 460
  temporomandibular, 317–318
Frey's syndrome, 325
Frontal sinus infection, 289–290
Functional adaptation complex, 89
Functional biomechanical deficit, 89, 90
Functional capacity
  assessment of, 736–739
  definitions of, 4
  development of, 704
    at home, 5
    at work, 5
Functional limitation, 4
Functional progression, 105, 106
Functional restoration, 706–708
  program outcome for, 708
  psychological evaluation in, 19–20

G proteins, opioid receptors and, 156–157
GABA. *See* Gamma-amino butyric acid
Galvanic stimulation, 565
Gamma-amino butyric acid, 163
  in neurotransmitter inhibition, 197
  neurotransmitter systems of, 582–583
Ganciclovir, 507
Gap junctions, odontoblastic zone, 311
Gastrocnemius muscle
  pain in with myofascial syndromes, 554
  weakness of, 362
Gate control theory, 18, 117–118, 136–137
  evidence against, 75–76
  first clinical application of, 74–75
  introduction of, 74
  in phantom pain, 498–499
  transmission cells in, 310
General Education Development (GED)
  Scale, 717–718t, 720
Geniculate neuralgia, 284
  neurosurgical treatment of, 299
Giant cell arteritis, 537
  blindness with untreated, 537–438

Giant cell tumor, cervical spine, 371
Glans penis, 410
Gliomas, spinal, 338–339
Glisson's capsule, infiltration of, 461
Glossodynia, 291, 323
  treatment of, 323–324
Glossopharyngeal nerve, 239
Glossopharyngeal neuralgia, 250, 284–285
Gluteus maximus pain, 552
Gluteus medius pain, 552
Gluteus minimus pain, 552
Glycerol, 296–297
Gold compounds, 531
Gonadotropin-releasing hormone agonists,
  403
Gonadotropin-releasing hormone analogs,
  405
Gout, 533
  cervical spine, 342
  treatment of, 533–534
Graphic Rating Scale, 24
Grasp, repeated or sustained, 564
Gravity, center of, 389–390
Grid classification, 8f
Grief, 596
Group approaches, 685
Group psychotherapy, 383
Group therapy, 690
Guided reactivation, 701–702
*Guides to the Evaluation of Permanent
  Impairment* (AMA), 732–733, 735–739, 747
Guillain-Barre syndrome, 465, 466
Guyon's canal
  masses in, 474, 475
  ulnar nerve compression at, 43–44
Gynecologic pain, 401
  diagnostic tools in, 401–402
  with ectopic pregnancy, 402
  with endometriosis, 404–405
  infectious causes of, 406
  ovarian causes of, 403–404
  unexplained causes of, 406–407
  uterine causes of, 402–403

H reflex, 39
Halazepam (Paxipam), 207
Halban's syndrome, 404
Hallucis longus muscle pain, 554
Haloperidol (Haldol)
  for chronic pain, 206
  for neurologic disorders, 194
Hamilton Rating Scale for Depression, 26
Hamstring jerk, change in, 362
Hand
  pain in with myofascial syndromes, 548
  repetitive motions of, 657–658
Handicap, definition of, 86
Handling, 718
Hansen's disease, 380
Hazards, work, 719
Head
  computed tomographic scan of, 243
  pain in single-muscle myofascial
    syndromes, 541–542
  pain-sensitive structures of, 239, 240t

Head, Henry, 11
Head-forward posture, 563
Headache
  Ad Hoc Committee on the Classification
    of, 253
  allergies and, 241
  assessment of, 270–272
  associated symptoms of, 240–241
  benzodiazepines and hydroxyzine for,
    195
  cervical origin, 101
  in children, 262–263
  chronic, 253
  classification of, 244–251
  cluster, 300
  differential diagnosis of, 239–251, 270–
    272
  factors in, 241
  imaging studies for, 243–244
  incidence of, 239
  in inpatient units, 264–265
  laboratory studies for, 242–243
  location of, 240
  lower-half, 286, 300
  medical management of, 253–265
  medication overuse and dependency in,
    264
  multiple medication regimens for, 265
  neuroleptics for, 194
  ocular causes of, 251
  onset of, 239
  patient history of, 239–241
  physical and neurologic examination for,
    241–242
  positional, 241
  post-traumatic, 263
  precipitating factors in, 241
  prodromal symptoms and signs of, 240
  psychological management of, 268, 272–
    277
  radiation palliation of, 460–461
  rebound, 264
  severity and pain characteristics of, 240
  special drug techniques for, 263–264
  with temporomandibular joint disease,
    316
  tension, 240–249, 253, 262, 541
  time, course, and frequency of, 239–240
  treatment of
    general considerations in, 254
    medical, 254–265
  tricyclic antidepressants for, 186–187
  types and defining characteristics of,
    268–270
  tyramine and, 242t
Headache questionnaire, 271
Health studies, ergonomic, 641
Hearing, 718
Heavy work, 716, 738
Helplessness, learned, 31
Hemiplegic migraine, 246
Hernias, obturator, 45
Herniated disk, 335
  manipulation for, 101
  MRI of, 365f
  radiculopathy with, 40
  risk of, 387
Herniated nucleus pulposus, 357
  location of, 358f
  neuritis from, 378
Herpecin-L, 324

Herpes infections, gynecologic, 406
Herpes simplex viruses
  orofacial pain with, 324
  type 1, 560–261
Herpes virus type 1, 560
Herpes zoster, 503. *See also* Post-herpetic
  neuralgia
  clinical manifestations of, 504–505
  complications of, 505
  diagnosis of, 505
  distribution of lesions of, 504t
  treatment of, 505–509
Herpes zoster neuritis, 379–380
Herpesvirus varicellae, 503
High-voltage pulsed galvanic
  stimulation, 91
Hip joint arthropathy
  diagnosis of, 374
  hip arthroplasty for, 375–376
  pathology of, 373–374
  total hip revision for, 376
  treatment of, 374–376
Hip pathology, 354
Histamine desensitization, 261
History-taking, 673
HLA-B27, in joint fluid, 526
Ho-Ku point, 118
Home, functional status at, 5
Homeostasis, in care for elderly, 220
Homework, cognitive-behavioral treatment,
  148–149
Horner's syndrome, 251
  incomplete, 286
Hospital-based inpatient treatment
  programs, 686–687
  behavioral management in, 690–691
  cost-effectiveness of, 692
  description of, 687
  ergonomics in, 691–592
  goals and objectives of, 687–688
  nursing care in, 692
  objective findings in, 691
  patient profile in, 688–689
  physical medicine and rehabilitation in,
    9–690
  vocational rehabilitation in, 690
Hospital consultations, 670
Hospitalization, criteria for, 686–687
Human chorionic gonadotropin assays, 402
Human immunodeficiency virus (HIV)
  infection, 465
Human papilloma viruses, condylomata
  with, 417
Hunt's syndrome, 504
HVPGS. *See* High-voltage pulsed galvanic
  stimulation
Hydrocele, scrotal, 416
Hydrocortisone, 263
Hydrodynamic theory, 312
Hydromorphone (Dilaudid), 159
  for cancer pain, 451
  efficacy of, 161
Hydrostatic pressure, 390–391
Hydroxyapatite deposition disease, 533
Hydroxychloroquine, 536
Hydroxyzine (Vistaril)
  for acute pain, 195

  as analgesic adjunct, 606
  for chronic pain, 195–197
  interaction with lithium, 204
  mechanism of action of, 197
  for migraine, 256
Hyperanalgesia mechanical, 489, 491
Hyperemia, 52
Hyperextensive trauma, 325
Hyperintensity density areas, 244
Hypermobility, 98
Hyperpathia, 70
Hyper-reflexia, 337
  with spinal cord compression, 339
Hypersensitivity, thermal, 492
Hypertension, relaxation training with, 116
Hypnoanalgesia, 108, 109
  direct hypnotic suggestion in, 109–110
  hypnotic dissociation in, 110
  hypnotic time disorientation in, 110
  indirect hypnotic suggestion in, 110
  mechanism of, 111–112
  techniques of, 110–111
Hypnoanesthesia, 108
Hypnoplasty, 110–111
Hypnosis, 108–112, 582
  for cancer pain, 439–440
  efficacy of, 116–117
  for phantom pain, 500
  susceptibility to, 108–109
Hypnotic amnesia, 111
Hypnotic displacement, 110
Hypnotic dissociation, 110
Hypnotic reinterpretation, 110
Hypnotic suggestion
  direct, 109–110
  indirect, 110
Hypnotic time disorientation, 110
Hypochondria, 270
Hypochondriac, 585
Hypochondriasis, 593–594, 751
Hypoglycemia, 560
Hypometabolism, 560
Hypomobility, 98
Hyponosedatives, detoxification protocols
  for, 229–235
Hypophysectomy
  for cancer pain, 450
  chemical, 71–72
Hypothalamic autonomic centers,
  stimulation of, 602
Hypothalamic-pituitary-adrenal (HPA) axis
  suppression, 528–529
Hypothalamotomy, posteromedial, 71
Hypothyroidism, 116
Hypoventilation, 602
Hysteria, 596
  physical disease and, 23–24

IASP. *See* International Association for the
  Study of Pain
Ibuprofen (Motrin), 168–169
  in children, 216
  for connective tissue disease, 536
  lithium interaction of, 204
  for migraine, 256
  pharmacology of, 605–606
  for rheumatic disease, 527

Ice therapy, 517
Idoxuridine, 507–508
Ileostomy, 157
Illness
    acute model of, 139
    severity of, 686
Illness Behavior Questionnaire, 26, 29
Imagery training, 582
    in cancer pain treatment, 441
    in cognitive-behavioral treatment, 148
Imaging, 573
Imipramine (Tofranil)
    for acute pain, 182
    for arthritic disorders, 188
    in benzodiazepine detoxification, 233
    depressive symptoms with, 186
    for headache, 186
    for low back pain, 188
    for mixed chronic pain, 188
    selection of, 199–200
Immobilization
    for cervical spine infection, 345
    side effects of, 106
Impairment
    definition of, 4, 86
    determination of, 732–734
    psychological, 742–756
Incentive programs, in cancer pain
    treatment, 442
Independence, fostering of, 680
Individualized care, 678–680
Indoleacetic acids, 170
Indomethacin (Indocin)
    for crystal-induced arthritis, 533
    headache with, 241
    for migraine, 258
    for rheumatic disease, 527
Indoprofen, 605–606
Industrial athletic therapy, 700–701
Industrial rehabilitation, stage model of,
    696–698
Industrial Rehabilitation Program,
    Massachusetts General Hospital, 706
Infections
    cervical spine, 344–345
    chronic, 560–561
    with deep brain stimulation, 79
    gynecologic, 406
Infestations, chronic, 560–561
Inflammation
    NSAIDs in, 166–167
    penile, 417
Inflammatory disease
    cervical spine, 371
    joint, corticosteroids for, 528t, 529
    vascular, orofacial pain with, 300
Inflammatory headaches, 249–251
Inflammatory mediators, pain-producing,
    157
Infraspinatus muscle pain, 545–546
Injury
    accidental, 725–727
    job-related, 727–728
    musculoskeletal, 732
    personal, 724–725, 744–745
Inpatient treatment programs, 686–692
Insertional activity, 37
Insulinoma, 466

Insurance carriers, 709
Integrative relaxation training, 113–116
Intercostal nerve blocks, 57, 616–617
Intercostal pain, manipulation for, 104
Interdisciplinary pain management
    program, 676–677
    consistent care in, 678–680
    evaluation of, 682
    follow-up planning in, 681–682
    models of, 677–678
    patient satisfaction measures for, 682–685
    vocational rehabilitation in, 680–681
Interdisciplinary team, 145–147
Interferon, 508
Intermittent distraction technique, 102
Internal capsule, 15–16
International Association for the Study of
    Pain
    definition of, 3–4
    journal of, 7
    pain classification of, 7–10, 144
    Subcommittee on Taxonomy,
        Classification of Chronic Pain of, 280
    taxonomy of, 141
International Headache Society
    classification system, 244, 268–269
Interossei muscles pain, 548, 554
Interosseous space subluxation, 97
Interpersonally Distressed patient, 144
Interpleural analgesia, 516
Intervertebral disk
    degeneration of, 372
    lumbar, disease of, 373
    manipulation of, 102
Intracranial hemorrhage, 79
Intravenous pyelogram, 414
Iron deficiency, 324
Ischemic compression, 565
Isometheptene mucate (Midrin), 255–256
Isometric exercises, 92
Isopropyl alcohol, 515
Isotonic saline injection, 565–566

JAMAR hand dynamometer, 737
Jaw muscle fatigue, 287
Job design, 642
    ergonomic approach to, 641, 642–664
    faulty, 654–656
Job enlargement/enrichment, 653
Job modification, 705
Job-related injury, compensation formula
    for, 727–728
Job restructuring, 738
Job simulation, 690
Joint
    dysfunction of with muscle dysfunction,
        568
    pain, treatment of, 523–524. See also
        Arthritis; Rheumatic disease
    passive mobilization techniques for, 92
    protection of during rehabilitation, 91–92
    taping of, 651

Kappa receptors, 156
Ketamine, 156
Ketoprofen, 168–169
Ketorolac (Toradol), 170

for migraine, 256
    pharmacology of, 605–606
Kidney
    male, 409
    pain in, 412–413
Kinesthetic sensations, 498
Kinetic sensations, 498
Kinins, 459
Klippel-Feil syndrome, 342
Knee reflex, depressed, 362
Kneeling, 718
Krusen, Frank H., 85
Krute, Aaron, 635
KTP laser urethrotomy, 414

L4 radiculopathy, 41
L5 radiculopathy, 41
Laboratory tests, for myofascial pain
    syndrome, 573
Lamellae, 386
Laminar flow, frontal resistance, 391f
Laparoscopy
    in gynecology, 401–302
    for pelvic pain, 404
Lateral cutaneous nerve entrapment, 481
Lateral femoral cutaneous nerve
    blockade of, 57–58
    entrapment of, 45
Lateral flexion subluxation, 97
Lateral funiculus, 12–13
Lateral medullary syndrome, 14
Laterolisthesis subluxation, 97
Latissimus dorsi pain, 546
Lawsuits. See Legal system; Litigation
Leg pain
    anatomic level of, 361–363
    chronic, 7
    distribution of, 361
    motor loss with, 362–363
    muscle wasting with, 362
    neurologic signs of, 362
    neurologic symptoms of, 361–362
    radicular distribution of, 357f
    referred, 356
    reflex activity changes with, 362
    sensory impairment with, 363
Legal disincentives, 636
Legal system
    impact on prevention/early intervention,
        634–636
    psychological disability in, 746–747
    psychological impairment in, 742–745
    Social Security disability and, 712–721
Leiomyoma, of uterus, 403
Lemniscus, medial, 15
Leukotrienes, 166
Levator scapulae pain, 544–545
Levorphanol, 159
Lewit stretch technique, 565
Lidocaine
    in nerve blockage, 52
    for peripheral neuropathy, 467
    for post-herpetic neuralgia, 515
Lifestyle, cumulative trauma disorder and,
    648
Lifting, 716

education for, 628
testing of, 737–738
Ligamentous cervical spine injuries, 343
Light work, 716, 738
Limb, phantom, 499; *See also* Phantom limb pain
Limbic system, 581
in emotional dimension of pain, 157
orofacial nociceptive information and, 310
Line of drive, 103
Lipoxygenase pathway, 166
Lissauer's tract, 13, 581
List classification, 8f
Lithium, 203
for acute and chronic pain, 191
interactions of, 204
mechanism of action of, 191
pretreatment evaluation with, 204
properties and side effects of, 203
treatment outcomes with, 190t
treatment techniques for, 204
Lithium battery technology, 81
Lithium carbonate (Eskalith, Lithobid, Lithane), 181, 260–261
Litigation
chronic pain and, 147
functional improvement and, 570
personal injury, 744–745
Litigation reaction, 348–349, 351
Liver cancer, 461
Loading
in patient-controlled analgesia, 611
static, 642–645
Lobotomy
for phantom pain, 500
for post-herpetic neuralgia, 517
prefrontal, for thalamic pain, 71
Lock-out interval, 611
Long thoracic nerve lesions, 479
Lorazepam (Ativan), 207
for acute pain, 207–208
in alcohol withdrawal detoxification, 234
Low back disability syndrome, 87
Low back pain
assessment method for, 347
category I, 99–100
category II, 100–101
chronic, 581
clinical approach to, 347–363
diagnostic trap of, 353–355
differential diagnosis of, 347–368
disability syndrome, 87
documenting structural lesion in, 363–368
indicating spinal manipulation, 99–101
mechanical, 355–361
structural lesions in, 363t
syndromes in, 356
nonmechanical, 354t
occupational rehabilitation for, 701
physical disability with, 348–353
tricyclics for, 187–188
Lower extremities, in myofascial pain syndromes, 552–554
Lumbago-mechanical instability, 356
Lumbar nerve root blockade, 55–56
Lumbar paraspinal muscles pain, 549–550

Lumbar sacral plexus, malignant invasion of, 460
Lumbar spine
anatomy, pathoanatomy, and biomechanics of, 386–387
aquatic rehabilitation of, 386–398
arthropathy, 372–373
management of, 373
ligaments and muscles of, 387
manipulation of, 103–104
pain of
clinical work-up and diagnosis of, 387–388
treatment of, 92–93
Lumbar sympathetic block, 59
Lumbosacral spine arthropathy, 372–373
Luschka's joints, 332
Luteinizing hormone, 403
Lysine acetyl salicylate, 605

Mabumetone, 170
Machine design, improper, 659–660
Magnetic resonance imaging
cervical spine, 337–338, 343
for headache, 243–244
for low back pain assessment, 347
of lumbar disk herniation, 365f
for mechanical low back pain, 366
of temporomandibular joint, 316–317
Magnetic stimulation studies, 40
Maladaptive behaviors, 138–139
Male genitalia. *See also* specific organs
anatomy of, 409–412
pain in, 409, 412–417
Malignancies
individualized pharmacologic tailoring for, 421–422
ovarian, 404
pain management algorithm for, 421f
pain of
neurosurgical treatment for, 447–452
psychological management of, 431–444
physical management of, 419–428
radiation therapy for, 454–461
prevalence of, 454
Malingering, 753–754
with back pain, 349
Malnutrition, alcohol-related, 465
Malocclusion, 294
Man-machine interface, faulty, 653
Man-machine system, 640, 641f
Mandible
neoplastic activity in, 289
range of motion of, 320
Manipulation
versus mobilization, 96
in pain relief, 96–97
Manual for Orthopaedic Surgeons in Evaluating Permanent Physical Impairment, 734
MAOIs. *See* Monoamine oxidase inhibitors
MAP-based taxonomy, 144
Maptazinol, 161
Massage, deep muscle, 565
Masseter muscle pain, 542–544
Masticatory muscles
pain in, 541–542
referred pain areas from, 313t

Material handling, 642
Maxillary nerve, branches of, 308
McGill Pain Inventory, 626
McGill Pain Questionnaire, 26, 27f, 420
Mechanoreceptors, low-threshold, 491
Mechanothermal nociceptors, 157
Meclofenamate, 170
for rheumatic disease, 527
Median nerve
anatomy of, 470–471
entrapment of
electrodiagnosis of, 42–43
neuropathy of, 470–472
proximal, 472
Medical benefits, 729–730
Medical decision-making, 674
Medical electrodiagnostics, 36–47
Medical examination, for headache, 271
Medical Examination and Diagnostic Information Coding System (MEDICS), 143
Medical-physical findings, quantification of, 141–143
Medical procedures, rank-ordering of, 142t
Medical witnesses, 723–724
Medication
issues of, 669
scheduling in cancer pain treatment, 442
Meditation, 113
Medium work, 716, 738
Medullary cervical junction, 67–68
Medullary tractotomy, 284
for post-herpetic neuralgia, 517
Melzack, Ronald, gate control model of, 136
Meningioma, midbrain, 15
MENS. *See* Minimal electrical noninvasive stimulation
Menstrual cycle
migraine with, 264
pain during, 402–403
Mental disorders
diagnostic and statistical manual of, 750–756
Social Security evaluation of, 748–750
Mental-mental injury, 725
Mental-physical injury, 725
Meperidine (Demerol), 159, 191
for acute pain, 182
in children, 217
efficacy of, 161
interaction with MAOIs, 202
intravenous, 607
in patient-controlled analgesia, 610
pharmacology of, 603–605
Mephenesin carbamate, 295
Meralgia paresthetica, 45, 481
nerve blockade for, 57–58
Merskey, Dr. Harold, pain classification of, 7
Mesencephalotomy, rostral, 450
Metabolism
dysfunction of, 560
first-pass, 609
Metacentric principle, 390

Metastasis
  bone, 459–460
  to brain, 460–461
  cervical spine, 371
Metatarsal, long second, 563
Metaxalone, 177
Met-enkephalin, 156
  levels of with acupuncture, 118
Methacrylate, 375–376
Methadone (Dolophin), 159–160
  with antidepressants, 189
  in children, 217
  efficacy of, 161
  intravenous, 606–607
  for malignancy pain, 428
  in opiate detoxification, 225–226, 229t
Methocarbamol, 177–178
  dosage and side effects of, 178
Methotrexate
  for rheumatoid arthritis, 532
  for spondyloarthropathies, 535
Methotrimeprazine (Levoprome)
  analgesic activity of, 191
  efficacy of, 186
  for postsurgical pain, 191–193
Methylergonovine (Methergine)
  for cluster headache, 261
  for migraine, 257
Methylphenidate, 209
  for pain, 197
Methylprednisolone, 515
Methylprednisolone acetate (Depo-Medrol,
  Depo-Predate), 53
Methysergide, 261
  for migraine, 257–258
Metoclopramide (Reglan), 263–264
Metoprolol (Lopressor), 257
Metronidazole, 465–466
Mickel's cave tumor, 281
Microvascular decompression
  for glossopharyngeal neuralgia, 299
  trigeminal nerve, 281
  for trigeminal neuralgia, 297–298
Midrin. See Isometheptene mucate (Midrin)
Migraine, 244–245
  basilar artery versus migraine with aura,
    246t
  characteristics of, 269
  classifications of, 269
  complicated, 246–247
  cyclic, 189
  description of, 245
  distinguishing features of, 248t
  hallmark of, 245
  hormonal factors in, 245
  menstrual, 239–240
    treatment of, 264
  neurogenic theory of, 245–246
  ocular prodromata of, 240t, 246
  pathogenesis of, 245
  pathophysiology of, 269
  precipitating factors in, 241
  prevalence of, 245
  preventive treatment of, 256–259
  special drug techniques for, 263–264
  symptomatic treatment of, 254–256
    versus preventive treatment, 254t
  tension headache and, 253
  tricyclic antidepressants for, 186
  visual prodromata of, 240t, 246

Migraine accompagnee, 246
Millon Behavioral Health Inventory
  (MBHI), 28–29, 625–626, 691
Minimal electrical noninvasive
  stimulation, 91
Minnesota Multiphasic Personality
  Inventory, 24–26, 593, 691
  for chronic pain prevention, 630
  scales in predicting treatment outcome,
    29
  for surgical prediction in chronic pain,
    625–626
Minnesota Multiphasic Personality
  Inventory 2, 436
Minnesota Rate of Manipulation Test, 737
Misonidazole, 465–466
Mixed headache syndrome, 249
MMPI. See Minnesota Multiphasic
  Personality Inventory
Mobilization, 96
Monakow's area, 14
Monoamine oxidase, 490
Monoamine oxidase inhibitors, 181
  for acute and chronic pain, 189–190
  for depression, 595
  interactions of, 202–203
  mechanism of action of, 191
  for migraine, 258
  pretreatment evaluation for, 203
  properties and side effects of, 202
  selection of, 203
  treatment techniques with for chronic
    pain, 203
Mononeuropathies, multiple, 466
Mood States, Profile of, 630
Morphine, 155
  adverse effects of, 158–159
  ceiling dose of, 158
  in children, 217
  clearance of, 604–605
  effects of, 158
  efficacy of, 161
  endogenous, 582
  intrathecal, 612–613
  for malignancy pain, 428
  oral, 609
  in patient-controlled analgesia, 610
  for post-herpetic neuralgia, 512
  spinal, 451
  value of, 163
May T. Morrison Center for Rehabilitation
  program, 696
Motion cascade, 398
  in swimming therapy, 93
Motion restriction, in single-muscle
  myofascial syndromes, 540
Motivation, 679–680
Motor disorders, cervical spine, 339
Motor horn cell loss, anterior, 334
Motor loss, with leg pain, 362–363
Motor unit
  action potentials of, 46
  definition of, 36
Movement therapy, 690
MPI. See Multidimensional Pain Inventory
MRI. See Magnetic resonance imaging
Mu receptors
  localization of, 156

stimulation of, 155–156, 157
  types of, 156
Mucosal disease, orofacial pain with, 290–
  291
Multiaxial Assessment of Pain (MAP), 28
Multiaxial pain assessment, 141
Multidimensional Pain Inventory, 143
Multidimensional pain tests, 27–28
Multidisciplinary team, 146
Multiple sclerosis, cervical spine and, 342
Munchausen syndrome, 595–596
Muscle
  atrophy of, 92
  lengthening of, 565
  strain, cervical spine, 342–343
  stretching of, 689; See also Stretching
  voluntary contraction of, 38
  wasting of with leg pain, 362
Muscle contraction headache. See also
Tension headache
  characteristics of, 269–270
  vascular headache and, 270
Muscle fiber
  intracellular potentials of, 36–37
  resting potential of, 36, 37–38
Muscle relaxants, 173–179; See also specific
  drugs
  central-acting, 173, 174t, 174–179
  detoxification protocol for, 235
Muscle spasm, 601
  back, 358
  cycle of anxiety and pain with, 174f
Muscle-specific weakness, 540
Muscle syndromes, manipulation for, 100
Musculocutaneous nerve entrapment, 478–
  479
  electrodiagnosis of, 45
Musculoskeletal disorders, 86
  cardinal signs of, 96
  orofacial pain with, 324–325
Musculoskeletal injury, 732
  case presentation of, 89–93
  rehabilitation goals for, 88–89
Musculoskeletal pain
  physiatrist in management of, 85–93
  rehabilitation model for, 87–93
Myeloceles, traumatic, 64–65
Myelography
  in assessing low back pain, 347
  cervical, 64–65
  for mechanical low back pain, 364–365
  oil-soluble contrast, 364f
Myeloma, multiple, 340
Myelotomy, commissural, 449
Myocardial infarctions, silent, 30
Myofacial pain dysfunction, 315
Myofascial contracture, 689
Myofascial pain syndromes, 288
  chronic, 556–557
    identifying pieces of, 570–573
    inactivation of trigger points in, 564–
      566
    management of, 568–570, 573–575
  mechanical factors in, 562–564
  patient information questionnaire for,
    571–572f
  perpetuating factors in, 557–564
  similar conditions to, 566–568

single-muscle, 539–554
Myofascial trigger points, 288, 539–340
  location of, 543f, 545f, 547f, 549–550f,
    551f, 553f
  pathogenesis of, 541
  single-muscle syndrome due to, 567
Myopathies, 46
Myospasm, 318
Myospastic cycle, 319
Myotoxins, 261

Nabumetone, 169
  for rheumatic disease, 527
Nadolol (Corgard), 257
Nail brittleness, 492
Nalbuphine, 161
  in patient-controlled analgesia, 610
  pharmacology of, 605
  side effects of, 616
Naloxone (Narcan)
  MAOI drug interactions and, 202
  in opiate detoxification, 229
Naloxone opiate physical dependent test,
  227t
Naltrexone, 229t, 231t
Naproxen, 168–169
  in children, 216
  pharmacology of, 605–606
  for rheumatic disease, 527
Naproxen sodium (Anaprox), 256, 258
Narcissistic personality disorder, 596
Narcotic agonists
  biophase concentrations of, 603–604
  pharmacology of, 602–603
Narcotic analgesics
  in children, 218t
  individualized tailoring of, 421–422
  interaction with MAOIs, 202–203
  interaction with neuroleptics, 205
  for malignancy pain, 423
  for migraine, 256
Narcotics, 155. *See also* Analgesics; Opioids
  with antidepressants, 189
  in children, 217
  for chronic back pain, 631
  continuous spinal/epidural infusion of,
    424–425
  continuous subcutaneous infusion of, 424
  dosage of, 591
  effectiveness of, 590–591
  elimination of, 605
  epidural administration of, 613–614
  guidelines for use of, 590t
  individual tailoring of, 428
  intramuscular, 608
  intrathecal administration of, 612–613
  intraventricular, 451–452
  new techniques in administration of,
    424–425
  pharmacokinetics of, 603–604
  pharmacology of, 602–605
  for renal and ureteral pain, 412–413
  for severe pain, 592t
  sublingual administration of, 424
  tolerance to, 614
  transdermal delivery of, 424
  underuse of, 590
  unpredictability of in elderly, 222
National Institute of Neurological Disease

and Blindness, Ad Hoc Committee
  diagnostic criteria of, 268–269
Nausea and vomiting, with neuraxial
  opioids, 615
NCS. *See* Nerve conduction studies
Neck
  acute trauma to, 371
  anatomy and biomechanics of, 331–334,
    336
  pain in
    with cervical osteophytes, 370–371
    clinical examination for, 335–337
    diagnostic studies of, 337–338
    differential diagnosis and management
      of, 331–346
    incidence of, 331
    management of, 371–372
    medical history of, 335
    radiation to shoulder, 344–345
    in single-muscle myofascial
      syndromes, 541–542
Needle electrodes, 36
Needles, in nerve blockage, 52
Neospinothalamic tract, 13
Neotrigeminothalamic pathway, 310
Nerve blocks
  autonomic nervous system, 58–60
  basic equipment for, 52–53
  in chronic pain management, 51–52
  diagnostic and therapeutic, 51–60, 668–
    669
  facet joint, 60
  for herpes zoster, 508–509
  for intractable pain, 583
  peripheral, 54–58, 616–619
  for post-herpetic neuralgia, 515–516
  prognostic and diagnostic, 420–421
  for renal and ureteral pain, 413
  spinal, 53–54
  for trigeminal neuralgia, 321
Nerve compression, 431
Nerve conduction studies, 36, 38–39
  for mechanical low back pain, 367
  proximal, 39–40
Nerve conduction velocity testing, 338
Nerve ending, unencapsulated, 11
Nerve root infiltration
  for mechanical low back pain, 366
  patient response to, 367
Nerve roots
  irritations of, 341–342
  neuritis from compression of, 378
  reflex components of, 98–99
  section of for cancer pain, 447–449
  selective blockage of
    purpose of, 54–55
    technique for, 55–56
  spinal, 333–334
  stimulation of, 39
Nervous system. *See* Autonomic nervous
  system; Brain; Central nervous system;
  specific nerves; Sympathetic nervous
  system
Neural decompression, 321
Neural foramina, 333
Neural pain signaling, central transmission
  of, 74
Neural stimulation devices, totally
  implanted, 81
Neural stimulation techniques, 74–82. *See*

also Electrical stimulation; specific
  techniques; Transcutaneous electrical
  nerve stimulation
Neuralgia, 377, 381–383
  atypical facial, 187, 250
  benzodiazepines and hydroxyzine for,
    195
  definition of, 381
  geniculate, 284, 299
  glossopharyngeal, 250, 284–285
  of head and face, 280–286
  management of, 320–322
  versus neuropathy, 380
  occipital, 101, 285–286
    nerve blockade for, 56
  penis pain in, 417
  post-herpetic, 250, 283–284, 300–301,
    379–380, 403–418
  post-traumatic (postsurgical), 320–322
  preherpetic, 504
  signs and symptoms of, 250t
  trigeminal, 14, 240, 249–250, 280–283,
    294–298
    atypical, 298
    clonazepam for, 208
    sensory epilepsy and, 381
  vagoglossopharyngeal, 298–299
Neuralgic syndromes, 383
Neurectomy
  peripheral, 281, 447
  for peripheral denervation, 296
Neuritis
  definition of, 377–378
  herpes zoster, 379–380
  mechanisms of, 378–379
  versus neuropathy, 380
  peripheral, 378
Neuritis, Sensory Neuritis and Neuralgia, 377
Neuroablative techniques. *See also* Ablative
  neurosurgery
  for intractable pain, 583
  for malignancy pain, 426
  for post-herpetic neuralgia, 516–517
Neuroanatomic pain pathways, 581
Neuroanatomy, pain, 581–584
Neurobiotaxis law, 13
Neurogenic claudication, 361
Neuroleptics
  with antidepressants, 201
  commonly used, 204t
  drug therapy outcomes of, 191–194
  interactions of, 205
  pretreatment evaluation for, 205
  properties and side effects of, 204–205
  selection of, 205–206
  treatment techniques with
    for acute pain, 206
    for chronic pain, 206
  tricyclic interactions with, 199
Neurologic disorders, 86
  benzodiazepines and hydroxyzine for,
    195
  neuroleptics for, 194
  tricyclic antidepressants for, 182–186
Neurologic examination, for neck pain,
  336–337
Neurolysis
  complications of, 427
  intrathecal and epidural, 427
  for malignancy pain, 426–427
Neurolytic blocks, 516

Neurolytics, 53

Neuroma
neural decompression for, 321
pressure on, 314
traumatic, 314
trigeminal, 283

Neuromuscular disease,
temporomandibular, 318–320

Neurons
first-order, 308–309
second-order, 309–310
third-order, 310

Neuropathy
causes of, 380–381
compression, 470–482
definition of, 377, 379–380
entrapment, 470–482
low back pain with, 355
peripheral, 463–467
radiation palliation of, 460
syndromes of, 380

Neuropeptides, 18

Neurosurgery
ablative, 447–451
augmentative, 451–452
for cancer pain, 447–452
for deafferentation pain, 62–72
for malignancy pain, 426

Neurosynaptic transmitters, 490

Neurotic bodily pain, 381, 382

Neurotransmitters, 582
noxious, 12
in pain pathway, 166

Neurovascular bundle, 410

Neurovascular compression syndrome, 56

Nicotine, detoxification protocol for, 235

Nifedipine, 258

Nitrofurantoin, 465–466

Nociception, 136
definition of, 165, 307
modulation of, 601
orofacial, 306–307
of tooth dentin, 311–312

Nociceptive fibers, 307
in opioid action, 157

Nociceptive impulses, stratification of
response to, 602t

Nociceptive neurons, of subnucleus
caudalis, 309–310

Nociceptor afferents, 488

Nociceptor fibers, orofacial, 308

Nociceptors, 165

Noncontact manipulation techniques, 102

Nonsteroidal anti-inflammatory drugs, 162,
165, 170–171
adverse effects of, 168, 170–171, 527–528
analgesic, 167–168, 605–606
antiprostaglandin effect of, 89
for arthritic disorders, 188
categories of, 168–170
in children, 216
for cluster headache, 261
for connective tissue disease, 536
for crystal-induced arthritis, 533–534
in elderly, 171
for headache in children, 263
in inflammation and analgesic processes,
166–167
for inflammatory joint disease, 523–524

interactions of, 168
for malignancy pain, 423
for migraine, 256, 258–259
for myofascial pain syndrome, 574
for osteoarthritis, 530
pain production and, 165–166
in patient-controlled analgesia, 610
for peripheral neuropathy, 467
pharmacokinetics of, 528t
for post-herpetic neuralgia, 515
for post-traumatic headache, 263
for rheumatic disease, 527–528
for rheumatoid arthritis, 531
for soft tissue injury, 91
for spondyloarthropathies, 535
for temporomandibular joint
derangement, 316
for tension headache, 262

Norepinephrine, reuptake blockade of, 512

Normeperidine, 161

Nortriptyline (Aventyl)
for migraine, 258
for post-herpetic neuralgia, 513
selection of, 199–200

Nose, lesions of, 289–290

Noxious stimulus, 11

NSAIDs. *See* Nonsteroidal anti-inflammatory drugs

Nuclear medicine studies, cervical spine,
338

Nucleus caudalis dorsal root entry zone
lesions, 301

Numbness, in peripheral neuropathy, 463

Numerical Rating Scale, 24

Nuprin Pain Report, 268

Nursing care, 692

Nutrition, inadequacy of, 557–559

Objective findings, 691

Obturator nerve entrapment, 45

Occipital nerve, greater, 56

Occipital neuralgia, 101, 285–286

Occupational Access System (OASYS), 715

Occupational rehabilitation
California program of, 694–695
equipment in, 698
historical perspective of, 695–696
primary treatment of, 699–701
process of, 696–698
program models for, 698–709
secondary treatment of, 701–706
services of, 697f
tertiary treatment of, 706–708
treatment programs for, 694–709

Occupational Safety and Health
Administration (OSHA), 645

Occupational therapy, 690

Odontalgia, 290

Odontoblastic zone, 311

Odontogenic pain, 290

On-Demand Analgesia Computer (ODAC),
610

Operant conditioning, 138

Operant pain-control techniques, 276

Ophthalmoplegia syndromes, painful, 251

Ophthalmoplegic migraine, 246–247

Opiate receptors, 582
in substantia gelatinosa, 618

Opiates, 155
addiction to, 155
in children, 217
detoxification protocols for, 224–229,
230t, 231t
dosage of, 591–592
for post-herpetic neuralgia, 516
for rheumatic pain, 524
tricyclic interactions with, 199

Opioid peptides, 155

Opioid receptors, 155–157

Opioids. *See also* Analgesics; Narcotics
action of, 157
clinical use of, 157–158
continuous spinal/epidural infusion of,
424–425
definition of, 155
epidural, with local anesthetics, 616
intrathecal and epidural, 611–616
issues in use of, 669
neuraxial, 611–614
side effects of, 614–616
partial agonists and partial agonist-
antagonists, 605
pharmacology of, 602–605
for post-herpetic neuralgia, 512
single-dose injection of, 425
types of, 158–162

Opium, 155

Oral cavity, lesions of, 289–290

Oral contraceptives, dysmenorrhea and,
403

Orchialgia, 415

Orchitis, 416

Ordiazepam, 208

Organic mental syndromes, 754

Orofacial analgesic systems, 312

Orofacial central pathways, 308–310

Orofacial pain
dental management of, 306–326
differential diagnosis and management
of, 280–291
epidemiologic studies of, 307–308
medical/neurosurgical management of,
294–302
of mucosal origin, 290–291
of odotogenic origin, 290
pathologies of, 314–326
of psychological origin, 291
temporomandibular dysfunction causing,
314–320

Orofacial peripheral nerves, 308

Orphenadrine, 178
dosage of, 178–179
side effects of, 179

Orthosis, 345

Osler, Sir William
on acupuncture, 117
on morphine, 163

Osteoarthritis, 529–530
cervical, 340–341, 380
temporomandibular joint, 288–289, 317
treatment of, 530

Osteoid osteoma, vertebral body, 371

Osteophytes, 370–371
mechanical and biochemical changes
with, 371

Osteophytosis, 387

Osteoporosis, 528

Otolaryngologic disease, 322
Outpatient chronic pain management
  programs, 676–677
    characteristics of excellence in, 678–685
    treatment models in, 677–678
Ovary
  cancer of, 461
  in gynecologic pain, 403–404
Overload muscle injury, 87
  rehabilitation of, 87–88
  vicious cycle of, 89f
Overprescribing, in elderly, 215
Oxacams, 169, 170
Oxazepam (Serax), 207
Oxycodone, 159
Oxygen therapy, 260

Pacinian corpuscle, encapsulated, 11
Pagets' disease, spinal, 335
Pain. *See also* Chronic pain; Pain behavior;
  Psychogenic pain
    acute and chronic, 307t
    adaptive nature of, 584
    altered perception of in elderly, 215
    anatomy of, 11–17
    approach to, 586
    assessment of, 18–33
      behavioral and observational, 22–24
      in cancer patient, 433–438
      in children, 31–32
      in elderly, 30–31
      integration of findings in, 143–144
      with malignancy, 420
      misconceptions in, 18–19
      multiaxial, 141
      multidimensional tests of, 27–28
      psychological, 19–33
      psychophysiologic, 28
      quantification of medical-physical
        findings in, 141–143
      quantification of psychosocial and
        behavioral data in, 143
      questions to guide, 141
      referral process in, 20
      specific devices for, 24–29
      unidimensional devices for, 25f
    "blockability" of, 668–669
    brainstem systems of, 13–15
    cerebral cortex and, 16
    chemical mediators of, 459
    classification systems for, 632–634
    cluster analysis of, 143–144
    cognitive-behavioral conceptualization
      of, 136–149
    deafferentation, 62–72
    definitions of, 3–6, 165, 307
    descending pathways of, 17
    diagnosis of
      by location, 672t
      by presumed etiology, 673t
      and primary care treatment of
        disorders of, 587–589
    in disability, 86–87
    early reporting of, 645
    emotional factors in, 5
    ergonomic analysis of, 645
    etiology of, 9
    fast and slow, 582
    first component of, 157
    functional capacity and, 4
    gate control model of, 136–137
    gynecologic, 401–407

induction of, 111
intensity and time since onset of, 9f
internal capsule and, 15–16
legal aspects of, 712–721
in male genitalia, 409–417
malignant, 419–428
  psychological management of, 431–444
management of
  with acupuncture, 117–120
  hypnosis in, 108–112
  pharmacologic, special considerations
    in, 215–223
  placebos in, 120–124
  relaxation response in, 112–117
  spinal surgery for, 328–330
maps of, 24
mechanisms of production of, 165–166
multidimensional nature of, 20–21, 181
musculoskeletal, physiatrist in
  management of, 85–93
neural stimulation techniques for, 74–82
neuroanatomy and physiology of, 581–
  584
nonpharmacologic management
  considerations in, 597
operational definition of, 4–6
perception of, 136–137, 602
peripheral mechanism of, 167f
peripheral structures in, 11–12
personality and secondary gain factors,
  586–587
phantom, 497–501
physiologic and behavioral changes in,
  18
postoperative
  anatomy and neurophysiology of, 600–
    602
  management of, 600–619
in primary care medicine, 581–597
projected, 313–314
proneness to, 594
versus psychiatric disorder, 3
psychoanalytic schematization of, 382f
psychogenic, 634
psychological evaluation and testing of,
  18–33
psychological significance of, 583
psychopharmacologic agents for, 181–210
rating of intensity of, 24
"real" vs. psychogenic, 669
referred, 12, 353, 370, 372, 412
  myofascial, 539–541
  orofacial, 312–313
requiring consultations, 667–668
sensation of, 4–5
spinal cord and, 12–13
subjective intensity of, 678
subjectivity of, 3
sympathetically maintained, 486
syndromes of by group, 9t
taxonomy and classification of, 7–10
temporal characteristics and pattern of
  occurrence of, 8f
temporal classification of, 378t
thalamus and, 15
thresholds of, 28
tolerance of and manipulation, 96–97
Pain, Disability and Chronic Illness
  Behavior Committee, Institute of
  Medicine, functional capacity definition
  of, 4
Pain behavior, 5
  with cancer, 433–434
  determinants of, 523

evaluation of, 21–22
  overt, 433–434
  prediction of, 625–626
  sociocultural variables affecting, 584–586
Pain Behavior Scale, University of
  Alabama, 22, 23f
Pain-blocking feedback endorphin system,
  378–379
Pain clinics, 589
  chronic pain management programs in,
    676–685
Pain cocktails, 574
Pain-conducting afferent fibers, 12
Pain-conducting fibers, 11, 581
  to cerebral cortex, 15–16
Pain consultations
  appropriate response to, 670–672
  Current Procedural Terminology codes
    in, 672–674
  reasons for initiating, 667–670
  role of, 674–675
  services of, 667
  unsatisfactory, 671–672
Pain diary, 626–627
Pain drawings, 24
Pain gait control mechanism, 582–583
Pain inhibitory pathways, orofacial, 312f
Pain intensity scales, 24, 25f
Pain pathways, 12–13
  central nervous system, 309–310
  modulation of, 425–426
  pain production and, 165–166
Pain precipitators, cancer, 434–435
Pain-prone disorder, 634
Pain receptors, 11
  in viscera, 12
Pain Research Group, Wisconsin Brief Pain
  Inventory of, 436
Pain Severity Index, 630
Pain shock, 593
Pain specialist, 730–731
Pain stimuli, 581–582
Pain thermometers, 32
Pain triad, 625
Pain Visual Analog Scale, 420
Paleospinothalamic tract, 13, 601
  in opioid action, 157
Paleotrigeminoreticulothalamic pathway,
  310
Pampiniform plexus, 411
Pancreas, cancer of, 461
Papaverine, 155
Paracelsus, 155
Paraphimosis, 416
Paraplegia, deafferentation pain in, 62,
  65–66
Parasitic infestations, chronic, 261
Parasympathetic system, stimulation of,
  600–601
Parasympathetic vagus nerve, 12
Paratrigeminal neuralgia, 286
Paresthesias, 463
Paresthetic discomfort, leg, 361–362
Pariental operculum, 16
Parovarian cysts, 404

Paroxetine (Paxil), 188
  efficacy of, 186

Paroxysmal hemicrania, chronic, 247
  treatment of, 259

Parzepam (Centrax), 207

Passive motion, 690

Patient
  communication with, 670–671
  fostering independence in, 680
  profile of for inpatient program, 688–689

Patient-controlled analgesia, 609–610
  bolus demand-dose in, 611
  choice of agents in, 610
  loading in, 611
  lock-out interval in, 611
  route of administration in, 610

Patient education, myofascial pain syndrome, 574

Patient history, in chronic pain prevention, 628–629

Patient satisfaction parameters, 630, 682–685

Pectoralis muscles pain, 548

Pediatrics Clinics of North America, 215

Pelvic inflammatory disease, 406

Pelvis
  autonomic innervation to, 412
  chronic pain of, 407
  female, 401
  male, 409

Pemoline, 209

Penicillamine, 531–532

Penis, 410
  innervation of, 410–411
  pain from, 416–417

Pentazocine, 156, 160–161
  pharmacology of, 605

Percocet, 428

Performance evaluations, ergonomic, 692

Performance rate, 647

Performance standards, 653–654

Periapical periodontitis, 290

Periaqueductal gray
  electrical stimulation of, 79, 81
  in pain amelioration, 17

Periarticular pain syndromes, 524

Pericarditis, 535–536

Pericarotid syndrome, 300

Perineum, male, 412

Periodontitis, 291

Peripheral joints, dysfunction of, 398

Peripheral nerve block, 54–58, 616–619
  for post-herpetic neuralgia, 515

Peripheral nerve entrapment syndromes, 42–46

Peripheral nerves
  inflammation of, 378
  stimulation of, 74–75

Peripheral neuropathy, 463
  causes of, 464t
  differential diagnosis of, 464–466
  symptoms and signs of, 463–464
  treatment of, 466–467

Peripheral polyneuropathy, 46

Peripheral structures, 11–12

Periventricular gray-periaqueductal gray matter stimulation, 452

Peroneal nerve
  entrapment of, 45–46
  lesions of, 479–480

Peroneus brevis muscle pain, 554

Peroneus longus muscle pain, 554

Perphenazine (Trilafon), 191

Personal factors, in cumulative trauma disorder, 647–648

Personal injury
  compensation formula for, 724–725
  lawyers for, 147
  psychological impairment with, 744–745

Personality
  in cumulative trauma disorder, 648–649
  disorders of, 749–750
  pain and, 586–587

Personality traits, premorbid, 455

Peyronie's disease, 416–417

Phantom limb syndrome, 86, 380
  prevention of, 629

Phantom pain, 497
  clinical cases of, 497–498
  theories of, 498–499
  treatment for, 499–501

Phantom tooth syndrome, 313, 322–323

Pharmacodynamics, 603

Pharmacokinetics, 603
  in elderly, 220

Pharmacologic pain management
  in children, 215–219
  in elderly, 219–222
  special considerations in, 215–223

Pharmacotherapy, issues of, 674

Phencyclidine (PCP), 156

Phenelzine (Nardil), 189–190
  in benzodiazepine detoxification, 233
  interactions of, 202
  for migraine, 258
  selection of, 203

Phenobarbital, 233t

Phenothiazines
  for acute pain, 191–193
  for chronic pain, 193–194
  efficacy of, 186
  for headache, 263
  for herpes zoster, 508
  mechanisms of action of, 194
  for migraine, 256
  for neurologic disorders, 194
  for post-herpetic neuralgia, 512–513

Phentolamine, 486

Phenylbutazone (Butazolidin)
  for crystal-induced arthritis, 533
  development of, 165
  lithium interactions with, 204
  for rheumatic disease, 527

Phenytoin (Dilantin)
  analgesic effect of, 163
  for migraine, 259
  for post-herpetic neuralgia, 513
  for post-traumatic headache, 263
  for trigeminal neuralgia, 295

Phimosis, 416

Physiatrist
  definition of, 85
  history of, 85–86

in musculoskeletal pain management, 85–93
  rehabilitation model of, 87–93
  training of, 86–87

Physical activity, pain with, 525

Physical capacities evaluation, 734

Physical demands, 716–719
  strength rating for, 720–721

Physical disability
  assessment of, 732–740
  with low back pain, 348–353

Physical examination
  in consultation, 673
  in preventing chronic pain, 629–630

Physical medicine, 689–690

Physical Medicine and Rehabilitation, 85–86

Physical-mental injury, 725

Physical reconditioning, 687

Physical therapy
  individualized, 679
  for osteoarthritis, 530
  for phantom pain, 500
  for rheumatoid arthritis, 532

Physician
  as analgesic, 596–597
  primary, 146
  psychological disability and, 745–746
  referring, 146

Physician monitoring, 686

Physiologic assessment devices, 24

Pimozide, 295

Piriformis muscle pain, 552

Piroxicam, 169, 170
  for rheumatic disease, 527

Pituitary gland, removal of, 450

Placebo response, 121–122

Placebos
  analgesic, 120–124
  definition of, 120
  ethical considerations with, 123
  mechanisms of action of, 122–123
  pain relief studies with, 121
  uses of, 120

Plain radiography
  cervical spine, 343
  for mechanical low back pain, 363–365

Platelet aggregation, inhibition of, 168

Pleuritic pain
  in connective tissue disease, 535
  radiation palliation of, 461

Poker Chip Tool, 32

Polio, spinal degeneration with, 334

Polycystic ovarian syndrome, 404

Polymyalgia rheumatica, 537

Polymyositis, 325

Polypharmacy, 221, 222

Porphyritic neuropathy, 466

Positive flip test, 359f

Postconcussion syndrome, 263

Posterior facet syndrome, 99–100

Posterior interosseous nerve syndrome, 44, 475–476

Post-herpetic neuralgia, 379–380, 503
  acute herpes zoster infection and, 503–509
  differential diagnosis of, 283–284

management algorithm for, 514f
management of, 284
medical/neurosurgical management of, 300–301
pain of, 509–510
pathophysiology of, 510–511
symptoms and pain characteristics of, 511
treatment for, 511–518
Post-herpetic pain, 67–68
 neurosurgery for, 68–70
Post-isometric relaxation, 565
Post-laminectomy syndrome, 76
Postlumbar puncture headache, 249
Postoperative pain
 analgesics for, 602–611
 anatomy and neurophysiology of, 600–602
 intrathecal and epidural opioids for, 611–616
 neuroleptics for, 191–193
 pathophysiology of, 601–602
 peripheral nerve blocks for, 616–619
Post-traumatic cephalgia, 263
Post-traumatic headaches, 250, 251t
Post-traumatic hyperirritability syndrome, 261
Post-traumatic stress disorder, 596, 754–755
Post-traumatic sympathetic dystrophy, 58
Post-traumatic syndrome, 27
Postural stress
 seated, 563
 standing, 563
Posture
 extreme, 642, 646
 sitting, 655t
Prednisone
 for cluster headache, 260
 for connective tissue disease, 536
 for rheumatoid arthritis, 532
Pre-employment strength testing, 628
Preganglionic neurons, stimulation of, 600–601
Pregnancy, ectopic, 402
Pressure
 painful, 11
 perception of, 14–15
Prevention
 aspects of, 628
 behavioral approach in, 637
 tertiary, 628, 631, 636–638
Prevention/early intervention, 623
 chronic back pain as paradigm of, 630–631
 in chronic pain syndrome, 623–638
 with chronic pain syndrome-prone patient, 625–628
 education campaigns for, 624–625
 impact of compensation, disability and law on, 634–636
 legal disincentive and, 636
 patient history and examination in, 628–630
 state of art of, 623–624
Prevocational programs, 696
Priapism, 417
Primary care
 common pain disorders in, 588t
 pain problems in, 581–597

Principles and Practice of Medicine, 117
Probenecide, 534
Problem-solving perspective, 149
Problem-solving skills, 140
Prochlorperazine (Compazine), 191
Product design, 642
Productivity, 698
Proenkephalin A, 157
Profile of Mood States (POMS), 436–437
Progressive muscle relaxation, 113, 114
 for cancer pain, 441
Progressive reorientation, 105
Projected pain, orofacial, 313–314
Promazine (Sparine)
 analgesic activity of, 191
 for cancer pain, 194
Promethazine (Phenergan), 191
 as analgesic adjunct, 606
 for migraine, 256
Pronator syndrome, 473
Propiomazine (Largon), 191
Propionic acids, 168–169
 new, 169–170
Propoxyphene, 160
 for post-herpetic neuralgia, 512
 for rheumatic disease, 526
Propranolol (Inderal)
 for migraine, 186, 257
 in opiate detoxification, 228
 tricyclic interactions with, 199
Proprioceptive neuromuscular facilitation techniques, scapular and glenohumeral, 92
Prosopalgia, 291
Prostaglandin synthetase inhibitors, 402–403
Prostaglandins, 162
 in endometrium, 402–403
 for inflammatory joint disease, 523–524
 inhibition of, 168
 in pain production, 165–166
 in pain relief, 459
 peripheral, 378–379
 for rheumatic disease, 528
Prostate, 410
 pain from, 413–414
Prostatitis, 413–414
Prostatodynia, 414
Prosthetic replacement
 of proximal femur, 375
 total hip, 375–376
Protopathic pain, 11
 nerve roots and, 12
Proximal conduction studies, 39–40
Pruritis, 615
Pseudodementia, 594
Pseudogout, 533
Pseudounipolar cells, descending fibers of, 14
Psoriatic arthritis, 534
 treatment of, 535
Psychiatric disorders
 monoamine oxidase inhibitors for, 202
 versus pain, 3
 primary care chronic pain with, 593–597
Psychiatric dual diagnosis, 233–235

Psychoactive substance abuse, 754
Psychogenic headache, 270
Psychogenic pain, 20, 381, 634
 disorder, 291
 spinal, 348, 350
Psychologic assessment, 691
Psychological evaluation/testing, 18–33
Psychological factors
 affecting physical condition, 753
 in pelvic pain, 407
 in phantom pain, 499
Psychological impairment/disability
 evaluation of under Social Security, 747–750
 factors influencing, 745–747
 in medical-legal system, 742–745
 nosology of, 750–756
 permanent, AMA evaluation guidelines of, 747
Psychological management
 of headache pain, 268, 272–277
 issues in, 277, 443
 of malignant pain, 431–444
 for post-herpetic neuralgia, 517–518
Psychological pain theories, 676
Psychological stress, 561–562
Psychomimetic effects, 156
Psychopathologic profile, 25–26
Psychopharmacologic agents, 181. *See also* specific drugs
 drug therapy outcomes of, 181–199
 treatment approaches with, 199–210
Psychophysiologic assessment, 28
Psychophysiologic evaluation, 271–272
Psychosis, with pain delusions, 629
Psychosocial/behavioral data, quantification of, 143
Psychosomatic disorder, 753
Psychosomatic pain, 377
 spinal, 348, 350
Psychostimulants
 common used, 209t
 for depression, 595
 mechanism of action of, 197–199
 for pain, 197, 209
 treatment outcome of, 198t
Psychotherapy
 for cancer pain, 439
 for chronic pain, 383
 features of, 122–124
 for phantom pain, 500
Psychotomimetics, detoxification protocol for, 235
Pterygoid muscle, lateral, pain, 544
PTS Program, Tacoma, Washington, 706
PTSD. *See* Post-traumatic stress disorder
Pulling, 716
Pulpitis, 290
Punishment, 584
Purdue Pegboard Test, 737
Pushing, 716
Pyridoxine
 inadequacy of, 558–559
 intoxication with, 466

Quadratus lumborum muscle pain, 548–549
Quadriceps femoris pain, 552–553

Quadriceps weakness, 362–363
Quality of working life, 649
Quality programs, 679
Quebec Task Force on Spinal Disorders, 695, 699

Radial nerve
  compression of below elbow, 475–476
  entrapment of, 44
  high entrapment and compression of, 475
Radial sensory neuropathy, 476
Radiating leg pain, 354–355
Radiation
  acute morbidity scoring criteria for, 455, 456–457t
  in cancer treatment, 455
  for cervical spine tumors, 340
  dose fractionation, 457–459
  forms of, 455
  for pain secondary to malignancy, 454–461
Radiation morbidity scoring scheme, late, 458–459t
Radiation oncology, 454–461
  toxicity of, 455–457
Radicular pain
  with cervical nerve root disorders, 336
  cervical origin, 101
Radicular syndrome
  acute
    by age group, 361t
    bilateral, 360
    complaint in, 357
    diagnostic criteria for, 360t
  chronic
    bilateral, 361
    unilateral, 360–361, 366
  unilateral acute, 356
    history in, 356–357
    physical examination in, 357–360
Radiculopathies
  cervical, 41, 341
  electrodiagnostic studies of, 40–42
  evaluation of, 39
  lumbosacral, 41–42, 74
  management of, 372
  with myofascial trigger points, 568
  with spinal arthropathy, 370
  thoracic, 42
Radioculitis, cervical, 341
Radiofrequency electrocoagulation
  for glossopharyngeal neuralgia, 299
  with glycerol injection, 296–297
  for trigeminal neuralgia, 296
Radiofrequency electrode, 53
Radiofrequency lesion, 321
Radiography, 363–364
Raeder's paratrigeminal syndrome, 251
Raeder's syndrome, 286
Rationale restructuring, 140
Raynaud's phenomenon, 525
  carpal tunnel syndrome and, 471
Reaching, 718
  avoidance of, 652–653
Rebound, 231
Receptors
  opioid, 155–157
  pain, 11

in viscera, 12
Recommended dietary allowance (RDA), 558
Recreational therapy, 690
Referred pain, 12
  in cervical region, 372
  low back, 353
  in male genitalia, 412
  orofacial, 312–313
  single-muscle myofascial
    distribution of, 539–540
    reproduction of, 541
  with spinal arthropathy, 370
Reflex activity, changes in with leg pain, 362
Reflex sympathetic dystrophy, 300
  clinical signs and symptoms of, 484–486, 494–495t
  complication of, 493
  diagnostic considerations for, 487t
  theory of, 486–488
Refraction, 392
Reglan (metoclopramide hydrochloride), 256
Rehabilitation
  acute phase of, 91–92
  benefits for, 730
  of chronic pain syndrome patient, 636–638
  goals and objective of, 687–688
  hospital-level, 687
  in inpatient program, 689–690
  lumbar spine aquatic, 386–398
  maintenance phase of, 92
  for musculoskeletal pain, 87–93
  occupational, 694–709
  physical process of, 105
  proper modalities of, 105–106
  recovery phase of, 92
  spinal manipulation and, 96–106
  vocational, 680–681, 690
Reimbursement, CPT codes and, 672–675
Reiter's syndrome, 534
  corticosteroids for, 529
  diagnosis of, 525
  treatment of, 535
Relapse prevention, 149
Relaxation response, 112–117
Relaxation skills, 140
Relaxation techniques, 582
  for cervical pain, 371–372
  for phantom pain, 500
Relaxation training, 113
  adverse patient reactions in, 116
  for cancer pain, 440–441
  efficacy of, 116–117
  for headache pain, 272–273
  home-based, 276
  integrative approach in, 113–116
Renal failure, NSAID-related, 168
Renal pain, male, 412–413
Repetitive task, 642
  avoidance of, 653
  cumulative trauma disorders and, 645
Rescue fantasies, 586
Reserpine, 241
Residual functional capacity, 713
Respiratory depression, 614–615
Reticular formation, 13

Reticular nuclei, 15
Retrolisthesis subluxation, 97
Rexed layers, 63, 64f
  DREZ lesions in, 69f
Rheumatic disease
  diagnostic approaches to, 524–526
  drug therapy for, 526–529
  extra-articular manifestations of, 525
  forms of, 529–538
  laboratory analysis for, 525–526
  pain associated with, 523
  pain management in, 523
  treatment of, 523–524
Rheumatoid arthritis, 530–531
  of cervical spine, 371
  in cervical spine arthropathy, 370
  drug treatment for, 531–532
  neck pain with, 343–344
  physical therapy for, 532
  step-care approach to, 532–533
  of temporomandibular joint, 317
Rheumatoid factor, 525
  high titers of, 530
Rhizotomy
  for cancer pain, 447–449
  for carcinoma, 302
  dorsal, 516–517
  for glossopharyngeal neuralgia, 285
  for malignancy pain, 426
  for phantom pain, 500
  for post-herpetic neuralgia, 515–517
  sacral, 448–449
Rib cage, supine position manipulation of, 104–105
Ribs
  intercostal nerve injury with fracture of, 57
  manipulation for pain of, 101–102
Rochester Rehabilitation Center work evaluation program, 695
Role-playing, 148
Role-reversal, 148
Root compression, L5, 362
Root tension, 358
Rotational subluxation, 97
Rotator cuff tendinitis, 536
  causes of, 90–91
Rusk, Howard, physiatric interventions of, 85–86

S1 radiculopathy, 41–42
Sacral nerve root
  avulsion of, 64f
  blockade of, 56
Sacroiliac joint arthropathy, 369, 373
Sacroiliac subluxation, 98
Sacroiliac syndrome, 100
Safety, 641
  in occupational rehabilitation program, 698
Salicylates
  for connective tissue disease, 536
  for osteoarthritis, 530
  for rheumatic disease, 526–527, 527
Salivary gland, pain from, 323
Salpingostomy, 402
Saphenous nerve entrapment, 481
Satisfaction

measures of, 682–685
  parameters of, 630
Saturday night palsy, 44
Scaleni muscles pain, 544
Scapular winging, 479
Schizophrenia, pain with, 595
Sciatic nerve, lesions of, 480
Sciatic scoliosis, 357–358
Sciatica
  differential diagnosis of, 354t
  reflex changes with, 362
Sclerotome, 12
Scrotum, 411
  pain from, 415–416
Secondary gain, 586–587
Sedative-hypnotics
  lithium interaction with, 204
  MAOI interaction with, 203
  tricyclic interactions with, 199
Sedatives
  as analgesic adjuncts, 606
  drug therapy outcomes of, 194–197
Sedentary work, 716, 737
Selective block, 611
Self-care regimen, 145
Self-hypnosis, 111
  efficacy of, 116–117
Self-monitoring, 22
  of cancer pain management, 435
  in cognitive-behavioral approach, 140
  for headache, 271, 276
Self-observation, 140
Self-pity, 689
Self-reporting, 440
Self-statements, 433
Self-therapies, 589
Seminal vesicles, 411–412
Sensations, hypnotic replacement or
  substitution of, 110
Sensory assessment devices, 24
Sensory conduction studies, 39
Sensory disorders, cervical spine, 339
Sensory-evoked potentials, 367
Sensory impairment, with leg pain, 363
Sensory-physiologic response, 434
Sensory substitution, cancer pain, 439–440
Sequential evaluation process, 712–713
Sequestra, 289
Serial functional testing, 704–705
Serologic studies, 525
Serotonergic mechanisms, 18
Serotonin, 162
  in reflex sympathetic dystrophy, 490
  reuptake blockade of, 512
  reuptake inhibitors of
    efficacy of, 186
    selective, 188
Serratus anterior muscle pain, 548
Serratus posterior superior muscle pain,
  548
Sertraline (Zoloft), 188
Serum
  complement levels in rheumatic disease,
    526
  protein abnormalities of, 466

Service, intensity of, 686–687
Sewing machine, ergonomic improvement
  of, 660
Sexual Functioning Index, 630
Sexually transmitted disease
  gynecologic, 406
  penis involvement in, 417
  urethral pain with, 414
Sharp waves, positive, 37
Shingles, 69. *See also* Herpes zoster
Shoulder pain
  with myofascial syndromes, 544–545
  rehabilitation model of, 90–91
Sialogogues, 324
Sick role, 145
Sickness Impact Profile (SIP), 29
Sight, evaluation of, 718–719
Sigma receptors, 156
Simulated movement testing, 353f
Simultaneous Interview Technique (SIT), 29
Single-muscle myofascial syndromes, 539
  acute forms of, 541–554
  history of onset of, 539–540
  recognition of, 539–541
  trigger points in, 539, 541
Sinus disease, 301
Sinusitis
  acute, 290
  chronic, 261, 289–290
Sitz bath, 414
Sjögren's syndrome, 536
  neuropathy with, 466
Skeletal muscle, energy storage in, 557
Skilled performance, 641
Skills
  acquisition of in cognitive-behavioral
    treatment, 148
  transferability of, 713, 715
Skills training
  in cancer pain treatment, 442
  in cognitive-behavioral approach, 140
Skin conductance biofeedback, 441
SLE. *See* Systemic lupus erythematosus
Sluder's syndrome, 286
Social Security
  chronic pain and, 714–715
  disability for, 712–721
  evaluation of impairment and disability
    under, 747–750
  physical disability benefits of, 742
  psychological disability benefits of, 744
  sequential evaluation process of, 712–713
Social Security Act, 712
  Titles II and XVI of, 712, 715
Social Security Administration, disability
  and impairment guidelines of, 733–734
Social Security Commission on the
  Evaluation of Chronic Pain, 744
Social Security Disability Benefits Reform
  Act, 744
Sociocultural factors, in pain behavior, 584–
  586
Sodium valproate, 295
Soft tissue injury
  chronic, 91
  inflammatory response to, 87–88
  key components of, 89

managing local effects of, 89
  rehabilitation of, 91
Soft tissue masses, 461
Soleus pain, 554
Somatic dysfunction, 96
Somatic pain, 381
  classification of, 11
Somatic preoccupation, 5–6
Somatization, depression with, 629
Somatization disorders, 593–594, 751–752
  diagnostic criteria for, 752t
Somatoform disorders, 593–594, 749
  DSM categories of, 750–753
  undifferentiated, 752–753
Somatoform pain disorder, 752
  diagnostic criteria for, 753t
Somatosensory-evoked potentials, 40
Spastic torticollis, 325
Specific Vocational Preparation (SVP), 720
Spermatic cord, 411
Sphenopalatine neuralgia, 286
Spinal anesthesia, 52
Spinal arteries/veins, 334
Spinal arthropathy, 369
  cervical, 370–372
  diagnosis of, 369
  lumbar and lumbosacral, 372–373
  pathophysiology of, 369–370
  thoracic, 372
Spinal blocks, 53–54
Spinal canal, narrowing of, 100
Spinal cord
  afferent connections and Rexed layers of,
    63f
  anatomy and biomechanics of, 333–334
  compression of, 338–339
    with cancer, 420
    radiation palliation of, 460
    syndromes of, 334
  cysts on, 66f, 334
  dorsal horn of, 157
  electrical stimulation of, 452
  epidural masses of, 335
  extradural processes of, 335
  extrinsic neoplasms of, 339–340
  ischemia of, 339
  pain transmission and, 12–13
  pathology of, 334–335
  Rexed layers and physiology of, 64f
  stimulation of, 76–79
    electrode placement in, 78–79
    indications for, 77
    technical difficulties with, 78
Spinal electrode system, 78f
Spinal fixation, 98
Spinal Function Sort, 704
Spinal manipulation, 96
  contraindications for, 104
  indications for, 99–102
  lumbar, 103–104
  pain tolerance and, 96–97
  rehabilitation goals of, 105–106
  short-lever, high-velocity, 103
  spinal biomechanics and, 97–99
  types of, 102–103
  variations of techniques in, 103–104
Spinal pain
  psychogenic, 348
  clinical description of, 350

Spinal pain,
psychogenic—*continued*
modification of, 348, 350
psychosomatic, 348
clinical description of, 349–350
situational, 348
exaggeration reaction with, 351–353
litigation reaction with, 351
Spinal root avulsion
causes of, 63
neurosurgery for, 63–65
Spinal root ganglia, 11–12
Spinal surgery, 328–330
evaluation for, 329
perioperative support for, 328
types of, 328
Spine
cervical, differential diagnosis and
management of pain in, 331–346
hypo- and hypermobility of, 98
peripheral joints and, 398
vascular supply of, 334
Spinocerebellar tract, 67–68
Spinothalamic pathways, 13
in brainstem, 13–14
Spinothalamic system, 601
Spleen, cancer of, 461
Splenii muscle pain, 544
Splenomegaly, 461
Splints, 651
Split Seconds, 486
Spondyloarthropathies, 534–535
corticosteroids for, 529
treatment of, 535
Spondylolisthesis, 100
structural lesions of, 356
Spondylosis
anterolisthesis subluxation with, 97
cervical, 341
Sports medicine, lumbar spine aquatic
rehabilitation in, 386–398
Sprain, cervical spine, 101, 342–343
Staff education, in cancer pain treatment,
442
Stanford Hypnotic Clinical Scale, 109
Staphylococcal infection, cervical spine, 344
Static loading, 642–645
Static posture, avoidance of, 653
Stellate ganglion block, 58–59
for herpes zoster, 509
Stenosis, 100
Step-care treatment, for rheumatoid
arthritis, 532–533
STEPS Rehabilitation Center, 706
Stereotaxic mesencephalotomy, 71
Sternocleidomastoid muscle, 332
pain of, 542
Steroids
epidural, 54
for herpes zoster, 506
Stiff neck syndrome, 544–545
Stimulants, detoxification protocol for, 235
Stimulation waveforms, 81–82
Stimulus, noxious, 11
Stoic type, 585
Stomatitis, herpetic, 324

Stomatognathic system, 315f
Stooping, 718
Straight leg raise (SLR) test, 352f
false-positive and false-negative, 358
positive, 358
reduced movement in, 351
Strains, cervical, 101
Strength Rating, Physical Demands, 720–
721
Streptococcal infection, cervical spine, 344
Stress
concentration of, 642
avoidance of, 653
coping training, for headache pain, 275–
276
headache and, 241
myofascial pain syndrome with, 561–562
seated postural, 563
standing postural, 563
vocational, 563–564
Stretch and spray treatment, 564–565
Stretching, 652
Struthers ligament entrapment, 473
Styloid process, elongated, 301
Subarachnoid hemorrhage, 250–251
Subarachnoid nerve block, 53–54
Subchondral cysts, hip joint, 374
Subdural hematomas, 249
Subluxation
description of, 96
rehabilitative, 97–98
Subnucleus caudalis, nociceptive neurons
of, 309–310
Suboccipital craniectomy, 297–298
Suboccipital muscle pain, 544
Subscapularis muscle pain, 546
Substance P, 162, 581
in pain pathway, 166
in placebo response, 123
release of, 514
Substantia gelatinosa, 583
extent and merging of, 68f
opiate receptors in, 618
Substitute activity complex, 90
Suffering, 468–469
intensification of, 570
Suicidal thoughts, 517–518
Sulfinpyrazone, 534
Sulindac, 170
for rheumatic disease, 527
Sumatriptan (Imitrex), 255
for cluster headache, 260
Supinator muscle pain, 546–547
Supine position manipulation, 104–105
Supine swimming, 396, 397f
Support groups, 685
Suprascapular nerve
blockade of, 56–57
entrapment of, 45, 56–57
Suprascapular neuropathy, 478
Supraspinatus muscle pain, 546
Surgery
for cluster headache, 261
for cumulative trauma disorder, 652
for endometriosis, 405
for geniculate neuralgia, 284

for occipital neuralgia, 285–286
for phantom pain, 500
for post-herpetic neuralgia, 284, 516
spinal, 328–330
for trigeminal neuralgia, 281
Surgical wound perfusion, 617
Swimming
biomechanics of, 90
freestyle stroke in, 92–93
Swimming stroke phases, 90t
Sympathectomy
for causalgia, 486, 491
for post-herpetic neuralgia, 516
for reflex sympathetic dystrophy, 491–
492, 493
surgical approaches in, 493–495
Sympathetic blocks
for herpes zoster, 509
for post-herpetic neuralgia, 516
Sympathetic denervation, 488
Sympathetic hyperactivity, 491
Sympathetic nerves, 12
blockade of, 58–59, 509, 516
Sympathetic nervous system
in peripheral neuropathy, 464
stimulation of, 600–601
Sympathetic outflow, hyperactivity of, 58
Sympathomimetic agents, 202
Sympathomimetic amines, 199
Symptom Checklist 90-revised
(SCL-90R), 29
Symptom magnification syndrome, 706–707
Symptom negotiation, 704
Synapses, in reflex sympathetic dystrophy,
489–490
Synovial fluid analysis, 525–526
Syringomyelia, 13, 342
pain and, 66–67
symptoms of, 67
Syringoperitoneal shunting, 67
Syrinx, surgical drainage of, 67
Syrinx-to-subarachnoid shunting, 67
Systemic lupus erythematosus, 535–536
corticosteroids for, 529

T-cells, 581
in pain control, 583
Talking, 718
Tardive dyskinesia, 205
Tardy ulnar nerve palsy, 43, 380, 473–474
Tarsal tunnel syndrome, 46, 481–482
Task time/frequency, 646
Taste, loss of, 504
Taut muscle bands
with myofascial syndromes, 550
in single-muscle myofascial syndromes,
540
Team approach, in physiatric care, 86–87
Telescoping, 499
Temporal arteritis, 249
Temporal artery, biopsy of, 300
Temporalis muscle pain, 542–544
Temporomandibular disorder, 286
classification of, 144
Temporomandibular dysfunction, 306, 315
with arthritides, 317

differential diagnosis and treatment of, 314–316
  internal derangements of, 316–317
    with osteoarthritis, 317
    with rheumatoid arthritis, 317
    with traumatic arthritis, 317
Temporomandibular joint
  click in, 316
  closed lock of, 316
  components of, 315
  degeneration of with malocclusion, 294
  disease of, 301–302, 315
    referred pain from, 313
    treatment of, 302
  fracture of, 317–318
  inflammation of, 325
  internal derangements of, 315–316
  normal function of, 315
  osteoarthritis of, 288–289
  pain in, 541
  tumors of, 317
Temporomandibular neuromuscular disease, 318
  etiologic theories of, 318–319
  myospastic cycle and, 319
  work-up for, 319–320
Temporomandibular pain and dysfunction syndrome, 286–287
Tendinitis
  Achilles, 537
  bicipital, 536
  de Quervain's, 537
  rotator cuff, 90–91, 536
Tennis elbow
  causes of, 44
  posterior interosseous nerve syndrome and, 476
Tenosynovitis
  carpal tunnel syndrome and, 472
  corticosteroids for, 529
TENS. *See* Transcutaneous electrical nerve stimulation
Tension headache, 240, 541
  chronic, 248
  description of, 248
  migraine and, 253
  stress and, 241
  syndromes of, 248–249
  treatment of, 262
  tricyclic antidepressants for, 186
Testicles, 411
  pain from, 415
  trauma to, 415
Tetracaine (Pontocaine), 52
Thalamic infarction, 301
Thalamic neural stimulation, 517
Thalamic syndrome, 15
  chemical hypophysectomy for, 71–72
  pain with, 70–71
Thalamogeniculate stalk, 70–71
Thalamotomy, 302, 451
  for phantom pain, 500
Thalamus
  cell bodies of, 310
  electrode placement in, 79
  in pain perception, 15, 17
  ventrobasal nuclear complex of, 13
Thallium intoxication, 465
Theophrastus, 155

Therapeutic modalities. *See* specific techniques
Therapeutic orphan, 215
Thermal biofeedback, 273, 274–275
Thermal hypersensitivity, 492
Thermography
  for mechanical low back pain, 368
  for reflex sympathetic dystrophy, 493
Thiamine, inadequacy of, 558
Thioridazine (Mellaril)
  cardiotoxicity of, 205–206
  for post-herpetic neuralgia, 512
THIP, 163
Third-party payers, 146–147
Thoracic muscle pain, 549–550
Thoracic nerve root block, 55
Thoracic outlet, 477
Thoracic outlet syndrome, 43, 324, 477
  definition of, 44
  neurogenic, 477–478
  treatment of, 477–478
  vascular, 477
Thoracic pain, 101–102
Thoracic spine
  arthropathy of, 372
    management of, 372
  manipulation of, 104
Thoracoabdominal pain, 69–70
Thoracolumbar presacral neurectomy, 495
Thoracotomy, 57
Thumb therapy, 565
Thymidine analogs, 508
Thyroid function, 560
  tests for, 204
Thyroid supplementation, 560
Tibial H reflex, 39
Tibial nerve entrapment, 481–482
  electrodiagnosis of, 46
Tibialis anterior muscle pain, 554
Tic douloureux. *See* Trigeminal neuralgia
Time distortion, hypnotic, 111
Timolol (Tenormin), 257
Tinel's sign, positive, 44
Tissue injury
  complex, 89, 90
  model of cycle of, 89–91
Tissue overload complex, 89, 90
Title II benefits, 712
Title XVI benefits, 712
Tizanidine, 179
Tolmetin, 170
  in children, 216
  for rheumatic disease, 527
Tolosa-Hunt syndrome, 251
Tongue, burning, 291, 323–324
Tool modification, 705
Tooth
  anatomy of, 311f
  dentin of, 311–312
  innervation of, 310–311
  pain following extraction of, 321
  referred pain from, 313
Tooth pulp
  afferent fibers of, 309
  electrophysiologic recordings of, 311
  nerve fibers of, 311

pain in, 310
Toothache, 290
Topical preparations, 514–515
Toricollis, 101
Tort system, 722–723
  personal injury in, 744–745
Touch, perception of, 14–15
Toxins, peripheral neuropathy with, 465–466
Traction, 689
  cervical spine, 372
Traction headache, 249–251
Tractotomy, medullary, 450
Tranquilizers
  for herpes zoster, 508
  for post-herpetic neuralgia, 512–513
Transcendental meditation, 272
Transcutaneous electrical nerve stimulation, 75. *See also* Electrical stimulation
  acupuncture and, 118–119
  analgesic effects of, 75–76
  applied physiology in, 618
  for cancer pain, 452
  contraindications and precautions for, 75
  in pain pathway modulation, 425–426
  for peripheral neuropathy, 467
  for phantom pain, 500
  placebo response to, 637–638
  for post-herpetic neuralgia, 301, 517
  for postoperative pain, 617–618
  practical considerations in, 618–619
  in rehabilitation, 689–690
  for soft tissue injury rehabilitation, 91
  for temporomandibular pain, 287
  trial of, 74–75
Transdermal drug administration, analgesic, 609
Transdermal patch, clonidine-alone, 230t
Tranylpromine, 203
Trapezius muscles, 332
  pain of, 542
Trauma
  cervical, 342–343
  headache with, 250, 251t
Travell, Janet G., 557
Treatment
  adjunctive techniques of, 108–124
  hospital-based inpatient, 686–692
  occupational rehabilitation, 694–709
  outcome predictors for, 29–30
  outpatient chronic pain management, 676–685
Treatment Helpfulness Questionnaire, 683–684
Trendelenburg lurch, 362
Triamcinolone, 515
Triceps brachii muscle pain, 546
Triceps reflex, 99
Trichomoniasis, 406
Tricyclic antidepressants
  for acute pain, 182
  in children, 217–218
  for chronic pain, 182–189
  in depressed pain patients, 202
  for depression, 595
  for fibrositis-like symptoms, 524
  for herpes zoster, 508

Tricyclic antidepressants—*continued*
  interactions of, 199
  for malignancy pain, 424
  mechanism of action of, 189
  for migraine, 258
  with monoamine oxidase inhibitors, 203
  neuroleptics and, 206
  for post-herpetic neuralgia, 512–513
  pretreatment evaluation for, 199
  properties and side effects of, 199
  selection of, 199–200
  for tension headache, 262
  treatment outcomes with, 183–185t
  treatment techniques with, 200–202
Trifluoperazine (Stelazine), 191
Trigeminal brainstem neurons, 312
Trigeminal fibers, 15
Trigeminal gangliolysis, 281
Trigeminal ganglion, percutaneous
  microcompression of, 297
Trigeminal innervation, 308f
Trigeminal nerve, 239
  ablation of, 302
  decompression of, 297–298
  denervation of, 295–296
  divisions of, 308
  herpes zoster involvement of, 505, 509
  neuropathy of, 298
  nociceptors of, 308–309
  postsurgical damage of, 320–322
  processes of, 309
Trigeminal neuralgia, 280
  atypical, 281, 298
  clonazepam for, 208
  conditions associated with, 283t
  glycerol treatment for, 296–297
  headache with, 249–250
  idiopathic, 280–281
  incidence of, 294
  management of, 281–282
  medical treatment of, 294–295
  microvascular decompression for, 297–298
  percutaneous microcompression for, 297
  peripheral denervation for, 295, 296
  radiofrequency electrocoagulation for, 296
  secondary, 282
  sensory epilepsy and, 381
  severity of pain in, 240
  symptomatic, 281–282
Trigeminal neuropathic pain, 282–283, 283
Trigeminal nucleus caudalis, 67–69
Trigeminal thalamic pathways, 15
Trigeminal tract, 14–15, 67–68
Trigeminal tractotomy, stereotaxis, 284
Trigger points
  desensitization of, 689
  of extensor digitorum muscles, 569–570
  injection and stretch of, 565–566
  muscles most likely to develop, 569t
  myofascial, 288, 539–541, 556–557
    inactivation of, 564–566
    location of, 543f, 545f, 547f, 549–550f, 551f, 553f
  of spinal pain, 350
Trimipramine (Surmotil), 186
Trunk, pain in with myofascial syndromes, 548–552
L-Tryptophan, 162–163

with monoamine oxidase inhibitors, 203
  in reflex sympathetic dystrophy, 490
Tumors
  cervical spine, 371
  invasion of bone by, 431
  orofacial, 289
  ovarian, 404
  spinal cord, 335, 339–340
  temporomandibular joint, 317
  of temporomandibular joint, 317
  uterine, 403
Tunica albuginea, 411
Tunica vaginalis, 411
Twitch response, 540–541
Tyramine-free diet, 242t
Tzanck smear, 505

Ulcerative lichen planus, 291
Ulnar nerve
  entrapment and compression of, 473–474
    below elbow, 474–475
    treatment of, 474
  entrapment of, 43–44
Ultrasonography
  in gynecology, 401
  low-intensity, 565
  for mechanical low back pain, 368
  for post-herpetic neuralgia, 517
  of testicle, 415
  thermal effects of, 85
  vaginal, 402
Underprescribing, in children, 215
Upper extremities, pain in with myofascial
  syndromes, 544–548
Uremic neuropathy, 466
Ureter, 409
  colic in, 412
  pain in, 412–413
Urethra
  male, 409, 410
  pain from, 414
Urethral strictures, 414
Uric acid, normalization of serum levels, 533–534
Uricosuric agents, 534
Urinary bladder, 409
  innervation of, 409–410
  pain in, 413
Urinary drainage, 413
Urinary retention, 615
Urinary tract pain, 401–407
Urodynamic study, 414
Uterus
  in gynecologic pain, 402–403
  tumors of, 403

Vagoglossopharyngeal neuralgia, 298–299
Vagus nerve, 239
Vail's syndrome, 286
Valpar Whole Body Range of Motion Test, 737
Valproate (Depakote)
  for cluster headache, 261
  for migraine, 259
Valproic acid (sodium valproate), 163
  in alcohol withdrawal detoxification, 235
Vapocoolant
  in rehabilitation, 689

spray, 564
Varicella-zoster virus, 503
Varicoceles, 416
Varni/Thompson Pediatric Pain
  Questionnaire, 33f
Vas deferens, 411
Vascular disease/dysfunction, orofacial
  pain with, 300, 322
Vascular headache
  muscle contraction headache and, 270
  types of, 244–248
Vascular occlusion, 300
Vasculitis, systemic, 300
Vasomotor instability, 492
Vasospastic ischemia, 601–602
Venography, epidural, 367–368
Ventrobasal nuclear complex, 13
Verapamil (Isoptin, Calan), 258
Vertebral artery, 334
Vertebral disk
  composition of, 386–387
  L5-S1 protrusion of, 362
  manipulation for, 100–101
  rupture and degeneration of, 332, 356–357
Vertebral facets, 387
Vertebral ligament, innervation of, 369
Vertebral motor distortions, static, 97–98
Vertebral motor unit subluxations, kinetic, 98–99
Vidian neuralgia, 286
Viral infections, chronic, 560–561
Viral myalgia, 101
Virtuous circle, 149
Visceral afferent blockade, 59–60
Visceral efferent blockade, 58–59
Visceral pain, 12, 13, 381
  to cerebral cortex, 16
  radiation palliation of, 461
Visual analog scales, 24, 25f
Vitamins. *See also* specific vitamins
  deficiency and inadequacy of, 557–559
  fat-soluble, 559
  studies of for myofascial pain syndrome, 573
  water-soluble, 558–559
Vocational evaluation protocols, 715
Vocational feasibility, 697
  improved, 702–704
Vocational rehabilitation, 680–681, 690
  for myofascial pain syndrome, 574–575
  patient profile for, 689
Vocational Rehabilitation Act, 695
Vocational relevance concept, 713
Vocational retraining benefits, 730
Vocational stress, 563–564

Wait-and-*see* approach, 586
Wall sit, 393f
Water
  properties of, 389–392
  sensory overload in, 392–393
  temperature of, 392
Watson-Schwartz test, 466
Weber's syndrome, 14

Wegener's granulomatosis, 291
  vasculitis with, 300
Wellness program, 652
Westhaven Yale Multidimensional Pain
  Inventory (WHYMPI), 27–28, 143
Whiplash injury, 348–349
White noise generators, 583
Whole patient concept, 219
Withdrawal syndrome. *See also* Drug
  detoxification protocols
    hypnosedatives, 229–231
    opiate, 224
      management principles for, 224–225
Work
  assessment of, 734
  categories of, 737–738
  conditions in, 719
  environment of, 647
  environmental demands of, 698
  functional status at, 5
  physical demands of, 716–719
  procedural demands of, 698
  procedure modification in, 628
  return to, 680–681
Work Assessment and Rehabilitation
  Program, 706
Work Capacities evaluation, 734
Work conditioning, 690, 702

Work Employment Rehabilitation Center,
  Loma Linda University, 706
Work evaluation program, 695
Work function theme development, 704
Work hardening, 696, 702–704
  outcome of, 706
  program accreditation for, 705–706
  programs for, 707f
  strategies of, 704–705
Work Hardening Program, Washington
  University, 706
Work physiology, 640–641
Work processes, obsolete, 656–657
Work Recovery Center, 706
Work simulation, 681
Work therapy program, 696
Work tolerance screen, 734
Workers' Compensation, 722
  American with Disabilities Act and, 731
  benefits of, 728–730
  in California, 700, 701f
  for chronic back pain, 630
  compensation formula in, 724–728
  disability, pain, and chronic pain
    specialist and, 730–731
  follow-up in, 681–682
  impact on chronic pain prevention/early
    intervention, 634–636

  medical witnesses in, 723–724
  occupational rehabilitation and, 694–695,
    709
  for psychological impairment, 743–744
  versus tort-based systems, 722–723
Workplace
  cumulative trauma disorders in, 645–652,
    660–664
  design of, 642
  early reporting of pain in, 645
  ergonomic conditions in, 640–664
  improvements of, 654, 661f
  inadequacies of, 647
  physical demands of, 716–719
  poorly designed, 659f
  risk assessment in, 660
  tolerance of, 698

X-ray, cervical spine, 337, 343, 345

*The Yellow Emperor's Classic of Internal
  Medicine*, 117
Yin-Yang theory, 117

Zimeldine, 512
Zoster immune globulin, 508
Zoster sine herpete, 504
Zung Depression Index, 26
Zygapophyseal joints, 332, 333
  overgrowth of, 370